HANDBOOK OF
Child and
Adolescent
Psychiatry

Volume One

HANDBOOK OF
Child and Adolescent Psychiatry

Joseph D. Noshpitz / Editor-in-Chief

VOLUME ONE

Infants and Preschoolers:
Development and Syndromes

STANLEY GREENSPAN, SERENA WIEDER, AND JOY OSOFSKY

EDITORS

John Wiley & Sons, Inc.
New York • Chichester • Weinheim • Brisbane • Singapore • Toronto

ISBN 0-471-55079-5 (vol. 1)
    0-471-55075-2 (vol. 2)
    0-471-55076-0 (vol. 3)
    0-471-55078-7 (vol. 4)
    0-471-17640-0 (set)

Printed in the United States of America

10 9 8 7 6 5 4 3 2

DEDICATION

This set of volumes grows out of an attitude that reflects the field itself. To put it succinctly, the basic theme of child and adolescent psychiatry is hope. Albeit formally a medical discipline, child and adolescent psychiatry is a field of growth, of unfolding, of progressive advance; like childhood itself, it is a realm of building toward a future and finding ways to better the outcome for the young. But within the field, an even greater theme inspires an even more dominant regard. For, beyond treating children, child and adolescent psychiatry is ultimately about rearing children. This is literally the first time in human history that we are on the verge of knowing *how* to rear a child. While people have reared children since we were arboreal, they did it by instinct, or by cultural practice, or in keeping with grandma's injunctions, or by reenacting the memories, conscious and unconscious, of their own childhood experiences. They did what they did for many reasons, but never because they really knew what their actions portended, what caused what, what was a precondition for what, or what meant what.

At this moment in history, however, things are different. The efforts of researchers, neuroscientists, child developmental specialists—in short, of the host of those who seek to understand, treat, and educate children and to work with parents—are beginning to converge and to produce a body of knowledge that tells us what children are, what they need, what hurts them, and what helps them. Hard science has begun to study the fetus, rating scales and in-depth therapeutic techniques have emerged for the mother with the infant in her arms, increasing precision is being achieved in assessing temperament, in measuring mother/infant

fit, and in detecting the forerunners of personality organization. Adolescence and the intricacies of pubertal transformation are being explored as never before. Indeed, a quiet revolution is coming into being: the gradual dissemination of knowledge about child rearing that, within a few generations, could well alter the quality of the human beings who fall under its aegis.

If children—all children—could be reared in a fashion that gave them a healthier organization of conscience, that preserved the buds of cognitive growth and helped these to flower (instead of pinching them off as so many current practices do), that could recognize from the outset any special needs a child might have in respect to impulse control or emotional stability—and could step in from the earliest moments in development with the appropriate tactics and strategies, anodynes and remedies, techniques of healing and practices of enabling to allow the youngster to better manage his or her inner life and interpersonal transactions—consider what fruit this would bear.

Today this is far more than a dream, far more than a wistful yearning for a better day to come. The beginnings are already accomplished, much of the initial work has been done, the directions of future research are becoming ever more evident. The heretofore cryptic equations of development are beginning to be found and some of their solutions to be discerned, the once-mystical runes are being read—and are here inscribed in page after page of research report and clinical observation.

Some of the initial changes are already well under way. As with all science first a process of demystification must occur. Bit by bit, we have had

v

to unlearn a host of formulaic mythologies about children and about parenting that have been part of Western civilization for centuries.

We have indeed begun to do so. We have been able to admit to the realities of child abuse, first to the violence directed toward children and then to their sexual exploitation. And we have had to admit to children's sexuality. Simply to allow those things to appear in print, to become part of common parlance, has taken immense cultural energy, the overcoming of tremendous defensiveness; after all, such things had been known but not spoken of for generations. Right now the sanctity, the hallowed quality of family life, is the focus of enormous cultural upheaval. There is much to suggest that the nuclear family set in the bosom of a body of extended kin relationships that had for so long served as the basic site for human child rearing is no longer the most likely context within which future generations of our children will grow. The quest is on for new social arrangements, and it is within this milieu that the impact of scientific knowledge, the huge and ever-increasing array of

insights into the nature of childhood, the chemistry of human relationships, the psychodynamics of parent-child interplay—in short, within the area of development that this work so carefully details—that we find the wellsprings of hope. As nursery schools, kindergartens, grade schools, and high schools become more sophisticated, as the psychiatric diagnostic manuals become more specific and more differentiated, as doctors become better trained and better prepared to address human issues with dynamic understanding, as what children need in order to grow well becomes ever more part of everyday cultural practice, the realization of this hope will slowly and quietly steal across the face of our civilization, and we will produce children who will be emotionally sounder, cognitively stronger, and mentally healthier than their parents. These volumes are dedicated to advancing this goal.

Joseph D. Noshpitz, M.D.
Editor-in-Chief

PREFACE

Some 16 years ago the first two volumes of the *Basic Handbook of Child Psychiatry* were published, to be followed shortly by volumes III and IV, and then, in 1985, by the fifth volume. More than a decade has passed since that volume was released, during which time the field of child psychiatry has advanced at a remarkable pace. Indeed, it has even changed its name to be more inclusive of the teenage years. New advances in neuroscience, in genetics, in psychoanalytic theory, in psychopharmacology, in animal studies—new findings in a host of areas have poured out during these years. It is therefore necessary to revise the handbook, to reorganize it, to update many of the clinical accounts, and to bring it to the level where the active practitioner can use its encyclopedic format to explore the enormous variety of clinical possibilities he or she may encounter.

The focus of this work is on development. It is no exaggeration to look on child development as the basic science of child and adolescent psychiatry. Development is so vital a concern that in this revision, we have abandoned the classical way of presenting the material. Rather than following tradition, wherein development, diagnosis and assessment, syndromes, treatment, and so on are discussed for a variety of related topics, in these volumes the bulk of the material is presented developmentally. Thus, volumes I, II, and III focus on development and syndromes of infancy and preschool, of grade school, and of adolescence, respectively. Within each of these larger sections, the material on development comes first, followed by chapters on syndromes, conceptualized as disturbances of development. While syndromes are

described in depth, they are discussed only within the framework of the developmental level under study. Volume IV, entitled "Varieties of Development," explores a host of ecological niches within which children are reared.

Volumes V and VI will contain sections on consultation/liaison, emergencies in child and adolescent psychiatry, the prehistory of child and adolescent psychiatry, current cultural issues that impinge on young people, forensic issues involving children and youth, and professional challenges facing the child and adolescent psychiatrist. Volume VI will include a most unusually rich banquet of studies on the assessment and evaluation of children, adolescents, and their families, plus reports on the basic science issues of the field and the current status of the various treatment techniques.

The intention of the work is to be as comprehensive and as readable as possible. In an encyclopedic work of this sort, concerns always arise as to how much space to allot to each topic and to which topics should be covered. To deal with such questions, a number of readers reviewed each submission. One editor had primary responsibility for each section; a coeditor also reviewed submissions. Then the editor of another section reviewed the submissions, exchanging his or her chapters with the first colleague so that someone outside the section read each chapter. In addition, one editor reviewed all submissions with an eye to contradictions or excessive overlap. Finally, the editor-in-chief reviewed and commented on a large proportion of the materials submitted. In short, while the submission process was not juried, a number of readers reviewed each chapter. Each

vii

author was confronted with the in cumulative critiques and asked to make appropriate changes. Most did so cheerfully, although not always with alacrity.

The writing and review process lasted from about 1990 to 1996. For much of this time, a host of authors were busy writing, revising, and polishing their work. The editors worked unstintingly, suffering all the ups and downs that accompany large projects: many meetings, huge expenses, moments of despair, episodes of elation, professional growth on the part of practically all the participants (a couple of authors who never came through with their material may be presumed to have shrunk), profound disappointments and thrilling breakthroughs, lost causes that were snatched from the jaws of defeat and borne aloft to victory, and, ultimately, the final feeling that we did it!

I speak for all the editors when I say that it was our purpose and it is our earnest wish that these volumes make for better understanding of young people, greater access to knowledge about children and adolescents, a richer sense of what this field of human endeavor entails, and a better outcome for the growth, development, mental health, and happiness of all the young in our land and of those who would help them.

Joseph D. Noshpitz, M.D.
Editor-in-Chief

CONTENTS

ix

Contents

SECTION III / Clinical Syndromes of Infancy and Early Childhood

CONTRIBUTORS

LEILA BECKWITH, PH.D.
Professor Emeritus of Pediatrics, University of California, Los Angeles, California.

ANNI BERGMAN, PH.D.
Clinical Professor of Psychology, The City University of New York; Clinical Associate Professor of Psychology, New York University; Training and Supervising Analyst, New York Freudian Society; Faculty, Institute for Psychoanalytic Training and Research, New York, New York.

JANICE BROWN, PH.D.
Instructor, Vanderbilt University, Nashville, Tennessee.

JUDE CASSIDY, PH.D.
Associate Professor, Department of Psychology, University of Maryland, College Park, Maryland.

IRENE CHATOOR, M.D.
Professor of Psychiatry and Behavioral Sciences, George Washington University School of Medicine; Vice Chair, Director of Infant Psychiatry, Children's National Medical Center, Washington, D.C.

ROBERT B. CLYMAN, M.D.
Research Scientist and Director, Developmental Psychiatry, Children's National Medical Center; Assistant Professor of Psychiatry, Behavioral Science, and Pediatrics, The George Washington University Medical Center, Washington, D.C.

SUSAN COATES, PH.D.
Director, Childhood Gender Identity Center, St. Luke's-Roosevelt Hospital Center, New York, New York.

LEON CYTRYN, M.D.
Clinical Professor of Psychiatry and Pediatrics, George Washington University Medical School, Washington, D.C.

GEORGIA A. DeGANGI, PH.D., OTL, FAOTA
Director of Research, Reginald S. Lourie Center for Infants and Young Children, Rockville, Maryland.

KENNETH A. DODGE, PH.D.
Professor of Psychology and Psychiatry; Director, Developmental Psychopathology Research Training Program; Director, Institute on Development and Psychopathology, Vanderbilt University, Nashville, Tennessee.

JANE A. DOUSSARD-ROOSEVELT, PH.D.
Research Associate, Institute for Child Study, University of Maryland, College Park, Maryland.

ROBERT N. EMDE, M.D.
Professor of Psychiatry, University of Colorado School of Medicine; Adjunct Professor of Psychology, University of Denver, Denver, Colorado.

STANLEY I. GREENSPAN, M.D.
Clinical Professor of Psychiatry and Behavioral Science and Pediatrics, George Washington University Medical School, Washington, D.C.

ROBERT M. HODAPP, PH.D.
Associate Professor of Educational Psychology (Special Education), Graduate School of Education and Information Studies, University of California, Los Angeles, California.

JUDY HOWARD, M.D.
Professor of Pediatrics, University of California, Los Angeles, California.

JEROME KAGAN, PH.D.
Professor of Psychology, Harvard University, Cambridge, Massachusetts.

CONNIE KASARI, PH.D.
Associate Professor of Educational Psychology (Special Education), Graduate School of Education and Information Studies, University of California, Los Angeles, California.

Contributors

JOHN H. KENNELL, M.D.
Professor of Pediatrics, Case Western Reserve University; Rainbow Babies and Childrens Hospital, Cleveland, Ohio.

MARSHALL H. KLAUS, M.D.
Adjunct Professor of Pediatrics, University of California, San Francisco, California.

AMI KLIN, PH.D.
Assistant Professor of Child Psychology, Yale Child Study Center, New Haven, Connecticut.

CLAIRE B. KOPP, PH.D.
Visiting Professor of Psychology, Claremont Graduate School, Claremont, California.

SHELLY J. LANE, PH.D., OTR/L, FAOTA
Chair, Department of Occupational Therapy, Virginia Commonwealth University, Richmond, Virginia.

ALICIA F. LIEBERMAN, PH.D.
Professor in Residence, Department of Psychiatry, University of California, San Francisco; San Francisco General Hospital, San Francisco, California.

ANN S. MASTEN, PH.D.
Professor of Child Psychiatry, University of Minnesota Institute of Child Development, Minneapolis, Minnesota.

JEANNE M. MCINTOSH, PH.D.
Los Angeles, California.

DONALD H. MCKNEW, JR., M.D.
Clinical Professor of Psychiatry and Pediatrics, George Washington School of Medicine, Washington, D.C.

KLAUS MINDE, M. D., F.R.C.P. (C)
Head, Division of Child Psychiatry, Professor of Psychiatry and Pediatrics, McGill University; Director, Department of Psychiatry, Montreal Children's Hospital, Westmount, Quebec, Canada.

DAVID A. MRAZEK, M. D., F.R.C.P.
Chairman, Department of Psychiatry, Children's National Medical Center; Professor of Psychiatry and Behavioral Sciences and Pediatrics, George Washington University School of Medicine, Washington, D.C.

JOSEPH D. NOSHPITZ, M.D.
Clinical Professor of Psychiatry and Behavioral Science, The George Washington University; Private Practice, Washington, D.C.

JOY D. OSOFSKY, PH.D.
Professor of Pediatrics and Psychiatry, Louisiana State University School of Medicine, New Orleans;

Adjunct Professor of Psychology, University of New Orleans, New Orleans, Louisiana.

RHEA PAUL, PH.D., CCC-SPL
Professor and Program Director, Speech and Hearing Sciences, Portland State University, Portland, Oregon.

JEREE H. PAWL, PH.D.
Clinical Professor, Department of Psychiatry, University of California, San Francisco; Director, Infant-Parent Program, San Francisco General Hospital, San Francisco, California.

STEPHEN W. PORGES, PH.D.
Professor, Department of Human Development and Psychology, University of Maryland, College Park, Maryland.

BARRY M. PRIZANT, PH.D.
Professor, Division of Communication Disorders, Emerson College, Boston, Massachusetts.

HOLLY A. RUFF, PH.D.
Professor of Pediatrics, Albert Einstein College of Medicine, Bronx, New York.

BERTRAM A. RUTTENBERG, M.D.
Medical Director, Center for Autistic Children, Philadelphia, Pennsylvania; Professor (Honorary) of Psychiatry and Human Behavior, Jefferson University College of Medicine, Philadelphia, Pennsylvania; Private Practice, Child Psychiatry, Merion Station, Pennsylvania.

ARNOLD J. SAMEROFF, PH.D.
Professor of Psychology, Research Scientist, Center for Human Growth and Development, University of Michigan, Ann Arbor, Michigan.

LOUIS W. SANDER, M.D.
Professor of Psychiatry Emeritus (Retired), University of Colorado School of Medicine, Denver, Colorado; Visiting Professor of Psychiatry, Boston University School of Medicine, Boston, Massachusetts.

ARIETTA SLADE, PH.D.
Associate Professor, Doctoral Program in Clinical Psychology, The City College and Graduate Center of The City University of New York, New York, New York.

SUSAN K. THEUT, M.D., M.P.H.
Clinical Associate Professor of Psychiatry and Behavioral Sciences, Children's National Medical Center and George Washington University School of Medicine; Private Practice, Washington, D.C.

EDWARD Z. TRONICK, PH.D.
Associate Professor of Pediatrics, Harvard Medical

xii

Contributors

School; Chief, Child Development Unit, Children's Hospital, Boston, Massachusetts.

FRED R. VOLKMAR, M.D.
Harris Associate Professor of Child Psychiatry, Pediatrics, and Psychology, Yale Child Study Center, New Haven, Connecticut.

M. KATHERINE WEINBERG, PH.D.
Instructor in Pediatrics, Harvard Medical School; Research Associate in Medicine, General Pediatrics, Children's Hospital, Boston, Massachusetts.

AMY M. WETHERBY, PH.D.
Professor, Department of Communication Disorders, Florida State University, Tallahassee, Florida.

SERENA WIEDER, PH.D.
Private Practice, Infant Emotional, Developmental, and Learning Disorders, Silver Spring, Maryland.

G. GORDON WILLIAMSON, PH.D.
Associate Clinical Professor of Occupational Therapy, Columbia University College of Physicians and Surgeons, New York, New York; Director, Project ERA, Pediatric Rehabilitation Department, John F. Kennedy Medical Center, Edison, New Jersey.

SABRINA WOLFE, PH.D.
Co-Director, Childhood Gender Identity Center, St. Luke's-Roosevelt Hospital Center, New York, New York.

MARGARET O'DOUGHERTY WRIGHT, PH.D.
Associate Professor of Psychology, Miami University, Oxford, Ohio.

SECTION I
Normal Development in Infancy and Early Childhood

1 / The First Year of Life

Alicia F. Lieberman and Arietta Slade

The emotional life of the infant has long been a topic of profound fascination to students of human nature. Incontestably a person, yet unable to use adult language to tell us about his or her inner life, the baby becomes a projection object, one in which we are ready to see what we believe or what we already know.

The history of theoretical and clinical descriptions of the baby presents a kaleidoscope of contrasting images. Freud (1920/1955) thought of infants in the first weeks of life as protected by a stimulus barrier that shielded them from the bombardment of internal and external stimuli. Margaret Mahler expanded this hypothesis by formulating a normal autistic phase where newborns perceive very little outside their body (Mahler, Pine, & Bergman, 1975). William James, on the other hand, imagined newborns as subjected to a world of "blooming, buzzing confusion." These two views represent poles in a continuum from withdrawal to overexposure to stimuli as the predominant experience of the infant. In contrast, recent research on the capabilities of infants has led to an emphasis on their amazingly well developed skills to engage in synchronous interactions with the outside world. (See Stern, 1985, and Field, 1990, for comprehensive reviews.)

Current conceptions of the first year of life tend to focus on the epigenetic unfolding of physical, cognitive, and social capabilities in a predictable sequence of stages. These progress in time through differentiation and organization of parts (Erikson, 1950). Different models have been offered that emphasize specific aspects of this sequence (Greenspan, 1981, 1989; Mahler, Pine, & Bergman, 1975; Sander, 1975; Sroufe, 1979; Stern, 1985). These models have in common a recognition of three complementary processes of organization: the biological processes of the body, the psychological processes that organize individual experience, and the social processes that regulate the relationship of the individual with other people in the community.

The Developmental-Structuralist Framework

The developmental-structuralist framework proposed by Stanley Greenspan will be used in this chapter to describe the ways in which infants and young children organize experience (Greenspan, 1981, 1989).

This approach is based on two major assumptions. One is the epigenetic premise that the capacity to organize experience is present from birth and evolves to higher levels as the individual matures. This increasing organization is manifested in phase-specific patterns that emerge from the interplay between the maturation of the central nervous system and the child's involvement with age-appropriate environmental experiences. In Greenspan's model, the organizational level of experience is characterized by parameters that include phase-appropriateness, range, depth, stability, and personal uniqueness.

The second assumption of this framework is that each organizational level gives rise to characteristic types of affective experience, which involve age-specific interests, wishes, fantasies, curiosities, and fears.

The interplay between organizational levels and the kinds of affective experiences that characterize each of these levels can be described using a theatre metaphor (Greenspan, 1989). The organizational level is compared to a stage on which the drama of specific affective experiences is performed. This stage (or organizational level) may be so restricted that it cannot sustain a rich and complex drama with a variety of themes. Alternatively, the stage may be large and sturdy, with the capacity to house a rich and varied production. Some stages may have hidden deficits that emerge while a drama is in progress. Ultimately, these deficits may restrict or distort the unfolding of the play.

3

The theater metaphor highlights a particular strength of the structuralist-developmental approach: its simultaneous attention to sensory and affective-thematic domains of experience. The integration of these domains is crucial for a comprehensive understanding of normal development as well as developmental deficits and deviations.

In the following sections, the unfolding of development in the first year of life is described in terms of phase-specific tasks. These achievements emerge through the child's neurophysiological maturation and through the negotiation of salient interactional issues posed to the infant and caregiver by the attainment of new skills. The phases of infancy proposed by Greenspan are (1) homeostasis, (2) attachment, (3) somatopsychological differentiation (i.e., purposeful communication and symbolic representation), and (4) internalization. All of these processes are ongoing from birth, but each of them gains ascendancy at a particular developmental phase.

HOMEOSTASIS: SELF-REGULATION AND INTEREST IN THE WORLD

In recent years, knowledge about the development of the fetus and about the capacities of the neonate has accumulated rapidly. These data provide powerful evidence for the assumption that, from the very beginning of life, behavior becomes organized at increasingly higher levels.

Learning begins in utero. Our understanding of this phenomenon has been considerably enhanced by the development of fetal ultrasonography, a technique that allows for detailed monitoring of fetal movements and even facial expressions. The growing fetus not only shows reflexes such as soothing, sucking, and grasping but is capable of increasingly more controlled movements in the course of gestation. As it develops, the fetus shows more reliable responses to tactile, visual, and auditory stimulation. Eventually it can discriminate between different tasks, as shown in facial expressions denoting pleasure or disgust. The fetus also learns to habituate to repetitive stimulation. For example, it responds to a sound by accelerated heart rate and increased movements; these reactions decline when the stimulus is repeated but increase once again when a new sound is introduced (Field, 1990). Such findings indicate that the fetus is attuned to its environment and capable of the basic learning processes of discrimination and habituation.

At least some of the learning that occurs in utero persists after birth. This is true, for example, of the ability to recognize and prefer the mother's voice. In an experimental setup, newborns were offered the choice of eliciting either their mother's voice or another woman's voice by differentially sucking on a pacifier hooked to a tape recorder. It turned out that they consistently activated the recording of their mother's voice (De Casper & Fifer, 1980). In addition, the newborns tended to activate the version of a story that they heard in utero rather than another version that was new to them. These responses indicate both that babies remember what they learn in utero and that they have an early preference for familiarity (De Casper & Spence, 1986).

Given this prenatal background of learning, it is not surprising that newborns are equipped with a remarkably rich repertoire of behaviors that enables them to seek out and respond to environmental stimulation. These abilities pave the way toward the development of differentiated emotional relationships (Field, 1990; Stern, 1985).

Infants' readiness for interaction is particularly apparent in relation to the caregiver (usually the biological mother). Early preference for mother has been shown in studies of olfactory, visual, and auditory perception. Newborns root toward their mothers' breast pads; they do not turn either towards an unused breast pad or towards one worn by an unfamiliar woman (Cernack & Porter, 1985; MacFarlane, 1975). The mother's face is discriminated and preferred within hours after birth, and this tendency is strengthened when the mother's voice is added (Field, 1990). The studies by De Casper and colleagues cited earlier provide evidence of early preference for the mother's voice.

Taken together, these studies speak to the existence of a specific early connection between baby and mother. This bond is mediated by the infant's sensory capacities and developed through repeated affectively colored interactions between infant and caregiver.

Early interactive readiness notwithstanding, it is also true that newborns spend most of the day eating, sleeping, drowsing, and fussing or crying. They are alert mostly around feedings; these occur at 3- to 4-hour intervals for periods lasting between 5 and 10 minutes (Wolff, 1965). During about 20 hours of each day, newborns face the developmental task of regulating cycles of hunger and satiation, elimination, sleep and wakefulness, and comfort and distress. These are the regulatory efforts Greenspan (1989) refers to as characterizing the phase of homeostasis, and that other authors describe in terms of regulation of psychophysiological processes (Sander, 1962; Sroufe, 1979).

Young infants can be alert and socially responsive only when they have achieved a relative measure of homeostatic balance. This means that newborns need to cope with body-centered processes while simultaneously engaging and learning about the world outside of themselves. Many of the processes leading to physiological stability take place in the context of caregiving routines such as feeding, diapering, and being put to sleep. Such seemingly prosaic daily activities become the setting for important social exchanges between mother and child. This is what Winnicott (1965) meant when he suggested that the baby's experience of bodily processes is intricately connected with the mothering experience.

Each baby's individuality is present from the very beginning and is manifested both in his or her constitutional makeup and in the baby's idiosyncratic ways of responding to the mother's ministrations. Infants differ along parameters such as activity level, irritability, soothability, alertness, and ability to regulate arousal (Brazelton, 1973; Escalona, 1968; Thomas & Chess, 1977). These characteristics—referred to as temperament—simultaneously color the child's responses to the parent's ministrations and influence the parental responses to the child.

The functioning of the sensory pathways—the neurophysiological foundations of vision, audition, olfaction, touch, and taste—affects the range and quality of the experiences available to the infant. Each sensory pathway may be normally reactive; alternatively, it may be hyperarousable, hypoarousable, or have some subtle form of deficit in processing that profoundly influences how the infant perceives stimulation and responds to it (Greenspan, 1989).

When a sensory pathway is hyperarousable, the information processed through that channel may easily become overwhelming. Depending on the specific sensory pathway involved, the baby may overreact and become distressed and disorganized in response to experiences of taste, sound, touch, smell, visual stimulation, or movement. On the other hand, when a sensory pathway is hypoarousable, babies may show only muted responses or even no response to stimuli in the normal range of intensity. The third type of deficit involves qualitative rather than quantitative disorders of processing; this group of disturbances may be earlier versions of the perceptual-motor or auditory-verbal processing problems identified in older children. These disorders may involve distortions in the perception and modulation of the stimulus. There may be deficits in the integration of a given stimulus with other elements of the child's experience that is with other stimuli impinging simultaneously on the child, with stimuli stored in memory, or with appropriate motor responses.

The quality of caregiving may alleviate or exacerbate a baby's constitutional difficulties. Infants cannot thrive without the consistent and committed care of a parental figure (Bowlby, 1969; Emde, 1989; Mahler et al., 1975; Winnicott, 1965). The affective development of healthy, intact, normal infants may be seriously derailed by abrupt, inconsistent, or inappropriate care (Bowlby, 1969; Fraiberg, 1980; Greenspan et al., 1987). On the other hand, babies with constitutional challenges such as excessive irritability, or with sensory handicaps such as blindness, may be helped to achieve harmonious functioning when their mothers learn to respond sensitively to their signals (Crockenberg, 1981; Fraiberg, 1977).

The infant's reliance on the mother figure as a container, modulator, and shaper of affective experiences led Winnicott (1965) to quip that "there is no such thing as a baby." The quality of the mother-infant interaction colors the infant's expectations and serves as an organizer of experience from the very beginning. A series of classic experiments by Sander (1975, 1980) illustrates the early interconnection between the rhythms of mother and child in establishing a "specificity of regulatory fittedness between a particular infant and a particular caregiver" as early as the tenth day of life (p. 383). As Sander (1975) concludes: "One of the features most idiosyncratic during the first three months is the extent to which the infant is helped or compromised in beginning to determine aspects of his own regulation ... [and the mother's] feeling of confidence that she knows her baby's needs and can specifically meet them" (p. 137).

Affective responses tend to be global in nature in the first weeks of life. Newborns express anger and pleasure by moving the whole body in characteristic ways (Bennett, 1971; Lipsitt, 1976). Similarly, there is likely to be little differentiation of perceptions, cognition, and actions, and only rudimentary differentiation between self, others, and the physical world (Greenspan, 1989; Stern, 1985).

During the first two months of life, the infant is capable of substantial feats of recognition and discrimination. However, these capacities are not reliably manifested in the infant's performance, and tend rather to be mobilized only when the infant is in homeostatic balance. The capacities employed when the infant needs to process and organize deeply felt emotional experiences tend to lag behind those available for organizing affectively neutral experiences.

For this reason, it is quite plausible that infants in intense need states or in states of blissful satisfaction experience a lack of differentiation between self and mother that is akin to Mahler's early concept of symbiosis (Greenspan, 1989; Mahler, Pine, & Bergman, 1975; Pine, 1985). This interval of merger may give way to periods of recognition of the mother as a separate object when the infant is quiet and alert, a state that enhances receptivity to outside stimulation. Both processes—the experience of merger and the experience of separateness—while different, are likely to be equally fundamental and complementary ways of organizing experience.

ATTACHMENT

Perhaps the most famous statement about the importance of the attachment between a baby and his mother was made by Sigmund Freud (1940/1965) when he wrote that the child-mother relationship is "unique, without parallel, laid down unalterably for a whole lifetime, as the first and strongest love object and as the prototype of all later love relations . . ." (p. 188). This section will elaborate on current knowledge about how such a strong relationship is formed.

The onset of the social smile by about 2 months of age may be considered a transition point from more body-centered processes to a more active, autonomous interest in the outside world. At around 4 months infants begin to show general signs of hilarity and, for the first time, respond with hearty laughter when tickled. This reaction indicates a significant shift in the baby's awareness of self and other as separate agents. The tickler needs to be perceived as different in order to induce laughter, which is the reason that adults cannot tickle themselves (White, 1975).

The interactional patterns gradually become organized around the relationship with the mother or primary caregiver; by 6 to 8 months she has become the center of the infant's emotional life. This developmental milestone has its onset at about 8 months; its hallmark is baby's separation protest upon the mother's departure along with baby's refusal to be readily consoled by a substitute (Bowlby, 1969; Schaffer, 1977). Concomitant with this development is the onset of wariness to strangers.

These two behaviors appear almost simultaneously and indicate a dramatic increase in the baby's ability to appraise and respond actively to events of emotional significance, such as changes in the caregiver's physical availability. There is now a focal attachment to a particular caregiver. In contrast to the 4-month-old baby who engages primarily in synchronistic interactions, the 8-month-old is capable of taking the initiative in "wooing" the mother. Baby actively asserts his desire for her presence, protests her departure, and shows unmistakable reserve, displeasure, or emotional withdrawal in response to the social overtures of a stranger.

The onset of fear as a discrete facial expression is first identified at about 6 months (Cicchetti & Sroufe, 1978), and signals a new capacity to recognize and anticipate danger. This is symptomatic of a higher level of thematic affective organization, in which several discrete emotions—pleasure, joy, assertiveness, curiosity, fear, protest, and anger—become organized around an intensely specific emotional relationship with the mother. From about 6 months of age, infants use the voice and facial expression of the mother to appraise whether a novel situation is dangerous or safe. This phenomenon, called "social referencing"

(Sorce, Emde, Campos, & Klinnert, 1985), highlights the baby's use of the mother as a source of protection. The baby's perception of the parent as a reliable protector is a paramount feature in defining attachment (Bowlby, 1969).

Attachments differ in their emotional quality. A dimension of security versus anxiety has been particularly fruitful in investigating patterns of individual differences in infant-mother attachment in the first year of life (Ainsworth, Blehar, Waters, & Wall, 1978).

Protection and safety are central emotional issues in the development of relationships. In keeping with this, secure attachments are defined as the infant's expectation that the mother will be emotionally available and responsive to her signals of need. Securely attached infants show this expectation behaviorally through a tendency to use the mother as a "secure base." They set off to explore the environment with interest and curiosity, then, when wary, fatigued, or simply in need of reestablishing the connection with her, they return to her unambivalently for comfort and reassurance.

Securely attached babies also show a predominance of positive affects (such as interest, pleasure, and curiosity) over negative affects (fear, withdrawal, anger, and avoidance) in the presence of the mother. After separation and the stress of being away from her, they greet her readily, seeking to restore proximity and contact.

Anxious attachments, on the other hand, involve the infant's uncertainty that the mother will respond contingently to his or her social and need signals. As a result of this uncertainty, infants may tend to avoid their mothers, resist proximity and contact, or show emotional disorganization characterized by contradictory signals or odd, idiosyncratic behaviors (Ainsworth et al., 1978; Main & Solomon, 1986).

Instead of using the mother as a secure base from which to explore, anxiously attached infants may be inhibited in their exploration and show excessive dependence on the mother's presence. Alternatively, they may avoid the mother and become overly absorbed in the exploration of the inanimate world. Avoidant infants tend to use exploration not as a source of autonomy and pleasure, but rather as a defense against or compensation for the deficiencies in their emotional experiences with their attachment figures.

What factors contribute to the formation of secure or anxious attachments? There is substantial research evidence that maternal sensitivity to the infant's signals during the first year of life plays a major role in shaping the quality of the relationship (Ainsworth et al., 1978; Belsky & Isabella, 1988). The underlying assumption is that when the mother responds contingently to the baby's communications, her infant develops a sense of inner competence about his ability to make himself understood, to secure the fulfillment of his needs, and to derive pleasure and a feeling of well-being from his social overtures. This interactional history, in turn, creates a sense of trust in the mother's emotional availability.

Conversely, maternal insensitivity, abruptness, or lack of contingency to the infant's signals convey that intimate human connections cannot be trusted to create an inner sense of well-being. The infant experiences intimate emotional relationships as feelings of incompetence, anger, and emotional withdrawal rather than as a source of pleasure, comfort, and relief.

The infant is also an active contributor to the quality of attachment. Some infants have predictable physiological rhythms, are easy to soothe, have low levels of irritability and show pleasure in social interaction; such babies are able to facilitate the mother's caregiving task because they engage more readily in reciprocal, mutually contingent, and pleasurable interactions. In contrast, babies with "difficult" temperaments—those who are unusually irritable, unpredictable in their responses, and difficult to soothe and engage—may tax the average mother's emotional resources by making her feel incompetent and unappreciated by her baby (Chess & Thomas, 1978).

The "goodness of fit" between infant and caregiver is as important as each partner's individual contributions to the formation of secure, emotionally satisfying attachments (Chess & Thomas, 1978; Sameroff & Emde, 1989). Attachments are intrinsically relational, and parent and baby continually influence each other. The same infant characteristics may have a different emotional impact on different mothers. For example, excessively irritable newborns can be helped to surmount their fussiness and to form secure attachments by the end of their first year when the mother is empathic to their distress and appropriately responsive to their crying (Crockenberg, 1981).

Attachments do not exist in a developmental vacuum. The quality of the relationship influences the infant's functioning in other areas as well. Longitudinal studies are particularly valuable in delineating the influence of early quality of attachment on later development. By the time they reached their second birthday, securely attached 1-year-olds were found to have longer attention spans, to show more pleasure in free play, to be more persistent at attempting to solve an age-appropriate task, and to be less easily frustrated than their anxiously attached counterparts (Main, 1973; Matas, Arend, & Sroufe, 1978). Waters, Wippman, and Sroufe (1979) found that securely attached infants became highly competent pre-schoolers, both with peers and in their exploration of their surroundings. Sroufe (1983) reported that preschoolers who had been classified as securely attached during infancy scored higher than anxiously attached peers on a variety of mental health and socioaffective measures, including self-esteem, expression of affect and impulses, social competence, classroom deportment, and empathy. These children were also independently rated by their teachers as less dependent than children who had been anxiously attached. In a study of 6-year-olds focusing on the links between early quality of attachment and psychopathology, Lewis, Feiring, McGoffog, and Jaskir (1984) found that anxious attachment at 12 months was significantly related to later psychopathology (as defined by behavioral problems) for males, although no such relationship was observed for females.

While early quality of attachment can influence the course of development, it should not be considered as a fixed attribute in the child's evolving personality structure. Changing life circumstances can alter the quality of attachment, leading to improvement or deterioration in the relationship, depending on how these life changes affect the mother's emotional availability to her child (Thompson, Lamb, & Estes, 1982; Vaughn, Egeland, Sroufe, & Waters, 1979). Moreover, intervention with anxiously attached mother-infant dyads that which focuses on enhancing the mother's empathic responsiveness has been effective in enhancing the quality of the relationship between mother and child (Lieberman, Weston, & Pawl, 1991).

INITIATIVE AND INTERNALIZATION

In the last 3 months of the first year, behavioral sequences show increased richness and complexity. Infants deliberately seek to share experiences about events with the people that are closest to them.

This eagerness to share experiences first becomes notable at about 9 months of age, and has been called by different names; the best-known are "innate interpersonal relatedness" (Fairbairn, 1949); "interpersonal field" (Sullivan, 1953); and "intersubjectivity" (Trevarthan & Hubley, 1978). All these terms have in common an appreciation of the infant's increased ability to understand that people have minds whose functioning can be engaged with and understood—that infants develop a theory of "interfaceable separate minds" (Bretherton & Bates, 1979).

Language is not needed for the experience of intersubjectivity. Stern (1985) proposed that three nonlinguistic mental states are of great importance in interpersonal communication: sharing joint attention, sharing intentions, and sharing affective states.

Shared attention occurs when the baby and his or her social partners have a joint focus of attention. This is achieved nonverbally through two major behaviors: pointing and following the direction of the partner's attention. Both of these behaviors emerge at about 9 months of age; before then, babies do not point, and, when the mother does so, they stare at her finger and do not follow her line of vision.

Joint attention in turn elicits social referencing. Nine-month-olds not only point and look in the direction the mother points to, but they also check back and forth between the target and the mother's face. This behavior indicates that the baby may be checking whether her intention in pointing is being met by a congruent maternal response, and vice versa: whether the baby's perception matches the mother's intention when she initiates the pointing.

Intentions also can be shared. Babies persist in a communicative behavior until its purpose is achieved. Perhaps the most ubiquitous example is the preverbal 9-month-old's use of "Eh! Eh!" with an unmistakable imperative intonation, as he tries to grasp a cookie or cherished object out of the mother's hand (Dore, 1975). This behavior indicates the infant's belief that the mother can understand and respond to his intention.

Sharing affective states is the most complex form of early intersubjectivity, and the phenomenon of social referencing described earlier illustrates it well. When babies are placed in a situation in which they are uncertain about what is the safe course of action, they look at the mother's face for clues about what to do. If she smiles encouragingly, the infant sets forth and explores; if she looks wary, the child holds back with a worried expression (Emde, Klingman, Reich, & Wade, 1978; Emde & Sorce, 1983).

The emergence of the capacity for subjective relatedness is most likely the result of interaction between maturational social and cognitive skills and affective transactions with the parents and other caregivers. When infants experience responsive care, they show an exuberant trust that their communications will be understood and that they, in turn, can trust the adult's social cues as a guide to behavior. In contrast, normal infants who have been neglected may show delayed or impoverished versions of the behavioral sequences involved in sharing attention, intention, and affective states. Such different responses indicate that the babies have internalized important as-pects of their interactive history with the caregiver. These internalizations, in turn, serve as a filter that colors and shapes infants' perceptions and expectations of the world.

Conclusions

The first year of life is the period of fastest growth in the human life span. Babies come to unfold their potential for differentiated, organized behavior through affectively colored exchanges with the caregiver and through exploration of the inanimate world. By the time of their first birthday, babies are remarkably able to engage in subtle affective communications where attention, intention, and emotions are clearly conveyed and accurately understood. These acquisitions allow babies to give social meaning to the two major behavioral milestones that mark the transition from the first year to the second year of life: the beginnings of language and the onset of locomotion. Language as a form of communication is built on an infrastructure of preverbal communicative gestures that babies have learned to produce and decode. Similarly, it is infants' ability to understand and respond to social communications that enable them to harness autonomous locomotion to an affective network of expectations and demands that will keep them safe and interpersonally related even while engaged in the process of taking off.

REFERENCES

Ainsworth, M. D. S., Blehar, M., Waters, E, & Wall, S. (1978). *Patterns of attachment: A psychological study of the Strange Situation.* Hillsdale, NJ: Erlbaum.

Belsky, J., & Isabella, R. (1988). Maternal, infant and social-contextual determinants of attachment security. In J. Belsky & T. Nezworski (Eds.), *Clinical implications of attachment* (pp. 41–94). Hillsdale, NJ: Lawrence Erlbaum.

Bennett, S. (1971). Infant-caretaker interactions. *Journal of the American Academy of Child Psychiatry, 10,* 321–335.

Bowlby, J. (1969). *Attachment and loss: Vol 1. Attachment.* New York: Basic Books.

Brazelton, T. B. (1973). The neonatal behavioral assessment scale. *Clinics in Developmental Medicine, 50.*

Bretherton, I., & Bates, E. (1979). The emergence of intentional communication. In I. Uzgiris (Ed.), *New directions for child development,* Vol. 4. San Francisco: Jossey-Bass.

Cernack, J. M., & Porter, R. H. (1985). Recognition of maternal axillary odors by infants. *Child Development, 56,* 1593–1598.

Chess, S., & Thomas, A. (1978). *Temperamental indi-*

9

viduality from childhood to adolescence. Annual Progress in Child Psychiatry & Child Development, pp. 489–497.

Cicchetti, D., & Sroufe, A. (1978). An organizational view of affect: Illustration from the study of Down's syndrome infants. In M. Lewis & L. Rosenblum (Eds.), The development of affects. New York: Plenum Press.

Crockenberg, S. (1981). Infant irritability, mother responsiveness and social support influences on the security of infant-mother attachment. Child Development, 52, 857–869.

De Casper, A. J., & Fifer, W. P. (1980). Of human bonding: Newborns prefer their mothers' voices. Science, 208, 1174–1176.

De Casper, A. J., & Spence, M. J. (1986). Prenatal maternal speech influences newborns' perception of speech sounds. Infant Behavior and Development, 9, 133–150.

Dore, J. (1975). Holophrases, speech acts and language universals. Journal of Child Language, 2, 21–40.

Emde, R. N. (1989). The infants' relationship experience: Developmental and affective aspects. In A. J. Sameroff & R. N. Emde (Eds.), Relationship disturbances in early childhood (pp. 3–14). New York: Basic Books.

Emde, R. N., Klingman, D. H., Reich, J. H., & Wade, J. D. (1978). Emotional expression in infancy: I. Initial studies of social signaling and an emergent model. In M. Lewis & L. Rosenblum (Eds.), The development of affect. New York: Plenum Press.

Emde, R. N., & Sorce, J. E. (1983). The rewards of infancy: Emotional availability and maternal referencing. In J. D. Call, E. Galenson, & R. Tyson (Eds.), Frontiers of infant psychiatry, Vol. 2 (pp. 17–30). New York: Basic Books.

Erikson, E. H. (1950). Childhood and society. New York: W. W. Norton.

Escalona, S. (1968). The roots of individuality. Chicago: Aldine.

Fairbairn, W. R. D. (1949). Steps in the development of an object-relations theory of personality. British Journal of Medical Psychology, 22 (1,2), 6–31.

Field, T. (1990). Infancy. Cambridge, MA: Havard University Press.

Fraiberg, S. (1977). Every child's birth right: In defense of mothering. New York: Basic Books.

Fraiberg, S. (Ed.) (1980). Clinical studies in infant mental health. New York: Basic Books.

Freud, S. (1955). Beyond the pleasure principle. In J. Strachey (Ed.), (hereafter Standard edition) Complete Psychology Works of Sigmund Freud Standard edition of the Vol. 18, (pp. 7–65). London: Hogarth Press, (Originally published 1920.)

Freud, S. (1965). An outline of psychoanalysis. Standard edition, Vol. 23, London: Hogarth (pp. 141–208). (Originally published 1940.)

Greenspan, S. I. (1981). Psychopathology and adaptation in infancy and early childhood: Principles of clinical diagnosis and preventive intervention. New York: International Universities Press.

Greenspan, S. I. (1989). The development of the ego. Madison, CT: International Universities Press.

Greenspan, S. I., Wieder, S., Lieberman, A. F., Nover, R., Lourie, R., & Robinson, M. (1987). Infants in multirisk families. Madison, CT: International Universities Press.

Lewis, M., Feiring, C., McGoffog, C., & Jaskir, J. (1984). Predicting psychopathology in six-year-olds from early social relations. Child Development, 55, 123–126.

Lieberman, A. F., Weston, D., & Pawl, J. H. (1991). Preventive intervention and outcome with anxiously attached dyads. Child Development, 62, 199–209.

Lipsitt, L. P. (1976). Developmental psychobiology comes of age. In L. P. Lipsitt (Ed.), Developmental psychobiology: The significance of infancy. Hillsdale, NJ: Lawrence Erlbaum.

MacFarlane, J. (1975). Olfaction in the development of social preferences in the human neonate. In M. Hofer (Ed.), Parent-infant interaction. Amsterdam: Elsevier.

Mahler, M., Pine, F., & Bergman, A. (1975). The psychological birth of the human infant. New York: Basic Books.

Main, M. (1973). Exploration, play and cognitive functioning as related to child-mother attachment. Unpublished doctoral dissertation, The Johns Hopkins University, Baltimore, MD.

Main, M., & Solomon, J. (1986). Discovery of disorganized & disoriented attachment pattern. In T. B. Brazelton M. W. Yogan (Eds.), Affective development in infancy (pp. 95–124). Northvale, NJ: Ablex.

Matas, L., Arend, R., & Sroufe, L. A. (1978). Continuity of adaptation in the second year: The relationship between quality of attachment and later competence. Child Development, 49, 547–556.

Pine, F. (1985). Developmental theory and clinical process. New York: Basic Books.

Sameroff, A. J., & Emde, R. N. (1989). Relationship disturbances in early childhood. New York: Basic Books.

Sander, L. (1962). Issues in early mother-child interaction. Journal of the American Academy of Child Psychiatry, 1, 141–166.

Sander, L. (1975). Infant and caretaking environment: Investigation and conceptualization of adaptive behavior in a system of increasing complexity. In E. J. Anthony (Ed.), Explorations in child psychiatry (pp. 129–166). New York: Plenum Press.

Sander, L. (1980). New knowledge about the infant from current research: Implications for psychoanalysis. Journal of American Psychoanalytic Association, 28, 181–98.

Schaffer, H. R. (1977). Studies in infancy. London: Academic Press.

Sorce, J. F., Emde, R. N., Campos, J. J., & Klinnert, M. D. (1985). Maternal emotional signaling: Its effect of the visual cliff behavior of 1-year-olds. *Developmental Psychology, 21,* 195–200.

Sroufe, L. A. (1979). The coherence of individual development. *American Psychologist, 34,* 834–841.

Sroufe, L. A. (1983). Infant-caregiver attachment and patterns of adaptation in preschool: The roots of maladaptation and competence. In M. Perlmutter (Ed.), *Minnesota Symposium in Child Psychology* (Vol. 16, pp. 41–83). Hillsdale, NJ: Lawrence Erlbaum.

Stern, D. N. (1985). *The interpersonal world of the infant.* New York: Basic Books.

Sullivan, H. (1953). *The interpersonal theory of psychiatry.* New York: W. W. Norton.

Thomas, A., & Chess, S. (1977). *Temperament and development.* New York: Brunner/Mazel.

Thompson, R., Lamb, M. E., & Estes, D. (1982). Stability of infant-mother attachment and its relationship to changing life circumstances in an unselected middle class sample. *Child Development, 53,* 144–148.

Trevarthan, C., & Hubley, P. (1978). Secondary inter-subjectivity: Confidence, confiders and acts of meaning in the first year. In A. Lock (Ed.), *Action, gesture and symbol.* New York: Academic Press.

Vaughn, B., Egeland, B., Sroufe, L. A., & Waters, E. (1979). Individual differences, in infant-mother attachment at twelve and eighteen months: Stability and change in families under stress. *Child Development, 50,* 971–975.

Waters, E., Wippman, J., & Sroufe, L. A. (1979). Attachment, positive affect, and competence in the peer group: Two studies in construct validation. *Child Development, 50,* 821–829.

White, B. (1975). *First three years of life.* Englewood Cliffs, NJ: Prentice-Hall.

Winnicott, D. W. (1965). *The maturational process and the facilitating environment.* New York: International Universities Press.

Wolff, P. (1965). The development of attention in young infants. *Annals of the New York Academy of Sciences, 118,* 815–830.

2 / Cognitive Development in the First Year of Life

Holly A. Ruff

The study of cognitive development is the study of how individual children come to adapt to the demands of reality, gather knowledge, learn age-appropriate skills, and solve the problems that challenge them. The underlying processes involve attention, perception, learning, memory, abstraction, and generalization. These processes can be understood, however, only as part of a functional adaptation to the inanimate and social worlds, both of which change dynamically over time just as the developing child does. Brown, Bransford, Ferrara, and Campione (1983) distinguish between everyday cognition and academic cognition. Everyday cognition takes place in the context of social relationships, and there is little concern about whether it is efficient or systematic; academic cognition occurs in formal settings such as school. Here I focus on everyday cognition, which is most relevant for children in the preschool years.

Cognitive development, although discussed in isolation for heuristic reasons, is only one aspect of the complex system we know as the child; advances in cognition are intimately related to social, emotional, and motoric development. To understand the development of cognition, we must see how all aspects of the system are interrelated, not only in underlying processes but also at different levels, such as neurological and behavioral.

The chapter begins with a section that revolves around *what* develops over time—knowledge and skills. The next section is concerned with *how* specific knowledge and skills develop; the discussion is framed in terms of some developmental principles and includes examples relevant to the first year. The third section deals with the major trends and advances in cognition during the first year and emphasizes play, problem-solving, and representation. The final section deals with the formal assessment of development and specifically compares the psychometric approach to intellectual development with a process-oriented approach.

11

What Develops in Early Cognitive Development?

Advances toward adult cognition begin in the first year and are based on the growth of knowledge (Mandler, 1983) and the emergence of new skills (Fischer, 1980). To begin with, cognitive development involves both an accumulation and a reorganization of knowledge about the world. Infants learn about the social aspects of the world; they learn to recognize and differentiate among individuals in their environment (Barrera & Maurer, 1981; Cohen, DeLoache & Strauss, 1979; Ellsworth, Muir, & Hains, 1993); they learn to differentiate among a variety of emotional expressions and to respond to them appropriately (Serrano, Iglesias, & Loeches, 1995; Walker, 1982); and they learn to interact with others in mutually satisfying ways (Lewis, 1987; Stern, Hofer, Haft, & Dore, 1985). Infants also learn a great deal about the object world, about the physical properties of objects and what can be done with those objects (Ruff, 1982, 1984b). They learn about events—how objects move (Bertenthal, Profitt, & Kramer, 1987; Ruff, 1980), what happens to objects as a result of their own actions (Rovee-Collier, 1987), what the constraints are on the motion and relationship of different objects (Kellman & Spelke, 1983), and how other people move and act in situations that do not involve them. The foundations of the complex and extensive knowledge base of the adult are in infancy, a period during which an amazing amount of information is picked up and incorporated into the infant's own activity and expectations.

The gathering of information from the environment is made possible by several perceptual systems working in concert (Gibson, 1966). These systems are discussed in more detail later. It is assumed here that there is adequate information in the objective environment for veridical perception; the child does not have to interpret ambiguous information but perceives the world directly. However, no matter how accurately the world is perceived, only a small portion of it can be apprehended at any one time. An important aspect of the growth of knowledge therefore is the development of selective attention (Pick, Frankel, & Hess, 1975; Ruff & Rothbart, 1996).

Knowledge has been categorized into *knowing how* to do something and *knowing that* something is the case. These two forms of knowledge also have been referred to as procedural and declarative (Mandler, 1983). The infancy period often is thought of as a time in which the development of procedural knowledge dominates; Piaget (1954) refers to infancy as the sensorimotor period. Certainly infants gradually learn *how* to obtain objects that they want, including those that have temporarily disappeared, *how* to put two objects together, and *how* to interact with their parents and other social partners. Infants, however, also learn a great deal about the properties of both the inanimate and animate aspects of the world in the first year—*knowing that*. For example, they come to differentiate and recognize people, household objects, and toys. More important, these objects are perceived and known in the context of dynamic events and in terms of the actions they afford. Through observation, infants soon learn that events (which may or may not involve their own actions) proceed in a predictable manner, and they thereby develop expectations about what things look like and how they act or are acted upon. These expectations in turn serve as the basis for understanding physical and social principles (Baillargeon, 1994).

Cognitive development is also a matter of the emergence of skills. Skill might be subsumed under procedural knowledge, but the notion of cognitive advances depending on skill development deserves specific treatment (Fischer, 1980; Fischer & Hogan, 1989). Infants may, for example, *know* how to find objects hidden under covers, but finding hidden objects requires several skills—careful observation of objects and their trajectories, the ability to reach and grasp, and the ability to uncover or reverse the action of covering. Many skills developed in infancy are sensorimotor in that they involve the coordination of perception and action; these skills include such actions as sucking, reaching, exploring, observing, and imitating. Bruner (1973) suggests that the early development of a skill is effortful, but with practice, it becomes more automatic; the automaticity releases attention for new observations and new activities. In addition, specific skills, when well practiced, serve as modules that can be combined into more complex skills. The major skills developed in the first year are observational skills, such as learning what to attend to in different contexts; exploratory and manipulative skills; social skills such as imitation and joint attention; and regulatory skills such as state control and inhibition of prepotent responses.

How Do Knowledge and Skills Develop?

Before discussing specific developmental changes in detail, I briefly review some important principles of development to serve as an overall framework. The principles are based on recent discussion about dynamic systems approaches to development (Sameroff, 1983; Thelen & Fogel, 1989; Thelen & Smith, 1994).

The first principle is that the causes of development are multiple, interactive, and nonobvious. To account for development with a concept such as neural maturation is to beg the question. There may indeed be some behavioral developments that cannot occur without the development of given brain structures (Diamond, 1987). However, the specific nature of the child's experience with people and objects interacts with such neurological changes and may, in fact, contribute to them. Given activities are best conceived of as assemblages of components, some of which may be ready long before the activity actually emerges in the course of development. The appearance of a behavior may be delayed because some critical component is either missing or not fully developed. This component, however, albeit a limiting factor, is not more important than other components. For example, Thelen (1984; Thelen & Ulrich, 1991) has analyzed the components of independent walking. She suggests that the emergence of independent walking cannot occur until there is sufficient strength in the legs; equally important, although ready earlier, are the pattern of alternating leg movements, the motivation to move forward, postural control and balance, and the appropriate body proportions, such as head/body ratio. Some causes of development, therefore, may not be obvious because they are present long before the behavior in question is observed.

They also may not be obvious because they are hidden to observation. Hofer (1981) suggests, for example, that, embedded in the observable interactions between parent and newborn are many processes that regulate the behavior and physiology of the developing infant, processes that are critical to the initial attachment of young to parent. We must consider, therefore, how multiple components interact to produce particular behavior once they are all available.

The second principle is that development involves periods of instability and reorganization (Thelen & Smith, 1994). Some developments can be characterized as a gradual accumulation. For example, learning to recognize the distinctive features of objects seems to occur simply with increased exposure to the objects (Gibson & Gibson, 1955). The infant's knowledge about objects expands with every experience that involves observing events or manipulating objects (Gibson, 1988). On the other hand, development often involves periods of disorganization and reorganization at more complex or more advanced levels. Immediate and temporary perturbations disrupt current patterns of functioning; adaptation to these disruptions requires some accommodation. For example, once infants start to manipulate objects, parents will introduce new, more complex toys or will demonstrate new ways of handling objects; the children then have to change their usual mode of manipulation to accommodate to the novel structures and functions or to match the parents' actions. Imitated actions may not continue when infants then resume independent play (Lockman & McHale, 1989), but when infants are challenged frequently by adults, their accommodation eventually will be permanent.

While most perturbations and reorganizations occur at this level, there are some major transition points in development as well (McCall, Eichorn, & Hogarty). One of these transitions in the first year is around 2 months of age (Emde, Gaensbauer, & Harmon, 1976). At this time infants become more attentive to qualitative features of the environment (Ruff & Turkewitz, 1975), their recognition memory becomes more robust (Cohen et al., 1979), and they are better able to regulate arousal level (Dittrichova & Lapackova, 1964). Another transition occurs at 8 to 9 months, just after independent locomotion emerges with crawling and creeping. Bertenthal

13

and Campos (1990) argue that independent loco-motion fosters a reorganization of spatial cogni-tion. The children's own movement through the environment increases attention to objective spa-tial relationships and leads to new experiences with restrictions and frustrations. Moreover, chil-dren exhibit a growing dependence on distal emo-tional cues from parents to gather information about the safety or danger of new situations.

The third principle is that development occurs in a social context. This principle incorporates two meanings. One is that development occurs in part because relatively unsophisticated infants interact with more mature, experienced members of the society (Rogoff, 1990; Rogoff, Mistry, Göncü, & Mosier, 1993; Valsiner, 1987; Wertsch, 1979). Ro-goff (1990) speaks of guided participation, with the more experienced older child or adult guiding the younger and less experienced child in specific ways that facilitate the child's development and change in accord with his or her growing com-petence. That is, before specific knowledge and skills are consolidated, given activities may re-quire attention-directing, encouragement, and in-struction (Tomasello, Savage-Rumbaugh, & Kru-ger, 1993); after those skills are firmly in place, the child and the older members of society work to-gether on the less well formed aspects of cognitive functioning. It is important to note that this coop-erative effort is based as much on the child's seek-ing out help as it is on the readiness of the older partners to provide it.

The second meaning of social context stems from the fact that development occurs in the framework of a society's goals and standards for adult behavior. These will vary in different cul-tures, and we need to be mindful of the extent to which a child's development is determined by the parents' ideas (implicit and explicit) of what it is important for the child to learn or master. Rogoff (1990) provides a striking example of infants in New Guinea being able, with supervision, to han-dle knives and fire by the time they are able to walk; in American culture, we consider infants and toddlers incapable of handling either knives or fire without risking serious injury. In part, this attitude reflects the peripheral role that knives and fire have in our lives; but, more to the point, the example illustrates the importance of those at-titudes for development.

Major Developments in the First Year

PLAY

Play is sometimes considered the work of chil-dren because it appears to be a major avenue for development and learning. In the first year, play serves two major functions: exploration and learn-ing; and practice of motor and social skills. Thus, during play, knowledge is expanded and emergent skills are consolidated.

Infants in our culture spend considerable time playing alone. After about 6 months, this play usu-ally involves manipulation of toys and household objects. During manipulative play, infants engage in exploration of novel objects and motor play with familiar objects. Exploration of objects in-volves visual inspection and specific manipula-tions that provide particular kinds of information (Ruff, 1984b); these include fingering to explore texture and detail, turning the object around to provide different visual perspectives, and trans-ferring the object from hand to hand, an activity that provides global information about shape and size. Some aspects of mouthing also serve an im-portant role in exploration, providing the infant with tactual or haptic information about the ob-ject being mouthed (Ruff, Saltarelli, Capozzoli, & Dubiner, 1992). Exploring is intimately connected to attention; when exploring objects, infants show signs of concentration, such as a facial expression of interest, a reduction in irrelevant physical activ-ity, and a lower level of distractibility (Oakes & Tellinghuisen, 1994; Ruff, Capozzoli, & Saltarelli, in press; Ruff & Lawson, 1990).

Manipulative play with objects changes dramat-ically over the first year. It cannot occur, of course, without the skills of reaching and grasping, and infants do not reliably reach out and grasp nearby objects until 4½ or 5 months. From that time on, certain more refined activities, such as finger-ing, increase, as infants attain ever greater control over the fine muscles. Exploratory mouthing de-creases. Separate components become integrated into more complex activities so that the visual, haptic, and auditory systems reinforce and direct each other in gathering information about the ob-ject (Ruff, 1989).

Much play during infancy occurs in a social context with other people participating. The infants' initial play with others is usually face to face with one of the parents, although it can be with siblings and other adults as well. During this early play, infants learn a great deal about people; they learn to discriminate mother from stranger in terms of touch, voice, and sight; they learn to expect the predictable aspects of their mother's interchanges with them and to be distressed when these expectations are violated (Gusella, Muir, & Tronick, 1988; Toda & Fogel, 1993); and they learn to discriminate and recognize facial expressions of emotion (Walker, 1982). Later in the first year, infants start to play simple games with parents and, as they learn the "rules," they begin to take the initiative (Bruner & Sherwood, 1976; Gustafson, Green, & West, 1979).

After 5 or 6 months, infants' attention tends to focus more on elements in the environment outside the immediate dyad, in part because of the emerging ability to reach out and manipulate nearby objects. Play with others now includes joint play with objects in which the children gradually assume more initiative. By the end of the first year, children are somewhat adept at attending to and accommodating to the focus of another's attention (Adamson & Bakeman, 1991). At the same time, they are able to initiate episodes of play by persuading the partner to join in something that they themselves have started (Hubley & Trevarthen, 1979). The requisite skills include careful observation of the partner, being able to share a focus of attention, and imitation.

Imitation is important to cognitive development because it represents a means by which novel actions can emerge and become part of infants' behavioral repertoires. Uzgiris, Benson, Kruper, and Vaser (1989) suggest that imitation has three functions. One is the sharing of affective states where facial expressions and actions may be matched in face-to-face play. Later, the imitation of one partner by another constitutes taking a turn so that reciprocal and repeated imitation may be one form of "dialogue" between infant and adult. The third function of imitation is its role in learning new actions. During joint play with objects, mothers frequently demonstrate what can be done with objects; this often serves a training or didactic function (Bornstein, 1989; Lawson, Parri-

nello, & Ruff, 1992). Meltzoff (1988) found that 50% of a group of 9-month-olds imitated actions in both immediate and deferred conditions, and that for the whole group, these actions occurred significantly more often than the baseline frequency. The point at which infants are capable of imitation is a subject of controversy. Piaget (1951) considered that imitation did not occur until the latter half of the first year; others suggest that newborn infants may have a rudimentary ability to match facial expressions and actions (Field, Woodson, Greenberg, & Cohen, 1982; Meltzoff & Moore, 1977). In either view, initially adults assume the burden, demonstrating actions that are already in the infants' repertoire though perhaps in a new context; later children are able to imitate more novel and complex actions (Tomasello et al., 1993).

In summary, independent play and social play introduce children both to novel objects and events and to familiar objects and events in new situations. Both provide infants with an opportunity to explore these novel aspects of the environment and to practice and master emerging skills. Adults and older children play an important cooperative role in sharing and directing attention and in providing stimulation and information as they play jointly with infants.

PROBLEM SOLVING

An important aspect of cognitive development is the increasing ability to find solutions for everyday problems. Solving problems is largely a matter of overcoming obstacles to a goal. A problem that looms large in infancy is how to retrieve objects that have disappeared temporarily or to obtain visible objects that are out of reach. In these situations, the goal is a tangible object and the obstacles, physical ones; the skills and strategies developed for dealing with these physical obstacles, however, lay the foundation for the later ability to deal with more abstract problems.

Piaget (1954) dealt in detail with the problem of finding hidden objects. In his classic framework, the infant begins to retrieve partially hidden objects at approximately 5 months, then to find objects that have been covered as the infant watches at around 8 months, and to find an object when there are two possible hiding places even after a delay at around 10 to 11 months. Piaget considered only the situation in which objects could be retrieved by manual search. More recently, Baillargeon (1987, 1994) has argued that the understanding that this retrieval implies, often referred to as object permanence, is present earlier in the first year, at about 4 months. In one of her paradigms, infants simply watch displays in which a moving screen occludes an object. If the screen appears to move through the object rather than having its movement blocked by the object, the infants look longer than if the screen stops upon reaching the object. According to Baillargeon, infants are surprised or puzzled by the "impossible" event; that is, they have some expectation that objects will continue to exist at the location where they were last seen. Although there are limitations to the methods used, the disagreement between Piaget and Baillargeon in the age at which object permanence is considered to exist is a good example of how knowledge and skills are intertwined. At any given time, the perceptions and expectations of infants are based on the infants' particular skills; the emergence of new skills will lead to a reorganization of existing knowledge. Accordingly, when infants learn to reach and grasp, their perception and expectations about objects change. On the other hand, knowledge constrains the extent to which new skills can be formed and mastered; an infant whose understanding of objects is limited may not search for hidden objects, even when such search is physically possible.

The search for hidden objects is part of the general problem of finding the appropriate means for particular ends. Consider the problem of how to obtain something that can be seen but cannot be reached by a direct route; for example, a desired toy lies behind a transparent Plexiglas barrier. The skills and knowledge involved in the successful retrieval of the object in this case are (1) perceiving the situation correctly, (2) understanding the relationship between action and consequences, (3) inhibiting the inappropriate response of reaching directly, and (4) reaching around the barrier. The ability to modify activity in accordance with the consequences is present very early in development (Rovee-Collier, 1987), and infants readily repeat actions that are followed by interesting events (Piaget's [1952] secondary circular reactions). In the case of a transparent barrier, it might be argued that the infant does not perceive the Plexiglas as a solid surface. In unsuccessful infants, however, direct and ineffective reaching can occur even if the information for the Plexiglas as a solid surface is emphasized (Ruff, 1982). On the other hand, infants will reach correctly around or under an opaque surface before they will reach correctly with regard to a transparent barrier (Diamond, 1989; Gratch, 1972); the sight of the object seems to elicit a strong impulse to reach for it directly, an impulse that must be inhibited to achieve success.

On the basis of results from both human infants and young monkeys, Diamond and Goldman-Rakic (1989) have argued that the prefrontal cortex develops around 1 year of age and that its functioning in particular underlies infants' emerging ability to inhibit a strongly elicited, but inappropriate, response. If a strongly competing response is not activated by the situation, as may be the case in Baillargeon's method, then infants may attend to the relevant features of the environment. That is, a situation may be perceived accurately before it is acted on effectively (Baillargeon, 1994).

Along with the increasing ability to inhibit prepotent responses comes the ability to plan. Planning requires that there be a goal before the means are developed. Piaget (1952) suggests that, before 8 months, the infant is not truly goal directed. The infant acts, notices interesting consequences, and then can repeat the action in order to make the interesting consequences occur again. That is, the goal does not exist before the original action brought it to the infant's attention. After 8 months, however, the infant can have a goal and adapt activity in order to reach the goal; later the infant can experiment to find novel means of reaching the goal. Using one- and two-step problems, Willats and Rosie (1991) suggest that, after 9 months, infants show evidence of planning and not simple trial and error in reaching the desired end.

REPRESENTATION/MEMORY

Some researchers consider how children represent the external world in an abstract internal form to be the most important issue in early cognitive development. (See Mandler, 1983, for an extended discussion.) One approach to the study of representation is to investigate the development of memory. The simplest form of memory is recognition of an object or event to which the individual was exposed earlier. Fantz (1964) and Fagan (1971) developed one recognition memory paradigm. When an infant is repeatedly exposed to an event, that event loses its novelty and the infant becomes less responsive—a process known as habituation. Then when a different event is presented along with the now-familiar one, a stronger response to the novel event is taken as a sign that the infant differentiates between the novel and familiar events, recognizes the familiar event, and prefers the novel one. Care must be taken, of course, to avoid spontaneous preferences for certain types of events, but a systematic manipulation of the degree of discrepancy between the two events demonstrates the grossness or precision with which the familiar event has been perceived and recognized. Work with this paradigm shows that as they develop, infants can discriminate even smaller changes; beyond that, as they grow, they attend to more and somewhat different aspects of the events that they are exposed to (Cohen, DeLoache, & Strauss, 1979; Gibson & Spelke, 1983). Furthermore, after 3 or 4 months, recognition memory appears to be robust across time and interference (Cohen, DeLoache, & Pearl, 1977; Fagan, 1977; McCall, Kennedy, & Dodds).

When does the infant's behavior go beyond accurate perception and recognition and come to be based on some abstract representation of the world? A variation of the paradigm just described has been used to study concept formation. Different objects, which the experimenter judges to be in a single category, as presented to the child for familiarization. The experimenter can then test for categorization by presenting a novel exemplar of that category along with an object from a novel category. If the infant responds more to the novel category, the inference is that the infant is responding at the level of category rather than to specific objects. Although there are reasons to be cautious about the differentiation between perception and conception as it is studied with this method (Ruff, 1984a), a number of interesting developments do seem to occur. One is that from 4

to 7 months, the infant's ability to attend to the relationship among attributes in objects increases, and, from 7 to 10 months, the ability to abstract invariant relationships from a group of objects increases (Younger, 1985, 1993; Younger & Cohen, 1986). Under some circumstances, infants respond to prototypical objects as more familiar than the objects that actually were presented (Strauss, 1979)! This process of abstraction is a fundamental part of perception; it involves the detection of properties of objects that are invariant across changes in position, lighting, and general situation (Gibson, 1979). When we expose infants to multiple objects with a feature or a configuration of features in common, they readily attend to and remember the common characteristic (Ruff, 1978; 1984a). This process appears to be facilitated by being exposed to pairs of objects that differ along irrelevant dimensions, as if the invariant aspects are being emphasized (Ruff, 1978). At times, infants can respond to two categories where the characteristics differentiating between them are themselves quite abstract—birds versus airplanes, for example (Mandler & McDonough, 1993). Infants' ability to appreciate the nonobvious properties of objects can be seen as early as 9 months if the objects can be actively explored (Baldwin, Markman, & Melartin, 1993). Thus, knowledge grows with increasing exposure to objects and events in the world and is manifested in memory for specific events as well as in responses to categories of objects.

The ability to recall something that is not present is sometimes considered the hallmark of true representation and is generally not considered to be present in the first year. Mandler (1983) and Ashmead and Perlmutter (1980), however, argue that infants at around 9 months demonstrate recall of specific objects and can search for those objects in both permanent and temporary locations. For example, at 9 months, when asked "Where is your teddy?" infants begin to search for objects in their usual locations. This indicates that the infants know what object is being referred to and remember where it usually is kept. By 11 months, infants can remember temporary locations, that is, where an object was last seen. Ashmead and Perlmutter (1980) give an example of an 11-month-old girl playing with a toy baby bottle in the kitchen where it rolled partway under the refrigerator. The little girl then left the bottle and went to play elsewhere. Twenty minutes later she brought her doll to the kitchen, picked up the bottle, and took both back to her room. It is no accident that these examples come from infants acting in the home environment; a familiar setting increases the likelihood that they will demonstrate their maximum skills. The important point is that during the first year, infants begin to act on the basis of events that are no longer available to direct perception.

Assessment of Development

Although the discussion so far has revolved around specific issues, it has necessarily been general and has dealt with the average child. One concern of developmental psychologists and child psychiatrists, however, is how to understand the development of *individual* children. Formal, standardized means of assessing cognitive functioning exist, but a number of new techniques may help us to understand more about the processes underlying the cognitive development of individual infants.

The psychometric approach to developmental evaluation consists of items that the infant is judged to pass or fail. These items are linked to specific age ranges, and the final score is the number of items passed relative to the number passed by children of the same age in the normative sample. Although a clinician makes note of the manner in which items are passed or failed and thereby adds a qualitative element to the account, the score itself reflects specific criteria for correct performance.

The most widely used standardized cognitive test for infants is the Bayley Scale of Mental Development (Bayley, 1969, 1993). It is commonly said that the test has no predictive validity. McCall (1979) summarized the results of a number of studies and concluded that there was no clinically meaningful predictive value because correlations between infant test scores and later performance were typically in the range of 0.30. Kopp and McCall (1982) pursued this argument with regard to children at risk for developmental delays and

drew the same conclusion. On the other hand, a number of systematic longitudinal studies of low-birthweight infants have yielded substantial correlations between earlier and later tests (Lawson, Koller, Rose, & McCarton, 1994; Feldman, Wallace, & McCarton, 1989, 1991; Siegel, 1981), especially in infants at risk; these results support the usefulness of the early tests, but enough variance is left unaccounted for that we need to consider other possibilities.

Looking at development in terms of prediction is problematic because any single observation of a child gives us only a small window on a dynamic process. Also, different individuals reach the same endpoint by different paths; they may therefore look quite different from each other at earlier points. Finally, as valuable as the standardized instrument may be, it will not necessarily cover all the important aspects of development that may distinguish individuals.

For all of these reasons, process-oriented approaches have received more attention in recent years and are based on the large body of empirical work on infant development (Vietze & Vaughan, 1988). Two general issues must be considered. One is a concern about the context in which behavior is observed. Skills and knowledge are not things that infants "have." Instead, they are the results of an interplay among several factors, including the state of the organism, the capacities of the receptors, the specific psychological and physical aspects of the environment that support or interfere with the expression of a given behavior, and the immediate goal or purpose. Behavior that is elicited readily in one context may be completely absent in another. The pattern of responses in different situations, therefore, provides us with information about the processes that underlie behavior in a given situation.

A second aspect of a process-oriented approach is not so much a focus on outcome, but rather a concern with the manner in which the individual succeeds or fails particular items. This concern also raises the possibility that entirely new methods are required to illuminate important processes such as attention, learning, and memory. Ruff and Lawson (1991) have suggested some simple procedures to be used to assess attention during a developmental evaluation. The assessment involves the observation of the infant during manipulative play with objects and the measurement of focused attention (Ruff & Lawson, 1990). Focused attention represents those episodes during play that reflect effort and concentration and that usually occur when infants are examining novel objects. When assessed while infants play alone, the duration of focused attention provides a picture of the infants' tendency to mobilize spontaneously attention and effort for exploration. When assessed during infants' play with mother or other adult, it provides a picture of infants' ability to focus on an object with the help of an adult (Lawson et al., 1992; Parrinello & Ruff, 1988). There is wide variation in the amount of focused attention that normal infants show, and clinicians are concerned mainly with those who show extremely low levels, even with adult guidance. Recent work with a group of developmentally delayed toddlers, however, suggests that infants occasionally show so much focused attention to a single object that it could be described as perseverative (Saltarelli, Fulter Weit, & Ruff, 1991). The duration of focused attention is related at once to current risk status and later cognitive development (Ruff, 1988), to later attention (Ruff et al., 1990), and to some aspects of temperament (Ruff, 1990). Hence these simple procedures can add important information about the quality of the infant's activity in a context quite different from that of the standardized evaluation.

There has been a concerted effort to develop methods of assessing learning and memory in infancy. The most prominent example is the work of Fagan (Fagan & Shepherd, 1987; Fagan, Singer, Montie, & Shepherd, 1986), who has translated his experimental findings on recognition memory into an instrument that is now widely used. The Fagan Test of Infant Intelligence familiarizes infants with a picture and then presents that picture along with a novel one; the relative amount of time that infants look at the novel picture serves as an index of their interest in novelty and their recognition of and lower interest in the familiar object; the novelty index is continuous, not simply a pass/fail score. Premature infants and other infants at risk tend to spend less time looking at the novel picture (Rose, Feldman, McCarton, & Wolfson, 1988); the percent of time spent looking at the novel picture is related to later cognitive status (Fagan, Thompson & Fulker, 1991; Rose et al., 1989). Probing the issue of underlying processes, Rose, Feldman, McCarton, and Wolfson (1988) have shown that high-risk infants will learn and remember as much as full-term healthy infants only after longer periods of familiarization time. The high-risk infants also tend to be less efficient in gathering information during the familiarization period; that is, they turn away more often and take longer to accumulate the same degree of exposure. Rose et al. advocate that the number and length of individual looks be recorded in order to examine efficiency during familiarization (the learning period) as well as responsiveness during the test trial. McCall and Mash (1995) speculate that these tasks assess inhibitory capacity, a factor important in later intelligences.

In summary, enough research has been conducted on the cognitive development of infants that we can think seriously about applying the results to the problem of evaluating individual infants. In addition, the importance of context in contributing to the expression of knowledge and skills makes it essential that we observe individual infants in different situations. In that way, we can describe more adequately the infant's ability to gather information, solve problems, and adapt to the cognitive demands of everyday life.

REFERENCES

Adamson, L. B., & Bakeman, R. (1991). The development of shared attention during infancy. In R. Vasta (Ed.), *Annals of child development* (Vol. 8, pp. 1–41). London: Kinsley

Ashmead, D. H., & Perlmutter, M. (1980). Infant memory in everyday life. *New Directions for Child Development, 10*, 1–16.

Baillargeon, R. (1987). Object permanence in 3½- and 4½-month-old infants. *Developmental Psychology, 23*, 655–664.

Baillargeon, R. (1994). How do infants learn about the physical world? *Current Directions in Psychological Science, 3*, 133–140.

Baldwin, D. A., Markman, E. M., & Melartin, R. L.

(1993). Infants' ability to draw inferences about non-obvious object properties: Evidence from exploratory play. *Child Development, 64,* 711–728.

Barrera, M., & Maurer, D. (1981). The perception of facial expressions by the three-month-old. *Child Development, 52,* 203–206.

Bayley, N. (Ed.). (1969). *Bayley Scales of Infant Development.* New York: The Psychological Corporation.

Bayley, N. (1993). *Bayley scales of infant development* (2nd ed.). San Antonio, TX: Psychological Corporation.

Bertenthal, B. I., & Campos, J. J. (1990). A systems approach to the organizing effect of self-produced locomotion during infancy. In C. Rovee-Collier & L. P. Lipsitt (Eds.), *Advances in infancy research* (Vol. 6, pp. 1–60). Norwood, NJ: Ablex.

Bertenthal, B. I., Proffitt, D. R., & Kramer, S. J. (1987). Perception of biomechanical motions by infants: Implementation of various processing constraints. *Journal of Experimental Psychology: Human Perception and Performance, 13,* 577–585.

Bornstein, M. H. (1989). Between caretakers and their young: Two modes of interaction and their consequences for cognitive growth. In M. H. Bornstein & J. S. Bruner (Eds.), *Interaction in human development* (pp. 197–214). Hillsdale, NJ: Erlbaum.

Brown, A. L., Bransford, J. D., Ferrara, R. A., & Campione, J. C. (1983). Learning, remembering, and understanding. In P. H. Mussen (Ed.), *Cognitive development. Handbook of child psychology* (Vol. 3, pp. 79–166). New York: John Wiley & Sons.

Bruner, J. S. (1973). Organization of early skilled action. *Child Development, 44,* 1–11.

Bruner, J. S., & Sherwood, V. (1976). Peekaboo and the learning of rule structures. In J. S. Bruner, A. Jolly, & K. Sylva (Eds.), *Play—Its role in development and evolution* (pp. 277–285). New York: Basic Books.

Cohen, L. B., DeLoache, J. S., & Pearl, R. A. (1977). An examination of interference effects in infants' memory for faces. *Child Development, 48,* 88–96.

Cohen, L. B., DeLoache, J. S., & Strauss, M. S. (1979). Infant visual perception. In J. D. Osofsky (Ed.), *Handbook of infant development* (pp. 393–438). New York: John Wiley & Sons.

Diamond, A. (1991). Frontal lobe involvement in cognitive changes during the first year of life. In K. Gibson & A. Petersen (Eds.), *Brain and behavioral development* (pp. 127–180). New York: Aldine Press.

Diamond, A. (1989). Development as progressive inhibitory control of action: Retrieval of a contiguous object. *Cognitive Development,* 223–249.

Diamond, A., & Goldman-Rakic, P. S. (1989). Comparison of human infants and rhesus monkeys on Piaget's AB task: Evidence for dependence on dorsolateral prefrontal cortex. *Experimental Brain Research 74,* 24–40.

Dittrichova, J., & Lapackova, V. (1964). Development of the waking state in young infants. *Child Development, 35,* 365–370.

Ellsworth, C. P., Muir, D. W., & Hains, M. J. (1993).

Social competence and person-object differentiation: An analysis of the still-face effect. *Developmental Psychology, 29,* 63–73.

Emde, R. N., Gaensbauer, T. G., & Harmon, R. J. (Eds.). (1976). Emotional expression in infancy: A biobehavioral study. *Psychological Issues Monograph Series, 10* (37).

Fagan, J. F. (1971). Infants' recognition memory for a series of visual stimuli. *Journal of Experimental Child Psychology, 11,* 244–250.

Fagan, J. F. (1977). Infant recognition memory: Studies in forgetting. *Child Development, 48,* 68–78.

Fagan, J. F., & Shepherd, P. A. (Eds.). (1987). *The Fagan Test of Infant Intelligence Training Manual* (Vol. 4). Cleveland: Infantest Corp.

Fagan, J. F., Singer, L. T., Montie, J. E., & Shepherd, P. A. (1986). Selective screening device for the early detection of normal or delayed cognitive development in infants at risk for later mental retardation. *Pediatrics, 78,* 1021–1026.

Fantz, R. L. (1964). Visual experience in infants: Decreased attention to familiar patterns relative to novel ones. *Science, 146,* 668–670.

Field, T. M., Woodson, R., Greenberg, R., & Cohen, D. (1982). Discrimination and imitation of facial expressions of neonates. *Science, 218,* 179–181.

Fischer, K. W. (1980). The theory of cognitive development: The control and construction of hierarchies of skills. *Psychological Review, 87,* 477–531.

Fischer, K. W., & Hogan, A. E. (1989). The big picture for infant development: Levels and variations. In J. J. Lockman & N. L. Hazen (Eds.), *Action in social context: Perspectives on early development* (pp. 275–305). New York: Plenum Press.

Gibson, E. J. (1988). Exploratory behavior in the development of perceiving, acting, and the acquiring of knowledge. *Annual Review of Psychology, 39,* 1–41.

Gibson, E. J., & Spelke, E. S. (1983). The development of perception. In P. H. Mussen (Ed.), *Cognitive development. Handbook of child psychology* (Vol. 3, pp. 1–76). New York: John Wiley & Sons.

Gibson, J. J. (Ed.). (1966). *The senses considered as perceptual systems.* Boston: Houghton-Mifflin.

Gibson, J. J. (Ed.). (1979). *The ecological approach to visual perception.* Boston: Hougton-Mifflin.

Gibson, J. J., & Gibson, E. J. (1955). Perceptual learning: Differentiation or enrichment? *Psychological Review, 62,* 32–41.

Gratch, G. (1972). A study of the relative dominance of vision and touch in six-month-old infants. *Child Development, 43,* 615–623.

Gusella, J. L., Muir, D., & Tronick, E. Z. (1988). The effect of manipulating maternal behavior during an interaction on three- and six-month-olds' affect and attention. *Child Development, 59,* 1111–1124.

Gustafson, G. E., Green, J. A., & West, M. J. (1979). The infant's changing role in mother-infant games: The growth of social skills. *Infant Behavior and Development, 2,* 301–308.

Hofer, M. A. (1981). The parent-infant relationship. In

The roots of human behavior (pp. 193–233). San Francisco: W. H. Freeman.

Hubley, P., & Trevarthen, C. (1979). Sharing a task in infancy. In I. C. Uzgiris (Ed.), *New directions for child development* (Vol. 4, pp. 57–80). San Francisco: Jossey-Bass.

Kellman, P. J., & Spelke, E. S. (1983). Perception of partly occluded objects in infancy. *Cognitive Psychology, 15,* 483–524.

Kopp, C. B., & McCall, R. B. (1982). Predicting later mental performance for normal, at-risk and handicapped infants. In P. B. Baltes & O. G. Brim (Eds.), *Life span development and behavior* (Vol. 4, pp. 33–61). New York: Academic Press.

Lawson, K., Koller, H., Rose, S. A., & McCarton, C. (1994). *Relationships between early developmental assessments and IQ scores in very low birth weight children.* Unpublished manuscript.

Lawson, K. R., Parrinello, R., & Ruff, H. A. (1992). Maternal behavior and infant attention. *Infant Behavior and Development, 15,* 209–229.

Lewis, M. (1987). Social development in infancy and early childhood. In J. D. Osofsky (Ed.), *Handbook of infant development* (pp. 419–493). New York: John Wiley & Sons.

Lockman, J. J., & McHale, J. P. (1989). Object manipulation in infancy: Developmental and contextual determinants. In J. J. Lockman & N. L. Hazen (Eds.), *Action in a social context: Perspectives on early development* (pp. 129–167). New York: Plenum Press.

Mandler, J. M. (1983). Representation. In P. H. Mussen (Ed.), *Handbook of child psychology* (4th ed., Vol. 3, pp. 420–494). New York: John Wiley & Sons.

Mandler, J. M., & McDonough, L. (1993). Concept formation in infancy. *Cognitive Development, 8,* 291–318.

McCall, R. B. (1979). The development of intellectual functioning in infancy and the prediction of later I. Q. In J. D. Osofsky (Ed.), *Handbook of infant development* (pp. 707–741). New York: John Wiley & Sons.

McCall, R. B., Eichorn, D. H., & Hogarty, P. S. (1977). Transitions in early mental development. *Monographs of the Society for Research in Child Development, 42* (171).

McCall, R. B., Kennedy, C. B., & Dodds, C. (1977). The interfering effects of distracting stimuli on the infant's memory. *Child Development, 48,* 79–87.

McCall, R. B., & Mash, C. W. (1995). Infant cognition and its relation to mature intelligence. In R. Vasta (Ed.), *Annals of child development* (Vol. 10, pp. 27–56). London:Kingsley.

Meltzoff, A. N. (1988). Infant imitation and memory: Nine-month-olds in immediate and deferred tests. *Child Development, 59,* 217–225.

Meltzoff, A. N., & Moore, M. K. (1977). Imitation of facial and manual gestures by human neonates. *Science, 198,* 75–78.

Oakes, L. M., & Tellinghuisen, D. J. (1994). Examining in infancy: Does it reflect active processing? *Developmental Psychology, 30,* 748–756.

Parrinello, R. M., & Ruff, H. A. (1988). The influence of adult intervention on infants' level of attention. *Child Development, 59,* 1125–1135.

Piaget, J. (Ed.). (1951). *Play, dreams and imitation in childhood.* New York: W. W. Norton.

Piaget, J. (Ed.). (1952). *The origin of intelligence in children.* New York: International Universities Press.

Piaget, J. (Ed.). (1954). *The construction of reality in the child.* New York: Basic Books.

Pick, A. D., Frankel, D. G., & Hess, V. L. (1975). Children's attention: The development of selectivity. In E. M. Hetherington (Ed.), *Review of child development research* (Vol. 5, pp. 325–383). Chicago: University of Chicago Press.

Rogoff, B. (1990). *Apprenticeship in thinking.* New York: Oxford University Press.

Rogoff, B., Mistry, J., Göncü, A., & Mosier, C. (1993). Guided participation in cultural activity by toddlers and caregivers. *Monographs of the Society for Research in Child Development, 58* (8, Serial No. 236).

Rose, S. A., Feldman, J. F., McCarton, C., & Wolfson, J. (1988). Information processing in seven-month-old infants as a function of risk status. *Child Development, 59,* 589–603.

Rose, S. A., Feldman, J. F., Wallace, I. F., & McCarton, C. (1989). Infant visual attention: Relation to birth status and developmental outcome during the first 5 years. *Developmental Psychology, 25,* 560–576.

Rose, S. A., Feldman, J. F., Wallace, I. F., & McCarton, C. (1991). Information processing at 1 year: Relation to birth status and developmental outcome during the first 5 years. *Developmental Psychology, 27,* 723–737.

Rovee-Collier, C. (1987). Learning and memory in infancy. In J. D. Osofsky (Ed.), *Handbook of infant development* (pp. 98–148). New York: John Wiley & Sons.

Ruff, H. A. (1978). Infant recognition of the invariant form of objects. *Child Development, 49,* 193–206.

Ruff, H. A. (1980). The development of perception and recognition of objects. *Child Development, 51,* 981–992.

Ruff, H. A. (1982). The role of manipulation in infants' responses to invariant properties of objects. *Developmental Psychology, 18,* 682–691.

Ruff, H. A. (1982). Unpublished data.

Ruff, H. A. (1984a). An ecological approach to infant memory. In M. Moscovitch (Ed.), *Infant memory* (pp. 49–73). New York: Plenum Press.

Ruff, H. A. (1984b). Infants' manipulative exploration of objects. Effects of age and object characteristics. *Developmental Psychology, 20,* 9–20.

Ruff, H. A. (1988). The measurement of attention in high risk infants. In P. Vietze & J. H. G. Vaughan (Eds.), *Early identification of infants with developmental disabilities* (pp. 282–296). Philadelphia: Grunne & Stratton.

Ruff, H. A. (1989). The infants' use of visual and haptic

information in the recognition of objects. *Canadian Journal of Psychology, 43,* 302–319.

Ruff, H. A. (1990). Individual differences in sustained attention during infancy. In J. Colombo & J. W. Fagen (Eds.), *Individual differences in infancy: Reliability, stability, and prediction* (pp. 247–269). Hillsdale, NJ: Erlbaum.

Ruff, H. A., Capozzoli, M., & Saltarelli, L. M. (In press). Focused visual attention and distractibility in 10-month-old infants. *Infant Behavior and Development.*

Ruff, H. A., & Lawson, K. R. (1990). Development of sustained, focused attention in young children during free play. *Developmental Psychology, 26,* 85–93.

Ruff, H. A., & Lawson, K. R. (1991). Assessment of infants' attention during play with objects. In C. E. Schaefer, K. Gitlin, & A. Sandgrund (Eds.), *Play diagnosis & assessment* (pp. 115–129). New York: John Wiley & Sons.

Ruff, H. A., Lawson, K. R., Parrinello, R., & Weissberg, R. (1990). Long-term stability of individual differences in sustained attention in the early years. *Child Development, 61,* 60–75.

Ruff, H. A., & Rothbart, M. K. (1996). *Attention in early development: Themes and variations.* New York: Oxford University Press.

Ruff, H. A., Saltarelli, L. M., Capozzoli, M., & Dubiner, K. (1992). The differentiation of activity in infants' exploration of objects. *Developmental Psychology, 28,* 851–861.

Ruff, H. A., & Turkewitz, G. (1975). Developmental changes in the effectiveness of stimulus intensity on infant visual attention. *Developmental Psychology, 11,* 705–710.

Saltarelli, L., Capozzoli, M., & Ruff, H. A. (1990, April). Focused attention and distractibility. Paper presented at the International Conference on Infant Studies, Montreal, Canada.

Saltarelli, L. M., Futterweit, L. R., & Ruff, H. A. (1991). *Focused attention: A clinical measure of individual differences in attention during play.* Unpublished manuscript.

Sameroff, A. J. (1983). Developmental systems: Contexts and evolution. In P. H. Mussen (Ed.), *Handbook of child psychology* (Vol. 1, pp. 237–294). New York: John Wiley & Sons.

Serrano, J. M., Iglesias, J., & Loeches, A. (1995). Infants' responses to adult static facial expressions. *Infant Behavior and Development, 18,* 477–482.

Siegel, L. S. (1981). Infant tests as predictors of cognitive and language development at 2 years. *Child Development, 52,* 545–557.

Stern, D. N., Hofer, L., Haft, W., & Dore, J. (1985). Affect attunement: The sharing of feeling states between mother and infant by means of inter-modal fluency. In T. Field & N. Fox (Eds.), *Social perception in infants* (pp. 249–268). Norwood, NJ: Ablex.

Strauss, M. S. (1979). Abstraction of prototypical information by adults and 10 month old infants. *Journal of Experimental Psychology: Human Learning and Memory, 6,* 618–632.

Thelen, E. (1984). Learning to walk: Ecological demands and phylogenic constraints. In L. P. Lipsitt & C. Roxee-Collier (Eds.), *Advances in Infancy Research* (Vol. 3, pp. 213–264). Norwood, NJ: Ablex.

Thelen, E., & Fogel, A. (1989). Toward an action-based theory of infant development. In J. Lockman & N. Hazen (Eds.), *Action in social context: Perspectives on early development* (pp. 23–63). New York: Plenum Press.

Thelen, E., & Smith, L. B. (1994). *A dynamic systems approach in development of cognition and action.* Cambridge, MA: MIT Press.

Thompson, L. A., Fagan, J. F., & Fulker, D. W. (1991). Longitudinal prediction of specific cognitive abilities from infant novelty preference. *Child Development, 62,* 530–538.

Toda, S., & Fogel, A. (1993). Infant response to the still-face situation at 3 and 6 months. *Developmental Psychology, 29,* 532–538.

Tomasello, M., Savage-Rumbaugh, S., & Kruger, A. C. (1993). Imitative learning of actions on objects by children, chimpanzees, and enculturated chimpanzees. *Child Development, 64,* 1688–1705.

Uzgiris, I. C., Benson, J. B., Kruper, J. C., & Vasek, M. E. (1989). Contextual influences on imitative interactions between mothers and infants. In J. J. Lockman & N. L. Hazen (Eds.). *Action in social context: Perspectives on early development* (pp. 103–127). New York: Plenum Press.

Valsiner, J. (Ed.). (1987). *Culture and the development of children's action.* New York: John Wiley & Sons.

Vietze, P. M., & Vaughan, H. G., Jr. (Eds.). (1988). *Early identification of infants with developmental disabilities.* Philadelphia: Grune & Stratton.

Walker, A. S. (1982). Intermodal perception of expressive behaviors by human infants. *Journal of Experimental Child Psychology, 33,* 514–535.

Welsh, M. C., & Pennington, B. F. (1988). Assessing frontal lobe functioning in children: Views from developmental psychology. *Developmental Neuropsychology, 4,* 199–230.

Wertsch, J. V. (1979). From social interaction to higher psychological processes. A clarification and application of Vygotsky's theory. *Human Development, 22,* 1–22.

Willats, P., & Rosie, K. (1991, April). A longitudinal study of planning in infants. Paper presented at the biennial meeting of the Society for Research in Child Development, Seattle, Washington.

Younger, B. A. (1985). The segregation of items into categories by ten-month-old infants. *Child Development, 56,* 1574–1583.

Younger, B. (1993). Understanding category members as "the same sort of thing": Explicit categorization in ten-month infants. *Child Development, 64,* 309–320.

Younger, B. A., & Cohen, L. B. (1986). Developmental change in infants' perception of correlation among attributes. *Child Development, 57,* 803–815.

3 / Normal Language Development: The First Year

Rhea Paul

The first year of life is a time in which infants, though not yet using words, nonetheless engage in a great deal of communication. From the moment of birth, this communication is an active process between child and the social environment. The infant is far from being either a blank slate on which language is impressed by adults or a passive recipient of adult speech. Instead, the infant engages in behaviors that rivet the adult's attention and elicit social interaction. For the infant, these abilities to attract the adult's notice, to initiate and maintain social contact, and to evoke positive emotions have powerful survival value. Helpless, troublesome, noisy individuals who did not possess these winning traits might soon appear to be more bother to their social group than they were worth. In addition, these capacities are ideally suited to eliciting for the infant a rich array of linguistic stimulation. In the following sections, we examine the perceptual and communicative skills that lay the basis for the development of language.

The Newborn's Equipment for Language Learning

Crying is the newborn's principal form of vocal behavior. Crying is primarily involuntary, a response to the infant's internal distress. Although crying is an important form of communication for the infant and is effective in soliciting adult attention, language probably does not evolve out of cry behavior. Lenneberg (1967) has argued that infant crying develops into adult crying and that language has different roots in some of the infant's other vocal behaviors.

It does appear that newborns begin life with attentional preferences for human, linguistic interaction and that they are endowed with a set of social behaviors that can elicit this stimulation. Because of their emergence so soon after birth, these abilities would appear to be innately programmed. As such, they provide a great deal of economy in the task of mastering language. Certain propensities are present from the first days of life; these include a preference for sounds in the frequency range of the human voice (Hutt, Hutt, Leonard, Benuth, & Muntjewerff, 1968) and a preference for speech over other rhythmic or musical sounds (Butterfield & Siperstein, 1974). When newborns hear a voice, they look for the source of that sound, register pleasure with facial expression when they identify the source, and remain quiet, inhibiting their movements, until the voice ceases (Owens, 1992). They do not show this kind of recognition when a nonhuman auditory stimulus is heard. Three-day-old infants have been shown to be able to recognize their own mother's voices as opposed to the voices of other women (DeCasper & Fifer, 1980); this is probably a result of prenatal experience with the mother's voice heard through the amniotic sac. Newborns also are attracted to and prefer to look at faces (Kagan & Lewis, 1965). Parents, conveniently, interpret this preference as a sign of willingness to interact. The newborn would appear, then, to be biologically organized to attract language input and to attune to the linguistic environment.

The Infant's Perceptual Skills

Babies have been shown to have some special capacities for processing language that are present from very early in life (Eimas et al., 1971). Nonnutritive sucking paradigms have been used to study the ability of infants as young as 4 weeks of age to discriminate among the sounds of speech. In these studies, the infant is given a pacifier attached to a pressure-measuring device, which is used to control a stimulus, such as a tape-recorded speech sound. If the stimulus is reinforcing or pleasant to the child, the infant will suck at a high rate, which makes the stimulus available continuously. After a while, the infant tires of the stimulus or habituates to it, and slows down the sucking rate. When this happens, the experimenter can switch the stimulus. If the child hears a difference in the new stimulus, he or she will again suck faster. If the child does not perceive the new sound as different from the old one, the sucking rate will not increase. In this way it is possible to tell whether infants 1 to 4 months of age can discriminate one sound from another.

Using this paradigm, babies as young as 4 weeks have been able to discriminate among a variety of speech sounds, including /pa/ vs. /ba/, /ta/ vs. /da/, and /ba/ vs. /ga/, to name a few (Aslin, Pisoni, & Juscyck, 1983; Eimas, Siqueland, Juscyck, & Vigorito, 1971). Of even greater interest is the observation that infants make these distinctions along the same categorical boundaries as do adults. For example, /b/ and /p/ sounds differ, essentially, only in what phoneticians call voice-onset time, or the period between the silent stoppage of air behind the lips and the onset of voicing at the larynx. Adults perceive a sound as /ba/ when voice-onset time is less than about 40 milliseconds. Adults hear a /pa/ when voice-onset time exceeds about 50 milliseconds. Babies in the nonnutritive sucking paradigm experiments ignored differences in voice-onset time that adults would consider to be within the /ba/ or /pa/ category but responded to changes of the same magnitude when those changes resulted in the voice-onset time's going over the boundary between the two sounds.

The fact that such distinctions can be made at 1 month of age can be interpreted to mean that the ability to make them is innate. Alternatively, it can suggest that this perceptual learning happens very quickly. Researchers have attempted to address this question by looking at sound discriminations that infants could not have learned from their environment because they never heard them made. For example, Werker and Tees (1984) found that infants in English-speaking environments were able to distinguish sounds that are not used in English but are used in Hindi. By 1 year of age, though, this ability to discriminate sounds not heard in the native language had all but dis-

appeared. These findings suggest that the infant does have some "built-in" capacity to make discriminations among sounds that are important in speech but that this ability is modified with experience. Rather than learning to make these distinctions from the language they hear, however, it seems that the infant comes to the task of language with some discriminations "preset." Depending on what particular distinctions are used by the ambient language, some of these innately programmed distinctions will be maintained by the child's experience, while others will be extinguished.

Young babies also appear to be able to coordinate acoustic information about speech with visual information about oral posture. Kuhl and Meltzoff (1988) showed babies 18 weeks of age two pictures of the face of the same woman articulating two different sounds: /a/ and /i/. They played one of these sounds through a loudspeaker located midway between the two pictures. They were able to show that the infants looked for a significantly longer time at the picture of the face whose oral gesture corresponded to the vowel the babies were hearing at the time (retracted lips for /i/; open lips for /a/). This surprising finding suggests a very early ability to integrate visual and auditory cues in the perception of speech, and would seem to provide children with an excellent foundation for learning the articulatory movements associated with the speech sounds they eventually will learn to produce.

Although children do not understand words per se until near the end of the first year, they appear to begin to develop the bases for the semantic categories with which these words will be associated much earlier. Colombo, O'Brien, Mitchell, Roberts, and Horowitz (1987) showed slides of various kinds of birds to babies 6 to 7 months of age; this was continued until the children habituated to these stimuli and reduced their visual fixation time. The investigators then showed two new slides simultaneously, one of a parakeet and one of a horse, for example. Babies reliably looked longer at the horse, suggesting that it was more novel to them than the parakeet, which they had also not seen before. Thus it appears that the children included the parakeet in the category they had formed for the objects viewed previously—birds. These findings suggest that even at this early age, babies are able to organize their perceptions into conceptual categories that eventually can be mapped onto words.

Recent studies of speech perception in 7-month-olds suggest that they also are sensitive to auditory information that is associated with syntactic boundaries. Hirsh-Pasek, Golinkoff, and Cauley (1987) showed that babies of this age preferred to look toward a speaker that played sentences containing pauses at clause or phrase boundaries (Cinderella lived in a great big house/ but it was sort of dark/because she had a mean/ stepmother), as opposed to sentences with pauses in the middle of a clause (Cinderella lived in a great big house but it was/sort of dark because she had/a mean/stepmother). These results suggest that babies as young as 7 months can detect syntactic boundaries, an ability that would greatly economize the amount of information they ultimately will need to acquire in order to understand sentences.

Although parents act as if they believe their child understood speech almost from the first day of life, true lexical comprehension does not emerge until about 8 months of age. Babies as young as 6 months will inhibit their behavior if told "no" in a loud, sharp voice, but they will do the same if they hear "yes" spoken in the same tone (Spitz, 1957). Around the last quarter of the first year, though, babies begin to respond to certain words that they hear as part of familiar routines; they will, for example, clap hands when mother says, "Let's play patty-cake." This early comprehension is contextually bound, however. If the baby is used to playing patty-cake on the changing table but is told to clap hands in the bathtub, the youngster probably will not comply.

Chapman (1978) points out that this contextually bound comprehension often leads parents to believe that babies at 8 to 12 months understand much more language than they actually do. Chapman describes a set of strategies for comprehension that are frequently used by infants of this age to comply with parental requests and that give the parent the impression the child is actually understanding language. Babies look at what mother looks at, which can give the impression that the baby understands what the mother is saying. In fact, though, all the baby has to do is follow the mother's line of regard.

Babies also tend to do something to the objects they notice. Since their repertoire of actions is fairly limited at this stage, by judiciously choosing their instructions, parents can heighten the likelihood that the child will comply. For example, a mother might say to the baby, "See the pretty ball!" Following her line of gaze, the baby looks at the ball. Once noted, baby is very likely, then, to move toward it. If the mother says at the same time, "Go get the ball for Mommy," the baby can appear to comply with the instruction, when, in fact, that was what the child was going to do anyway.

Another strategy infants employ at this stage is to imitate ongoing action. Mother says, "Give me a kiss" and purses her lips. The baby smacks his lips, too. Is the baby really comprehending the mother's sentence, or only doing what she is doing? Evidence from presenting similar sentences without nonverbal cues suggests that the baby is imitating action rather than comprehending language.

What is the function of these comprehension strategies? Are the mother and baby trying to deceive someone? Hardly. What the baby is trying to do is to participate successfully in an interaction, and is using every means at his or her disposal to do so. Mothers, on the other hand, also are trying to get the baby to participate and succeed. They unconsciously behave in such a way as to give the baby ample cues, both linguistic and nonlinguistic, as to their meaning. When the baby responds appropriately, two things happen. First, the child experiences the pleasure of a positive social interaction. And second, the child gets another example of the way in which language works to encode what he or she already knows about the world. In this way the baby moves closer to truly linguistic comprehension.

Infant Sound Production

The quality of infant vocalization changes drastically throughout the first year of life. Stark (1979) has presented a framework for describing infant vocal behavior. According to this framework, from birth to 2 months of age, the infant produces primarily reflexive cries and other vegetative sounds. Part of the reason for the small range of sounds produced during this period is anatomical (Sachs, 1989). The newborn's oral cavity is small, and the tongue takes up most of the space in it. The vocal folds are relatively high in the pharynx, so that there is little ability to modify the shape of the resonating chamber. Although the infant's cries have a profound effect on the adults who hear them, the infant is not using the crying in any intentional way to attract the adults' notice. Rather the cry is an instinctual response to an internal state such as hunger, cold, or boredom. Vegetative sounds such as burps, coughs, and sneezes are also reflexive, but adults will respond to these noises as if they were communicative. This willingness on the part of adults to attribute intentionality to the infant's early reflexive sound production may be one of the ways in which infants are "taught" to use sound to communicate.

As the baby grows, the head and neck anatomy changes, resulting in a greater diversity of sounds that can be produced and a more speechlike resonance associated with vocalization. Between 2 and 5 months of age, babies begin two behaviors that are important for the development of speech and communication. One is the pleasant, somewhat speechlike sound that babies produce primarily in response to social interactions, known as cooing, or "comfort" sounds. The name arises from the "oo"-like quality of most of the vowels heard during this type of vocalizing and from the fact that most of the consonants produced sound like /k/ and /g/. Again, the reasons for the "coo" quality of these vocalizations are anatomical. As the baby lies in a prone or semiprone position, gravity operates most strongly on the relatively large posterior portion of the tongue, pulling it back toward the roof of the mouth. This oral posture produces the consonants we recognize as /g/ and /k/ as well as the vowel we recognize as "oo." Cooing is highly rewarding to people who elicit it, and adults will work hard to get babies to respond to them with coos and goos.

A second vocal behavior that adults find highly reinforcing is the infant's laugh, which emerges around the same time as cooing. Usually accompanied by a social smile, infant laughing is produced in response to an interaction the infant perceives as pleasurable, very often because it is a known routine whose components are predictable. Thus babies may laugh when mother plays "peek-a-boo" for them, or when she assumes a posture as if ready to tickle them. Crying becomes less frequent during this period of increasingly diverse and speechlike vocalization.

The next stage of vocal development begins at about 4 months of age and extends to about 8 months. Stark refers to this period as "vocal play." In this phase the infant begins to pronounce what sounds like single syllables with vowel- and consonantlike components. Though not approximations of words, and not meant to convey any referential meaning, these early forms of babbling continue the infant's progress toward increasingly speechlike sounds. The consonants produced tend to be made more toward the front of the mouth than were those used for cooing.

Vocal play, unlike cooing, does not appear principally in response to social interactions. Although infants do use vocal play as a means of responding to or initiating contact with adults, babies also engage in vocal play when alone. Vocal play may, then, function as a means for infants to "practice" the new sound production abilities they are acquiring. As Mattingly (1972) suggests, the configuration of the infant's growing vocal tract is changing rapidly at this time. As infants engage in vocal play, at the same time they are exploring the spatial properties of this chamber and updating sensory and proprioceptive information about it. In addition, the feedback, both proprioceptive and acoustic, that infants receive from this sound play may help to associate particular articulatory behaviors with acoustic consequences.

Prior to the vocal play stage, the babbling of deaf babies resembles that of their normal hearing counterparts. Lenneberg (1967) was the first to note that it is during the vocal play stage that the deaf baby's babbling begins to differ from that of the normal hearing infant. More recently, Stoel-Gammon and Otomo (1986) substantiated these observations, showing that at this age level, hearing-impaired babies had smaller repertoires of consonants than normal-hearing peers and that, in fact, the size of the hearing-impaired babies' inventories decreased from 4 to 18 months, while those of the normal-hearing babies increased. Thus the ability to derive auditory feedback from vocal play appears to be important in the development of the babbling repertoires and their eventual transition to speech.

Stark (1979) reports that a new form of vocal behavior, which she refers to as "reduplicated babbling," appears in the second half of the first year of life. This type of vocalization includes consonant-vowel combinations, such as /bababa/ or /nanana/, in which the same syllable is repeated over and over. Consonants most likely to appear include /b/, /p/, /t/, /d/, /m/, /n/ and the glide *y*. Like vocal play, reduplicated babbling often occurs when the baby is alone. Stark points out that at this stage, gestures carry most of the communicative value of the interaction; only later are babbled vocalizations coordinated with gestures in the service of communication.

Toward the end of the first year of life, many babies begin to use "vocables," or phonetically consistent forms. These are productions that are unique to the child in that they do not closely resemble any adult word but are used reliably in certain situations (Owens, 1992). For example, Carter (1978) reported that one child consistently used an /m/ sound along with reaching to indicate that he wanted something. These early consistent forms are sometimes referred to as "proto-words."

Infant Interaction and Communication

An infant as young as 1 month of age will, when wide awake and held in an appropriate position, look intently at an adult and vocalize (Bullowa, 1979). Babies also may begin to imitate some of the parent's intonation patterns (Trevarthen, 1979); by 3 months of age, they will show more vocal responsiveness to their mothers than to other adults. Although infants can distinguish their mothers from other adults at a very early age, they do not show any fear or distrust of strangers in this early period. Rather in their gaze and facial expression they evidence mild surprise and interest on seeing a new face. These new faces are often a stimulus for vocalization, leading the baby's cooing to increase (Wolff, 1963).

As babies get older and the face becomes more familiar, their preference for faces decreases and the babies become attracted to more complex stimuli (Brennan, Ames, & Moore, 1966). When infants are about 3 months of age, parents begin to modify their behavior, providing greater stimulation in order to maintain their baby's attention. Parents exaggerate their facial expressions, talk more, and exaggerate the intonational contours of the voice. Infants, for their part, respond with vocalization more frequently to the parent's speech than to touch (Lewis & Cherry, 1977). For their part, after their own vocalizations, parents give the child longer pauses as if waiting for the infant to take a turn (Schaffer, Collis, & Parsons, 1977). This back-and-forth vocalization pattern is thought to lay the basis for conversational turn-taking and is sometimes referred to as "proto-conversation." It is not, however, the only pattern of vocalization between parents and infants. The two often will vocalize together, with the parent imitating the baby's sounds, as if singing in unison (Stern, Jaffe, Beebe, & Bennett, 1975).

Babies use gaze extensively to regulate these interactions. Babies look at the parent when they are interested in interacting and avert their gaze when they become tired or overstimulated (Stern, 1977). Babies can follow their parent's gaze to attend to an object the adult points to; later, babies begin to direct the parent's attention by looking at objects themselves. Parents will follow the infant's line of regard and look at what the baby looks at. Frequently, parents will comment on this object of the baby's gaze. These interactions, in which the parent and child share focus on an object, have been called "joint attention routines" (Bruner, 1977). Such routines are thought to be very important in laying the foundation for the basic topic-comment structure of language an organization in which one speaker directs the other's attention to a focus of interest, on which the conversation then elaborates.

Snow (1977) points out that in babies of 3 months of age, mothers respond to whatever the infant does, including to burps and coughs, and treats these behaviors as if they were communicative. Mothers also spend a great deal of time and energy trying to get young babies to take their conversational turn by cooing or smiling. (This is in contrast to what we do as adults in conversation, which is to try to get as much time for our own turn as possible.) As noted, mothers pause after an utterance to give the baby a chance to respond. If they fail to get a response, they may repeat themselves, or use a questioning intonation, such as "hmm?" In young infants, parents accept almost any behavior as fulfilling the child's conversational obligation to take a turn. Later, the requirements for what constitute the child's turn become more stringent.

Within these communicative interactions, the quality of speech directed to infants has some distinctive properties. Adults from a variety of cultures (not all) speak to babies with a higher pitch than they use for other listeners (Snow & Ferguson, 1977). In addition, the intonational patterns of adult speech to babies have more exaggerated contours and a "singsong" quality (Sachs, 1989). These features appear to match the babies' perceptual preferences and may function to attract their attention to the speech, making it easier for parents and babies to interact. Parents may use a special "baby talk" lexicon, such as calling the baby's stomach a "tummy" or referring to toes as "toesie-toes." They may even produce speech that contains "errors" similar to the type children make when they first begin talking; so, for example, a parent may call the child a "toot [cute] widdo [little] baby." Sachs (1989) points out that this special quality of speech directed to infants has not only a perceptual but an affective salience. It is a way that we express affection to babies, and this special speech style is just one aspect of the adult's effort to establish a strong affective bond with the infant. These types of infant-directed speech are extremely common across of a range of cultures and are in no way detrimental to the child's development.

At about 8 months of age, babies enter the cognitive stage of intentionality (see Chapter 2), the point at which mental development allows them to hold goals in mind long enough to pursue them through action. Cognitive development at this time also supports the ability to understand actions as a means to an end. Now babies begin to use communication as a means to the outcomes—in the form of parental attention or the acquisition of objects—that they desire. Such communicative acts usually become manifest at about the same time that other forms of intentional behavior emerge—about 8 to 10 months of age.

At this stage communication is accomplished primarily with gestures, such as holding objects up for the mother to view or pointing. Acredolo and Goodwyn (1988) reported that the use of idiosyncratic symbolic gestures to communicate is quite common during the last half of the first year of life. These investigators found that some children as young as 11 months of age used relatively stable gestures, motions that resembled manual signs, to stand for objects or actions for the purpose of communication. For example, a child might bounce up and down to indicate "rabbit" or press on the eyes to indicate "sun." Often these gestures are accompanied by a look at the parent to see that she is attending.

Based on their communicative function, Bates (1976) categorizes these early intentional behaviors into two broad types: proto-imperatives and proto-declaratives. Proto-imperative speech acts are those in which children attempt to get the listener to do something for them or to stop doing something; these would appear to evolve into linguistic imperatives or commands. Proto-imperative speech acts include requests for objects that the child can indicate by pointing or reaching. Requests for actions, also fall into this category; the child can convey these by miming some part of a familiar ritual. For example, a frequent part of interactive routines at this stage is the "body-part-naming-game." The child might climb on the mother's lap and touch his nose to indicate that he wants his mother to play this. Protests or rejections also occur, in the course of which the child communicates the desire to turn down some object or activity the mother is attempting to offer by pushing away or turning away.

Proto-declarative speech acts direct the mother's attention to an object of the child's interest by pointing to it, holding it up, showing, or giving it. These acts are thought to lay the basis for the later use of referential language. Proto-declarative speech acts are thought to evolve out of the earlier-established joint attentional routines that appear to be very important for later language development. Several studies of language-impaired individuals (Paul & Shiffer, 1991 Wetherby, Yonclas & Bryan, 1989); suggest that proto-declarative speech acts are less frequently used by children with various types of language disorders.

As babies begin to evidence this intentional communication, parents "up the ante" (Bruner, 1978), requiring a more sophisticated form of response in order for it to "count" as the child's contribution. Whereas we saw earlier that mothers accepted any child behavior, such as a burp or a cough, as a communicative response, when true intentionality does develop, the mother requires the child to do something more sophisticated in order to fulfill a turn. The child is now expected to imitate the mother, to produce a conventional gesture, and, eventually, to vocalize. In this way, the baby's communication is "shaped" into language.

Summary

The first year of life is a time in which the foundation for the development of language is laid down. Perceptual and attentional processes apparent from birth render human, linguistic stimulation particularly salient. Parents tune their input to the changing needs and interests of the child, requiring more and more sophisticated responses as the baby's repertoire of social and linguistic behaviors expands. Vocal behavior becomes increasingly speechlike and is used both in solitary play and for interaction. At the same time, the ability to use communication as a means toward a desired end is shaped by the parent's early attribution of communicative intent to the child's behavior. Eventually, in the last part of the first year, this intent does emerge, and the child uses primarily gestural means to express a small range of communicative functions. The child's desire to participate successfully in interactions and the parent's desire to see the child do so converge. Together, they result in the appearance of linguistic comprehension that is, in fact, the product of the child's use of interactive strategies for responding to adult input. As the child moves into the second year of life, all these abilities—perceptual, social, vocal, communicative, and receptive—come together and take form in the child's use and understanding of the first true words.

REFERENCES

Acredolo, L., & Goodwyn, S. (1988). Symbolic gesturing in normal infants. *Child Development, 59,* 450–466.

Aslin, R. N., Pisoni, D. B., & Jusczyk, P. W. (1983). Auditory development and speech perception in infancy. In M. M. Haith & J. J. Campos (Eds.), *Handbook of child psychology: Vol. 2. Infancy and developmental psychobiology* (pp. 107–112). New York: John Wiley & Sons.

Bates, E. (1976). *Language and context: The acquisition of pragmatics.* New York: Academic Press.

Brennan, W., Ames, E., & Moore, R. (1966). Age differences in infants' attention to patterns of different complexities. *Science, 151,* 354–356.

Bruner, J. (1977). Early social interaction and language acquisition. In R. Schaffer (Ed.), *Studies in mother-infant interaction* (pp. 4–36). New York: Academic Press.

Bruner, J. (1978). Learning how to do things with words. In J. Bruner & A. Gurton (Eds.), *Wolfson College lectures 1976: Human growth and development* (pp. 255–287). Oxford: Oxford University Press.

Bullowa, M. (1979). Infants as conversational partners. In T. Myers (Ed.), *The development of conversation and discourse* (pp. 72–85). Edinburgh: Edinburgh University Press.

Butterfield, E., & Siperstein, G. (1974). Influence of contingent auditory stimulation upon non-nutritional suckle. *Proceedings of the Third Symposium on Oral Sensation and Perception: The Mouth of the Infant* (pp. 313–334). Springfield, IL: Charles C. Thomas.

Carter, A. (1978). From sensori-motor vocalizations to words: A case study of the evolution of attention-directing communication in the second year. In A. Lock (Ed.), *Action, gesture and symbol: The emergence of language* (pp. 310–349). New York: Academic Press.

Chapman, R. (1978). Comprehension strategies in children. In J. F. Kavanaugh & W. Strange (Eds.), *Speech and language in the laboratory, school and clinic* (pp. 308–327). Cambridge, MA: MIT Press.

Colombo, J., O'Brien, M., Mitchell, D., Roberts, K., & Horowitz, F. (1987). A lower boundary for category formation in preverbal infants. *Journal of Child Language, 14,* 383–385.

De Casper, A. J., & Fifer, W. P. (1980). Of human bonding: Newborns prefer their mothers' voices. *Science, 208,* 1174–1176.

Eimas, P., Siqueland, E., Jusczyk, P, & Vigorito, J. (1971). Speech perception in infants. *Science, 171,* 303–306.

Hirsh-Pasek, K., Golinkoff, R., & Cauley, K. (1987). *The verb's the thing: Therein to catch the origins of grammar.* Paper presented to Society for Research in Child Development, Baltimore, MD.

Hutt, S., Hutt, C., Leonard, H., Benuth, H., & Muntjewerff, W. (1968). Auditory responsivity in the human newborn. *Nature, 218,* 888–890.

Kagan, J., & Lewis, M. (1965). Studies of attention. *Merrill-Palmer Quarterly, 11,* 92–127.

Kuhl, P., & Meltzoff, A. (1988). Speech as an intermodal object of perception. In A. Yonas (Ed.), *Perceptual development in infancy* (pp. 235–266). Hillsdale, NJ: Erlbaum.

Lenneberg, E. (1967). *Biological foundations of language.* New York: John Wiley & Sons.

Lewis, M., & Cherry, L. (1977). Social behavior and language acquisition. In M. Lewis & L. Rosenblum (Eds.), *Interaction, conversation, and the development of language* (pp. 112–127). New York: Wiley.

Mattingly, I. (1972). Reading, the linguistic process, and linguistic awareness. In J. Kavanaugh & I. Mattingly (Eds.), *Language by ear and eye* (pp. 133–148). Cambridge, MA: MIT Press.

Owens, R. E., Jr. (1992). *Language development* (3rd ed.), Columbus, OH: Merrill.

Paul, R., & Shiffer, M. (1991). Communicative initiations in normal and late-talking toddlers. *Applied Psycholinguistics, 12* (4), 419–431.

Sachs, J. (1977). The adaptive significance of linguistic input to prelinguistic infants. In C. Snow & C. Ferguson (Eds.), *Talking to children: Language input and acquisition* (pp. 51–62). New York: Cambridge University Press.

Sachs, J. (1989). Communication development in infancy. In J. B. Gleason (Ed.), *The development of language* (pp. 39–64). New York: Merrill.

Schaffer, H., Collis, G., & Parsons, G. (1977). Vocal interchange and visual regard in verbal and pre-verbal children. In H. Schaffer (Ed.), *Studies in mother-infant interaction* (pp. 291–324). New York: Academic Press.

Snow, C. (1977). Mothers' speech research: From input to interaction. In C. Snow & C. Ferguson (Eds.), *Talking to children: Language input and acquisition* (pp. 31–50). New York: Cambridge University Press.

Snow, C., & Ferguson C. (1977). *Talking to children: Language input and acquisition.* New York: Cambridge University Press.

Spitz, R. (1957). *No and yes: On the genesis of human communication.* New York: International Press.

Stark, R. (1979). Prespeech segmental feature development. In P. Fletcher & M. Garman (Eds.), *Language acquisition* (pp. 57–70). New York: Cambridge University Press.

Stern, D. (1977). *The first relationship.* Cambridge, MA: Harvard University Press.

Stern, D., Jaffe, J., Beebe, B., & Bennett, S. (1975). Vocalizing in unison and in alternation: Two modes of communication within the mother-infant dyad. In D. Aaronson & R. Rieber (Eds.), *Developmental psycholinguistics and communication disorders* (pp. 7–202). New York: New York Academy of Science.

Stoel-Gammon, C., & Otomo, K. (1986). Babbling development of hearing-impaired and normally hearing subjects. *Journal of Speech and Hearing Disorders, 51,* 33–41.

Trevarthen, C. (1979). Communication and cooperation in early infancy: A description of primary intersubjectivity. In M. Bullowa (Ed.), *Before speech.* New York: Cambridge University Press.

Werker, J. F., & Tees, R. C. (1984). Cross-language speech perception: Evidence for perceptual reorganization during the first year of life. *Infant Behavior and Development, 7,* 49–64.

Wetherby, A., Yonclas, D., & Bryan, A. (1989). Communicative profiles of pre-school children with handicaps: Implications for early identification. *Journal of Speech and Hearing Disorders, 54,* 148–158.

Wolff, P. (1963). Observations on the early development of smiling. In B. Foss (Ed.), *Determinants of infant behavior II* (pp. 113–138). New York: John Wiley & Sons.

4 / Motor Development: Birth to One Year

Shelly J. Lane

Motor development is most often viewed as the predictable attainment of a series of motor skills during the early years of life. Many clinicians will reach for a text addressing development and search for the motor section in which they can be reminded that a child should sit independently by 5 months or roll prone to supine at 4 months. The characterization of motor development into attainable milestones has served a worthwhile pur-

pose, and the work of investigators such as McGraw (1943), Gesell (1945), and Piaget (1952) is to be lauded. Investigations of developmental sequence continue, and the application of a normal developmental framework to development in children with disabilities may further our understanding of strengths and needs within these groups of children (Green, Mulcohy, & Pountney, 1995). Nonetheless, while developmentalists have docu-

30

mented the existence of age/stage task attainment, they have not clearly addressed important issues such as motivation for movement, movement quality, transitional patterns, and the planning of motor skills. Furthermore, the role of sensory input in motor development has not been clarified. These knowledge areas reside in studies of sensory integration, perceptual motor development, and motor learning and control (Ayres, 1972; Fisher & Murray, 1991; Schmidt, 1988). Inherent in these theories is the concept that the central nervous system is the system that is critical to the processing of sensory input and is the storehouse of programs for motor output. Successful production of complex movement is seen as the ability to process sensory input from the environment and combine this input with prior developmental skills to plan and execute a motor response. Even with these conceptualizations, the potential role of environmental or task context in successful task completion has not been explored adequately.

More recently a "dynamical theory" of motor development has been posited that takes into account the contributions of environment and task context, along with physical and neurological development (Thelen, 1987, 1995). This theoretical perspective of motor development suggests that the central nervous system is but *one* subsystem that must be called upon for the successful production of motor skill. Other subsystems, such as behavioral state, motivation, physical development, the mechanical aspects of the movement system, and environmental constraints, also are seen as major determinants in motor performance. All subsystems are seen as equal in their influence on the production of a motor behavior. von Hofsten (1989) suggests that this conceptualization poses a problem in that the role of the brain is overly simplified. However, viewing motor development as some combination of these factors offers a broader perspective that is useful in understanding the variability in normal motor development. Dynamical systems theory of motor development is in many ways similar to general systems theory as applied to the developmental process as a whole (O'Brien, 1993). It encourages the viewer to consider a more complete picture and as such is useful in understanding the variability inherent in the developmental process.

In this chapter I combine information from classical developmental perspectives and dynami-

cal or general systems theory perspectives to present an overall picture of motor development from birth to the first birthday. A simple listing of developmental milestones accomplishes only a component of the task of presenting motor development. Tables delineate expected skills and associated ages of emergence of the skills. However, my focus is on interaction between the various subsystems and the processes thought to underlie motor development and the expression of motor skills.

Reflexes

What role do reflexes play in the process of motor development? They are present in the infant prior to birth and can be seen at varying times during the first year of life. These behaviors are considered innate and species-specific (Fischer & Hogan, 1989). While the existence of such behaviors in the infant is not questioned, the purpose of these motor behaviors is controversial. Fischer and Hogan suggest that reflexes form the basis for all voluntary motor activities. In this view, reflexes are considered voluntary, although specific postures or body positions must be present to allow the infant control. The infant incorporates and combines reflexes in the process of establishing voluntary motor skills. Other investigators suggest that reflexes are behaviors that inhibit the onset of voluntary movement and must disappear before related voluntary motor movement can be established. McDonnell, Corkum, and Wilson (1989) posit that reflex development may facilitate voluntary motor development but that reflexes are not necessarily components of voluntary movement. Whichever view is promoted, it is important to realize that the infant is not solely a reflexive being. That is, the infant is not merely reactive to sensory input. According to Towen (1984): "The infant's brain has two main properties: it generates motor patterns, both rhythmical (sucking, breathing, stepping movements) and phasic; and it can react to stimulation. The interaction between these two properties leads to the complex and very individualized and variable display of the infant's (motor) behavior" (p. 119).

Reflexes have been categorized as primitive or

TABLE 4.1

Reflex Development

Reflex	Onset	Integration (months)
Rooting	Birth	3–4
Suck	Birth	replaced by voluntary suck
Palmar Grasp	Birth	3–6
Moro	Birth	3–6
Asymmetrical Tonic Neck	Birth	6–7
Stepping	Birth	3–5
Placing	Birth	12+

postural (Gallahue, 1982). Examples of primitive reflexes include the moro, sucking, rooting, and grasp reflexes. They have been considered to have two primary functions: nourishment seeking and/or protective (Gallahue, 1982). The term *primitive* has been called into question, as it implies low-level function in the infant brain, rather than giving credit to the infant brain for these age-specific behaviors adapted to meet current need (Towen, 1984).

Postural reflexes act to maintain balance by regulating muscle tone when body position changes. They also serve to provide stability in body parts, allowing other parts to be mobile (McDonnell et al., 1989). Postural reflexes include such skills as tonic neck and labyrinthine reflexes, righting reactions, protective extension, crawling, and stepping. McDonnell and colleagues (1989) suggest that while early postural reflexes limit an infant's motor options, mature postural reflexes are essential for the development of volitional skill.

Reflexes are assessed based on intensity and quality of response to stimulus, with too brisk or too soft a response considered problematic (Keogh & Sugden, 1985). In addition, the presence of *obligatory* reflexes that persist is reason for concern. Table 4.1 lists commonly assessed reflexes, time of expected emergence, and time of expected diminishing influence on behavior. It is again important to note that variability in development may alter the emergence and dissolution of reflexes, and the method of eliciting the reflex (e.g., initial body posture, environmental context

behavioral state) may influence results (Fischer & Hogan, 1989; Towen, 1971).

RHYTHMIC STEREOTYPIES

If the infant is indeed more than a reactive being, even early in the first year, what skills can be expected? Although some authors state that early movements appear to be random, diffuse, and extraneous, Thelen (1981) suggests that in the early postnatal weeks, "rhythmic stereotypies" become observable. She characterized such movements throughout the course of the first year and identified logical groupings of movements (e.g., leg kicking, foot rubbing, rocking). The age of movement onset and peak activity differed for each grouping. These movements are characterized by repetitious movement of body parts or the entire body. They may be preprogrammed, and serve to facilitate motor development. Movements with similar characteristics have been identified by Prechtl and Hopkins (1986). These investigators identified a change in the quality of movement at approximately 2 months of age from "writhing" movements to "fidgety" movements. Writhing movements are described as general movements with variable intensity, force, and speed and no specific sequence of extremity, trunk, or head motion, "which have a writhing appearance because of contraction of the antagonist muscles" (p. 234). In contrast, fidgety movements are "continual small and elegant movements" (p. 237) that occur spontaneously and may involve the extremities, the head, or the body. Prectyl and Hopkins suggest that these later movements are necessary to calibrate the proprioceptive system. Regardless of whether such movements serve to facilitate later development or to calibrate the proprioceptive system, they are not stimulus dependent. As such, the infant is not merely a stimulus-response being; he or she can generate such movements in the absence of an external stimulus.

Thus, given an appropriate environment, motivational factors, and behavioral state the infant can control simple motor expression in the form of reflexes. The precise role of such skills is equivocal. However, because normally developing infants exhibit motor reflexes, they constitute an important aspect of first year development.

Gross Motor Development

Beyond reflexes, the first year of life is a busy time for motor skill development. Table 4.2 presents a list of significant gross motor skills associated with the first year, along with a range of expected ages for attainment. It is important to note that expected ages for attainment are averages that do not necessarily take into account the vast variability in development that can be expected from a single child, nor do they account for intercultural variability (Broadhead & Church, 1985; Capute, Shapiro, Palmer, Ross, & Wachtel, 1985; Cintas, 1989, 1995). Developmental attributes, such as child's strength and body size, can influence the attainment of developmental skills. Gender differences for at least some tasks in early motor development have been both reported (Capute et al., 1985; Largo, Molinari, Weber, Comenale Pinto, & Duc, 1985; Thomas & French, 1985) and refuted (Espenschade & Eckert, 1980; Kopp, 1971; Streit & Hanzlik, 1991). Eaton and Enns (1986) also have reported early gender differences in motor activity level. Finally, it has been noted that differences in motor performance can be related to behavioral state (Streit & Hanzlik, 1991; Rothbart, 1986).

TABLE 4.2

Gross Motor Development

Skill	Age Range of Onset (month)
Head turns to one side	Birth–4
Lifts chin in prone	Birth–3
Head held steady upright, still	1–4
Head held steady upright, moving	1–5
Head held at 90 degrees—Prone	1–3
Chest up prone	2–4
Sits momentarily without support	2–6
Sits steadily, good coordination	4–10
Gets into sitting position independently	5–10
Rolls prone to supine	3–5
Rolls supine to prone	4–10
Crawls (prone locomotion)	6
Creeps	9
Pulls to stand	5–12
Stands holding on	5–10
Sits down from standing	7–14
Walks with one hand for support	6–12
Cruising	7–13
Climbs stairs	13
Stands independently	9–16
Stoops and recover	10–14
Walks independently	8–17

POSTURAL DEVELOPMENT

Outside the womb, the newborn immediately strives to conquer the force of gravity and gain control of his or her own body. This drive takes the form of development of, first, head control, then trunk control, both within the first several months of life. Next, more refined trunk movements, righting and equilibrium reactions, and locomotion develop during the first year. In fact, the fight against gravity continues throughout childhood and adult lives as we attempt climbing, running, jumping, and later skills such as skating and skiing. Gravity is a powerful motivator. However, it is an insufficient motivator in and of itself, as can be demonstrated by considering infants with blindness. These infants exhibit delays in the accomplishment of basic motor skills not through a default in their response to gravity but rather because they do not have the drive of visual stimuli. Thus vision, too, is a powerful driving force behind the development of motor skill.

Keogh and Sugden (1985) discuss movement problems or challenges for the infant striving to gain postural control during the first 24 months of life. The initial challenge is the maintenance of a steady position relative to gravity. According to these authors, this problem is addressed via the development of head and trunk control and righting and equilibrium reactions. As noted, head control begins to develop at birth as the neonate lifts his or her head momentarily to turn it from one side to the other. By 3 weeks of age the neonate can raise the head in prone, clearing the chin, and maintain this position for a moment. With this new control the infant can gaze momentarily at people and objects within the environment. Vision then serves as a motivator for the infant to repeat this new skill. Repetition promotes the development of muscular strength and stability, leading to the ability to hold the head upright and steady while being held and moved. This skill is a major accomplishment notable between 1 and 5 months of age. Trunk control also begins to be exhibited in the prone position as the infant lifts both head and upper trunk off the surface beginning at approximately 2 months. Rolling first from side to supine and later supine to prone are further indications of the development of trunk control. Rolling supine to prone occurs in conjunction with the development of trunk control in sitting, with the average age of appearance of 5 to 6 months of age. At this point in development, infants have relatively stable heads and trunks in an upright posture.

The second of the postural challenges facing the infant is that of maintaining a posture and changing to a new position (Keogh & Sugden, 1985). Righting and equilibrium responses aid in the maintenance of position, as do the development of head and trunk control. This challenge will continue to be present throughout the life span as we work, and sometimes struggle, to maintain an upright posture. Changing positions relies on the previously noted skills of righting and equilibrium and requires the development of *transitional movements* or patterns. Such transitional movements require coordination of head and trunk along with the extremities. Supine-to-prone rolling provides an example. This skill may be motivated by visual tracking and reach. The pattern of early rolling often is initiated by pushing up off the surface, head turning leading to trunk twisting, a leg push, and possibly a reach to complete the task. Initial rolling in this manner seems to occur by chance, and the infant likely will have difficulty replicating the movement immediately, unless encouraged to do so with a new visual tracking activity. Thus, it becomes apparent very early that motor skill development is tied closely to the influences of environment, sensory input, and motivation. The infant may be seen to practice the transitional movements repeatedly while developing the rolling skill. That is, the infant may push up on the arms, turn the head, and

reach around over and over again before completing the roll to supine. In some cases the opposite arm may be poorly positioned, preventing the roll, but in other instances the infant simply may be practicing this transition for the sake of practice.

Meeting the challenge of changing positions is begun between the fourth and fifth month of the first year and continues throughout the first 24 months as the infant discovers the variety of positions available to him or her in the environment (Keogh & Sugden, 1985). Although traditional developmental perspectives place the emphasis on the attainment of a new and stable position, it is transitional movements that allow the new positions to have functional significance to the infant. For instance, although stable sitting is an admirable skill to have attained, the utility of this skill comes into play when the child realizes that he or she can successfully push back from prone and use trunk rotation with arm extension to get into such a position in order to examine a newly found toy. For some children this occurs by the age of 7 months (Keogh & Sugden, 1985). A child who must be placed in a sitting position in order to use this position for object manipulation has a limited repertoire of motor options. Other critical transitional movements occur during the first year of life as the infant learns to rotate into quadruped from sitting and back into sitting from quadruped, at approximately 8 months, and uses lateral trunk movements and weight shifting to pull to stand.

What is the drive to meet this second postural challenge? Once again the environment and its components as a motivator must be considered. The desire to see an object, reach for it, and bring it to the mouth for exploration is strong in normally developing infants. Although antigravity responses are not well developed early in the first year, the infant's drive to move pits his or her antigravity muscles and equilibrium responses against gravity, using vestibular input to facilitate further development. Given the opportunity, typically developing children will challenge themselves and their motor skills to explore both the environment and objects within it.

The third postural control challenge facing the infant is that of developing a dynamic equilibrium (Keogh & Sugden, 1985)—that is, maintaining balance while moving. Keogh and Sugden believe this entails attaining motion stability, which refers to the ability we all develop to maintain what would be an unstable body position due to the fact that we are in motion. According to these authors, ". . . unstable body positions at rest can be maintained when the body is in motion" (p. 36). Such motion stability is needed during walking, running, and other mobile activities in which we will engage throughout life. It can be seen in its most rudimentary form at the close of the first year of life as the infant begins to walk. Walking requires moving the center of gravity outside the base of support and relies on adequate dynamic equilibrium. It is easy to see that when we are new at it, as in the later part of the first year of life, we struggle and often fall as our stability fails us and we give in to the power of gravity. Motion stability is thus dependent on the infant's ability to utilize successfully play skills such as righting, equilibrium, weight shift, and trunk rotation, and coordinate head, trunk, and extremities to meet the demands of the environment.

Thus, by the close of the first year of life, the infant has met and at least partially conquered three significant movement challenges: The infant has head and trunk control, can assume and maintain a variety of positions, and has at least rudimentary motion stability. In addition to upright locomotion, most infants of this age successfully have accomplished creeping in quadruped. An impressive factor inherent in normal development is the infant's ability to transfer learned skills to unfamiliar environments, environments that will require adaptations of established motor patterns.

THE DEVELOPMENT OF MOBILITY

Initially babies stay put when placed. While this may make caring for infants easy, few caregivers wish for this situation to continue and eagerly await the moment when babies begin to move on their own. Early mobility patterns take the form of changing position of the head in prone and pushing up on the arms. Some arm and leg movements may take place, but they are largely ineffective in locomoting, although they may serve to change the angle of the prone position to some degree (Keogh & Sugden, 1985). The motivator for this movement likely lies in sound and visual input from the environment and the motivation to search for the source of such entertainment.

A major achievement in the drive toward locomotion is rolling, which usually becomes a functional skill by about 6 months (Keogh & Sugden, 1985). As noted in Table 4.2, prone-to-supine rolling occurs in advance of supine-to-prone rolling. Both movements may be combined with pivoting in prone, all of which serve to change the location and the position of the baby relative to the environment. When sitting, some infants engage in rocking behavior, tilting the pelvis forward and back. This not only provides enjoyment to the infants, it also can serve to move the children slightly, if the support surface does not provide too much resistance. Mobility is further enhanced in some infants by 7 to 8 months as they can get into and out of sitting and may begin to pull to stand. Gallanue (1982) suggests that standing is an important milestone in the development of stability. It is at time that caregivers must become wary about the environment in which the child is to be placed. It is no longer adequate to make just the child's personal space safe; the home must now be child-proofed in anticipation for the explosion of locomotion and exploration to come.

True locomotion emerges after the infant has developed trunk and neck stability. Locomotion relies on prior stability in order to be functional (Gallahue, 1982). The first form of movement into the environment is generally prone belly crawling, emerging during the sixth and seventh month (Gallahue, 1982; Keogh & Sugden, 1985). The pattern of belly crawling is quite variable from child to child and may involve only arms, only legs, or a combination of arms and legs. Such patterns often seem clumsy or unrefined, but they effectively serve the purpose of mobility. Some infants choose "hitching," or movement on their bottoms, as a form of early locomotion. Creeping, or movement on all fours with the chest held off the floor, emerges at approximately 9 months. This skill requires dynamic balance around a midline, but the center of gravity is low to the ground and the base of support quite wide. Thus early experience with dynamic balance is likely to be successful (Keogh & Sugden, 1985). Creeping is often preceded by hours of practice in getting into and out of the creeping position from sitting. Creeping also may be preceded by rocking on hands and knees. Practice of transitional patterns serves to provide the infant with additional sensory input from proprioceptive and vestibular sources. Rocking in sitting or on hands and knees, and movement into and out of sitting, prone, and all fours are examples of such transitional movement patterns. These patterns may promote better stability for the head and trunk muscles and provide for increased stability at shoulder and hip joints via coactivation of flexor and extensor muscles surrounding these joints.

Using a dynamical systems analysis of rocking and creeping, Goldfield (1989) suggested that orienting, reaching, and kicking play critical roles in the development of these locomotor skills. Orienting to persons and objects in the environment provides the infant with the motivation to move, reaching assists in the steering component of creeping, and kicking leads to forward movement of the body. These skills, present early in development, come together with the development of the postural skills and muscle mass. They allow the infant to weight shift and release arms and legs from weight bearing at the time of creeping.

Controversy has existed for some time over the importance of creeping on all fours to the development of later skills. It has been suggested that the process of creeping provides tactile, proprioceptive, and kinesthetic sensory input that may be important to the later development of body scheme and the quality of upper extremity function (Farber, 1982). This suggestion has found some support in the work of McEwan, Dihoff, and Brosvic (1991), but additional study is necessary to confirm such views. Further, some theorists believe that the absence of creeping may be related to the later development of learning disabilities. This appears to be an erroneous conclusion. According to Snow (1989) ". . . crawling and creeping are not essential for normal development" (p. 112).

Following on the heels of creeping is the development of upright locomotion, or walking. Pulling to stand is the first step toward this major accomplishment. This transitional skill generally is accomplished using a pattern that entails reach and grasp on a stable object, bringing one leg forward in flexion and placing the sole of this foot on the ground, and pushing with this support leg while pulling with the hands. Cruising, or walking sideways while holding on, develops soon thereafter, and is a pattern that may be used for some time in conjunction with creeping. Thus, the child will creep to a stable object, pull to stand, cruise until

there is no longer a stable surface for assistance, then lower to sit and creep again. Lowering to sit becomes an important transitional movement associated with this advanced locomotor skill, as it allows the child the ability to get out of the upright posture and into a different position from which to continue his or her mobility. Controlled lowering to sit from upright is itself a skill dependent on the development of leg strength and balance and the environmental motivation to move out of upright (Keogh & Sugden, 1985).

True independent walking generally is expected by the close of the first year of life, although many children will not be independent walkers until sometime in the second year. Initially, independent walking is characterized by a wide base of support in the lower extremities, knees slightly bent and toes turned out, arms held high and out to the sides (Gallahue, 1982). Upright mobility presents the child with many new challenges: The base of support has been greatly decreased, the center of gravity is high, and the child must move the center of gravity outside of the support base in order to move in a forward direction. Initially the pattern is one of discontinuous steps without reciprocal arm movements, but it changes rapidly (Gallahue, 1982). This is another pattern from which children seem to derive joy in repetition (Keogh & Sugden, 1985). The walking pattern continues to refine and develop throughout the preschool years, and children will attain a mature walking pattern between the ages of 4 and 7 (Espenschade & Eckert, 1980).

What is the functional significance of self-produced locomotion? It of course marks the child's first foray into parts unknown and the beginning of the child's ability to separate from the caregiver. Development of the fear of heights occurs only after the onset of crawling (Campos & Bertenthal, 1989). Full appreciation of the skills needed to manage ascending and descending slopes appears to develop even later, after the onset of walking (Adolph, Eppler, & Gibson, 1993). In addition, independent locomotion is considered integral in the reorganization of spatial concepts by the infant. Bai and Bertenthal (1992) have suggested that with the onset of independent locomotion, the baby must learn to monitor his or her own actions, increasing vigilance of the physical surroundings and leading to the ability to detect changes in body position relative to other objects. Once mobile, infants alter their search strategies for objects in the environment. Mobility also affords infants the opportunity to develop spatial maps of the environment (Campos & Bertenthal, 1989; McEwan, Dihoff & Brosvic, 1991).

Incorporating concepts important in dynamical theory, what role will environment, task context, and physical development play in the attainment of gross motor skill? Thelen and Fogel (1989) suggest that walking is the result of dynamic interaction of many subsystems. These include the motivational system; the perceptual system, which gives infants the knowledge of what surfaces may be walked upon and what may not be; the mechanical system of muscles and joints, which must be able to support the body in upright; and balance and dynamic equilibrium systems. In addition, the early dominance of flexor tone in the legs must diminish, allowing the legs to extend with gravity (Thelen & Ulrich, 1991). Furthermore, infants must be able to initiate voluntary movement toward the goal and be able to evaluate and regulate emotional and motivational states. Some aspects of environmental motivators have been presented already in that it is the children's interest in discovery that drives the early motor system. Children see an object of interest and attempt to attain it at all costs. Initial attempts may be met with bumps and bruises as the children challenge their motor skills beyond their capabilities. However, the long-term benefit of such persistence is the development of mobility as the various subsystems integrate. Thelen and Fogel suggest that early in the first year, infants do not walk because they do not have the muscle mass or strength to support body weight on one leg, to allow the other to swing forward, nor do they have adequate balance and equilibrium reactions to stay in upright. If these shortcomings are somehow facilitated— for example, if the body is supported and assisted in balancing—walking can be achieved earlier given the proper assortment of environmental motivators.

What happens to the normally mobile and explorative child in a new environment? Some inhibition of activity is to be expected, at least until the child warms to the new environment. The basic skills needed for exploration are still present, but a change has occurred in the perceptual subsystem, and until a new "balance" is reached, mobility cannot be demonstrated.

The importance of task context can be seen as the skill a parent reports in a child's ability to pull to stand at the coffee table at home is not demonstrated on the very different table in the doctor's examining room. Although the two tables may be approximately the same height, other qualities of environment and task context may be interfering with the child's ability to express the skill or to generalize it to this new environment without some practice.

Finally, it is relatively easy to see that behavioral state is a major player in the expression of motor skill. Sleepy, fatigued, hungry babies are much less aware of environmental motivators and much less able to meet the new challenges with skill that may be apparent at other times during the day. Thus, all systems must interact appropriately to permit the identical expression of skill the parent may observe in the mornings at home. As skills become more ingrained, their adaptability to environmental changes, state alterations, and motivation will broaden, permitting their expression perhaps "against all odds."

Fine Motor Development

The assumption has been made that the development of skill in upper-extremity function is dependent on earlier development of postural stability (Case-Smith, Fisher, & Bauer, 1989). This concept supports a proximal-to-distal, or gross-to-fine motor developmental framework. Recent work has indicated that while proximal stability and distal skill are not *developmentally dependent*, they are likely to be functionally related. That is, in cases where proximal stability is inadequate but distal skill is present, the expression of distal skill is dependent on the individual's ability to fix or stabilize the arms (Case-Smith et al., 1989). Thus, functionally, fine motor skill is closely related to the development of head and trunk stability, and skill in the fine motor area becomes apparent as that in the gross motor area improves.

Table 4.3 summarizes important achievements in fine motor development within the first year of life. Fine motor, or manipulative, development during the first year is characterized by reach,

TABLE 4.3

Fine Motor Development

Skill	Age Range of Onset (month)
Reflexive grasp	Birth
Global reaching	1–4
Reach in supine	2–6
2 hand ulnar-palmar grasp	2–6
Hands to mouth	2
Hands to midline	3
Finger play with own hands	4–5
Hands across midline	4.5–5
Bangs objects	4–7
Transfers objects	4–8
Sit with reach	5
Mouthing—exploratory	5
Holds two objects	6
Rake grasp	5–9
Purposeful release	5–11
Inferior pincer grasp	7–9
Radial digital grasp	7
Neat pincer grasp	8–11
Thumb opposition	9
Poke with index finger	10

grasp, and release: the rudiments of environmental exploration. Manipulative development is difficult to separate from the development and influence of vision since this sensory input is a critical factor. Visually directed manipulation as a component of environmental exploration, plays an important role in cognitive and perceptual development (Ruff, 1984). Thus, although for simplicity manipulative development can be examined alone, it is intricately tied to several other aspects of development. In addition, fine motor skill expression is subject to the same subsystem constraints as discussed for gross motor skill expression. That is, not only must sufficient central nervous system maturation have taken place but behavioral state, mechanical functions of the body, and muscular development all must be appropriate to support the expression of a fine motor skill.

REACH

Some researchers view neonatal hand-to-mouth movements as early, goal-oriented reaching (Butterworth & Hopkins, 1988). That such very early movements do not usually result in successful contact between hand and mouth implies that they are unskilled, but not that they are random or haphazard. It has been suggested that such a pattern is an early precursor of later self-feeding. Other early reaching movements present prior to 4 months of age are driven by visual attraction to an object. They are characterized by global arm movements in the general direction of the object of interest rather than by accurately directed reach. In addition, in order to express these skills, the infant must be alert and positioned with proper head and trunk support. These early movements, sometimes called prereaching (Snow, 1989; von Hofsten, 1984) rarely result in tactile contact with the object and certainly do not lead to manipulation. In fact, von Hofsten (1982) stated that such early eye-hand coordination serves the function of orienting to objects of interest within the environment. Furthermore, such orienting lays the foundation for later manipulative eye-hand coordination. According to Sherick, Greenman, and Legg (1976), "The child's approach to his outer world begins first with the asymmetry of the tonic neck reflex" (p. 175). Utilizing this posture, the infant gazes at his or her hand and, as the reflex becomes less predominant, the infant develops hand-to-mouth skills, object manipulation, and bilateral hand skills.

Refinement of the reaching pattern develops as looking at and reaching for an object become coordinated (Fischer & Hogan, 1989). At this point reach may be interrupted by visual interest in the hands themselves (Snow, 1989; Williams, 1983). Bushnell (1985) states that prior to 4 months of age, reaching is *visually elicited*, while between 4 and 8 months of age, reaching is *visually guided*. The visual guidance of reaching is what improves accuracy as the infant attends not just to the object of interest but also to his or her hand as it moves toward the object in space. This early visually motivated reach is often associated with hand grasp *as the reach is taking place*. Although this makes actual *object grasp* impossible, it is an early sign of the relationship among seeing, reaching, and grasping (Fischer & Hogan, 1989). It is generally agreed that by 4 months of age a baby can make contact with the object of interest with fair consistency. It is of interest to note that it is between 3 and 4 months that the asymmetrical tonic neck reflex is waning, and the infant becomes able capable of bilateral movements of the hands and engagement of the hands at midline (Sherick, Greenmam, & Legg, 1976). At this age reach is associated with an open hand and grasp of an object can take place, although it may not as grasp is still not well coordinated (Fischer & Hogan, 1989). Recent research indicates that infants can lean and reach to obtain more distant object by 8 months of age, and can further extend their reach using a mechanical aid by 12 months of age (McKinzie, Skouteris, Hartman, & Yonas, 1993). Toward the close of year one the visual guidance in reaching is becoming less important, perhaps due to skill mastery (Bushnell, 1985).

GRASP AND RELEASE

Grasp begins as a reflex elicited by tactile contact and traction on the fingers. Elicited in this way, early grasp lacks the associated ability to release at will. However, if traction is not applied, grasp can be released.

Grasp early in the first year is bimanual and not associated with in-hand manipulation to any great degree, as the infant explores objects more often by mouth. Early grasp is palmar, with the thumb and fingers holding the object into the palm (Eckert, 1987), with little strength (Gallahue, 1982). Such early grasp places the object being grasped closer to the little finger then to the thumb, thus classifying this grasp as ulnar (Erhardt, 1974). Rochat (1989) has stated that between 2 and 5 months of age, manual exploration is primarily grasp, serving the function of transporting the object to the mouth. However, at about 4 months of age, fingering begins to emerge as an early form of bimanual, in-hand manipulation. This occurs in conjunction with an increase in vocalization as the mouth is "freed" from the task of exploration and can go on to develop other skills. Further bimanual differentiation occurs between 4 and 5 months of age as the infant begins to transfer objects from hand to hand. The development of this manipulative skill in young infants depends on, and is organized by, visual guidance (Rochat, 1989). Finally, as early as 3 months of age, infants demonstrate the ability to alter manual exploration, based on the novelty and qualities of the object of interest (Rochat, 1989). In fact, Ruff (1989) suggests that a critical criterion of exploratory behavior is that it varies with object novelty. Another interesting aspect of exploration is that it will vary with the qualities of the table surface upon which the object of interest is placed (Palmer, 1989). Thus, infant actions with a toy will depend on the sound-making potential of both the toy and the available surface for toy manipulation. Both of these aspects of early exploration have important implications for assessment of manipulative ability.

Erhardt (1982) states that visual input is important to bring eye-hand coordination to higher levels. The coordination of manipulation with perception can be seen between the ages of 6 and 8 months when the infant can begin to use manipulation to explore objects in their environment during play (Fischer & Hogan, 1989). Actual appreciation for the information gained by exploration activities increases as the infant gets older (Ruff, 1989). After 6 months of age, grasp begins to refine and thumb opposition becomes more apparent. Although coordination of thumb and fingers is still minimal at 7 months (Gallahue, 1982), between 8 and 9 months of age true thumb opposition is noted and objects are held "radially," or closer to the thumb side of the hand (Erhardt, 1974; Gallahue, 1982). Pincer grasp can be seen in most children by 9 months of age, although it may not be refined to a "neat pincer" grasp with true index finger/thumb opposition for another couple of months (Erhardt, 1974; Keogh & Sugden, 1985). The pattern of reach/grasp appears well coordinated by 10 months. Work by Fontaine and le Bonniec (1988) has indicated that reach and grasp are determined by postural maturity of the infant. Visually directed grasp occurs between the ages of 4 and 6 months, but the infant must be positioned in such a manner that grasp is possible. If placed in sitting without external support at this age, the infant must use his/or her hands to prop. Seeing an object of interest for reach and grasp, the infant is faced with dual tasks of reach/grasp and regaining balance. As such, reach/grasp is produced inaccurately and manipulation of the object is minimal. Between the ages of 6 and 8 months, the infant demonstrates the ability to sit somewhat independently. Fontaine and le Bonniec have suggested that postural development is at least as important as age in the expression of grasp and manipulation skills. Independent sitting frees the hands for manipulation during play, and manipulative skills progress from this point onward.

Midline skills have been suggested to follow a predictable developmental trend (Sherick, Greenham & Legg, 1976). As noted earlier, with the disappearance of the tonic neck reflex between 3 and 4 months of age, the hands are available to work bilaterally and explore body midline. Work of Fraiberg (1968) with infants with blindness indicates that early midline hand play is visually directed and requires vision for maintenance. Furthermore, it is considered to be an important component in the development of prehension. Between 3 and 4 months of age, the infant develops the ability to hold an object and visually explore it, and by 5 months an infant can reach out in a bilateral manner. Given trunk stabilization via an infant seat, Provine and Westerman (1979) demonstrated that the ability to contact objects at midline becomes apparent between 9 and 17 weeks of age, and precedes the ability to cross midline, which may develop between 18 and 20 weeks of age. These investigators have suggested that the use of the infant seat prevented the infant from using other skills to reach an object of interest, notably midline reorienting coupled with a unilateral reaching response. Interestingly, the infant will resort to unilateral reaching again by 7 months of age, when he or she becomes able to hold one object while approaching another with the other hand. At 10 months of age, bilateral reach and manipulation again become apparent as the child learns to hold and use two objects at midline (e.g., bang two objects together) (Sherick, Greenham, & Legg, 1976).

Purposeful release movements develop during the second half of the first year. Until this time the infant may be seen to shake and bang objects, but release is accidental and inaccurate. As release is developed, Gallahue (1982) suggests that the child now manipulates objects to discover more about his or her environment rather than to merely touch, feel, or mouth the object itself.

Thus, reach and grasp/release and object manipulation are dependent on development of postural control or support. In addition, they are environmentally motivated and related to the development of cognitive functions. Over the course of the first year, the manipulative skills available to the infant change and the infant develops the capacity to use skills appropriately for given tasks (Ruff, 1984). Hence, while between 6 and 8 months of age dropping and throwing indicate the development of purposeful release, by the end of this year such behaviors indicate that the infant has lost interest in an object, that the object is no longer novel and has ceased to offer the infant motivation for exploration (Ruff, 1984). Depending on object characteristics, transferring, fingering, and rotating may be used to explore new objects. Thus, given proper motivation and support, reach, grasp, and manipulation of objects in normally developing children should take on different characteristics, depending on task context. Therefore, examining the development of reach and grasp in context and using cognitively appropriate objects becomes critical in determining the existence of skills. The complexity of fine motor development is limited by age/stage explanations. Dynamical theory, or general systems theory as applied to motor development, expands upon this basic view by calling attention to the various systems that interact.

Summary

The first year of life is full of motor challenges and accomplishments. Historically, these accomplishments have been looked at as motor milestones that unfold on a predictable timetable. More recent perspectives on motor skill attainment offer insight into the variability with which children develop skills, by considering all systems that impact on skill expression. Given expected developmental and environmental parameters, 1-year-olds typically are stable in mobility, able to get into and out of many positions, and able to use multiple means of mobility. In addition, the postural stability they have developed provides the foundation needed for fine motor skills underlying object exploration and manipulation. At this point, infants become mobile, active toddlers, intent on exploring their world.

REFERENCES

Adolf, K. E., Eppler, M. A., & Gibson, E. J. (1993). Crawling versus walking infants' perception of affordances for locomotion over sloping surfaces. *Child Development, 64,* 1158–1174.

Ayres, A. J. (1972). *Sensory integration and learning disorders.* Los Angeles: Western Psychological Services.

Bai, D., & Bertenthal, B. I. (1992). Locomotor status and the development of spatial search skills. *Child Development, 63,* 215–226.

Broadhead, G. D., & Church, G. E. (1985). Movement characteristics of preschool children. *Research Quarterly for exercises and sport, 56* (3), 208–214.

Bushnell, E. W. (1985). The decline of visually guided reaching during infancy. *Infant Behavior and Development, 8,* 139–155.

Butterworth, G, & Hopkins, B. (1988). Hand-mouth coordination in the new-born baby. *British Journal of Developmental Psychology, 6,* 303–314.

Campos, J. J., & Bertenthal, B. I. (1989). Locomotion and psychological development in infancy. In F. J. Morrison, C. Lord, & D. P. Keating, (Eds.), *Applied developmental psychology* (pp. 230–258). San Diego: Academic Press.

Capute, A. J., Shapiro, B. K., Palmer, F. B., Ross, A., & Wachtel, R. C. (1985). Normal gross motor development: The influences of race, sex and socioeconomic status. *Developmental Medicine and Child Neurology, 27,* 635–643.

Case-Smith, A., Fisher, A. G., & Bauer, d. (1989). An analysis of the relationship between proximal and distal motor control. *American Journal of Occupational Therapy, 43* (10), 657–662.

Cintas, H. M. (1989). Cross-cultural variation in infant motor development. *Physical & Occupational Therapy in Pediatrics, 8* (4), 1–20.

Cintas, H. M. (1995). Cross-cultural similarities and differences in development and the impact of parental expectations on motor behavior. *Pediatric Physical Therapy, 7,* 103–111.

Eaton, W. O., & Enns, L. R. (1986). Sex differences in human motor activity level. *Psychological Bulletin, 100* (1), 19–28.

Eckert, H. M. (1987). *Motor development* (3rd ed.). Indianapolis: Benchmark Press.

Erhardt, R. P. (1974). Sequential levels in development of prehension. *American Journal of Occupational Therapy, 28* (10), 592–596.

Erhardt, R. P. (1982). *Developmental hand dysfunction.* Laurel, MD: Ramsco Publishing.

Espenschade, A. S., & Eckert, H. M. (1980). *Motor development.* Columbus, OH: C. E. Merrill.

Farber, S. D. (1982). *Neurorehabilitation. A multisensory approach.* Philadelphia: W. B. Saunders.

Fischer, K. W., & Hogan, A. E. (1989). The big picture for infant development. In J. J. Lockman, & N. L. Hazen, (Eds.), *Action in social context. Perspectives on early development* (pp. 275–305). New York: Plenum Press.

Fisher, A. G., & Murray, E. A. (1991). Introduction to sensory integration theory. In A. G. Fisher, E. A. Murray, & A. C. Bundy (Eds.), *Sensory integration theory and practice* (pp. 3–26). Philadelphia: F. A. Davis.

Fontaine, R., & le Bonniec, G. P. (1988). Postural evolution and integration of the prehension gesture in children aged 4 to 10 months. *British Journal of Developmental Psychology, 6,* 223–233.

Gallahue, D. L. (1982). *Understanding motor development in children.* New York: John Wiley & Sons.

Gesell, A. (1945). *The embryology of behavior.* New York: Harper.

Goldfield, E. C. (1989). Transition from rocking to crawling: Postural constraints on infant movement. *Developmental Psychology, 25* (6), 913–919.

Green, E. M., Mulcahy, C. M., & Pountney, T. E. (1995). An investigation into the development of early postural control. *Developmental Medicine and Child Neurology, 37,* 437–448.

Keogh, J., & Sugden, D. (1985). *Movement skill development.* New York: Macmillan.

Kopp, C. B. (1971). *Readings in early development, for occupational and physical therapy students.* Springfield, IL: Charles C. Thomas.

Largo, A. H., Molinari, L., Weber, M., Comenale Pinto, L., & Duc, G. (1985). Early development of locomotion: Significance of prematurity, cerebral palsy and sex. *Developmental Medicine and Child Neurology, 27,* 183–191.

McDonnell, P. M., Corkum, V. L., & Wilson, D. L. (1989). Patterns of movement in the first 6 months of life: New directions. *Canadian Journal of Psychology, 43* (2), 320–339.

McEwan, M. H., Dihoff, R. E., & Brosvic, G. M. (1991). Early infant crawling experience is reflected in later motor skill development. *Perceptual and Motor Skills, 72,* 75–79.

McGraw, M. B. (1943). *The neuromuscular maturation of the human infant.* New York: Columbia University Press.

McKinzie, B. E., Skouteris, H., Day, R. H., Hartman, B., & Yonas, A. (1993). Effective action by infants to contact objects by reaching and leaning. *Child Development, 64,* 415–429.

O'Brien, S. P. (1993). Human occupation frame of reference. In P. Kramer & J. Hinojosa (Eds.), *Frames of reference for pediatric occupational therapy* (pp. 309–310). New York: Williams & Wilkins.

Palmer, C. F. (1989). The discriminating nature of infants' exploratory actions. *Developmental Psychology, 25* (6), 885–893.

Piaget, J. (1952). *The origins of intelligence in children* (M. Cook, Trans.) New York: International Universities Press.

Prechtl, H. F. R., & Hopkins, B. (1986). Developmental transformations of spontaneous movements in early infancy. *Early Human Development, 14,* 233–238.

Provine, R. R., & Westerman, J. A. (1979). Crossing the midline: Limits of early eye-hand behavior. *Child Development, 50,* 437–441.

Rochat, P. (1989). Object manipulation and exploration in 2- to 5-month-old infants. *Developmental Psychology, 25* (6), 871–884.

Rothbart, M. K. (1986). Longitudinal observation of infant temperament. *Developmental Psychology, 22* (3), 356–365.

Ruff, H. A. (1984). Infants' manipulative exploration of objects: Effects of age and object characteristics. *Developmental Psychology, 20* (1), 9–20.

Ruff, H. A. (1989). The infant's use of visual and haptic information in the perception and recognition of objects. *Canadian Journal of Psychology, 43* (2), 302–319.

Schmidt, R. A. (1988). *Motor control and learning* (2nd ed.). Champaign, IL: Human Kinetics Publishers.

Sherick, I., Greenman, G., & Legg, C. (1976). Some comments on the significance and development of midline behavior during infancy. *Child Psychiatry and Human Development, 6,* 170–183.

Snow, C. W. (1989). *Infant development.* Englewood Cliffs, NJ: Prentice-Hall.

Streit, J. M., & Hanzlik, J. R. (1991). Gross motor development and testing implications according to the pilot edition III of the Miller Infant and Toddler Test. *Occupational Therapy Journal of Research, 11* (1), 40–53.

Thelen, E. (1987). The role of motor development in developmental psychology: A view of the past and an agenda for the future. In N. Eisenberg (Ed.), *Contemporary topics in developmental psychology* (pp. 3–33). New York: John Wiley & Sons.

Thelen, E. (1981). Rhythmical behavior in infancy: and ethological perspective. *Developmental Psychology, 17* (3), 237–257.

Thelen, E. (1995). Motor development. A new synthesis. *American Psychologist, 50,* 79–95.

Thelen, E., & Fogel, A. (1989). Toward an action-based theory of infant development. In J. J. Lockman & N. L. Hazen (Eds.), *Action in social context. Perspectives on early development* (pp. 23–63). New York: Plenum Press.

Thelen, E., & Ulrich, B. D. (1991). Hidden skills: A dynamic systems analysis of treadmill stepping during the first year. *Monographs of the Society for Research in Child Development, 56,* 1–98.

Thomas, J. R., & French, K. E. (1985). Gender differences across age in motor performance: A meta-analysis. *Psychological Bulletin, 98,* 260–282.

Towen, B. C. L. (1971). A study on the development of some motor phenomena in infancy. *Developmental Medicine and Child Neurology, 13,* 435–446.

Towen, B. C. L. (1984). Primitive reflexes—conceptional or semantic problem? In H. F. R. Prechtl (Ed.), Continuation of neural functions from prenatal to postnatal life. *Clinics in Developmental Medicine* (No. 94) (pp. 115–125). Philadelphia: J. B. Lippincott.

von Hofsten, C. (1982). Eye-hand coordination in the newborn. *Developmental Psychology, 18* (3), 450–461.

von Hofsten, C. (1984). Developmental changes in the organization of prereaching movements. *Developmental Psychology, 20* (3), 378–388.

von Hofsten, C. (1989). Motor development as the development of systems: Comments on the special section. *Developmental Psychology, 25* (6), 950–953.

Williams, H. G. (1983). *Perceptual and motor development.* Englewood Cliffs, NJ: Prentice-Hall.

5 / Sensory Patterns in Infants and Young Children: Introduction and Infancy

Georgia A. DeGangi

Introduction

Infants and children with developmental, learning, and emotional problems are often burdened with problems related to the processing and integration of basic sensory information. When there is an underlying deficit in the capacity to synthesize the range of sensory experiences (e.g., tactile, proprioceptive, vestibular, visual, or auditory inputs), the child may be unable to organize purposeful actions in areas including communication, movement, and play. Often perceptual thinking and the regulation of affects are impaired, as well.

The early symptoms of sensory processing disorders in infancy often are related to regulatory problems, such as sleep difficulties, poor self-calming, very low or high activity level, atypical muscle tone with slowness in attaining motor milestones, and under- or overresponsiveness to sensory stimulation (DeGangi, 1991; DeGangi & Greenspan, 1988). By the preschool years, delays often become apparent in fine and gross motor skills, balance, the planning and sequencing of motor actions, and coordination (DeGangi, Berk, & Larsen, 1980). Distractibility, sensitivities to touch and movement stimulation, language delays, and visual-spatial problems may be present (Ayres, 1979; Fisher, Murray, & Bundy, 1991). By the school-age years, handwriting problems, dyslexia, attention deficits, and reading disabilities often emerge (DeQuiros & Schrager, 1979).

This chapter describes sensory integrative disorders in infants. The first section focuses on the various types of sensory integrative dysfunction. The following section highlights common sensory integrative problems in the young infant. Assessment strategies are discussed and a case example is presented to illustrate key points.

Overview of Sensory Integration: Incidence and Typical Problems

Sensory integrative disorders have been documented among children and adults with learning disabilities, autism, and schizophrenia. It has been estimated that approximately 70% of learning disabled children have sensory integrative disorders (Carte, Morrison, Sublett, Uemura, & Setrakian, 1984). Developmental dyspraxia, a disorder involving the sequencing of motor actions, is the most common type of sensory integrative disorder, occurring in about 35% of these children (Schaffer, Law, Polatajko, & Miller, 1989). Deficits in the processing of vestibular and tactile information are also common among children with learning disorders and motor incoordination (Ayres, 1972; DeQuiros, 1976; Fisher, Mixon, & Herman, 1986; Horak, Shumway-Cook, Crowe, & Black, 1988) and in autistic children and schizophrenic adults (Maurer & Damasio, 1979; Ornitz, 1970, 1974; Ottenbacher, 1978). Since the most typical types of sensory integrative dysfunction involve tactile-proprioceptive problems, vestibular dysfunction, and motor planning deficits, this chapter emphasizes these areas.

THE CONCEPT OF SENSORY DEFENSIVENESS AND SENSORY DORMANCY

In order to understand the notion of sensory integrative dysfunction, it is useful to review the concepts of sensory defensiveness and sensory dormancy. *Sensory defensiveness* is a term used to describe children who are hypersensitive to sen-

Sensory dormancy	Modulation	Sensory defensiveness
Underrespond		Overrespond

FIGURE 5.1

Continuum from sensory dormancy to sensory defensiveness.

sory stimulation (e.g., olfactory, visual, tactile, auditory, movement) (Knickerbocker, 1980). In most cases, several sensory modalities are involved; children are rarely overly responsive to only one sensory channel. As a result, children thus burdened tend to be overly active, distractible, and disorganized in motor actions.

On the other end of the continuum is a condition described as sensory dormancy (Knickerbocker, 1980). This describes a lack of sensory arousal due to an excessive inhibition of incoming sensory inputs. Typically, children freighted with this problem will be passive and inactive and will fail to orient to important sensory stimuli. Figure 5.1 depicts the continuum from sensory dormancy to sensory defensiveness.

Normal children experience some variation over the course of the day as they respond to state of arousal, activity level, and sensory, cognitive, or motor demands of a task or situation. Most individuals with sensory integrative dysfunction, however, will be either hyperresponsive (sensory defensive) or hyporesponsive (sensory dormant). Some children have such severe sensory modulation problems that they fluctuate from one extreme to the other within the course of a very short time. Indeed, it has been speculated that sensory modulation problems underlie both sensory defensiveness and dormancy (Cermak, 1988; Royeen, 1989). The concepts of sensory defensiveness and dormancy are useful in considering the various types of sensory integrative dysfunction that are described in the following sections.

TACTILE SYSTEM FUNCTIONS

The Development of Touch and Tactile Dysfunction: The somatosensory system is a primal receptive system that responds to various touch stimuli on the surface of the skin. It is the predominant sensory system at birth and remains critical throughout life as a major source of information for the central nervous system. An infant's first movements are in response to tactile input (e.g., rooting reflex, palmar grasp reflex, stepping response). Early learning is dependent on making contact with the external world and is important in guiding experiences and interactions with the environment (Collier, 1985; Gottfried, 1984; Reite, 1984; Satz, Fletcher, Morris, & Taylor, 1984; Suomi, 1984).

The sense of touch involves the ability to receive and interpret sensations and stimuli arising from contact with the skin. Tactile receptors are activated by touch, pressure, pain, and temperature. Movement of the body and limbs stimulates the proprioceptors, which interact closely with the touch system. Since exploration through the sense of touch typically is combined with limb movement, the tactile and proprioceptive systems have overlapping neural mapping (Kandel & Schwartz, 1981). Children's responses to tactile input give us a great deal of information about the degree of integration in their nervous system. Problems in the tactile system affect not only motor and reflex development; there is a critical link between tactile perception, motor planning, and emotional stability (Ayres, 1972; Montagu, 1978).

The tactile system serves functions of both protection and discrimination. Table 5.1 presents the tactile system functions. The anterolateral system, or tactile protective system, is activated by temperature changes of the skin, light touch, and general contact with the skin. It acts as a protective mechanism to the central nervous system by giving warning if an outward stimulus is too close for safety. In the newborn child, this protective reaction predominates until the baby becomes accustomed to being touched and learns to discriminate between tactile experiences that are dangerous versus those that are enjoyable. Children who are unable to tolerate light touch and are highly sensitive to tactile experiences such as standing next to another child, wearing a long-sleeved shirt, or

TABLE 5.1

Functions of the Tactile System

Component of Tactile System	Functions
Tactile protective system (anterolateral)	Protection and survival General awareness of environment linked with touch Emotional responses to touch
Tactile discriminative system (lemniscal system)	Tactile discrimination of shape, contour, weight, texture Perception of touch pressure Perception of touch with motion (e.g., moving object in hand) Precise localization of touch Important for initiation and planning of movement

even sitting on a chair surface are termed *tactually defensive*. Often this problem is associated with hyperactivity.

A second important function of the tactile system is discrimination. The development of tactile discrimination (e.g., the ability to differentiate various textures, contours, and forms by feel) plays an important role in adaptive motor behaviors, particularly in the initiation and planning of movement as well as in exploration of the environment (Ayres, 1972). Tactile discrimination is important for localization of touch, two-point discrimination, finger identification, shape recognition, and stereognosis (Sinclair, 1981). Since hand skills involve many discrete manipulations of objects, fine motor skills often are compromised in children with poor tactile discrimination (Haron & Henderson, 1985; Nathan, Smith, & Cook, 1986). If children are unable to manipulate an object due to muscle tone abnormalities, the problem is compounded. If the tactile discriminative system is not functioning properly, children will have difficulty orienting to and organizing tactile input in time and space in a meaningful manner. This is why many children with poor tactile discrimination cannot sequence movements in the course of practicing such skills as dressing.

When the tactile discriminative system is not functioning properly, children often link a negative emotional meaning to touch. As a result, social interactions and the regulation of emotions often are maladaptive in children with poor tactile discrimination. For example, in the course of social interactions, children learn to interpret different types of touch and to link emotions to pleasant or aversive contacts of this kind (e.g., aggression, love). The mother who playfully burrows her face into her baby's tummy should elicit smiling and laughter from her baby. An infant or child with poor tactile discrimination may avert gaze, pull away from the contact, or even cry. Later on, such a toddler or preschooler may not tolerate close proximity with others and may well respond by fleeing or by engaging in aggressive actions.

In order for normal development to occur, this protective and discriminative system must be balanced. When the central nervous system malfunctions, as seen in learning disabled and developmentally delayed children, the nervous system tends to regress to a developmentally earlier response that has greater survival value. In these children, the protective system is overaroused, and they experience normally pleasant tactile stimulation as irritating or threatening. When the child is unresponsive or avoidant of touch, there is a negative impact on emotional development.

Somatosensory Dysfunction: The tactile dysfunctions most commonly observed are tactile defensiveness and tactile hyposensitivities. Reactions to somatosensory stimuli can range from overresponsivity to underresponsivity. Overresponsiveness is more commonly characterized by feelings of discomfort and, typically, is responded to by physical withdrawal from certain types of tactile stimuli. Ayres has described this as tactile defensiveness (1972, 1979, 1985).

Sensitivities to touch may be environmental (e.g., the child may flee from contact with furniture or complain of discomfort because of contact with clothing), other-initiated (e.g., the child may withdraw from mother's attempts at hugging or avoid being in groups of children), or self-initiated (e.g., the child avoids touching textured objects).

45

Faced with the stress of contact, children may respond aggressively by hitting or kicking, or may physically retreat (e.g., by hiding under furniture). Emotional responses, including hostility, are not uncommon.

Tactile defensiveness is a severe sensitivity to being touched and usually involves an adverse reaction to initiating touch with non-noxious tactile stimulation. It has been suggested that the phenomenon of tactile defensiveness results from a failure of the central nervous system to modulate and inhibit incoming tactile stimuli (Fisher & Dunn, 1983). Children with tactile defensiveness will express feelings of discomfort and asset a desire to escape from situations involving touch. The symptoms are much worse in situations where touch is thrust on rather than initiated by the child. Typically, a child will respond by attempting to remove himself from the situation and will state, "I hate this game, it hurts," or "It tickles." He may pull away from being touched, run away from the adult, hit or kick aggressively, or hide under furniture. Even if he is touched slightly, he may exclaim "Don't push me!" or "Watch where you're going!" Anxiety, discomfort, a need to withdraw, and hostility are common behavioral manifestations of tactile defensiveness.

The phenomenon of tactile defensiveness is characteristic of some children with learning disorders and has been correlated with hyperactivity and distractibility (Ayres, 1964; Bauer, 1977). It also has been documented in autistic children (Ayres & Tickle, 1980). Inadequate cortical inhibition of sensory processing and poor regulation in the reticular activating system have been speculated to cause symptoms of increased activity level, sleep/wake disturbances, tactile defensiveness, or withdrawal from sensory stimulation (Royeen, 1989).

Decreased tactile awareness or a hyporeactivity to touch is seen less often than tactile defensiveness. Children experiencing hyporeactivity to touch suffer from a decrease in tactile awareness and are not aware of touch unless the contact is very intense. Such children may laugh and actually enjoy a firm pat on the buttocks when being disciplined. It is as if their threshold for noticing or reacting to tactile stimuli is very high. Often these children do not seem to experience pain; moreover, they are slow to initiate movement for tactile exploration and therefore suffer from a

type of sensory deprivation. It is common for such children to seek touch-pressure input. Some self-abusive behaviors may be interpreted as a means to trigger very high thresholds (e.g., biting, head banging). Some children may bite themselves hard, actually breaking the skin, without reacting. Another problem seen in children with diminished tactile awareness is that they are slow to initiate movement and explore objects by feel.

Because of the inefficient use of touch in exploring objects, children with either tactile defensiveness or tactile hyporeactivity often exhibit a lag in motor development. Frequently, children with tactile dysfunction have low muscle tone, perhaps related to poor sensory support for movement experiences. For instance, an afflicted child may sit half on and half off a chair or sit with one arm caught under the body with no apparent discomfort. It is important to note that the same child may exhibit elements of both tactile hyper- and hyporeactivity to tactile experiences (e.g., crave deep-pressure contact on the hands but express an aversion to light touch or certain textures on the palms).

VESTIBULAR SYSTEM FUNCTIONS

Early Development: The vestibular system develops early, enabling the fetus and infant to receive and respond to specific movement stimuli. At birth, the vestibular system is predominantly sensory. Investigators of fetal development have found that the vestibular nerve myelinates at 28 weeks of gestational age. It is thus the second earliest sensory system to develop, the first being oral tactile sensation (Erway, 1975). In utero, the fetus receives constant vestibular stimulation from movement of the amniotic fluid as well as from the mother's own body movements.

Vestibular System Functions: The vestibular system plays a major role in assisting infants to orient themselves in space and to initiate exploratory and adaptive movements. As a result, the vestibular system and the tactile system are particularly critical for the development of basic functions in young infants (Naunton, 1975). The vestibular system has an impact on the development of body posture, muscle tone, oculo-motor control, reflex

TABLE 5.2

Primary Purposes of the Vestibular System

1. Detect motion
2. Detect and respond to the earth's gravitational pull
3. Detect motion within the visual field
4. Influence muscle tone and posture
5. Influence motor coordination including bilateral motor control and sequencing
6. Affect the formation of body scheme
7. Provide gravitational security during body movement
8. Modulate arousal and alertness for attention and calming

TABLE 5.3

Common Vestibular-based Disorders

• Vestibular-postural deficits
• Postural-ocular movement disorder
• Gravitational insecurity
• Intolerance or aversive response to movement
• Under responsiveness to movement in space

integration, and equilibrium reactions (Keshner & Cohen, 1989). These vestibular-based functions have a strong impact on the development of motor skills, visual-spatial and language abilities, hand dominance, and motor planning (Ayres, 1972; Clark, 1985). Evidence also suggests that vestibular-proprioceptive functioning may be the basis for bilateral motor integration and sequencing (Ayres, 1989).

Another important function of the vestibular system is to provide gravitational security when moving in space. A secure sense of where the body is in space contributes to the development of emotional stability. Children who lack adequate vestibular functioning may be insecure in their body movements and fearful of movement in space (particularly when the feet leave the ground). Moreover, they are likely to exhibit emotional instability.

Additionally, the vestibular system plays a role in arousal and alertness. Vestibular-proprioceptive stimulation has been found to increase visual alertness and attention (Gregg, Haffner, & Korner, 1976) and to be more effective in consoling babies than tactile contact alone (Korner & Thomas, 1972; Pederson & Ter Vrugt, 1973). Table 5.2 summarizes the primary purposes of the vestibular system.

Vestibular-based Problems: Here I describe the various clinical populations exhibiting vestibular-based problems. The anatomy and neurophysiology of the vestibular system is complex, and ac-

cordingly, there are many types of vestibular-based problems (Fisher, Murray, & Bundy, 1991). Table 5.3 presents the most common vestibular-based disorders.

Vestibular-postural problems are among the most common type of vestibular-based deficits. Frequently children with minor neurological impairments have difficulty with postural reactions including balance, ocular-motor control, and visual-spatial skills (Steinberg & Rendle-Short, 1977). Children with severe emotional and behavioral problems also have been reported to display deficient equilibrium and postural responses, decreased postrotary nystagmus, and an absence of autonomic responses such as dizziness and nausea following vestibular stimulation (Ottenbacher, 1982).

The primary problem underlying a vestibular-postural problem is inadequate postural control. The neck and trunk muscles provide stability in movement, and their development provides the foundation for postural control. If the proximal musculature is not well developed, the child is often unstable in maintaining body postures, has poor balance, and may have poor fine manipulation and locomotor skills.

Postural or gravitational security seems to play an important role in the development of emotional stability as well as balance, postural mechanisms, and spatial perception (Fisher & Bundy, 1989; Matthews, 1988). Children who are hypersensitive to movement usually are overwhelmed by intense movement stimuli such as spinning, frequent changes in direction and speed, or unusual body positions (e.g., inverted). Typically, such youngsters are fearful about leaving the earth's surface and are thus called gravitationally insecure (Ayres, 1979). Often they display considerable autonomic reactivity (dizziness, nausea) during and after any type of vestibular stimulation. Increased sensitivity to vestibular stimulation can result in motion sickness (Baloh & Honrubia, 1979).

The gravitationally insecure child demonstrates an extreme fearfulness of moving in space. These children typically have a strong preference for maintaining an upright position and seek to avoid rotational movement patterns such as rolling. They prefer close-to-ground positions (i.e., W-sitting posture), "lock" the body and neck in rigid postures to avoid movement stimulation, and tend to avoid movement activities. Not only are they fearful of body movement in space, but they resist any change in position that they may perceive as threatening. Movement that is imposed is particularly upsetting to them. The emotional response that accompanies gravitational insecurity is evoked by any sudden change of head position, a displacement in the body's center of gravity, or the feet suddenly leaving the ground. As a result of insecurities associated with moving in space, children with gravitational insecurity tend to be emotionally unstable. They frequently display fearfulness of new situations, rigidity, and a resistance to change. It has been hypothesized that gravitational insecurity may be due to poor modulation of otolithic inputs (Fisher & Bundy, 1989). These infants evidence a strong preference for sameness in routines with crying and agitated behavior appearing when routines vary. In addition, they have a strong need to be held and carried constantly, along with a fearfulness of certain body positions (e.g., lying on the back or stomach).

Some individuals are intolerant of movement, and experience considerable autonomic discomfort during movement activities. These children may exhibit gravitational insecurity as well. Typically the youngster will feel nauseated and dizzy, particularly during rapid movement activities such as spinning. It is not infrequent for such an individual to experience motion sickness in a car or boat ride. It is hypothesized that the individual with intolerance for movement is hyperresponsive to semicircular canal stimulation—spinning, for example (Fisher & Bundy, 1989). Since gastrointestinal symptoms are common, vestibular-vagal connections are also involved. Sometimes children exhibiting intolerance for movement have visual motion sensitivity (i.e., are troubled while watching spinning or swinging objects, or watching motion pictures that assimilate movement

or flight in space) without feeling autonomic responses (Fisher, Mixon, & Herman, 1986).

Underresponsiveness

When children have a high tolerance for vestibular input (underresponsiveness to movement in space), the behavioral response pattern is different. These children may seek movement experiences and yet do not seem to profit from them. They may exhibit explosive movement quality, poor judgment in starting and stopping movement activities, or difficulty with transitional movements. Children with vestibular problems typically exhibit low muscle tone and may not be able to move against gravity easily enough to stimulate the vestibular system in a variety of movement planes. Because they do not move as much as other children, they experience a poverty of movement and, as a result, they have fewer opportunities for developing vestibular output for postural control and balance. Children who are hyporeactive to movement usually crave being moved by others, yet they do not display any evidence of autonomic responses such as dizziness associated with movement.

SENSORY-BASED MOTOR PLANNING DISORDERS

Developmental dyspraxia, also known as a motor planning disorder, is a sensory processing deficit often related to tactile and/or vestibular processing disorders. The problem lies not so much in the processing of sensory input or the ability to produce the movement skill but in the intermediary process of planning the movement. Children with developmental dyspraxia have significant problems in planning and directing goal-directed movement, skilled, or nonhabitual motor tasks. Because dyspraxic children lack internal cognitive organization to focus thoughts and actions, they are often vulnerable to distraction (Ayres, Mailloux, & Wendler, 1987). Table 5.4 presents the distinct types of motor plan-

TABLE 5.4

Types of Motor Planning Problems

Postural dyspraxia	Inability to plan and imitate large body movements and meaningless postures
Sequencing dyspraxia	Difficulty making transitions from one motor action to another and in sequencing movements (e.g., thumb-finger sequencing)
Oral and verbal dyspraxia	Inability to produce oral movements on verbal command or in imitation, a skill that affects speech articulation
Constructional dyspraxia	Inability to create and assemble three-dimensional structures (e.g., block bridge)
Graphic dyspraxia	Inability to plan and execute drawings
Dyspraxia involving symbolic use of objects	Inability to use objects symbolically

ning problems. Children with vestibular or tactile dysfunction may exhibit any of these types of dyspraxia (Ayres, 1985; Cermak, 1985; Conrad, Cermak, & Drake, 1983).

The underlying problem in developmental dyspraxia is the inability to maneuver through the three stages of organizing a purposeful plan of action. The stages include ideation, planning the action, and executing the plan.

Stage 1—Ideation. In this first stage of motor planning, children must develop the conceptual organization of the skill or task. They need to link the feeling of enacting the motion or action with the concept of which actions lead to task completion. In treatment, the therapist may move such children through the action while describing what is happening. Sometimes children are more ready to try a difficult task if they have experienced what it feels like to move through the motions. Once they have understand and performed it successfully a few times, it is important to then vary the task demands slightly in order to present a new challenge. In this way, children learn to self-correct and to execute new movement patterns.

Stage 2—Planning the action. Before children can plan out what they want to do, they must be prepared to act. In order to undertake an action, they need to be motivated to do the action; therefore, it is important to find activities that excite them and elicit their interest and involvement. The first step in learning to plan an action is to be able to experience it and to verbalize or conceptualize what needs to happen. Once children have enacted the action with the help of a model or with the therapist's assistance, they need to under-

stand what the end goal will be and how to get there. Selecting activities that give sensory feedback throughout the sequence helps the children to construct a plan. For example, if an obstacle course is used, children may crawl through an opening in a large foam tunnel, then pull themselves onto the scooter board by holding a resistive rope, and last, swing while pushing over the large sandbag man. Each of these movements would have distinctly different sensory inputs that would help the children mark each event in time and space.

Stage 3—Executing the plan. This is often the easiest stage of praxis. An important component of plan execution is self-correction and verbal mediation. The therapist may help children to articulate what they are doing in order to help them link language with motor actions. While the children are engaged in a task, verbal commands from the therapist help to organize the sequence for them. Once they have consolidated their actions with verbal guidance from the therapist, they should then be helped to articulate what they are going to do next.

The most common types of motor planning disorders observed in children with somatosensory and vestibular-based problems are related to postural, sequencing, bilateral motor coordination, constructional, and praxis to verbal commands (Ayres, 1985). An emphasis of therapy is on the ability to plan whole-body movements in space and to combine the body with objects. Through the use of postural patterns of flexion and extension against gravity, trunk rotation, and diagonal rotary patterns, children can learn to map simple body movements in space. These postural patterns are combined with functional activities so that the movement pattern has a purpose for the child. Therapy focuses on the use of sensory stimulation in combination with a strong visual component to help children become aware of what they are doing in space and to visualize the effect their actions have on objects. For example, having a child sit in a hammock and swing across the room to kick over a tower of cardboard blocks will maximize vestibular, proprioceptive, and visual feedback. This will help to consolidate this particular motor plan, which may not have occurred if the child simply tried to kick over the tower while standing. The major emphasis therefore is placed on orienting the body in space in relation to objects.

Infants with Sensory Processing Dysfunction

The early manifestations of sensory processing dysfunction often are discernible in how an infant regulates sleep-wake cycles, feeds, self-calms, and tolerates such everyday activities as being dressed and bathed. Among infants with regulatory problems (i.e., disorders of sleep, feeding, and self-calming), hypersensitivities to touch, movement, visual, or auditory stimulation are prevalent (De-Gangi & Greenspan, 1988). Infants who show signs of early sensory processing dysfunction often continue to experience problems; if left untreated, they are all too likely to develop more serious developmental disorders by the preschool years (DeGangi, Porges, Sickel, & Greenspan, 1993).

Young infants who experience distress from sensory input show their discomfort by grimacing, yawning, hiccoughing, sneezing, and averting their gaze. In an effort to "shut-down" the level of stimulation, they may be drowsy and sleep most of the time. Or they may become hyperaroused and sleep fewer hours than expected at that age.

The next sections describe common regulatory problems associated with both sensory processing disorders and with tactile and vestibular dysfunction observed in the first year of life. Assessment strategies to evaluate sensory processing in infants are discussed. Finally, a case example is presented to depict the common problems observed in young infants with sensory processing dysfunction.

SENSORY-BASED REGULATORY PROBLEMS

Sleep problems (difficulties falling and staying asleep) are common among infants with sensory processing problems. By observing what help the infant seeks and needs in order to fall and to stay asleep, it is possible to distinguish a sensory-based sleep problem from other types (e.g., parental mismanagement, separation problems). A high need for vestibular stimulation often is observed. For example, parents may find that driving the infant around in the car, bouncing the child at their shoulder, or swinging the baby in an infant swing for long periods of time helps to make him or her drowsy. Sleeping in a crib hammock or on a water bed sometimes helps babies with this type of sleep disorder. In contrast, other infants have a high need for prioprioceptive input and become drowsy when exposed to vibration such as that provided by a clothes dryer or crib vibrator. Or the infant may be calmed by white noise (e.g., rotating fan, or audiotape of heart beat, or ocean waves).

Many infants with sensory processing dysfunction are highly irritable; they cry excessively and have difficulties self-calming. For example, children with this problem may be delayed in bringing a hand to their mouths for sucking or in holding their hands in midline as a means to self-calm. Some babies require intense vestibular stimulation (e.g., swinging, bouncing vigorously) in order to calm, while others need more soothing types of movement experiences (i.e., slow rocking, riding in a car). Some infants can quiet if they suck on a pacifier or are swaddled tightly in a blanket, thus using their tactile senses to organize themselves.

TACTILE DYSFUNCTION

When infants are underreactive to tactile input, they may appear very passive and content to be

TABLE 5.5

Symptoms of Tactile Defensiveness in Infants

- Arch away when held (not high muscle tone)
- Make fists of the hands to avoid contact of objects
- Curl the toes
- Dislike cuddling
- Reject nipple and food textures (not oral-motor problem)
- Strong preference for no clothing or tight swaddling
- Preference for upright or sitting position rather than lying on back or stomach
- Dislike face or hair being washed
- Aversion to car seat and other confining situations

left alone. Often such a baby does not cry during physically painful medical procedures and a low activity level is commonly present. It is important to differentiate these behaviors from other medical problems or severe cognitive delay.

Tactile defensiveness, the more typical type of tactile dysfunction, can be easily identified in young infants by noting the manner in which they tolerate everyday handling experiences such as being dressed and bathed. Table 5.5 presents common symptoms of tactile defensiveness in infants up to 1 year of age. Because tactile perception is learned within the context of social interactions (e.g., parent-child interactions), it is important to consider not only the infant's tactile functioning but what the caregiver and environment bring to the experience. Consider the effects of a tactually defensive parent on the infant's emotional development. For example, the parent who is defensive to touch may avoid holding and cuddling the infant. Traumas early in life, such as child abuse or poor mother-infant bonding, may shape the child's affect throughout life in interactions involving touch. Likewise, the environment may induce a state of sensory deprivation such as that experienced by the very premature infant who suffers a prolonged hospitalization with a minimum of holding and carrying from a loving caregiver. This may be complicated by invasive medical procedures (e.g., oral intubation, heel sticks).

VESTIBULAR DYSFUNCTION

Infants with vestibular hypersensitivities typically show an intolerance for low-to-ground positions (e.g., prone or supine), a strong preference for upright postures, low muscle tone, slowness in developing motor skills, delayed balance, and/or fear of irregular or unexpected movement (DeGangi & Greenspan, 1988).

The infant who is underresponsive to movement in space seems to crave movement; indeed, such a baby may become very fussy and demanding unless the parents provide a great deal of movement stimulation. Once the baby is more adept at moving about, he or she may rock vigorously while sitting or on hands and knees. The infant may seek to be swung for long periods of time and particularly enjoy roughhousing with parents.

CLINICAL ASSESSMENT OF SENSORY PROCESSING DYSFUNCTION IN INFANTS

One tool that can be used to assess sensory processing in infants is the Test of Sensory Functions in Infants (TSFI) (DeGangi & Greenspan, 1989). This 24-item test focuses on evaluation of responses to tactile deep pressure, visual-tactile integration, adaptive motor skills, ocular-motor control, and reactivity to vestibular stimulation. It was constructed as a criterion-referenced test and has been validated on developmentally delayed and regulatory-disordered infants from 4 to 18 months of age. The reactivity to tactile deep pressure subtest measures infant's capacity to tolerate firm deep pressure applied in the form of a systematic massage to body parts. The visual-tactile integration subtest measures the infant's ability to tolerate contact with textured objects placed on various body parts. The adaptive motor skills subtest assesses the infant's capacity to plan motor actions when presented with a problem (i.e., yarn tie wrapped around hands in midline). Ocular-motor control is observed in visual tracking and lateralization of the eyes. The vestibular subtest focuses on the infant's responses to being moved in space by the examiner or parent in a systematic roughhousing routine.

The TSFI is intended to be used in combination with neuromotor assessments that include observations of muscle tone, reflex maturation, and postural mechanisms. The infant's motor skills also should be assessed. When sensory processing problems are identified using the TSFI, it is important to validate these findings with observations of the child's functional play using sensory materials (e.g., textured toys, movement equipment). For example, if the child showed hypersensitivities to tactile deep pressure and avoided handling the textured toys on the TSFI, it is important to determine if these same behaviors occur during play with textured toys (e.g., dislikes being touched, avoids sitting in close proximity to mother, bangs toys but does not manipulate them in the palms of the hands, and avoids touching certain types of textured toys).

In addition, the Infant-Toddler Symptom Checklist (DeGangi, Poisson, Sickel, & Wiener, 1995) may be used with infants from 7 through 30 months to determine how the parents view the child's sleep, self-calming, feeding, sensory processing, and emotional regulation. This checklist contains 6 versions with specific questions pertinent to each age range (e.g., 7 to 9, 10 to 12, 13 to 18, 19 to 24, and 25 to 30 months). Combining information from this checklist with formal observation measures helps provide a comprehensive profile of the infant's overall sensory processing and regulatory functions.

CASE EXAMPLE

The following case describes an infant with sensory hypersensitivities. Some details are presented of the assessment and treatment strategies employed for this particular child.

Tommy was referred by his parents at 12 months of age because of extreme irritability. When seen for the initial interview session, Tommy was crying uncontrollably in his mother's arms in the waiting room. He cried throughout most of the session, only quieting down occasionally to wander about and explore the toys in the office. Even when spoken to softly, he began once again to cry inconsolably.

Mother's chief concerns were that Tommy was different from other babies and that he was very hard to handle. Tommy was recognized as different soon after birth. On his second day of life, a nurse from the new-

born nursery approached his mother saying, "Mrs. G., you are going to have to do something about Thomas. He's keeping all the other babies awake." When he first came home from the hospital he slept approximately 12 out of 24 hours: most of the time that he was not asleep, however, he was screaming. The earliest interventions occurred when he was 4 weeks old; a pediatrician diagnosed the baby as having "colic" and prescribed Donnatol. Neither parent wanted their baby to be medicated, so mother instead got a referral to a nurse practitioner and explained that Tommy was very easily overstimulated—even by such things as faces, lights, and noises. The nurse recommended decreasing stimulation by doing such things as holding him facing away from her when feeding and soundproofing his sleeping environment.

Mother reported that during Tommy's first year, he had otitis media about five times, which was then regarded as the explanation for his persistent crankiness. There was no evidence of chronic ear pathology, and the remainder of his medical history was negative. He had good weight gain on breast-feeding but was weaned at 3½ months of age because he kicked and punched, which the mother interpreted as his way of fighting being held. Once on bottle feedings, he slept through the night. He now goes to bed, gets to sleep, sleeps through the night, and awakens in the morning on his own.

When he was 3½ months old, mother tried to return to work part time. Tommy was placed in a family day care, where he was the only child. The caregiver described the child as "sensitive" and often reported to his mother that he was "cranky all day." Mother gave up going to work when the baby-sitter decided to take in other children. Although mother wanted to work, she felt that Tommy's fussiness could cause a caregiver who did not love him to abuse him. The parents have a support system that is too limited to provide much respite. Father's sister and brother-in-law have watched Tommy briefly on a few occasions, and a teenage baby-sitter has been employed for a few hours in the daytime.

Mother reported that she felt that father had always been able to soothe Tommy a little better than she could and that he was the baby's preferred person. Whenever she felt frustrated with Tommy, she gave him to her husband. At times, she reported, her husband pointed out that she was acting irritable and/or tense with the child. Mother admitted having a great personal struggle with her current feelings about this child, who made her doubt her capacity to be a mother. She reported having such concerns even before Tommy was born, mainly because she felt she lacked the experience to be a good mother. She felt embarrassed by his unsoothable crying in public and had experienced an exacerbation of psychophysiological problems since his birth—a spastic colon had reoccurred.

Developmental testing was conducted, using the Bayley Scales of Infant Development, Mental Scale (Bayley, 1969), and Tommy was found to be functioning at age level. Despite his age-appropriate cognitive level of functioning, he exhibited evidence of an expressive language delay with absence of babbling or sounds, but no receptive language difficulties. On the Test of Sensory Functions in Infants, Tommy demonstrated severe hypersensitivities to touch and movement and an inability to plan simple motor actions in response to a sensory stimulus (i.e., textured mitt placed on his foot). His balance was poor so that he fell over when standing at furniture, and his muscle tone was low with a slumped body posture in sitting. Overall, Tommy exhibited delays in expressive language, in balance and muscle tone, and was hypersensitive to touch, sound, and movement.

On parent-child interaction measures, when Tommy played quietly, the mother was observed to be understimulating and at times nonparticipating and withdrawn. Mother's interactions involved assisting Tommy to obtain a toy out of reach or introducing a new toy when he became fussy or distracted. No symbolic play or reciprocal interactions were observed.

Traditional developmental intervention would have been directed toward Tommy's needs in the areas of sensory hypersensitivities, emotional regulation, poor balance and low muscle tone, and expressive language; moreover, it would typically have been therapist- or teacher-directed. However, if Tommy were required to respond to a prescribed developmental program, his needs to engage with another person while tolerating sensory stimulation would have been overlooked. The ability to desensitize himself to sensory stimulation, organize sensorimotor experiences, create a motor plan, communicate needs through gestures and words, and take pleasure in reciprocal interactions during self-initiated play can be accomplished only using an approach where parent-child interactions are the medium.

The treatment sessions focused on developing initiative, reciprocal interactions, purposeful manipulation of toys, regulation of mood state, and desensitizing responses to touch and movement. During the child-centered activity, Tommy spent a considerable amount of time lifting objects and pounding and pushing carts, thus providing himself with heavy proprioceptive input and desensitizing his responses to loud noises. Mother discovered that when she gently imitated him, his pleasure and length of playing time increased. In the first week of treatment, Mother was encouraged to allow Tommy to play in a large bin of balls and to explore textured objects (i.e., a textured Slinky, rough hairbrushes), tactile activities that Tommy soon began to crave.

Within a short period of time, Tommy developed a strong interest in interacting with both his parents. He appeared to derive enormous pleasure out of reciprocal interactions with them. His father began to attend our sessions and shared more excitement and involvement with his son. By the third week of treatment, Tommy's crying behavior was greatly diminished. The break point appeared to occur once Tommy was able to express himself through gestures, and he could then tolerate touch, sounds, and movement. Tommy became much less reliant upon his close-to-the-ground positions, the W-sitting posture, and the use of trunk rotation in transitional movements; in addition he fell much less often when standing. Moreover, his gestures of pointing became clear. The greatest change was in Tommy's ability to organize sensorimotor experiences for himself, to be able to plan and initiate play interactions, and to communicate through gestures.

Conclusion

Sensory integrative disorders involve a dysfunction in children's capacity to modulate incoming sensory input to allow for purposeful adaptation to the environment. These disorders are common among learning disabled and emotionally disturbed children and may be observed as early as infancy. The tactile system is important for protection and survival; it affects motor and reflex development, tactile perception, motor planning, and emotional stability. The tactile dysfunctions most commonly observed are tactile defensiveness and tactile hyposensitivities. Tactile defensiveness is a severe sensitivity to being touched that may be environmental, other-initiated, or self-initiated. On the other hand, children with tactile hyposensitivities do not experience touch unless it is very intense.

The vestibular system influences the development of body posture, muscle tone, ocular-motor control, reflex integration, and equilibrium reactions. The vestibular system is important in motor planning, arousal and alertness, and security when moving in space. The common vestibular-based problems include gravitational insecurity, under-responsiveness to movement in space, intolerance for movement, postural-ocular movement disorder, and vestibular-postural deficits.

Developmental dyspraxia is a disorder in the

planning and direction of goal-directed movements that are skilled or nonhabitual in nature. Motor planning problems typically are based in the somatosensory and vestibular systems and affect postural movements, sequencing movements, language, spatial constructions, drawing, and symbolic use of objects.

Identifying infants with sensory processing disorders is crucial in light of recent research suggesting that these infants are at high risk for later perceptual, language, sensory integrative, and emotional/behavioral difficulties in the preschool and school-age years. A comprehensive assessment should include formal and informal observations of sensory processing in conjunction with parent report of the child's regulatory and sensory processing abilities.

REFERENCES

Ayres, A. J. (1964). Tactile functions: Their relations to hyperactive and perceptual motor behavior. *American Journal of Occupational Therapy, 18,* 6–11.

Ayres, A. J. (1972). *Sensory integration and learning disorders.* Los Angeles: Western Psychological Services.

Ayres, A. J. (1975). *Southern California Postrotary Nystaqmus Test Manual.* Los Angeles: Western Psychological Services.

Ayres, A. J. (1979). *Sensory Integration and the Child.* Los Angeles: Western Psychological Services.

Ayres, A. J. (1985). *Developmental dyspraxia and adult onset apraxia.* Torrance, CA: Sensory Integration International.

Ayres, A. J. (1989). *Sensory Integration and Praxis Tests.* Los Angeles, CA: Western Psychological Services.

Ayres, A. J., Mailloux, Z. K., & Wendler, O. L. (1987). Developmental dyspraxia: Is it a unitary function? *Occupational Therapy Journal of Research, 7* (2), 93–110.

Ayres, A. J., & Tickle, L. S. (1980). Hyper-responsivity to touch and vestibular stimuli as a predictor of positive response to sensory integration procedures by autistic children. *American Journal of Occupational Therapy, 34,* 375–381.

Baloh, R. W., & Honrubia, V. (1979). *Clinical neurophysiology of the vestibular system.* Philadelphia: F. A. Davis.

Bauer, B. (1977). Tactile-sensitive behavior in hyperactive and non-hyperactive children. *American Journal of Occupational Therapy, 31,* 447–450.

Bayley, N. (1969). *Bayley Scales of Infant Development.* New York: Psychological Corporation.

Carte, E., Morrison, D., Sublett, J., Uemura, A., & Setrakian, W. (1984). Sensory integration therapy: A trial of a specific neurodevelopmental therapy for the remediation of learning disabilities. *Developmental and Behavioral Pediatrics, 5* (4), 189–194.

Cermak, S. (1985). Developmental dyspraxia. In E. A. Roy (Ed.), *Advances in psychology: Vol. 23. Neuropsychological studies of apraxia and related disorders* (pp. 225–248). New York: Elsevier Science Publishers.

Cermak, S. (1988). The relationship between attention deficits and sensory integration disorders (Part I). *Sensory Integration Special Interest Section Newsletter, 11* (2), 1–4.

Clark, D. L. (1985). The vestibular system: An overview of structure and function. *Physical & Occupational Therapy in Pediatrics, 5,* 5–32.

Collier, G. (1985). *Emotional expression.* Hillsdale, NJ: Lawrence Erlbaum.

Conrad, K., Cermak, S. A., & Drake, C. (1983). Differentiation of praxis among children. *American Journal of Occupational Therapy, 37* (7), 466–473.

DeGangi, G. A., & Greenspan, S. I. (1988). The development of sensory functions in infants. *Physical & Occupational Therapy in Pediatrics, 8* (3), 21–33.

DeGangi, G. A., & Greenspan, S. I. (1989). *Test of Sensory Functions in Infants.* Los Angeles: Western Psychological Services.

DeGangi, G. A., Berk, R. A., & Larsen, L. A. (1980). The measurement of vestibular-based functions in preschool children. *American Journal of Occupational therapy, 34* (7), 452–459.

DeGangi, G. A. (1991). Assessment of sensory, emotional, and attentional problems in regulatory disordered infants. *Infants and Young Children, 3* (3), 1–8.

DeGangi, G. A., Porges, S. W., Sickle R., & Greenspan, S. I. (1993) Four-year follow-up of a sample of regulatory disordered infants. *Infant Mental Health Journal, 14 (4),* 330–343.

DeGangi, G. A., Poisson, S., Sickel, R. Z., & Wiener, A. S. (1995). *Infant-Toddler Symptom Checklist.* Tucson, AZ: Therapy Skill Builders.

DeQuiros, J. (1976). Diagnosis of vestibular disorders in the learning disabled. *Journal of Learning Disabilities, 9* (1), 50–58.

DeQuiros, J. B., & Schrager, O. L. (1979). *Neuropsychological Fundamentals in Learning Disabilities* (rev. ed.). Novato, CA: Academic Therapy Publications.

Dunn, W. (1981). *A guide to testing clinical observations in kindergartners.* Rockville, MD: American Occupational Therapy Association.

Erway, L. C. (1975). Otolith formation and trace elements: A theory of schizophrenic behavior. *Journal of Orthomolecular Psychiatry; 4,* 161–26.

Fisher, A. G., Murray, E. A., & Bundy, A. C. (1991). *Sensory integration theory and practice.* Philadelphia,: F. A. Davis.

Fisher, A. G., & Bundy, A. C. (1989). Vestibular stimulation in the treatment of postural and related disorders. In O. D. Payton, R. P. DiFabio, S. V. Paris, E. J. Protas, & A. F. VanSant (Eds.), *Manual of physical therapy techniques* (pp. 239–258). New York: Churchill Livingstone.

Fisher, A. G., & Dunn, W. (1983). Tactile defensiveness: Historical perspectives, new research: A theory grows. *Sensory Integration Special Interest Section Newsletter, 6* (2), 1–2.

Fisher, A. G., Mixon, J., & Herman, R. (1986). The validity of the clinical diagnosis of vestibular dysfunction. *Occupational Therapy Journal of Research, 6,* 3–20.

Gottfried, A. W. (1984). Touch as an organizer for learning and development. In C. C. Brown (Ed.), *The many facets of touch* (pp. 114–122). Skillman, NJ: Johnson & Johnson Baby Products.

Gregg, C., Haffner, M., & Korner, A. (1976). The relative efficacy of vestibular-proprioceptive stimulation and the upright position in enhancing visual pursuit in neonates. *Child Development, 47,* 309–314.

Haron, M., & Henderson, A. (1985). Active and passive touch in developmentally dyspraxic and normal boys. *Occupational Therapy Journal of Research, 5,* 102–112.

Horak, F. B., Shumway-Cook, A., Crowe, T. K., & Black, F. O. (1988). Vestibular function and motor proficiency in children with impaired hearing, or with learning disability and motor impairments. *Developmental Medicine and Child Neurology, 30,* 64–79.

Kandel, E. R., & Schwartz, J. H. (1981). *Principles of neural science.* New York: Elsevier Science Publishing.

Keshner, E. A., & Cohen, H. (1989). Current concepts of the vestibular system reviewed: 1. The role of the vestibulospinal system in postural control. *American Journal of Occupational Therapy, 43* (5), 320–330.

Knickerbocker, B. M. (1980). *A holistic approach to learning disabilities.* Thorofare, NJ: C. B. Slack.

Korner, A. F., & Thomas, E. B. (1972). The relative efficacy of contact and vestibular-proprioceptive stimulation in soothing neonates. *Child Development, 43,* 443–453.

Matthews, P. B. C. (1988). Proprioceptors and their contribution to somatosensory mapping: Complex messages require complex processing. *Canadian Journal of Physiology and Pharmacology, 66,* 430–438.

Maurer, R. G., & Damasio, A. R. (1979). Vestibular dysfunction in autistic children. *Developmental Medicine and Child Neurology, 21,* 656–659.

Montagu, A. (1978). *Touching: The human significance of the skin.* New York: Harper & Row.

Nathan, P. W., Smith, M. C., & Cook, A. W. (1986). Sensory effects in man of lesions of the posterior columns and of some other afferent pathways. *Brain, 109* (pt. 5), 1003–1041.

Naunton, R. (Ed.). (1975). *The vestibular system.* New York: Academic Press.

Ornitz, E. (1970). Vestibular dysfunction in schizophrenia and childhood autism. *Comparative Psychiatry, 11,* 159–173.

Ornitz, E. M. (1974). The modulation of sensory input and motor output in autistic children. *Journal of Autism & Childhood Schizophrenia, 4,* 197–215.

Ottenbacher, K. (1978). Identifying vestibular processing dysfunction in learning disabled children. *American Journal of Occupational Therapy, 32* (4), 217–221.

Ottenbacher, K. J. (1982). Vestibular processing dysfunction in children with severe emotional and behavioral disorders: A review. *Physical & Occupational Therapy in Pediatrics, 2* (1), 3–12.

Pederson, D., & Ter Vrugt, D. (1973). The influence of amplitude and frequency of vestibular stimulation on the activity of two-month-old infants. *Child Development, 44,* 122–128.

Reite, M. L. (1984). Touch, attachment and health—Is there a relationship? In C. C. Brown (Ed.), *The many facets of touch* (pp. 58–65). Skillman, NJ: Johnson & Johnson Baby Products.

Royeen, C. B. (1989). Commentary on "tactile functions in learning-disabled and normal children: Reliability and validity considerations." *Occupational Therapy Journal of Research, 9,* 16–23.

Satz, P., Fletcher, J. M., Morris, R., & Taylor, H. G. (1984). Finger localization and reading achievement. In C. C. Brown (Ed.), *The many facets of touch* (pp. 123–130). Skillman, NJ: Johnson & Johnson Baby Products.

Schaffer, R., Law, M., Polatajko, H., & Miller, J. (1989). A study of children with learning disabilities and sensorimotor problems or let's not throw the baby out with the bathwater. *Physical & Occupational Therapy in Pediatrics, 9* (3), 101–117.

Sinclair, D. (1981). *Mechanisms of cutaneous sensation.* New York: Oxford University Press.

Steinberg, M., & Rendle-Short, J. (1977). Vestibular dysfunction in young children with minor neurological impairment. *Developmental Medicine & Child Neurology, 19,* 639–651.

Suomi, S. J. (1984). The role of touch in rhesus monkey social development. In C. C. Brown (Ed.), *The many facets of touch* (pp. 41–50). Skillman, NJ: Johnson & Johnson Baby Products.

6 / The Second Year of Life

Alicia F. Lieberman and Arietta Slade

The second year of life is ushered in by two momentous achievements: the beginning of internal representation, marked by language and symbolic play, and the onset of locomotion. The developmental agenda of the second year is shaped primarily by the changes in both the sense of self and the nature of relationships that follow from these developments. There is a consolidation and expansion of the ability to move autonomously, to communicate verbally with others, and to their use symbols in order to encode and express subjective experience. This waxing of capacities changes children's relationships to their world and to themselves in numerous ways.

The Psychological Meanings of Locomotion

Autonomous walking has a profound effect at once on the toddler's self-concept and on the way she is regarded by others: the child has now become an "upright person," someone "standing on her own two feet" who has the potential to "go far" (Erikson, 1950). Between 13 and 18 months, movement becomes an end in itself: Walking is followed quickly by the ability to climb and to run, which opens new vistas in the exploration of previously unreachable realms. In portraying the exuberant mood of this period, Mahler and her colleagues describe children of this age as having a "love affair with the world" (Mahler, Pine, & Bergman, 1975).

The mastery of locomotion develops hand in hand with a new sense of personal will. Children of this age can now determine when and where to go, and toddlers often take off without consulting the parent and without looking back. At the same time, they expect that they will be followed and retrieved. Young toddlers seem to assume that the protective parent is always at their side. When about to lose their balance, they automatically reach back as if to hold on to their mothers, who may have been left far behind.

This behavior indicates that the patterns and dynamics of interaction have begun to be internalized: children show an expectation that the parent will be there whenever needed, an expectation based on many previous exchanges where this was indeed the case. The internalized images serve to give children a sense of safety and protectedness in their personal initiatives. However, the conflicting pulls of autonomy versus the wish for closeness are not always easy to integrate. The effort to find a solution finds symbolic expression in a favorite game: to run away from mother again and again, only to squeal in delight when pursued and scooped up in her arms. This game helps toddlers to consolidate and internalize an understanding that mobility need not mean abandonment or alienation, and that independence and togetherness can go hand in hand (Lieberman, 1993).

The Representational Capacity

The ability to use symbols serves as a vehicle for the expression of inner experience and social communication. It is a remarkable but meaningful coincidence that the onset of independent motion overlaps with the beginnings of this new attainment. Whereas locomotion promotes distance from people, symbols bridge this gap and help toddlers stay connected while engaging in the very process of taking off.

The use of language and the capacity for symbolic play are hallmarks of the representational capacity. In the second year of life, children begin to imagine objects that are not present, and these youngsters can evoke such objects verbally or through the use of signs and symbols that are understood by others. Toddlers may observe someone perform an action they have never seen before, and hours or even days later they imitate the same behavior. This deferred imitation is another manifestation of the capacity to represent because it involves the retrieval of images stored in long-term memory even in the absence of external cues (Piaget, 1954).

Optimally, the mental representation of objects is multisensory and includes levels of affective meaning abstracted from repeated experiences with a given object. In other words, toddlers internalize the visual, auditory, olfactory, tactile, and functional features of an object. These features are usually retrieved according to the demands of the situation. When there is constriction in the range, depth, and integration of these sensory experiences, the quality of the mental representation of the object will suffer as well (Greenspan, 1989).

At the level of sensory organization, children need to process auditory-verbal and visual-spatial patterns in accordance with physical, temporal, spatial and affective qualities. Children need to decode what objects and events are "real" and "pretend," "me" and "no me"; familiar and unfamiliar; past, present, and future; near and far; safe and dangerous; permitted or forbidden. Information needs to be categorized in the sequential order in which it occurs. The intactness of the sensory pathways (i.e., the capacity to perceive and process visual, auditory, olfactory, tactile, taste, and kinetic stimuli) enable children to keep up with this formidable array of tasks. Conversely, compromises in any of the sensory domains lead to difficulty in processing incoming information through the particular sensory channel involved.

The thematic-affective organization of experience during this period involves the attribution of meaning at a higher level than before through language and symbolic play. The affective-thematic domain undergoes a process of elaboration and differentiation that begins in the second year and gains momentum in children of 3, 4, and 5 years of age. As children develop, increasingly subtler, more varied and complex affective themes are represented in symbolic play; these themes include pleasure, fear, mastery, anger, assertiveness, empathy, and love. By the end of the second year, children can use symbolic play simultaneously to elaborate and differentiate their experiences, ushering in the stage of "representational differentiation" (Greenspan, 1989).

THE USE OF LANGUAGE

Using words also gives concrete evidence that children have internalized experience and that they are joining in the human community at a new level by using symbols with a shared social meaning. The choice of specific words reflect the emotional preoccupations of children. The first words give a name to the cherished caregivers ("mama," "dada") and to objects which are central to the baby's sense of well-being ("baba" for bottle). Only later, at about 18 months or so, will words be used to convey their concern with establishing and protecting a separate identity through the use of "no," "me," and "mine."

Behavioral sequences of increased richness and complexity help toddlers to supplement the inevitable linguistic deficits, and give evidence of their growing ability to have an internal agenda that can be systematically implemented. Greenspan (1989) offers the example of a 14-month-old who can take the mother's hand, walk her to the refrigerator, bang on the door to signal that she wants it open, and then point to the food she desired since the beginning of the sequence (p. 31). It is likely that she will have been saying some (unintelligible to others) version of her word for that food all along. In this chain of behaviors, the child is using wish and intentionality as the organizers of a complex behavioral pattern where each component is causally linked to the next. Language may be present, but it is still insufficient to convey intentionality all by itself.

Between 15 and 18 months, toddlers try very hard to make themselves understood. Children of this age attempt to say any word that they hear and amuse themselves with vocal play. They understand and obey simple directions such as "Bring me your doll" or "come here." The use of language to indicate their own intentions and to respond to the intentions of others acquires new momentum.

At the same time, during the first half of the second year, gestures are a prevalent form of communication. Facial expressions, motor movements, body gestures, and vocal patterns say more at this age about toddlers' inner experience than their meager vocabulary can possibly convey. A 16-month-old cannot say "I am angry," but his narrowing eyes, stretched lips, clenched fists, stiff posture, and loud, defiant vocalizations convey this emotion eloquently indeed.

Between the middle and the end of the second year, toddlers are stringing together phrases made up of two or more words that greatly enhance their capacity to say what they mean. Emotions ("sad," "mad," "happy") can be conveyed through words in addition to gestures. Two-year-olds can use pronouns such as "I," "me," and "you," indicating the evolution of a more advanced sense of self as the agent of behavior; "mine" conveys a rudimentary though intense sense of ownership. Although there are very great individual differences in verbal fluency and sophistication in the second year, toddlers become ever more skilled communicators and are increasingly creative in finding ways to convey their wishes and intentions.

SYMBOLIC PLAY

Play has important cognitive, social, and emotional functions. It enables children to experiment in a safe setting with the physical, functional, and symbolic properties of objects (including children's own bodies) and with their relationship to other objects. Social roles—being the mommy or the daddy, serving a meal—are practiced and learned through symbolic play.

Play is also a major avenue for mastering anxiety. Erikson (1950) proposed that play enables children to set up model situations to work out different ways of controlling reality. In play, children become the master of what happens to them rather than passive recipients. Children can set up a different version of a painful event, giving it a "happy ending." A difficult experience can be processed emotionally by playing it out again and again in different forms until they can finally master it.

Much as they use objects as symbolic vehicles, toddlers use their bodies as symbolic instruments. For example, the anxieties over separation (the "darker side" of autonomy) may be symbolically expressed and mastered through games of hide and seek. Here a child experiences in manageable doses the fear of losing the parent, a fear that in the game is quickly relieved through a joyous reunion. The fear that moving away from the parent (i.e., exercising one's autonomy) can lead to being lost is enacted and alleviated through games of darting away and being scooped up in the parent's arms—a reassurance that the parent will not allow the child to be lost (Mahler et al., 1975).

Another anxiety of toddlerhood—fear of body damage through loss of balance or loss of a body part—is worked out by breaking things apart and then putting them together again. Here, objects are used as symbolic representations of the body. For example, at this age, games such as building towers only to make them collapse and then rebuilding them again are a common pastime.

In the course of the second year and thereafter, representational use of objects in play and in "real" life evolves in evermore complex fashion. Three levels have been identified (Greenspan, 1989; Piaget, 1962). The first level involves description (i.e., labeling objects) and the performance of single acts of "pretend," such as drinking from a toy cup or talking on a toy telephone. The second level involves rudimentary elaboration of affective themes through a small number of sequences. The child may say: "me hungry; need cookie," establishing an implicit causal connection between the two statements. In symbolic play, the child may kiss a doll and then put it to bed. At the third level, a number of representational units are linked together into a coherent drama that unfolds in orderly fashion, such as a tea party where tea is ceremoniously prepared, served, and enjoyed by the guests.

Toddlers' capacity to engage pleasurably in autonomous play—whether of a physical or symbolic nature—is closely linked to the quality of the mother-child relationship. Children secure in their mother's availability explore the world around them with evident interest and enjoyment, without either overconcern or indifference to her whereabouts. Their physical play tends to be free and exuberant, their symbolic play is rich, coherent, and diverse, and they are more likely than anxiously attached children to play at their highest level of cognitive ability.

In this sense, securely attached children are better able to make the most of their own abilities and of the world around them (Slade, 1986, 1987).

They use symbols to make bridges toward others rather than away from them, or away from the symbolic realm altogether. Children with secure relationships to their mothers are both better able to use their mothers as collaborative play partners, and to show less regression when left to play alone (Slade, 1987).

By the end of the second year, toddlers who are unable to engage in meaningful, expressive, symbolic play for a reasonable length of time are often in some kind of developmental difficulty. It can be a symptom of emotional disturbance or of problems in sensory regulation and modulation. Only observation, testing, and developmental history can give clues to the etiology of the condition, but the consistent failure to play is almost certainly a symptom of an underlying difficulty.

Self-Recognition, Body Awareness, and Sexual Curiosity

Awareness of oneself as an objectively recognizable individual develops gradually in the course of the second year. Toddlers' response to their mirror image is a telling indication of how this awareness progresses. Amsterdam (1972) and Lewis and Brooks-Gunn (1979) conducted experiments in which infants had their noses dabbed with lipstick and were then encouraged to look at themselves in the mirror. Before 13 months, the infants tended to establish social interactions with their images as if they were playing with another child, laughing, babbling, and patting at the image. Between 13 and 14 months, this behavior changed to involve a clear search for the image in the mirror: the toddlers tried to enter the mirror, and, when this behavior did not succeed, they looked and reached behind the mirror. Some children at this age responded with fear when they could not find the image; they turned away from the mirror and avoided looking at it.

Self-conscious behavior emerged at 14 months, and consisted of coyness, clowning, clear admiration (such as in a girl who looked at herself with evident pleasure while stroking her hair), and embarrassment. By 18 months, the toddlers began to show unmistakable recognition of their image: Whereas before this age they tended to touch the dab of lipstick in the mirror image, after 18 months they touched their own noses and tried to rub the lipstick off.

This age sequence shows an increasing consolidation of the sense of self recognition in the course of the second year. By the time they recognize themselves in the mirror, toddlers also begin to incorporate "I," "me," and "mine" in their speech, and they use their own name to refer to themselves.

These observations suggest that after 18 months, toddlers are able to experience themselves objectively, as people who can be seen from the outside as well as felt from the inside. In other words, they acquire a "categorical" self that coexists with a "subjective" or "experiential" self (Greenspan, 1989; Stern, 1985). The question of how the "inside" and the "outside" fit together becomes a new area of exploration.

Consistent with this interest in who one is and how one's body is put together, curiosity about fecal and urinary matters looms large in the toddler years. Toddlers experience increasingly differentiated sensations in the anal and urethral areas, and they gradually become better able to control the muscles responsible for those sensations. The readiness for toilet training is in part dependent on this maturation, although family and community values play an important role as well.

Bodily products—feces and urine—are objects, and, as such, they become a feature of children's internal representational world. The visual, olfactory, and textural qualities of these objects are internally represented, as well as their functional significance (bodily pressure and relief from it) and the affective experiences associated with them.

Erik Erikson (1950) has pointed out that the bodily sensations involved in withholding and expelling body products set the stage for the child's experimentation with two sets of social modalities: holding on and letting go. Toddlers experiment with mastery over the body functions by playing with symbolic representations: clay, wet sand or soil, paint, water. They practice the social modalities of holding on and letting go in many contexts. Some of these contexts are the patterns of secure base behavior, where toddlers hold on to the parent when wary or tired but let go in order to explore when feeling confident and strong; defiance (holding on to one's wishes) versus cooperation; keeping for oneself versus sharing with others.

Another aspect of the symbolic meaning of body products involves children's emotional association of their behavior with the approval or disapproval of those they love. In the second year of life there is a rapid development of representational skills. In keeping with this, toddlers become aware of social standards of right and wrong (Kagan, 1981) in the context of the relationship between cause and effect. In toilet training, cause (i.e., producing or withholding feces at a particular time) is linked to effect (parental praise or displeasure). In this way, anal and urethral activities become associated with family and community values about being dirty (bad, reprehensible, cast off) and being clean (good, lovable, accepted by the group). Through these associations, concrete body functions acquire a powerful symbolic and emotional meaning.

The maturation and differentiation of the muscles and accompanying sensations in the anal-urethral area also bring about a new interest in the genitals. Toddlers explore themselves with a purposefulness that is qualitatively different from the casual genital play of infants. They scrutinize their bodies to find out how they are made, how the "inside me" (subjective self) and the "outside me" (objective, external self) fit together. They associate their actions with the different kinds of pleasure they feel as a result.

The self-recognition that begins to crystallize at about 18 months applies to genital identity as well. Girls learn that they have vulvas and vaginas and are girls; boys learn that they have penises and scrotums and are boys. They compare themselves to each other, sometimes being proud of their own attributes, at other times feeling envy that they do not have what the other sex has.

The psychoanalytic concepts of "penis envy," "womb envy," and "breast envy" emerged originally from reports of children and adults undergoing psychoanalysis. More recently, observations of nonclinical samples have confirmed the existence of strong feelings about one's own genitals and how they compare with the other gender's genitals as a normal part of toddlers' development (Roiphe & Galenson, 1981). These feelings are experienced in a more rudimentary form in the second year and become elaborated and incorpo-

rated into the age-specific issues of the third, fourth, and fifth years of life.

The process of representational differentiation described by Greenspan (1989) applies to gender identity as well. Toddlers learn about their gender but they simultaneously believe that they also have the features of the opposite sex. Three-year-old boys declare they can have babies and will grow breasts to suckle them; girls believe that they have penises as well as vaginas. The knowledge that each gender has only one set of sexually specific attributes and functions does not consolidate until about age four, when it gives way to strong interest in the relationship between the sexes and how babies are made. The pronounced sexual curiosity of these years does not subside until the so-called latency age, beginning at about 6 years of age.

Opposition and Negativism

In the popular imagination, negativism and defiance have become the hallmark of toddlerhood, earning this age the rather undeserved label of the "the terrible twos."

Toddlers' newfound ability to say "no" can be understood in the context of their rapidly consolidating representational and motor skills and their more solid sense of self as distinct and separate from others. They can now envision new possibilities, work out the sequence of actions that are needed to attain a goal, and literally move toward that goal by walking, running, or climbing. The "I" is self-aware, active, and determined to achieve its goals.

In this process toddlers encounter many parental prohibitions because their level of socialization lags greatly behind their capacity to take action. The second year of life marks the beginning of a protracted and painstaking process of differentiating right from wrong, learning what is allowed and what is forbidden, and testing the limits of the rules set down by the parents. The toddler's "no" can be understood as the mirror of the many parental "nos" he must hear and abide by.

This "battle of the nos" has an important role in the regulation of the toddler's self-esteem. When a parent can remain firm but loving in depriving a child of something he or she wants but should not have, toddlers learns that disappointment, frustration, and anger are bearable emotions that do not lead to emotional alienation (Fraiberg, 1959; Mahler et al., 1975). On the other hand, toddlers may experience chronic and pervasive lack of parental empathy, intrusiveness, or excessive efforts to control as assaults on their sense of self (Kernberg, 1975; Kohut, 1971).

The Anxieties of Toddlerhood

The anxieties of the second year have specific, phase-appropriate themes that reflect the affective organization of behavior during this period. At this age, toddlers become capable of *imagining* situations, are gradually more aware of standards of right and wrong, and are exquisitely sensitive to the relationship between cause and effect caused by their own behavior. These capacities coalesce to make fear of losing the parent the central anxiety of this age.

Separation anxiety begins at about 8 months, but it becomes most acute at around 18 months. It may seem paradoxical that separation anxiety increases just as toddlers delights in their emerging autonomy and capacity to move away from the parent. This polarity becomes understandable when it is viewed as a struggle *within the child* about wanting the safety of the mother's presence while relishing the freedom of moving away (Mahler et al., 1975).

The key issue here is the toddler's desire to be in charge of the decision. When she wants to move away, all is well in her own mind. The anxiety emerges when she is the passive recipient of the parent's decision to go out on her own.

As toddlers become increasingly aware of standards of right and wrong, anxiety over loss becomes more specific: Children are afraid not only of losing the mother's physical presence but also of losing her approval. Fear of losing the parent's love looms large towards the end of the second year and continues well into the third year.

The central organizing theme of children's increasing differentiation of feeling is this fear of losing love. Older toddlers (30 months and up) pay close attention to feelings and are very interested in what feelings are experienced in different situations. They are particularly concerned about anger (the parent's and their own), and whether anger will lead to abandonment and loss. Toddlers know that they can't feel love and anger at the same time. As a result, they worry that the parent doesn't love them when he or she is angry at them. The integration of positive and negative feelings into the acceptance of ambivalence is a key component of object constancy, an achievement which occurs gradually between the middle of the second year and into the third and fourth years (Mahler et al., 1975).

Body-centered anxieties are also prevalent during toddlerhood. Anxiety over loss is interwoven with still-rudimentary logic to generate fears that seem irrational from an adult point of view. Fears about bodily integrity originate in misconceptions about the source of anatomical differences between the sexes. Fears of losing a part of the body may be manifested in refusal to have one's hair cut, in constipation, or in other idiosyncratic forms.

Temperamental Differences

No two children are alike. Their unique individuality is manifested along many dimensions. Some are outgoing and ebullient, others reserved; some are physically active, others prefer sedentary pursuits; some relish adventure, others crave familiarity; some are seemingly impervious to frustration, others collapse in tears when faced with stress. Many parents report that from the time they were born, their children had strongly maintained and clearly recognizable ways of responding to the world.

The concept of temperament is a useful construct to organize the observation that even very young children differ markedly in their behavior in spite of being reared in similar environments. But what is temperament? There have been many efforts to define it and to describe the dimensions most likely to explain current functioning and predict future development (Escalona, 1968; Goldsmith et al., 1987; Thomas, Chess, & Birch, 1968).

While there is some debate abut the specific parameters involved, scholars agree that the hallmarks of temperament are emotionality and activity level. In this sense, temperament can be defined as the "how" of behavior—its intensity, rhythmicity, adaptability, and mood quality, in contrast to the content or "what" of behavior (i.e., individual talent or ability), or motivation (its reason, or "why" it occurs [Thomas et al., 1968]).

One example of a temperamentally based personality style is shyness, which has emerged as a stable individual response to novelty beginning in the second year of life and continuing at least into middle childhood (Kagan, Reznick, Snidman, Gibbons, & Johnson, 1988). Shyness, which may be defined as a reliable slowness to engage in novel situations, has an identifiable physiological profile involving higher-than-average arousal of the sympathetic nervous system in unfamiliar settings. A group of toddlers was identified as shy on the basis of their response to novelty. When faced with mildly stressing stimuli, they tended to show larger increases in heart rate and pupil dilation than did a group of outgoing age mates (Kagan, Reznick, & Snidman, 1987).

In spite of this tendency toward stability, temperament is not immutable. Indeed, depending on the characteristics of the caregiving environment and on the course of maturation, it can in fact, be modified.

The "goodness of fit" between the parents' own child-rearing styles and the child's temperament is considered a key variable in facilitating or hampering his or her healthy development (Thomas & Chess, 1977). When parents are able supportively to redirect children's more problematic tendencies in more adaptive directions, negative temperamental propensities may be modulated by children's more positive traits and become integrated in constructive ways.

Conclusion

The second year of life brings about the onset and consolidation of autonomous locomotion and the capacity for symbolic representation. These developmental milestones have profound effects on toddlers' sense of self and on their relationships with parents. Autonomous movement brings about a new independence, while the rapid development of language, symbolic play, and deferred imitation give children new tools to store information, organize experience, and engage in higher levels of interpersonal communication. It is at this time that issues of control, with the concomitant themes of cooperation versus defiance and negativism, become central. At the same time, toddlers still rely on parents for a basic sense of safety and well-being. The efforts to integrate intimacy with autonomy set the stage for the affective themes of the third year of life.

REFERENCES

Amsterdam, B. K. (1972). Mirror self-image reactions before age two. *Developmental Psychology, 5,* 297–305.

Erikson, E. (1950). *Childhood and society.* New York: W. W. Norton.

Escalona, S. (1968). *The roots of individuality.* Chicago: Aldine.

Fraiberg, S. (1959). *The magic years.* New York: Charles Scribner's Sons.

Goldsmith, H., Buss, A., Plomin, R., Rothbart, M., Thomas, A., Chess, S., Hinde, R., & McCall, R. (1987). Roundtable: What is temperament? *Child Development, 58,* 505–529.

Greenspan, S. I. (1989). *The development of the ego.* Madison, CT: International Universities Press.

Kagan, J., Reznick, J. S., & Snidman, N. (1987). The physiology and psychology of behavioral inhibition in children. *Child Development, 58,* 1459–1473.

Kagan, J., Reznick, J. S., Snidman, N., Gibbons, J., & Johnson, M. D. (1988). Childhood derivatives of inhibition and lack of inhibition to the unfamiliar. *Child Development, 59,* 1580–1589.

Kernberg, O. F. (1975). *Borderline conditions and pathological narcissism.* New York: Jason Aronson.

Kohut, H. (1971). *The analysis of the self.* New York: International Universities Press.

Lewis, M., & Brooks-Gunn, J. (1979). *Social cognition and the acquisition of self.* New York: Plenum Press.

Lieberman, A. F. (1993). *The emotional life of the toddler.* New York: The Free Press.

Mahler, M., Pine, F., & Bergman, A. (1975). *The psy-*

chological birth of the human infant. New York: Basic Books.

Piaget, J. (1926). *The language and thought of the child.* London: Routledge, Kegan & Paul.

Piaget, J. (1954). *The origins of intelligence in children.* New York: International Universities Press.

Roiphe, H., & Galenson, E. (1981). *Infantile origins of sexual identity.* New York: International Universities Press.

Slade, A. (1986). Symbolic play and separation-individuation: A naturalistic study. *Bulletin of the Menninger Clinic, 50,* 541–563.

Slade, A. (1987). A longitudinal study of maternal involvement and symbolic play during the toddler period. *Child Development, 58,* 367–375.

Stern, D. N. (1985). *The interpersonal world of the infant.* New York: Basic Books.

Thomas, A., Chess, S., & Birch, H. (1968). *Temperament and behavior disorders in children.* New York: New York University Press.

Thomas, A., & Chess, S. (1977). *Temperament and Development.* New York: Brunner/Mazel.

7 / Cognitive Development in the Second Year of Life

Holly A. Ruff

The focus in this chapter is on the knowledge and skills acquired by the child in the context of everyday life, with an emphasis on the social aspects of that context. In the first section, I summarize the major cognitive advances that occur in the second year of life. In the second section, I discuss specific developments in play, problem solving, and representation or memory in detail. Finally, I briefly present alternatives to the standard assessments for this period of development.

Major Advances in Skill and Knowledge

The second year of life is characterized by several major transitions. The most salient of these is the beginning of speech, which, for most normal children, blossoms around 18 months, as they come to understand that words refer to objects, actions, and events in the world around them (Anisfeld, 1984). Shortly thereafter, children typically produce two-word utterances. On the other hand, several studies have shown that children understand words long before they produce them. For example, in her longitudinal study, Benedict (1979) found that the children understood 50 words at about 13 months but were not producing 50 words until 18 months. Furthermore, although children initially tend to extend words beyond their conventional definitions, overextension seems to be limited to production and appears rarely in comprehension (Harris, 1983); that is, children may understand the word-referent relationship better than their own speech would suggest. Thus, both general knowledge and comprehension of language are precursors and important components of spoken language. Speech, however, involves other skills, and immaturities in attention and motor coordination may delay its appearance relative to knowledge and understanding.

The emergence of language, in both its receptive and productive forms, is inextricably woven into the child's social interactions. During both play and routine activities, it is the child's interactions with older siblings, parents, and other adults that make the initial connection between objects and their referents possible (Baldwin, 1991; Baldwin & Markman, 1989; Schmidt, in press; Tomasello & Barten, 1994). On the other hand, growing comprehension of language increases the degree to which young children are able to cooperate in social situations. Kaler and Kopp (1990) independently measured comprehension and compliance with directives; they found that with age, there was a significant increase in both comprehension and compliance.

These were directly linked, so that children rarely complied when they did not understand the constituents (nouns, verbs) of a command, and they rarely failed to comply when they did. As with imitation, children's ability to follow directions may lead to actions outside their current repertoire, thereby adding to their experience and expanding their understanding of themselves and of the world. Also, when children begin to communicate effectively with other people, they are expected to behave more maturely in other areas as well; these expectations then challenge the children's emerging capacity to function in both social and inanimate environments.

Although the beginnings of language stand out as the most salient accomplishment of this year, other related and equally important transitions are occurring. According to Piaget (1952), the development of language is part of the onset of general symbolic functioning; This is manifested by delayed imitation (but see Meltzoff, 1988), pretend play, and fully developed object permanence (the ability to find hidden objects that have been displaced in ways that are not visible to the child). For Piaget, the significance of all of these activities is that they require the child to have some representation of absent objects—absent models and actions in the case of delayed imitation, substitutes for absent objects in the case of pretend play, and invisible displacements and search for absent objects in the case of object permanence. The issue of the relationship among these different forms of symbolic functioning has led to considerable research (Corrigan, 1978; Harris, 1983; McCune, 1995; McCune-Nicolich, 1981a). Some synchrony in development has been found; for example, in some studies, the word "allgone" tends to appear at about the same time that the child has mastered the final level of object permanence (Corrigan, 1978). McCune-Nicolich (1981a) interprets the available data as showing that the last stage of object permanence is not a *necessary* precursor to the use of such terms; rather, such relational words develop in parallel with nonverbal manifestations of representation. Other work suggests that children come to relate two components at about the same age, whether the components are words or blocks (Case & Khanna, 1981). There is also considerable asynchrony (Fischer & Bullock, 1981), however, as would be expected given that the emergence and manifestation of

particular skills depends, in part, on the context and the nature of the supports available for that skill (Fischer, 1980).

It is not until the latter part of the first year that we see evidence of planning; this development is attributed, in part, to development of the frontal cortex (Diamond, 1991). The development of the frontal cortex continues for a long period thereafter (Goldman-Rakic, 1987; Welsh & Pennington, 1988), and so does behavioral evidence for planning ahead. The ability is still primitive in the second year, but toddlers do look ahead to problem solutions and are able to plan in ways that seem to be impossible for infants. Where younger infants will solve problems only through an extended period of trial and error, toddlers may solve problems by perceiving the solution before effecting it (Piaget, 1952). An example is Piaget's daughter Lucienne, who attempted to put a chain into a matchbox; her first try at putting one end of the flexible chain into the box was unsuccessful, but she paused briefly and then rolled the chain up into a ball that could be put into the box with a single movement (Observation 179). Such problem solving involves both some ability to represent the solution before acting and the capacity to inhibit the more obvious, but ineffective, action.

In the second year, young children continue to gather prodigious amounts of information about the physical and social environment. They also learn more about themselves in relation to the environment. At the same time, children's knowledge is being linked to a symbolic system that allows them to comprehend language and to begin to produce it. This particular achievement introduces new possibilities for learning and for acquiring new actions. A reorganization takes place in the form of a shift from perceptual- and action-based knowledge to more generalized and abstract knowledge. With this, children begin to separate events in the world from their own actions.

Examples in Specific Domains

The changes observed in the second year arise from multiple causes: expansion of knowledge, comprehension in context, skills in following the

64

motion of objects and finding objects that are out of view, insight into the connection between objects and events and the symbols for them, and challenges imposed by both the child and the older members of the child's social world (Rogoff, Mistry, Göncü, & Mosier, 1993).

PLAY

Since one of the major advances in the second year is the emergence of symbolic functioning, it is not surprising that the child's play begins to show evidence of pretend. Late in the first year or early in the second, infants show what Leslie (1987) calls sophisticated functional play; they show by their actions on objects that they understand the purpose of those objects—putting a brush to the hair, drinking from an empty cup, or pushing along a toy car while making a motor sound. Initially, these actions may be engaged in for an extended period of time, but their duration soon becomes very brief, a more abstract indication of the child's knowledge or "enactive naming" (Belsky & Most, 1981). These behaviors, however, may not be truly symbolic because they do not involve object substitution or an object that is absent, but whose presence is implied. According to McCune-Nicolich (1981b) and Belsky and Most (1981), object substitution emerges around 13 to 14 months but does not become a typical part of play until 18 to 21 months. Examples that stem from this period tend to involve nondescript objects that do not have salient functions of their own, such as a block of wood. The criteria for scoring truly symbolic play in a research or clinical setting include some evidence that children know that they are pretending, perhaps by virtue of a knowing look or exaggerated sounds (McCune, 1995).

Construction in play can be seen as children begin to combine blocks and other types of objects. At this age, children do not build elaborate structures, both because they have difficulty conceiving of such structures and because they do not have the fine motor skill to execute them. In line with this, children in the second year show, on average, fairly short periods of focused attention (Ruff & Lawson, 1990). On the other hand, because of the simplicity of their activity, at this point they may not need long episodes of focused attention. Also, the failure to plan ahead leaves the child with no goal around which to organize activity and maintain it over time; if the goal of an activity, such as putting blocks together, is fuzzy, then there is no particular reason not to move on to another activity, if something else catches the child's interest (Ruff & Rothbart, 1996). We might consider such behavior as showing a lack of sustained attention, but, from a functional point of view, the child's behavior is perfectly adaptive.

Much play occurs in the context of interaction with others. The phenomenon of joint attention—that is, the sharing of attention to the same object or task with another person—develops in two ways. One, the child comes more readily to follow the direction of someone else's gaze. Butterworth and Jarrett (1991) have shown that 12-month-old infants will locate an object that the mother looks at *if* the target is already in the visual field. If the mother looks at a target behind the infant, the infant does not locate it but tends to look ahead. By 18 months, however, a child will turn around to look at something behind, providing that there is no competition within the visual field at the time. The mother's pointing increases the probability that infants of 12 and 18 months will turn to the target, suggesting that they understand the directing function of that gesture as well (Butterworth, 1991; Murphy & Messer, 1978).

The second development is that, from 12 to 18 months, the child is better able simultaneously to coordinate attention to the object or task and to the partner. Bakeman and Adamson (1984) document the increase in what they call "coordinated joint attention" that is, the child and partner are not only attending to the same object but also are aware of each other and the direction of each other's attention. At this age, there is less joint attention with peers than there is with mothers; this suggests that mothers play an important role in maintaining such attention, probably because they tend to follow the infant's lead. On the other hand, infants gradually take more initiative and try actively to get the partner to share the target of their attention—"showing" or "taking the partner's hand," for example.

The role of joint attention is important to cognitive development in a number of ways. First, when a parent follows the infant's direction of attention, the infant may not have to devote as much effort to maintaining joint attention and has resources left to learn from the playful interaction with the parent. For example, when the parent demonstrates some new action with a toy that already has been focused on, the infant may be more likely to watch the action and imitate it (Tomasello, Savage-Rumbaugh, & Kruger, 1993). Second, being able to follow the adult's line of sight helps the infant to establish word-referent relationships and to comprehend new words (Baldwin, 1991; Dunham, Dunham, & Curwin, 1993; Schmidt, in press). Third, within episodes of joint attention to toys, at 21 months the number of references mothers make to objects within the child's focus of attention is positively related to size of the child's productive vocabulary (Tomasello & Farrar, 1986). Interestingly, in a comparison of joint attention episodes involving toddler, sibling, and mother versus joint attention between toddler and mother, Barton and Tomasello (1991) found that the triadic conversations were longer than the dyadic ones, and that the toddler took more turns. These results suggest that the young language learner may not profit only from situations in which the mother is sharing her attention with two children, but that in that context, the linguistic environment may be enhanced in some ways compared to dyadic interaction.

The child's linguistic and cognitive experiences vary across various play situations. O'Brien and Nagle (1987), for example, observed toddlers, 18 to 24 months of age, playing with their mothers or fathers in three situations—with dolls, toy vehicles, or a shape sorter. The investigators found that parents spoke the most, used the most nouns, asked the most questions, and gave the children the greatest opportunity to respond during play with the dolls as compared to play with the vehicles or the shape sorter. The shape sorter elicited more directives and commands for attention, and the dyads were generally more goal-oriented than in the other settings.

A number of studies have shown that the linguistic experience is richer and more elaborate during book reading, a common joint activity in the second year, than in other play settings (Dunn, Wooding, & Herman 1977) or during routine caretaking (Hoff-Ginsberg, 1991). Results reported by Lewis and Gregory (1987) suggest that increased elaboration (longer utterances and more complex words) is more characteristic of book reading in the second year than it is in the first year. Thus it may be an important way that parents both acknowledge the child's cognitive and linguistic progress and stimulate it further. (See also Whitehurst et al., 1994.) Moreover, book reading takes on special significance in any society that values educational achievement, and this value is communicated to the child by the parents' enthusiasm for an activity that emphasizes language and the medium of the written word.

PROBLEM SOLVING

Finding the means to reach particular goals involves accurate perception of the objective situation, attention to the relevant details, and certain motor skills. It may or may not involve planning. In Chapter 2, it was noted that before about 9 months, infants may not have goals clearly enough in mind to be said to be planning; there is more evidence for such planning by 12 months (Willats & Rosie, 1989). In the second year, the child is increasingly able to think of solutions to a problem rather than groping for and then stumbling on the solution by trial and error. This more thoughtful approach is sometimes referred to as "insightful" problem solving. It has been shown, however, that such problem solving is dependent on previous experience, often having the character of playful interaction, with the objects that are involved in the problem and its solution (Birch, 1945; Rubin, Fein, & Vandenberg, 1983). For example, consider a situation in which a desired object is out of reach. However, a stick is in the vicinity and could be used to bring the object within reach. Under these circumstances, children, as well as animals and older humans, are more likely to see the relationship between the desired object and the stick if they are already familiar with the stick from other situations.

Piaget (1952) richly illustrated his theoretical account of the development of the child's understanding of means-ends relationships throughout the first two years. One of his illustrations was his son's groping attempts to retrieve an object that was on one tier of a table with revolving circular tiers. Using a very similar problem, Koslowski and Bruner (1972) systematically observed children in three age groups—12 to 14 months, 14 to 16 months, and 16 to 24 months. A toy was attached to a rotating lever and the children were given 15 to 20 minutes to retrieve it. The solution was to push the lever away from the body in order to rotate the end of the lever with the toy on it into reaching distance. In the course of the study, the children employed several approaches, which varied in sophistication and in the age at which they appeared. The most common approach among the 12-month-olds was a direct reach for the object. Failing to reach it, some children walked around the table in order to grasp the object directly. When foiled by the experimenters, they tried again or switched to a second approach—moving the lever back and forth, but always bringing it back to midline. That is, they seemed to appreciate the fact that the lever rotated but not that rotation would bring the object close enough to reach for it directly. In the third approach, the 14- to 16-month-olds rotated the lever partway or even all of the way but made no attempt to reach for the object even when it was close. Possibly the children were attending to the relationship of lever and toy and were, as the authors put it, "operationally preoccupied." The last approach, used only by the 16- to 24-month-olds, was, of course, to rotate the lever until the toy was within reach and then to grasp it.

A preoccupation with the means rather than the end suggests that the use of an unpracticed skill takes considerable effort; until the skill becomes more practiced or automatic, the child may not be able to devote resources to combining the various components required to solve the problem. In the study by Koslowski and Bruner (1972), reaching and grasping the object would have already been a well-polished action pattern, but, until the first and necessary component of rotation had been mastered, the children either could not attend to the goal or could not integrate means and goal. In the course of development, this aspect of skill development is repeated over and over again; when children are required to use new skills, attention and resources are co-opted and may not be available for other requirements of the task.

The problem of finding objects continues to be a practical problem that children have to solve. Sophian (1984) suggests that several underlying skills are involved. One is to use selected sources of information correctly in order to guide the search. Thus, a relevant kind of information may be previous experience—the child's blanket is usually in the bedroom where it is a comfort at bedtime. Another source of information is being told that the object is elsewhere: "Your blanket is in the kitchen." In this case, the child has to choose between prior and current data where the information is conflicting; the child will search most effectively if the parent's statement is used as the basis for action. Whether the source of current information is verbal or nonverbal, 16-month-olds use it much more consistently than younger children (Sophian, 1984). A second relevant skill is the ability to follow the movements of an object even if some movements have to be inferred rather than perceived directly. For example, 20-month-olds can find an object after it has been hidden under one of three cups and the location of the cups is changed, but 13-month-olds have difficulty if the cup that hides the object does not itself remain stationary. The kinds of errors children make may change with age as well. For example, if children have difficulty following the movements of an object—that is, if they do not pick up adequate information through observation—they do not search randomly but tend rather to have biases for one location or another. As might be expected, the degree of response bias decreases from 9 to 16 months for the same problem, suggesting that the older children pick up the necessary information more readily.

REPRESENTATION/MEMORY

Understanding the development of representation involves understanding how the child's knowledge of the world is organized and reorganized with experience. Declarative, as opposed to procedural, knowledge becomes relatively more important with development (Mandler, 1983). What kinds of declarative knowledge do children have in the second year? How do they represent their worlds? Nelson and Gruendel (1981) suggest that young children's initial representations or abstractions from concrete experiences revolve around the familiar routines of their lives, hence the terms *event representation* and *scripts*. Specific experiences lead to and are incorporated into generalized schemes of what we do at mealtime, at bedtime, and so forth. Although at this age children may not be able to verbalize these scripts, their knowledge is manifest in their ability to initiate and participate in these routines; by word, gesture, or action they anticipate the appropriate sequence of steps. For example, if a mother says "Bathtime!" to her 18-month-old, the child may collect bath toys, throw them in the tub, and try to turn on the water faucet.

Also, in the course of observing events, children begin to extract certain physical regularities that some have referred to as principles. Keil (1979), for example, presented 18-month-olds with a simple construction, one block resting on top of two other blocks. The children were then surprised to see the top block remain in place (by a trick of the experimenter!) when the two supporting blocks were removed. A more complex problem was presented that involved a structure's standing after the removal of a single support and a loss of balance. The children accepted this, however, suggesting that their expectations were not precise or highly specific. Another expectation that young children have is that an object that is hidden will remain the same object, and that it will not change locations without intervention. LeCompte and Gratch (1972) hid objects for infants of 9, 12, and 18 months to find. On two trick trials, the object was surreptitiously replaced by a different one. Although children at all ages expressed some puzzlement and searched more in the trick trials than in the regular trials, the puzzlement and degree of search were higher for the 18-month-olds than for the two groups of younger children. The change over age was linear, suggesting that the children's expectations did not change abruptly but were gradually held with more confidence.

As noted before, infants may respond to their perceptual experiences categorically; in the second year there is evidence that the organization of categories is more active and spontaneous (Sugarman, 1981). For example, an 18-month-old may sequentially touch or pick up all of the little people in a farm set, leaving the animals and buildings alone, thus showing by action that the category of people is being acted upon. It has been argued that the initial categories are formed on a basic level—more abstract than a representation of an object itself, but more concrete than a superordinate category. Mandler and Bauer (1988) probed the level at which children spontaneously organized objects of two different classes. In one condition, the two classes were basic level—cars versus dogs; in another condition, the classes were superordinate ones—animals versus vehicles. The procedure involved scattering several objects from each category in front of the seated child; the child's behavior was then coded for the number of sequential touches on members of one class or the other. There were four items in each category. Exhaustive categorizing was considered to occur if the child sequentially touched three or four of them. At 12, 15, and 20 months, more children met the criteria for exhaustive categorizing in the basic level condition than in the superordinate condition. At the same time, some children at 15 and 18 months exhaustively categorized the objects at the superordinate level. While the data do not show that children understand superordinate categories in the sense of hierarchical classification, Mandler and Bauer conclude that young children's activity with and responsiveness to objects is based on a somewhat abstract level of organization. (See also Mandler, 1993.)

Internal or mental representation also involves the use of symbols. Development of symbolic activity is reflected in the emergence of both language and symbolic or pretend play (McCune, 1995; Tamis-LeMonda & Bornstein, 1994). In pretend play with substitute objects, the child has "double knowledge" (McCune-Nicolich, 1981b, p. 790)—an awareness of the object's real function as well as the role that it plays in the pretend scheme. Also, as Leslie (1987) points out, for adequate functioning, the pretending child must be able to separate behavior from knowledge of the world without losing track of reality and also must recognize the pretend behavior of others. Symbols therefore are abstractions shared by people and allow communication between them; in order to understand and use them, however, the child must be able to achieve some distance between the physical object and the word or substitute object that symbolizes it (Werner & Kaplan, 1963). DeLoache (1991) suggests that it is the child's awareness of an object as a symbol that allows the child to operate flexibly and to guide activity by means of symbols.

Representation is also manifest in children's memory for objects and events. As was noted in Chapter 2, infants' recognition memory for objects and pictures is robust, even over quite long delays. Daehler and Bukatko (1977) found that, at 19 months, children's recognition memory for pictures was good, even after 50 intervening pictures; it did not improve substantially at later ages. In contrast, recall or recollection shows marked changes. In Piaget's (1952) theory of the development of intelligence, recall of objects and events can occur only at the end of the sensorimotor period, or about 18 months, when the child is capable of internally representing the object or event in its absence. Although there is anecdotal evidence for recall as early as 9 months, there is far more evidence for it in the second year. Nelson and Ross (1980) studied children of 21, 24, and 27 months of age, using well-trained parents as observers. They found that 21% of the memories documented at 21 months involved verbal recall of an earlier event. The most common aspect (54%) of the recalled events was the spatial location of a valued object or person. These memories were likely to be recalled when the location was seen again (73%) or by seeing the person or object in some other context (27%). The longest lag between the original experience and the recall was 6 months. Children who were 2 years and older recalled more events and events from longer ago than did younger children, and were less likely to be dependent on location as a cue. Nelson and Ross (1980) suggest that children's experiences, especially those involving routine events in familiar settings, are likely to be incorporated into their general fund mass of knowledge. As a result, children may find it hard to remember specific instances of these events; that is, their experiences are represented in their minds as familiar event sequences or scripts rather than as memories of specific events. On the other hand, Bauer and Dow (1994) show that 16- to 20-month-olds sometimes acquire generalized representations of events without necessarily forgetting specific details of those events.

The Assessment of Development

The standardized tests of cognitive development (e.g., Bayley, 1969, 1993) for this second year include many perceptual-motor items, such as imitating strokes and scribbles with a crayon, putting shapes into form boards and pegs into a peg board, and simple means-ends problems. In contrast to the array of items for the first year, the items for second-year include a number of language items that require the child to name objects and pictures or to comprehend words and simple commands. Few items assess processes such as sustained attention, learning, or problem solving. Yet we know that there are individual differences along these lines and that these differences are likely to affect cognitive functioning.

In a study of children from 12 to 24 months, Power, Chapieski, and McGrath (1985) examined the short-term stability of three sets of measures covering developmental level, attention span, and diversity of exploratory play. The measures of developmental level—pegs placed in a peg board and highest level of pretend activity—were highly correlated with age, as they should have been, while measures of attention and exploration were not. Stability of behavior in individual children over a 2-week period appeared to be good for some measures in all categories; correlations for the measures of attention span were consistently high. The intercorrelations among the sets of measures show that measures of attention span and persistence are related much more highly with each other than with measures of developmental level or exploratory diversity. Such a pattern suggests that attention span and persistence are constructs independent of our standardized measures of children's mental development. This fact underscores the value of obtaining information about attention separately from the standardized evaluation.

Besides observing the child's attentiveness during free play, there are other alternatives or supplements to standardized developmental assessments. Nonverbal measures of recognition memory could be obtained easily, just as they can be during the first year of life (Daehler & Bukatko, 1977). In addition, a number symbolic or pretend play scales become useful in the second year (e.g., Lowe, 1975; Westby, 1991). These involve the presentation of a standard set of toys and observation of the level of pretend behavior. These levels include functionally appropriate use of an object directed to the self, the same activities directed to a doll, object substitution, and so on. One advantage of using such play measures is that toddlers may be shy about using their beginning language skills in an unfamiliar setting but are much freer about playing with toys. A child, for example, may not utter a word during the administration of the Bayley Mental Development scale; during play, however, the same child will pretend that one object is another and pretend to feed the doll and put it to bed. The child may even use some language in this less demanding situation. The overall evaluation of such a child would be quite different from another child who achieved the same Bayley Mental Development Index but provided no evidence of symbolic activity during free play.

In summary, all of these measures of attention, learning, and pretend involve the observation of spontaneous activity and thereby provide information quite different from the more structured tests. In addition, the emphasis is on the process by which the child deploys its attention or organizes play materials. Thus, these techniques provide a window on the processes important in cognition during this period of rapid development.

REFERENCES

Anisfeld, M. (1984). *Language development from birth to three.* Hillsdale, NJ: Erlbaum.

Bakeman, R., & Adamson, L. B. (1984). Coordinating attention to people and objects in mother-infant and peer-infant interaction. *Child Development, 55,* 1278–1289.

Baldwin, D. A. (1991). Infants' contribution to the achievement of joint reference. *Child Development, 62,* 875–890.

Baldwin, D. A., & Markman, E. M. (1989). Establishing word-object relations: A first step. *Child Development, 60,* 381–398.

Barton, M. E., & Tomasello, M. (1991). Joint attention and conversation in mother-infant-sibling triads. *Child Development, 62,* 517–529.

Bauer, P. J., & Dow, G. A. (1994). Episodic memory in 16- and 20-month-old children: Specifics are generalized but not forgotten. *Developmental Psychology, 30,* 403–417.

Bayley, N. (1993). *Bayley Scales of Infant Development* (2nd ed.). San Antonio, TX: Psychological Corporation.

Bayley, N. (Ed.). (1969). *Bayley Scales of Infant Development.* New York: The Psychological Corporation.

Belsky, J., & Most, R. K. (1981). From exploration to play: A cross-sectional study of infant free play behavior. *Developmental Psychology, 17,* 630–639.

Benedict, H. (1979). Early lexical development and production. *Journal of Child Language, 6,* 183–200.

Birch, H. G. (1945). The relation of previous experience to insightful problem solving. *Journal of Comparative Psychology, 38,* 267–283.

Butterworth, G. (1991, April). Evidence for the "geometric" comprehension of manual pointing. Paper presented at a meeting of the Society for Research in Child Development, Seattle, Washington.

Butterworth, G., & Jarrett, N. (1991). What minds have in common is space: Spatial mechanisms serving joint visual attention in infancy. *British Journal of Developmental Psychology, 9,* 55–72.

Case, R., & Khanna, F. (1981). The missing links: Stages in children's progression from sensorimotor to logical thought. *New Directions for Child Development, 12,* 21–32.

Corrigan, R. (1978). Language development related to stage six object permanence development. *Journal of Child Language, 5,* 173–189.

Daehler, M. W., & Bukatko, D. (1977). Recognition memory for pictures in very young children: Evidence from attentional preferences using a continuous presentation procedure. *Child Development, 48,* 693–696.

DeLoache, J. S. (1991). Symbolic functioning in very young children: Understanding of pictures and models. *Child Development, 62,* 736–752.

Diamond, A. (1991). Frontal lobe involvement in cognitive changes during the first year of life. In K. Gibson & A. Petersen (Eds.), *Brain and behavioral development* (pp. 127–180). New York: Aldine Press.

Dunham, P. J., Dunham, F., & Curwin, A. (1993). Joint-attentional states and lexical acquisition at 18 months. *Developmental Psychology, 29,* 827–831.

Dunn, J., Wooding, C., & Hermann, J. (1977). Mother's speech to young children: Variation context. *Developmental Medicine and Child Neurology, 19,* 629–638.

Fischer, K. W. (1980). The theory of cognitive development: The control and construction of hierarchies of skills. *Psychological Review, 87,* 477–531.

Fischer, K. W., & Bullock, D. (1981). Patterns of data: Sequence synchrony, and constraint in cognitive development. *New Directions for Child Development, 12,* 1–20.

Goldman-Rakic, P. S. (1987). Development of cortical circuitry and cognitive function. *Child Development, 58,* 601–622.

Harris, P. L. (1983). Infant cognition. In P. H. Mussen (Ed.), *Infancy and developmental psychobiology. Handbook of child psychology* (Vol. 2, pp. 689–782). New York: John Wiley & Sons.

Hoff-Ginsberg, E. (1991). Mother-child conversation in different social classes and communicative settings. *Child Development, 62,* 782–796.

Kaler, S. R., & Kopp, C. B. (1990). Compliance and

comprehension in very young toddlers. *Child Development, 61,* 1997–2003.

Keil, F. (1979). The development of the young child's ability to anticipate the outcomes of simple causal events. *Child Development, 50,* 455–462.

Koslowski, B., & Bruner, J. S. (1972). Learning to use a lever. *Child Development, 43,* 790–799.

LeCompte, G. K., & Gratch, G. (1972). Violation of a rule as a method of diagnosing infants' levels of object concept. *Child Development, 43,* 385–396.

Leslie, A. (1987). Pretense and representation: The origins of "Theory of Mind." *Psychological Review, 94,* 412–426.

Lewis, C., & Gregory, S. (1987). Parents' talk to their infants: the importance of context. *First Language, 7,* 201–216.

Lowe, M. (1975). Trends in the development of representational play in infants from one to three years—An observational study. *Journal of Child Psychology and Psychiatry, 16,* 33–47.

Mandler, J. M. (1983). Representation. In P. H. Mussen (Ed.), *Handbook of Child Psychology* (4th ed., Vol. 3, pp. 420–494). New York: John Wiley & Sons.

Mandler, J. M. (1993). On concepts. *Cognitive Development, 8,* 141–148.

Mandler, J. M., & Bauer, P. J. (1988). The cradle of categorization: Is the basic level basic? *Cognitive Development, 3,* 247–264.

McCune, L. (1995). A normative study of representational play at the transition to language. *Developmental Psychology, 31,* 198–206.

McCune-Nicolich, L. (1981a). The cognitive basis of relational words in the single word period. *Journal of Child Language, 8,* 15–34.

McCune-Nicolich, L. (1981b). Toward symbolic functioning: Structure of early pretend games and potential parallels with language. *Child Development, 52,* 785–797.

Meltzoff, A. N. (1988). Imitation, objects, tools, and the rudiments of language in human ontogeny. *Human Evolution, 3,* 45–64.

Murphy, C. M., & Messer, D. J. (1978). Mothers, infants and pointing: A study of a gesture. In H. R. Schaffer (Ed.), *Studies in mother-infant interaction* (pp. 325–354). London: Academic Press.

Nelson, K., & Gruendel, J. (1981). Generalized event representation: Basic building blocks of cognitive development. In A. Brown & M. Lamb (Eds.), *Advances in developmental psychology* (Vol. 1, pp. 131–158). Hillsdale, NJ: Lawrence Erlbaum.

Nelson, K., & Ross, G. (1980). The generalities and specifics of long-term memory in infants and young children. *New Directions for Child Development, 10,* 87–101.

O'Brien, M., & Nagle, K. J. (1987). Parents' speech to toddlers: The effect of play context. *Journal of Child Language, 14,* 269–279.

Piaget, J. (Ed.). (1952). *The origin of intelligence in children.* New York: International Universities Press.

Power, T. G., Chapieski, L., & McGrath, M. P. (1985). Assessment of individual differences in infant exploration and play. *Developmental Psychology, 21,* 974–981.

Rogoff, B., Mistry, J., Göncü, A., & Mosier, C. (1993). Guided participation in cultural activity by toddlers and caregivers. *Monographs of the Society for Research in Child Development, 58* (8, Serial No. 236).

Rubin, K. H., Fein, G. G., & Vandenberg, B. (1983). Play. In E. M. Hetherington (Ed.), *Handbook of Child Psychology* (Vol. 4, pp. 693–774). New York: John Wiley & Sons.

Ruff, H. A., & Lawson, K. R. (1990). Development of sustained, focused attention in young children during free play. *Developmental Psychology, 26,* 85–93.

Ruff, H. A., & Rothbart, M. K. (1996). *Attention in early development: Themes and variations.* New York: Oxford University Press.

Schmidt, C. L. (In press). Scrutinizing reference: How gesture and speech are coordinated in mother-child interaction. *Journal of Child Language.*

Sophian, C. (1984). Developing search skills in infancy and early childhood. In C. Sophian (Ed.), *Origins of cognitive skills* (pp. 27–56). Hillsdale, NJ: Lawrence Erlbaum.

Sugarman, S. (1981). Transitions in early representational intelligence: Changes overtime in children's production of simple block structures. In G. Forman (Ed.), *Action and thought: From sensorimotor schemes to symbolic operations* (pp. 65–93). New York: Academic Press.

Tamis-LeMonda, C. S., & Bornstein, M. H. (1994). Specificity in mother-toddler language-play relations across the second year. *Developmental Psychology, 30,* 283–292.

Tomasello, M., & Barton, M. (1994). Learning words in nonostensive contexts. *Developmental Psychology, 30,* 639–650.

Tomasello, M., & Farrar, M. J. (1986). Joint attention and early language. *Child Development, 57,* 1454–1463.

Tomasello, M., Savage-Rumbaugh, S. S., & Kruger, A. C. (1993). Imitative learning of actions on objects by children, chimpanzees, and enculturated chimpanzees. *Child Development, 64,* 1688–1705.

Welsh, M. C., & Pennington, B. F. (1988). Assessing frontal lobe functioning in children: Views from developmental psychology. *Developmental Neuropsychology, 4,* 199–230.

Werner, H., & Kaplan, B. (Eds.). (1963). *Symbol formation.* New York: John Wiley & Sons.

Westby, C. E. (1991). A scale for assessing children's play scales. In C. E. Schaefer, K. Gitlin, & A. Sandgrund (Eds.), *Play diagnosis & assessment* (pp. 131–161). New York: John Wiley & Sons.

Whitehurst, G. J., Arnold, D. S., Epstein, J. N., Angell, A. L., Smith, M., & Fischel, J. E. (1994). A picture book reading intervention in day care and home for children from low-income families. *Developmental Psychology, 30,* 679–689.

Willats, P., & Rosie, K. (1989, April.). Planning by 12-month-old infants. Paper presented at the biennial meeting of the Society for Research in Child Development, Kansas City, MO.

8 / Normal Language Development: The Second Year

Rhea Paul

During the second year of life, the child moves from being a communicator to being a talker. The pace of language growth during this time is enormous. At the beginning of this year, the average child will be saying 3 to 5 words and understanding 50. By the end, he or she will be producing over 300 words, many of which will be combined into 2- and 3-word sentences, while the size of the receptive vocabulary will be two to three times as large. Not only the sophistication but also the amount of speech increases dramatically, as does the range of ideas and the interactional functions expressed. This chapter outlines the patterns of this growth.

Words and Sounds

The average child says his or her first word around the time of the first birthday, close to the time he or she takes the first step. The normal age range for first words is 9 to 18 months. First words of children learning to speak any language share some properties in common. They tend to be words for objects and activities with which the child has direct contact. So, *shoe* which children can put on and take off by themselves is more likely to be one of the first words than *shirt*. First words also tend to be those used very frequently in social interactive routines, such as *hi* and *bye-bye*. Although most first words are nouns, or names of things, not all are. *More, up,* and *no* are frequent entries in lists of early words.

First words tend to have sounds and syllable shapes that correspond to the babbling patterns children are using at this time. Stark (1979) discusses "nonreduplicative babbling" or "expressive jargon" as being prevalent in the first half of the second year. This babbling is more varied than the earlier, reduplicated form. It involves new types of consonants, particularly those known as *fricatives,* that involve constriction rather than complete obstruction of the airway. The /s/ sound is one common early fricative. In addition, more than one consonant may appear within an utterance. So instead of /babababa/ a child may produce /pata/. Syllable structures that are produced also become more complex. Reduplicated babbling primarily contains consonant-vowel sequences, such as /ba/. But jargon babbling also may contain vowel-consonant-vowel sequences—/aba/—as well as consonant-vowel-consonant productions—/bap/. Still missing from this form of babbling are the liquid sounds, /l, such as r/, and any combination of consonants, such as the *pl* in *play.* Sounds made in the front of the mouth, such as /b/, /p/, and /m/, are more frequent than those made in the back, such as /k/ or /g/. Jargon babbling co-occurs with early speech, and the sound sequences present in both are similar. During the 12- to 18-month period, children use some words but continue to use jargon extensively, both to communicate and as a form of vocal play. Jargon babble begins to take on the intonation contours of the ambient language at this time, so that the child's vocalizations sound as if the child is speaking, but the listener is unable to understand the words.

Between 18 and 24 months of age, children's repertoire of sounds and syllable shapes expands with their expanding vocabulary. Stoel-Gammon (1987) found that by 24 months of age, normal children produce 9 to 10 different sounds in word-initial position, 5 to 6 different in word-final position, and at least a few words with consonant clusters, like the *pl* in *play.* Paul and Jennings (1992) report that by 24 months, normal children produce many syllables that contain two different consonants as well as some multisyllabic words. Stoel-Gammon (1987) also showed that 70% of the consonants produced by normal 24-month-olds were correct according to the adult target word.

Children, like adults, understand many more words than they say. What determines which of these comprehended words will be produced?

One characteristic that seems to be a factor is the sound structure of the word. Children are more likely to produce words that have at least a beginning sound that is already in their repertoire than they are to produce a word with sounds that are not under their control (Leonard, Schwartz, Folger, Newhoff, & Wilcox, 1979). This active process of selection and avoidance of words based on their sound structure is typical of children in this very early stage of language acquisition (Ferguson & Farwell, 1975).

Average expressive vocabulary size at 12 months is 3 words; at 15 months, it is 10 words (Templin, 1957). By 18 months, most children are producing more than 50 words (Nelson, 1973), and average number of different words produced is about 100 (Fensun, Dale, Reznick, Hartung, & Burges, 1990). By 20 months, average expressive vocabulary size is about 150 words (Dale, Bates, Reznick, & Morisset, 1989). The average 24-month-old says 300 different words (Dale, 1991). Still, there is a great deal of individual variation in expressive vocabulary size. Fensun et al. (1990) report a standard deviation of 111 at 18 months, larger than the mean of 100 words. Even at 24 months the standard deviation in vocabulary size is 176, a smaller proportion, but nonetheless more than half as large as the mean of 300 words (Dale, 1991). Despite this variation, recent studies suggest that children of 24 months of age who produce fewer than 50 words can be considered to be performing below the normal range of expressive language and are at risk for chronic linguistic handicap (Paul, 1991; Rescorla, 1989).

The rate of growth of vocabulary during the second year of life is not linear. Typically, there is slow acquisition of the first 50 words, with points at which new acquisition appears to halt for a time. Some words may drop out of the vocabulary temporarily. But about the time the child acquires the 50th word or so, around 18 months, a spurt in vocabulary acquisition is seen, and vocabulary size increases suddenly and sharply. The failure of a child to undergo this spurt in vocabulary growth during the second year of life may be another warning signal of risk for chronic delay.

The meanings that children attach to their first words are not identical to the meanings of those words in the adult lexicon. Studies of vocabulary acquisition suggest that children use a "fast-mapping" strategy (Carey & Bartlett, 1978) to acquire an incomplete notion of the meaning of a word. This allows them to use the word and refine its definition through subsequent feedback. This kind of strategy could help to explain the exponential rate at which words are acquired during this second year.

Children's use of words during this period also may not always conform to adult usage. One frequent type of error is *overextending* a word to exemplars the adult would not consider to be in its conceptual category. So, for example, the child may call a cow a *dog*. Overextension is common in children's early word use, but it may not be the only way in which children make naming errors. Some words may be *underextended,* that is, used for fewer referents than adults would use them. For example, a child may use *flower* only to refer to pictures of flowers in a picture book and not for flowers growing outside. It is important to note, too, that words are overextended in production much more often than in comprehension. Rescorla (1976) reports that children who label both a truck and a plane with the word *car* can very often point to pictures of the correct items when *truck* and *plane* are named for them.

The Development of Sentences

When children are using their first 50 words, their "sentences" consist of one word at a time. These early 1-word sentences are sometimes called "holophrases" because they seem to carry the force of a whole sentence within the compass of one word. So if a 15-month-old says "Open!" it may mean "Please open this for me because I can't do it myself."

But at about the time the child produces the 50th word, usually around 18 months of age, another important language milestone appears. The child begins to combine words into "telegraphic" sentences (Brown, 1973). These utterances resemble telegrams in that they include the most important words of the adult sentence, while leaving out the little function words and word endings. So instead of saying "I want two cookies," the 18-month-old may say, "Want cookie" or "Two cookie."

The ideas that children relate in their telegraphic sentences generally revolve around the concepts they are developing at the time (Bloom, 1970). They talk about ideas related to the permanence of objects (see Chapter 7), by commenting on the appearance, disappearance, and reappearance of things ("There cookie!" "Allgone cookie!" "More cookie!"). They also talk about people doing actions to other people or things, as they develop their notions of causality (see Chapter 7). They might say "Daddy throw," "Throw ball," or "Daddy ball" to express a wish that their father toss them a ball. Two-word utterances tend not to encode ideas for which the child has not yet developed the cognitive underpinnings. So, for example, children do not construct telegraphic sentences about concepts of time, even though they could do so with two words (Go soon).

Children at this age can produce some simple sentence variations. Negative sentences, for example, are produced by putting a *no* or *not* at the beginning or end of a two-word phrase (Klima & Bellugi, 1966). So the child may say "No daddy go," meaning "Don't leave, Daddy," or "Go bed no," meaning "I don't want to go to bed." Some questions are also produced, although these tend to be routines that are limited to a few memorized forms such as "Wazzat?" and "Where (X) going?" A rising intonation contour is used to express questions that require a yes/no answer (Have cookie?), as it sometimes is by adults, as well (Klima & Bellugi, 1966).

By the end of the second year of life, most children are beginning to produce some 3- and 4-word sentences. These early longer forms tend to include the most meaningful elements that were left out of the telegraphic sentences. So while the telegraphic child might say "Daddy ball," to indicate that the father should toss the ball, the slightly older child may say "Daddy throw ball." Many small function words and word endings are still omitted (Owens, 1992).

Understanding Language

When children produce sentences of only 1 or 2 words in length, are they able to understand much longer ones? Many parents believe so and will often claim that children as young as 12 months "understand everything" said to them. However, linguistic comprehension is still quite limited in this period (Chapman, 1978; Paul, 1991); unlike the large gap that is typically seen between receptive and expressive vocabulary size, the difference between the number of sentence elements that can be processed receptively and produced in speech may not be very great. Just as they did at the end of the first year, children manage to convince adults that they understand more than they do by employing a series of strategies, or shortcuts for responding to the language that they hear. In the second year, however, their strategies integrate emerging linguistic knowledge with the understanding of contexts and interactions.

Chapman (1978) characterizes the 12- to 18-month-old's comprehension as demonstrating the use of "lexical guides to context-determined responses." Here children pair their newly acquired knowledge of the meaning of single words with knowledge about what usually happens in interactive situations. This integration allows children to act on objects the parent mentions by name, even if the parent does not look at them. Knowledge of how objects are conventionally used (see Chapter 7) gives children access to a do-what-you-usually-do strategy. This results in children's using the mentioned object for its intended purpose, without having to understand the full linguistic force of an instruction. Thus, if told "Brush your hair," toddlers are able to comply without fully understanding the instruction, simply by recognizing the word *brush* and knowing for what brushes are used.

In the latter half of the second year, as noted, children begin to combine 2 words in their own speech. The ability to understand 2-word combinations also emerges, but comprehension probably is limited to not much more than 2 words per sentence. More than that, newly solidified object permanence skills (see Chapter 7) allow children to respond to directions involving objects not present in the immediate environment. Eighteen-month-olds can fetch objects named by the parent from the next room, for example, whereas 12-month-olds would need to have an object in view in order to comply with an instruction to retrieve it. Understanding 2 words in a sentence also allows children to respond to apparently complex instructions without having to process their full linguistic form. For example, children in this stage might comply successfully with the request "Why don't you go and close that door for me?" not because they understand the whole question, but because they were able to pick out the words *close* and *door* and know that adults usually ask children to do things (Shatz, 1978).

Parents' Speech to Toddlers

Parents continue to use a special speech style in talking to their 1-year-olds, as they did to their infants. Many properties of this "motherese" or "baby talk" style are similar to those used by parents during the first year. Speech to 1-year-olds continues to have exaggerated intonation contours and may even contain the speech sound changes discussed earlier. But in the second year, parents concentrate on mapping with simple, concrete words what children see in their immediate experience. Speech to toddlers is slower, more fluent, and contains fewer grammatical errors than does speech to adults or older children (Chapman, 1981). More emphatic stress is used, and vocabulary is restricted to concrete words that refer to ongoing events in the children's environment. Lengthwise, sentences are only about 2 words longer than the children's own sentences (Paul & Elwood, 1991). A large portion of adults' utterances are questions, designed to attempt to solicit a response from children, whereas speech to adults contains primarily declarative sentences (Newport, Gleitman, & Gleitmon, 1977). Few sentences directed to toddlers contain complex or embedded constructions (Chapman, 1981). Adults tend to focus the topic of their remarks to toddlers on what the children currently are doing, or to make a request of the children to do something to the objects to which they are already attending. Thus adults' speech to toddlers would seem to be ideally suited to the task of teaching them about language.

Several aspects of adults' speech to toddlers have been investigated to determine whether these changes, in fact, accomplish the teaching function they would seem to imply. Owens (1992) points out that the aspects of mothers' speech that seem to be most closely associated with acceleration of language acquisition are those that elicit some form of imitation from the children. Adults repetition of children's utterances frequently encourage children to repeat it yet again. Adults' expansion of children's telegraphic utterance to a more fully grammatical form—Child: Daddy ball. Mother: Yes, Daddy has the ball—also frequently results in children's attempt to imitate and add a new element to their own rendition. Adults' extensions of the child's remark with a semantically related comment—Child: Juice allgone. Mother: Yes, your juice is all gone and your cup is empty—give children the opportunity to imitate a remark that is contingent on their own. Certain types of questions on the adults' part also have been shown to increase language growth. Hoff-Ginsberg (1986) reports than mothers' use of questions to which they really do not know the answer and questions that repeat some part of children's previous utterance were predictive of accelerated language.

All these strategies on adults' part appear to facilitate children's linguistic growth by providing input that is related to the child's expression and serves as a stimulus for child imitation or response. This response can make use of the adult's prior utterance, using it as a syntactic framework or scaffold on which to build a meaningful sentence. While these parental strategies appear to be used quite commonly and have been shown to be effective in facilitating language (Owen, 1992), it might seem surprising to learn that parents rarely explicitly correct their children's grammar; moreover, explicit correction seems to play little role in grammatical acquisition (Brown & Hanlon, 1970). When parents do correct their toddlers, they are much more likely to correct them on the basis of the utterance's truth value than on syntactic accuracy.

Child Communication

By the end of their first year, children used gestures and vocalization to express proto-declarative and proto-imperative functions. These forerunners to language are transformed into true linguistic expression in the second year, with requests and comments now expressed with the child's newly developing words. At 12 to 18 months, just as words are coexisting with jargon babble, these intentions are expressed both with words and with nonconventional vocalizations. By 18 months, though, the use of words begins to predominate, and, by the end of the second year, most communication is taking place through the medium of language.

As the form of communication matures during the second year, the quantity of communication also increases. Wetherby, Cain, Yonclas, and Schaffer (1988) show that the average 12-month-old produces about one communicative act per minute, while the 24-month-old produces an average of five acts. The increase in the rate of communication probably is related to the child's developing knowledge of the conversational obligation to respond to speech. Although younger children can respond to adult speech with the communicative means they have available—gestures, vocalizations, or words—they are not very reliable about doing so and often need coaxing to speak when spoken to. The realization of this obligation, besides increasing the frequency of communicative acts, also leads to some new communicative functions that emerge after 18 months of age. Chapman (1981) reports that at this age children begin to answer questions more reliably, at first responding primarily to routine questions, such as "What does a doggy say?" and "Where is your nose?" In addition, toddlers show their compliance with the conversational obligation to speak when spoken to by acknowledging their partner's comments. They may do this at first by simply repeating 1 or 2 words from the interlocutor's utterance. Later they learn the more conventional devices for acknowledging, such as "um-hm."

Another new communicative function emerges in the second half of the second year. Halliday (1975) refers to this as the "mathetic" or heuristic function of language. Children at 12 to 18 months of age generally talk about the here and now, making comments on objects and events that are obvious in the immediate context and that add little new information to the listener's knowledge base. Older toddlers, however, begin to use language both to learn about the world and to provide the listener with new information. One of the first heuristic uses of language is asking questions. "Whazzat?" is a frequent early question, with which toddlers request the names of objects. The use of this function is a manifestation of children's developing understanding that language can be used to learn about the world.

The toddler's communication skill is also evident in word choice when the number of words that can be produced in one utterance is limited. In the holophrastic stage, children tend to produce the most informative word they have available in their vocabulary in order to encode a comment (Greenfield & Smith, 1976). For example, suppose a child has both the words *ball* and the *doggie* in vocabulary. If that child has been playing ball with the father, and the family dog suddenly appears in the room and takes the ball in its mouth, the child is more likely to express a comment by saying "Doggie!" since this is the new element in the situation than by saying "Ball!"

In the telegraphic stage, too, toddlers choose which 2 words to produce on the basis of sociocommunicative considerations. For example, children learn very quickly in this period that the 2-word utterance "Cookie please" is much more likely to achieve the desired result than is "Gimme cookie!"

One-year-olds have difficulty maintaining any topic of conversation for more than two or three conversational turns, particularly if they did not initiate the topic themselves (James, 1990). They may attempt to maintain a topic simply by imitating an adult remark or may fail to provide any contingent response. Children of this age still require extensive scaffolding and support from a more mature speaker in order to keep a conversation going.

Summary

By 24 months of age, normal children have an expressive vocabulary of several hundred words, can produce 2- to 3-word sentences, are correct in the great majority of the speech sounds they produce, and use language as their primary mode of communication to express not only wants and needs but to direct adults' attention and engage in social conversation. Although children's comprehension of sentences may not be far ahead of production, they continue to advance their use of comprehension strategies in order to participate in interactions. The normal 2-year-old is on the way to becoming a skilled and engaging conversationalist.

REFERENCES

Bloom, L. (1970). *Language development: Form and function of emerging grammars*. Cambridge, MA: MIT Press.

Brown, R. (1973). *A first language: The early stages*. Cambridge, MA: Harvard University Press.

Brown, R., & Hanlon, C. (1970). Derivational complexity and order of acquisition. In J. Hayes (Ed.), *Cognition and the development of language* (pp. 133–151). New York: John Wiley & Sons.

Carey, S., & Bartlett, E. (1978). Acquiring a single new word. *Papers and Reports on Child Language Development, 15*, 17–29.

Chapman, R. (1978). Comprehension strategies in children. In J. F. Kavanaugh & W. Strange (Eds.), *Speech and language in the laboratory, school and clinic* (pp. 308–327). Cambridge, MA: MIT Press.

Chapman, R. S. (1981). Exploring children's communicative intents. In J. F. Miller (Ed.), *Assessing language production in children* (pp. 111–138). Baltimore: University Park Press.

Dale, P. (1991). The validity of a parent report measure of vocabulary and syntax at 24 months. *Journal of Speech and Hearing Research, 34*, 565–571.

Dale, P., Bates, E., Reznick, S., & Morisset, C. (1989). The validity of a parent report instrument of child language at twenty months. *Journal of Child Language, 16*, 239–250.

Fensun, L., Dale, P., Reznick, S., Hartung, J., & Burges, S. (1990). *Norms for the McArthur Communicative Development Inventories*. Poster presented at the International Conference on Infant Studies, Montreal, Quebec.

Ferguson, C., & Farwell, C. (1975). Words and sounds in early language acquisition: English initial consonants in the first fifty words. *Language, 51*, 419–439.

Greenfield, P., & Smith, J. (1976). *The structure of communication in early language development*. New York: Academic Press.

Halliday, M. (1975). *Learning how to mean: Explorations in the development of language*. New York: Arnold.

Hoff-Ginsberg, E. (1986). Function and structure in maternal speech: Their relation to the child's development of syntax. *Developmental Psychology, 22*, 155–163.

James, S. L. (1990). *Normal language acquisition*. Boston: College-Hill Press.

Klima, E., & Bellugi, U. (1966). Syntactic regularities in the speech of children. In J. Lyons & R. Wales, *Psycholinguistic papers* (pp. 55–68) Edinburgh: Edinburgh University Press.

Leonard, L., Schwartz, R., Folger, M., Newhoff, M. &

Wilcox, M. (1979). Children's imitation of lexical items. *Child Development, 50*, 19–27.

Nelson, K. (1973). Structure and strategy in learning to talk. *Monographs of the Society for Research in Child Development, 38*.

Newport, E., Gleitman, A., & Gleitman, L. (1977). Mother I'd rather do it myself: Some effects and non-effects of maternal speech style. In C. Snow & C. Ferguson (Eds.), *Talking to children: Language input and acquisition*. New York: Cambridge University Press.

Owens, R. E., Jr. (1992). *Language development* (3rd ed.). Columbus, OH: Merrill.

Paul, R. (1991). Profiles of toddlers with slow expressive language development. *Topics in Language Disorders, 11*, 1–13.

Paul, R., & Elwood, T. J. (1991). Maternal linguistic input to toddlers with slow expressive language development. *Journal of Speech and Hearing Research, 34*, 982–988.

Paul, R., & Jennings, P. (1992). Phonological behavior in toddlers with slow expressive language development. *Journal of Speech and Hearing Research, 35*, 99–107.

Pease, D. B., Gleason, J. B., & Pan, B. A. (1989). Gaining meaning: Semantic development. In J. B. Gleason (Ed.), *The development of language*. New York: Merrill.

Rescorla, L. (1976). *Concept formation in word learning*. Unpublished doctoral dissertation, Yale University, New Haven, CT.

Rescorla, L. (1989). The language development survey: A screening tool for delayed language in toddlers. *Journal of Speech and Hearing Disorders, 54*, 587–599.

Shatz, M. (1978). Children's comprehension of their mothers' question-directives. *Journal of Child Language, 5*, 39–46.

Stark, R. (1979). Prespeech segmental feature development. In P. Fletcher & M. Garman (Eds.), *Language acquisition* (pp. 57–70). New York: Cambridge University Press.

Stoel-Gammon, C. (1987). Phonological skills of two-year olds. *Language, Speech, and Hearing Services in Schools, 18*, 323–329.

Templin, M. (1957). *Certain language skills in children*. Minneapolis: University of Minnesota Press.

Wetherby, A., Cain, D., Yonclas, D., & Walker, V. (1988). Analysis of intentional communication of normal children from the prelinguistic to the multiword stage. *Journal of Speech and Hearing Research, 31*, 240–252.

9 / Motor Development: The Second Year

Shelly J. Lane

With the achievement of mobility, the child's world opens up. Now that some control over body actions has been acquired, the child seeks in turn to control the environment. As environmental and behavioral variables assume increasing importance, the interaction among the various subsystems takes on new complexity. The child has more energy and a developing drive for independence; add mobility to these characteristics and now, more than ever, the child needs a safe environment for play and exploration.

The major tasks that emerge in the second year of life center around the refinement of previously attained skills (Gallahue, 1982; Hempel, 1993). Walking improves and gives way to running and jumping and to other challenges of the upright position. Hand skills refine and tool use becomes a fact of life. By the end of the second year, children have attained great freedom of movement and can select among many movement options for environmental exploration. Their bodies are relatively stable with respect to gravity, and they have developed manipulative skills capable of some precision (Gallahue, 1982). Specific skills associated with this developmental time span are listed in Tables 9.1, 9.2, and 9.3. The processes associated with development during the second year will be discussed.

Gross Motor Development

BALANCE

Attainment of balance or equilibrium reactions is a complex process requiring interaction of several sensory input and feedback systems, central nervous system mechanisms, muscle strength, environmental factors, and motivation. Further, the establishment of equilibrium is not fixed; the requirements for maintaining equilibrium change as the child grows, gains height and weight, develops new strength, challenges him-/or herself, and faces environmental changes (Barsch, 1967; Palisano, 1988). As the child progresses, he or she attains different positions relative to gravity; as a result, balance and movement are often precarious. Equilibrium reactions are not present at birth and lag behind the ability to maintain posture. Thus, as discussed in Chapter 4, a highly motivated 5-month-old infant may be able to sit independently for a brief period due to the development of strength in neck and trunk musculature. If, however, the infant should be displaced from this stable posture, equilibrium reactions are insufficient to regain the sitting posture, and he or she will fall out of this position. This makes sitting only marginally functional for the young infant (Palisano, 1988). The toddler between 1 and 2 years of age can both attain and maintain upright stance with some degree of independence. Nonetheless, equilibrium reactions during this year are at best tenuous. The toddler will stumble, move too quickly and trip over his or her own feet, turn too quickly in pursuit of a person or object, and fall as his or her equilibrium reactions are insufficient to maintain the upright posture.

Functionally, the toddler is better off than was the 5-month-old. The toddler has increased strength in the trunk and legs and a broader range of motor options from which to choose. When equilibrium fails, the toddler can regain the standing position. At first this is achieved by creeping to a stable object and pulling to stand; later it is accomplished by pushing to stand from the fallen position. Thus, although equilibrium development has not kept pace with the drive to explore the environment, changes in other subsystems continue to make it possible for the energetic toddler to engage in appropriate activities. Equilibrium reactions become essentially mature during late preschool age, and it is then that the components needed to maintain balance become available (Palisano, 1988; Williams, 1983). The application of equilibrium skills to everyday demands will continue to be met with successes and failures throughout life.

TABLE 9.1

Gross Motor Development, 1–2 Years

Skill	Average age of appearance (months)
Stands up from supine by rolling to prone	9–18
Stands up from supine by rotating to side	11–30
Goes from standing to sitting by falling	12–18
Throws ball in forward direction	13–18
Stoops to obtain toy, recovers	15–18
Stands on 1 foot with help	12–22
Stands briefly on 1 foot, no help	15–30
Walks sideways/backward	10–24
Creeps up stairs	15–18
Runs stiffly on flat feet	18–24
Walks up stairs, marking time with help	12–23
Squats in play	18–24
Kicks ball	21–27

TABLE 9.2

Fine Motor Development, 1–2 Years

Skill	Age of appearance (months)
Tools (spoon, cup, comb)	12
Controlled release	12–18
Turns book pages	8–18
Throws ball	13
Builds 2-cube tower	12–20
Scribbles spontaneously	18–22

WALKING, RUNNING, AND CLIMBING

If the child is not walking at the start of the second year, this skill will soon emerge. Most children develop this ability by 18 months of age (Keogh & Sugden, 1985). Shirley (1931) authored a comprehensive analysis of the development of walking skill in 25 infants. Her work has laid the foundation for other developmental analyses of locomotion. Walking progresses from cruising, to walking without support forward, sideways, and finally backward. By the end of the second year, the child is fairly adept at this task (Eckert, 1987; Keogh & Sugden, 1985; Williams, 1983). These changes in the walking pattern are due to a combination of developments in several subsystems: balance and equilibrium, as already discussed; lower extremity strength; the drive for independence; and a supportive environment. Sideways walking can be seen as the child edges around a piece of furniture to examine what is on it or be-

yond it. Backward walking may be more difficult to elicit in the course of an assessment, but can be evoked in play by providing a toy to pull. Initially, walking is penguinlike, and it is for that reason that the name *toddler* is applied to children at this stage. "Toddling" has a stiff quality with a wide base of support; the feet are flat, and there is lateral weight shift but minimal trunk rotation. Steps are short and unsteady. Arms are held in "high guard," and there is no coordinated interaction between legs and arms in stride (Keogh & Sugden, 1985; Williams, 1983).

Concurrent with the development of equilibrium reactions, the early toe-out position is replaced by a toe-straight position, and the wide base of support is decreased. At this point the child's arms are held at the sides in a more relaxed position (Williams, 1983). "High guard" posturing of the arms makes functional arm use difficult. As the arms lower, the child begins to carry objects around the environment. The skill of walking is thus significantly refined, at least on even and flat surfaces, and now provides a sophisticated gross motor base upon which the child can expand the development of visual-motor and spatial organization skills (Mullen, 1989).

Through the use of righting reactions and associated trunk rotation, the child transitions from sitting to weight-bearing on hands and feet. Upright stance can then be assumed from this bear-walking position. Initially this complicated and inefficient pattern is necessary, as balance and leg strength are not sufficiently developed at this stage to allow the child to move from sitting directly into the erect stance. As both improve, the transitional pattern of getting into an upright stance becomes more efficient. The child uses the

TABLE 9.3

Self-Help Skills, 1–2 Years

Skill	Age of appearance (months)
Finger feeds	10+
Helps to self-feed	16–20
Removes loose garments	18–24
Pulls on simple garments	24+
Good with cup	21+
Begins to use spoon	10–15

more mature pattern of rotating from sitting into side sitting and pushing up to upright stance from there. The child also develops a new play position: squat (Folio & Fewell, 1983). This new position allows the child to move about the environment, stoop to examine an interesting object, and play in the squatted position until diverted by or drawn to another object or person. The ability to walk, squat to play, and recover to walking entails complex interactions among muscle strength, motivation, and balance reactions.

Walking gives way to running almost immediately. Early running is not true running in that the feet are not both off the ground simultaneously. Instead, it is stiff and, like walking, does not incorporate trunk rotation and arm movements to any great extent. Even the child who is not using the arms in the "high guard" position for walking will resort to this position of the arms when running (Eckert, 1987; Palisano, 1988). This apparent regression may relate to the fact that the child is providing a greater challenge to the maturing balance and strength systems. Old patterns provide comfort in movement in that they represent earlier adaptations to environmental challenges that have proven to be successful. The reversion to this early pattern of movement when challenged is, in fact, a very adaptive response. As the child practices running, and as equilibrium and strength continue to develop, the "high guard" position is again abandoned, leaving the arms free for other activities.

As strength increases in the legs (evident in the squat-to-play position), the child will begin using this new strength to navigate stairs. Within the second year of life, strength and one-foot balance reactions are such that the child will need some assistance on stairs with a hand hold or railing and will "mark time" (put two feet on each step) in the course of his or her ascent (Folio & Fewell, 1983; Williams, 1983).

Thus, during the second year of life, the interacting subsystems work together to enable the child to develop independence and explore his or her environment. Central nervous system maturation, increasing muscle strength, the development of balance and equilibrium, and the child's internal drive or motivation integrate, and the child develops new gross motor skills and new motor options with which negotiate the environment. Behavioral state also must be factored into the expression of motor skill. A fatigued toddler may creep up the stairs rather than walk, or he or she may not squat in play and recover to erect stance. If gross motor skill is being clinically evaluated, all component subsystems must be considered.

Fine Motor Development

Eckert (1987) reports that "The manipulative activity of the young child is as constant and all encompassing as time and circumstances will permit. Children want to touch, feel, pick up, carry, and play with every object on which they can get their hands" (p. 185). This author maintains that while gross motor skills will continue to develop within the ordinary course of a child's life, the refinement of fine motor skills is dependent on opportunity and influenced by instruction and encouragement. Thus, for fine motor skill, subsystems beyond biomechanical, physical, and the central nervous system assume a major role in determining developmental progress.

Controlled and graded release develops between 12 and 18 months of age, permitting the child to use fine motor skills for more effective interaction with toys (Gallahue, 1982; Keogh & Sugden, 1985). Thus, the child can control release and coordinate it with visual guidance in a manner sufficient to allow put a raisin into a small bottle. In addition, arm movements and grasp/release are now such that the child can begin to develop stacking skills. Until this point the visual system was able to direct the arm and hand in stacking, but the upper extremity control was insufficient to allow for controlled release. Thus, any actual stacking that might have occurred was more by chance than volition. Children will practice these visually guided fine motor skills in play, adapting the skills to meet the demands of specific tasks and specific play situations. What 2-year-old can resist putting his or her Cheerios, one by one, through the small holes in a heater grate?

Tool use—that is, use of a spoon, crayon, or scissors—is a major accomplishment during the second year. This function, which is considered a sign of intellect (Connolly & Dalgleish, 1989), has been suggested as a criterion that separates humans from other animals. In humans, tool use evolves from rather gross total arm/hand movements at the outset of the second year, to the ability to use a spoon with some accuracy in feeding, and to hold a crayon in the fingers and direct movement of this tool using arm and shoulder movements. By 24 months of age, crayon use and visual motor control have developed to the point where the child enjoys scribbling, does so spontaneously, and can imitate a vertical stroke.

Initial tool use patterns are likely to be characterized by a variety of tool positions in the hand and a variety of motor patterns in using the tool. The 12-month-old may practice several grip patterns on a spoon and bang, mouth, dip, or drop the spoon. Even prior to 12 months the child will have shown an interest in the spoon, which often makes feeding difficult. Basic tool use is a highly motivating activity. Connolly and Dagleish (1989) indicate that spoon skill develops over the course of the second year in such a manner that there is increasing consistency in grip patterns, increasing preference for one hand, changes in patterns of action from less to more productive, smoother and more direct hand movement to bowl and mouth, and increased visual monitoring of the spoon as it moves from dish to mouth. In addition, as the second year progresses, there is an increased involvement of the contralateral hand to assist in the eating process. The nonpreferred hand is first used to put food on the spoon in order to assist an unskilled scooping pattern. Gradually, as scooping improves, the nonpreferred hand becomes a stabilizer for bowl or plate (Connolly & Dagleish, 1989). Similar skill progressions occur with other tools (e.g., crayons, scissors) and with

toy manipulation, as well. By the end of the second year, the child is sufficiently skilled with the spoon to be considered a self-feeder (albeit a somewhat messy one) and an accomplished designer of abstract art.

Thus, fine motor development is tied to physical and central nervous system maturation. According to Towen (1995), efficiency of fine motor skills such as prehension develops as the child coordinates postural skills and arm/hand motility. However, opportunity, in an environment that permits trial-and-error practice and encourages adaptation of skills, is equally critical. The *potential* for skill attainment is made possible by physical and neurologic development. The *expression and refinement* of skill depends on exposure and practice.

HAND PREFERENCE

The development of hand preference has been a topic of considerable investigation and discussion. Although some investigators have suggested that early hand preference can be determined by tonic neck reflex predominance or by head orientation during and shortly after birth, these concepts have not generally received much support (Eckert, 1987; Michel, 1985). Rather, a great deal of hand-preference switching occurs during infancy and childhood, along with shifts from unilateral to bilateral hand-use patterns. Thus, identification of a preference has been suggested to be task and culturally dependent (Eckert, 1987). Connolly and Dagleish (1989) note hand preference in tool use (defined as using one hand at least 80% of the time) as early as 12 months of age, prior to the actual development of skill with the tool. By 17 months of age, these authors note that for some activities, hand preference reaches nearly 100%. Other investigators report the development of preference between 12 and 18 months of age (Archer, Campbell, & Segalowitz, 1988; Bates, O'Connell, Vaid, Sledge, & Oakes, 1986). Such repeated use of one hand may serve the function of preparing the hand muscles for skilled action. Archer et al. suggested that instability in handedness in young children may be a sign of immature motor control and motor skill development. Is the child who does not show such early preference doomed to uncoordinated tool usage? This is unlikely. Although establishment of a preferred hand results in more practice time by that hand and thus perhaps quicker skill development, concern in regard to establishment of hand preference is not generally expressed until school age. However, this issue, as with the issue of the importance of creeping prior to walking, remains a focus of discussion and research.

The Development of Motor Planning

An important concept that underlies motor development in all areas throughout the second year is the development and refinement of motor planning abilities. Such abilities are apparent in the first year as well, but become much more obvious during year 2. Imagine being 2 years old, with a strong desire to "do it yourself." Tightly hugging a new "baby," along with this baby's bottle and blanket, you are faced with the need to descend the stairs. How is this task to be mastered? You can go down the steps, but you know that you need at least one free hand for holding on. You are holding baby, blanket, and bottle, and in the current arrangement this requires two hands. You could ask for help, but you would rather do it yourself. Can you find a way? Faced continually with new motor "problems," the child is forced to design strategies for accomplishment of the task. Initially strategy options are limited, but, with the continued development of strength, balance, central nervous system maturity, and cognitive functions, the child finds a widening array of options from which to choose. Thus, the 12-month-old, without sufficient leg strength and balance to permit the squat/recover pattern, sees an interesting object

on the floor. He or she toddles to it but is perplexed by the task of retrieval. The solution: fall to a sitting position and play with the object in its current location. During play the child faces another dilemma; he or she cannot activate the toy without adult assistance. The 12-month-old may thereupon resort to crying to bring adult attention to his or her plight. These solutions involve problem solving and draw on the child's current capabilities. Six months later, with increased strength and equilibrium, the child will walk to the object, squat, play for a short time, stand, and this time bring the object to an adult for to turn it on or make it go. This new strategy is much more complex. It relies on the advances in the various subsystems noted earlier, as well as the development of body scheme and the ability to access, combine, and adapt previous motor strategies (Lane, 1991). This process is motor planning. Early in development, this demonstration of problem solving may provide observers with a window into cognitive development.

Summary

Second-year gross motor skills reflect the integration of increasing strength, developing equilibrium, and a motivating yet safe environment. Fine motor skills reflect continued interest in exploration along with the development of motor patterns such as wrist rotation and radially oriented grasp. Such skills are perfected through practice. The toddler is undaunted by environmental challenges and equilibrium, strength, and/or coordination failures. In normally developing toddlers, the internal drive to "conquer" the environment and objects within it is immediately obvious.

REFERENCES

Archer, L. A., Campbell, D., & Segalowitz, S. J. (1988). A prospective study of hand preference and language development in 18 to 30 month olds. *Developmental Neuropsychology, 4* (2), 85–92.

Barsch, R. H. (1967). *Achieving perceptual-motor efficiency.* Seattle: Special Child Publications.

Bates, E., O'Connell, B., Vaid, J., Sledge, P., & Oakes, L. (1986). Language and hand preference in early development. *Developmental Neuropsychology, 2,* 1–15.

Connolly, K., & Dalgleish, M. (1989). The emergence of a tool-using skill in infancy. *Developmental Psychology, 25* (6), 894–912.

Eckert, H. M. (1987). *Motor development* (3rd ed.). Indianapolis: Benchmark Press.

Folio, M. R., & Fewell, R. R. (1983). *Peabody Developmental Motor Scales.* Dallas: DLM Teaching Resources.

Gallahue, D. L. (1982). *Understanding motor development in children.* New York: John Wiley & Sons.

Hempel, M. S. (1993). Neurologic development during toddling age in normal children and children at risk of developmental disorders. *Early Human Development, 34,* 47–57.

Keogh, J., & Sugden, D. (1985). *Movement skill development.* New York: Macmillan.

Lane, S. J. (1991). Motor planning. In C. B. Royeen (Ed.). *AOTA self study series: Neuroscience foundations of human performance* (pp. 1–35) Bethesda, MD: AOTA.

Michel, G. F. (1985). Self-generated experience and the development of lateralized neurobehavioral organization in infants. In J. S. Rosenblatt, C. Beer, M. C. Busnel, & F. J. B. Slater (Eds.), *Advances in the study of behavior* (pp. 61–83). New York: Academic Press.

Mullen, E. M. (1989). *Infant MSEL Manual.* Cranston, RI: T.O.T.A.L. Child.

Palisano, R. J. (1988). Motor development. In M. A. Short-Degraff (Ed.). *Human development for occupational and physical therapists* (pp. 445–480). Baltimore: Williams & Wilkins.

Shirley, M. M. (1931). *Postural and locomotor development. Vol. 1. The first two years; A study of twenty-five babies.* Minneapolis: University of Minnesota Press.

Towen, B. C. (1995). The neurologic development of prehension: A developmental neurologist's view. *International Journal of Psychophysiology, 19,* 115–127.

Williams, H. G. (1983). *Perceptual and motor development.* Englewood Cliffs, NJ: Prentice-Hall.

10 / Sensory Patterns in Infants and Young Children: The Toddler

Georgia A. DeGangi

Introduction

Sensory processing disorders often are related to problems with self-regulation, such as difficulties sleeping and self-calming. In the first year of life, difficulties tolerating everyday activities involving touch and movement, such as being diapered or bathed, are evident. Often children experiencing sensory processing problems also have low muscle tone, unsteady balance, and poor posture and coordination. Difficulties coordinating the two body sides in skills such as creeping, climbing, and bringing the hands to midline are observed. Organization of gestures for communication and the ability to explore a range of sensory experiences in play are delayed as well.

By the second year of life, sensory processing problems have a greater impact on adaptive functioning. Delays in motor and language performance not present before may become apparent.

The capacity to organize attention and play becomes affected. Whereas in the first year of life sensory processing problems can affect attachment and the ability to maintain eye contact and sustain reciprocal interactions, the link between sensory and social-emotional problems becomes compromised in a different way in the second year of life. The child's sensory processing problems may impact the ability to play with peers, tolerate separations from the caregiver, and negotiate issues around aggression and control.

This chapter describes the sensory integrative problems typically observed in toddlers. Chapter 5 provides specific details about the types of sensory integrative dysfunction. Since no formalized assessments are available for children between 18 months and 3 years, common symptoms are described in detail. These may be used as an observational guide in determining if a toddler might have sensory processing problems. Finally, a case example is presented to illustrate key points.

Toddlers with Sensory Integrative Dysfunction

The symptoms of toddlers with sensory integrative dysfunction occur in relation to how children are developing autonomy, independence, and mastery of language and motor skills. Toddlers with hypersensitivities usually display discomfort by actively fleeing from the sensory stimulus, retreating to a safe space, or lashing out at the person or object that imposed the perceived "adverse" stimulus. Hitting, biting, and throwing are behaviors that may be related to hypersensitivities. Many normal toddlers will hit, bite, and throw in an effort to assert a sense of control and independence, however, in children with hypersensitivities, these behaviors occur more frequently and as a result of being overstimulated by sensory input. Toddlers who display the range of sensory hyper- and hyposensitivities (i.e., sensory modulation problems) often show mood difficulties with regulation. These toddlers may quickly escalate from a contented, happy mood to a full-blown temper tantrum, sometimes without warning or an attributable stimulus or event. Frustration tolerance is low; thus, toddlers with sensory integrative problems often become extremely upset when they are unable to discern how to manipulate or handle a particular toy. Although all normal toddlers show frustration and temper tantrums for a while, the frequency, duration, and intensity with which they occur differs in the toddler with sensory processing problems. Unlike the normal toddler, incidents of frustration and tantrums usually occur several times per day with little response to calming or limit-setting techniques. In children with sensory processing problems, tantrums and low frustration tolerance often continue beyond the toddler years.

The ability to self-calm is often a problem. Parents of toddlers with sensory integrative problems find that they must constantly warn the child about changes in activity (e.g., going somewhere, changing clothes, changing task). Toddlers with these difficulties rely on the parents to help them find ways to self-calm (e.g., holding a special toy in situations where impulse control is needed; constant verbal monitoring from parents). At the crux of the problem are the toddlers' difficulties with problem solving and organizing a planned motor action in response to task or situational requirements.

Increasing difficulties with separation often become apparent, particularly when the parent is the only person who provides a predictable sensory world for the child. Often toddlers with sensory integrative problems find it hard to enter into play groups or to function in either a day-care situation or, indeed, in any other context where they are expected to play with peers and/or separate from a parent. Parents may find that they avoid busy environments such as supermarkets, play groups, or shopping malls because their child becomes overwhelmed by the stimulation. For toddlers with sensory integrative problems, the unpredictable touch and movement of other children can be very threatening; as a result, merely playing with peers is a significant challenge. Some children react by becoming aggressive, whereas others become avoidant and withdraw to some safe haven (e.g., under a table).

In the following sections, I describe some of the common tactile and vestibular processing problems and motor planning difficulties of such toddlers. Since there are no formal standardized tests for the 18-month to 3-year-old, assessment of toddlers with sensory integrative problems is strictly observational. For this reason, comprehensive tables of behaviors that commonly occur in toddlers with sensory integrative problems are provided in this chapter. Finally, a case example is presented.

TACTILE PROCESSING PROBLEMS

As children with sensory integrative problems grow older and encounter more challenging and varied tactile experiences, their discomfort with tactile experiences heightens. For example, the children must be able to go beyond the parents' familiar touch and accommodate to the touch of playmates and other adults. Although the parents of these children may have found ways to approach and make contact with them in a manner that feels acceptable to the children, other children and adults have not made this accommodation. As a result, the children's tactile problems may appear worse.

TABLE 10.1

Symptoms of Tactile Dysfunction in the Toddler

1. Dislikes being touched or cuddled by others: pulls away from being held, cries or whines when touched, or hits back.

2. Is distressed when people are near, even when they are not touching (i.e., standing nearby, sitting in a circle).

3. Avoids touching certain textures. Hates getting hands messy (i.e., fingerpaints, paste, sand).

4. Likes firm touch best and may enjoy games where there is very intense high contact (e.g., jumping into stack of pillows from a height).

5. Prefers touch from familiar people.

6. Dislikes having face or hair washed. Especially dislikes having a haircut.

7. Prefers long sleeves and pants even in warm weather or prefers as little clothing as possible, even when it's cool.

8. Touches everything in sight.

9. Bumps hard into other people or objects.

10. Withdraws from being near others, particularly groups.

11. May hit, kick, or bite others and is aggressive in play.

12. Has a strong preference for certain food textures (i.e., only firm and crunchy, or only soft).

13. Dislikes being dressed or undressed.

14. Bites or hits self.

15. Likes to hang by arms or feet off of furniture or people.

16. Uses mouth to explore objects.

As the youngsters enter the second year of life, independence and mobility allow them to flee from uncomfortable tactile experiences or to approach and touch those that are pleasureable. Some parents begin to notice that their child seems unusually active as he or she moves from one unpleasant tactile experience to another. Some children are observed to mouth or bite toys, seeking hard, deep pressure in an area of the body that can adapt to incoming tactile sensations more easily. The children often prefer intense, deep pressure activities such as roughhousing with parents. Table 10.1 presents some of the common symptoms of tactile dysfunction in toddlers.

VESTIBULAR PROCESSING PROBLEMS

Vestibular processing problems in toddlers may take the form of hyper- or hyposensitivities to movement. Those toddlers who are gravitationally insecure, that is, are fearful of movement experiences with a strong preference for movement activities near to the ground, often have an accompanying separation anxiety disorder. Children rely heavily on the parent to provide safety in new situations, such as helping them to find a place to play where other children will not bump into them and cause them to fall. Since toddlers with gravitational insecurity usually dislike playing on playground equipment, these children usually stay close by an adult when outside, or prefer to play with small manipulable toys. Within a large space, the children's play is constricted and confined to a small area, even when engaged in play with cars and trucks on the floor.

When toddlers are underreactive to movement stimulation, different issues emerge. Toddlers are notorious for their desire to test limits and attempt activities that allow them to master new motor skills. In particular, children who are underreactive to movement are fearless and constantly test limits. Such children often challenge

TABLE 10.2

Symptoms of Vestibular Hyper- or Hyposensitivities in the Toddler

Vestibular Hypersensitivities

1. Is easily overwhelmed by movement (i.e., car sick).

2. Has strong fear of falling and of heights.

3. Does not enjoy playground equipment and avoids roughhousing play.

4. Is anxious when feet leave ground.

5. Dislikes having head upside down.

6. Is slow in learning to walk up or down stairs and relies on railing longer than other same-age children.

7. Enjoys movement that he or she initiates but does not like to be moved by others, particularly if the movement is unexpected.

8. Dislikes trying new movement activities or has difficulty learning them.

Underresponsiveness to Movement

1. Craves movement and does not feel dizziness when other children do.

2. Likes to climb to high, precarious places. No sense of limits or controls.

3. Is in constant movement, rocking or running about.

4. Likes to swing very high and/or for long periods of time.

5. Frequently rides on the merry-go-round while others run around to keep the platform turning.

6. Enjoys getting into an upside-down position.

---

parents by climbing onto dangerous surfaces, jumping from unsafe heights, or trying a movement activity that exceeds their motor capacity, such as climbing too high on a jungle gym. The youngsters may crave movement activities and become very upset when restrained from continuing to swing, climb, or spin. Parents often report that on days where their child is unable to engage in such movement activities, he or she becomes irritable, has frequent temper tantrums, and has difficulty with sleep. Table 10.2 presents many of the traits of toddlers with vestibular problems.

MOTOR CONTROL AND MOTOR PLANNING PROBLEMS IN TODDLERS

By the second year of life, motor control and motor planning problems become more evident. The toddler has difficulty coordinating the two hands in simple bilateral tasks such as putting together pop beads. Muscle tone may be diminished; for example, the child may sit or stand in a slumped body posture. Balance may be poor with difficulties in skills such as climbing and walking downstairs without holding a railing.

Motor planning problems become evident as the toddler experiences extreme frustration over tasks that he or she cannot problem solve. Because of the motor planning disorder, children often break toys, then become upset when they cannot fix them. Often children rely on the parents to guide them whenever an activity changes. Some parents find that they need to prepare their child several days in advance about upcoming events to prevent major emotional upsets. The parents often explain in detail what will happen; then, when the activity occurs, they provide elaborate verbal feedback to help organize their child. The children seem to struggle with how to get started on an activity. They may not understand how to carry out the necessary steps to complete the task. Activities with sequences such as undressing and dressing are struggles for such children. Tables 10.3 and 10.4 list some of the common symptoms of motor control and motor planning problems observed in toddlers.

TABLE 10.3

Motor Control Problems in the Toddler

1. Frequently breaks toys—cannot seem to judge how hard or soft to press when handling toys.

2. Trips over obstacles or bumps into them.

3. Falls frequently (after 18 months).

4. Slumped body posture when sitting or standing.

5. Leans head on hand or arm.

6. Prefers to lie down than to sit, or to sit rather than to stand.

7. Has a loose grip on objects such as a pencil, scissors, or spoon, or grip is too tight on objects.

8. Tires easily during physical activities.

9. Is loose jointed and floppy; may sit with legs in a W.

10. Has difficulty manipulating small objects, particularly fasteners.

11. Eats in a sloppy manner.

12. Does not use two hands for tasks that require two hands, such as holding down the paper while drawing, holding the cup while pouring.

Sensory Integrative Problems in Toddlers

CASE EXAMPLE

Tactile defensiveness in a child with motor and language delays: Michael was a 2-year-old with a moderate expressive language disorder who was normal in all areas of development except motor coordination. His parents were concerned that he still had not regulated his sleep cycles. He had difficulty falling asleep and could nap only if driven around in the car. Bedtime was typically a major ordeal with many ritualized manipulative types of behavior. The use of time-outs and behavioral procedures had not worked, due to Michael's strong fear of separation, being left alone, and his adverse reaction to being held. Calming techniques such as swinging in a hammock had been unsuccessful.

Michael was evaluated by an occupational therapist to determine if there were any sensory integrative problems underlying his sleep difficulties and motor incoordination. Throughout the testing, Michael was very fearful of being physically moved and touched by the examiner and, consequently, refused to attempt many tasks. An interview with the mother confirmed Michael's hypersensitivities to touch and movement. He hated having his face washed and avoided messy activities such as fingerpaints. He was very picky about the textures of clothing. In group situations, he tended to withdraw into hiding places (i.e., under a table or inside a tent) and became very irritable when in close quarters. He resisted being hugged and held, but would tolerate cheek-to-cheek contact with his mother on occasion. In addition, Michael avoided movement experiences such as swings or slides and was very cautious about heights and climbing. He preferred to initiate movement activities rather than being moved by others. Sometimes he enjoyed making himself dizzy, but he became fearful if he moved too fast.

The treatment program was directed toward alleviating his tactile defensiveness and sensitivities to movement through activities that Michael could self-initiate. The tactile activities emphasized firm deep pressure. He particularly enjoyed wedging himself between heavy mats, covering himself with pillows, and jumping into bins of plastic balls. Some of these activities were modified for use before bedtime to help Michael develop better self-calming.

Over the course of several months, Michael learned to fall asleep on his own while holding a stuffed animal. Irritability was no longer an issue. Michael seemed very happy, thriving on his interactions with parents and other children. Learning how to gesture and use simple words to communicate helped to diminish his frustration. Hypersensitivities to touch had resolved. He could tolerate having his face washed and being held by his parents while reading a book. He also enjoyed exploring different textured toys and sought sensory play. Michael

TABLE 10.4

Motor Planning Problems in the Toddler

1. Is afraid to try new motor activities. Likes things to be the same and predictable (i.e., routines).

2. Has difficulty making transitions from one activity to next.

3. Must be prepared in advance several times before change is introduced.

4. Cannot plan sequences in activities, needing structure from an adult.

5. Is easily frustrated.

6. Is very controlling of activities.

7. Has difficulty playing with peers.

8. Is aggressive or destructive in play.

9. Has temper tantrums easily.

10. Did not crawl before starting to walk.

11. Has difficulty with dressing and sequenced motor actions.

was able to overcome his fear of movement and began to enjoy climbing on small jungle gyms and riding on swings and slides. However, he continued to demonstrate low muscle tone and poor coordination in skills such as running around obstacles and jumping on a trampoline. The intervention provided helped to prepare Michael for treatment by a speech and language therapist. Prior to this intervention, she had difficulty focusing Michael's attention and engaging him in activities to promote communication.

Summary

Sensory integrative disorders in the toddler may be manifested by tactile hyper- or hyposensitivities, gravitational insecurity, underresponsiveness to movement in space, and other vestibular-based problems as well as deficits in motor planning and control. Although there are no formalized tests of sensory integration for toddlers between the ages of 18 months and 3 years, systematic observations of their play during sensory experiences and everyday activities that they find challenging can be used to delineate potential problems. If left untreated, toddlers with sensory processing disorders usually do not resolve in their problems. By the preschool and school years, these children are apt to develop delays in perceptual, language, and emotional/behavioral development as well. Early screening and intervention of sensory integrative dysfunction in the toddler years may help to prevent such long-term problems.

11 / Affective Development During the Third Year of Life

Arietta Slade and Alicia F. Lieberman

Developmental Overview

The establishment of representational intelligence during the second year of life provides the groundwork for what will be the truly extraordinary changes of the preschool years. The third year of life marks the beginning of a child's life as a "representational" being (Greenspan, 1989; Piaget, 1963). This is the period when "thinking" as we know it really begins: Children can speak their mind, they can remember, they can respond to events and feel them in their own right, and they begin to play a more central and active role in relationships and family interactions. Two-year-olds are increasingly able to express themselves in words and play, to communicate a wide and powerful range of emotions, to make themselves felt and understood in relationships, and to create meaningful narrative descriptions of their experiences. Just as walking transforms the world of the 1-year-old (Mahler, Pine, & Bergman, 1975), so do thinking, remembering, and developing rich modes of communication transform the world of the 2-year-old.

These developments will have an enormous impact on children's functioning, upon their capacity to understand and regulate their impulses and feelings, upon their relationships with family and peers and upon their ability to function competently and autonomously away from primary caregivers. As representation develops, so do children's abilities to modulate and monitor behavior and to test and comprehend reality (Greenspan, 1989). This is the period Freud (1905) designated as the anal phase, that Erikson (1950) termed the crisis of autonomy versus shame and doubt, and that Mahler (Mahler et al., 1975) believed was the crucial and final stage of the separation-individuation process, "on the way to object constancy." From the standpoint of attachment theorists, the autonomy of the late toddler period provides a crucial test of the stability and quality of a child's attachment to primary caregivers (Matas,

Arend, & Sroufe, 1978; Sroufe, 1983). Many psychoanalysts and researchers believe that one can meaningfully begin to speak of the emergence of a consolidated "self" during this period (Pine, 1985; Stern, 1985; Wolf, 1990). While these perspectives address different aspects of the young child's ego and object relations development (Pine, 1985), they are all linked to the development of representation, as it is manifested in children's increasing ability to put things into words, to think about and remember what they have experienced, and to use their imagination to transform the events of their life.

Affective Development—Phases and Themes

Anna Freud (1965) introduced the concept of developmental lines three decades ago. She described the child as maturing along a number of dimensions: from dependence to emotional self-reliance, from suckling to rational eating, from wetting and soiling to bladder and bowel control, from irresponsibility to responsibility in body management, from egocentricity to companionship, from the body to the toy, and from play to work. If we were to observe 2- to 3-year-old children along any of these lines, we would see children who have begun to be master of their own body, of their desires, their impulses, and their relationships. Two-year-olds have begun to function autonomously and have a rudimentary knowledge of human relationships and feelings; these will develop over the course of the third year, to the point that they will separate easily and tolerate longer separations with equanimity. They will be ready to enter nursery school. By the age of 2, children manifest their emerging sense of self in willfulness, possessiveness, and actively use the pronoun "I" to describe self and articulate desires. By 3, the verbal or narrative self is well developed and elaborate. Two-year-olds are feeding themselves and actively assert their will in relation to what goes into their body. Children of this age often become quite ritualistic and opinionated about food likes and dislikes. Children of 2 can control fine and large motor movements with increasing competence; wish to do much more for themselves and are able to do so. As a consequence, they are less at the mercy of their impulses and can control their actions and behavior more and more effectively. Whereas toddlers may kick and hit at the slightest provocation, 2-and-a-half-year-olds will not. Words and thought become substitutes for action. It is also at this age that bowel and bladder control become possible. Across a range of domains, the children of this age are assuming increasing control over their body.

Children of 2 also have begun to turn to others as collaborators and partners in their efforts. They can begin engage in dialogue in a way that invites input and exchange from the other; by the time they are 3, they will be truly social partners. Play begins to be more genuinely collaborative, and efforts can be shared and mutually understood. Three-year-olds can create worlds together with make-believe. Finally, while infants are concerned primarily with the sensations afforded them by the body and its exploration, 2-year-olds are genuinely interested in and curious about the world and the objects in it. Toys become a means of self-expression and a source of intense pleasure in mastery. They are people with a relationship to and interest in their environment. Issues of autonomy, separateness, control, and mastery comprise the emotional dilemmas and struggles of this period.

From the perspective of classical psychoanalysis, these issues become salient as a consequence of changes in bodily experience; concern about autonomy and control are viewed as the natural outgrowth of psychosexual development and shifting libidinal cathexes. Freud (1908/1959) designated the period between 2 and 3 as the anal phase, following his belief that the anal region as well as children's bodily products (feces and urine) become especially important to them at this time. Thus, a new and profound libidinal investment in their bodies' functionings leads to struggles for control. Although there continues to

be debate about the correctness of Freud's notions of the drives and of psychosexual development, there can be little question that the period between 2 and 3 is characterized by children's struggling for control in a range of domains: they want to control what they wear, when they leave and when they are left, who does what to whom, and what goes into and out of their bodies. They chafe at external control and struggle to establish their autonomy in numerous ways.

Freud characterized children of this age as "preoedipal." What this means, among other things, is that children define their primary relationships in dyadic, rather than triadic, terms. Children have a relationship with both parents, but they have not yet integrated or understood the complexities of their interrelationships as a triangle. It is the attainment of this level of awareness that will catapult a child into the oedipal stage, and that will unleash the feelings of rivalry, competition, anger, longing, and guilt that characterize this phase of development. Preoedipal children, by contrast, are still concerned with establishing themselves as separate, autonomous beings, free from the control of any and all of their primary caregivers. They are engaged in a series of dyadic struggles; in classical terms, the struggle is for bodily control and mastery. While there can certainly be seductive and eroticized elements to 2-year-olds' relationships with their parents, they have not yet been confronted cognitively with the profound reality of family triangles and necessarily divided loyalties.

Nevertheless, children of this age can be very "phallic" in the sense that they are tremendously interested in showing off their bodies, demonstrating their physical prowess, and pretending to be endowed with superhuman abilities. Greenspan (1989) suggests that phallic concerns may be even more apparent than anal ones at this stage. Two- to 3-year-olds are certainly very aware of anatomical differences between boys and girls, and of their own genitals. It is at this age that they learn the labels for their genitals, and speak openly (sometimes *too* openly for their parents!) about their functioning. Girls of this age often have a reaction to the discovery that they do not have a penis, although most latter-day analysts disagree with Freud's assumption that this reaction is necessarily distress or envy. Girls often ask their mothers to obtain a penis for them ("Mommy, I want you to go to the store and buy me a penis, NOW!"). However, as Bergman (1987) has beautifully described, the mother's response to the female child's sexuality will have far more to do with the child's developing feelings of femininity than will her discovery of anatomical differences per se.

Psychoanalytic theory has suggested that "conflict" is an oedipal development that follows from the emergence of the superego. However, as Greenspan (1989) has observed, "clinical observations of young children suggest that representational differentiation alone may be a sufficient condition" for the emergence of anxiety and internal conflict (p. 61). "Conflicts between self-object representations can occur in terms an 'internal debate' at the level of ideas (e.g., the good me and you versus the angry evil me and you). Conflicts between self-object representations and external expectations can also occur (the 'greedy' me and the 'strict' limiting other)" (p. 61). In his work on the second year of life, Kagan (1984) has suggested that even 2-year-olds compare themselves to internalized standards and are distressed when they fall short of these standards. Thus, internal divisions do lead to anxiety and bring about early forms of conflict and internalized struggle. While they lack the richness of later, oedipal conflicts, they are rightly thought of as preludes to these later manifestations.

Mahler and her colleagues (Mahler et al, 1975) offer a different explanation for the prevalence of concerns about autonomy and control during the third year of life, and describe the period between the second and third birthday as comprising the latter stages in the "separation-individuation" process. The separation-individuation process refers to children's gradually developing sense of themselves as separate from the mother (and her caregivers); this development hinges on their gradually differentiating themselves from their mother. Prior to the establishment of representational intelligence, children cannot truly recognize their and their mother's separateness. Thus, the achievement of object permanence provokes the rapprochement crisis. It is a crisis of representation and symbolization: Children are for the first time cognitively *aware* of their separateness, and the moods, storms, and separation anxiety of the terrible twos represent their efforts to come to terms with that awareness. As Mahler so bril-

liantly describes, children want to undo their separateness and maintain their intimacy with their mothers, while at the same time they bridle at her restraints and long to exercise their newfound autonomy. Children feel rage at the mother for her separateness, and long to return to their earlier closeness. They cling to her, struggle to keep her in their control, and shadow her movements. At the same time, they are enthralled by separateness, with its rewards and possibilities. They are full of themselves and their abilities, and vehemently make their needs and wishes known. They are quite aware of what is theirs, and vociferously defend it as "mine." These are the first signs of the emerging sense of a separate self.

The "ambitendency" of the rapprochement period gives way to more ideational conflicts as representation develops. The development of object and self constancy over the course of the third year allows children to carry mother with them as they move away and to heal the splits between feelings of rage and of love. Children bring together their loving and angry feelings toward mother and slowly come to understand that both the good and the bad mother are one. The consolidated, constant object represents such a fusion: Children must temper their anger with love and their longing with self-confidence. As these internalized representations develop and become more stable and more sustaining, 2-year-olds can tolerate separation more easily, can accept substitute caregivers once again, and begin to move more comfortably outside the "mother-child orbit." The libidinal object becomes a powerful and important modulator of affective and of self-experience. Children now carry the reality of their primary relationships internally, in a representation that is modulated and transformed by their own internal states (Slade & Aber, 1992).

By age 2, the storms and tantrums of the rapprochement crisis should be waning, as children become increasingly capable of representation and gradually establish the fundamentals of libidinal object constancy. It is significant that Mahler refers to the last stage as "on the way to object constancy," thus emphasizing the ongoing nature of this developmental task. For Mahler, the success of the resolution of both the rapprochement crisis and the beginning establishment of libidinal object constancy will determine the nature and quality of all later intimate relationships. The development of consolidated maternal and paternal representations will form the basis for more oedipally based conflicts. Whereas preoedipal conflicts are rooted in struggles between different parts of the self, oedipal conflicts will revolve around the struggle between different sets of feelings *in relation to* libidinal objects.

Attachment researchers view autonomy and mastery as issues intrinsically related to the quality of the early parent-child relationship. One of the concepts central to attachment theory is the "attachment/exploration balance." Bowlby (1969) and later Ainsworth (Ainsworth et al., 1978) believed that maternal emotional availability in infancy leads to the development of internal representations that sustain children in their move into autonomy. Thus, the quality of children's primary relationships will have a direct and distinct impact on the quality of their move into the world of play, of language, and of new relationships. The quality of attachment in infancy (see Chapter 1) has been found to predict numerous social competencies during the toddler period: positive affect, curiosity, sociability, symbolic play, problem-solving ability, perserverance, and mastery motivation (Belsky, Garduque, & Hrncir, 1984; Goldberg & Easterbrooks, 1984; Matas, Arend, & Sroufe, 1978; Pastor, 1981; Slade, 1987; Sroufe, 1983). Interestingly, attachment researchers have also found that children who are secure in their parents' availability are also more likely to ask for help when they need it. Thus, their forays into independence are modulated by returns to their parents for assistance and guidance. They are healthily self-reliant, but able to turn to nurturing figures when they are needed (Matas, Arend, & Sroufe, 1978). Only when parents become emotionally unavailable to their children as a consequence of significant stressors in their own lives (financial hardship, loss of a partner, etc.) do children who were secure as infants fare poorly as toddlers (Easterbrooks & Goldberg, 1990; Egeland & Farber, 1984). The converse also may be true. Thus, ongoing parenting along with historical factors influence toddlers' socioemotional adaptation (Sroufe, 1983). Researchers have recently begun using more "representational" approaches (Main, Kaplan, & Cassidy, 1985) to modify the infant Strange Situation procedure, so that it can be meaningfully administered to toddlers (Aber & Baker, 1990; Cassidy & Marvin, 1988).

The Emergence of Representation

It is impossible to understand the struggles for control and autonomy that characterize the third year of life without considering the dramatic role played by the development of representation. The period from 2 to 3 years of age is one in which distinctions between self and other; fact and fiction; past, present, and future are gradually solidified and organized as the narrative, representational "self" emerges. These changes in children's perception of themselves, their world, and their relationships will have far-reaching effects on both the ways they function in their relationships with others, and the ways they see themselves. They most certainly influence and shape the struggles for selfhood, individuality, and autonomy that characterize the "terrible twos."

Freud once noted that "where id is, ego shall be." The dawning of representational intelligence and its gradual unfolding over the course of the third year of life brings with it dramatic changes in ego functioning. For the first time, 2-year-olds have the capacity to mentally manipulate and thus "think" about what they have experienced. As a consequence, ego functions such as reality testing, impulse control, the capacity to plan and anticipate, as well as mood stabilization can be observed for the first time. Although differentiation and integration of these functions will continue throughout the preschool period (Greenspan, 1989), it is during the third year that we see children beginning to distinguish fantasy from reality, containing impulses, and tolerating frustration and delay. By the same token, 2-year-olds can plan actions and imagine their effects upon others. They are no longer prey to the affect storms of toddlerhood and can manage transitions and changes with more emotional equanimity and resilience. Representations provide the elements of rudimentary psychic structure and defense, and comprise the basic aspects of ego organization. We can begin to speak of the 2-year-old child as a person and a personality. And, with the advent of abstract representation, autonomy becomes a real possibility.

In her extraordinary memoir, *The Story of My Life*, Helen Keller (1902) describes—albeit from the vantage point of an adult—the moment she discovered the rich possibilities of representation. Rendered blind and deaf by illness at 18 months, she had lost what little language she had. Her teacher, Annie Sullivan, was trying to teach her to use sign language, but she first had to engage Helen in the process of using symbols.

One day, while I was playing with my new doll, Miss Sullivan put my big rag doll into my lap also, spelled "d-o-l-l" and tried to make me understand that "d-o-l-l" applied to both. Earlier in the day we had a tussle over the words "m-u-g" and "w-a-t-e-r". Miss Sullivan had tried to impress it upon me that "m-u-g" is mug and that "w-a-t-e-r" is water, but I persisted in confounding the two. In despair she had dropped the subject for the time, only it to renew it at the first opportunity. I became impatient of her repeated attempts, and seizing the new doll, I dashed it upon the floor. I was keenly delighted when I felt the fragments of the broken doll at my feet. Neither sorrow nor regret followed my passionate outburst. I had not loved the doll. In the still, dark world in which I lived there was no strong sentiment or tenderness . . . We walked down the path to the well-house, attracted by the fragrance of the honeysuckle with which it was covered. Someone was drawing water and my teacher placed my hand under the spout. As the cool stream gushed over one hand she spelled into the other "w-a-t-e-r", first slowly, then rapidly. I stood still, my whole attention fixed upon the motions of her fingers. Suddenly I felt a misty consciousness as of something forgotten—a thrill of returning thought; and somehow the mystery of language was revealed to me. I knew then that "w-a-t-e-r" meant the wonderful cool something that was flowing over my hand. That living word awakened my soul, gave it light, hope, joy, set it free! There were barriers still, it is true, but barriers that could in time be swept away. . .I left the well-house eager to learn. Everything had a name, and each name gave birth to a new thought. As we returned to the house every object which I touched seemed to quiver with life. That was because I saw everything with the strange, new sight that had come to me. On entering the door I remembered the doll I had broken. I felt my way to the hearth and picked up the pieces. I tried vainly to put them together. Then my eyes filled with tears; for I realized what I had done, and for the first time I felt repentance and sorrow. (pp. 23–24)

Her description of what it meant to be able to name and to express what she knew and felt is extraordinarily poignant. Her linking emotion with knowledge is especially germane to how dramatically life changes once representation replaces action as a means of discovery.

For most children, the third year of life brings discoveries that are no less momentous than those described by Helen Keller. Nevertheless, it will be a long time before representations are stable and coherent; the third year, in particular, is a year devoted to gradually making sense of this new view of the world. As will be described, children of 2 are in some respects quite competent; at the same time, there is much instability and uncertainty as their skills slowly take hold. Stability is much more in evidence by age 3; knowledge is less tenuous and concrete, memories and representations are more organized. Many of the struggles for control seen in children of this age undoubtedly have to do with instability, and children's efforts to diminish it in any way they can. The tenuous nature of early cognitive structures underlie developmental regressions as well, as such structures are particularly vulnerable to intense feelings and longings (Pine, 1985).

Language and play both develop dramatically during this period. In language, children move from simple labels and single words late in the second year to sentences that are syntactically meaningful and convey a range of meanings and relationships. Language develops more between the ages of 2 and 3 than in any other period in development. Children truly become communicators. They will begin to refer specifically to themselves, to their inner experiences and to their possessions. By the time they are 2 and a half, they will ascribe agency to play characters and place themselves and their wishes centrally in narrative formulations. Their emerging sense of self will be dramatically captured in their language. The emergence of syntactic forms such as subject, object, verb, and predicate are particularly significant, because they so clearly convey the children's efforts to struggle with the representation of relationships (between people and between objects).

The development of symbolic, representational language is accompanied by the emergence of symbolic or make-believe play. Two-year-olds can now begin to create a world of their own, one based on their own unique commingling of reality and wish. By their second birthday, they begin to use toys and objects in a way that is genuinely symbolic (Nicolich, 1977). They will pretend to feed themselves with a toy spoon, they will pretend to sweep the room with a toy broom, and they will converse happily on a toy telephone. They will soon make dolls and animals the recipients of such ministrations, and finally use them as active agents in imaginary play (Watson & Fischer, 1977; Wolf, 1982). The mother doll will feed the baby doll, the toy tiger will "fix" the broken car, and so on. Themes will gradually emerge in the middle of the third year, and play characters are endowed with increasing agency and individuality. Children begin to tell stories that link events together in meaningful ways and to create characters that have feelings and motivations. It is also a time of creative transformation, as children begin to play with reality in a new way, using whatever they can find to create their pretend worlds. A shell can be used as a cat, a cup as a hat, and a lump of clay can serve as chocolate chip cookies for a hungry crew of firemen. While 2-year-olds certainly can become confused by the distinction between fact and fiction, these boundaries are well established by the time children are 3. By this time, their appreciation of pretense is far more developed: They know that dolls cannot actually be thirsty, they know that an imagined monster cannot be seen publicly, and they know that giving a toy animal a pretend bath will not actually result in its getting wet (Harris, 1989).

Piaget thought that the process of constructing a representational world was just as complex and painstaking as was the process of constructing a world of known, acted upon objects. He viewed the "preoperational" or "preconceptual" period as dominated by children egocentrism; he was referring not to selfishness, but to children's inability to take another person's view into account. Piaget believed that only after several years of gradual "decentering" are children are capable of "operational" logic, where objects and ideas retain their identity despite changing contexts and circumstances. Although 2-year-olds are certainly susceptible to faulty logic, Piaget's pioneering studies of early play and language emphasize children's egocentrism to such an extent that their function as a means of *understanding* the world is obscured. He only partially recognized that children's make-believe play, along with their efforts at narrating and documenting experience, are aimed at figuring out how the world works and how people work. However, recent advances in the study of early play and language have demonstrated that children perceive relationships between objects from early infancy and that early internalized images include these relationships as part of the representation.

Children as young as 2 years of age have generalized event representations (GERs) of familiar, known events (Nelson & Gruendel, 1981; Schank & Abelson, 1977). Thus, a child asked

what happens at a birthday party or at McDonald's can provide a remarkably coherent and organized "script" of such events that contains all of the vital components of the event in proper order ("You sing 'Happy Birthday,' blow out candles, eat cake, open presents"). The advent of "script theory" and the discovery that children indeed have generalized representations of events in their lives led to a reexamination of what toddlers' language and play reveal about what they think about and understand. From this research effort emerged the view of the 2-year-old as someone trying to sort out and order numerous narrative and thematic possibilities rather than as someone trying to piece together diverse and discrete pieces of symbolic knowledge. This was particularly well demonstrated by Nelson and her colleagues' recent study of the nighttime monologues of 2-year-old Emily (Nelson, 1989). These monologues reveal an enormously sophisticated mind at work, recalling and reworking the scenarios in her life in order to make sense of them. Her narratives recall the past, anticipate the future, and—in some cases—belie her wish to try to change the present. They are derived and distinctly shaped from dialogues with significant others in Emily's world, with caregivers being re-envoiced (Dore, 1989) by Emily in her narratives. She takes in many relationships in the world—among people, among objects, within herself—and her play and language during this period reveal her effort to make sense of these many relationships. In this newer conceptualization, 2-year-olds are seen as vastly more competent in their basic understanding than in the decades following Piaget's discoveries. By the end of the third year, they have developed a voice that is uniquely theirs.

The understanding that is made possible by symbolic intelligence shapes the way children think about and understand their emotional lives. It also changes the way they experience their primary relationships. Emotions shape and inform representations of the self and others in critical ways. Bretherton and her colleagues (Bretherton & Beeghly, 1982; Dunn, Bretherton, & Munn, 1987) have found that by 2 years of age, children use words that indicate that they see themselves and others as able to perceive, to feel pleasure, pain, and a range of other emotions; to wish, to think, and remember. Whereas emotions and impulses had been internal, surging, cresting experi-

94

ences that happened within the course of events and interactions, during the third year of life they can be named, described, played with, and ultimately, anticipated. Just as children begin to explain and represent the external world, the inner life becomes a terrain to be known as well; here, too, there are dramatic changes between the second and third birthday. There are few words for internal experience in the vocabulary of a 2-year-old; there are many in the vocabulary of a 3-year-old.

The development of the ability to refer to emotion reflects children's increasingly dimensional and complex understanding of the way emotion "works" between people. Observing toddlers in normal interaction with younger siblings, Dunn and her colleagues (Dunn, 1988) found that "children from 18 months on understand how to hurt, comfort, or exacerbate another's pain; they understand the consequences of their hurtful actions for others and something of what is allowed or disapproved behavior in their family world; they anticipate the response of adults to their own and to others' misdeeds; they differentiate between transgressions of various kinds. They comment and ask about the causes of others' actions and feelings" (p. 169). In short, children are remarkably knowledgeable about how emotions function interpersonally. Although such knowledge is admittedly piecemeal and confined to the circumstances in which they are experienced, this knowledge of the social and emotional world becomes ever more explicit and detailed over the course of the third year, as children become able to make use of these abilities in increasingly diverse situations.

Harris (1989) proposes that the development of symbolic abilities, particularly the capacity to imagine, coupled with the emerging capacity to understand emotions, allows children to imagine themselves in another's experience, to enter the emotional reality of others. The intersubjectivity of infancy is now greatly enhanced and evolved. Imagination "allows the child to entertain possible realities, and, what is especially important, to entertain the possible realities that other people entertain. It is a key that unlocks the minds of other people and allows the child temporarily to enter into their plans, hopes and fears" (p. 71). The child of 2 can imagine what will make others happy, what will make them sad, and what will

make them angry. Nevertheless, as impressive as these rudimentary emotional understandings are, it will be another 2 years before children really can understand and articulate the complex processes underlying guilt, shame, and pride. It also will be some time before children can accept and integrate mixed emotions, or recognize and act upon the premise that emotions can be felt but hidden from others.

By the time children are 3, they can create a world of their own that incorporates an increasingly complex understanding of emotion and of relationships. Stern (1985) argues that the development of the "verbal self" allows children to establish new levels and types of intimacy with others, as the capacity to describe what they have seen and what they have known is vastly enriched by words and emerging syntax. On the other hand, language and play also allow children to distort experience and keep feelings secret in a way that inevitably creates a new kind of distance and separateness. In a related vein, Wolf (1990) has described the emergence at this age of what she terms the "authorial self: a self independent enough of any given situation to select which voices and what versions of experience to acknowledge. It is a new kind of self, one who can speak as object or subject, as observer or participant" (p. 185). Children take on different voices, genres, and stances in their play, and implicitly recognize that they can be the author of many realities. It is this heterogeneity, Wolf believes, that comes to constitute selfhood. There are many versions of our internal experience, and together they form the core of increasingly heterogeneous and dimensional self-experience. Pine (1985), too, writes of the special vulnerability that follows the emergence of such a clear and separate sense of the "me." While it allows for an increasingly rich, textured, and personal evocation of self experience and self feeling, it also allows for a particular and poignant kind of vulnerability, because only a self that has emerged can be hurt in a way that feels personal and—in that sense—meaningful.

Affective developments during the third year of life cannot be understood outside the context of representational development. The findings reported by developmental researchers have greatly expanded our understanding of the processes that account for the changes that occur in reality testing, affect regulation, impulse control, and integration during the third year of life. As mental representations of experience become more stable and elaborated through experience and maturation, both external reality as well as the internal realities of affects and impulses are understood and organized in an increasingly differentiated and coherent way. As these developments take place, struggles for control diminish, and autonomy and separateness become less threatening. Representation—as exemplified in the development of language and play—marks a thrilling and momentous developmental advance that will change the quality of children's experiences forever.

Individuality and Its Complexities

Children move through the third year in dramatically different ways from one another. Some children move through this period with what seems an almost incredible intensity. None of the crises of the twos—separation, toiletting, exploration—are accomplished without angst and turmoil. With some children, fights for control are intense, rebellions are powerful and prolonged, and rage and moodiness sometimes seem unmitigated. Other children, by contrast, may move through all these developmental challenges without incident. The "terrible twos" may never be terrible. These children may remain mellow about separations, toilet easily, comply without becoming passive and submissive; in short, for some, their vulnerability never takes on the painful cast that it does for other children. It is impossible to discuss the issue of individuality without considering the biological, temperamental differences among children. While there can be no doubt that some of these variations may be understood in terms of the quality of the caregiving environment (Sroufe, 1985), there can also be no doubt that children's temperament—the quality and dimension of their emotional responsiveness, their sensitivity to transitions and changes, their ability to contain and modulate internal states, and thus, to maintain homeostasis—plays a powerful role in organizing their response to the many changes that they must adapt to during the third year of life. The tempo of children's moves from one stage to another also

varies. Some children seem to come upon the awareness of separateness very suddenly; this may have to do with early walking or with early cognitive development. The speed of their cognitive development creates something akin to the experience of shock. Other children come upon these changes in consciousness more gradually; separateness is a slow dawning rather than a rude awakening. There are children whose physical prowess and general alertness are such that they find tremendous pleasure in mastery; these children pick things up quickly and easily. These factors will mitigate and temper their dependence upon mother in a myriad of ways. These are but a few of the ways that biology, cognitive development, and affective experience can interact; we mention them in order to make the important point that in development, there is never a simple cause-and-effect relationship between environment and behavior. The paths of influence are always complex and multiply determined.

Familial circumstances also must be considered. The third year of life poses particular challenges to parents; differences in parental response to these challenges affect the developing family system in a number of ways (Marvin & Stewart, 1991). Some parents welcome their children's newfound ability to communicate and welcome the move into a more verbal relationship. Others find it difficult to give up the days when their infants were malleable and distractible, and may feel drained and provoked by the demands, willfulness, and open aggression of the 2-and-a-half-year-old (Benedek, 1959; Sander, 1962). In intact families, husbands and wives are just beginning to find each other again after the long onslaught of infancy and toddlerhood (Belsky, 1984), and there are many subtle realignments that take place as the child moves from "dependence to relative independence" (Winnicott, 1965). In particular, the parents may begin to rediscover their intimate relationship. Ironically, it is often at this time of increased vulnerability and autonomy that children must adjust to the birth of a sibling and must cope with the feelings of loss and abandonment that this event inevitably engenders. Many children begin to turn to the father in a more direct and delineated way; Abelin (1971) saw this shift in the father-toddler relationship as facilitating the final phases of the separation-individuation process. This constellation of relationships will shift again once the child enters the oedipal phase. In any event, a child's move into representation demands a new set of adaptations in the parents and in the family. The more successful these adaptations, the more confident and whole 2-year-olds will feel, and the more sure they feel that their primary love objects welcome and applaud their emerging self.

Much of what is written about this period still makes a variety of assumptions about the culture of "normal" toddlers or preschoolers: They live at home, their mother is the primary caretaker, the father is the primary wage earner, and their social encounters usually take place in the domain of the playground or family living room. Children leave this protected environment only slowly, usually entering school at around the age of 3. But, as has been well documented in both the popular and academic press, fewer and fewer families can be described in these traditional terms. The past decade has seen a dramatic shift in fathers' involvement in parenting. Parenting is no longer the exclusive domain of women. In addition, a vast proportion of parents of children under 5 years old work, and indeed most children, are in some form of alternative care—either day care or nursery school—by the time they are 2. Even in middle- or upper-class families, both parents often work, for economic as well as personal reasons. Most children are separated from their parents repeatedly during the course of their early years in the course of daily, normal life. Many are placed in daycare and other child care settings that accommodate numerous children, exposing them to many diverse social experiences. Also, most children not only see both their parents off to work each day, but also must share their parents with one or more siblings. Families often space children 2 to 3 years apart, which means that for many children, the period between their second and third birthday brings a new, younger sibling into the home. Unfortunately, statistics attest to the fact that an increasing number of divorces take place in families where children are under 5. In some families, children must adjust to and then lose relationships with maternal companions. Many many women raise one or more children on their own, juggling the demands of childrearing and wage-earning without the support of a partner. Thus, for many children, cognitive instability is coupled with the demand that they adapt to life's exigencies at a time when this may be particularly difficult for them.

These challenges to personal equanimity and to smooth, unencumbered development are ubiquitous across social class and across diverse and culturally distinct members of the population. Challenge is not new to our time in history; these are simply the challenges faced by our children as they move through the preschool years. Thus, any theoretical, empirical, or even clinical views of this period must be adjusted and modified when a particular, individual child is considered. How he or she develops must be understood against the backdrop of the realities and challenges he\she faces in his\her particular life and in relationship to the particular family.

Interestingly, children often first come to the attention of mental health professionals between the ages of 2 and 3 (Slade & Bergman, 1988), and infant-parent psychotherapy is recommended with increasing frequency during the toddler period (Fraiberg, 1980; Lieberman & Pawl, 1993; Seligman, 1994). In part, this has to do with the parents' perception that the child is now an individual with problems that can be addressed outside the context of environmental ministrations. The basic physical and social adjustments of the period are those that most often concern parents, and most often lead them to seek psychiatric help: their child's ability to talk, play, sleep, eat, and eliminate properly; along with the child's ability to adjust, to sustain primary relationships and to make new ones outside the family. While such problems rarely are truly internalized at this age and usually require work with parents as well, consolidated difficulties in many of these areas are frequently seen in children of 2 or 3, and often benefit from intervention. Both dyadic treatment and developmental guidance for parents can be particularly helpful during this period, as the many changes of the period are as stressful and demanding for parents as they are for children and are likely to awaken parental conflicts and other "ghosts in the nursery" (Fraiberg, 1980).

Conclusion

The development of representation dramatically alters children's relationship to their entire world and presents a new set of challenges to both them and their families. It can be a period of discovery

97

and growth, and it can be a time of struggle, vulnerability, confrontation, and regression. For most children, it is both. There are dramatic developments in communicative competence, in physical competence, and in social competence. At the same time, the demands made upon children by their parents as well as the society at large increase just as substantially. They feel conscious of their separateness for the first time ever, and—

as exciting as this may be—it is also frightening. As such, it is often a period of regression and developmental imbalance (A. Freud, 1965). It is a time when past experience with others, both successes and failures, must be consolidated and become a part of the self. It is a period that will define how children see themselves and use their minds. It is truly a new beginning.

REFERENCES

Abelin, E. L. (1971). The role of the father in the separation-individuation process. In J. B. McDevitt & C. F. Settlage (Eds.), *Separation-individuation: Essays in honor of Margaret S. Mahler* (pp. 229–253). New York: International Universities Press.

Aber, J. L., & Baker, A. J. (1990). Security of attachment in todderhood: Modifying assessment procedures for joint clinical and research purposes. In M. T. Greenberg, D. Cicchetti, & E. M. Cummings (Eds.), *Attachment in the preschool years* (pp. 427–463). Chicago: University of Chicago Press.

Ainsworth, M. D. S., Blehar, M., Waters, E., & Wall, S. (1978). *Patterns of attachment: A psychological study of the Strange Situation.* Hillsdale, NJ: Erlbaum.

Belsky, J. (1984). The determinants of parenting: A process model. *Child Development, 55,* 83–96.

Belsky, J., Garduque, L., & Hrncir, E. (1984). Assessing performance, competence and executive capacity in infant play: Relations to home environment and security of attachment. *Developmental Psychology, 20,* 406–417.

Benedek, T. (1959). Parenthood as a developmental phase. *Journal of the American Psychoanalytic Association, 7,* 389–417.

Bergman, A. (1987). On the development of female identity: Issues of mother-daughter interaction during the separation-individuation. *Psychoanalytic Inquiry, 7,* 381–396.

Bowlby, J. (1969). *Attachment and loss: Volume 1. Attachment.* New York: Basic Books.

Bretherton, I., & Beeghly, M. (1982). Talking about inner states: The acquisition of an explicit theory of mind. *Developmental Psychology, 18,* 906–921.

Cassidy, J., & Marvin, R., with the Attachment Working Group of the John D. and Catherine T. MacArthur Network on the Transition from Infancy to Early Childhood (1988, April). *A system for coding the organization of attachment behavior in 3 and 4 year old children.* Paper presented at the International Conference on Infant Studies, Washington, D.C.

Dore, J. (1989). Monologue as reenvoicement of dialogue. In K. Nelson (Ed.), *Narratives from the crib* (pp. 231–263). Cambridge, MA: Harvard University Press.

Dunn, J. (1988). *The beginnings of social understanding.* Cambridge, MA: Harvard University Press.

Dunn, J., Bretherton, I., & Munn, P. (1987). Conversations about feeling states between mothers and their young children. *Developmental Psychology, 23,* 132–139.

Easterbrooks, M. A., & Goldberg, W. A. (1990). Security of toddler-parent attachment: Relation to children's sociopersonality functioning during kindergarten. In M. T. Greenberg, D. Cicchetti, & E. M. Cummings (Eds.), *Attachment in the preschool years* (pp. 221–245). Chicago: University of Chicago Press.

Egeland, B., & Farber, E. A. (1984). Infant-mother attachment: Factors related to its development and changes over time. *Child Development, 55.* 753–771.

Erikson, E. H. (1950). *Childhood and society.* New York: W. W. Norton.

Fraiberg, S. (1980). *Clinical studies in infant mental health.* New York: Basic Books.

Freud, A. (1965). *Normality and pathology in childhood.* New York: International Universities Press.

Freud, S. (1953). Three essays on the theory of sexuality. In J. Strachey (Ed. and Trans.), *The standard edition of the complete psychological works of Sigmund Freud* (Vol. 7, pp. 135–243). London: Hogarth Press. (Original work published 1905.)

Freud, S. (1959). Character and anal erotism. In J. Strachey (Ed. and Trans.), *The standard edition of the complete psychological works of Sigmund Freud* (Vol. 9, pp. 167–177). London: Hogarth Press. (Original work published 1908.)

Goldberg, W., & Easterbrooks, M. A. (1984). Toddler development in the family. Impact of father involvement and parenting characteristics. *Developmental Psychology, 55,* 740–752.

Greenspan, S. I. (1989). *The development of the ego.* Madison, CT: International Universities Press.

Harris, P. L. (1989). *Children and emotion.* Oxford: Basil Blackwell.

Kagan, J. (1981). *The second year: The emergence of self-awareness.* Cambridge, MA: Harvard University Press.

Keller, H. (1902). *The story of my life.* Garden City, NY: Doubleday.

Lieberman, A. (1994). *The emotional life of the toddler.* New York: Free Press.

Lieberman, A. F., & Pawl, J. (1993). Infant-parent psychotherapy. In C. H. Zeanah (Ed). *Handbook of infant mental health* (pp. 427–442). New York: Guilford Press.

Mahler, M., Pine, F., & Bergman, A. (1975). *The psychological birth of the human infant.* New York: Basic Books.

Main, M., Kaplan, N., & Cassidy, J. (1985). Security in infancy, childhood & adulthood: A move to the level of representation. *Monographs of the Society for Research in Child Development, 501* (1–2, Serial No. 209).

Marvin, R., & Stewart, R. B. (1991). A family systems framework for the study of attachment. In M. T. Greenberg, D. Cicchetti, & E. M. Cummings (Eds.), *Attachment in the preschool years* (pp. 51–87). Chicago: University of Chicago Press.

Matas, L., Arend, R. A., & Sroufe, L. A. (1978). Continuity of adaptation in the second year: The relationship between quality of attachment and later competence. *Child Development, 49,* 547–556.

Nelson, K. (1989). Monologue as representation of real-life experience. In K. Nelson (Ed.), *Narratives from the crib* (pp. 27–73). Cambridge, MA: Harvard University Press.

Nelson, K., & Gruendel, J. M. (1981). Generalized event representations: Basic building blocks of cognitive development. In A. Brown & M. Lamb (Eds.), *Advances in developmental psychology, Vol. 1* (pp. 131–158). Hillsdale, NJ: Lawrence Erlbaum.

Nicolich, L. M. (1977). Beyond sensorimotor intelligence: Assessment of symbolic maturity through analysis of symbolic play. *Merrill Palmer Quarterly, 23,* 89–101.

Pastor, D. (1981). The quality of mother-infant attachment and its relationship to toddlers's initial sociability with peers. *Developmental Psychology, 23,* 326–335.

Piaget, J. (1963). *The origins of intelligence in children.* New York: W. W. Norton. (Originally published 1952.)

Pine, F. (1985). *Developmental theory and clinical process.* New York: Basic Books.

Sander, L. (1962). Issues in early mother-child interaction. *Journal of the American Academy of Child Psychiatry, 1,* 141–166.

Schank, R. C., & Abelson, R. P. (1977). *Scripts, plans, goals and understanding.* Hillsdale, NJ: Erlbaum.

Seligman, S. (1994). Applying psychoanalysis in an unconventional context: Adapting infant-parent psychotherapy to a changing population. *Psychoanalytic Study of the Child, 49,* 481–500.

Slade, A. (1987). The quality of attachment and early symbolic play. *Developmental Psychology, 23,* 78–85.

Slade, A., & Aber, J. L. (1992). Attachments, drives and development: Conflicts and convergences in theory. In J. W. Barron, M. N. Eagle, & D. L. Wolitzky (Eds.), *Interface of psychoanalysis and psychology* (pp. 154–186). Washington, D.C.: American Psychological Association.

Slade, A., & Bergman, A. (1988). The clinical assessment of the toddler. In C. Kestenbaum & D. Williams (Eds.), *The assessment of children and adolescents* (pp. 180–196). New York: New York University Press.

Sroufe, L. A. (1983). Infant-caregiver attachment and patterns of adaptation in preschool: The roots of maladaptation and competence. In M. Perlmutter (Ed.), *Minnesota Symposium in Child Psychology* (Vol. 16, pp. 41–83). Hillsdale, NJ: Lawrence Erlbaum.

Sroufe, L. A. (1985). Attachment classification from the perspective of infant-caregiver relationships and infant temperament. *Child Development, 56,* 1–14.

Stern, D. N. (1985). *The interpersonal world of the infant.* New York: Basic Books.

Watson, M. W., & Fischer, K. W. (1977). A developmental sequence of agent use in later infancy. *Child Development, 48,* 828–36.

Winnicott, D. W. (1965). *Maturational processes and the facilitating environment.* New York: International Universities Press.

Wolf, D. P. (1982). Understanding others: The origins of an independent agent concept. In G. Forman (Ed.), *Action and thought: From sensorimotor schemes to symbol use* (pp. 297–328). New York: Academic Press.

Wolf, D. P. (1990). Being of several minds. In D. Cicchetti & M. Beeghly (Eds.), *The self in transition: Infancy to childhood* (pp. 183–213). Chicago: University of Chicago Press.

12 / Cognitive Development in the Third Year of Life

Holly A. Ruff

The third year in a child's life can be a fascinating time to observe behavior and development. Most children can talk in sentences, some very proficiently, and they can communicate to others their intentions and thoughts about people and events. At the same time, their knowledge of the world is still limited and their capacity to reason logically still immature. The combination of increased language skills and limited knowledge means that their misunderstandings are often more transparent than in the second year. A touching example offered by Fraiberg (1959) is the story of the child who became very distressed with the family discussion of flying to see Grandma; apparently afraid that he was going to be left behind, he finally burst out, "But I don't know how to fly!" On the other hand, we have to be careful not to assume that 2- to 3-year-old children can put into words everything that they know; the discrepancy between procedural and declarative knowledge is still very important as are considerations of context and function.

The structure of this chapter is like that of Chapters 2 and 7. After summarizing the major cognitive advances in the third year of life, I elaborate on specific developments in play, problem solving, and representation or memory. The final section presents alternative to standardized cognitive tests for this age range.

Major Advances in Skill and Knowledge

Piaget (1954) described the period from 2 to 6 years as preoperational; that is, the child is not capable of logical thought or logical operations but has advanced beyond the sensorimotor intelligence of the first 2 years. As was emphasized in Chapter 7, Piaget believed that the achievement of this period is the ability to represent reality internally and to manipulate these representations—whether as images, words, or other symbols. He describes the child from 2 to 4 years, however, as egocentric. Egocentricity manifests itself in children's failure to take another person's viewpoint into account and to see the world from a different perspective. One of the consequences of such a limitation is that children do not think about their own cognitive processes. They feel no need to justify their own thinking or to correct contradictions in their own reasoning. While children can now imagine and manipulate symbols, they still tend to be very concrete, focused on perceptually salient features of a situation. As Flavell (1963) writes, "Preoperational thought can scarcely be considered 'good' thought, relative to the conceptual forms into which it eventually evolves" (p. 156). On the other hand, he points out that Piaget's account of this period is his least well developed (see also Case & Khanna, 1981; Sugarman, 1981). Fortunately, in recent years many investigators have focused attention on this period and have provided us with much more information.

Perhaps the most important feature of this recent research is the appreciation of the extent to which 2-year-olds function intelligently in situations where their motivation is engaged and that draw upon their previous experiences. As a specific illustration of this, children as young as 2 years can be very systematic in keeping track of hidden objects in familiar, large-scale environments (DeLoache & Brown, 1983), even with long delays between seeing the object hidden and finding it, and they make many fewer errors in such tasks than in the laboratory-based delayed response tests. In their play and manipulation of objects, children in the third year are also systematic in spatially organizing objects according to a category (Sugarman, 1981, 1982), for example, putting all of the blue chips on one side of the table and all of the red on the other. They readily understand the content of pictures and use pictured information to guide action (DeLoache, 1991). They show the beginnings of an understanding of internal cognitive and emotional states, such as knowledge, intention, and motivation (Shatz, Wellman, & Silber, 1983).

The first year contains two to three major transition points, and the second year involves the transition to symbolic functioning. No major or global transitions have been identified in the third year. Case and Khanna (1981), however, argue that there are four substages in the period from the emergence of symbolic functioning in the second year to the emergence of logical reasoning at 4½ years. First of all, these authors characterize this period as one of "symbolically encoding—by means of words, images, gestures, and so forth—the relationship between two or more objects or people in the world" (p. 23). They then suggest that there are transition points at 2 years and again at 3 years; these transitions are marked by the number of relations that can be coordinated in a single task. For example, children of 1½ years may be able to build towers of blocks, but it is not until the next stage that they can create a structure that involves building in two directions. At about 3 years, children are able to manage three relations in such tasks as building from block models, assembling puzzles, repeating sentences, and obeying instructions. Data are presented that generally support their expectations. Although the investigators use tasks that may not engage the child maximally or provide typical environmental supports, the results still show that, during the third year, children's acting and thinking become more complex in systematic, if not perfectly synchronous, ways.

Sugarman (1981, 1982) contends that the shift in complexity involves the coordination of actions and categories, such that a 2½-year-old can consider two categories of objects simultaneously and refer to the relationship between these classes in both language and action. For example, when presented with a scattered set of objects representing two classes, children from 1½ to 3 years spontaneously organize them; the youngest children may simply touch objects in the same class sequentially; the older children are more likely to segregate the two classes of objects spatially. The 1½-year-olds tend to work with one class at a time, touching all of the dolls, perhaps ignoring the second class or touching the objects in that class later. The 2½-year-old, in contrast, will work with both sets, putting a doll on one side of the table and a boat on the other side, before picking up the next

doll. Likewise, the 1½-year-old is likely to refer to only one class at a time ("A lady . . . another lady . . . another lady") while the older child will refer to both ("She's a lady. That is a lady. That a boat. This is two [boats]"; Sugarman, 1982, p. 428). Sugarman argues that "by 2½ children impose . . . structure on what they see, do, and hear . . ."; they are able to coordinate relationships between elements as reflected in their counting, learning the grammar of the language, and simultaneously grouping classes of objects (pp. 446–447).

Although both Case and Khanna (1981) and Sugarman (1981) argue for an important reorganization of representational abilities from 2 to 3 years, the third year also might be considered a period of consolidation. Most children begin to talk in the second year, displaying a dramatic growth in vocabulary and the use of simple sentences; however their language becomes far more elaborate in the third year. As Anisfeld (1984) writes: "By the age of 3 years the typical child has gained entry into all domains of language, including vocabulary, phonology, syntax, and morphology. There is a great deal of specific material that remains to be learned, but the child will now be learning as an insider . . ." (p. 247). Observational learning or imitation and direct manipulation of objects are still major means by which new knowledge and skills are acquired (Tomasello, Savage-Rumbaugh, & Kruger, 1993). However, the consolidation of language skills, particularly comprehension, makes it possible for the child to learn more than previously by being verbally informed. Other skills, such as planning, also undergo an expansion and elaboration.

Although we see the beginning of planning ahead at 12 months (Willats & Rosie, 1989) and the emergence of "insightful" problem solving in the second year (Piaget, 1952), we find that children in the third year are able to plan farther ahead and to formulate more elaborate plans. Werner (1948) suggests that the growth of planning is intimately related to an increased differentiation of self from other. He writes:

. . . increasing subject-object differentiation involves the corollary that the organism becomes increasingly less dominated by the immediate concrete situation; the person is less stimulus-bound and less impelled by his own affective states. A consequence of this freedom is the clearer understanding of goals, the possibility of employing substitutive means and alternative ends. There is hence a greater capacity for delay and planned action. The person is better able to exercise choice and willfully rearrange a situation. In short, he can manipulate the environment rather than passively respond to the environment. (p. 126)

The differentiation between self and other is a process that begins in the first year as infants, during their own actions, simultaneously pick up information about their own bodies and the outside world (Gibson, 1979). In the second year, between 18 and 24 months, there is a marked increase in the children's ability to recognize their mirror images (Asendorpf & Baudonniere, 1993; Bertenthal & Fischer, 1978). The gradual increase in the use of "I" also is taken as evidence that, with advancing development, the children have a more complete sense of self. In the third year, children make this differentiation in an even more profound way; they are better able to delay responding (Golden, Montave, & Bridger, 1977; Vaughn, Kopp, & Krakow, 1984), to evaluate themselves (Stipek, Recchia, & McClintic, 1992), and to see or create goals to be achieved through planned action. These plans, even if rudimentary, are powerful organizers of behavior as they recruit basic processes such as attention and reasoning.

Examples in Specific Domains

The child's cognition is thus reorganized and consolidated in a number of ways in the third year. The causes of these changes stem from both the child's knowledge, previously acquired skills, and new challenges from the older members of the child's society. The immediate causes are likely to be newly mastered skills that thrust the child into new modes of action and thought. The important developments of this period can be illustrated in several specific ways.

PLAY

During free play with toys, we see increases in focused attention to the toys (Ruff & Lawson, 1990), very likely a consequence of the increasing complexity of play. For example, a 30-month-old, compared to an 18-month-old, is able to think of and plan to build a castle or a garage with blocks. Carrying out this plan and actually constructing the building takes time and concentration; the child's goal therefore may mobilize and maintain attention. A child in a study by Ruff and Lawson (1990) was working to combine several bristle blocks; although her initial actions seemed without a particular goal, it became clear at one point that she wanted to put three yellow blocks end to end; she concentrated and persevered in the face of difficulties and finally got them all lined up. At that point, she announced "I got it!" and went on to another activity. Her actions and words show that she had something in mind before she accomplished it; her attention was focused and sustained while she worked toward that goal; then, when the goal was finally reached, that episode of focused attention ended.

The increases in focused attention during play (Ruff & Lawson, 1990) are paralleled by increases in looking, specifically focused looking, at televised events (Anderson & Levin, 1976; Ruff, Weissberg, Lawson, & Capozzoli, 1992). As they become more able to comprehend the language and action sequences of the events being shown, children spontaneously, without instruction or encouragement, look longer at television programs (Anderson & Lorch, 1983).

Pretend play begins in the second year; for the 2- to 3-year-old, it becomes a major vehicle for trying out social roles and for expressing wishes and fears. There is no question at this age that children are aware that they are pretending. A young boy threw a scarf around his neck and marched up to his father and announced in a gruff and atypical voice, "I police!" His change of voice signals to himself and others that he is engaging in make-believe. This particular example also illustrates the extemporaneous nature of much pretend play; as the boy caught sight of the family cat coming into the room, he said gruffly, "That police kitty cat!" Pretend play at this age, however, also can involve planning and longer sequences, for example, in setting a table (the hassock) with utensils (Tinker Toys) and calling people to dinner. As McCune-Nicolich (1981) notes, the element of planning often can be seen when children stop and search for just the right prop to fit in with their intended schemes.

PROBLEM SOLVING

Search for hidden objects is still a real-life problem for children at this age, and its study has led to interesting information about the development of search strategies. DeLoache and Brown (1984) demonstrate that search for a toy hidden in the child's home is very accurate even at 24 months. If the object is not where they saw it hidden originally, children, at least by 27 months, tend to search for it around the location in which they last saw it; a young boy, for example, having seen a toy put into a desk drawer but not finding it there, wondered aloud whether it had fallen out and looked under and behind the desk (DeLoache & Brown, 1984). Children of 2½ years will search in a comprehensive and nonredundant fashion for an object that they have been told is in one of several identical containers, providing that there is some visual reminder, such as open lids, of where they have already searched (Wellman et al., 1984). By 3 years, children may spontaneously mark locations for the purpose of remembering where something has been put (Wellman, 1988). Children in the third year are less likely than younger children to show response biases to specific locations, but they act this way mainly because they understand the tasks better and search successfully more of the time (Sophian, 1984).

DeLoache and Todd (1988) examined the 2-year-olds' ability to sort and selectively retrieve containers that contained desirable M & M's as opposed to nondesirable sticks. As Sugarman (1981) and others have noted, children in the third year will spontaneously segregate different classes of objects in different spatial locations, presumably from a desire to organize objects and their own experiences. In the study by DeLoache and Todd, the child's task was to watch as either M & M's or sticks were put into the containers, take the containers one by one as they were filled, and then hand back only the ones that contained the candies. The question was whether they would spontaneously segregate the containers in order to keep track of which ones held the M & M's. They did not. DeLoache and Todd reasoned that the behavior of spatially segregating objects (in this task, a simple strategy for getting as much candy as possible) may at this age depend on visible differences between classes. Indeed, when the candy and the sticks were put into two different types of containers, the children were much more likely to sort them spatially as they were given them and were more likely to hand back only the candy containers or, at least, to hand those back first. The 2-year-olds in this study were more likely to engage in this type of categorization when they were told to remember where the candies were than were control children who were simply handed the two types of containers. This difference suggests that the behavior was guided by a desire to remember; it therefore qualifies as an early mnemonic strategy for solving this particular problem.

REPRESENTATION/MEMORY

Although symbolic functioning and mental representation emerge and are well documented in the second year, there are further advances in the third year of life. In the latter half of the third year, in particular, there are some rather significant changes. After hiding a stuffed animal in a room, DeLoache (1991) told 2½- to 3-year-old children who had not observed the hiding where to find the stuffed animal. She either put a small replica of the animal behind the same piece of furniture in a small-scale model of the room or pointed to the piece of furniture in a picture of the room. Surprisingly, the 2½-year-olds were far more accurate (78% errorless trials) in the picture condition than in the model condition (25%). The 3-year-olds, in contrast, were highly accurate in both conditions. This result, which has been replicated, occurs even if the experimenter simply points to the right piece of furniture in the model. DeLoache argues that, in order to understand what the experimenter is telling them with either picture or model, children must first understand the symbolic nature of the picture or model. The picture apparently is readily accepted as a symbol of the large room, while the model is not. The unfamiliarity of the model and its three-dimensionality may make it difficult for the 2½-year-olds to treat the model as a symbol rather than as an object. Pictures are a familiar form of representation, however, as would be expected on the basis of the amount of book reading that parents and children engage in. DeLoache suggests that the task requires a dual orientation to the scale model—it is an object that could be played with itself, and it is also a representation of another room. By 3 years, children apparently can assume this orientation and are therefore more flexible in their use of symbols than children just 6 months younger. Even so, they may have difficulty maintaining this orientation if a long delay is imposed before they are allowed to find the object (Uttal, Schreiber, & DeLoache, 1995).

Pederson, Rook-Green, and Elder (1981) found a similar developmental shift in the ability to substitute objects in pretend play. Children at 2½ and 3 years were presented with realistic objects, such as a toy hammer, and asked to show the experimenter what we do with them. All of the children performed appropriate actions. When given ambiguous objects, such as a flat piece of wood, they were able to pretend that it was another object and act accordingly. They also were willing and able to pretend that readily identifiable objects, such as a bowl or dustpan, were other objects. However, when it came to objects that strongly elicit particular actions on their own, such as a tennis ball or toy car, the 2½-year-olds, but not the 3-year-olds, had difficulty pretending that these objects were something else. The researchers, in this case, argue quite persuasively that the younger children had trouble inhibiting a prepotent response in order to perform one that was incompatible, even though fanciful. Like the De-Loache results, children at 2½ years had some difficulty responding to one object as a symbol of another when the first object was salient in its own right, while 3-year-olds were able to. The slightly older child seems to have achieved a significantly greater distance between symbols and their referents (Werner & Kaplan, 1963).

What is happening to representation as manifested by memory in this age range? As was noted in Chapter 7, recognition memory is good. Perlmutter and Myers (1974) found that 2-year-olds could correctly identify new and old items with 80% accuracy. These same investigators (1979) presented 2-year-olds with nine-item lists and asked them to recall all items. Although children were unlikely to name objects that had not been presented, their ability to name those they had seen was limited to an average of two. The last object presented was the most likely to be named. The authors found no evidence of deliberate use of strategies for remembering. On the other hand,

the conditions were restricted and somewhat artificial, so it is possible that recall was underestimated.

In contrast, Wellman (1988) suggests that even very young children show evidence of some deliberate attempts to remember. He reports that, when asked to remind their parents to do something in the future (take the wash out of the washing machine, buy milk at the store), even 2-year-olds did so at rates that were significantly above chance. The fact that they were less likely to do so after long delays suggests a typical forgetting function. Another study by DeLoache and her colleagues (DeLoache, Cassidy, & Brown 1985) showed that some 2-year-olds, while waiting to retrieve a hidden object, would name the hidden object along with its location, "Big Bird chair," or remind themselves of the task, "Find Big Bird," or point to the location. The fact that they did not engage in such behavior in other conditions where the object was visible or someone else was supposed to retrieve the object strongly suggests that the children were deliberately trying to remember.

There is also evidence of spontaneous rehearsal in the case of long-term memories (Nelson & Ross, 1980) where children verbally repeat an experience. Thus, a young boy became attached to an aunt at her vacation home, which was next door to his grandparents' home. A few months later, when his aunt was visiting him at his home, he was drawing a picture of water; he said, "There is water at Grandma's" and, looking at his aunt, "I see you there." At another visit some time later, he told his aunt, "You have a house at Grandma's." These verbal recollections reinforce the memory and keep it intact for longer. Such rehearsal is most likely to occur for salient events or situations in a child's life, ones that do not occur routinely enough to become part of the child's representation of familiar event sequences (Nelson & Gruendel, 1981).

Assessment of Development

For this age, items on standardized tests range deal much more with language and conceptual items than is true in the first year. This is in line with the expansion of declarative knowledge and the child's ability to answer questions verbally and to comprehend information that is presented verbally rather than concretely. Observing children during free play still serves as a supplement to standardized assessments and allows both symbolic functioning and sustained attention to be evaluated. As already indicated, Sugarman (1981) argues that spontaneous organization of objects during play also provides a window into the child's conceptual organization. Further work with specific sets of objects that fall into two or more classes could provide the clinician with a useful tool for evaluating conceptual development.

Since one of the developments of this period is the greater capacity for planning and organization, tools such as the Goodman Lock Box (Goodman & Field, 1991) now become appropriate. With the Lock Box, Goodman and her colleagues have tried to operationalize the concept of self-regulated organization of behavior. The apparatus is a panel of 10 doors, each one locked with a different device, such as padlock, hook, butterfly catch, sliding bolt, and so forth. Behind each door is a different toy designed to be of interest to children between 2 and 6 years, such as a baby doll, car, clay, and music box. The child is given 6.5 minutes to play freely with the box, and parents are asked not to interfere. During this time, the evaluator keeps a running record of all of the child's activities. Competence is measured by how many doors are opened and relocked successfully. Organization is determined by the sequence with which the doors are opened and the pattern of behavior once the door is open. Credit is given for opening adjacent doors and for systematically exploring or playing with the objects found inside. Credit is lost when doors are opened in a haphazard fashion and when the child goes back to doors that have been opened already. The organization measure is designed to determine the degree of efficiency that the motivated child brings to the problem of finding toys and playing with them. The degree of aimlessness is assessed separately by recording repetitive actions, such as repeatedly opening and closing the same door or putting the same toy in and out of the box without playing with it.

The test has obvious advantages. One is that it is a novel and stimulating situation for almost all children. Another is that no explicit demands are made on the children, so that their ability to organize and regulate themselves spontaneously is being assessed. No language is required either to understand the situation or to participate in it. As Goodman and Field (1991) note, the scores are not related to conventional IQ scores, a fact that suggests that the situation draws on abilities not usually assessed, even though they are clearly important for adaptive behavior. Used in conjunction with standardized tests, discrepancies may be illuminating, by pointing either to weaknesses in cognitive organization in children who otherwise are scoring within the normal range or to strengths in children who score below the average range. The Lock Box and other nonconventional tests may help us to assess a fuller range of skills, all of which may be important both to the children's adaptation to demands and to their ability to solve problems that face them in everyday life.

REFERENCES

Anderson, D. R., & Levin, S. R. (1976). Young children's attention to "Sesame Street." *Child Development, 47,* 806–811.

Anderson, D. R., & Lorch, E. P. (1983). Looking at television: Action or reaction? In J. Bryant & D. R. Anderson (Eds.), *Children's understanding of television. Research on attention and comprehension* (pp. 1–33). New York: Academic Press.

Anisfeld, M. (1984). *Language development from birth to three.* Hillsdale, NJ: Erlbaum.

Asendorpf, J. B., & Baudonniere, P.-M. (1993). Self-awareness and other-awareness: Mirror self-recognition and synchronic imitation among unfamiliar peers. *Developmental Psychology, 29,* 88–93.

Bertenthal, B. I., & Fischer, K. W. (1978). Development of self recognition of the infant. *Developmental Psychology, 14,* 44–50.

Case, R., & Khanna, F. (1981). The missing links: Stages in children's progression from sensorimotor to logical thought. *New Directions for Child Development, 12,* 21–32.

DeLoache, J. S. (1991). Symbolic functioning in very young children: Understanding of pictures and models. *Child Development, 62,* 736–752.

DeLoache, J. S., & Brown, A. L. (1983). Very young children's memory for the location of objects in a large-scale environment. *Child Development, 54,* 888–897.

DeLoache, J. S., & Brown, A. L. (1984). Where do I go next? Intelligent searching by very young children. *Developmental Psychology, 20,* 37–44.

DeLoache, J. S., Cassidy, D. J., & Brown, A. L. (1985). Precursors of mnemonic strategies in very young children's memory. *Child Development, 56,* 125–137.

DeLoache, J. S., & Todd, C. M. (1988). Young children's use of spatial categorization as a mnemonic strategy. *Journal of Experimental Child Psychology, 46,* 1–20.

Flavell, J. H. (1963). *The developmental psychology of Jean Piaget.* Toronto: Van Nostrand.

Fraiberg, S. H. (Ed.). (1959). *The magic years.* New York: Charles Scribner's Sons.

Gibson, J. J. (Ed.). (1979). *The ecological approach to visual perception.* Boston: Hougton-Mifflin.

Golden, M., Montare, A., & Bridger, W. (1977). Verbal control of delay behavior in two-year-old boys as a function of social class. *Child Development, 48,* 1107–1111.

Goodman, J. F., & Field, M. (1991). Assessing attentional problems in preschoolers with the Goodman Lock Box. In C. E. Schaefer, K. Gitlin, & A. Sandgrund (Eds.), *Play diagnosis and assessment* (pp. 219–248). New York: John Wiley & Sons.

Kopp, C. B., & Vaughn, B. E. (1982). Sustained attention during exploratory manipulation as a predictor of cognitive competence in preterm infants. *Child Development, 53,* 174–182.

McCune-Nicolich, L. (1981). Toward symbolic functioning: Structure of early pretend games and potential parallels with language. *Child Development, 52,* 785–797.

Nelson, K., & Gruendel, J. (1981). Generalized event representation: Basic building blocks of cognitive development. In A. Brown & M. Lamb (Eds.), *Advances in developmental psychology* (Vol. 1, pp. 131–158). Hillsdale, NJ: Erlbaum.

Nelson, K., & Ross, G. (1980). The generalities and specifics of long-term memory in infants and young children. *New Directions for Child Development, 10,* 87–101.

Pederson, D. R., Rook-Green, A., & Elder, J. L. (1981). The role of action in the development of pretend play in young children. *Developmental Psychology, 17,* 756–759.

Perlmutter, M., & Myers, N. A. (1974). Recognition memory development in two- to four-year-olds. *Developmental Psychology, 10,* 447–450.

Perlmutter, M., & Myers, N. A. (1979). Development of recall in 2- to 4-year-old children. *Developmental Psychology, 15,* 73–83.

Piaget, J. (Ed.). (1952). *The origin of intelligence in children.* New York: International Universities Press.

Piaget, J. (Ed.). (1952). *The construction of reality in the child.* New York: Basic Books.

Ruff, H. A., & Lawson, K. R. (1990). Development of sustained, focused attention in young children during free play. *Developmental Psychology, 26,* 85–93.

Ruff, H. A., Weissberg, R., Lawson, K. R., & Capozzoli, M. (1992). *Development and individuality in sustained visual attention in the preschool years.* Unpublished manuscript.

Shatz, M., Wellman, H. M., & Silber, S. (1983). The acquisition of mental verbs: A systemic investigation of the first reference to mental state. *Cognition, 14,* 301–321.

Sophian, C. (1984). Developing search skills in infancy and early childhood. In C. Sophian (Ed.), *Origins of cognitive skills* (pp. 27–56). Hillsdale, NJ: Lawrence Erlbaum.

Stipek, D., Recchia, S., & McClintic, S. (1992). Self-evaluation in young children. *Monographs of the Society for Research in Child Development, 57* (1, Serial No. 226).

Sugarman, S. (1981). Transitions in early representational intelligence: Changes overtime in children's production of simple block structures. In G. Forman (Ed.), *Action and thought: From sensorimotor schemes to symbolic operations* (pp. 65–93). New York: Academic Press.

Sugarman, S. (1982). Developmental changes in early representational intelligence: Evidence from spatial classification strategies and related verbal expressions. *Cognitive Psychology, 14,* 410–449.

Tomasello, M., Savage-Rumbaugh, S., & Kruger, A. C. (1993). Imitative learning of actions on objects by children, chimpanzees, and enculturated chimpanzees. *Child Development, 64,* 1688–1705.

Uttal, D., Schreiber, J. C., & DeLoache, J. S. (1995). Waiting to use a symbol: The effects of delay on children's use of models. *Child Development, 66,* 1875–1889.

Vaughn, B. E., Kopp, C. B., & Krakow, J. B. (1984). The emergence and consolidation of self-control from 18 to 30 months of age: Normative trends and individual differences. *Child Development, 55,* 990–1004.

Wellman, H. M. (1988). The early development of memory strategies. In F. W. Weinert & M. Perlmutter (Eds.), *Memory development: Universal changes and individual differences* (pp. 3–30). Hillsdale, NJ: Erlbaum.

Wellman, H. M., Somerville, S. C., Revelle, G. L., Haake, R. J., & Sophian, C. (1984). The development of comprehensive search skills. *Child Development, 55,* 472–481.

Werner, H. (Ed.). (1948). *The comparative psychology of mental development.* New York: International Universities Press.

Werner, H., & Kaplan, B. (Eds.). (1963). *Symbol formation.* New York: John Wiley & Sons.

Willats, P., & Rosie, K. (1989, April). Planning by 12-month-old infants. Paper presented at the biennial meeting of the Society for Research in Child Development. Kansas City, MO.

13 / Normal Language Development: The Third Year

Rhea Paul

We call 2-year-olds *toddlers*, people just getting on their feet. But we think of 3-year-olds as young *children*, persons who are on a firm footing and have started marching down the path of life. One of the things that causes us to change our perceptions of youngsters at these two ages is that 3-year-old sound much more like people rather than telegrams in the way they talk. This chapter explores how this change and others related to it take place.

Pronunciation

Although 2-year-olds are accurate in their production of speech sounds most of the time, they do tend to make some characteristic changes in pronunciation that serve to simplify the task of articulation. They may leave off unstressed syllables in long words, saying /nana/ for *banana*, make the sounds in a word more alike, pronouncing *doddie* for *doggie*, for example, change certain sounds that are hard to pronounce, as in *wabbit* for *rabbit; sair* for *chair;* or leave out one of the consonants in a consonant blend, using *pay* for *play*. These types of errors are very typical of children's speech in the 24- to 36-month period (Grunwell, 1982; Shriberg & Kwiatkowski, 1980).

Vocabulary

Both expressive and receptive vocabulary size continue to grow rapidly during the third year. Smith (1926) estimated expressive vocabulary size at 36 months to be about 900 words, a threefold increase over this size at 24 months. As children increase their vocabulary, they develop mastery over a range of semantic categories. Spatial terms including *in, on, under, beside, next to, on, off, out,* and *over* (Boehm, 1969) generally are mastered by 3 years of age. *Big* and *little* are the first pair of dimensional adjectives to be acquired, with *long* and *short* following soon after, both generally learned by age 3. Color terms are learned by 2-year-olds but are used first as a field rather than in association with specific hues (Pease, Gleason, & Pan, 1989). In other words, when 2-year-olds are asked, "What color is this?" they generally will reply with a color term, although it may not be the right one. By 36 months, most normal children will be naming two to three colors correctly. Children also learn to produce and understand question words *what* and *where,* and occasionally use *who* and *how* by age 3 (Tyack & Ingram, 1977). Pronouns including *I, me, my, mine, it* usually are used by age 3. Frequently *you, your, she, them, he, yours, we,* and *her* are mastered by age 3, as well (Haas & Owens, 1985).

Grammatical Production

An enormous amount of growth takes place in children's production of syntax between 24 and 36 months of age. Children move from producing primarily telegraphic utterances to the use of fully formed, though simple, grammatical sentences during the third year. This growth can be examined in three different contexts: the child's elaboration of telegraphic utterances through the use of inflectional markers and function words (*a, the,* etc.); elaboration of the basic units, or phrase structures, within simple sentences; and the production of various types of sentences.

GRAMMATICAL MORPHEMES

One means by which children express their increasing linguistic sophistication is by beginning to mark their utterances with the inflectional endings and function words that were left out of telegraphic speech. Children begin to produce these markers soon after their sentences include 3 words. Cazden (1968) studied the acquisition of these *grammatical morphemes*, the units of meaning that are expressed either as inflections on nouns and verbs, as function words such as articles (*a, an,* and *the*), or *be* verbs. She identified 14 of these morphemes that seemed to undergo substantial change in children's usage and for which the obligatory contexts were easy to establish. *Obligatory contexts* refer to those places in a sentence where a morpheme, if absent, would be considered to have been omitted, rendering the sentence grammatically incorrect by adult standards. So, for example, the sentence *The psychologist is dreaming* would be considered to contain an obligatory context for the *-ing* morpheme. If the *-ing* were omitted—The psychologist is dream—the sentence would be considered grammatically incorrect. Cazden, and other researchers who enlarged these studies, found that children learning English acquired the 14 morphemes in a relatively consistent order. Between the ages of 2 and 3, children were found to learn to produce the *-ing* ending, plural /s/ and possessive ('s), and the prepositions *in* and *on* in nearly all their obligatory contexts. Children learning other languages, however, do not acquire these morphemes in the same order as English-speaking children do (Kvaal, Shipstcad-Cox, Nevitt, Hodson, & Launer, 1988). The differences found across languages in the order of acquisition of grammatical morphemes are thought to reflect the fact that some languages have more difficult or complicated ways of expressing the meaning encoded by these morphemes. For example, in English, articles are learned relatively late, but in Spanish, children produce articles as one of their earliest morphemes. The relative ease of acquisition of articles in Spanish is thought to be a result of the fact that the English articles are somewhat harder to hear in running conversation, while the Spanish forms—*el, la, los, las,* and so on—are more acoustically salient. Although children begin using some grammatical morphemes between 2 and 3 years of age, children learning English and other languages continue to make morphological errors and omissions until at least the end of the preschool period.

SENTENCES STRUCTURES

A second aspect of syntactic development is seen in the expansion of the two basic units of simple sentences: the noun phrase (usually the subject or object of a verb) and the verb phrase, or sentence predicate (Miller, 1981). During the telegraphic period, the noun-phrase and verb-phrase segments of the sentence generally contain only 1 word. During the third year, however, child learns to elaborate these elements by adding additional words to each.

When noun-phrase elaboration begins, it generally is seen on nouns that occur alone rather than in a sentence context. Noun-phrase elaboration starts with the addition of a single element, usually an article or a modifier. Modifiers frequently used by 2-year-olds include *this, that, these, those, a, the, some, a lot, more, two, my,* and *your* (Miller, 1981). A child just beginning noun-phrase elaboration would, for example, be likely to say "My kitty!" but not "My big kitty." By the end of the third year, children are embedding elaborated noun phrases within sentences. When this occurs, the elaboration is most likely to occur on the object noun phrase at the end of the sentence rather than on the subject at the beginning (Miller, 1981). So the 3-year-old is apt to say "Mommy has a big ball" but not "My big mommy has a ball." Two-year-olds still frequently omit subject noun phrases; they might say "Want big ball" rather than "I want big ball."

Verb phrase development begins with the production of single verbs that are unmarked for person, tense, or number. The child may say, "He throw ball" to mean "Daddy threw the ball to me." One of the first forms of elaboration of the verb phrase, which appears around 2 years of age, is the use of forms called *catenatives* or *semiauxiliaries*. These are forms that function as unanalyzed wholes for the child but would be broken down into several parts according to adult grammar. They include such forms as *gonna* (going to), *gotta* (got to), *wanna* (want to), and *hafta* (have to), which children use almost like auxiliary or "helping" verbs (Owens, 1992). Two-year olds may say "I gonna help," or "I wanna watch." True auxiliary verbs appear toward the end of the third year; *can* and *will* are the earliest forms to be used. Forms of the auxiliary verb *be* also may emerge at this time but will not be used consistently or with correct subject-verb agreement (Miller, 1981). So the child may say "You am going" or "You going home." Some use of irregular past tense forms (*came, saw, went, fell*) may appear by age 3, although regular past tense forms, which are inflected with *-ed,* may continue to be produced without any inflection (Trantham & Pedersen, 1976). The child may use both "I came home" and "I help Daddy" to refer to events in the past.

SENTENCE TYPES

The third area in which syntactic development is seen is the production of the various sentence types available in the language. Two major sentence variants have been found to show significant development between 2 and 3 years in children acquiring English: negative sentences and questions. Negative intentions appear very early; one of the first preverbal intentions children express is the desire to reject, protest, or deny their their interlocutor's utterance. Early verbal expression of negation is also the rule in development. As we saw earlier, *no* is one of the first words almost every child says, and negative sentences also emerge early in the telegraphic period. Between 2 and 3 years of age, in addition to the already acquired *no* and *not,* the child learns some new negative markers; these include *can't* and *don't*. It is interesting to note that these early negative forms appear *before* their positive correlates *can* and *do* are used (Brown, 1973). When *can't* and *don't* are added to the repertoire of negative markers, the child also modifies the rule for placing them in sentences. Although negative forms were first placed at the beginning of the sentence, children between 2 and 3 years of age begin to move them inside, generally putting them in between the noun and the verb. So the 2-year-old may say "Daddy no eat my candy" or "I can't find it."

Children also ask questions early in their language development. As we saw in the telegraphic period, questions mark the emergence of the heuristic use of language. Between 2 and 3 years, children move beyond the first routine questions to produce novel *what* and *where* questions that are not the result of a learned formula. They can now, for example, not only ask "Whazzat?" but also

"What you eating?" Similarly, they can not only ask "Where Daddy going?" but also "Where my glass of milk?" Still, these questions usually leave out auxiliary and *be* verbs. In this period yes/no questions continue to be marked only by rising intonation (Klima & Bellugi, 1966).

Comprehension

As we saw earlier, children employ a variety of strategies for responding to linguistic input that is beyond their current level of comprehension ability. This process continues in the third year of life and, again, children integrate their newly acquired linguistic skill with prior knowledge to come up with more sophisticated strategies. Chapman (1978) discusses two strategies that are used in the third year of life: the "probable event" and "supplying missing information" strategies.

The probable event strategy allows children to respond correctly to passive sentences that encode events they know to be likely to happen in the world, even when they do not understand the passive structure. For example, 2-year-olds could correctly act out the sentence "The baby is fed by the mommy," not because they really understand the syntax of the sentence, but because they knows mommies usually feed babies, not the other way around. If asked to act out "The mommy is fed by the baby" or even "The baby feeds the mommy," though, 2-year-olds are likely to interpret the sentence according the probability of events, rather than according to its syntactic structure. Similarly, children use the probable event strategy to respond to sentences that contain prepositions they do not fully understand. A young 2-year-old, for example, if asked to put a spoon *under* a cup, would be most likely to put the spoon *in* the cup, because containers, like cups, are usually used to put things *in*.

The strategy of supplying missing information is used to respond to questions that contain question words children do not understand. For example, 2-year-olds usually do not comprehend *when* because of its temporal features. If asked a *when* question, 2-year-olds are likely to respond as if the question contained some other question word that they did understand. For example, if asked, "When did you have lunch?" 2-year-olds would be likely to reply "Hot dogs."

Parental Input

Parents talking to 2-year-olds continue to use a variety of strategies to help the children be successful at conversation. Martlew (1980) showed that mothers provide opportunities for children to make verbal contributions by asking questions about objects and events in the children's experience, talking about what the children have just talked about in a slightly different way, or adding a new idea to the children's comments.

Use of expansions decreases during this period, and mothers of 2-year-olds use a new strategy called "turnabouts" (Kaye & Charney, 1981). These are utterances that structure discourse for children by responding to what they said and at the same time requiring response. Thus these utterances model the back-and-forth structure of conversation and cue children to provide a remark that continues the topic of conversation. For example, the 2-year-old might say "Baby's shoe!" The mother using a turnabout would reply, "Yes, it's a baby's shoe, just like yours, isn't it?"

Picture book reading is another context in which much language facilitation goes on. Snow (1983) discusses book reading as an ideal context in which advanced syntactic and semantic structures are exemplified for children. Because picture books often are read to children over and over, the children have the opportunity to internalize these forms, store them, and use them for later imitation or analysis. Exposure to reading during the preschool years is known to be associated with successful performance in school, as well.

Child Communication

One way in which children's communicative skill advances in the third year of life is through an expansion of the purposes to which language can be put. Children learn to use language to convey new information, to talk about past events, and to imagine or pretend (Chapman, 1981) as well as to combine more than one intention within an utterance. Similarly, 2-year-olds learn to use of variety of forms to express their intentions. They may say either "I want cookie" or "I hungry," for example.

Two-year-olds also become more adept at managing conversation, although they still rely on adults to provide much of the conversation's structure for them. While the basic back-and-forth structure of conversation is mastered early, children between 2 and 3 are learning some of the subtle cues used by speakers to allocate the conversational floor. Children interrupt another speaker relatively infrequently, but when it does happen, it is most likely to occur at the end of a phrase or clause (Ervin-Tripp, 1979). By age 3 children recognize that a pause of more than one second between conversational turns means that the listener is not going to respond (Craig & Gallagher, 1983). During this period children are less likely to use imitation as a means of acknowledgment or as a strategy for fulfilling their turn than they were during the second year (Chapman, 1981), although to some extent they continue to use it.

Children's ability to stick to a topic improves in the third year, although by 36 months only 50% of child utterances still continue the topic of the previous utterance (Bloom, Rocissano, & Hood, 1976). Children of this age have difficulty sustaining a topic for more than one or two turns, particularly if the topic is one they did not initiate (Owens, 1992). Two-year-olds continue topics primarily by means of "adjacency pairs," structured by the mother's turnabouts.

Two-year-olds also begin to learn how to deal with conversational breakdowns. If an adult signals such a breakdown, by asking "What?" the 2-year-old typically responds by either repeating the utterance, usually with some phonetic change (Child: I kit ball. Mother: What? Child: I kick ball.) or by deleting an element (Child: I kick big ball. Mother: What? Child: I kick ball.). At this age, however, children rarely request another speaker to clarify an utterance.

Even at age 2 children realize that one talks differently to different people. Thus, 2-year-olds frequently talk differently to their mother than to their father, often using more polite language to the father. Two-year-olds frequently will speak to babies in a high-pitched voice, as adults do. Another determiner of how we choose to say things is the level of knowledge we believe the listener to possess. For example, if the speaker knows the listener is already looking at a picture of a baby, the speaker may comment "She's cute!" But if the listener is not already looking at the baby, the speaker will need to say something to direct attention to it, and might remark "Look at this picture of Patty's new baby. Isn't she cute!" Two-year-olds are not very good at making such judgments. Frequently they fail to provide necessary information, assuming that adults know everything. This tendency can lead, for example, to a 2-year-old telling his grandmother over the phone, "See, I got this for my birthday!"

Two-year-olds are still in the process of learning the obligation to say things, particularly to make requests, politely. Frequent parent reminders help facilitate this development, and politeness is one of the few aspects of language development that is explicitly taught. Two-year-olds have little flexibility in their range of politeness markers, and if told to "ask more nicely" will either add *please* to their request or produce it with a whining intonation (Bates, 1976). They also may produce problem or need statements, such as "I'm hungry"

or "I can't reach it" as forms of requests. Two-year-olds do understand some of the social parameters of polite requesting and are more likely to include *please* in their request if the listener is bigger, less familiar, or in possession of something they want (Ervin-Tripp & Gordon, 1986).

Summary

Between 24 and 36 months of age, children's language expands from primitive telegraphic sentences to simple grammatical communication. Although young 3-year-olds still make some mistakes in use of grammatical markers, syntactic forms, and speech sounds, their speech will be largely intelligible to people inside and outside the family and will communicate a range of ideas. By 36 months children are beginning to assimilate some of the social conventions for language use, keeping the conversation going, showing some limited topic coherence, talking differently to different people and in different situations. Although they still have much to learn, 3-year-olds are true linguists who have mastered the fundamentals of a first language.

REFERENCES

Bates, E. (1976). *Language and context: The acquisition of pragmatics*. New York: Academic Press.

Bloom, L., Rocissano, L., & Hood, L. (1976). Adult-child discourse: Developmental interaction between information processing and linguistic interaction. *Cognitive Psychology, 8*, 521–552.

Boehm, A. E. (1969). *Boehm test of basic concepts*. New York: The Psychological Corporation-Harcourt Brace Jovanovich.

Brown, R. (1973). *A first language: The early stages*. Cambridge, MA: Harvard University Press.

Cazden, C. (1968). The acquisition of noun and verb inflections. *Child Development, 39*, 433–438.

Chapman, R. (1978). Comprehension strategies in children. In J. F. Kavanaugh & W. Strange (Eds.), *Speech and language in the laboratory, school and clinic* (pp. 308–327). Cambridge, MA: MIT Press.

Chapman, R. (1981). Exploring children's communicative intents. In J. Miller, *Assessing language production in children* (pp. 111–138). Baltimore: University Park Press.

Craig, H., & Gallagher, T. (1983). Adult-child discourse: The conversational relevance of pauses. *Journal of Pragmatics, 7*, 347–360.

Ervin-Tripp, S. (1979). Children's verbal turn-taking. In E. Ochs & B. Schieffelin (Eds.), *Developmental pragmatics* (pp. 1–21). New York: Academic Press.

Ervin-Tripp, S., & Gordon, D. (1986). The development of requests. In R. Schiefelbusch (Ed.), *Language competence: Assessment and intervention* (pp. 22–40). San Diego: College-Hill Press.

Grunwell, P. (1982). *Clinical phonology*. Rockville, MD: Aspen System Corporation.

Haas, A., & Owens, R. (1985, November). *Preschoolers' pronoun strategies: You and me make us*. Paper presented at the American Speech-Language-Hearing Association annual convention. Boston, MA.

Kaye, K., & Charney, R. (1981). Conversational asymmetry between mothers and children. *Journal of Child Language, 8*, 35–49.

Klima, E., & Bellugi, U. (1966). Syntactic regularities in the speech of children. In J. Lyons & R. Wales,

Psycholinguistic papers (pp. 55–68). Edinburgh: Edinburgh University Press.

Kvaal, J. T., Shipstead-Cox, N., Nevitt, S. G., Hodson, B. W., & Launer, P. B. (1988). The acquisition of 10 Spanish morphemes by Spanish-speaking children. *Language, Speech, and Hearing Services in Schools, 19,* 384–394.

Martlew, M. (1980). Mothers' control strategies in dyadic mother/child conversations. *Journal of Psycholinguistic Research, 9,* 327–347.

Miller, J. (1981). *Assessing language production in children.* Baltimore: University Park Press.

Owens, R. E., Jr. (1992). *Language development* (3rd ed.). Columbus, OH: Merrill.

Pease, D. B., Gleason, J. B., & Pan, B. A. (1989). Gaining Meaning: Semantic Development. In J. B. Gleason (Ed.), *The development of language* (pp. 115–150). New York: Merrill.

Shriberg, L., & Kwiatkowski, J. (1980). *Natural process analysis: A procedure for phonological analysis of continuous speech samples.* New York: John Wiley & Sons.

Smith, M. E. (1926). An investigation of the development of the sentence and the extent of vocabulary in young children. *University of Iowa Studies in Child Welfare, 3* (5).

Snow, C. (1983). Literacy and language: Relationships during the preschool years. *Harvard Educational Review, 53,* 165–189.

Trantham, C., & Pedersen, J. (1976). *Normal language development.* Baltimore: Williams & Wilkins.

Tyack, D., & Ingram, D. (1977). Children's production and comprehension of questions. *Journal of Child Language, 4,* 211–224.

14 / Affective Development During the Fourth and Fifth Years of Life

Arietta Slade and Alicia F. Liebermann

Introduction

The period between a child's third and fifth birthday probably has been discussed and written about more extensively than any other period in infancy or early or middle childhood. For many years, this was virtually synonymous with what is widely described as the "oedipal" stage, the important developmental crisis that Freud (1905, 1909) believed spans these years and continues into the sixth and seventh years. For Freud, the move into the oedipal stage marked a vital transition in the process of early psychosexual development, and signalled the beginning of life as a rational, conflicted, reality-oriented, conscious, and sexual individual. Although recent research and developmental study have enlightened us as to the profound significance of the infant and toddler periods for social, emotional, and object relations development, there can be no doubt that Freud was correct in pointing to these years as vital to later psychological organization and adaptation. The 3- and 4-year-old has moved into a stage

that is dramatically different from those that preceded it and equally different from those that will follow it. It is a time of reorganization, of redefining relationships, of redefining the newly emergent self, and of deepening emotional experience and awareness. Oedipal development heralds the emergence of what can genuinely be called the epoch of regnant fantasy of conflict and of complex emotions such as guilt, pride, and desire.

The oedipal period is, of course, the time when children fall in love for the first time. This experience is quite distinct from earlier longings for closeness; it is a child's first experience of desire, incorporating genital sensations, longing, and the wish to possess another exclusively. Usually, the object of childrens affection is the opposite-sex parent—for the boy, his mother; for the girl, her father. The intense feelings of this stage, which some have maintained are among the most powerful a child will ever feel (Brenner, 1955), are accompanied by equally intense feelings of rivalry and competition with the same-sex parent. The child is catapulted from a dyadic to a triadic existence. He recognizes, also for the first time, that

112

not only does *he* desire his mother, but his father does too. The strains of this triangle, and of his awareness of its interrelationships, are what constitute the oedipal crisis. The child cannot solve his dilemma with action, as Oedipus himself did. He cannot do away with his rival, nor can he possess his desired object. Therefore, his resolution of this crisis of desire must be a psychological one: He must transform his longing into productive and acceptable activity, his rivalry into identification, and his guilt into a broader sense of conscience, morality, and compassion. Psychoanalysts believe that the individual child's resolution of this complex panoply of relationships, interrelationships, and emotion will determine the course of later relationships and will contribute significantly to the organization of defensive processes and the quality of adaptation. The individual's character style and his particular adult neurosis will be powerfully predicted by his resolution of what is known as his "infantile neurosis" (A. Freud, 1965, p. 149).

Time and again, close observers of preschool-age children have confirmed the essential truth of Freud's basic observations (Erikson, 1950; Fraiberg, 1969). However, as developmental research has recently begun to demonstrate, these fundamental changes in children's orientation to the world do not derive solely or even largely from changes in drive or psychosexual development. Rather, they are part of a larger set of developmental processes that underlie children's changing awareness of self, other, affect, and relationships; these changes dramatically alter their views of themselves and their relationships to their world. For our purposes, the term *oedipal* will be used to refer to the broad range of changes observed during these years, rather than to the more specific emergence of the individual child's familial attachment. Although these libidinal relationships certainly take center stage at points during these years and constitute what Pine (1985) calls "affectively supercharged moments," there are other—equally supercharged—moments that take place as well. Together these will lead to the changes that will make school entry and the development of a more rational, separate, and independent child possible.

Developmental transitions are the result of shifts in underlying organization, and usually follow maturational changes (Greenspan, 1989;

Stern, 1985); biological changes dramatically alter both cognitive and affective processes and herald the emergence of new modes of adaptation. The resolution of the rapprochment crisis and the establishment of object constancy during the latter phases of the separation-individuation process are made possible by the establishment and integration of early symbolic abilities. Ironically, the establishment and elaboration of these processes can be seen as triggering the next period of imbalance, leading to what Piaget termed *décalage* (Piaget, 1924). As will be described in this chapter children's ability to recognize and acknowledge new levels of complexity in their world triggers the moods and powerful affects that we characterize as oedipal. As time passes and maturation proceeds, the development of the means for coping with this awareness will permit him to resolve the dilemmas it poses.

The Oedipal Period—Classical Views

Freud (1905/1953) believed that the shift into the oedipal period is made possible by developmental changes in drive expression. The genital region is gradually libidinized, and both the pleasure and frustration of oral and anal gratification diminish; they will now be experienced via the "language" and modes of the genitals. As this phase begins, children become increasingly aware of their genitals and of genital sensations. He or she is intensely excited by genital stimulation; pleasure and excitement in a range of situations are often experienced in terms of these genital sensations. This shift in mode of expression, from anal to genital, changes the quality of children's concerns as well as their relationships. Thus, the concern with autonomous success that characterized the 2-year-old gives way to a new awareness of the body and its power. The interest that a children previously had paid to their feces and the investment they previously had made in independence are now transformed into the desire for initiative and prowess.

There is in every child at every stage a new miracle of vigorous unfolding, which constitutes a new hope and a new responsibility for all. Such is the sense and the pervading quality of initiative. The criteria for all these senses and qualities are the same: a crisis, more or less beset with fumbling and fear, is resolved, in that the child suddenly seems to "grow together" both in his person and in his body . . . Initiative adds to autonomy the quality of undertaking, planning and "attacking" a task for the sake of being active and on the move, where before self-will, more often than not, inspired acts of defiance or, at any rate, protested independence . . . The ambulatory stage and that of infantile genitality add to the inventory of basic social modalities that of "making," first in the sense of "being on the make." There is no simpler, stronger word for it; it suggests pleasure in attack and conquest. In the boy, the emphasis remains on phallic-intrusive modes; in the girl it turns to modes of "catching" in more aggressive forms of snatching or in the milder form of making oneself attractive and endearing. (Erikson, 1950, p. 255)

The distinction is frequently made between "phallic" and later "genital" modes of relating to the world. "Phallic" is a term that connotes these early, vulnerable efforts at conquest and struggle. This phase marks the first steps in evolving sexuality; the development of more mature, related, and dimensional sexuality awaits the development of more "genital" modes of relating, well into adolescence and early adulthood.

One of the first manifestations of the move into oedipal functioning is an interest in the body and its workings, and a new kind of concern with prowess and intactness. There is in boys an unabashed interest in genitals and genital stimulation. In girls, there is less concern with overt prowess, and more concern with genital stimulation. The awareness of anatomical sex differences takes on new meaning and intensity (Galenson & Roiphe, 1971). Accompanying this concern and power is a new kind of vulnerability. Castration anxiety often emerges in dramatic ways in children this age, who may be tremendously concerned with bodily injury. Three- and 4-year-olds can be terrified by the sight of their own blood and often need reassurance that they can survive small injuries. Children of this age are very sensitive to slights to their bodies, to their strength and abilities, and to the integrity of their ideas and feelings. These children evidence a kind of moodiness and sensitivity, a new kind of concern with boundaries and with right and wrong. Children's newfound investment in their body and in their powers lead them to become more aware of those around them and to wish to engage with them in

an entirely new way. Interactions now become proving grounds for their rightness and their desirability. One of the most dramatic features of this age is children's curiosity: "Why?" is asked relentlessly, as children try to come to terms with the many levels of their new awareness.

These developments set the stage for the oedipal romance, children's love affair with the opposite-sex parent. Freud maintained that the reasons behind developing such feelings are simple: Powerful libidinal strivings are experienced in relationship to the person children are is closest to. The universality of this fantasy has been well documented. Young children can be quite unabashed and articulate in their wishes, and often give direct voice to their wish to replace the rival parent: "Why can't Daddy just go away?" These fantasies often emerge in play, in spontaneous remarks, and in dreams. And although genital feelings certainly play a role in their longings—as can be confirmed by any parent who has been the object of such desire—children wish to possess and seduce but not bed their parent. Sexuality, in the adult sense, is not the issue; exclusive possession is. Feelings of hatred for the opposite-sex parent often can be as powerful as the desire to possess; but they are experienced within the context of a simultaneous ongoing love for the rival. As a result, these feelings cause tremendous guilt and anxiety, and are thought to account for many of the anxieties and phobias that are intrinsic to this period. Murderous fantasies toward one's rival are projected onto the external world and fill children with fear of imagined danger, such as monsters, fierce animals, and the like. Presumably this is the youngsters' only means of coping with their aggression, and parents are often astonished at the intensity of their children's aggression at this stage. Powerfully afraid of being excluded themselves, of being humiliated in their quest for intimacy or of being overwhelmed by their rivals, children can become strong-willed, articulate competitors.

It was this turning to the opposite-sex parent, Freud believed, in concert with feeling intense rivalry and competition toward the same-sex parent, that triggers the development of the sense of guilt, morality, conscience, and conflict that typifies modern man (Freud, 1930/1961). Children must translate their longing for the opposite-sex parent into activities that are less fraught with guilt and torment, and must transform their rivalries and jealousies into identification. These concerns must be "quieted" or sublimated and transformed into more productive, socially acceptable modes of learning. It is the sublimation of sexual aggressive energies that accounts for the tremendous investment in competence and learning that is the hallmark of the latency or postoedipal period. Although children may have felt remorse or shame at earlier points in their development, this period marks the first true emergence of guilt and internalized conflict. A child becomes—in essence—pitted against himself. This is the meaning of internalized conflict. He does not avoid killing his father because he is told not to, or is kept from doing so. He is kept in check by feelings of love for his father, by feelings of guilt, and by fears of retribution. These are internal experiences that are in direct opposition to his longings. For the first time in his life, he is at war with himself, *not* with his parents.

Oedipal developments, like the ones just described, appear to be universal; they take place even in families where the family triangle does not take the middle-class, Western form of mother, father, and child. The issues of initiative, desire, rivalry, and guilt do not confine themselves to such situations, but are translated in a variety of ways depending on the particular family and the particular possibilities for romance. An uncle or brother can serve as an oedipal rival, and humiliation from any source can wound. In today's modern "reconstituted" families, oedipal rivalries can be experienced toward new stepparents, regardless of their gender. A child raised by two adults of the same gender can "triangulate" these relationships in much the same way children in more traditional nuclear families do. Although it was long believed that children's later sexual orientation was a function of their resolution of the oedipal struggle, an individual's sexual orientation is now understood to originate from a more complex set of variables, many of which are likely biological. The quality and pattern of object relations, particularly those of this period, account only partially for an individual's later sexual development (Coates, 1992). Rather, the setbacks and accomplishments of the oedipal drama are thought to determine the individual's ability to relate to others in mature, dimensional ways, to balance his or her own feelings and wishes against the broader needs of the family and their interrelationships.

Freud discovered the oedipal phase largely through his work with adult patients. He had rela-

tively little experience working with children, although later psychoanalytic work with children documented many of his basic assumptions (Erikson, 1950; A. Freud, 1965). Freud suggested that oedipal concerns would emerge sometime around a child's fifth birthday. Although this is certainly a time when children are quite vocal about their wishes to possess and marry their beloved and about their fantasies of eliminating their rival, many children become aware of the family triangle well before they turn 4; in fact oedipally tinged play and fantasy often will color the later stages of the anal phase and the separation-individuation process. As the issues of the earlier stages wane, the concerns of the later stage emerge. Similarly, manifestations of oedipal yearnings, fantasies, and conflicts may be evident well into a child's seventh year and often intermingle with the concerns and interests of the next phase, latency.

Like any crisis or phase, the shape, intensity, and timing of the oedipal period are multidetermined and have much to do with the nature of a particular child's temperament, the quality of the caregiving environment, and the mesh between them. Many latter-day theories of temperament have, interestingly, much in common with Freudian notions of drive and instinct, in the sense that temperament is viewed as modulating experience in an individual way. In addition, the issues of this phase are resolved somewhat differently depending upon the gender of the child. Freud maintained that girls' oedipal development proceeded along a parallel—although obviously opposite—course to boys', but was inevitably compromised by her necessarily having to shift her libidinal investment from the preoedipal mother to the oedipal father. Boys do not have to shift their libidinal cathexis from one object to another; rather, their libidinal relationship to their mothers is simply transformed. Freud saw this complicating factor as invariably compromising female development. These views have continued to generate controversy for years and have led some feminists to dismiss Freud's contributions altogether. However, most scholars now agree that Freud's views on female oedipal development were considerably less developed than his views of male oedipal development; only recently have psychoanalysts and other theorists begun to describe the significant components of female oedipal development as these affect future relationships and self feeling (Benjamin, 1988; Chodorow, 1978; Gilligan, 1982; Mahler, Pine, & Bergman, 1975).

The Oedipal Period— Developmental Perspectives

Children's concern with the wonder of their bodies, with exclusive possession of the object of desire, and with feelings of rivalry along with fears of humiliation and retribution, are a hallmark of the fourth and fifth years of life. It is difficult, when observing 3- and 4-year-olds, not to be compelled by how concerned they are with their bodies, with their genitals, with doggedly asserting their strength and prowess, with wooing their chosen, and with defeating their rivals. Considerations of drive development take on new meaning and new veracity. Freud saw children's concerns with rivalry and competitiveness as the sequelae of enhanced libidinal investment in phallic functioning. However, these shifts in the nature and content of children's emotional experience must be understood as inextricably tied to developments in ego functioning, specifically to shifts in thinking, remembering, and understanding. Taken together, the many cognitive developments that occur over the course of this period dramatically alter their ability to test reality, to regulate impulses, and emotions, and, finally, to resolve the oedipal crisis. Children's increased awareness of the relationships in their world, their appreciation of the nuances of emotion and fantasy, and their use of increasingly sophisticated and ideational defenses must be seen as a function of these developmental changes. Recent advances in developmental study offer an important view of the processes that lead to new levels of awareness, and provide the means to cope with that awareness.

Developmental psychology, as exemplified by the work of Piaget, had for many decades emphasized the cognitive immaturity and egocentrism of children of this age. However, as studies of children in naturalistic settings have abounded and researchers have developed more sophisticated means of examining children's thought processes, considerable evidence of their many capacities has been amassed. In fact, cognitive developmentalists see the changes of this period as indicative of a major revision of children's frameworks for understanding emotion and therefore of their "theory of mind" (Harris, 1994). Studies of the way children represent their experience in spontaneous monologues and dialogues with others provide dramatic evidence of their emerging ability to perceive relationships in their world, and to communicate their knowledge of such relationships to others (Nelson, 1986, 1989). Researchers have discovered that children can provide narrative accounts of events in their lives that are remarkably nuanced and complex, and that convey their appreciation of their own and others' multiple relationships to reality and to each other.

Erikson (1950) used the word *initiative* to describe the child's relationship to the world during this stage. Interestingly, the correctness of his term is underscored by a wealth of research demonstrating a child's increasing ability to experience himself as a narrator and an agent in his life. No longer the passive recipient of the parents' ministrations, 3- to 4-year olds are moving quickly beyond autonomy to recognizing their role as people who can and want to make things happen. By the age of 3, children are usually enrolled in nursery school; they are speaking in complex sentences; they can make themselves understood easily; and they are eating, toiletting, and sleeping on their own. Children's make-believe offers dramatic evidence of this shift. Simple stories offered as accompaniements to action schemes become the essence of the play. They become layered and textured, with strands of different themes woven together in complex ways (Slade, 1986). The introduction of children's storytelling is one of the first and most compelling pieces of evidence for their emerging sense of agency. The action no longer dictates the play, the story does. Whereas a younger child given a group of trucks will be moved by the physical attributes of the trucks themselves, a child of this age will provide a story of truck repair and organize her play accordingly. Play figures can become agents in the play; characters are designated as able to make things happen (Watson & Fischer, 1977; Wolf, Rygh, & Altshuler, 1984). Finally, children will incorporate objects into their play that are not direct replicas of the referent (i.e., a youngster will use a toy telephone as a gas pump); this signals the child's awareness that she herself can take an active role in transforming reality.

Wolf (1990) has demonstrated this beautifully in her description of the emergence of the "authorial" self. *Authorship* is the ability to act independently of the facts of a situation. In children between the ages of 2 and 4, two abilities appear that make this separation possible. The first is the ability to "uncouple" lines of experience using "pretense, obfuscation, and deceit. In each of these situations, the self rearranges, edits or changes the 'facts' to align with some exogenous goal, hope, or wish. This cleavage essentially creates a new experience of self" (p. 185). Reality can be distorted in a deliberate way, either for play or for deception. The second ability to emerge is the acquisition of complex syntax, which allows children to make "articulate and public" the various stances they take toward experience. The children's use of linguistic markers provides evidence for the increasing heterogeneity of their perspective. The youngsters talk about the play and during the play reveal a number of stances, all of which reflect the recognition that any experience can be seen from a number of vantage points. These multiple stances make it possible for reality to be construed from a number of angles, based on an increasing appreciation of its many contrasts and complexities. Together, the ability to take heterogeneous stances toward reality and to be able to transform reality using a "whole range of editorial, fictional, and even deceitful behaviors" result in the emergence of the "authorial" self. This sense of authorship plays a pivotal role in both the drama and the ultimate resolution of this stage. Children of 2 take in events serially; they do not yet recognize the relationship *between* events. Children of 3 and 4, by contrast, have begun to develop an awareness of relationships in the world that are external to their desires. They have also begun to appreciate that there is no such thing as a single reality; rather, reality is defined by the stance and perspective they take in relationship to it. The joy and exhilaration of children's early autonomous strivings give way to a more nuanced awareness of life's complexity.

Much of the moodiness and vulnerability that is characteristic of the oedipal period must be understood in light of these changes in children's perception of the world. As cognitive development proceeds, they begin to be aware of the network or system of relationships among people in their human environment. Researchers have used the term *intersubjectivity* to describe the infant's awareness of others' mental states and affects (Stern, 1985; Trevarthen, 1979). At this stage, intersubjectivity extends beyond self and other to the self in relationship to numerous others and to the relationships that exist among them. At times, this awareness and the child's changing theory of mind cannot help but be threatening. Just as child in rapprochement experiences vulnerability in his new "I"-ness, so does the oedipal child experience the vulnerability inherent in her efforts to initiate and change events and relationships in her life. Suddenly aware of the world beyond the dyad she had grown so comfortable at navigating, she does not yet have a sense of how she will cope with the challenges posed by the complexity she must now acknowledge. Children's moodiness and concrete adherence to primitive moral principles provide evidence of their efforts to maintain their equilibrium in the face of these new and dramatic changes.

Some of children's vulnerability must be understood in terms not only of the extent of their new awareness, but in terms of its limitations as well. Children under 4 cannot coordinate or simultaneously maintain multiple representations of the same information (Wolf, 1990). It takes years for the gradual accretion of self-knowledge to translate into knowledge about the world of other people. Citing research by Fischer and his colleagues (Fischer, Hand, Watson, Van Parys, & Tucker, 1984) and Flavell (1986), Wolf (1990) notes that "it is improbable to think of children below school age understanding, as a matter of principle, how the several aspects of their selves are coordinated into a single, albeit multifaceted self. Similarly, before that time, it is unlikely that children realize that the multistranded quality of their own internal experiences is a general property of human minds" (p. 205). In this sense, children's moodiness and distress during the oedipal period must have as much to do with what they *don't* understand as with what they do. This is reminiscent of Kagan's (1981) account of the distress that often accompanies early self-awareness in 2-year-olds.

Naturally, cognitive changes also lead to developments in children's understanding of emotional processes. By the time they are 3 or 4, children show a remarkable ability to understand another's feelings and to respond to them, even if they do not (apparently) feel similarly themselves (Stewart & Marvin, 1984). This kind of perspective taking allows them to comfort others, as well as to understand what will disturb and provoke them. Children can now figure out what kinds of situations will evoke what kinds of emotions and to imagine themselves in the mental world of another. They also can imagine their responses to different situations, depending on their desires. Children can now pretend to want or to imagine wanting something "that another person wants. If the child now examines the reality facing that other person, he can anticipate what emotion will ensue when reality either satisfies or frustrates that desire. The child can use the outcome of that simulation to attribute to the other person the appropriate emotion, be it sadness or happiness" (Harris, 1989, p. 77).

Thus, children are not only aware of relationships and of interrelationships; they can imagine others' feelings and responses as well. Certainly, within the context of oedipal developments, this awareness will have important sequelae, and must be seen as contributing directly to the affective changes of the period. The child of 3 or 4 years now realizes that his father may be angry at his assaults; he also can envision and desire his mother's exclusive love. He can imagine his father's feelings for his mother as well. He is not simply trying to change the way he feels; he also is trying to change the way others feel. Oedipal guilt and anxiety must be seen as direct outgrowths of these changes in imaginative abilities. The child feels guilty for what he imagines will happen to his rival, and he feels anxious about his rival's imagined response.

According to Freud, superego or moral development was an outcome of the oedipal crisis. A 3- or 4-year-old child's wish to preserve parental relationships leads him or her to internalize their prohibitions; ultimately, these internalizations function to regulate id impulses and facilitate their transformation into other forms of expression. Recently, however, researchers have found that children as young as 3 years of age clearly know the difference between right and wrong, use parental prohibitions to inform their

behavior, and are able—albeit in a limited way—to grapple with moral dilemmas (Dunn, 1988; Buchsbaum & Emde, 1990; Emde & Buchsbaum, 1990; Smetana, 1985). Thus, children appear to be able to recognize and describe the difference between right and wrong; and more than that, they can act to adjust their behavior in accord with such knowledge much earlier than had originally been formulated by psychoanalysts. Emde and Buchsbaum (1990) suggest the possibility of biological preparedness; cognitive developmentalists, such as Smetana (1985) and Harris (1989), propose that the perception of right and wrong is an outgrowth of the child's ability to evaluate and understand his or her reality. Evidence of these developments raises the possibility that the development of a primitive moral sense is a trigger for, rather than an outgrowth of, the oedipal struggle. Children have a basic sense of right and wrong that antedates the development of fantasies of possession and rivalry. These fantasies cannot help but be evaluated in light of this moral sense, and are—to a greater or lesser extent—troubling to them.

Emde and Buchsbaum (1990) suggest that the development of moral narratives provides evidence of what they term "autonomy and connectedness." The emerging moral sense serves as a modulating, regulating voice; it is the voice of "we." It allows children to be at once autonomous and at the same time connected to the "developing sense of we and of the interpersonal world of shared meaning" (p. 45). Thus, the early establishment of libidinal object constancy (Mahler et al., 1975) is modified over time; it adds to the "I" and "you" a representation of "we." Interestingly, Emde and Buchsbaum (1990) also speak to the more dimensional quality of children's autonomy at this age: "We believe that the more sophisticated narrative responses provide evidence for a new sense of autonomy (with enhanced control and power) that emerges from the connectedness. This is what we have referred to as an executive sense of we" (p. 55). From this perspective, the sense of initiative and authorship described by Erikson (1950) and Wolf (1990) is directly related to children's developing awareness of interpersonal relationships and interrelationships.

Among other things, the resolution to the oedipal crisis is signaled by children's ability to temper anger toward their rivals with love; this is achieved through the establishment of positive identifications. The move into latency is signaled by a more mature emotionality, by the replacement of primitive defenses such as denial with more rational, flexible defenses such as sublimation and reaction formation. Developmental psychology has amply confirmed that denial is slowly replaced by a more dimensional appreciation of emotional reality (Harris, 1989). However, although Freud understood this shift as tied to superego development and an evolving pattern of defense, both psychoanalysts and developmental psychologists have tied these shifts to cognitive changes that are likely related to underlying neurological maturation (Harris, 1989, 1994; Shapiro & Perry, 1976). Latency-age children are able to use reason in an entirely new way and to understand that feelings are mental processes and not actions. While they may still feel guilty for their feelings (because they can now imagine their effects were they translated into action), they also are aware that these are internal experiences that can be kept to themselves (Harris, 1989).

Latency-age children also can begin to acknowledge that they have mixed feelings about many of the people and events in their life. To the child of 3 or 4, the possibility that he may have love as well as hate feelings seems overwhelming. To compare them, however, is virtually inconceivable, because these two experiences are considered contradictory and mutually exclusive. Although the toddler may express ambivalence in behavior (Ainsworth, Blehar, Waters, & Wall, 1978), the 3- and 4-year-old does not yet understand that he *can* feel two things at more or less the same time. In fact, there is considerable evidence that many children cannot acknowledge or recognize the existence of mixed feelings until they are 8- to 10-years-old (Harris, 1989; Harter & Whitesell, 1989), although some researchers (Donaldson & Westerman, 1986) find evidence of such acknowledgment in 6-year-olds. Harris (1989) suggests that the family context may be one of the earliest arenas in which the child both experiences and acknowledges mixed feelings. In families where emotional vacillation is unpredictable and frightening, cognitive processes may not be successfully applied to affectively charged situations.

Although attachment researchers have concerned themselves primarily with the periods of infancy and toddlerhood, a number of studies have demonstrated that the quality of early attachments has long-lasting effects that span the preschool years (Cicchetti, Cummings, Greenberg, & Marvin, 1990). Children whose early attachments were secure typically meet the challenges of this period with a wide array of competencies: they are able to approach tasks with enthusiasm and an eagerness to achieve mastery (although these do not override other relational pleasures) (Maslin-Cole & Spieker, 1990), they interact enthusiastically and positively with peers (Waters, Wippman, & Sroufe, 1979), they represent themselves in positive ways (Cassidy, 1990), they are more ego-resilient (Arend, Gove, & Sroufe, 1979), and they are able to describe their emotions in an open fashion. They can turn to teachers as facilitators, and do not revert to earlier, dependent modes of relating (Sroufe, 1983; Sroufe, Fox, & Pancake, 1983). They are self-sufficient and self-reliant. Interestingly, an early positive relationship with father is associated with adaptive levels of self-control in preschoolers (Easterbrooks & Goldberg, 1990). Children's success at navigating triangular relationships will be influenced by their having had prior positive relationships with both parents; then, both mother and father are perceived as positive figures during the period of oedipal turmoil.

Research in this area also has begun to investigate some of the factors underlying the fact that not all secure children are necessarily socially competent and well-adapted preschoolers (Easterbrooks & Goldberg, 1990; Erickson, Sroufe, & Egeland, 1985). Given the emotional and cognitive challenges of this period, such findings are not surprising. As Sroufe (1983) has pointed out, the quality of early care is not the only factor influencing adaptation during the preschool years. Equally important is the parent's ability to manage the aggressive impulses and feelings that are so much a part of the period. Other factors include the effects of parental stresses that mitigate emotional availability (Egeland & Farber, 1984). Erickson and her colleagues (Erickson et al., 1985) report that some children judged secure in infancy were found to have behavior problems at 4 years of age. Examination of parent-child interaction data suggested that children whose mothers were unable to help them negotiate subsequent developmental stages—by providing age-appropriate toys and guidance at 30 months and by providing support and encouragement alongside limits and consistency at 4 years—were those most likely to develop behavior problems. These same children were also less affectionate with their mothers. Similarly, anxiously attached children whose parents were able to provide support and structure during the preschool period did not develop behavior problems. Thus, ongoing patterns within the family play a vital role in determining children's adaptation (Marvin & Stewart, 1991).

We have described this phase primarily in terms of internal struggles and resolutions. However, both the parents' response and availability during the child's efforts to come to grips with the complexities he is facing, as well as the availability of ongoing stable, sustaining images of self and other are critical to successful adaptation. Children of this age demand that they be recognized in ways that can be very unsettling to parents, and are able to arouse feelings of rivalry and competition in the most mature adults. Parents must sometimes allow the child to feel that he has won without giving him the sense that he has outstripped them; at other times, they must curb his initiatives without arousing feelings of humiliation and guilt. The oedipal crisis often reawakens the memory of old battles (Benedek, 1959), and can provide new opportunities for the parents to re-solve some of their own neurotic conflicts and difficulties.

Conclusion

The period between a child's third and fifth birthdays is a time of tremendous change—for the child herself, for the parents, and for the family. The cognitive and emotional challenges of this era are many; it is a period of crisis and transition, and only gradually is internal stability achieved. Children must cope with an increasing awareness of themselves and of others alongside internal changes in their sense of their bodies and their powers. The clash of their own needs along with their emerging knowledge of the social world and its conventions provokes tremendous guilt and sharpens their moral strivings. Thus begins the gradual tempering of children's rigid superego and the advent of a new rationality. The ego develops dramatically during this period. Cognitive development will make possible the emergence of ego functions to help them cope with the intense feelings and longings that characterize these years. In their early manifestations, these changes create uncertainty and anxiety; ultimately, they give way to reason and productivity.

REFERENCES

Ainsworth, M. D. S., Blehar, M., Waters, E., & Wall, S. (1978). *Patterns of attachment: A psychological study of the Strange Situation.* Hillsdale, NJ: Erlbaum.

Arend, R., Gove, F., & Sroufe, L. A. (1979). Continuity of individual adaptation from infancy to kindergarten: A predictive study of ego-resiliency and curiosity in pre-schoolers. *Child Development, 50,* 950–959.

Benedek, T. (1959). Parenthood as a developmental phase. *Journal of the American Psychoanalytic Association, 7,* 389–417.

Benjamin, J. (1988). *The bonds of love.* New York: Pantheon Books

Brenner, C. (1955). *An elementary textbook of psychoanalysis.* Garden City, NY: Doubleday Anchor.

Buchsbaum, H. K., & Emde, R. N. (1990). Play narratives in 36 month-old children. *Psychoanalytic Study of the Child, 45,* 129–155.

Cassidy, J. (1990). Theoretical and methodological considerations in the study of attachment and self in young children. In M. T. Greenberg, D. Cicchetti, & E. M. Cummings (Eds.), *Attachment in the preschool years* (pp. 87–120). Chicago: University of Chicago Press.

Chodorow, N. (1978). *The reproduction of mothering: Psychoanalysis and the sociology of gender.* Berkeley: University of California Press.

Cicchetti, D., Cummings, M., Greenberg, M., & Marvin, R. (1990). An organizational perspective on attachment beyond infancy: Implications for theory, measurement and research. In M. T. Greenberg, D. Cicchetti, & E. M. Cummings (Eds.), *Attachment in the preschool years* (pp. 3–50). Chicago: University of Chicago Press.

Coates, S. (1992). The etiology of boyhood gender identity disorder: An integrative model. In J. W. Barron, M. N. Eagle, & D. L. Wolitzky (Eds.), *Interface of psychoanalysis and psychology* (pp. 245–265). Washington, DC: American Psychological Association.

Donaldson, S., & Westerman, M. (1986). Development

of children's understanding of ambivalence and causal theories of emotions. *Developmental Psychology, 22,* 655–662.

Dunn, J. (1988). *The beginnings of social understanding.* Cambridge, MA: Harvard University Press.

Easterbrooks, M. A., & Goldberg, W. A. (1990). Security of toddler-parent attachment: Relation to children's sociopersonality functioning during kindergarten. In M. T. Greenberg, D. Cicchetti, & E. M. Cummings (Eds.), *Attachment in the preschool years* (pp. 221–245). Chicago: University of Chicago Press.

Egeland, B., & Farber, E. A. (1984). Infant-mother attachment: Factors related to its development and changes over time. *Child Development, 55,* 753–771.

Emde, R. N., & Buchsbaum, H. (1990). "Didn't you hear my mommy?": Autonomy with connectedness in moral self-emergence. In D. Cicchetti & M. Beeghly (Eds.), *The self in transition: Infancy to childhood* (pp. 35–60). Chicago: University of Chicago Press.

Erickson, M. F., Sroufe, L. A., & Egeland, B. (1985). The relationship between quality of attachment and behavioral problems in preschool in a high risk sample. In I. Bretherton & E. Waters (Eds.), *Growing points in attachment theory and research: Monographs of the Society for Research in Child Development, 50* (1–2, Serial #209). 147–167.

Erikson, E. H. (1950). *Childhood and society.* New York: W. W. Norton.

Fischer, K. W., Hand, H., Watson, M. W., Van Parys, M., & Tucker, J. (1984). Putting the child into socialization. In L. G. Katz, P. J. Wagemaker, & K. Steiner (Eds.), *Current topics in early childhood education, Vol. 5.* Norwood, NJ: Ablex.

Flavell, J. (1986). The development of children's knowledge about the appearance-reality distinction. *American Psychologist, 41,* 418–425.

Freud, A. (1965). *Normality and pathology in childhood.* New York: International Universities Press.

Freud, S. (1953). Three essays on the theory of sexuality. In J. Strachey (Ed. and Trans.), *The standard edition of the complete psychological works of Sigmund Freud* (hereafter *Standard edition*) (Vol. 7, pp. 135–243). London: Hogarth Press. (Original work published 1905.)

Freud, S. (1955). Analysis of a phobia in a five-year old boy. In *Standard edition)* (Vol. 10, pp. 5–149). London: Hogarth Press. (Original work published 1909.)

Freud, S. (1959). Character and anal erotism. In *Standard edition* (Vol. 9, pp. 167–177). London: Hogarth Press. (Original work published 1908.)

Freud, S. (1961). Civilization and its discontents. In *Standard edition* (Vol. 21, pp. 59–145). London: Hogarth Press. (Original work published 1924)

Galenson, E., & Roiphe, H. (1971). The impact of early sexual discovery on mood, defensive organization and symbolization. *Psychoanalytic Study of the Child, 26,* 195–216.

Gilligan, C. (1982). *In a different voice: Psychological theory and women's development.* Cambridge, MA: Harvard University Press.

Greenspan, S. I. (1989). *The development of the ego.* Madison, CT: International Universities Press.

Harris, P. L. (1989). *Children and emotion.* Oxford: Basil Blackwell.

Harris, P. L. (1994). The child's understanding of emotion: Developmental change and the family environment. *Journal of Child Psychology and Psychiatry, 35,* 3–28.

Harter, S., & Whitesell, N. (1989). Developmental changes in children's emotion concepts. In C. Saarni & P. L. Harris (Eds.), *Children's understanding of emotion* (pp. 81–116). New York: Cambridge University Press.

Kagan, J. (1981). *The second year: The emergence of self-awareness.* Cambridge, MA: Harvard Universities Press.

Mahler, M., Pine, F., & Bergman, A. (1975). *The psychological birth of the human infant.* New York: Basic Books.

Marvin, R., & Stewart, R. B. (1991). A family systems framework for the study of attachment. In M. T. Greenberg, D. Cicchetti, & E. M. Cummings (Eds.), *Attachment in the preschool years* (pp. 51–87). Chicago: University of Chicago Press.

Maslin-Cole, C., & Spieker, S. J. (1990). Attachment as a basis of independent motivation: A view from risk and nonrisk samples. In M. T. Greenberg, D. Cicchetti, & E. M. Cummings (Eds.), *Attachment in the preschool years* (pp. 245–272). Chicago: University of Chicago Press.

Nelson, K. (1986). *Event knowledge: Structure and function in development.* Hillsdale, NJ: Erlbaum.

Nelson, K., (1989). Monologue as representation of real-life experience. In K. Nelson (Ed.), *Narratives from the crib* (pp. 27–73). Cambridge, MA: Harvard University Press.

Piaget, J. (1926). *The language and thought of the child.* London: Routledge, Kegan & Paul.

Piaget, J. (1962). *Play, dreams and imitation in childhood.* New York: Norton. (Originally published 1951.)

Pine, F. (1985). *Developmental theory and clinical process.* New York: Basic Books.

Shapiro, T., & Perry, R. (1976). Latency revisited. *Psychoanalytic Study of the Child.*

Slade, A. (1986). Symbolic play and separation-individuation: A naturalistic study. *Bulletin of the Menninger Clinic, 50,* 541–563.

Smetana, J. (1985). Preschool children's conceptions of transgressions: Effects of varying moral and conventional domain-related attributes. *Developmental Psychology, 21,* 18–29.

Sroufe, L. A. (1983). Infant-caregiver attachment and patterns of adaptation in preschool: The roots of maladaptation and competence. In M. Perlmutter (Ed.), *Minnesota symposium in child psychology* (Vol. 16, pp. 41–83). Hillsdale, NJ: Erlbaum.

Sroufe, L. A., Fox, N. E., & Pancake, V. (1983). Attachment and dependency in developmental perspective. *Child Development, 54,* 1615–1627.

Stern, D. N. (1985). *The interpersonal world of the infant.* New York: Basic Books.

Stewart, R. B., & Marvin, R. S. (1984). Sibling reltaions: The role of conceptual perspective-taking in the ontogeny of sibling caregiving. *Child Development, 55*, 1322–32.

Trevarthen, C. (1979). Communication and cooperation in early infancy: A description of primary intersubjectivity. In M. Bullowa (Ed.), *Before speech: The beginning of interpersonal communication.* New York: Cambridge University Press.

Waters, E., Wippman, J., & Sroufe, L. A. (1979). Attachment, positive affect, and competence in the peer group: Two studies in construct validation. *Child Development, 50*, 821–829.

Watson, M. W., & Fischer, K. W. (1977). A developmental sequence of agent use in later infancy. *Child Development, 48*, 828–36.

Wolf, D. P. (1990). Being of several minds. In D. Cicchetti & M. Beeghly (Eds.), *The self in transition: Infancy to childhood* (pp. 183–213). Chicago: University of Chicago Press.

Wolf, D. P., Rygh, J., & Altshuler, J. (1984). Agency and experience: Actions and states in play narratives. In I. Bretherton (Ed.), *Symbolic Play* (pp. 195–217). Orlando, FL: Academic Press.

15 / Cognitive Development During the Fourth and Fifth Years of Life

Holly A. Ruff

The period from 2 to 3 years of age has been described as an era of elaboration and consolidation of the skills that emerged previously. To some extent, the same can be said of the fourth and fifth years. On the other hand, within this period development advances on so many fronts that children who are 5 years of age can be said to be qualitatively different from children who are just 3. Five-year-olds are more rational individuals, beginning to interact with older children and with adults on a more equal footing. As children approach their fifth birthdays, the gaps in their knowledge and their mistakes in reasoning are less obvious than in the third year. Their language has reached adult standards in many respects, and the rate at which they acquire new words is starting to slow down. Most 5-year-olds are ready for formal schooling, or what Brown, Bransford, Ferrara, and Campione (1983) call "academic cognition." That is, they are ready to learn and think on a more abstract level and to do so in response to the explicit demands of a school setting. Not inconsequentially, their inhibitory skills have generally improved sufficiently to make possible the lower level of physical activity required for school. How do children reach this point?

Major Advances in Skills and Knowledge

Children's knowledge expands rapidly and continuously over the first few years. By 3 and 4 years of age, they have experienced many regularities in the events they observe or in which they participate, and they therefore understand something akin to the principles of the physical world. By 5 years of age, they can anticipate readily what the outcome of various events will be and can reason about physical causes. For example, Sophian and Huber (1984) asked children to make judgments about which car on a three-car train made the middle car move. The situation was such that the caboose could push or the engine could pull. The principles of contiguity and temporal priority, however, were sometimes redundant and sometimes in conflict with each other. Three to 4-year-olds did not respond correctly more than would be expected by chance; 5-year-olds, on the other hand were correct significantly more often than chance. Furthermore, the 5-year-olds were consistent in their use of the principle that the cause

122

must temporally precede the effect, even when concrete cues conflicted with it; as Sophian and Huber point out, this suggests a reliance on logical principles. These investigators hypothesize that young children first start reasoning about cause and effect on the basis of observed regularities, that is, on the basis of probability. As children develop, however, they begin to extract from repeated experiences more abstract principles, which in time gain the force of logical necessity.

Children also observe regularities in the social world and incorporate them into their understanding; this understanding includes an awareness of psychological or cognitive determinants of behavior. Words for internal states—such as believing, thinking, knowing, understanding, feeling, needing—develop in the second and third years, with words for emotions emerging before words for cognitive states (Miller & Aloise, 1989; Shatz, Wellman, & Silber, 1983). Three-year-olds can differentiate between the mental and physical realms and realize that mental events can be at variance with observable events. An example from Shatz et al. is a child's statement that "I thought there wasn't any socks but when I looked I saw them"—a contrast between a previous thought and a current reality. Children also know that someone can *think* that something is true when something else is actually true. This particular distinction, however, is much clearer to 4- to 5-year-olds than it is to 3-year-olds. For example, if children are told a story in which a man goes into a room and hides an object, and then someone else comes along when no one is around and moves the object to a new location, the 3-year-olds are likely to say that the man would come back and look in the *new* location, while 4-year-olds would predict that the man would look where he himself had hidden the object (Miller & Aloise, 1989; Perner, Leekham, & Wimmer, 1987). That is, 3-year-olds tend to confuse their own knowledge with that of others and fail to understand the consequences of a false belief, while 5-year-olds appreciate and anticipate the results of another's perspective or beliefs.

In general, the trend in the fourth and fifth years is toward a firmer understanding of cognitive functioning, including one's own. Children in this age range know that it is harder to learn and remember when there are distractions or when there is a great deal to remember (Wellman,

1977). They also know that motivation and effort are important determinants of performance (Miller & Zalenski, 1982; O'Sullivan, 1993; Wellman, Collins, & Glieberman, 1981). Three-year-olds understand the conditions necessary for someone else to see or not see an object that is always visible to them—for example, that the other person's eyes have to be open and the line of sight must be unobstructed. They may have difficulty, however, understanding that the other person has a different perspective and therefore does not see the object in the same way that they do. For example, they may show an adult a picture so that the adult can see it clearly, but they do not understand that the adult, who is opposite to them, will see the picture upside down while they see it right side up. In contrast, 4-year-olds manifest both types of understanding (Flavell, 1988). Even at 5 years, however, there are still limits on children's understanding of the mental state of others; for instance; they do not fully understand the "stream of consciousness" or appreciate how unlikely it is that a waking person will have an empty mind (Flavell, Green, & Flavell, 1993). These are examples of metacognition,—thinking about one's own or another's thought processes. Although there are signs of such metacognition before 3 years of age, children understand much more as they develop from 3 to 5 years and can use this knowledge more effectively.

This enhanced knowledge of the physical, social, and internal worlds is accompanied by the emergence or strengthening of a number of skills. These include reasoning, using strategies to improve memory, attention, and other cognitive processes, and planning; inhibitory skills. Hudson, Shapiro, and Sosa (1995) studied planning in 3- to 5-year-olds in the context of familiar events—shopping for groceries and going to the beach. They found that the verbal plans of 4-year-olds included more components than those of 3-year-olds, and the plans of 5-year-olds were more elaborate than those of 4-year-olds. In addition, the children were asked about how to remedy or prevent mistakes, such as forgetting to take lunch to the beach; plans for remedying and preventing mistakes increased over the age range, with younger children better at stating what to do when mistakes happened than in preventing them. The investigators conclude that 3- and 4-year-olds can plan for single goals, while 5-year-olds can flexibly manage multiple goals and new goals. In terms of inhibition, Reed, Pien, and Rothbart (1984; see also Kochanska, Murray, Jacques, Koenig, & Vandergeest, in press) hypothesized that internal inhibition (as measured in a spontaneous alternation task) would be related to development of verbally regulated inhibition. In a task that required turning one switch to see the same slide again and another switch to see a different slide, alternation is presumed to depend on an involuntary buildup of inhibition because there are no demands or instructions. In tasks where children are verbally instructed to delay or inhibit responding in the face of tempting situations, inhibition is more voluntary and presumably controlled by the verbal instructions. Reed et al. found that both forms of inhibition were related to age, with 3- to 3½-year-olds showing lower levels than 3½ to 4-year-olds, suggesting a specific shift that may be related to underlying neurological changes (Ruff & Rothbart, 1996).

Even so, the social situation and the systematic attempts by others to control the child's behavior are critical precursors of these later self-regulated inhibitory skills. This view is consistent with the emergence of private speech as a means of regulating behavior (Vygotsky, 1978; Wertsch, 1985). Self-regulation underlies increases in voluntary control of attention; it is related to children's use of strategies and systematic approaches to problem solving where inappropriate or inefficient responses have to be inhibited. It also may be important in allowing children to ignore salient perceptual features of an event in order to understand the logic of the event, as in conservation.

Reasoning is another skill that improves dramatically in this age range. One of the most interesting aspects of reasoning that can and has been studied in children of 3 to 5 years is their grasp of cause-and-effect relationships. Even though children in the second year of life show some anticipation of consequences when they perceive antecedent conditions (Keil, 1979), and even though 3-year-olds can correctly identify the cause of an observed effect under some circumstances (Bullock & Gelman, 1979; Shultz & Mendelson, 1975), children of this age still have some difficulty understanding the nature of causal relationships. By age 5, however, many of these difficulties in reasoning are no longer present.

The research on children's reasoning about "mental" causes also shows developmental trends toward more consistent, less vulnerable judgments about how intentions, motivation, effort, and emotion can influence behavior. Even 3-year-olds can predict behavior correctly from knowledge about the actor's mental state (Miller & Aloise, 1989). In fact, they tend to use intention as a cause to situations in which an individual's actions are involuntary or to situations involving inanimate objects, for example, ascribing the intention to go somewhere in a car. This overextension may be due to children's lack of knowledge about physical and biological processes (Miller & Aloise, 1989); as they learn more about these processes, they will no longer confuse intention, a mental cause, with physical or biological ones. In general, the evidence suggests that young children show accurate causal reasoning about social and cognitive causes earlier than they do about physical causes (Miller & Aloise, 1989); this may stem both from the central importance of social activity in children's lives and from an emphasis by the children's more sophisticated partners on such causes. Dunn Brown, Slomkowski, Tesla, and Youngblade (1991), for example, found that individual differences in children's understanding of social causality were related to the extent to which their families had engaged in earlier discussions of feelings and to the degree of earlier cooperation between the children and their siblings.

It is frequently said that 4-year-olds can be distinguished from younger children by the extent to which they use a strategic approach to problem solving both when they address challenges spontaneously and when they do so according to instructions. A number of specific examples will be discussed, but here it can be said that while strategic performances are seen in younger children, the use of such strategies is more explicit and probably more effective in older children. As DeMarie-Dreblow and Miller (1988) suggest, strategies are deliberate techniques that may require so much initial effort that performance on the task they are intended to facilitate is not improved. Thus, the evolution of problem solving requires that the components become well practiced; only then can attention can be freed from them and directed toward the goal. Moreover, from 3 to 5 years, there also is an increase in the number of strategies that children have available for dealing with any particular problem.

As with the development of causal reasoning, the use of strategies is likely to emerge and be facilitated within the context of social interactions. A mother and child may, for example, work together on a task or problem; if both partners understand the task in the same way, the more experienced mother can adjust her behavior to accommodate and challenge the child's interaction with the materials. She may let the child struggle with the problem for a short time and then suggest specific strategies either verbally or by example. The more efficiently the child is working, however, the more likely the mother is to adjust her activity downward and the more likely the child is to ask for or demand the chance to act independently. As Wertsch (1985) suggests, the social support and guidance the adult provides to the young child is intended to move the child toward taking responsibility for completion of the task or for solving the problem. Cognitive development, therefore, is in part a shift from an interpersonal or collective strategic approach to problems to self-directed strategies (Vygotsky, 1978; Wertsch, 1979, 1985).

Examples in Specific Domains

This period of development clearly involves some major reorganizations in and expansions of children's cognition. The more children learn, the more likely they are to run into situations that do not fit into their previous conceptions. Preschool peers and teachers are more likely than family members to challenge children's current understanding and to demand that children adjust their behavior and thought to fit new realities. Multiple factors determine the changes that we see in play, problem solving, and representation during the period from 3 to 5 years.

PLAY

Although even infants can participate in games and implicitly follow rules for taking turns (Bruner & Sherwood, 1976), only in the late pre-

school years do children begin to play structured games that involve explicit rules (Rubin, Fein, & Vandenberg, 1983). By 3 years of age, children show an interest in simple board games; while they may have a hard time emotionally accepting the consequences of playing by the rules, they are aware of them. In another two years, they will be better prepared cognitively to understand and accept the rules, because they can anticipate the consequences of particular moves and can see the advantages of all the participants playing fairly.

Book reading continues to be an important leisure activity shared by children and their parents. Sorsby and Martlew (1991) have shown that the demand on 4-year-old children's representational capacity is greater during reading than during the use of such materials as Play-Doh. That is, while reading parents are more likely to ask children questions about objects and events that are not currently present, such as "What is the same about an apple and an orange?" Such questions require children to think about things out of their immediate context, a skill that is essential for formal schooling and literacy. Interestingly, Sorsby and Martlew found that children's answers to abstract questions were significantly more likely to be fully adequate during book reading than during modeling with Play-Doh; the authors suggest that this is because the context of book reading does not require physical action, and the children are free to concentrate on symbolic activity. Just as in the earlier development of practical skills, it is harder to focus on representational skills in situations that require the coordination of several subskills or components. By limiting the number of components, book reading offers a better opportunity for practicing the emerging capacity for more abstract thinking.

During the fourth and fifth years, pretend play involves more elaborate scripts and dialogs. As Watson (1981) points out, children develop a greater concern with social roles along with an increasing capacity to represent those roles in play. An early step is to regard a role as a list of characteristic behaviors, what Watson calls a "behavioral role." For example, when asked to play with a doctor doll, a 3½-year-old may have the doll run through a series of appropriate actions, taking the temperature and listening to the heart of the patient. By 4 years, the child may be able to coordinate two roles in doll play and thereby create "social" roles for the dolls; now the child pretends that a patient doll says that it is sick, that the doctor doll respond appropriately by taking the patient's temperature and telling the patient to go to bed, whereupon the patient doll follows the doctor's instructions. By 5 years, the child can coordinate the social roles of three dolls so that a nurse now assists the doctor in treating the patient. At this point, the child is only beginning to represent in play the possibility of one doll playing more than one role, an understanding that increases after the preschool years. Settings that encourage pretend play allow more expression of children's understanding of the social world and provide them with opportunities to explore novel social as well as nonsocial possibilities.

As pretend play becomes more complex, there are advances in the nature of pretend. There are also important limits. O'Reilly (1995), for example, found that 3-year-olds both understood and produced pantomined pretend actions involving a body part (brushing teeth with a finger) more often than actions involving an imaginary object. In contrast, 5-year-olds understood the two types of action equally well and produced more acts with imaginary objects than with body parts. O'Reilly concludes that the 5-year-olds "demonstrate increasing independence from concrete environmental support in their knowledge about actions" (p. 999; see also Boyatzis & Watson, 1993). According to research by Lillard (1993), neither 4- nor 5-year-old children fully understand that a person, in order to pretend to be something else, must represent that something else symbolically and internally. That is, children at this age, if asked whether another child is pretending to be a rabbit, will say yes if the child is hopping. This is often the case, even if the children are specifically told that the other child is not thinking of a rabbit. Lillard suggests that children have an early working understanding of pretend as occurring when someone is "acting-as-if"; it is not generally until the school years that children revise this notion of pretend and consider it to be based on mental representations.

PROBLEM SOLVING

In this age range, the problems presented to children can be increasingly complex and abstract.

Klahr (1978) analyzes the skills that are involved in solving practical problems in everyday life and suggests that by the end of the preschool years, children have mastered a wide range of skills. He illustrates this with the following example:

Scene: Child and father in yard. Child's playmate appears on bike.
Child: Daddy, would you unlock the basement door?
Daddy: Why?
Child: 'Cause I want to ride my bike.
Daddy: Your bike is in the garage.
Child: But my socks are in the dryer. (pp. 181–182)

The sequence of steps involved here are analyzed as follows:

Top goal: Ride bike.
  Constraint: Shoes or sneakers on.
  Fact: Feet are bare.
Subgoal 1:   Get shod.
  Fact: Sneakers in yard.
  Fact: Sneakers hurt on bare feet.
Subgoal 2:   Protect feet (get socks).
  Fact: Sock drawer was empty this morning.
  Inference: Socks still in dryer.
Subgoal 3:   Get to dryer.
  Fact: Dryer in basement.
Subgoal 4:   Enter basement.
  Fact: Long route through house, short route through yard entrance.
  Fact: Yard entrance always locked.
Subgoal 5:   Unlock yard entrance.
  Fact: Daddies have all the keys to everything.
Subgoal 6:   Ask daddy. (p. 182)

The child in the example, presumably already 5 years old, shows her ability to assess what is needed to reach her main goal, but the underlying set of steps that Klahr suggests are not observable.

In an attempt to bring such processes to an observable level, Klahr and Robinson (1981) examined preschoolers' ability to plan ahead in solving a version of the Tower of Hanoi problem. This problem requires that a pyramid of three disks on one peg be transformed into an identical pyramid on another peg of a three-peg apparatus; the rules are that only one disk can be moved at one time, that each disk can be put down only on a peg, and that a larger disk can never be placed on top of a smaller disk. Klahr and Robinson modified the task to engage the interest of preschoolers more readily; the story line was that a monkey family (an arrangement of three cans) on one side of the river (child's side) wanted to move from one tree (peg) to another so that they were arranged in exactly the same way as the monkey family on the other side of the river (the experimenter's side). The rules were the same as the original problem, but the number of moves, and consequently the difficulty of the problem, was varied. Carrying out the instructions sometimes involved only one move and no obstructions, and sometimes involved as many as 7 moves, with the child having to remove one can from a peg in order to put another one in place first.

When the children could literally move the cans to solve the problem, most children between 4 and 5 years were able to succeed at 4-move problems, and some could solve 6-move problems (Klahr, 1978). Even more striking is that when the subjects were asked to tell the experimenter what moves they would make without actually touching the cans, 40% of 4-year-olds could solve 3-move problems and most 5-year-olds managed 4-move problems. In their analysis, Klahr and Robinson highlight the methods or strategies that the children use, such as means-ends analysis, search, evaluation, and planning. While the 4-year-olds solved only the simple problems, they still showed some ability to verbalize their plans in a systematic way.

REPRESENTATION/MEMORY

Play and problem-solving tasks reflect the child's growing base of knowledge about the inanimate and social worlds as well as the specific skills that have been acquired over the first few years. As already noted, the issue of knowledge, or how children represent and organize their understanding, has been investigated directly. The representation of events and familiar routines in the child's life can be studied more easily after the third year, because the child's language is so much more proficient. Nelson and Gruendel (1981) note that when children describe events in their lives, they do so accurately if not completely; that is, they report components of events in the order in which they typically occur or the order in which they must logically occur (you can't blow out the candles on a birthday cake until they are lit, and you can't cut the cake until the candles are blown out). They also take into account the roles and actions of different participants. These reports by children seem to be based on generalized representations because they are highly consistent over time and are reported in the present tense. In fact, children often have trouble answering specific questions, such as "What happened when you had dinner yesterday?" as opposed to general ones, such as "What happens when you have dinner?"

From 3 to 5 years, children's answers to general questions become structurally more complex and specific. Nelson and Gruendel (1981) provide examples. In response to "What do you do when you make cookies?" 3-year-olds are likely to say something like "Well, you bake them and eat them." A child at 4½ years, however, gives a more detailed answer: "My mommy puts chocolate chips inside the cookies. Then ya put 'em in the oven . . . Then we take them out, put them on the table and eat them."

In order to investigate the state of knowledge in infants, researchers must design experiments that do not require a verbal response on the part of the subject. Advances in our understanding of the development of knowledge during the preschool years, however, also have come from methods that allow children to act upon their knowledge without having to articulate it. For example, Gelman and Meck (1983) assessed 3- to 5-year-old children's knowledge of the principles of counting. Their understanding of the one-to-one principle—that each object should be counted once and only once—serves as an illustration. Children watched a puppet counting a line of 6 to 20 objects; the puppets counted correctly on some trials, skipped objects or counted the same object twice on other trials, or maintained one-to-one correspondence but did so in some unconventional way, such as counting every other object and then doubling back to count the rest. Both 3- and 4-year-old children were able to say with a high degree of accuracy whether the puppet had counted properly or not, even when the puppet counted in an unusual sequence. The number of objects to be counted did not seem to make any difference. In contrast, when children were asked to count a set of objects themselves, 3-year-olds were significantly less accurate than 4-year-olds, and all children counted less accurately as the size of the set increased. As Gelman and Meck point out, these data suggest that performance demands can obscure young children's knowledge of certain principles; when they have to do the counting themselves, children not only have to produce the numbers but also monitor their own performance for errors.

Monitoring one's own performance is a general skill that develops within this period; as already noted, the change revolves around a shift from implicit to explicit knowledge and also includes the further development of strategies. Children's ability to remember locations, objects, and facts has been studied extensively. Remembering is dependent upon the adequate pick of information in the first place, and children will attend more carefully when they have been asked to remember something (Baker-Ward, Ornstein, & Holden, 1984; Yussen, 1974). In this regard, the use of questions is also important. Shatz (1983) notes that, although early on children perceive questions as statements demanding a response, their own ability to ask questions for clarification develops more slowly. Three-year-olds will request information after ambiguous statements or requests from adults, but 4-year-olds are more likely to adapt their questions to the specific ambiguity involved. Older children are better at monitoring their own comprehension and are more likely to know what specific gaps need to be filled. The number of questions that children ask is positively related to their memory for information obtained in conversation with parents (Pierce, 1990).

Deliberate strategies for remembering have been studied extensively (Wellman, 1988), and Chapter 12 described some early forms of such strategic behavior in 2- to 3-year-olds. These strategies are used more often and more explicitly in the period from 3 to 5 years of age. Wellman (1988) notes that children in this age range spontaneously try harder, attend to the to-be-remembered object longer and more carefully, and use spatial organization or the association of specific cues to help them remember—general strategies advocated in self-improvement books! Five-year-olds use these techniques more efficiently than 3-year-olds. For example, 3-year-olds use all types of cues, some much less helpful than others for marking the location of hidden objects; 5-year-olds are more discriminating. By 4 years of age, children can judge whether certain situations facilitate or hinder remembering. They understand the role of distractors, the amount to be remembered, and the degree of effort. By 5 years they also understand the role of age, rehearsal, and the use of cues (Wellman, 1977; Wellman et

al., 1981). Importantly, 3-year-olds are less likely than 5-year-olds to ignore irrelevant factors such as a person's appearance or dress (Wellman, 1977). Wellman (1988) writes:

Remembering—storing and retrieving information for current or future use—is a complex, multifaceted job. Young children have only some, not all, of the job-related skills and understanding that they need and will eventually develop in order to do this job. It is sufficient, however, to claim that even preschoolers possess a relatively rich and reasonably accessible repertoire of memory strategies, rather than a severely limited one. (p. 18)

Miller and her colleagues (e.g., Miller & Harris, 1988) have investigated the use of attentional strategies in both preschool and school-age children. In a task that required children to say whether the pictures behind pairs of door were alike or different, 4-year-olds used the most efficient strategy, which was to open vertical pairs of doors systematically until they came to the end or to a mismatched pair. Furthermore, they showed more extensive use of that strategy over trials, suggesting that some children discovered the strategy through experience. Although the 3-year-olds were not as systematic as the older children, their responding was not random. Their patterns of door opening pointed either to partial strategies or to systematic, but inefficient, ones. As with memory, preschoolers can judge the effects of different factors, such as noise and effort, on the ability to concentrate (Miller & Zalenski, 1982).

Assessment of Development and Level of Functioning

Although there are many more standardized instruments available for use with children after age 3 than before, the emphasis of many still is on the child's *performance* rather than on the *process* by which the child comes to pass or fail particular items. Several developmental researchers have advocated a dynamic approach to evaluating children's cognitive functioning, using Vygotsky's notion of the zone of proximal development (Brown & French, 1979; Day, 1983). This zone represents those skills that the child may manifest with some assistance but would not display when working alone; it reflects both emergent skills and the child's ability to learn or profit from instruction. Thus, formal evaluations that focus on the zone of proximal development emphasize learning with assistance, maintaining information, generalization, and transfer to novel situations.

Such evaluations may be particularly helpful in the diagnosis of learning disabilities. Generally speaking, this includes children who in many ways are intelligent, but who have difficulty learning in a formal setting. Brown and French (1979) argue that such children have difficulty with developing strategic approaches to problems and with other aspects of self-regulation—one of the most salient features of normal cognitive development from 3 to 5 years. Casey, Tivnan, and Riley (1991) assessed preschoolers' ability to achieve organization, the degree to which the children used systematic approaches, and the children's efficiency in situations separate from the standardized evaluations of intelligence. Their results suggest that such skills are general ones, transferable to a num-

ber of tasks, and independent of the usual measures of intelligence. Therefore, one of the goals of an evaluation of the zone of proximal development should be to assess the child's ability to benefit from adult assistance in regulating behavior; the results of such an evaluation would have important implications for training of children with deficient skills.

This chapter has addressed the issue of everyday cognition from 3 to 5 years of age. The emphasis has been on children's ability to meet the demands and challenges that face them; these increase as children develop new skills and consolidate old ones. Even though children by 5 years of age may generally be ready for formal schooling in which academic cognition is dominant, assessment tools should measure skills and knowledge that will be as important for continuing adaptation to the nonacademic world as to the academic one. There is much divergence between what we know about the processes underlying cognitive development and the definitions of intelligence operationalized in our standardized instruments.

REFERENCES

Baker-Ward, L., Ornstein, P. A., & Holden, D. J. (1984). The expression of memorization in early childhood. *Journal of Experimental Child Psychology, 37,* 555–575.

Boyatzis, C. J., & Watson, M. W. (1993). Preschool children's symbolic representation of objects through gestures. *Child Development, 64,* 729–735.

Brown, A. L., Bransford, J. D., Ferrara, R. A., & Campione, J. C. (1983). Learning, remembering, and understanding. In P. H. Mussen (Ed.), *Cognitive development. Handbook of child psychology* (Vol. 3, pp. 79–166). New York: John Wiley & Sons.

Brown, A. L., & French, L. A. (1979). The zone of potential development: Implications for intelligence testing in the year 2000. *Intelligence, 3,* 255–273.

Bruner, J. S., & Sherwood, V. (1976). Peekaboo and the learning of rule structures. In J. S. Bruner, A. Jolly, & K. Sylva (Eds.), *Play—Its role in development and evolution* (pp. 277–285). New York: Basic Books.

Bullock, M., & Gelman, R. (1979). Preschool children's assumptions about cause and effect: Temporal ordering. *Child Development, 50,* 89–96.

Casey, M. B., Tivnan, T., & Riley, E. (1991). Differentiating preschoolers' sequential planning ability from their general intelligence: A study of organization, systematic responding, and efficiency in young chil-

dren. *Journal of Applied Developmental Psychology, 12,* 19–32.

Day, J. D. (1983). The zone of proximal development. In M. Pressley & J. R. Levin (Eds.), *Cognitive strategy: Psychological Foundations* (pp. 155–175). New York: Springer-Verlag.

DeMarie-Dreblow, E., & Miller, P. H. (1988). The development of children's strategies for selective attention: Evidence for a transitional period. *Child Development, 59,* 1504–1513.

Dunn, J., Brown, J., Slomkowski, C., Tesla, C., & Youngblade, L. (1991). Young children's understanding of other people's feelings and beliefs: Individual differences and their antecedents. *Child Development, 62,* 1352–1366.

Flavell, J. H. (1988). The development of children's knowledge about the mind: From cognitive connections to mental representations. In J. W. Astington, P. L. Harris, & D. R. Olson (Eds.), *Developing theories of mind* (pp. 244–270). Cambridge, MA: Cambridge University Press.

Flavell, J. H., Green, F. L., & Flavell, E. R. (1993). Children's understanding of the stream of consciousness. *Child Development, 64,* 387–398.

Gelman, R., & Meck, E. (1983). Preschoolers' counting: Principles before skill. *Cognition, 13,* 343–359.

Hudson, J. A., Shapiro, L. R., & Sosa, B. B. (1995). Planning in the real world: Preschool children's scripts and plans for familiar events. *Child Development, 66,* 984–998.

Keil, F. (1979). The development of the young child's ability to anticipate the outcomes of simple causal events. *Child Development, 50,* 455–462.

Klahr, D. (1978). Goal formation, planning, and learning by preschool problem-solvers. In R. S. Siegler (Ed.), *Children's thinking: What develops?* (pp. 181–212). Hillsdale, NJ: Erlbaum.

Klahr, D., & Robinson, M. (1981). Formal assessment of problem-solving and planning processes in preschool children. *Cognitive Psychology, 13,* 113–148.

Kochanska, G., Murray, K., Jacques, T. Y., Koenig, A. L., & Vandegeest, K. A. (In press). Inhibitory control in young children and its role in emerging internalization. *Child Development.*

Lillard, A. S. (1993). Young children's conceptualization of pretense: Action or mental representational state? *Child Development, 64,* 372–386.

Miller, P. H., & Aloise, P. A. (1989). Young children's understanding of the psychological causes of behavior. *Child Development, 60,* 257–285.

Miller, P. H., & Harris, Y. R. (1988). Preschoolers' strategies of attention on a same-different task. *Developmental Psychology, 24,* 628–633.

Miller, P. H., & Zalenski, R. (1982). Preschoolers' knowledge about attention. *Developmental Psychology, 18,* 871–875.

Nelson, K., & Gruendel, J. (1981). Generalized event representation: Basic building blocks of cognitive development. In A. Brown & M. Lamb (Eds.), *Advances in developmental psychology* (Vol. 1, pp. 131–158). Hillsdale, NJ: Lawrence Erlbaum.

Nelson, K., & Ross, G. (1980). The generalities and specifics of long-term memory in infants and young children. *New Directions for Child Development, 10,* 87–101.

O'Reilly, A. W. (1995). Using representations: Comprehension and production of actions with imagined objects. *Child Development, 66,* 999–1010.

O'Sullivan, J. T. (1993). Preschoolers' beliefs about effort, incentives, and recall. *Journal of Experimental Child Psychology, 55,* 396–414.

Perner, J., Leekam, S. R., & Wimmer, H. (1987). Three-year-olds' difficulty with false belief: The case for a conceptual deficit. *British Journal of Developmental Psychology, 5,* 125–137.

Pierce, J. W. (1990). The more they ask, the more they remember: Variables related to preschoolers' memory for answers to their own questions. *Child Study Journal, 20,* 279–286.

Reed, M. A., Pien, D. L., & Rothbart, M. K. (1984). Inhibitory self-control in preschool children. *Merrill-Palmer Quarterly, 30,* 131–146.

Rubin, K. H., Fein, G. G., & Vandenberg, B. (1983). Play. In E. M. Hetherington (Ed.), *Handbook of child psychology* (Vol. 4, pp. 693–774). New York: John Wiley & Sons.

Ruff, H. A., & Rothbart, M. K. (1996). *Attention in early development: Themes and variations.* New York: Oxford University Press.

Shatz, M. (1983). Communication. In J. H. Flavell (Ed.), *Handbook of child psychology* (Vol. 3, pp. 842–889). New York: John Wiley & Sons.

Shatz, M., Wellman, H. M., & Silber, S. (1983). The acquisition of mental verbs: A systematic investigation of the first reference to mental state. *Cognition, 14,* 301–321.

Shultz, T. R., & Mendelson, R. (1975). The use of covariation as a principle of causal analysis. *Child Development, 46,* 394–399.

Sophian, C., & Huber, A. (1984). Early developments in children's causal judgments. *Child Development, 55,* 512–526.

Sorsby, A. J., & Martlew, M. (1991). Representational demands in mothers' talk to preschool children in two contexts: Picture book reading and a modeling task. *Journal of Child Language, 18,* 373–395.

Vygosky, L. S. (Ed.). (1978). *Mind in society: The development of higher psychological processes.* Cambridge, MA: Harvard University Press.

Watson, M. W. (1981). The development of social roles: A sequence of social-cognitive development. *New Directions for Child Development, 12,* 33–41.

Wellman, H. M. (1977). Preschoolers' understanding of memory-relevant variables. *Child Development, 48,* 1720–1723.

Wellman, H. M. (1988). The early development of memory strategies. In F. W. Weinert & M. Perlmutter (Eds.), *Memory development: Universal changes and individual differences* (pp. 3–30). Hillsdale, NJ: L Erlbaum.

Wellman, H. M., Collins, J., & Glieberman, J. (1981). Understanding the combination of memory variables: Developing conceptions of memory limitations. *Child Development, 52,* 1313–1317.

Wertsch, J. V. (1979). From social interaction to higher psychogical processes. A clarification and application of Vygotsky's theory. *Human Development, 22,* 1–22.

Wertsch, J. V. (Ed.). (1985). *Vygotsky and the social formation of mind.* Cambridge, MA: Harvard University Press.

Yussen, S. R. (1974). Determinants of visual attention and recall in observational learning by preschoolers and second graders. *Developmental Psychology, 10,* 93–100.

16 / Normal Language Development: The Fourth and Fifth Years

Rhea Paul

The preschool years, between 3 and 5 years of age, are the time during which children move close to an adult level of language competence. Preschoolers are able to exploit most of the devices available in language for accomplishing communicative goals and become fully participating members in the human family of speakers.

Pronunciation

By age 4 the normal child is fully intelligible, producing nearly 100% of speech sounds correctly. If errors remain, they are likely to occur on the last sounds to develop: *l, r, th,* and possibly *s,* as well as on the production of several consonants that occur together within a word, as in *scrape.* Normal preschoolers also will continue to have difficulty with multisyllabic words, such as *spaghetti* or *aluminum.* About 5% of children enter school with phonological deficits (Shriberg, 1980), but most of these involve residual errors on one or two sounds.

Vocabulary

The average spoken vocabulary size at age 4 is about 1,500 words and at age five, about 2,100 words (Smith, 1926). Receptive vocabulary size continues to exceed these levels at each age. Vocabulary size continues to grow during the school years, as well. In addition to learning new words from conversations, though, school-age children begin to acquire many vocabulary items through their new language modality—written texts.

Children learn to use and understand a great many classes of words during the preschool period. They master the use of most pronouns, with the exception of the reflexives (himself, herself, ourselves, etc.), which are not learned until school age. Kinship terms in addition to *mother* and *father* or their diminutives, which are part of the child's earliest vocabulary, enter the lexicon. Depending on the child's experience, most terms for extended family members will be at least partially understood by age 5 (Haviland & Clark, 1974), but full comprehension is not achieved until age 10 or so. The preschooler, for example, may know that he has a brother but may not realize that he is a brother to someone.

Temporal terms enter the vocabulary at this time with *before, after, since,* and *until* coming in earliest. These are used first as prepositions (I'll go *after* school) and only later as subordinating conjunctions (I'll go *after* I get home from school). Question words *why, how,* and *when* are used with greater frequency during this period, and questions containing these words are answered correctly more often, although the context of the question has an influence on correct responding (James, 1990). Children are more likely to answer most types of wh- questions correctly when they can see the person, object, or event to which the question refers.

Children learn to refine their use of adjectives, adding more precise terms to their vocabulary during the preschool years. While a 3-year-old may know only *big* and *little,* by 5 children generally learn *large/small, tall/short, long/short, high/low, thick/thin, wide/narrow, deep/shallow* (Owens, 1992). The positive member of the pair is usually learned first. *More* and *less* and *same* and *different* are other pairs of dimensional adjectives usually learned during the preschool years. *More* and *less* may be used initially interchangeably. By age 5, most children use these terms correctly.

Grammatical Production

Between the ages of 3 and 5, children learning English acquire mastery of many grammatical morphemes (Cazden, 1968), including use of *be* verbs, articles, and third-person singular *s* marking on verbs (I run, you run, he runs). Children also master the use of past tense markers during this period. Typically, children start out by marking irregularly formed past tense verbs, such as *come/came*, *see/saw*, and *go/went*, correctly, before they begin using the regular past tense marker *-ed*. Children acquire the regular marker between the ages 3 and 5, and they very frequently overgeneralize it, marking incorrectly those irregular forms that were produced correctly earlier. This overgeneralization of past tense markers results in such productions such as, "I falled down and got hurted." This replacement of an early correct form by an error that is the result of a process of overregularization often is taken as evidence that children actually are inducing rules from the input language and not merely memorizing the forms heard, since, presumably, adults do not produce these overgeneralized forms. The use of overgeneralized past tense forms may persist to age 5 or 6. Some overgeneralized plural forms (foots, mouses) also may appear during this period. Other grammatical morphemes that are mastered during the preschool period include the comparative (small/small*er*) and superlative (small*est*) as well as the agentive *er* marker, used to denote one who performs as action (teach/teach*er*) (Carrow, 1973). Much learning about other morphological markers, particularly about prefixes and suffixes, which augment the meaning or modify the part of speech of a word, goes on during the school years (Wiig & Semel, 1984).

During the preschool years, children continue to increase both the elaboration of basic noun and verb phrases as well as the complexity of sentences types produced. Young 3-years-olds consistently include a subject noun phrase in sentences, no longer omitting it as 2-year-olds do. Noun-phrase elaboration becomes richer and more flexible throughout the preschool years by means of the ability to mark either the subject or the object noun phrase with a broader range and greater number of modifiers. Toward the end of the preschool period, children begin using clauses, rather than single words or phrases, to modify nouns. These relative clauses, again, usually are used first to modify nouns in object position (They're boys *that I know*). Modification of subject nouns with relative clauses (The boys *that I know* are big) is rare in children's speech until school age.

Verb-phrase elaboration during the preschool period consists of the mastery of the verb inflections for past and third singular marking, as we saw. In addition, new auxiliary verbs are acquired, including *could, would, should, must, might,* and *shall* and past tense forms of the verb *to be: was* and *were*. Auxiliary verbs *have, had,* and *has* are used very infrequently during the preschool period (Miller, 1981). When preschoolers do use auxiliary verbs, they use only one at a time. They rarely produce sentences with multiple auxiliaries, such as "I *could have* helped you." Use of semi-auxiliaries continues to be frequent during the preschool period. By this time, however, the semi-auxiliaries often are followed by a full clause (I *wanna* eat *what you're eating*) rather than by a single word (I *wanna* eat), as children used at age 2.

Sentence variations become more adultlike during the preschool period. Negative sentences are generally produced correctly by age 3. Instead of being able to use only *can't* and *don't* as negative markers, *isn't, aren't doesn't, didn't,* and *won't* appear. By age 4, children are also using past tense negative markers such as *wasn't wouldn't, couldn't* and *shouldn't*. By 4½, children use indefinite negative markers such as *nobody, no one, none* and *nothing* but may err by producing these forms in double negatives (Nobody didn't come) (Miller, 1981).

Auxiliary verbs begin to appear in both the yes/no and wh- questions of young 3-year-olds. At this time yes/no questions are produced with auxiliaries that are also appropriate when inverted, or placed before the subject (We *can* go./*Can* we go?). Rising intonation also remains an option for asking this type of question. Shortly after they begin using and inverting auxiliaries in yes/no questions, children begin to use auxiliaries in wh-questions, as well. At first, these questions are often produced without inverting the auxiliary (Tyack & Ingram, 1977). Instead of asking "Why *can't* I have a cookie?" preschoolers may say "Why I *can't* have a cookie?" They leave the auxiliary between the subject and the verb, as it would be placed in a declarative sentence, rather than moving it before the subject, as the rule for forming questions in English requires. Not all preschoolers make this mistake (Klee, 1985), although it is quite common. By age 5, most children will be producing all questions and negatives with auxiliary verbs appropriately placed.

A major addition to the child's repertoire of sentence forms appears at about age 3: Children begin producing complex sentences (Limber, 1973). These forms involve either joining two sentences together by means of a conjunction such as *and, if,* or *because* (I like ice cream because it tastes good) or embedding one sentence within another (I think *I'll have an ice cream cone*). These complex sentences are important not only because they allow children to make their utterances longer but also because they allow the combination of ideas within an utterance to produce a more condensed, elaborated statement. At age 3, 5 to 10% of the normal child's sentences will contain these conjoined or embedded clauses. This proportion increases to 20 to 30% by age 6 (Paul, 1981). The proportion of complex sentences continues to increase throughout the school years, although the most dramatic increases are seen not in children's speech but in their writing (Loban, 1976).

may make the baby feed the mommy doll, operating on the principle that the first noun is the agent of action (Chapman, 1978). Not all children adopt this strategy (Bridges, 1980), but at times it does occur. By age 7, most children understand that the passive sentence is an exception to normal word order rules (Paul, 1985).

Preschool children also have difficulty understanding complex sentences in which the order of mention of clauses does not correspond to the order of events, such as "Before you brush your teeth, turn off the water." And they have a hard time understanding sentences with conjunctions such as *unless* and *although,* which involve negative hypothetical propositions (Owens, 1992). Preschoolers and young school-age children typically misunderstand a few other specific sentence forms that violate the regular rules for sentence interpretation (Chomsky, 1969). Although preschoolers sound much like adult speakers in terms of the production of grammatical sentences, it is possible to trigger misinterpretations of sentences with forms that violate the general rules of the language.

Communication

Comprehension

Three-year-olds understand much of what is said to them, but some sentences types still cause problems. Children of this age have learned many of the basic grammatical rules of the language and, unlike 2-year-olds, can interpret improbable sentences such as "The baby feeds the mommy" correctly. Children of 3 or 4 have learned the basic word order rule of English: The first noun in a sentence is the doer of the action and the last noun is the receiver. But once this basic rule is learned, it tends, like the morphological rules learned around the same time, to be overgeneralized. Four-year-olds may now misinterpret the same passive sentence they interpreted earlier because of a probable event strategy. If asked to act out "The baby is fed by the mommy," 4-year-olds

In the preschool period, language begins to be put to use for the purpose of reasoning, solving problems, monitoring thought and actions, relating events, and constructing complex imaginative play (Tough, 1977). Rather than just a system for mapping what one sees and does into words, as it is primarily used by toddlers, language now becomes an instrument of thought. This new function of language is, of course, made possible by increasing cognitive development. But it also, in and of itself, contributes to children's intellectual skill, so that the growth of language and cognition become more closely entwined during the preschool years.

Preschoolers learn a broader range of devices for making requests politely during this time. Rather than merely adding *please,* they begin to use permission requests (Can I . . . ?), question requests with modals (Would you . . . ? Could you . . . ?), and indirect requests, such as "Why don't you . . . ?" and "Don't forget to . . ." (Garvey, 1975). By age 5, children are using hints and other forms in which the real object of the request is never mentioned explicitly at all. So they might request a snack by saying "Gee, Mom, those cookies you made sure smell good. You make the best cookies in the world." In addition, in playing with peers, preschoolers demonstrate knowledge that requests must fulfill certain conditions, such as that the speaker must have some reason for making the request rather than doing the action him- or herself. Garvey (1975) shows that preschoolers often make adjuncts in their requests to each other, in order to establish that these conditions have been met. They might say, for example, "Get that hammer for me. *I can't reach it.*" Despite this demonstration of the forms and conditions necessary for successful requests, preschool children still have much to learn about using verbal means to regulate others' behavior. They are not very efficient at getting others' attention when it is not already directed to them, or in persuading others to do something the listener is reluctant about. When attempting to get a parent to let her stay up later, for example, a 4-year-old might try "I want to stay up late because I need to see the dinosaur show," using only her own point of view as a basis for persuasion. A more sophisticated school-age child might attempt the same thing by addressing the parent's point of view in the argument, for instance: "I need to see the dinosaur show because we're doing a science essay tomorrow and it will give me something to write about."

During the preschool years children learn to increase the degree to which they can elaborate on a single topic of conversation. By age 5, children spend an average of five utterances on a single topic (Brinton and Fujiki, 1984), increasing the degree to which each utterance maintains the topic and adds new information.

Around 3 or 4 years of age children begin to use linguistic devices to provide links between the ideas they talk about in the conversations. One of these *cohesion devices* is the use of pronouns to link referents, as in "I have a *friend* at school. *He* builds blocks with me." Use of definite/indefinite articles (*a, the*) is another cohesive device that emerges during this time. The indefinite article *a* is used to signal that a referent is being introduced into the conversation for the first time (Alice saw *a* large cake). When the same referent is mentioned

again, the definite article *the* is used to signal the listener to retrieve the original referent from memory (Alice ate *the* cake). Ellipsis is another cohesive marker employed by preschoolers. This involves leaving out a part of the utterance that can be assumed because it was already mentioned. For example, in "I don't like spinach. Popeye does," *like spinach* is ellipted in the second sentence because it would be redundant. Leaving it out forces the listener to retrieve some of the meaning of the second sentence by looking for it in the first. This links the two propositions together into a cohesive unit. The ability to build these cohesive units, or *texts,* is one of the ways the child's discourse skills are advancing during the preschool years.

Children between ages 3 and 5 also become more adept at repairing conversational breakdowns. They are able to respond to requests for clarification of specific information, such as "You went where for dinner?" and can reply with just the piece being requested (Gallagher, 1981). Still, they rarely request clarification themselves when they misunderstand and cannot reformulate their message or provide missing background information when the listener looks confused.

With increasing linguistic competence, children are able to take advantage of many more communicative situations during the preschool years than they were as toddlers. Not only can the children engage in a carefully scaffolded conversation with Mother; now the preschooler can talk with peers, older children, and/or adults outside the family. Less conversational management is needed for the children's talk to succeed. But parent-child conversations at this time still play a very important role in structuring the child's social world, and much social learning goes on through the medium of language (Cook-Gumperz, 1979). Parents tell preschoolers what to do in different situations, how to behave, and what to expect, and they interpret situations verbally for children, providing reasons and explanations. Language itself becomes part of the experience of social relations, and preschool children are socialized linguistically as well as behaviorally into the community in which they will be expected to operate. Talk with peers, too, particularly in the context of cooperative play, teaches children how language can be used to initiate and construct social relations. Much preschool interactive play is done primarily through the medium of language, and by using language in this interactive fashion, children learn to exploit its flexibility.

Metalinguistic Development

One new area of language use that arises during the preschool years is the ability to use language to talk about language itself. This capacity is called *metalinguistic awareness.* One way in which preschoolers manifest this ability is in their play with language. Children begin to use words just for the fun of it, in interchanges like this one described by Garvey (1975):

Child 1:   It's snakey, because it has snakes.
Child 2:   And it's hatty because it has hats.

Interest in rhyme is another manifestation of metalinguistic awareness. Here children show that they are attending not only to what a word means but to other properties, independent of meaning, such as the word's sound and its similarity to the sounds of other words.

Use of language in role playing also demonstrates the child's metalinguistic skills. For example, preschoolers often correct each other's usage in role play, commenting on its appropriateness. A child might tell another "You can't call me 'Willy,' you're the baby. The baby has to call the father 'Daddy'!"

Metalinguistic awareness, particularly the awareness of print as a special form of language that has its own conventions, is greatly enhanced by the book-reading experience. Children whose parents read to them learn that the black marks on the page code language, because if a hand covers them up, parents will complain that they can't read the words. Children may even learn from this experience what a "word" is and may notice that words are separated from others on the page by a small space. They learn that books are held with a certain orientation, pages are turned in a certain direction, and when different people read the same book, they will say the same words. The youngsters, thus make the inference that print is a form of speech written down. This kind of knowledge often is referred to as "literacy socialization," and it is an important component of reading readiness in the early school years (Snow, 1983).

Despite these emerging metalinguistic and pre-literacy skills, preschoolers have much to learn in these areas. The school years are the time in which metalinguistic skills undergo their most rapid and extensive development. And with this burgeoning awareness, built on a solid foundation of oral language competence, comes the ability to acquire true literacy.

Summary

Between the ages of 3 and 5 children acquire the basic sounds, vocabulary, and grammar of the mother tongue. Although there is still a few sounds and many words to learn, and several sentence types may still confound the understanding, by the end of the preschool period children are flexible, voluble, competent communicators. Further, preschool children can manage conversations, adjust speech styles for different interlocutors, and use language in the service of play and other social relations. With this firm grounding in spoken communication, fostered by years of fine-tuned interactions with family and peers, 5-year-olds are ready to embark on a journey that will ultimately extend their world beyond their own space and time, ready to encounter and to master language in a new modality, the written word.

REFERENCES

Bridges, A. (1980). SVO comprehension strategies reconsidered: The evidence of individual patterns of response. *Journal of Child Language, 7,* 89–104.
Brinton, B., & Fujiki, M. (1984). Development of topic manipulation skills in discourse. *Journal of Speech and Hearing Research, 27,* 350–358.
Carrow, E. (1973). *Test of auditory comprehension of language.* Austin, TX: Urban Research Group.

Cazden, C. (1968). The acquisition of noun and verb inflections. *Child Development, 39,* 433–438.

Chapman, R. (1978). Comprehension strategies in children. In J. F. Kavanaugh & W. Strange (Eds.), *Speech and language in the laboratory, school and clinic* (pp. 308–327). Cambridge, MA: MIT Press.

Chomsky, C. (1969). *The acquisition of syntax in children from 5 to 10.* Cambridge, MA: MIT Press.

Cook-Gumperz, J. (1979). Communicating with young children in the home. *Theory into Practice, 18,* 207–212.

Gallagher, T. (1981). Contingent query sequences within adult-child discourse. *Journal of Child Language, 8,* 51–62.

Garvey, C. (1975). Requests and responses in children's speech. *Journal of Child Language, 2,* 41–63.

Haviland, S., & Clark, E. (1974). "This man's father is my father's son": A study of the acquisition of English kin terms. *Journal of Child Language, 1,* 23–47.

James, S. L. (1990). *Normal language acquisition.* Boston: College-Hill Press.

Klee, T. (1985). Role of inversion in children's question development. *Journal of Speech and Hearing Research, 28,* 225–232.

Limber, J. (1973). The genesis of complex sentences. In T. Moore (Ed.), *Cognitive development and the acquisition of language* (pp. 155–167). New York: Academic Press.

Loban, W. (1976). *Language development: Kindergarten through grade twelve* (Report no. 18). Urbana, IL: National Council of Teachers of English.

Miller, J. (1981). *Assessing language production in children.* Baltimore: University Park Press.

Owens, R. E., Jr. (1984). *Language development.* Columbus, OH: Merrill.

Owens, R. E., Jr. (1992). *Language development* (3rd ed.). Columbus, OH: Merrill.

Paul, R. (1981). Analyzing complex sentence development. In J. Miller, *Assessing language production in children* (pp. 36–40). Baltimore: University Park Press.

Paul, R. (1985). The emergence of pragmatic comprehension: A study of children's understanding of sentence-structure cues to given/new information. *Child Language, 12,* 161–179.

Shriberg, L. (1980). Developmental phonological disorders. In T. Hixon, L. Shriberg, & J. Saxman (Eds.), *Introduction to communication disorders* (pp. 263–310). Englewood Cliffs, NJ: Prentice-Hall.

Smith, M. E. (1926). An investigation of the development of the sentence and the extent of vocabulary in young children. *University of Iowa Studies in Child Welfare 3* (5).

Snow, C. (1983). Literacy and language: Relationships during the preschool years. *Harvard Educational Review, 53,* 165–189.

Tough, J. (1977). *The development of meaning.* New York: Halsted Press.

Tyack, D., & Ingram, D. (1977). Children's production and comprehension of questions. *Journal of Child Language, 4,* 211–224.

Wiig, E., & Semel, E. (1984). *Language assessment and intervention for the learning disabled* (2nd ed.). Columbus, OH: Merrill.

17 / Motor Development: Ages 2 to 4 Years

Shelly J. Lane

Observe Jeff, a 2½-year-old at play with the neighborhood children. The older children are playing a game of climb on and jump off a stoop that stands about two feet high. They are able to climb onto the stoop using upper extremity strength to pull and lower extremity strength to climb and push. Jeff is not as strong in either area. However, being creative and highly motivated, this younger child rests his chin on the top of the stoop and uses neck and upper trunk muscles to assist in the pulling. The need to expend a great deal of energy to accomplish this task is irrelevant; what counts is that the task is accomplished successfully and Jeff reaches the top of the stoop.

Now comes the jumping down. For this youngster, balance is not as dependable as it is for the older children. Seeming to know this, Jeff "walks" off the stoop rather then jumps and curls into a ball to roll out of the fall. Thus, balance is not significantly challenged, and the entire process is experienced as a success. What we have seen in this child is a combination of prior skills (holding on, pulling up, walking, rolling), developing strength, creativity in combining skills and strength (e.g., the ability to motor plan), and intense motivation. Because of the sense of success Jeff experienced, it is likely he will perform the task again, altering it slightly and leading to the development of more efficient motor patterns. What this observation indicates is that both during this era and in subsequent years, the influence of motivation and environment continue to play major roles in the expression of motor skill.

Motor planning, discussed in Chapter 9, continues to develop and becomes more obvious as the child faces and conquers new challenges. According to Towen, Hempel, and Westra (1992):

. . . between two and three years of age the child develops the ability to select the most appropriate strategies for specific activities and to use them automatically. The result is well-adapted, individually characteristic motor behavior, in which general detailed motor patterns can be applied at will. (p. 414)

These authors call this the beginning of "motor-cognition," and see it as an important precursor of motor skill development for the school-age child. Thus, during this stage of development the task of caregivers and other adults in the environment is to present the child with a milieu that requires the adaptation of prior skills.

During the second and third years, motor skills continue to refine and, in normally developing children, changes in performance become more difficult to discern by means of casual observation (Keogh & Sugden, 1985). Along with the previously noted influence of motivation and environment, experience and practice significantly influence motor development in the coming years. This process, called motor learning, will play a role in the further development of eye-hand skills, sequencing of tasks, and combining skills to produce new movements (Palisano, 1988). During an evaluation it is not uncommon to find a mother reporting that a child cannot color or cut; presently one learns that the child has never been exposed to these activities. Similarly, even at age 4 a child who has never been on a tricycle will not be able to coordinate his or her legs in the needed reciprocal pattern to move the bike forward. The venue for experience and practice that incorporates both motivation and an enticing environment is play. That play is the occupation of the child (Kielhofner, 1985) was never more true than during this developmental time period. Observing a child at play at this, or any, age may be the best means of assessing both motor skills and cognitive skills.

Tables 17.1, 17.2, and 17.3 list major developmental accomplishments during the years from 2

TABLE 17.1

Gross Motor Skills, 2–4 Years

Skill	Age of Appearance (month)
Goes up stairs, marking time, no support	22–29
Goes down stairs, marking time, no support	28–34
Goes up stairs, alternating feet, with support	29–35
Goes down stairs, alternating feet, with support	48+
Goes up stairs alternating feet, no support	31–41
Kicks a stationary ball	24–27
Jump from raised step	24–27
Throws small ball	24–29
Walk on tiptoes	28–31
Catches large ball with arms straight	30–35
Arms scoop in catch	32–36
Rides a tricycle using pedals	32–35
True running (both feet leave the ground and arms move reciprocally)	32–36
Walks with reciprocal arm swing	32–35
Balances 5 seconds on 1 foot	35–40
Gallops forward	40–46
Hops on one foot	36–47

to 4. These accomplishments represent refinements of skills that emerged earlier (e.g., stair climbing, running, tool use, dressing, etc.). Thus, fewer new skills are listed here than in Chapter 4 or 9. Adapting skills to suit the situation occurs now. Such adaptation may involve moving faster, making an activity more difficult, combining movements, or using skills in different contexts (Gutteridge, 1939). What subsystems are involved in development in these two years, and which of these are the primary players? As suggested, exposure, experience, and motivation take on major roles now. In normally developing children, physical constraints may hold them back from the accomplishment of tasks they are highly motivated to attempt. In fact, it is not uncommon to find a

TABLE 17.2

Fine Motor Skills, 2–4 Years

Skill	Age of Appearance (month)
Holds an object steady with one hand while other performs skilled motions	24–27
Draws with circular movements	24–27
Imitates vertical, horizontal lines	19–36
Removes screw on cap	24–29
Builds block tower of 9 cubes	28–35
Strings large beads	30–35
Snips with scissors	24–36
Cuts paper with scissors	32–48
Puts together simple puzzles	35–40
Strings small beads	36–41
Holds large crayon with static tripod grasp	36–47

TABLE 17.3

Self-Care Skills, 2–4 Years

Skill	Age of Appearance (month)
Eats an entire meal with a spoon, little spilling	24–35
Begins to use a fork	24–35
Dons simple clothing (hat, pants, shoes, socks); may need assistance	24–35
Dons all clothes except for buttoning	32–35
Buttons accessible buttons	36–48
Washes/dries hands	19–48
Puts on shoes, not always on correct foot	30–46
Turns doorknobs of most doors	36–48
Undoes fastenings that are accessible (large buttons, snaps, shoelaces)	32–44
Brushes teeth	48+

child greatly frustrated in his or her attempts to accomplish a task as well or as quickly as desired. Thus, central nervous system development, physical development, muscle strength, coordination, and balance are still making significant contributions to the expression of motor skills.

Gross Motor Development

WALKING, RUNNING, AND CLIMBING

Between the ages of 2 and 3 walking becomes automatic, and little attention to this task is needed even on uneven surfaces. Changes in the quality of walking, which include greater shoulder movement and trunk mobility, a narrowing of gait width, and improved agility, take place in typical children between 2 and 3 years of age (Hempel, 1993). There is a uniformity to the length, height, and width of each step taken, and reciprocal arm movements emerge, as well. Skill in this pattern continues to develop so that the child can walk on tiptoe and, given the proper motivation and play environment, can add a silliness to the walking pattern (e.g., the child can waddle, toe-in, etc.) (Keogh & Sugden, 1985). Thus, music and games that ask the child to walk like a bear or an elephant are great fun at this age; they provide the child with an accomplishable challenge that he or she can elaborate from the well-developed skill of walking.

With increasing confidence, the child can walk, talk, and manipulate a carried toy with ease. Although walking skills appear quite mature, the 4-year-old does not show adultlike anticipatory postural movements, such as those needed to maintain balance while reaching for an object. Such anticipatory postural adjustments are present, but slower to "kick-in" than in adult movements (Riach & Hayes 1990). Still the speed of walking can also be altered by age 4, and children can walk either rapidly or slowly, or can adjust their own cadence to that of another. Walking at the age of 4 is very adultlike (Eckert, 1987; Keogh & Sugden, 1985; Palisano, 1988). It has become an easily adapted pattern that can be relied upon when environmental challenges increase and motivation drives the child to meet the new challenges.

Between ages 3 and 4 running becomes "true" running, in that there is a period of "free flight" (Palisano, 1988). In addition, trunk rotation and arm swing are present, which add to the coordination of this pattern. The child has been motivated to increase speed in movement for quite some time now, and the added skill of running provides much enjoyment for the energetic 2- and 3-year-old. Although a smoother running stride develops between the ages of 2 and 3, balance and equilibrium are such that the child still cannot change directions while running (Eckert, 1987). When the terrain becomes steep, uneven, or otherwise unfamiliar, running may be abandoned in favor of the more comfortable skill of walking. However, motivation to "get there first" or to "keep up" may supersede caution, and the 3-year-old will challenge his or her running skills even in unfamiliar territory. Falls may not only produce bruised knees; they may lead to frustration and anger as the drive toward movement is subverted by the less mature physical subsystem.

Climbing appears to be a skill that is intrinsically motivating to children and heavily dependent on experience. In addition, physical attributes of the object to be climbed will influence the success of the climb (Williams, 1983). This task requires increasingly complex interactions between sensory input and feedback systems, physical development, visual-motor skill, and motor planning, as children tackle tables, stairs, and playground equipment. Managing stairs was begun the previous year using a pattern of marking time on each step; it now becomes more skilled as balance and strength are increased (Williams, 1983). Generally, by age 3, a child has sufficient leg strength to support the weight of the body and sufficient dynamic balance to stand on one foot for a movement and move the other without support (Eckert, 1987; Williams, 1983). As such, ascending stairs can now be accomplished using alternating feet, without holding onto a railing or the hand of another person. Descent is still challenging for the strength system; thus, it is not accomplished independently for several more months (Palisano, 1988).

On the playground, the 2-year-old can climb the slide ladder with perseverance and effort. This upward climb requires not only greater leg strength and balance, but also increased upper extremity strength due to the steepness of the ladder (Eckert, 1987). Parents of 2-year-olds often ascend the slide ladder behind the child to protect against a lack of strength or balance. By age 3, an alternating foot pattern will likely emerge due to improvements in strength and balance, and parents now to watch rather than trail.

JUMPING, HOPPING, GALLOPING, AND SKIPPING

Adequate strength and dynamic balance generally are developed close to the second birthday, permitting the child to jump in place with both feet (Keogh & Sugden, 1985; Palisano, 1988). Poe (1976) noted great variability in 2- to 3-year olds' jumping, such that attempts to describe a "typical" 2-year-old jump and reach pattern held little meaning. A child with adequate strength but insufficient balance may make a game out of jumping up and falling to the ground. This playfulness allows the child to challenge him- or herself in this motor task, while simultaneously practicing the skills needed to accomplish the task at a more complex level. Jumping down from a step or other small elevation develops shortly thereafter, and many children constantly challenge themselves (and perhaps the patience of their caregivers) by finding higher and higher ledges from which to jump. Long jumping is more difficult and often is not seen until after the age of 3. The initial pattern is clumsy, with the trunk held upright and little assistance from knee flexion or arm swing (Keogh & Sugden, 1985). Jumping over a barrier presents an even greater challenge for some children and may not be sufficiently interesting until after the age of 4 (Eckert, 1987; Gutteridge, 1939).

Hopping on a single foot requires a further increase in strength and dynamic balance. A 3-year-old may be able to produce a single hop on one foot, but repeated hops on one foot are much more difficult (Williams, 1983). This movement requires the maintenance of balance during movement, considerable trunk and leg strength, and the ability to modulate the height for push-off (Keogh & Sugden, 1985). As such it may not be seen until close to age 4. Early hopping is in a forward direction, since this helps to use the momentum generated by the hopping pattern. Hopping in place is not as inherently rewarding as forward movement, and it is more difficult due to increased balance demands. Thus, it may not be developed until later in the preschool period.

Galloping combines the basic patterns of walking and hopping forward, or leaping, and requires dynamic balance at the level of hopping or better (Eckert, 1987). It provides children with a means of moving forward quickly, and, because it incorporates "free flight" along with movement, most children generally view it as fun. Thus, it is a pattern that may be practiced often and consequently perfected. This unilateral "step, leap" pattern may be a precursor to skipping. It is easier since it uses one pattern repeatedly and does not require the skill of reciprocal movements (Palisano, 1988). Skipping may be seen as early as 3½ to 4 years of age, depending on the level of development in many subsystems. Initially it is often a very exaggerated pattern in which is easy to see the cognitive processing at work; the child slowly produces the alternating "step-hop" with a great deal of extraneous arm, head, trunk, and leg movements. Rhythmical, coordinated skipping will not appear for another year or more (Williams, 1983).

BALL SKILLS

Children younger than age 2 take an interest in balls and throw and chase them with glee. Kicking a ball seems to be at once a natural extension of locomotion and the desire to work on cause and effect. As such, it is a highly motivating childhood task. Catching presents more of a challenge to children as they need to overcome a protective response and develop the eye-hand skills needed to catch a moving target. Even so, the intrigue of the ball is sufficiently motivating to the child that such challenges generally are met and conquered.

Although throwing is apparent as soon as the infant has some control over release, aimed throwing develops between ages 2 and 3. Even then the pattern of throwing is immature. In spite of the fact that the child has developed good trunk

rotation skills that can be used in many motor patterns by this age, early throwing is accomplished without rotation. The child stands facing the target, the legs assume a wide stance, and the arm pattern in more a push than a throw (Palisano, 1988). This pattern provides a great deal of stability upon which the child can then impose some mobility. The result is forward motion of the ball. The child does not fall, but accuracy and power suffer. With practice, trunk rotation is added to this pattern, with the legs continuing in a stationary, wide base stance to offer the needed stability. By the age of 4, most children will decrease the base of their stance and as throwing occurs, the beginning of weight shift from the back to the front leg can be seen (Williams, 1983). This is accompanied with the reward of longer throwing distance and greater accuracy. Throwing continues to be refined in the ensuing years.

Catching is at first more like lucky corraling, with the body used to trap the ball and the arms used to stop its motion. Large balls are conquered before small balls. Initially a visual protective response is elicited, and, although the arms are outstretched, the child will turn the head away from the oncoming object. If the ball lands appropriately on the somewhat stiffly outstretched arms, the child will be able to flex the elbows and perhaps hold onto the ball, much to his or her surprise and delight (Palisano, 1988; Williams, 1983). Just prior to the fourth birthday, a child will begin to use some elbow flexion in preparation for catching, and the eyes will be able to follow the ball as it approaches the hands. However, skilled and consistent catching does not generally develop until later (Eckert, 1987; Williams, 1992). In fact, Loovis and Butterfield (1993) demonstrated continued improvement of catching skills between the ages of 4 and 14 years. Gender differences have been reported (Loovis & Butterfield, 1993), but this finding is not consistent (Williams, 1992). When seen, boys are more skilled at catching than are girls.

Kicking becomes refined as strength, balance, and visual-motor coordination develop. A 2-year-old will be able to kick at a ball while moving but often will not make contact with the ball (Eckert, 1987; Espenschade & Eckert, 1980). If contact is made, it may be so high that the foot merely skims the ball so that its forward movement is minimal. At age 3 the skills of strength, balance, and visual direction of the foot may interact to allow the child some backswing on the kick as well as to add some force to the movement and contact with the ball. Coordination with trunk rotation and reciprocal arm movements usually do not occur until after age 4 (Eckert, 1987; Palisano, 1988).

Thus, the gross motor challenges during the years from 2 to 4 are met with continued increases in physical skills and ever improving biomechanics. As these subsystems interact with the child's continued high energy and drive to conquer the environment, coordination improves. With this, the motivation to practice a task is stimulated, and a cycle develops. The child learns that with practice comes improved skill. Context is important, and during this age, children may begin to compete with others and strive to be the best at various activities. Thus, while a child may not throw a ball 15 feet during an evaluation, the same child may be able to accomplish this task outside with friends as they try to see who can throw the farthest. During this interval, gross motor activities may serve other functions: They allow the child an appropriate means for expending energy, and they promote the continued development of neck and trunk stability. Both of these functions may facilitate the continued development of fine motor skills as well.

Fine Motor Development

TOOL USE

The attainment of fine motor skills often is viewed as an expression of cognition. However, there is a great deal of variability in a child's interest in writing, cutting, and other fine motor tool-use activities. Thus, motivation will be an important subsystem in the development of tool-use skills during this period. Stability of the neck and trunk are also important in the coordinated use of tools. Between the ages of 2 and 4, environment may play an integral role in determining what fine motor skills will be expressed. The child enrolled in a day care or preschool program may be exposed to coloring, cutting, self-feeding, and tying: such exposure can serve to enhance the development of tool use skills. On the other hand, the child may find the environment so stimulating that the refinement of such skills is not possible. Alternatively, if the child is not enrolled in such a program, he or she may not be exposed to scissors, crayons, markers, and strings and may not have the opportunity to develop these tool-based skills. As a result, in the following discussion of fine motor skills, it is important to keep in mind that beyond cognition other subsystems are critical to the expression of such skills.

Hand preference is continuing to be refined, and recent reports suggest that 4- to 6-year-olds with continued mixed-hand preference are not inferior in fine motor performance to children with an established preference (Gabbard, Hart, & Gentry 1995; Gabbard, Hart, & Kanipe, 1993). Crayon grasp evolves from an overhand pattern to a "static tripod" pattern by the age of 3. This pattern holds the crayon between the thumb and first two fingers but does not allow for wrist and/or forearm movement (Exner, 1992; Palisano, 1988). Thus, the child uses the entire arm, from shoulder to wrist, for stability, as the hand attempts to move the tool and develop the requisite skill. Needless to say, this pattern results in some inaccuracy in direction of the writing tool, and the process is fatiguing. Children at this stage of development may have little tolerance for drawing/writing activities. The wrist and forearm are not likely to be "freed" for a more dynamic grip until between 5 and 6 years of age (Exner, 1992; Keogh & Sugden, 1985).

The drawing of lines begins with curved lines, progresses to "up and down" and then to "back and forth" (Keogh & Sugden, 1985). Vertical and horizontal lines can be drawn between the ages of 2 and 3; circles and squares are accomplished by a 4-year-old as perceptions of vertical and horizontal begin to integrate; more complex forms and diagonals appear between 5 and 6 years of age (Palisano, 1988). Although it is possible to teach these writing skills to younger children, they can become frustrated as their perceptual and motor skills may not be keeping pace with their cognitive abilities.

Similar to crayon use, scissors use develops slowly. The child of 2 or 3 understands what scissors can do and how they work; this can be seen as the child uses both hands to manipulate the scissors in an up-and-down pattern and produces a snip on the paper. Some 3-year-olds may be able to make the snip using one hand on the scissors, but these children likely will need assistance holding the paper, as associated movements in the nonpreferred hand may interfere with this ability (Palisano, 1988). Moving the fingers in the alternating pattern needed to produce a cut line and holding the paper with the other hand are a combination more consistent with later development (Palisano, 1988). The emphasis in some preschool and early learning programs on preacademic skills thus may lead to extreme frustration and anxiety. While the children may be able to understand conceptually what is being asked of them, they may lack sufficient motor and/or perceptual maturity to produce the desired response. In addition, if the response can be produced, it is likely to be inefficient, require a great deal of energy and concentration, and be less skilled than the children would like. At this age many children can see that their product only marginally resembles their goal, and frustration often ensues. Given this combination of difficulties, the children will not see this activity as play. An observer may view the children as having a short attention span and low frustration tolerance, when in reality they are being asked to perform at a level inconsistent with the interaction of all subsystems with which these children are working. Once again, it becomes imperative to look at all the elements that must be available to produce the desired response.

SELF-HELP SKILLS

A further example of the development of fine motor, manipulative skills can be seen in the attainment of self-help skills. Donning simple pieces of clothing can be accomplished by age 2, as long as the shirt or pants is oriented in the correct direction. By age 3 a child usually can manage to unbutton, and may be able to button larger, accessible buttons. Washing and drying activities can be accomplished between the ages of 3 and 4, although the process may not actually result in "clean" or "dry" hands. At this age children encounter great difficulty when the task requires repetitive motions. For example, tooth brushing is a challenge to the 3-year-old because of the repeti-

tive nature of the movements required (Keogh & Sugden, 1985).

LATERALITY

Handedness continues to increase through the preschool and school years (Gudmundsson, 1993). The issue of lateral preference for use of foot, eye and ear, and the consistency of these preferences, has come under investigation. Gudmundsson reported right-side preferences for all behaviors in most preschool-age children showing a high foot/hand consistency. This supports to some extent earlier findings of Gabbard (1992), at least for right-handed children. Left-handed children may not demonstrate as strong a hand/foot congruence. To further complicate this picture, Gabbard et al. (1995) were not able to demonstrate greater foot skill by the foot on the same side as the dominant hand. Thus, the picture of overall lateral preference remains muddy. The functional significant of such congruence also remains obscure.

BIMANUAL MANIPULATION

Throughout the period between ages 2 and 4, the child develops increasingly refined skill at bimanual manipulation. The nonpreferred hand is used more and more to stabilize as the preferred hand draws, unscrews, winds up, pushes in, pulls out, scoops up, and so on. According to Williams (1983), there is a progression from crude bilateral movements, to some degree of skill in unilateral movements, and onto the integration of unilateral movements into coordinated bilateral patterns. The latter may not occur until 5 or 6 years of age. During the preschool years, the hands are used in a number of complex patterns, both unilateral and bilateral. The child continues to improve his or her ability to capitalize on the trunk and shoulders as stabilizers, permitting skill to develop in the arms and hands (Keogh & Sugden, 1985).

Thus, the development of fine motor skills during the 2- to 4-year-old age range and beyond requires the interaction of appropriate environmental context, physical maturation notable in postural stability, bimanual hand use, eye-hand coordination, and motivation. Practice and experience are imperative. While making tool use or self-help tasks playful enough to motivate a child to practice may present a challenge to the caregiver or teacher, it is needed to prepare the child for continued development and readiness for school.

Summary

Environment and motivation are major players in the achievement of motor skills from this point forward, with experience and practice influencing the expression of skills. In addition, play is the best venue within which to promote and observe motor development. Why did Jeff attempt the task described at the beginning of the chapter, challenging his skills beyond what might be expected? His motivation was high, he had the capability to call into action his existing skills and combine them in a way which resulted in success, and he was playing with the other children. Had he been presented with the task in another environment, and asked to accomplish it by an adult, it is likely that he would not have taken the risk. We can learn a great deal about both existing and potential skills in children by simple observation of the child at play in a natural environment. We can facilitate the development of gross and fine motor skills by providing the appropriate setting for their expression and practice. The skills discussed here, and many more difficult skills, are most likely to be developed and refined if the child is allowed the freedom to try in a safe yet challenging environment.

REFERENCES

Eckert, H. M. (1987). *Motor development* (3rd ed.). Indianapolis: Benchmark Press.

Espenschade, A. S., & Eckert, H. M. (1980). *Motor development.* Columbus, OH: C. E. Merrill.

Exner, C. E. (1992). In-hand manipulation skills. In J. Case-Smith & C. Pehoski (Eds.), *Development of hand skills in the child* (pp. 35–46). Rockville, MD: AOTA.

Gabbard, C. (1992). Associations between hand and foot preference in 3 to 5 year olds. *Cortex, 28,* 497–502.

Gabbard, C., Hart, S., & Gentry, V. (1995). A note on trichotomous classification of handedness and fine-motor performance in children. *Journal of Genetic Psychology, 156,* 97–104.

Gabbard, C., Hart, S., & Kanipe, D. (1993). Hand preference consistency and fine motor performance in young children. *Cortex, 29,* 749–753.

Gudmundsson, E. (1993). Lateral preference of preschool and primary school children. *Perceptual & Motor Skills, 77* (3, part 1), 819–828.

Gutteridge, M. V. (1939). A study of motor achievements of young children. *Archives of Psychology, 34* (Serial No. 244), 5–178.

Hempel, M. S. (1993). Neurologic development during toddling age in normal children and children at risk of developmental disorders. *Early Human Development, 34,* 47–57.

Keogh, J., & Sugden, D. (1985). *Movement skill development.* New York: Macmillan.

Kielhofner, G. (1985). *A model of human occupation.* Baltimore: Williams & Wilkins.

Loovis, E. M., & Butterfield, S. A. (1993). Influence of age, sex, balance, and sport participation on development of catching by children grades K–8. *Perceptual & Motor Skills, 77* (3, part 2), 1267–1273.

Palisano, R. J. (1988). Motor development. In M. A. Short-Degraff (Ed.), *Human development for occupational and physical therapists* (pp. 445–480). Baltimore: Williams & Wilkins.

Poe, A. (1976). Description of the movement characteristics of two-year-old children performing the jump and reach. *Research Quarterly, 47,* 260–268.

Riach, C. L., & Hayes, K. C. (1990). Anticipatory postural control in children. *Journal of Motor Behavior, 22,* 250–266.

Towen, B. C. L., Hempel, M. S., & Westra, L. C. (1992). The development of crawling between 18 months and four years. *Developmental Medicine and Child Neurology, 34,* 410–416.

Williams, H. G. (1983). *Perceptual and motor development.* Englewood Cliffs, NJ: Prentice-Hall.

Williams, J. G. (1992). Catching action: Visuomotor adaptations in children. *Perceptual & Motor Skills, 75,* 211–219.

18 / Sensory Patterns in Infants and Young Children: The Preschool Child

Georgia A. DeGangi

Introduction

As children reach the preschool years, sensory integrative problems interfere with development of play skills, perceptual abilities, and fine and gross motor skills. Some children develop associated learning and emotional problems secondary to the sensory integrative disorder. This chapter describes the symptoms of preschool children with tactile, vestibular, and motor control and motor planning deficits. Chapter 5 provides for a desorption of the different types of sensory integrative dysfunction. By the time children reach the preschool years, more definitive testing is available to examine the nature of their disorder. The various tests that are available are described. Finally, case descriptions are presented that depict typical sensory integrative problems observed in the preschool years.

Tactile Dysfunction in Preschoolers

Preschool children with tactile hyper- or hyposensitivities lack the tactile discrimination to handle and manipulate objects within the palm and fingertips for refined use; as a result, they often display fine motor difficulties. For them, such commonplace tasks as drawing with a pencil or buttoning are very difficult. The children tend to look at their hands when manipulating objects. They may still mouth toys, and they often avoid touching new textures, preferring firm, hard toys. These children may insist on certain types of clothing, complain about clothing tags, and dislike having their hair and face washed. More advanced tactile discriminative skills, such as stereognosis (i.e., detection of objects by feel alone) and graphesthesia (i.e., identification of letter or num-

ber drawn on a body part while vision is occluded), are usually delayed, as well.

Play difficulties are common among preschoolers with tactile hypersensitivities. When they are required to play in close proximity with other children, destructive or aggressive play frequently follows. They may touch other children with force even when trying to be gentle. If given a choice, some children withdraw from other children or find spaces to play that provide them with tactile security, such as a corner of the room.

Vestibular and Bilateral Sequencing Problems in Preschoolers

In addition to gravitational insecurity and vestibular hyporeactivity, preschool children with vestibular problems often have problems in postural control, balance, and sequencing and coordination of movement. They may have poor equilibrium reactions in different body positions. When sitting at a desk, they may be fidgety with extraneous body movements due to weak trunk stability. When asked to engage in activities such as walking on hands in a wheelbarrow walk or climbing a trapeze bar, they may show weakness of the trunk and neck. As a result of weakness at the shoulders, they may have poor distal prehension, holding small objects with the pads rather than the tips of the fingers. It is not unusual for these youngsters to have ocular-motor problems, as well, such as difficulties looking up from paper to the chalkboard and then back down again.

Vestibular dysfunction often is observed in combination with bilateral integration problems, particularly in children who have postural deficits. Bilateral motor integration involves the ability to coordinate the two body sides and develop lateralization (Magalhaes, Koomar, & Cermak, 1989). Children with problems in this area frequently do not establish hand dominance by school age. Such children often will interchange hands with no consistent preference for either one. Bilateral assistive skills, where one hand acts as a specialized hand and the other as an effective stabilizer, are difficult. For example, the mastery of such simple tasks as buttoning and scissor cutting are delayed. Reciprocal bilateral movements such as skipping, jumping, or alternating the hands in a drumming pattern are difficult. Oftentimes children with this problem lack precision in hand function and cannot sequence hand movements. In addition, there may be a lack of symmetry and control in large body movements. As a result, they often are clumsy and stiff in gross motor tasks such as rolling and walking, since these movements require coordination of the two body sides. The children lack flexibility in rotating the trunk, and there is also a strong resistance to crossing the body midline. Consequently, when required to cross the midline, they may turn their entire body rather than rotating the trunk.

Motor Planning Deficits in Preschoolers

Some of the common symptoms of children with dyspraxia are delays in the ability to dress themselves and in acquiring fine and gross motor skills involving imitation, sequenced movements (i.e., lacing, skipping), and construction (i.e., building from a block model). Poor accuracy of movement is observed and skilled hand movements such as handwriting are very difficult for dyspraxic children. Movement quality may be explosive, with poor judgment of force, speed, and aim. Speech articulation may be poor, since this is also a planned, skilled motor activity. Nonhabitual tasks are very difficult for such children, who therefore prefer routines and strongly resist changes. Transitions from one activity to the next may cause behavioral upset.

Initiation of new movement sequences or new organized plans of behavior are difficult. For in-

stance, children may not be able to tell anyone what they plan to do because they lack an internal plan. As a result, dyspraxic children may become either very disruptive and aggressive, particularly when there is no external structure for organize around, or they may become very passive and prefer to repeat certain favorite activities, while resisting any that are new and different. Overall, tantrums, aggressive behavior, poor play skills with peers, frustration, and a strong resistance to change are common. Some children become very controlling and manipulative because of their inability to control and affect their environment. Needless to say, poor self-concept is a major problem of dyspraxic children.

Assessment Strategies for Preschoolers

Formal assessment of preschool children with sensory integrative dysfunction should include examination of vestibular reactivity, somatosensory functioning, postural control and muscle tone, balance, motor planning, and bilateral motor coordination. Not only should the assessment evaluate children's performance in sensorimotor processes affecting functional learning and behaviors; it also should incorporate behavioral observations of how the children function within the home and school environment. Clinical observations of the children in natural play contexts are useful (i.e., observations of them on the playground equipment or on mobile and suspended equipment) to substantiate standardized testing.

Once children reach the preschool years, several testing instruments may be used. The DeGangi-Berk Test of Sensory Integration (TSI) (Berk & DeGangi, 1983) may be used with preschool-age children with mild motor handicaps. This criterion-referenced test was designed either to measure overall sensory integration in 3- to 5-year-old children with delays in sensory, motor, and perceptual skills or to evaluate children suspected of being at risk for learning problems. Its focus is primarily on the vestibular-based functions and includes subtests measuring postural

TABLE 18.1

Behaviors Assessed by the DeGangi-Berk Test of Sensory Integration

Subtest	Task	Behaviors Assessed
Postural control	Money task	Antigravity flexion
	Side sit—cocontraction	Cocontraction of upper extremities and trunk
	Prone on elbows	Cocontraction of neck
	Wheelbarrow walk	Stability of neck, trunk, and upper extremities
	Airplane	Antigravity extension
	Scooter board—cocontraction	Cocontraction of upper extremities
Bilateral motor	Rolling pin activity	Symmetrical bilateral coordination control of arms, trunk rotation, crossing midline
	Jump and turn	Bilateral control of lower extremities, trunk rotation
	Diadokokinesis	Bilateral motor control and motor planning of hands
	Drumming	Bilateral coordination in alternating pattern
	Upper-extremity control in drawing task	Motor accuracy, trunk-arm disassociation, crossing midline
Reflex integration	Asymmetrical tonic neck reflex (ATNR)	Integration of ATNR in quadruped
	Symmetrical tonic neck reflex (STNR)	Integration of STNR in quadruped
	Diadokokinesis	Associated reactions

control, bilateral motor integration, and reflex integration. The TSI should be administered in conjunction with measures of functional motor performance (e.g., Peabody Developmental Motor Scales). Table 18.1 presents the domains of vestibular-based functions assessed by the TSI.

In addition to the TSI, Dunn (1981) developed *A Guide to Testing Clinical Observations in Kindergartners* for 5- to 6-½-year-olds. It contains a set of clinical observations for postural mechanisms, postural security, balance, and basic motor planning. Some clinical observations of attention, social interaction, and sensory reactivity accompany the Miller Assessment for Preschoolers (Miller, 1982), although these have not been standardized. The Touch Inventory for Preschoolers (TIP) (Royeen, 1987) measures tactile defensiveness. It is a rating scale with 46 questions to be completed by the parents. The questionnaire has been validated on a sample of preschoolers and is useful in delineating children who have sensitivities to touch.

Once children reach the age of 5, more definitive testing of sensory integrative functions can be conducted. The Sensory Integration and Praxis Tests (Ayres, 1989) were designed to identify sensory integrative disorders involving form and space perception, praxis, vestibular-bilateral integration, and tactile discrimination. The tests are intended primarily for 4- to 8-year-olds with learning disabilities; they are also particularly useful in delineating areas of treatment for children with sensory integrative disorders (Fisher, Murray, & Bundy, 1991).

Last, the Southern California Postrotary Nystagmus Test (SCPNT; Ayres, 1975) is a clinical test often used to measure vestibular functioning. The SCPNT is designed to measure the normalcy of postrotary nystagmus in 5- to 9-year-old children. It can be administered in a short period of time; however, the examiner must be very experienced in its administration and knowledgeable about conditions that may affect test results (e.g., visual fixation, arousal level, and lighting) (Ottenbacher, 1978). The examiner also must have a great deal of experience in the interpretation of test results, which may be confounded by the examiner's reaction time, movement of the subject's head during rotation of the board, and inaccuracies in observing the onset and cessation of nystagmus (Cohen, 1989; Cohen & Keshner, 1989). The SCPNT can be used with children with learning disabilities, autism, or mental retardation as well as children with vestibular dysfunction, but only where children are able to follow the test directions and maintain the test position. Test results of autistic and mentally retarded children should be interpreted with caution, since there are no reliability studies on these populations. Since 20% of the normative sample is likely to demonstrate hypo- or hyperreactive nystagmus, it is important to administer other measures of vestibular function in conjunction with the SCPNT to make a definitive diagnosis of vestibular dysfunction.

CASE EXAMPLES

This section includes three case examples involving preschool children with different tactile, vestibular, and motor planning deficits.

Tactile Defensiveness in an Autisticlike Child: Andrew was a 5-year-old with developmental delay and tendencies toward autisticlike behavior. Developmental skills were largely at the 3- to 4-year level. His underlying tactile defensiveness was considered to be the predominant problem affecting his development. Behaviorally, he exhibited a very short attention span and could apply himself to a teacher-directed task only for a few minutes at a time. When sitting in a chair, he constantly assumed bizarre positions and contortions. Andrew engaged in many self-stimulatory behaviors, including finger flapping, humming, fast spinning, and hanging and swinging on any apparatus that lent itself to this behavior.

Andrew would not permit others to touch him at all, including his family. If he were touched, he responded by pinching, biting, or kicking. At school, he was a severe behavior problem; these, too, he would scream and kick when touched. Once upset, it took a long time for Andrew to be calmed. He often withdrew into places where he could avoid being touched, such as under a table or in a corner of the room; it would then be very difficult to get him out of his hiding place. Andrew did not like other people to be too close to him; if placed in a group, he would kick, bite, and scream. Another aspect of this tactile defensiveness was his inability to tolerate having his face or hair washed. All of his clothing tags had to be cut out. On one occasion, the tag was accidentally left in a new shirt. Andrew began fidgeting with the tag and scratching his whole body, until, over the course of the morning, he began to rip his clothing off and could not be controlled.

Andrew's tactile problems are characteristic of a child with severe tactile defensiveness. Although his problems are not solely attributable to his tactile disorder, this does affect his capacity to develop appropriate interactional skills, attentional behaviors, and self-calming. In planning for him, this trait needs to be addressed as a major component of his classroom and home management program.

The Gravitationally Insecure Child with Developmental Dyspraxia: Emily was a 4½-year-old with low muscle tone, fearfulness in new movement activities, and poor balance. She fell frequently at school and avoided any playground activities. Although her fine and gross motor skills were at age level, she had difficulty with dynamic balance. Emily was a very shy and withdrawn child. When presented with motor tasks, she tended to cry silently even during very appealing activities. At tabletop tasks, Emily was very anxious, sitting with her shoulders in a tense, elevated posture. Emily was not sensitive to touch; in contrast, she would seek close proximity with the examiner or her mother whenever she was required to move.

When assessed, Emily demonstrated weakness in postural control (e.g., lifting her body up against gravity in flexed or extended body postures). She would sit in a W-sitting posture and preferred close-to-ground activities. Low muscle tone was observed in her winged scapula and rounded trunk posture when standing upright. She often yawned and complained of feeling tired. Emily was very slow and deliberate in her movement patterns, and her movement quality was stiff, awkward, and lacked fluidity. When placed in a sitting position on the therapy ball, Emily clung to the examiner and was extremely fearful. In addition to definite indicators of gravitational insecurity, she showed some evidence of motor planning difficulties. She displayed much fear and anxiety when approached with a new motor challenge, particularly when it included sequenced, unfamiliar movement patterns such as galloping.

Emily received sensory integrative therapy that focused primarily on her gravitational insecurity. Like other children with this problem, she responded best when movement was linear, such as forward-back or side to side. Coupling movement with firm deep-pressure activities helped her to organize movement experiences through the sense of touch. A very gradual approach was used, starting with activities that were close to the ground. It was important not to impose vestibular stimulation on her, because that could be more disorganizing than integrating. Slow, rhythmical movements were used. Helping Emily to anticipate where her body was moving in space by providing visual or auditory cues also helped her to learn where she was about to move. During the first weeks of treatment, it was necessary to entice Emily just to touch moving equipment or to put a favorite toy on the swing. In this way, she gradually learned to tolerate the visual component of watching the movement before she herself was expected to move in space. After several months of therapy, she spontaneously climbed on playground equipment and did not display the fear that she had originally manifested. Her balance and motor-planning skills began to improve through continual occupational therapy intervention.

Child with Sensory Integrative and Emotional Problems: Fred is a 5½-year-old who had been seeing a psychologist for several months because of significant behavioral problems at home and school. The psychologist felt that an impasse had been reached in treatment and that a new approach might be necessary in order for continued progress to occur. His kindergarten teacher reported that he was very bright and knew all the answers. However, he didn't do what was asked of him in school, didn't finish assignments, frequently jumped around, and had difficulty sitting still. In addition, he sometimes got stuck on one activity and found it hard to make transitions to anything else. His mother's concerns centered around his tendency to fight her about everything all day long, his aggressiveness with other children, and his destructive nature. She also was worried about his poor judgment regarding his own safety. For example, he would jump off the top of the shed or, when in a car, he would jump out the window unless restrained in a car seat. At home, Fred preferred to play alone rather than with other children in the neighborhood.

As an infant, Fred would scream whenever lying down. If driven, he was prone to car sickness. On the other hand, he liked to swing very high and for long periods of time, enjoyed fast-moving carnival rides, and never became dizzy. He only liked movement that he could initiate and resisted being moved by others. Fred enjoyed vibration created by power saws and drills, although he was sensitive to their noise.

During the occupational therapy evaluation, Fred showed normal postural reactions, good balance, and very slight motor-planning problems. Gross and fine motor skills were well developed. In this one-to-one situation, Fred could sit still for 45 minutes and attend the various activities presented to him. However, when permitted to play on the suspended equipment (i.e., swings), Fred's activity level increased dramatically. On the swing, he continually asked to go faster and higher, then would suddenly jump or dive off. He exhibited no fear of any activity or piece of equipment. In addition to these observations, Fred exhibited depressed nystagmus on the postrotary nystagmus test.

In sum, these findings suggested that Fred was having difficulty processing and appropriately using vestibular input. His vestibular system appeared to be underresponsive to many forms of vestibular sensory stimulation, compelling him to seek dangerous thrills and to overlook the consequences of his actions. It is likely that problems in this area were affecting his ability to develop appropriate behavioral limits and social interactions. He also seemed overly sensitive to being moved by others, suggesting that he was both under- and overresponsive to vestibular stimulation. By responding aggressively, he could control situations and therefore avoid unexpected movement by others.

Intervention directed toward his underlying sensory integrative deficits helped Fred with both his sensory and behavioral problems. If he had received traditional psychotherapy or behavioral interventions without therapy to address his sensory problems, these changes may not have occurred. This case provides an example of how emotional problems may be impacted by sensory integrative deficits.

Summary

Sensory integrative problems in preschoolers affect a range of skills including fine and gross motor, perceptual, self-care, and social-emotional functioning. These problems often are seen in children with learning disabilities, motor delays, and autism. In the preschool years, several formal assessments are available to evaluate the different types of sensory integrative dysfunction. It is important, however, to interpret evaluation findings in relation to functional, adaptive, and social-emotional skills so that appropriate interventions may be provided. Children identified with or suspected of having sensory integrative deficits should be referred to an occupational therapist skilled in the assessment and treatment of sensory integration deficits.

REFERENCES

Ayres, A. J. (1975). *Southern California Postrotary Nystagmus Test manual*. Los Angeles: Western Psychological Services.

Ayres, A. J. (1989). *Sensory Integration and Praxis tests*. Los Angeles: Western Psychological Services.

Berk, R. A., & DeGangi, G. A. (1983). *DeGangi-Berk Test of Sensory Integration*. Los Angeles: Western Psychological Services.

Cohen, H. (1989). Testing vestibular function: Problems with the Southern California Postrotary Nystagmus Test. *American Journal of Occupational Therapy, 43* (7), 475–477.

Cohen, H., & Keshner, E. A. (1989). Current concepts of the vestibular system reviewed: 2. Visual/vestibular interaction and spatial orientation. *American Journal of Occupational Therapy, 43* (5), 331–338.

Dunn, W. (1981). *A guide to testing clinical observations in kindergartners*. Rockville, MD: American Occupational Therapy Association.

Fisher, A. G., Murray, E. A., & Bundy, A. C. (1991). *Sensory integration theory and practice*. Philadelphia,: F. A. Davis.

Magalhaes, L. C., Koomar, J. A., & Cermak, S. A. (1989). Bilateral motor coordination in 5- to 9-year old children: A pilot study. *American Journal of Occupational Therapy, 43* (7), 437–443.

Miller, L. J. (1982). *Miller Assessment for Preschoolers*. Littleton, CO: Foundation for Knowledge in Development.

Ottenbacher, K. (1978). Identifying vestibular processing dysfunction in learning disabled children. *American Journal of Occupational Therapy, 32* (4), 217–221.

Royeen, C. B. (1987). Test-retest reliability of a touch scale for tactile defensiveness. *Physical and Occupational Therapy in Pediatrics, 7* (3), 45–52.

SECTION II

Theoretical and Clinical Perspectives in Infancy and Early Childhood

19 / Paradox and Resolution: From the Beginning

Louis W. Sander

Among the dynamic forces that shape organization in the developing infant and in the infant-caregiver system, a number of apparent paradoxes can be discerned. This brief chapter on early human development addresses only one of these paradoxes. The viewpoint is one that has emerged from nearly 40 years of experience with the subjects of the Boston University Longitudinal Study in Personality Development (Sander, 1984). As with a wide range of research on both the animal and human levels, this study has revealed the singularity, the uniqueness of each newborn, each family system, and each individual's own particular pathway of development. The other side of the apparent paradox emerges from the extensive research on the minutiae of events within the flow of interaction between infant and caregiver; these studies have been carried out at the level of microsecond film and video analysis (Condon & Sander, 1974; Stem, 1974; Trevarthen, 1979). From this viewpoint, the now well-established concepts of intersubjectivity and attunement have been defined—that is, how infant and caregiver can function rhythmically and synchronously with each other.

The paradox is that we begin with two biological "givens": the requirement for self-regulation (the agency to initiate action to self-regulate within the context of one's unique life support system must be the individual's own agency to initiate; the "being distinct from" pole) and the capacity for microsecond synchrony and attunement with an "other" (not cognitively managed by the individual; the "being together with" pole). Both givens are there from the beginning of life and provide the essential conditions for the experience of "connection with" another and for the positive affects that are the basis of motivational systems underlying healthy relationships, including the experiences of loving and being loved as we come to encounter, and then "know," them in later life. It is in the sharing of a focus of attention in these "moments of meeting" that sets the stage

for the microsecond tuning, the capability for which we are born with. The experiencing of such "attunement" organizes positive affects, their motivational role, and the organization of consciousness.

It seems evident from the diversity of possible developmental pathways that integration of these two poles is a relative matter, ranging from the derailments of gross pathology at the one extreme to what we consider "health," are the optimization of potential that lies within both the new individual and the system, at the other. Indeed, many of the difficulties in child rearing relate to the confusion and indefiniteness that obscure the presence of each pole of the paradox, the very essential role that each pole plays, and the awareness that it is their integration that lies at the heart of the early developmental process.

Infant research is intended to explore, identify, and comprehend the essential principles that govern the early developmental process. It is hoped that such findings can and will be assimilated into the way caregivers both think and feel as they begin to construct an environment for their newborn. "Essential" principles of the developmental process exist from conception and persist throughout life. This chapter offers two brief clinical vignettes and notes their relation to the highly complex, but centrally vital, task of integration that confronts caregiver and infant from the moment of conception. The real problem is the *translation* from the discovery of principles governing the developmental process to their incorporation within the exchanges and interactions that will be the shaping forces in new infant-caregiver systems.

Every field, infant research included, has its own language. If space allowed, it would be appropriate to consider here how that language applies to how caregivers think about early development. What would it mean for caregivers to think in terms of systems instead of individuals; in terms of process instead of structure; in terms of a flow

153

of sequence, recurrence, and expectancy within the recurring exchanges between themselves and their charges instead of thinking in terms of isolated events. How does one think in terms of temporal organization (e.g., the 24-hour day and its regular recurrences, whether reflecting change or stability), or in terms of the distribution of "moments of meeting" between components of the system and the specificity such meetings convey? Space limitations preclude a discussion of the necessary background biology brings to our thinking.

In psychology, we sometimes fail to address that underlying yet unavoidable mystery of biology, *organization* which is essential for life itself. Biology constantly confronts this mystery driven on the one hand to analyze the unending process of engagement between organism and environment on a scale or hierarchy of levels—subsystems within larger systems—yet always constrained, on the other, by the vital necessity of maintaining the coherence, or unity, required for the enduring existence of both the living organism and the living system.

From such an effort at translation could emerge a way of thinking about the early developmental process—about the role of time, place, and movement in the organization of the infant-caregiver system and its processes of regulation, adaptation, and integration; about the central issue of where the impetus for initiation of action lies in the exchanges between infant and caregiver, or why the essential features of self-regulation and self-organization that are required of every living organism cannot be bypassed when dealing with the developing human infant. In exactly the same way, translation from the language of the neurosciences would enrich our thinking about longer-term consequences of infants' experiences. Relevant here are current concepts of the way anatomical and functional organization of the brain itself is being shaped, while regulatory and adaptive modifications of behavior are taking place between infant and caregiver. In the presence of this broader perspective, our thinking could be extended to include the role of conscious experience in shaping the early developmental pathway. This is especially relevant in the place being given now to experiences of awareness and self-awareness; as a result, brain organization constantly is being revised and updated through processes of categori-

zation, mapping, and, especially, reentry (Edelman, 1992). Translation at this point from neuroscience to psychology would open the door to discussing the experience of "recognition" (Sander, 1991) as being one of specificity in a "moment of meeting" between the complexities of two unique subsystems—the infant and the caregiver. Recognition can be thought of as a way of representing how one individual comes to savor the wholeness of another—that is, the experiencing by one of some configuration of the whole, some gestalt of the state of coherence of the other (Sander, 1995a, b). I propose that the experience of recognition represents a specificity in the meeting of such gestalts, one that provides the critical condition for the reorganization of both interacting partners as they progress toward new integration. Recognition, as a process moving toward increasingly precise specificity, serves as an essential operational metaphor for both developmental process and therapeutic process. It also provides a broader base upon which coherence in the larger infant-caregiver system can be built (Sander, 1995a).

Obviously, this chapter cannot provide the necessary theoretical framework required to integrate philosophies from among the complexity of disciplines involved. But it is important to recognize that such an integration can open us up to new ways of thinking. Next I illustrate and enlarge upon the two poles of the paradox and the diversity of possible developmental pathways that are available to provide resolution.

Illustrative Example of "Being Together With"

The first case example illustrates the first "being together with" pole, and opens consideration of the powerful place of intersubjectivity in comprehending the glue that binds together infant and caregiver as a living system. The following description is an example of the way that "primary intersubjectivity" (Trevarthen, 1979) can enter the caregiving situation, shape it, and yet remain quite outside the awareness of either participant. The scene, drawn from some 3 minutes of movie film,[1] can be described as follows.

CASE EXAMPLE

The research team was filming one of our new neonatal subjects on the 8th postdelivery day out on the lawn in front of the parents' house. In those days (1958), that was 3 days after mother and baby had returned from the hospital. One of the team was standing on the lawn talking with the father. The mother was sitting nearby with the new baby talking with another member of the team. The baby became increasingly fussy, with mother trying unsuccessfully to quiet her. The mother became a bit embarrassed and decided it was time to bring out refreshments, so she gave the baby to the father, who was standing nearby talking, and went into the house. The next 2 or 3 minutes of film shows the father standing on the lawn, holding the baby in his left arm, continuing to talk to the researcher, during which time the baby simply falls asleep and the two go on talking. Run at normal film speed of 30 frames per second, this is all that can be seen.

When, however, the film is rerun frame by frame over the same few minutes, it can be seen that the father glances down momentarily at the baby's face. Strangely enough, in the same frames, the infant looked up at the father's face. Then the infant's left arm, which had been hanging down over the father's left arm, began to move upward. Miraculously, in the same frame, the father's right arm, which had been hanging down at his side, began moving upward. Frame by frame the baby's hand and the father's hand moved upward simultaneously. Finally they met over the baby's tummy. The baby's left hand grasped the little finger of the father's right hand. At that moment the infant's eyes closed and she fell asleep, while the father continued talking, apparently totally unaware of the little miracle of specificity in time, place, and movement that had taken place in his arms.

This example makes clear immediately the first pole of our dynamic: The principle of intersubjectivity. *Webster's Dictionary* defines "relation" as "connection." We begin life "connected," as part of each other. We begin in relationship. Intersubjectivity as a principle of first relationships has

[1] The film sequence being described was first demonstrated to me by Daniel Stern some 25 years ago. The film itself was taken in 1958.

been demonstrated richly, both empirically and conceptually, by both Stern (1974) and Trevarthen (1979), in Stern's "attunement" and Trevarthen's "primary and secondary intersubjectivity." Opportunities for the engagements of intersubjectivity hinge largely upon the way the caregiver's attention is organized and available. As Murray (1987) points out, it is here, in the organization of attention, that postpartum depression in the mother plays such a critical role. In Trevarthen's "secondary intersubjectivity"—in the extension of the role of intersubjective organization to the enacting of play, games, and all forms of cooperative engagement between individuals—we realize that we have a further elaboration of the way each participant assimilates aspects of the complex organization of the other in order to achieve new integration at the systems level. A game represents the integration of a system; in this it is akin to the achievement of a relative stability in regulation of infant states of sleeping and waking as the case example illustrated.

Illustrative Example of "Being Distinct From"

At the same time, Tronick, Als, Adamson, Wise, and Brazelton (1978) have demonstrated vividly just how vulnerable the infant in the first months of life is to derailment of this elementary experience of connection by showing the infant's collapse in both mood and engagement when confronted with a caregiver's unresponsive, still face. This brings us to the second pole of our paradox.

Almost from the very outset, an infant begins to organize his or her own unique set of expectancies, which emerge from the diversity among recurring engagements with the caregivers; this organization is apparent in the system of the infant as "being distinct from" the caregiver. Throughout the 24-hour day, as expectancy probabilities are becoming established for both, a dynamic field of forces begins and surrounds the recurrent moments of meeting between the infant and the caregiver. Exchanges of intersubjectivity, along with their positive emotional amplification, are being balanced by negative emotions as the infant meets a mismatch of expectancy, as when he or she encounters the still face or some equivalent interdiction. A dynamic balance emerges between initiatives for approach or for avoidance; this, in turn, begins to constrain the flow of behavior in the infant-caregiver system. The essential requirement that each living organism be self-regulating means that the initiative to choose a direction must arise from within the organism itself, not from an extrinsic source. We are all too familiar with avoidance and negative affects, but we also are beginning to track and appreciate the irreplaceable inward-motivating role played by positive affects in the initial adaptive encounters that make up "the first relationship."[2] Inasmuch as positive affects also energize, amplify, and motivate the infant as the "agent-to-initiate" in organizing his or her own goals, we can begin to describe both poles of the paradox as contained within the framework of positive affects. In the language of chaos theory (Gleick, 1987), rather than represent opposition and conflict, this would constitute a "strange attractor." We understand adaptation as a "fitting together" over time between infant and caregiver that constructs a new and enduring system; this builds on the idea that positive affects must embrace both the pole of "being together with" (intersubjectivity) and that of "being distinct from" (singularity). The singularity of an infant as he or she initiates action in his or her own self-organization is experienced by both the baby and the caregiver. It has been demonstrated (Papousek, 1967) that the early infant's realization of an expectancy, or the achievement of a goal is accompanied by positive affects. At such moments, the caregiver can express positive affects that match and amplify those of the infant; whether she does so depends in large measure on the extent to which she has, in her own psychological organization, already granted the infant this essential role as agent to initiate the action re-

quired for his or her own self-regulation and self-organization.

To glimpse how this all "works" in the earliest relationships brings us to our second case example: A state of relative stability in the regulation of the infant-caregiver system is established by means of mutual adaptations. The example illustrates an initial adaptation of this kind between the two. Biology has long pointed out that systems maintained in states of relative stability of regulation begin to show new, or "emergent" properties. The conditions under which sleep states gain 24-hour organization in the infant-caregiver system is one such emergent property that will be described. A second example illustrates the way we can think of the infant as a self-regulating subsystem. It demonstrates how the infant becomes loosely coupled or disembedded within the broader stability of regulation achieved within the larger system—that is, new, emergent property of the infant-caregiver system appears. Such loose coupling or disembedding of infant as self-organizing agent would represent the "being distinct from" pole of our paradox.

Before recounting case examples, I should clarify just what is meant by loosely coupled or disembedded ("disjoined," as Ashby [1952] has described it). Ashby introduced this concept in describing the significance of reaching the adapted state in a richly complex system. When there is a stable equilibrium in regulatory balance among a requisite variety of component functions, a selected function can itself (within its own phase-space) interact with the context—the organism's network of engagement—without a perturbation in the selected function spreading to or upsetting the stability of the rest of the system. On the other hand, a system may not be in such a state of regulatory equilibrium, or it may be trying desperately to maintain its coherence. Under such circumstances, component functions remain tightly coupled with the system as a whole, so that a slight perturbation of one part spreads at once to the rest of the system. To illustrate this Ashby uses the metaphor of someone learning to drive a stick-shift automobile:

---

[2]By adaptive encounter (Sander, 1962), I am referring to the epigenetic, selective process of mutual modification required to reach an essential specificity of coordination over time between the uniquely organized infant and the uniquely organized caregiver. This is a "fitting together," long described in biology as that coherence in organization of exchange at the level of both the infant and the system that provides the conditions necessary for continuity of existence. The failure-to-thrive infant attests to this necessity.

Adaptation may demand independence as well as interaction. The learner-driver of a motor car, for instance, who can only just keep the car in the center of the road, may find that any attempt at changing gears results in the car apparently trying to leave the road. Later, when he is more skilled, the act of changing gears will have no effect on the car's travel. Adaptation thus demands not only the integration of related activities, but the independence of unrelated activities. (p. 157)

In systems language, within the coherence of a stably regulated infant-caregiver system, conditions should allow the infant to function as a "self-as-agent," self-organizing, subsystem that becomes loosely coupled, or disjoined. Within yet another framework, would describe the systems condition under which Winnicott's "true self" development could begin (Winnicott, 1965b).

THEORETICAL BACKGROUND

The case example sheds light on this assumption. It is drawn from my work with associates some 30 years ago (Sander, 1979) on continuous, 24-hour, noninvasive, neonatal bassinet monitoring. With this instrument, it was possible to compare different infant-caregiving systems over the first months of life. Continuous, around-the-clock, real-time recording was made of states of infant sleep and wakefulness, including quiet sleep, active sleep, transitional states, infant crying, and movement patterns. Also recorded were timing of approach of caregiver and removal of and return of infant to bassinet. These measurements were coupled with regular daily observation and recording of feedings, and a weekly visual perceptual test of infant response to 1-minute presentations of the human face in still, nodding, and social conditions. Care was taken to select only normal newborns with normal prenatal and delivery histories. All were bottle-fed and monitored one at a time over the first 2 months of life. This array of variables gave us a rich empirical basis for comparing the process of state regulation and the way infant functions developed under different caregiving conditions. Three samples of 9 infants each were compared: Sample A infants were cared for in the neonatal nursery by a changing assortment of different nurses and fed every 4 hours around the clock, regardless of the state of the infant. This continued until the 11th day of life, when each began 24-hour rooming-in with one individual—a surrogate mother nurse who

fed only on demand—only contingent to a prior state change in the infant. Sample B infants, however, roomed-in from the day of birth similarly, with the same surrogate mother nurse, feeding only on demand until day 11, when a second surrogate mother nurse continued the rooming-in until day 30. Sample C roomed-in with their own mother until day 5, then went home and were also bottle-fed only on demand. All the mothers in group C had had at least one previous baby. Needless to say, there were great differences in the 24-hour picture of state regulation and change over days in the 3 groups.

The first illustration involves a system that is maintained in relative stability of regulation. An emergent property is drawn from the data of the first 10 postnatal days. The investigators compared samples in regard to the distribution of sleep and waking states over each 24 hours, whether located in the daytime 12 hours (6:00 A.M.–6:00 P.M.) or in the nighttime 12 hours (6:00 P.M.–6:00 P.M.). Between postnatal days 4 and 6 the infants of Samples B and C, those who were fed only contingent to a prior state change in the infant (fed "on demand"), showed the spontaneous emergence (and persistence) of a 24-hour circadian rhythm of sleep and wakefulness. That is, between days 4 and 6 they began (and then continued) to sleep more in the nighttime 12 hours and to be awake more in the daytime 12 hours. This was a new 24-hour organization of the infant-caregiver system as a whole. No such rhythm appeared in Sample A infants, for which a feeding was given every 4 hours around the clock, regardless of the state of the infant. Thus, caregiving intervention in Sample A was often an intrusion into the self-regulatory property of the infant organism. Crying and motility in Sample A far exceeded that in Samples B and C, denoting that regulation in Sample A was highly unstable. One might say that in Samples B and C the role of "infant-as-agent" in initiating his or her own self-regulation had been granted by the caregiver from the outset.

Illustration of a second emergent property was provided by the visual perceptual tests carried out twice weekly by Stechler (Sander et al., 1979) on all the infants. For the neonate, confrontation with the human face is an exciting stimulus. The 1-minute presentation turned out to be a test of limits for the Sample A infants. These infants broke down and cried before the minute was up; for them, regulation of this state of excitement was accomplished by the collapse of the state of the infant as a whole. For the sample C infant, however, regulation was achieved by means of the visual system alone. The infants could look directly at the face, become excited, look peripherally to chin or hair, quiet down, look back, then away repeatedly, maintaining their composure over the stimulus minute. On an initial level, we can think of this as the infants exercising their own agency for self-regulation under conditions of relative regulatory stability. These conditions have allowed a loose coupling or disjoin of the visual system; this was necessary to achieve the specificity—and hence adequacy—of regulation not available to the more precariously regulated, tightly coupled, Sample A neonates.

This example can be considered a systems metaphor for the state of regulation in the infant-caregiver system, one that allows the loose coupling of a self-as-agent, self-organizing subsystem. Such a loose coupling, or disembedding, would make possible the pole of "being distinct from" in the dialectic tension or polarity central to this discussion. Conditions of stability of regulation over time in the holding environment (Winnicott, 1965c) allow both poles to be organized together in a new coherence. Such an ordering would allow positive affects to be contingent on the activation of either pole.

Resolution of Paradox

The bassinet-monitoring study illustrated another emergent property of a system maintained in a state of relatively stable regulation—the appearance over the course of an infant's awake period of an "open space" (Sander, 1977) in time, one that allows the endogenously activated, self-organizing initiative of the infant to emerge and begin the process of constructing its own idiosyncratic goals—the pathway to be pursued in "being distinct from." Integration at this point, clearly, must be thought of in terms of process within a system.

Open space, as I have formulated it, begins to become recognizable during the course of an awake period toward the end of the first month of postnatal life. The mother feels she is coming to "know" her infant within what is now a relatively stable 24-hour framework of expectable states in her infant's cycling and sequencing. During an awake period, after the infant has been picked up, changed, fed, and socially interacted with, the baby still is in an awake-active or quiet-alert state, not yet ready to return to sleep. The mother puts the infant in a reclining chair where the baby can see and hear her and goes about her other work or interests. This is a moment of disengagement but one in a state of regulatory stability, a coherence in the infant-caregiver system as a whole. During this open space in time, the infant's "primary activity," his or her agency for generating self-organization, can take off and initiate and organize an idiosyncratic network of proximal engagement of his or her own. This may involve grasping his or her own fingers, or watching mother, or banging against a mobile hanging before the infant. The infant is free from the need to manage or restore the regulation of his or her own state as a whole, and self-regulation can be carried out within a specific component sensorimotor subsystem. The infant's agency can pursue its own interests in a variety of ways; the child can engage in active selective exploration either of self or the low-intensity stimuli or discrepancies in the surroundings. Feedback and self-correcting action become related specifically to the goals of the infant's own interests and action.

Here we have a systems model, then, of equilibrium constructed by an enduring coordination between infant and mother over time, a balance that provides containment without impingement. We can apply this model to our understanding of succeeding tasks for new adaptive coordination that will arise within the system as the infant matures over the ensuing months.

In the open space segment of the awake period, there is documentation for Winnicott's paradox: "The basis of the capacity to be alone is a paradox; it is the experience of being alone while someone else is present" (Winnicott, 1965a, p. 30). And, further "it is only when alone (that is to say in the presence of someone) that the infant can discover his own personal life. The pathological alternative is a false life built on reactions to external stimuli" (p. 34). The open space segment can be thought of as a first level of Winnicott's "intermediate area" and "true self" engagement with it. As Winnicott describes it: "The infant is able to become unintegrated, to flounder, to be in a state in which there is no orientation, to be alone, to exist for a time without being either a reactor to an external impingement, or an active person with a direction of interest or movement. The stage is set for an inner experience. In the course of time there arrives a sensation or an impulse. In this setting the sensation or impulse will feel real and be truly a personal experience" (p. 34).

If we think of the first relationship from the perspective provided by basic biological principles that govern the interactive-exchange process in all living systems, we begin to appreciate that the integration of dynamic polarities inherent within such systems is their essential direction. The idea of stages in development has provided important descriptive markers but tends to ob-scure such common, essential, underlying dynamics. For example, the process of separation-individuation has long been conceptualized and studied as part of the early developmental process, but it has been assumed to enter the picture at some later point, after initial "togetherness" has been established. As I have tried to illustrate, if we can translate from the biological level and think in terms of systems and process, it becomes evident that the same fundamental dynamic is there in the system from the first relationship. This suggests that we can view the progress of the developmental process as one of integration, one that brings together apparently contrasting poles on levels of new and increasing complexity. Ultimately it is this process that constructs the wide spectrum of pathways that, at the same time, preserve the uniqueness of the individual.

REFERENCES

Ashby, W. R. (1952). *Design for a brain.* London: Chapman and Hall.

Condon, W. S. & Sander, L. W. (1974). Neonate movement is synchronized with adult speech: Interactional participation and language acquisition. *Science, 183,* 99–101.

Edelman, G. M. (1992). *Bright air and brilliant fire: On the matter of the mind.* New York: Basic Books.

Gleck, J. (1987). *Chaos: Making a new science.* New York: Viking-Penguin.

Murray, L. (1988). Effects of post-natal depression on infant development: Direct studies of early mother-infant interaction. R. Kumar & I. Brockington (Eds.), *Motherhood and mental illness (Vol. 2).* London: John Wright.

Papousek, H. (1967). Experimental studies of appetitional behavior in human newborns and infants. In H. W. Stevenson, E. H. Hess, & H. L. Rheingold (Eds.), *Early behavior: Comparative and developmental approaches.* New York: John Wiley & Sons.

Sander, L. W. (1962). Issues in early mother-child interaction. *Journal of the American Academy of Child Psychiatry. 1,* 141–166.

Sander, L. W. (1977). The regulation of exchange in the infant caretaker system and some aspects of the context-content relationship. In M. Lewis, & L. A. Rosenblum (Eds.), *Interaction, conversation, and the development of language* (pp. 133–156). New York: John Wiley & Sons.

Sander, L. W. (1984). The Boston University Longitudinal Study—Prospect and retrospect after twenty five years. In J. Call, E. Galenson, & R. Lyson (Eds.),

Frontiers of infant psychiatry (Vol. 2, pp. 137–145). New York: Basic Books.

Sander, L. W. (1991). *Recognition process—organization and specificity in early human development.* Paper presented at the 1991 University of Massachusetts Amhurst Conference.

Sander, L. W. (1995a). Identity and the experience of specificity in a process of recognition. *Psychoanalytic Dialogues, 5* (4), 579–595.

Sander, L. W. (1995b, April 29). *Wholeness, specificity and the organization of conscious experiencing.* Paper presented at the meeting of the American Psychological Association, Division 39, Santa Monica, CA.

Sander, L. W., Stechler, G., Burns, P., & Lee, A. (1979). Change in infant and caregiver variables over the first 2 months of life: Integration of action in early development. In E. Thoman (Ed.), *Origin of the infant's social responsiveness* (pp. 349–407). New York: Lawrence Erlbaum.

Stern, D. N. (1974). Mother and infant at play: The dyadic interaction involving facial, vocal and gaze behaviors. In M. Lewis & L. A. Rosenblum (Eds.), *The effect of the infant on its caregiver* (pp. 187–213). New York: John Wiley & Sons.

Trevarthen, C. (1979). Communication and cooperation in early infancy: A description of primary intersubjectivity. In M. M. Bllowa (Ed.), *Before speech: The beginning of interpersonal communication* (pp. 321–347). New York: Cambridge University Press.

Trevarthen, C., & Hubley, P. (1978). Secondary intersubjectivity: Confidence, confiding, and acts of meaning in the first year. In A. Lock (Ed.), *Action, gesture, and symbol* (pp. 183–229). New York: Academic Press.

Tronick, E., Als, H., Adamson, L. Wise, F., Brazelton, T. B. (1978). The Infant's response to entrapment between contradictory messages in face-to-face interaction. *Journal of Child Psychiatry, 17,* 1–13.

Winnicott, D. W. (1965a). The capacity to be alone. In *The maturational processes and the facilitating envi-*ronment (pp. 29–37). New York: International Universities Press.

Winnicott, D. W. (1965b). Ego distortion in terms of true and false self. In *The maturational processes and the facilitating environment* (pp. 140–153). New York: International Universities Press.

Winnicott, D. W. (1965c). The theory of the parent-infant relationship. In *The maturational processes and the facilitating environment* (pp. 37–56). New York: International Universities Press.

20 / High-Risk Environments and Young Children

Claire B. Kopp and Jeanne M. McIntosh

Risk, by dictionary definition, is a hazard, something that has potential for negative consequences. Developmentalists use the term *high risk* to refer to biological or social conditions that increase the probability of adverse outcomes for children. Down syndrome is an example of a high-risk biological factor; virtually every child with the condition has intellectual and language impairments. A high-risk social condition is multigenerational criminality. Children from such backgrounds show antisocial behavior as early as elementary school (Rutter, 1988). A combination of biological-social risk for an infant is exemplified by preterm delivery of a drug-addicted adolescent mother who dropped out of school. This particular constellation of risks and vulnerabilities often is associated with long-term developmental disorders (Furstenberg, Brooks-Gunn, & Morgan, 1987).

High-risk environments include settings, events, and situations that produce child experiences that are detrimental to well-being and development. Children who grow up in high-risk environments are exposed to many imbalances: too much violence, too little nurturance and care, too much poverty, too little sensitivity to needs, too much unsupervised time, too little exposure to ideas and values that foster cognitive and social growth. No childhood age period is immune to these imbalances: When risks are pervasive and major, there may be cumulative effects across age periods.

This chapter is specifically concerned with the effects of high-risk environments on the develop-ment of very young children. The emphasis is on the early years, with special attention paid to the preschool period because of the importance of this developmental phase. The chapter begins with a useful framework for categorizing environmental risks. A review of additional issues relevant to attempts to sort out the effects of risks on development follows. The chapter continues with an in-depth examination of two pervasive risk environments, those associated with divorce and child maltreatment. The outcomes associated with these factors are noted in terms of both general research findings and those specific to young children.

As will be seen throughout this chapter, despite considerable information available about risk factors and development, causal associations between specific risk factors and specific child outcomes are complicated and difficult to delineate. As a consequence, causal statements often are couched in generalizations rather than particulars. The chapter closes with a brief discussion of research and clinical implications.

Categorizing Risks

The phrase *high-risk environment* is a designation of convenience that allows a nominal grouping of the various conditions and factors that adversely affect children. However, an understanding of the environmental forces and processes that are responsible for childhood developmental problems requires additional specificity. To this end, a useful approach draws upon Bronfenbrenner's (1979) ecology of human development. (Also see Bronfenbrenner & Crouter, 1983.) The ecological perspective provides a means to characterize particular environments: the child's proximal environments and the larger social context that surrounds child and family. Moreover, two central themes of the ecological perspective are interaction and influences. The child has interactions with others in his or her immediate environment just as the child's parents have interactions with others in their own immediate environment. Interactions lead to influences that affect each participant albeit some interactions lead to greater influences than others (e.g., a child with his or her parents).

Bronfenbrenner characterizes the ecological system as comprised of embedded subsystems—macrosystem, exosystem, microsystem, and mesosystem—that surround the child. As noted, the degree of mutual influence varies according to proximity to the child. Figure 20.1 provides a schematic of the ecology. The *macrosystem* represents the social context that is most distal to the child. It refers to the overall culture of a social group including its attitudes, ideologies, social conventions, and laws. Garbarino (1990) describes the macrosystem as a reflection of sociocultural institutions. Macrosystem factors are not static, because cultural values change over time. The *exosystem,* one step closer to the child, reflects those contexts and contacts that indirectly affect a him or her. These influences are indirect because they are mediated by caregivers who themselves are the recipients of direct influences. For example, a stressful workplace has an immediate effect upon a wage-earner; however, job-related stress often is brought home and colors the nature of parent/child interactions. Exosystem factors are varied and include: a parent's friends, neighbors, employers; the type and extent of a parent's involvement with the workplace, recreational facilities, places of worship; and a parent's ability to access social and legal services, support systems, and other resources. The exosystem perspective facilitates analysis of the positive and negative ways that individuals who play a significant role in a child's life interact with their own

cultural, social, and economic institutions. Positive and empowered interactions of parents are usually associated with good child outcomes.

The *microsystem* refers to direct relations the child has with his or her immediate environment. These can include interactions with parents, peers, and teachers as well as access to situations beyond the family, such as neighborhood centers and playgrounds. Also included in microsystem variables are family emotional climate, family structure and routines, and marital relationships (Belsky, 1984; Goodnow & Collins, 1990). The fundamental quality of the microsystem is "its ability to sustain and enhance development" (Garbarino, 1990, p. 81). Last, the *mesosystem* refers to the relationships between systems.

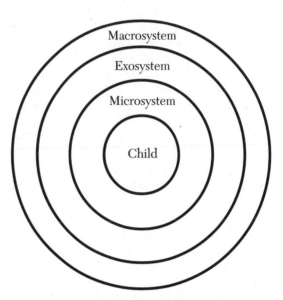

MACROSYSTEM: attitudes, mores, beliefs, ideologies of a culture

EXOSYSTEM: social settings that affect the child but do not directly influence him or her (e.g., parent's job site, coworkers, friends, support system)

MICROSYSTEM: relations and settings in which child takes part (e.g., family members, peers, teachers, neighborhood play setting, health system)

CHILD: age, sex, health, competencies, etc.

FIGURE 20.1

The ecological system

NOTE: From U. Bronfenbrenner (1979), *The Ecology of Human Development,* Cambridge, MA: Harvard University Press. Drawing adapted from C. B. Kopp, & J. B. Krakow, (Eds.), *The child: Development in a social context.* Reading, MA: Addison-Wesley, 1982.

Macrosystem risks can stem from cultural and social disasters—war, famine, political upheavals and strife, chronic and unrelenting poverty (Garbarino, Kostelny, & Dubrow, 1991). In contrast to highly visible disasters, some macrosystem risks are more subtle. For example, Americans as a group have participated in a major reconstruction of the family (Cherlin, 1988; Spanier, 1989). This cultural drift of norms includes a surge in female-headed households often with marginal economic resources as well as the attenuation of father involvement with children (Furstenberg & Harris, 1992). Although the adverse economic effects of father-absent households have been well documented, other consequences for the child are beginning to be explored in detail (e.g., Teachman, 1992).

Data on exosystem risks and their general effects are plentiful. As just one example, long-standing family poverty has been linked to psychopathology in children (Duncan, Brooks-Gunn, & Klabanov, 1994; Tarnowski & Blechman, 1991), conduct disorders (Offord, Boyle, & Racine, 1991), juvenile delinquency (Zigler, Taussig, & Black, 1992), and cognitive difficulties (Deutsch & Deutsch, 1963). Economic stress in general has been related to family disorganization, child abuse, and neglect (Kadushin & Martin, 1981).

Microsystem risks often arise because of abusive, insensitive, and inadequate parenting (Cicchetti & Carlson, 1987; Dishion, Duncan, Eddy, Fagot, & Fetrow, 1994; McCarthy, 1990; Patterson & Capaldi, 1991). Although some maladjusted parents are intentionally abusive, others simply do not understand the developmental and nurturant needs of children, still others are so preoccupied with their own stresses (e.g., illness, job, divorce) they unwittingly ignore the child, and some are simply authoritarian tyrants. As important as parental input is, Bates and colleagues offer a caveat that resonates with Bronfenbrenner's perspective. Parental behaviors should not be overemphasized as *the* unitary and pervasive influence upon children. Rather parent factors ought to be considered as one part of intertwined biological, psychological, and sociological factors that affect a child (Bates, Bayles, Bennett, Ridge, & Brown, 1991). While recognizing Bates et al.'s precaution, inadequate parental caregiving still often is the most powerful direct risk that adversely influences young children's development.

The reason is simply that infants, toddlers, and preschoolers are captive audiences for their caregivers; they have limited access to resources outside of their immediate milieu.

Despite the profound and ubiquitous nature of external forces upon development, children are not merely passive recipients of experiences. They bring their own competencies (e.g., temperament, intelligence, language skills) as well as their vulnerabilities (e.g., poor health) to family relationships, peer interactions, and other social and educational relationships (Rutter, 1987). These resources and vulnerabilities mean that children are differentially vulnerable to risks in their environments (Garmezy, 1991). Thus, risks must be considered in relation to a particular child; humans are adaptable and some children ". . . live, if not thrive, in many environments that are purely and simply hostile" (Garbarino & associates, 1982, p. 668).

Identification of Causal Agents within the High-Risk Environment

Identifying those who will thrive and those who will succumb is a major challenge for both researcher and clinician. Moreover, even though environmental risk factors are obvious, it is still difficult to define the specific process or condition that relates to a particular child outcome. Many factors are involved.

One factor has to do with the developmental process itself. Development even under optimal rearing conditions rarely shows a linear incremental path. Rather, development consists of periods where major behavioral reorganizations occur (e.g., the cognitive shift after the preschool years) and other periods when behavioral change is incremental (e.g., the growth in children's memory). Once in a while the specific processes that account for one or another developmental change can be identified; most times they cannot (Wohlwill, 1973). We do know, however, that behavioral reorganizations can work to a child's advantage by facilitating the growth of skills that potentially help him or her become less vulnerable to adverse

162

environmental forces. As an example, the blossoming of friendships that often occurs during the school years can help a child learn to cope with an uncaring parent. Alternatively, the developmental process itself also can *create* stresses for the child. Consider early and midadolescence, which is often a time of self-doubt, inordinate self-directed criticism, and worry about the future. These normal developmental growth crises can be exacerbated by nonsupportive family environments. Behavioral scientists do not have a magic lens that will allow them to predict how developmental reorganizations will modify a particular child's functioning and how changes in the child will intersect with the chain of events that simultaneously occur in the environment.

As a corollary, there is a complicated interaction among the maturing child, his or her characteristics, and the nature of the environment the child is exposed to. Thus, at times children's development shows a logical consistency within and across transition periods; other times it does not. Data from the Berkeley and Oakland longitudinal studies (of essentially normal children) provide telling examples of vastly different, and sometimes extremely variable, developmental trajectories (Honzik, MacFarlane, & Allen, 1948; MacFarlane, Allen, & Honzik, 1954). Sometimes family crises appeared to be an influence; other times there was no discernible event that foreshadowed a child who faltered or one who blossomed after a period of relative nonoptimal development. When risk factors enter the picture, it becomes even more of a challenge to understand the forces behind developmental trajectories and outcomes.

Relatedly, data are sparse about particulars of developmental transitions and the intellectual, temperamental, and social resources that are available to children who are not at the extreme for developmental resiliency or vulnerability. It is apparent, however, that across age periods, some children are able to negotiate their way through environmental "minefields" because someone provides effective psychological support and the child has increasing intellectual, social, emotional, and motivational resources to cope with hurtful stresses within the environment. (See Earls, Beardslee, & Garrison, 1987; Werner & Smith, 1977, 1982.)

Still another complicating factor related to

causal mechanisms pertains to issues of measurement technology. As noted recently by Horowitz (1992), measurement of the child's environment is still relatively unrefined. The field lacks a sufficient number of sensitive recording procedures that can be used to portray different kinds of environmental events as well as the nature of the rearing environment. Parenthetically, it seems that this measurement challenge holds little interest for many researchers. In contrast, witness the extensive efforts currently being expended on devising sophisticated measurement technologies for measuring genetic risk factors and gene-environment interactions (Rowe, 1994).

Despite these challenges, research efforts are slowly yielding gains. For example, data unequivocally show that faulty parent-child communication patterns are associated with children's emotional and social problems. (See, e.g., Patterson & Bank, 1989. Zahn-Waxler, Cummings, Iannotti, & Radke-Yarrow, 1984.) Nonoptimal communication is frequently found among parents who are domineering and aggressive, those who psychologically withdraw from the child because of emotional illness or some other condition, or parents whose frequent disagreements create uncertainties for the child (Jouriles et al., 1991). Other conditions, some of which are beyond a parent's direct control, also have been identified as contributors to negative developmental growth. Overcrowding within a household is an example (Goduka, Poole, & Aotaki-Phenice, 1992); in high-density living conditions, noise and confusion probably interfere with processes involved in attending and learning (Deutsch & Deutsch, 1963).

Other interesting research recently has addressed the role of timing, that is, the abrupt onset of a negative risk event and its subsequent effects on children's psychosocial development. Elder and colleagues maintain that the more abrupt the onset of a risk event, the less chance the individual has to make anticipatory adjustments and to cope (Elder, 1991; Elder & Caspi, 1988). Data reveal a complex interaction between development and timing. In a study of behavioral effects of sudden and substantial family income loss, findings revealed adolescent males showed better adjustment and maturity than younger boys. The former became more mature because of responsibilities they had to assume to assist their families. In contrast, economic adversity fostered immaturity and family dependence among young boys because they were unable to assist in meeting family needs (Elder & Caspi, 1988; Elder, Caspi, & Van Nguyen, 1986). Supporting data about adjustment problems were reported in another study of young adolescent males whose families also faced sudden economic hardship (Conger et al., 1992).

Notably, the issue of developmental effects as a function of *long-term* versus *sudden onset* of environmental risks does not appear to have been empirically investigated. Elder's findings are provocative because intuitively it seems that child problems that stem from a sudden event, such as income loss, should seem less pervasive that those that occur in the face of a long-standing, unrelenting risk, such as poverty. In support of this perspective, Haskins (1986) points out that children reared in chronic poverty undergo a different form of socialization than children reared in more advantaged households. Economically poor children are at considerable risk for retarded intellectual and adaptive behavior (Ramey & Finkelstein, 1981; Ramey & McPhee, 1986). In contrast, children whose families suffered a sudden economic downturn presumably had a reasonable exposure to the values and ideals of the larger community. While economic hardship may make life hard for them, they probably have a sense of what they have lost and what they may aim for again. This is not the situation for many children who are reared in chronic and deep poverty.

High-Risk Environments, Young Children, and Developmental Considerations

Age per se is not a risk factor; however, age interacts with high risk environments leading to greater or lesser vulnerability for a child. Very young children, for example, may be particularly vulnerable to adverse experiences because the toddler and the preschool years are a time of major growth in cognition, social interactions skills, compliance to family and social standards, com-

municative abilities, the sense of selfhood, and emotion control (e.g., see Kopp, 1982, 1989). These are foundation skills that caregivers help young children acquire. Of equal importance, these are skills that underlie long-term intellectual, social, and emotional competencies. Because preschoolers are a captive audience for their caregivers (unlike their school-age peers), they are unable to go beyond the immediate family to find psychological and social supports among peers, with teachers, and with others in the neighborhood. When caregiving goes awry, child problems tend to surface.

Developmental problems (e.g., cognitive delays, behavior problems) that become prominent during early childhood would be inconsequential if they were of limited time duration, disappearing with the onset of the elementary school years. Unfortunately, this tends not to be the rule. With the exception of a few emotional and social difficulties that are linked to developmental transitions (e.g., fears during the preschool years, see MacFarlane et al., 1954), developmental problems of the preschool period continue, particularly when high-risk environments do not improve (Campbell, 1990; Goodman, 1992; McGuire & Richman, 1986; Richman, Stevenson, & Graham, 1982). Rutter (1989) suggests that continuities are found because children maintain memories of earlier learning and maintain aspects of earlier structural and functional changes. Rutter further states that it is unlikely that individual characteristics will predict the type of later change but is likely to predict levels of functioning because of incorporation of earlier levels.

Overall, continuity data are most conclusive for preschool children's cognitive and language problems, attentional difficulties, and child discipline (see Bates & Bayles, 1988; Richman et al., 1982) and somewhat more ambiguous for the preschooler's social and emotional disorders (see Bates et al., 1991; Campbell, 1990). In part the ambiguity about the incidence of social and emotional disorders may be a function of imprecision of diagnosis with young children (Campbell, 1990).

In sum, despite some inconsistencies in the data, there is agreement that what happens in the preschool years has major implications for later childhood competencies. Because so many factors have been implicated, researchers have tried to enumerate those that indicate risk and those that speak to protective forces. Table 20.1 lists many of these factors using an ecological perspective as an organizational framework.

Microsystem Risks and Outcomes

We have just provided a brief overview of salient characteristics of high-risk environments, potential outcomes for children, and the complexity inherent in trying to link risks and outcomes precisely. The following sections focus on two common microsystem risks for children, divorce and abuse. We recognize that it is artificial to separate microsystem risks from the ecological unit as a whole. Nonetheless, it is easier to review the literature using this approach. General outcomes are mentioned, and where data are available, outcomes for young children are discussed.

The two risks we discuss reflect disparate processes. One risk, divorce, reflects a dissolution of a structural relationship namely the family. A family breakup invariably signifies *separation and changes in routine* for the child; clearly, these are risk events. However, the child of divorce is not

TABLE 20.1

Risks and Buffers Associated with Early Childhood Behavior Problems

Risks	Buffers
Child Characteristics	
Biological risk (e.g., preterm birth; sensor motor impairment; developmental delay due to genetic disorder)	Good physical health
	Resiliency to stress
	Ability to utilize aggression adaptively
Gender	Successful resolution of stage-salient
Irritability	developmental tasks
Language delay	Good cognitive and language skills
Low interest in social contacts	Adaptive temperament
Deficits in social skills	High threshold for frustration
Cognitive delays	Sensitivity to social norms/conventions
	Self-control
Ecological Factors Microsystem: Parenting Skills	
Insensitivity	Supportive siblings
Unavailability	Sensitive older kin
Limited or negative affective involvement	Interventions for parent training
Overly harsh or very permissive control	
Inappropriate developmental expectations	
Microsystem: Family Constellations and Routines	
Single parents	Access to multiple individuals: for nurturance,
High-density living quarters	positive experiences
Haphazard routines	Access to other settings; e.g., day care
Argumentative household	
Limited psychological resources	
Exosystem Variables	
Economic distress	Economic opportunities
Limited access to formal and informal supports	Job training skills
Limited access to neighborhood child care facilities	Opportunities for family services, interventions
Macrosystem Variables	
Cultural support of "violence" to children	Government-sponsored health and social supports
Economic depression	Legislation directed to children's well-being
Limited national and state supports for working mothers	

SOURCE: Adapted from Campbell, 1990, and Cicchetti and Aber, 1986.

the recipient of action directed solely and explicity to the child per se. The child is an innocent and unwilling bystander. In contrast, in the second risk we discuss, child maltreatment, a parent acts out against a child. Here a child is drawn into adverse interactions in which a parent repeatedly informs the child of physical and psychological unworthiness. Although direct comparisons of these two risks are unavailable, it seems that child maltreatment has more profound and lasting consequences for development than does divorce.

To some extent the data also will emphasize a point made earlier: Certain kinds of risks are differentially associated with certain kinds of outcomes. For example, we mentioned that children exposed to pervasive and entrenched poverty and attendant other stresses often have their greatest limitations in intellectual and language functioning (e.g., Haskins, 1986). Acting-out behaviors also are noted. In contrast, the data show that divorce, for example, is a risk condition that tends to have greater links to children's social and emotional problems than to major cognitive limitations.

DIVORCE

Divorce affects families' relationships, routines, and material resources and is usually difficult and stressful (Hetherington & Stanley-Hagen, 1995). A divorce typically forces parents to take on unfamiliar roles and maintain preexisting ones while experiencing extreme personal conflict and crisis. The complex changes and stresses associated with divorce and marital conflict often affect parents and children for years (Johnston & Campbell, 1988; Wallerstein & Blakeslee, 1989).

Family Effects: Wallerstein and Blakeslee (1989) describe three phases of family adjustment to divorce. During the first phase—before, during, and immediately after the divorce—parents may be overcome with powerful emotions and cognitions that temporarily impair their judgment. This results in uncharacteristic maladaptive behaviors that lead to less effective parenting (Hess & Camera, 1979; Hetherington, 1979; Long & Forehand, 1987; Wallerstein, 1985a, b, c). In addition, family conflict may be aggravated by

child custody and financial disputes and hostility between parents during and after the divorce (Wallerstein & Kelly, 1982). Children's behavior suffers under these circumstances (Wolkind & Rutter, 1985).

Parents define their separate lives during the second phase of divorce. This transition period involves new living arrangements and possibly new jobs and new relationships. The resulting experience of continual change within the family often is associated with significant stress upon all family members. Although briefly diminished parenting competence is common, some situations lead to chronic parenting deficits. In extreme cases, the parent devotes time and emotional resources previously available to the child to a new relationship or becomes unavailable for some other reason, such as depression or drug involvement. In such cases, the children are put in the position of parenting themselves and caring for their parents, as well (Wallerstein, 1985c).

During the final phases of divorce, parents often establish stable identities and household routines that provide both benefits and disadvantages for the child. Diminished family income, a frequent result of divorce, often occurs because the noncustodial parent (usually the father) does not provide child support (National Center for Children in Poverty, 1991). Relatedly, the child may find that contact with the noncustodial parent is infrequent.

Even the quality of the custodial parent's relationship with the child becomes compromised. Hetherington, Cox, and Cox (1978, 1982) identify disorganization, deterioration of discipline, increased anger, and lower expectations for a child's appropriate behavior as some of the problems that custodial mothers experience. Other findings suggest that parent-child conflict and tension will increase if the custodial parent is the opposite sex of the child (Santrock et al., 1982).

General Consequences of Divorce: As noted, the volatile and distressing context of divorce frequently results in negative consequences for children. Continued exposure to parental conflicts before, during, or after divorce has been associated with negative psychological and developmental outcomes for children of all ages, many of which continue into or appear in young adulthood (Cummings & Davies, 1994; Katz & Gottman,

1993). These may include traumatic memories and dreams that continue for years and the development of similarly conflictual intimate adult relationships (Emery, 1982, Wallerstein & Corbin, 1991). Disproportionate numbers of children of divorce are found in outpatient psychiatric, family agency, and private practice populations (Gardner, 1976; Kaltener, 1977; Tessman, 1977; Tooley, 1976). Sadness, shock, and intense anxiety are common responses of children of all ages, even under circumstances when they were aware of high marital conflict (Wallerstein & Corbin, 1991).

Gender differences are apparent in young children's reactions to divorce. Young boys display loud, aggressive, and acting-out behavior, often paralleling the climate of conflict in the home prior to the divorce, while girls may display internalizing behaviors. It is believed that the behavioral differences in boys and girls do not reflect differential levels of distress (anger, guilt, or rejection) resulting from the divorce (Hetherington et al., 1986). Rather, distress shows itself in different ways.

Early Childhood Consequences of Divorce: Diverse outcomes have been reported for children age 3 and older. Overall, however, Hetherington's (1991) data reveal that children's ability to cope with divorce depends on numerous factors, including gender, family relations, remarriage, child temperament, and stress.

Findings are mixed with respect to the age at time of divorce that places the child at most risk, in part because the behavioral and emotional patterns that children display following divorce differ in accordance with developmental periods. Some data indicate that latency-age and older children demonstrate the most effects of parental conflict, perhaps because of more mature expressive abilities (Emery, 1982). Preadolescents and teenagers also may suffer more long-term trauma because of longer exposure to marital problems (Wallerstein & Blakeslee, 1989). Other studies report that young children are most distressed immediately following divorce (Allison & Furstenberg, 1989; Emery, 1988; Wallerstein & Blakeslee, 1989; Wallerstein & Kelly, 1982). Again, it is difficult to reach definitive conclusions because studies are not always comparable with respect to length of time since divorce; compounded effects

may be observed for children several years postdivorce (Allison & Furstenberg, 1989).

Developmental regressions, separation anxieties, and sleep disturbances (Wallerstein & Corbin, 1991) as well as tearfulness, irritability, aggression, and less peer interaction (Cole & Cole, 1989) are common postdivorce responses among preschoolers. Because preschoolers have limited ability to express their emotions verbally, they may respond to the divorce by acting out or by withdrawing. Further, their ability to understand the reasons for divorce is limited by their level of cognitive development. They frequently have inflated hopes of parental reconciliation (Hetherington, 1979; Wallerstein & Kelly, 1974). Many preschoolers also blame themselves for the divorce of their parents or believe that they are "bad" and therefore drove the absent parent away (Neal, 1983). A belief that courses through these studies seems to be that although the preschooler's reactions to divorce are profound, younger children show fewer long-term effects than do older children. However, systematic comparison studies have not been made.

Developmental effects as a function of gender also have been investigated. Findings reveal that preschool girls' behavioral reactions to divorce are not as extreme or as observable as the responses of boys. However, Allison and Furstenberg (1989) note that use of different behavioral measures may account for variable findings with regard to sex differences. In any event, girls tend to react more adaptively and adjust faster to the stresses of changes in routine following the divorce (Hetherington et al., 1982; Wallerstein & Kelley, 1980), a finding that may relate to their customary placement with the same-sex parent (Wallerstein & Corbin, 1991). However, difficulties in girls' adjustment may appear in later adolescence or early adulthood (Allison & Furstenberg, 1989; Wallerstein & Corbin, 1989). In contrast, preschoolage boys often develop dependent, clinging (less traditionally masculine) behavior toward their mothers. These behaviors are thought to be related to insufficient opportunities for sex-role identification with the father. Yet even this can be counterbalanced. Young boys adapt well when their mothers portray their fathers positively, demonstrate positive attitudes toward men in general, and encourage independence (Hetherington et al., 1978). Overall, it is clear, however, that for both young boys and girls, the primary identification figure may shift or become unclear during different stages of the divorce (Wallerstein & Corbin, 1991) at a time when identification with parents influences personality development, identity formation, and social learning (Cole & Cole, 1989).

In sum, divorce must be considered a serious microsystem risk. For a while the popular press and the scientific community treated divorce as a benign factor. Research from the past decade points to a different picture. However, should the child's family situation improve—that is, both parents remain involved, a caring role model surfaces—the outlook may be encouraging over the long term.

CHILD MALTREATMENT

While child abuse is primarily a microsystem risk, most often occuring in the immediate family context, protective intervention such as detection of abuse and parent education usually occur at the exosystem level. Macrosystem influences are present as well. For example, child abuse reporting has increased dramatically due to increasing social awareness of the problem (Russell & Trainor, 1984). Despite this increased awareness, social attitudes against reporting known abuse prevent some people from doing so (Dhooper, Royse, & Wolfe, 1991). Clearly, attitudes against reporting child abuse pose a direct danger to abused children, by allowing the abuse to go undetected by child protection agencies. This interdependence among the child, child protective agencies, and social attitudes illustrates mesosystem risk.

The absolute causes of child maltreatment have yet to be identified; however, factors associated with increased risk for maltreatment have been recognized among children (e.g., high levels of irritability), among adults (usually parents) (e.g., social isolation), and within the environment (e.g., major economic downturns). Child maltreatment is a risk factor for children of all ages. Maltreatment has been linked to numerous serious and undesirable outcomes for children in the domains of cognitive, social, emotional, behavioral, and physical development and functioning.

Risk Factors Associated with Child Maltreatment: By way of background, findings with regard to incidence and prevalence rates and risk factors for maltreatment vary with the type of investigation (e.g., prospective or retrospective, and the operational definitions used) and sampling characteristics (e.g., general public survey vs. child protective services data). Starr, Dubowitz, and Bush (1990) provide a comprehensive explanation of these potential sources of bias.

Some risk factors are intrinsic to the child and may include child age; however, findings have been inconclusive with respect to ages that pose the most risk for children. According to some sources, younger children are more likely to be reported as victims of abuse than are older children (Starr et al., 1990). In contrast, a national incidence survey found the rate of reported sexual and physical abuse for children newborn to 2 years of age to be lower than abuse rates for older children. By age 3, however, abuse rates are comparable to those of older children (Cappilleri, Eckenrode, & Powers, 1993). One survey found that 7% of 3- to 4-year-olds were physically abused, compared to 4% of older children (Gelles, 1978). Young children are at the highest risk of abuse-related fatalities, because a blow to their fragile bodies is more likely to cause fatal injury (Starr et al., 1990).

Child gender differentiates types of maltreatment. Boys are more likely to be abused in general, except in the case of sexual abuse (Starr et al., 1990). Boys are also more likely to be injured seriously (Rosenthal, 1988). In contrast, girls are 3 to 4 times more likely than boys to be sexually abused (National Center on Child Abuse and Neglect [NCCAN], 1988). A child's behavioral characteristics are another risk factor: Oppositional and defiant children often provoke abusive episodes from caregivers who are frustrated, angry, or have little energy for coping with an intractable child (Ammerman, Hersen, Van Hasselt, McGonigle, & Lubetsky, 1989; Loeber, Felton, & Reid, 1984).

Other risk factors have been identified. Ethnicity is an example: more reports of abuse, as well as higher fatalities, are reported for black children (Cappelleri, 1993; Starr et al., 1990). However, race and ethnicity were found to be unrelated to rates of maltreatment in a national incidence survey (NCCAN, 1988), and family size is positively associated with both abuse and neglect. Income is an important factor; children from families earning less than $15,000 a year have substantially higher rates of physical abuse, sexual abuse, and serious physical injury (Cappelleri et al., 1993). Lastly, geographic location is unrelated to prevalence of sexual abuse (Cappelleri et al., 1993; Wyatt & Peters, 1986).

The search for adult correlates of child maltreatment has been an important avenue of research. Parent psychopathology has been researched extensively. Wolfe (1985) found that severe parental psychopathology is not the sole factor in most cases of child abuse, although low frustration tolerance, inappropriate expression of anger, social isolation (also cited by Garbarino, 1977), impaired parenting skills, unrealistic expectations of children, and low sense of parenting competence have been associated with abusive parenting (LaRose-Wolfe, 1987).

One reason that identification of parent correlates of child maltreatment has been difficult may relate to the complex roles and responsibilities that parents bring to child rearing. Researchers have tended to pay substantial attention to the most obvious parental contributions of psychopathology, isolation, and incompetence. Table 20.2 lists variables that also could be part of Bronfen-brenner's (1979) parent-child microsystem. For the most part, these variables have not been studied as additional parental contributors, along with the perpetration of actual abuse, to adverse child outcomes.

Parents' gender differentiates the type of maltreatment they perpetrate, but there is an interaction with child age. In a survey of the general public, Gelles (1978) found that 4% of fathers and 6% of mothers were abusive. Mothers are more likely to abuse younger children, and fathers abuse older children (Rosenthal, 1988). Females are more likely to murder, neglect, or psychologically maltreat their children (American Association for Protecting Children, 1988). Investigators have theorized that the apparent discrepancy between rates of abuse by fathers and mothers is related to mothers' greater contact with children (Starr et al., 1990).

Despite repeated evidence for the association of these factors to children's development, investigative limitations frequently result in inaccurate or inconclusive links to risk factors and outcomes. Convergent research support for the aforementioned factors is required in order to reach definitive conclusions. By way of support for this statement, consider the following: In one of the few prospective, longitudinal investigations of risk factors for abuse, Egeland and Brunnquell (1979) re-

TABLE 20.2

The Needs of Children—The Responsibilities of Parents

Children's Needs	Parents' Responsibilities
Nurturance	Affiliation Social support Caring
Physical care	Food, shelter, clothing Hygiene Health care
Teaching	Information facts, "how to" Family "dos" and "don'ts" Procedural knowledge "what," "when" Emotion and social norms Moral and legal systems
Temporal/spatial structure	Routines and schedules Time demands Opportunities for child within family schedules

ported no statistically significant risk factors for child outcome. In a related vein, Aber, Allen, Carlson, & Cicchetti (1989) note that much of the research on behavioral consequences of maltreatment is confounded by socioeconomic factors that have been empirically associated negative with behavioral symptomology. These findings illustrate the point made earlier about the difficulty of determining causal associations.

What conclusions can be drawn? Overall, it appears that the developmental sequelae of maltreatment are determined by the type of maltreatment the child has experienced (physical abuse, sexual abuse, physical neglect, psychological neglect, and psychological abuse, see Starr et al., 1990, for definitions, length of maltreatment, severity, frequency, child's age, and situational context). Consequences also are influenced by whether a single type of maltreatment occurred or whether different types co-occurred. The severity and nature of outcomes for maltreated children are therefore heterogeneous (Hoffman-Plotkin & Twentyman, 1984). Chronic, less severe physical or emotional abuse may produce more serious emotional and physical damage than a single severely abusive event (Herrenkohl, 1990). The numerous risk factors mentioned demonstrate that child, family, and sociocultural characteristics, in addition to demographic factors, are related to negative outcomes.

General Consequences of Maltreatment: Although outcome findings vary due to type of maltreatment examined, definitions employed, type of study, and sampling, there is consensus that all types of maltreatment are associated with detrimental outcomes. In addition to the physiological damage that is most often obvious (Ammerman, Cassisi, Hersen, & Van Hasselt, 1986), the consequences of maltreatment appear in social, cognitive, emotional, and behavioral domains. The social consequences of child maltreatment include agression (particularly for physically and sexually abused children; Egeland, Sroufe, & Erickson, 1983; Tong, Oates, & McDowell, 1987) and poor peer relations (Bousha & Twentyman, 1984; Martin & Beezley, 1977; Oates, Peacock, & Forrest, 1984; Tong et al., 1987). Peer relations in turn, predict present and future mental health problems, including psychiatric disorders (Coie, 1992; Cowen, Pederson, Babigan, Izzo, & Trost, 1973;

Roff, Sells, & Golden, 1972). Neglected children may fail to develop normally in the areas of social maturity, language development, and verbal ability (Oates et al., 1984; Polansky, Chalmers, Buttenweiser, & Williams). A long-term consequence of sexual abuse is lack of trust and difficulties with heterosexual relationships (Wolfe, Wolfe, & Best, 1988). Emotional problems include poor self-esteem, depression (Egeland et al., 1983; Kazdin, Moser, Colbus, & Bell, 1985; Oates et al., 1984; Tong et al., 1987) and anxiety (Green, 1978).

Behaviorally, maltreated children in general are found to be more aggressive/rejecting or withdrawn/isolated than their nonmaltreated peers (Aber et al., 1989; Burgess & Conger, 1978; Galdston, 1971; George & Main, 1979; Green, 1978; Martin, 1980; Martin & Beezley, 1977; Reidy, 1977; Straker & Jacobson, 1981). Physical abuse has been associated to both withdrawal and agression (Martin & Beezley, 1977), while neglected children are likely to be socially and emotionally withdrawn (Kent, 1976). Additional behavior problems include noncompliance, distractability, low ego control, and low creativity (Egeland et al., 1983). Conduct disturbances are disproportionately represented in samples of maltreated children (McCord, 1983). Various psychopathological outcomes have been reported for maltreated children, but no pattern of symptoms is evident for the group as a whole (Ammerman et al., 1986).

Common cognitive effects of maltreatment include intellectual deficits (Hoffman-Plotkin & Twentyman, 1984; Kent, 1976), poor academic performance (Martin & Beezley, 1977; Tong et al., 1987), problems with self-regulation (Aber et al., 1989), and less readiness to learn in terms of motivation, curiosity, and cognitive maturity (Aber et al., 1989). Although lack of empathy has been reported as a consequence of maltreatment (Straker & Jacobson, 1981), under certain circumstances maltreatment promotes empathy for social problems. Smetana, Kelly, & Twentyman (1984) found that physically abused children had higher awareness of the wrongness of psychologically harmful acts and that neglected children were more condemning of acts of unfair resource distribution.

Consequences of Maltreatment to Early Childhood Adaptation: Insecure attachment formation with the primary caregiver (Egeland & Sroufe, 1981; Schneider-Rosen, Braunwald, Carlson, & Cicchetti, 1985), delayed separation and individuation, and reluctance to explore the environment and relate to others (Sroufe & Rutter, 1984) are possible consequences of disruption during early childhood stages. Some findings indicate that preschoolers and early school-age children who have been maltreated demonstrate higher levels of dependence on unfamiliar adults (Aber et al., 1989), while others indicate internalizing behaviors with both peers and caregivers in day-care settings (George & Main, 1979). These early faltering steps along the path of psychosocial development may give rise to additional problems in later development, such as difficulty building trusting relationships (Kinnard, 1980). Verbal and cognitive dysfunctions also have been documented.

This overview focuses on child abuse as an early childhood risk that involves each level of Bronfenbrenner's ecological model and on the negative consequences of this major risk. These consequences are sometimes moderated by buffers or protective factors, as illustrated earlier. When protective factors outweigh the influence of risks in the child's environment, child abuse can be prevented, or the negative effects can be mitigated (Belsky, 1993; Cicchetti & Toth, 1995). The development and implementation of interventions designed to provide the right combination of protective factors is exceedingly difficult, due to the complex interactions between multiple risk and protective factors, and to the variation in the pattern of factors for each child and his or her family. Research that addresses the interplay of multiple risk and protective factors as well as the problem of specificity is needed to improve upon the effectiveness of current interventions. Cognitive problems often exacerbate social and emotional problems.

the nature of risks and related consequences requires recognition of factors that obscure their relationships, such as the variability of normal developmental patterns, individual differences in coping ability, and measurement limitations. Numerous risk factors have been identified across a range of relevant literatures. However, due to the typical complexity of multiple contributing factors, the precise determination of causal relationships has seldom been achieved.

Conclusions from two areas of investigation for which data predominate, divorce and child maltreatment, exemplify the important position of microsystem risk factors as contributors to child outcomes. Some connections between these factors and macro- and exosystem influences are also evident. The range of domains in which negative outcomes are observed parallels the multidimensional quality of the risk environments themselves. The consequences of divorce that have been reported commonly relate to emotion, self-concept, and conduct. Outcomes associated with intellectual functioning, social interaction, emotional state, conduct, and physiological state are indicated for various subcategories of child maltreatment. Despite problems of causal specificity, data resoundingly indicate that divorce and child abuse adversely affect children's development. The data on cognitive effects are less conclusive, but the social and emotional findings are clear. Moreover, it seems that if family economic status is controlled statistically, children's social and emotional functioning would be most affected. Just how many children are affected for the short or long term is unknown. Rutter (1989) provides a possible explanation for long-term continuity: "... the impact of some factor in childhood may lie less in the immediate behavioral change it brings about than in the fact that it set in motion a chain reaction in which one 'bad' thing leads to another ..." (p. 27).

SUMMARY

This discussion of risk environments and consequences to young children illustrates the multidimensional, interactional nature of environmental risks. Bronfenbrenner's ecological model delineates a framework for categorizing and evaluating risk factors. However, a careful interpretation of

Concluding Comments

APPLIED FACTORS

Macrosystem risks are not remediated easily and quickly, yet concerted actions by groups of concerned individuals can lead to change. Legislation enacted in the past three decades on behalf of children bear witness to this point; laws have been passed that mandated free and equal education irrespective of ethnic status or presence of a handicapping condition. Numerous programs have been initiated to deal with exosystem risks, some oriented to parents (e.g., education and training), to children both for prevention and remediation, and to both parents and children, as for example in Head Start programs. (See, e.g., Zigler et al., 1992.) It is likely that massive efforts will have to be directed to all levels of the exosystem in order to ameliorate the untoward effects of environmental risks. Promising efforts in this direction include the multidimensional Vaughn Street School Model, which provides comprehensive services to children and families in an easily accessible, familiar setting. This model shows that although risks will never disappear, they can be reduced.

RESEARCH ISSUES

This chapter has highlighted some of the unresolved questions about high-risk environments and child development. In situations where it is ethical and feasible, additional prospective, longitudinal investigations can help disentangle the complex web of risks and consequences, especially in the areas of child maltreatment and poverty, where such studies are scarce. Innovative methods for further differentiating the contribu-

tions of poverty from other risks are needed (Aber et al., 1989). Additionally, the protective factors that allow some children to succeed despite economic disadvantage (e.g., Werner & Smith, 1982) merit further inquiry.

As methodological advancements continue, research priorities should increasingly be directed to specification of findings with respect to ethnic and cultural factors. It is possible that adaptiveness varies as a function of culture because the "norms" of behavior, emotions, and cognitions vary culturally. Stated another way, this means that certain responses may be present in some populations without being associated with developmental risk. The point is that outcomes may vary considerably when different groups are studied. Caucasian samples often are used in studies of divorce. Are effects similar for non-Caucasian samples of children? Similarly, people of color are overrepresented in poverty. Thus, there is a need to disentangle influences from poverty per se with ethnic factors.

Overall, more representative sampling is needed in future research in order to compensate for the overrepresentation of ethnic subjects in some investigations (e.g., maltreatment prevalence reports based on welfare agency data) and their underrepresentation in others (e.g., divorce, sudden-onset poverty). Multisite and epidemiological research, although costly, is needed to address these issues.

The challenge of understanding causes and effects in high-risk environments is daunting. However, as has been shown in this chapter, progress is being made.

REFERENCES

Aber, J. L., Allen, J. P., Carlson, V., & Cicchetti, D. (1989). The effects of maltreatment on development during early childhood: Recent studies and their theoretical, clinical, and policy implications. In D. Cicchetti & V. Carlson (Eds.), *Child maltreatment: Theory and research on the causes and consequences of child abuse and neglect.* (pp. 579–619). New York: Cambridge University Press.

Allison, P., & Furstenberg, F., Jr. (1989). How marital dissolution affects children: Variations by age and sex. *Developmental Psychology, 25,* 540–549.

American Association for Protecting Children. (AAPC). (1988). *Highlights of official child neglect and abuse*

reporting, 1986. Denver: American Humane Association.

Ammerman, R. T., Cassisi, J. E., Hersen, M., & Van Hasselt, V. B. (1986). Consequences of physical abuse and neglect in children. *Clinical Psychology Review, 6,* 291–310.

Ammerman, R. T., Van Hasselt, V. B., McGonigle, J. J., & Lubetsky, L. (1989). Abuse and neglect in psychiatrically hospitalized multihandicapped children. *Child Abuse and Neglect, 13* (3), 335–343.

Bates, J. E., & Bayles, K. (1988). Attachment and the development of behavior problems. In J. Belsky and T. Nezworski (Eds.), *Clinical implications of attach-*

ment (pp. 253–299). Hillsdale, NJ: Lawrence Erlbaum.

Bates, J. E., Bayles, K., Bennett, D. S., Ridge, B., & Brown, M. M. (1991). Origins of externalizing behavior problems at eight years of age. In D. J. Pepler & K. H. Rubin (Eds.), *The development and treatment of childhood aggression* (pp. 93–120). Hillsdale, NJ: Lawrence Erlbaum.

Belsky, J. (1984). The determinants of parenting: A process model. *Child Development, 55,* 83–96.

Belsky, J. (1993). Etilogy of Child Maltreatment: A Developmental-Ecological Analysis. *Psychological Bulletin, 114* (3), 413–434.

Bousha, D. M., & Twentyman, C. T. (1984). Mother-child interactional style in abuse, neglect, and control groups: Naturalistic observations in the home. *Child Development, 93,* 196–214.

Bronfenbrenner, U. (1979). *The ecology of human development: Experiments by nature and design.* Cambridge, MA: Harvard University Press.

Bronfenbrenner, U., & Crouter, A. C. (1983). The evolution of environmental models in developmental research. In P. H. Mussen (Ed.), *Handbook of child psychology* (4th ed., pp.). New York: John Wiley & Sons.

Burgess, R. L., & Conger, R. D. (1978). Family interaction in abusive, neglectful, and normal families. *Child Development, 49,* 1163–1173.

Campbell, S. (1990). *Behavior problems in preschool children.* New York: Guilford Press.

Cappelleri, J. C., Eckenrode, J., & Powers, J. L. (1993). The epidemiology of child abuse: Findings from the Second National Incidence and Prevalence Study of Child Abuse and Neglect. *American Journal of Public Health, 83,* 1622–1624.

Cherlin, A. J. (1988). The weakening link between marriage and the care of children. *Family Planning Perspectives, 20* (6), 302–306.

Cicchetti, D., & Aber, J. L. (1986). Early precursors of later depression: An organizational perspective. In L. P. Lipsitt & C. Rovee-Collier, (Eds.), *Advances in infancy research* (Vol. 4, pp. 87–137). Norwood, NJ: Ablex.

Cicchetti, D., & Carlson, V. (1987). *Child maltreatment: Theory and research on the causes and consequences of child abuse and neglect.* New York: Cambridge University Press.

Cicchetti, D., & Toth, S. L. (1995). A developmental psychopathology Perspective on Child Abuse and Neglect. *Journal of the American Academy of Child and Adolescent Psychiatry, 34* (5), 541–565.

Coie, J. D., Lochman, J. E., Terry, R., & Hyman, C. (1992). Predicting early adolescent disorder from childhood aggression and peer rejection. *Journal of Consulting and Clinical Psychology, 60* (5), 783–792.

Cole, M., & Cole, S. (1989). *The development of children.* New York: Scientific American.

Conger, R. D., Conger, K. J., Elder, G. H., Jr., Lorenz, F. O., Simons, R. L., & Whitbeck, L. B. (1992). A family process model of economic hardship and adjustment of early adolescent boys. *Child Development, 63,* 526–541.

Cowen, E. L., Pederson, A., Babigian, H., Izzo, L. D., & Trost, M. (1973). Long-term follow-up of early detected vulnerable children. *Journal of Consulting and Clinical Psychology, 41* (3), 438–446.

Cummings, E. M., & Davies, P. (1994). *Children and marital conflict: The impact of family dispute and resolution.* New York: Guilford Press.

Deutsch, M., & Deutsch, C. (1963). *Disadvantaged children.* New York: Guilford Press.

Dhooper, S. S., Royse, D. D., & Wolfe, L. C. (1991). A statewide study of public attitudes toward child abuse. *Child Abuse and Neglect, 15* (1), 37–44.

Dishion, T. J., Duncan, T. E., Eddy, J. M., Fagot, B. I., & Fetrow, R. (1994). The world of parents and peers: Coerceive exchanges and children's social adaptation. *Social Development, 3,* 255–268.

Duncan, G. J., Brooks-Gunn, J., & Klebanov, P. K. (1994). Economic deprivation and early childhood development. *Child Development, 65,* 296–318.

Earls, F., Beardslee, W., & Garrison, W. (1987). Correlates and predictors of competence in young children. In E. J. Anthony & B. Cohler (Eds.), *The invulnerable child.* New York: Guilford.

Egeland, B., & Brunnquell, D. (1979). An at-risk approach to the study of child abuse. *Journal of the American Academy of Child Psychiatry, 18,* 219–236.

Egeland, B., & Sroufe, L. A. (1981). Attachment and early maltreatment. *Child Development, 52,* 44–52.

Egeland, B., Sroufe, L. A., & Erickkson, M. (1983). The developmental consequences of different patterns of maltreatment. *Child Abuse and Neglect, 1,* 459–469.

Elder, G. H., Jr. (1991). Family transitions, cycles, and social changes. In P. A. Cowan & M. Hetherington (Eds.), *Family transitions.* Hillsdale, NJ: Lawrence Erlbaum.

Elder, G. H., Jr., & Caspi, A. (1988). Economic stress in lives: Developmental perspectives. *Journal of Social Issues, 44* (4), 25–45.

Elder, G. H., Jr., Caspi, A., & Van Nguyen, T. (1986). Resourceful and vulnerable children: Family influences in hard times. In R. Silbereisen & H. Eyferth (Eds.), *Development in context.* Berlin: Springer.

Emery, R. E. (1982). Interparental conflict and the children of discord and divorce. *Psychological Bulletin, 92,* 310–330.

Emery, R. E. (1988). *Marriage, divorce and children's adjustment.* Beverly Hills, CA: Sage Publications.

Furstenberg, F. F., Brooks-Gunn, J., & Morgan, S. P. (1987). *Adolescent mothers in later life.* New York: Cambridge University Press.

Furstenberg, F. F., & Harris, K. M. (1992). The disappearing American father? Divorce and the waning significance of biological parenthood. In S. J. South & S. E. Tolnay (Eds.), *The changing American family.* Boulder, CO: Westview Press.

Galdston, R. (1971). Violence begins at home: The parents center for the study and prevention of child abuse. *Journal of the American Academy of Child Psychiatry, 10,* 336–350.

Garbarino, J. (1977). The human ecology of child maltreatment: A conceptual model for research. *Journal of Marriage and the Family, 39,* 721–735.

Garbarino, J. (1990). The human ecology of early risk. In S. J. Meisels & J. P. Shonkoff (Eds.), *Handbook of early childhood intervention.* New York: Cambridge University Press.

Garbarino, J., & associates. (1982). *Children and families in the social environment.* New York: Aldine.

Garbarino, J., Kostelny, K., & Dubrow, N. (1991). *No place to be a child: Growing up in a war zone.* Lexington, MA: Lexington Books.

Gardner, R. A. (1976). *Psychotherapy and children of divorce.* New York: Jason Aronson.

Garmezy, N. (1991). Resiliency and vulnerability to adverse developmental outcomes associated with poverty. *American Behavioral Scientist, 34* (4), 416–430.

Gelles, R. J. (1978). Violence toward children in the United States. *American Journal of Orthopsychiatry, 48,* 580–592.

George, C., & Main, M. (1979). Social interactions of young abused children: Approach, avoidance, and aggression. *Child Development, 50,* 306–318.

Goduka, I. N., Poole, D. A., & Aotaki-Phenice, L. (1992). A comparative study of Black South African children from three different contexts. *Child Development, 63,* 509–525.

Goodman, J. (1992). *When slow is fast enough.* New York: Guilford Press.

Goodnow, J., & Collins, A. (1990). *Development according to parents: The nature, sources, and consequences of parents' ideas.* Hillsdale, NJ: Lawrence Erlbaum.

Green, A. H. (1978). Psychopathology of abused children. *Journal of the American Academy of Child Psychiatry, 17,* 92–103.

Haskins, R. (1986). Social and cultural factors in risk assessment and mild mental retardation. In D.C. Farran & J. D. McKinney, *Risk in intellectual and psychosocial development.* Orlando, FL: Academic Press.

Herrenkohl, R. C. (1990). Research directions related to child abuse and neglect. In R. T. Ammerman & M. Hersen (Eds.), *Children at risk.* New York: Plenum Press.

Hess, R. D., & Camera, K. A. (1979). Post-divorce family relationships as mediating factors in the consequences of divorce for children. *Journal of Social Issues, 35,* 79–96.

Hetherington, E. M. (1979). Divorce: A child's perspective. *American Psychologist, 34,* 851.

Hetherington, E. M. (1991). The role of individual differences and family relationships in children's coping with divorce and remarriage. In P. A. Cowan & M. Hetherington (Eds.), *Family transitions.* Hillsdale, NJ: Lawrence Erlbaum.

Hetherington, E. M., Cox, M., & Cox, R. (1978). The aftermath of divorce. In J. H. Stevens & M. Matthews, M. (Eds.), *Mother/child, father/child relation-*

ships. Washington, DC: National Association for the Education of Young Children.

Hetherington, E. M., Cox, M., & Cox, R. (1982). Effects of divorce on parents and children. In M. Lamb (Ed.), *Nontraditional families: Parenting and child development.* Hillsdale, NJ: Lawrence Erbaum.

Hetherington, E. M., Cox, M., & Cox, R. (1986). Long-term effects of divorce and remarriage on the adjustment of children. *Annual Progress in Child Psychiatry and Child Development,* 407–429.

Hetherington, E. M., & Stanley-Hagen, M. M. (1995). Parenting in divorced and remarried families. In M. H. Bornstein (Ed.), *Handbook of parenting: Vol. 3. Status & social conditions of parenting* (pp 233–254) Mahweh, NJ: Lawrence Erlbaum.

Hoffman-Plotkin, D., & Twentyman, C. T. (1984). A multimodel assessment of behavioral and cognitive deficits in abused and neglected preschoolers. *Child Development, 55,* 794–802.

Honzik, M. P., MacFarlane, J. W., Allen, L. (1948). Stability of mental test performance between two and eighteen years. *Journal of Experimental Education, 17,* 309–320.

Horowitz, F. D. (1992, August). Symposium conducted at the annual meeting of the American Psychological Association, Washington, DC.

Johnston, J. R., & Campbell, L. E. G. (1988). *Impasses of divorce the dynamics and resolution of family conflict.* New York: Free Press.

Jouriles, E. N., Murphy, C. M., Farris, A. M., Smith, D. A., Richters, J. E., & Waters, E. (1991). Marital adjustment, parental disagreements about child rearing, and behavior problems in boys: Increasing the specificity of the marital assessment. *Child Development, 62* (6), 1424–1433.

Kadushin, A., & Martin, J. A. (1981). *Child abuse: An interactional event.* New York: Columbia University Press.

Kaltener, N. (1977). Children of divorce in an outpatient psychiatric population. *American Journal of Orthopsychiatry, 47,* 40–51.

Katz, L. F., & Gottman, J. M. (1993). Patterns of marital conflict predict children's internalizing and externalizing behaviors *Developmental Psychology, 29,* 940–950.

Kazdin, A. E., Moser, J., Colbus, D., & Bell, R. (1985). Depressive symptoms among physically abused and psychiatrically disturbed children. *Journal of Consulting and Clinical Psychology, 94,* 298–307.

Kent, J. (1976). A follow-up study of abused children. *Journal of Pediatric Psychology,* 1, 24–31.

Kinnard, E. M. (1980). Emotional development in physically abused children. *American Journal of Orthopsychiatry, 4,* 686–696.

Kopp, C. B. (1982). The antecedents of self-regulation: A developmental perspective. *Developmental Psychology, 18,* 199–214.

Kopp, C. B. (1989). Regulation of distress and negative emotions: A developmental view. *Developmental Psychology, 25,* 343–354.

Loeber, R., Felton, D. K., & Reid, J. (1984). A social

learning approach to the reduction of coercive processes in child abusive families: A molecular analysis. *Advances in Behavior Research and Therapy, 6,* 29–45.

Long, N., & Forehand, R. (1987). The effects of parental divorce and parental conflict on children: An overview. *Developmental and Behavioral Pediatrics, 8,* 292–297.

MacFarlane, J. W., Allen, L., & Honzik, M. (1954). *A developmental study of the behavior problems of normal children between twenty-one months and fourteen years.* Berkeley: University of California Press.

Martin, H. P. (1976). *The abused child.* Cambridge, MA: Ballinger.

Martin, H. P. (1980). The consequences of being abused and neglected: How the child fares. In C. H. Kempe & R. E. Helfer (Eds.), *The battered child* (3rd ed.). Chicago: University of Chicago Press.

Martin, H. P., & Beezley, P. (1977). Behavioral observations of abused children. *Developmental Medicine and Child Neurology, 9,* 373–387.

McCarthy, J. B. (1990). Abusive families and character formation. *American Journal of Psychoanalysis, 50* (2), 181–186.

McCord, J. (1983). A 40-year perspective on effects of child abuse and neglect. *Child Abuse and Neglect, 7,* 265–270.

McGuire, J., & Richman, N. (1986). Screening for behavioral problems in nurseries: The reliability and validity of the preschool behavior checklist. *Journal of Child Psychiatry, 27,* 7–32.

National Center for Children in Poverty. (1991). *Five million children: 1991 update.* New York: Columbia University School of Public Health.

National Center on Child Abuse and Neglect. (NCCAN). (1988). *Study findings: Study of national incidence and prevalence of child abuse and neglect: 1988.* Washington, DC: U.S. Department of Health and Human Services.

Neal, J. (1983). Children's understanding of their parent's divorce. In L. Kurdek (Ed.), *New directions for child development: Vol. 19. Children and divorce.* San Francisco: Jossey-Bass.

Oates, R. K., Peacock, A., & Forrest, D. (1984). Development in children following abuse and nonorganic failure to thrive. *American Journal of Disorders in Children, 138,* 764–767.

Offord, D. R., Boyle, M. H., & Racine, Y. A. (1991). The epidemiology of antisocial behavior in childhood and adolescence. In D. J. Pepler & K. H. Rubin (Eds.), *The development and treatment of childhood aggression.* Hillsdale, NJ: Lawrence Erlbaum.

Patterson, G. R., & Bank, L. (1989). Some amplifying mechanisms for pathologic processes in families. In M. R. Gunnar & E. Thelen (Eds.), *Systems and development: The Minnesota symposia on child psychology* (Vol. 22). Hillsdale, NJ: Lawrence Erlbaum.

Patterson, G. R., & Capaldi, D. M. (1991). Antisocial parents: Unskilled and vulnerable. In P. A. Cowan &

M. Hetherington (Eds.), *Family transitions.* Hillsdale, NJ: Lawrence Erlbaum.

Polansky, N. A., Chalmers, M. A., Buttenweiser, E., & Williams, D. P. (1981). *Damaged parents: An anatomy of child neglect.* Chicago: University of Chicago Press.

Ramey, C. T., & Finkelstein, N. W. (1981). Psychosocial mental retardation: A biological and social coalescence. In M. Begab, H. C. Haywood, & H. Garber (Eds.), *Psychosocial influences and retarded performance: Vol. 1. Strategies for improving competence.* Baltimore: University Park Press.

Ramey, C. T., & McPhee, D. (1986). Developmental retardation: A systems theory perspective on risk and preventive intervention. In D.C. Farran & J. D. McKinney, *Risk in intellectual and psychosocial development.* Orlando, FL: Academic Press.

Reidy, T. J. (1977). The aggressive characteristics of abused and neglected children. *Journal of Clinical Psychology, 33,* 1140–1145.

Richman, N., Stevenson, J., & Graham, P. J. (1982). *Preschool to school: A behavioral study.* London: Academic Press.

Roff, M., Sells, S. B., & Golden, M. M. (1972). *Social adjustment and personality development in children.* Minneapolis: University of Minnesota Press.

Rosenthal, J. A. (1988). Patterns of reported child abuse and neglect. *Child Abuse and Neglect, 12,* 263–271.

Rowe, D.C. (1994). *The limits of family influence: Genes, experience, and behavior.* New York: Guilford Press.

Russell, A. B. & Trainor, C. M. (1984). *Trends in child abuse and neglect. A national perspective.* Denver: American Humane Association.

Rutter, M. (1981). Stress, coping, and development: Some issues and questions. *Journal of Child Psychology and Psychiatry, 22,* 256–323.

Rutter, M. (1987). Psychosocial resilience and protective mechanisms. *American Journal of Orthopsychiatry, 57* (3), 316–331.

Rutter, M. (1988). Epidemiological approaches to developmental psychopathology. *Archives of General Psychiatry, 45,* 486–495.

Rutter, M. (1989). Pathways from childhood to adult life. *Journal of Child Psychology and Psychiatry, 30* (1), 23–51.

Santrock, J. W., Warshak, R., Lindbergh, C., et al. (1982). Children's and parents' observed social behavior in step-father families. *Child Development, 53,* 472–480.

Schneider-Rosen, K., Braunwald, K, Carlson, V., & Cicchetti, D. (1985). Current perspectives in attachment theory: Illustration from the study of maltreated infants. *Monographs of the Society for Research in Child Development, 50* (1–2, Serial No. 209).

Smetana, J. G., Kelly, M., & Twentyman, C. T. (1984). Abused neglected and nonmaltreated children's conceptions of moral and social-conventional transgressions. *Child Development, 55* (1), 227–287.

Spanier, G. B. (1989). Bequeathing family continuity. *Journal of Marriage and the Family, 51* (1), 3–13.

Sroufe, L. A., & Rutter, M. (1984). The domain of developmental psychopathology. *Child Development, 55,* 17–29.

Starr, R. H. Jr., Dubowitz, H., & Bush, B. A. (1990). The epidemiology of child maltreatment. In R. T. Ammerman, & M. Hersen (Eds.) *Children at risk: An evaluation of factors contributing to child abuse and neglect.* (pp. 23–53). New York: Plenum Press.

Straker, G., & Jacobson, R. S. (1981). Aggression, emotional maladjustment and empathy in the abused child. *Developmental Psychology, 17,* 762–765.

Tarnowski, K. J., & Blechman, E. A. (1991). Introduction to the special section: Disadvantaged children and families. *Journal of Clinical Child Psychology, 20* (4), 338–339.

Teachman, J. D. (1992). Intergenerational resource transfers across disrupted households: Absent fathers' contributions to the well-being of their children. In S. J. Scott & S. E. Tolnay (Eds.), *The changing American family.* Boulder, CO: Westview Press.

Tessman L. H. (1977). *Children of parting parents.* New York: Jason Aronson.

Tong, L., Oates, K., & McDowell, M. (1987). Personality development following sexual abuse. *Child Abuse and Neglect, 11,* 371–383.

Tooley, K. (1976). Antisocial behavior and social alienation post divorce: The "man of the house" and his mother. *American Journal of Orthopsychiatry, 46,* 33–42.

Wallerstein, J. S. (1985a). Changes in parent-child relationships during and after divorce. In E. J. Anthony & G. H. Pollock (Eds.), *Parental influences in health and disease.* Boston: Little Brown.

Wallerstein, J. S. (1985b). Children of divorce: Emerging trends. *Psychiatric Clinics of North America, 8* (4), 837–855.

Wallerstein, J. S. (1985c). The overburdened child: Some long-term consequences of divorce. *Social Work, 30,* 116–123.

Wallerstein, J. S., & Blakeslee, S. (1989). *Second chances: Men, women, and children a decade after divorce.* New York: Ticknor & Fields.

Wallerstein, J. S., & Corbin, S. B. (1989). Daughters of divorce: Report from a ten-year followup. *American Journal of Orthopsychiatry, 59* (4), 593–604.

Wallerstein, J. S., & Corbin, S. B. (1991). The child and the vicissitudes of divorce. In M. Lewis (Ed.), *Child and Adolescent Psychiatry.* Baltimore: Williams & Wilkins.

Wallerstein, J. S., & Kelly, J. B. (1974). The effects of parental divorce: The adolescent experience. In E. Anthony & A. Koupernik (Eds.), *The child in his family: Children as a psychiatric risk (Vol. 3).* New York: John Wiley & Sons.

Wallerstein, J. S., & Kelly, J. B. (1975). The effects of parental divorce: Experiences of the preschool child. *Journal of the American Academy of Child Psychiatry, 14,* 600–616.

Wallerstein, J. S., & Kelly, J. B. (1980). Effects of divorce on the visiting father-child relationship. *American Journal of Psychiatry, 137* (12), 1534–1539.

Wallerstein, J. S., & Kelly, J. B. (1982). *Surviving the breakup: How children and parents cope with divorce.* New York: Basic Books.

Werner, E. E., & Smith, R. S. (1977). *Kauai's children come of age.* Honolulu: University of Hawaii Press.

Werner, E. E., & Smith, R. S. (1982). *Vulnerable, but invincible: A longitudinal study of resilient children and youth.* New York: McGraw-Hill.

Wohlwill, J. F. (1973). *The study of behavioral development.* New York: Academic Press.

Wolfe, D. A. (1985). Child abusive parents: An empirical review and analysis. *Psychological Bulletin, 97,* 462–482.

Wolfe, D. A., Wolfe, V. V., & Best, C. L. (1988). Child victims of sexual abuse. In V. B. Van Hasselt, R. L. Morrison, A. S. Bellack, & M. Hersen (Eds.), *Handbook of family violence.* New York: Plenum Press.

Wolkind, S., & Rutter, M. (1985). Separation, loss and family relationships. In M. Rutter & L. Hersov (Eds.), *Child and adolescent psychiatry.* Oxford: Blackwell.

Wyatt, G. E., & Peters, S. D. (1986). Methodological considerations in research on the prevalence of child sexual abuse. *Child Abuse and Neglect, 10,* 241–251.

Zahn-Waxler, C., Cummings, E. M., Iannotti, R. J., & Radke-Yarrow, M. (1984). Young offspring of depressed parents: A population at risk for affective problems. In D. Cichetti & K. Schneider-Rosen (Eds.), *New directions for child development: Vol. 26. Childhood depression.* San Francisco: Jossey-Bass.

Zigler, E., Taussig, C., & Black, K. (1992). Early childhood intervention. *American Psychologist, 47* (8), 997–1006.

21 / Maternal Depression and Infant Maladjustment: A Failure of Mutual Regulation

M. Katherine Weinberg and Edward Z. Tronick

Unipolar maternal depression has been associated with impaired social, emotional, and cognitive development in children and adolescents (Downey & Coyne, 1990; Gelfand & Teti, 1990). More recently, a growing body of studies are demonstrating a similar association in infants and toddlers (Field, 1995; Rutter, 1990). If for the moment we suspend the complexity of thought that a phenomenon like depression demands and simply depict the depressed mother as sad, withdrawn, and uncommunicative, we might well ask how is it that these qualities compromise her child's development. Unfortunately, the answer to this question is not simple.

Figure 21.1 presents a scheme for understanding the many pathways that may lead to dysfunction or even psychopathology in young children of depressed mothers. Genetic factors may predispose or directly transmit problems to the child (Zuckerman & Beardslee, 1987). Physiological or temperamental characteristics evident at birth may lead to disorganized infant behavior that compromises mother-infant interactions (Hopkins, Campbell, & Marcus, 1987; Zuckerman, Bauchner, Parker, & Cabral, 1990). Maternal competence and availability may be affected by marital problems, lack of social support, and economic stress (Downey & Coyne, 1990; Frankel & Harmon, 1996; Teti, Gelfand, & Pompa, 1990). These processes are often interlocked. For example, maternal depression may affect newborn neurobehavioral functioning directly through prenatal physiological and hormonal changes associated with depression (Zuckerman et al., 1990).

Support for this project was provided by Grant No. R01 MH43398 and Grant No. R01 MH45547 from the National Institute of Mental Health. We gratefully acknowledge the assistance of Henrietta Kernan, Marjorie Beeghly, and Karen Nelson in the preparation of this manuscript.

Alternatively, infant difficulties could result indirectly from risk factors that are known to compromise infant development regardless of the mother's psychiatric status. These risk factors include smoking and drinking during pregnancy and lack of prenatal care, all of which have been reported to be associated with depression (Wolkind, 1981). Physiological changes and/or poor health habits during pregnancy may lead to difficult infant temperament, which in turn may increase the degree of stress experienced by the mother, lead to or exacerbate depressive symptoms, and compromise mother-infant interactions (Campos, Barrett, Lamb, Goldsmith, & Stenberg, 1983; Cutrona & Troutman, 1986; Field, 1987). If one then adds marital discord, lack of social support, and economic hardship, it is easy to see that double-jeopardy situations are created that affect both the mother's and the young child's functioning.

Although there are many pathways to child dysfunction, we believe that the final common pathway is the social-affective interchange that takes place between the child and the mother or other caregivers (Tronick, 1989; Tronick & Gianino, 1986a). Tronick (1986) has argued that social interchanges are mutually regulated. The child and the mother jointly regulate affective and behavioral states during social interactions in order to facilitate the child's goals of communicating and connecting with others and acting on the world (Sander, 1962; Trevarthen, 1979). The process of mutual regulation operates throughout development. Thus, although developmental issues change with the child's age, the basic process of mutual regulation remains the same. Our hypothesis is that disruptions of mutual regulation during social interactions account for many of the effects observed in young children of depressed mothers (Beeghly & Tronick, 1994; Tronick, 1989; Tronick & Gianino, 1986a).

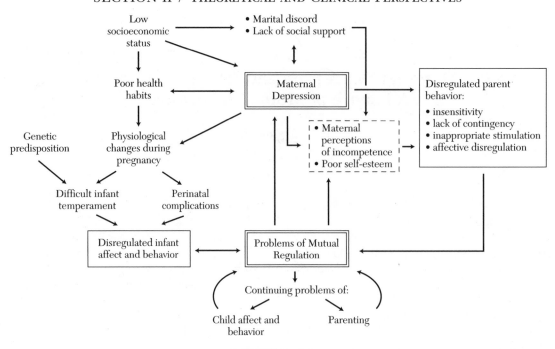

FIGURE 21.1

Pathways to infant dysfunction

The Normal Process of Mutual Regulation

What goes wrong in the mutual regulatory process of depressed mothers and their infants? The answer requires first knowing what goes right in the normal process of mutual regulation. Early models of mutual regulation argued that mother-infant interactions were characterized by large proportions of shared positive affect. Although infants experienced some negative affect, mothers rarely did, and negative affective states were not shared. Mothers, but not necessarily the infant, responded to their infant's signals in such a sensitive manner that both partners moved like dancers simultaneously changing interactive states, creating an interaction characterized by positive affect, reciprocity, synchrony, and attunement (Beebe et al., 1982; Brazelton, Koslowski, & Main, 1974; Stern, 1985). It was argued that good interactions had more of these qualities than poor interactions. Scales were developed that rated the interaction on a dimension of synchrony, attunement, or contingency. Underlying these scales was the widely accepted assumption that the more synchronous and contingent the interaction, the more positive

the affect, the better the interaction, and the more optimal the outcome of the child.

Subsequent research depicts a less idealized picture. Cohn and Tronick (1987) have shown that infants and mothers spend only about 30% of the time in synchronous or matching states. Modest proportions of negative affect expressed by the infant occasionally are shared by the mother. Changes in the affect and behaviors of the mother and infant are nonsimultaneous and bidirectional, with both partners responding to each other's communicative signals (Cohn & Tronick, 1988).

Recent research also demonstrates gender differences in infant affective and regulatory behavior as well as differences in interactive coherence. Weinberg, Tronick, Cohn, and Olson (1996) found that 6-month-old infant boys were more emotionally reactive than girls during face-to-face interactions with their mother. Boys displayed both more negative affective behaviors (e.g., crying, fussing, pick-me-up gestures, attempts to physically distance themselves from the mother, facial expressions of anger) and positive affective behaviors (e.g., facial expressions of joy, positive vocalizations). By contrast, girls were more likely than boys to focus on objects and to display facial expressions of interest. Weinberg (Weinberg et al., 1996) hypothesized that the boys' greater emotional reactivity suggest that they have greater difficulty regulating affective states on their own and that they may need to rely more on maternal regulatory scaffolding than girls. Gender differences in interactive coherence also have been demonstrated with mother-son dyads, evidencing more coherence than mother-daughter dyads (Tronick & Cohn, 1989; Weinberg et al., 1996). In particular, mothers and sons had higher synchrony scores than mothers and daughters, suggesting that mother-son dyads more carefully tracked each others' behavior and facial expressions than mother-daughter dyads. This greater coordination, which takes place at a subtle microtemporal level, may function to help boys maintain self-regulation (Weinberg et al., 1996). By carefully monitoring and responding to their sons' communicative messages, mothers provide structure to the interaction. These gender differences reflect normal variants of interactive and regulatory style and may be critical to our understanding of the effects of maternal depression, particularly if boys, as we would suggest, are more dependent on regulatory input from the mother than girls.

Tronick and his colleagues (Tronick & Cohn, 1989; Tronick & Gianino, 1986a; Weinberg & Tronick, 1996) have characterized the typical mother-infant interaction as one that moves from coordinated to miscoordinated states and back again over a wide affective range. The miscoordinated state is referred to as a normal interactive error (or miscommunication) and the transition from a miscoordinated state to a coordinated state as a repair. Interactive errors occur for a number of reasons. Infants are often difficult and demanding social partners. Their capacities are immature and limited, and it is impossible for the mother, however well intentioned, to be alert and sensitive to infant cues at all times. Interactive errors in normal dyads, however, are quickly repaired. In studies of face-to-face interaction at 6 months of age, repairs occur at a rate of once every 3 to 5 seconds, and more than one-third of all repairs occur by the next step in the interaction (Tronick & Gianino, 1986b). Observations by Beebe and Jaffe (1992) and Isabella and Belsky (1991) demonstrating that maternal sensitivity in the midrange, rather than at the high or low end, is associated with security of attachment also can be seen as reflecting this mutually regulated reparatory process.

From a perspective of mutual regulation, both the mother and infant bring their social capacities to the interaction, and both are responsible for the interaction's structure. Thus, reparation is fundamentally dyadic and the critical component of "good" interactions is both partners' ability to repair or negotiate interactive errors successfully. Regardless of age, developmental task, or stage, the child is motivated to maintain internal regulation in the service of communicating and connecting with others and acting on the world (Sander, 1962; Trevarthen, 1979). Successful achievement of these goals depends in part on the infants' ability to cope with and regulate physiological and affective disruptions and interactive errors on their own and to communicate their needs clearly to the caregiver by coordinating expressive modalities (i.e., face, voice, gaze, and gestures) into coherently organized communicative configurations (Weinberg & Tronick, 1994). Left to their own coping devices, however, infants would consistently fail and experience negative emotions and disregulation on a chronic basis. Fortunately, the infant's regulatory system is not "located" only in the infant. It has evolved as a dyadic system in which the other component is the mother (or other caregiver). The mother's behavior scaffolds the infant's regulatory capacities and is used by the infant in the service of his or her goals. The success or failure of the mother's regulatory input is dependent on her capacities to read her infant's communicative signals and to integrate this information with her knowledge of her infant. When the mother's scaffolding is effective, when reparation predominates, the infant experiences positive emotions and a sense of relatedness. When her regulatory input is ineffective, the infant experiences negative emotions and a sense of aloneness.

Normal infant functioning depends to a large extent on the successful resolution of interactive errors that typically occur in routine mother-infant interactions (Gianino & Tronick, 1988; Tronick & Cohn, 1989; Tronick & Gianino, 1986b). The experience of successfully coping and repairing interactive errors enhances the infant's development. The infant learns which communicative and coping strategies are effective and when to use them. This allows for the elaboration of communicative and coping skills, and the development of an understanding of interactive rules and conventions. With the accumulation of successful reparations and transformations of negative affect into positive affect, the infant establishes a positive affective core (Emde, 1983). The infant also learns that he or she has control over social interactions. Specifically, the infant develops a representation of him- or herself as effective, of his or her interactions as positive and reparable, and of the caregiver as reliable and trustworthy. These representations are crucial for the development of a sense of self that has coherence, continuity, and agency (Tronick, 1989).

It is our hypothesis that there is a failure in the process of mutual regulation between the depressed mother and her child. This regulatory failure can be caused by many different factors. Whatever the cause, the failure results in the infant experiencing negative emotions and a sense of disconnectedness with others on a chronic basis. In attempting to cope with this negative experience, the infant develops a negative affective core, primarily characterized by anger or sadness, a defensive coping style, and a distrust of the caregiver and of his or her own actions. These affective states and forms of dysfunction develop because of the ways infants experience and cope with failure, not because the infants are passively mirroring their mothers (Kohut, 1971, 1977). Thus, infants in unintended dyadic collusion with their mothers create in themselves affective states and forms of dysfunction that are similar to their mother's states and dysfunctions.

In this chapter we focus on the process of mutual regulation during social interchanges between mothers with unipolar depression and their infants. We review the literature on the quality of the caregiving of depressed mothers, the effects of maternal depression on the functioning and experiences of the infant, and the disrupted nature of the mutual regulatory process and how it may lead to developmental disturbances. Since our focus is on issues of regulation during the infant's first year of life, we direct the reader to several excellent reviews that examine the nature of maternal depression (Hopkins, Marcus, & Campbell, 1984; Zuckerman & Beardslee, 1987) and the effects of maternal depression on older children (Downey & Coyne, 1990; Gelfand & Teti, 1990; Rutter, 1990).

It should be noted that the term "depression" has been used to refer either to a continuum of depressive mood and psychological distress or to a discrete diagnostic entity. The prevalence of depressive disorder, based on diagnostic criteria and instruments such as the Research Diagnostic Cri-

teria (RDC) and the Schedule of Affective Disorders and Schizophrenia (SADS), has been estimated at approximately 10% (Campbell & Cohn, 1991; O'Hara, Zekoski, Phillips, & Wright, 1990). Interestingly, this rate has not been found to be higher for postpartum women as compared to nonpostpartum women (O'Hara et al., 1990). In comparison to diagnostic evaluations, the putative cut-offs for depression on self-report instruments such as the Beck Depression Inventory (BDI) or the Center for Epidemiologic Studies-Depression Scale (CES-D) may overidentify depression. Campbell and Cohn (1991) found that 58% of women with levels of depressive symptomatology above the cut-off did not meet RDC for depression. Furthermore, Campbell and her colleagues (Campbell, Cohn, Flanaghan, Popper, & Meyers, 1992) found that at 6 months postpartum, 76% of mothers were no longer depressed on the basis of the RDC but that 44% continued to report subclinical symptoms of depression. As has been suggested by Lyons-Ruth (1995), this continuity of symptoms of dysphoria even in the absence of a diagnosis of depression may help explain findings indicating that mothers continue to show parenting difficulties even after the resolution of a depressive episode (Weissman & Paykel, 1974). Thus, different assessment tools make the interpretation of results difficult. In future studies it will be important to use both self-report measures and diagnostic instruments to facilitate the definition of samples and clarify the relation between different types of assessment. As Seifer (1995) points out, there is a need for researchers to use similar operational definitions in order for us to comprehend more fully the phenomenon of maternal depression.

Maternal Depression and Infant Maladjustment: A Failure of Mutual Regulation

It is clear from the literature that many aspects of parenting are affected by a mother's depression. On a simplest level, depression appears to have a dampening effect on maternal behavior and affect

(Downey & Coyne, 1990). More specifically, as will be elaborated later, depression affects the mother's ability to respond sensitively to her infant's needs, affective states, and goal-directed activities. The depressed mother is less likely to provide her child with appropriately modulated levels of stimulation and to express positive affect. She is more likely to express flat or negative affect and to disrupt her child's states and ongoing engagements with objects and people.

The evidence suggesting that depression has a dampening effect on maternal behavior has led a number of researchers to question depressed mothers' ability to tend adequately to their infants' basic physiological needs (Dodge, 1990; Fleming, Ruble, Flett, & Shaul, 1988; Livingood, Daen, & Smith, 1983). Dodge (1990) suggested that the mother's depression may be so time-consuming and absorbing that it interferes with feeding and other caregiving activities. However, studies have generally found that, although depressed mothers feel less efficacious in the maternal role than other mothers (Teti & Gelfand, 1991), they engage in functionally adequate caregiving (Cohn, Matias, Tronick, Connell, & Lyons-Ruth, 1986; Cohn & Tronick, 1989; Fleming et al., 1988; Livingood et al., 1983).

Few studies have evaluated the behavior and affect of depressed mothers with newborn infants. Social and affective problems associated with depression have been studied more extensively in mothers of older infants. Findings on depressed mothers taken as an homogeneous group (an approach that we consider inadequate because research indicates that depressed mothers form an heterogeneous group) demonstrate that depressed mothers have difficulties providing adequate levels of social stimulation to their infants. When asked to interact with their infants, depressed mothers typically are described as less involved than control mothers. They slouch back in their chair, turn away from the infants, and touch their infants less often than other mothers (Cohn et al., 1986; Field, 1984; Fleming et al., 1988). They engage in fewer activities, games, and imitative behaviors (Field, 1984; Field et al., 1985; Field, Healy, Goldstein, & Guthertz, 1990). Their speech is less focused on the infant and shows less acknowledgment of infant agency (Murray, Kempton, Woolgar, & Hooper, 1993). Furthermore, they vocalize less often, fail to modify their speech in response to infant vocalizations, and take considerably longer to respond to vocalizations than nondepressed mothers (Bettes, 1988). Because infants are unable to detect a relation between their own and their mother's vocalizations if these delays are too long, Bettes suggests that depressed mothers fail to provide structure and predictability to their vocalizations.

Depressed mothers' affective tone and their capacity to regulate affect is compromised, as well. Depressed mothers are consistently described as sad, depressed, and anxious-looking during interactions with their young infants (Field et al., 1985; Sameroff, Seifer, & Zax, 1982). They show negative, flat, angry, and tense facial expressions (Field et al., 1985) both in the laboratory and during naturalistic observations (Cohn et al., 1986; Cohn, Campbell, Matias, & Hopkins, 1990; Cohn & Tronick, 1989). Cohn and his colleagues (Cohn et al., 1986; Cohn & Tronick, 1989) also have found that they are more likely to poke their infants in an intrusive and hostile fashion. Furthermore, the content and emotional tone of their speech is more negative than the speech of other mothers (Murray et al., 1993), and they are less likely to imbue their language with affective signals and the exaggerated and high-pitch intonations that typically characterize motherese (Bettes, 1988). Thus, in each communicative domain—voice, face, and touch—the quantity, quality, and timing of depressed mothers' affective behavior is distorted in ways that contrast sharply with the affective behaviors of control mothers.

Maternal depression has been associated with a number of infant problems. Although few studies have evaluated the functional status of newborn infants of depressed mothers, evidence suggests that these infants may be difficult interactive partners. Newborn infants of hospitalized or very high-risk depressed mothers evidence poor tonus, self-quieting ability, and responsivity to social stimulation on the Brazelton Neonatal Behavioral Assessment Scale (Field et al., 1985; 1988; Sameroff et al., 1982). Zuckerman et al. (1990) have further found that the newborn infants of depressed mothers cry excessively and are difficult to console. This research suggests that the newborn infants of depressed mothers are at risk for interactive and temperamental difficulties from birth even prior to interacting with their mother.

One interpretation of these findings is that these behavioral difficulties are related to the mother's depressed state through some unspecified genetic effect. There is little evidence, however, to support or refute this genetic hypothesis. Alternatively, we can hypothesize that changes in maternal hormonal functioning and disruptions associated with depression (e.g., sleeplessness, appetite loss) might change the physiologic milieu of the developing fetus and produce behavioral disorganization. This hypothesis suggests that there is a failure in maternal-fetal regulation that results in newborn disregulation. This hypothesis, also, however, remains unevaluated in part because the current evidence often is confounded by the high-risk status of the mothers studied. Furthermore, although newborns of depressed mothers experience a higher incidence of perinatal complications (Hopkins, et al., 1987), at the present time there is no indication that newborn status is related specifically to maternal depression. A study during the perinatal period of maternal-fetal and maternal-newborn regulation in a low-risk sample is needed if we are to learn whether depression compromises newborn infants' functioning. These studies need to take into account whether mothers were prescribed psychotropic medication during the pregnancy. At this point, there is minimal research on the effects of in utero exposure to psychotropic drugs on newborn functioning.

Maternal regulatory failures are associated with a wide range of infant affective problems. It is now well documented that infants of depressed mothers show fewer affectively positive facial expressions and vocalizations, more fussiness, more withdrawal, less attentiveness to the mother, and lower activity levels than control infants (Cohn & Tronick, 1989; Cohn et al., 1986; Field, 1984; Field et al., 1985, 1988, 1990). While these studies were compromised because the samples were high risk, studies by, for example, Hoffman and Drotar (1991), Cohn and Campbell (Cohn et al., 1990), Murray (1992), and Teti and Gelfand (Teti, Gelfand, Messinger, & Isabella, 1995) have found effects of maternal depression on maternal and infant functioning using low-risk samples.

The infants of depressed mothers also show limited engagement with people and objects. Cohn and Tronick (Cohn & Tronick, 1989); Cohn et al., 1986; have found that 6-month-old infants of depressed mothers engage in positive social play less than 5% of the time and explore objects only 13% of the time. These percentages are significantly lower than those of control infants, who

play more than 15% of the time and explore objects 30% of the time. Furthermore, in contrast to control infants, the infants of depressed mothers spend a substantial amount of the time looking away and being upset. Similar results have been reported by Field in 3-month-old infants (Field et al., 1990). Thus, it appears that the infants of depressed mothers have difficulty maintaining engagement with both objects and people. One interpretation of these findings is that compromises in object and social engagement reflect permanent cognitive impairment. An alternative interpretation suggested by a model of mutual regulation is that these compromises reflect defensive coping strategies developed by the infant to control disruptive affective states experienced in interaction with the mother. These coping strategies curtail the infant's engagements with the world of people and objects and deprive the infant of experiences necessary for normal cognitive development. If the situation with the mother persists, cognitive development will be compromised. If the situation resolves, cognitive development may proceed normally. This interpretation emphasizes the interplay among affect, coping, and cognition. Whatever the reason may be, there is evidence that the older infants of depressed mothers show some cognitive impairment. Murray (Murray, 1992; Murray et al., 1993) has found that these infants perform less well on Piagetian object concept tasks at 9 and 18 months; Lyons-Ruth (Lyons-Ruth, Zoll, Connell, & Grunebaum, 1990; Lyons-Ruth, Zoll, Connell, & Grunebaum, 1986) has shown that they have poorer scores on the Bayley Mental Scale at 1 year than the infants of asymptomatic mothers.

Infant and maternal regulatory failures are evident in the dyadic qualities of the interaction. Field (1984) described the affect of depressed mothers as unchanging, implying that they were unresponsive to their infants. Cohn (Cohn et al., 1986) noted that depressed mothers and their infants were unlikely to share affective states. In a later study, however, Cohn (Cohn et al., 1990) found that the interactions of depressed mother-infant dyads were contingent but that the mothers and infants consistently responded to and reinforced each other's negative displays. Similarly, Field (Field et al., 1990) found that depressed mothers and their infants match each other's level of expression but that they spend more time together in negative states than nondepressed dyads. Thus, it appears that depressed mothers and their infants are stuck in affectively negative states. The effect is that their interactions are not mutually regulated and the infants are deprived of the experience of reparation of negative into positive affect. We would expect that eventually this situation would compromise the infant's sense of self-agency and that the mother and infant would fail to establish primary interconnectedness.

It is important to consider infant gender when evaluating the effects of maternal depression on maternal and infant functioning. Weinberg (1996) found that mothers with a history of depression were more affectively negative (e.g., angry) with their 3- and 6-month-old sons than with their daughters during face-to-face social interaction. At 6 months of age, the sons as compared to the daughters of these mothers appeared more vulnerable to their mothers' depressive status. Boys expressed less joy, gestured more, and were less likely to self-comfort (e.g., suck on a thumb) than girls. Weinberg (Weinberg et al., 1996) has argued that boys are more demanding social partners than girls, that they have a more difficult time regulating affective states, and that they may need their mothers' help to regulate affect. The mothers with a history of depression appeared to have difficulties giving their sons the regulatory scaffolding that they needed, making the regulatory task of the mother-son dyads more difficult. In this way, a cycle of mutual regulatory problems between mothers and sons may become established. Murray (Murray, 1992; Murray et al., 1993) also has found that the male infants of depressed mothers experience greater difficulties than the female infants of these mothers. She found that male infants of mothers with a postnatal depression were more likely than female infants of mothers with a postnatal depression to be insecurely attached to the mother (Murray, 1992) and to have lower Bayley scores at 18 months (Murray et al., 1993).

Young infants' behavior reflects their interactive history with the mother. Field (1984) found that infants of depressed mothers are less reactive to their mothers in Cohn and Tronick's (1983) simulated depression paradigm. She interpreted this to mean that the infants had developed an expectation that the mother would act "depressed" and so were less distressed by the simulation of depression than control infants. The hypothesis that young infants establish particular interactive styles as a result of their interactive history with the mother is supported by Cohn's (Cohn et al., 1986) finding that infants of depressed mothers who are more negative during laboratory face-to-face interactions are also more negative during periods of naturalistic observation. It is further supported by a finding by Field (Field et al., 1988) that the negative interactions of the infants of depressed mothers generalize to their interactions with unfamiliar female adults. Pelaez-Nogueras, Field, Cigales, Gonzalez, and Clasky (1994), however, have found that infants' behavior is more positive when they interact with a familiar female nursery teacher than with their mother. Thus, the data suggest that negative interactions with the mother generalize to unfamiliar but not to familiar social partners.

Heterogeneity of Depression and the Process of Mutual Regulation

Most of the research evaluating the behavior and affect of depressed mothers has treated these women as if they form a homogeneous group. This research, however, needs to be qualified because data suggest that the behavior of depressed mothers is heterogeneous. Several researchers have found that the behavior and affect of some depressed mothers appear quite normal, whereas the behavior and affect of mothers with similar levels of depressive symptomatology are compromised (Cohn et al., 1986; Cohn & Tronick, 1989; Field et al., 1990; Lyons-Ruth et al., 1986; Radke-Yarrow, 1987). Cohn and Tronick (1989) have proposed a typology of 4 different styles of maternal affective and social behavior of mothers with high levels of depressive symptoms on the CES-D. They labeled one group of depressed mothers "intrusive." These mothers engaged in rough handling, spoke in an angry tone of voice, poked at their babies, and actively interfered with their infants' activities. A second group of depressed mothers, labeled "withdrawn," were disengaged, withdrawn, unresponsive, affectively flat, and unable to support their infants' activities. A third group of mothers, labeled "positive," evidenced a distribution of affective behavior that was similar to that of control mothers, although they looked away from their infants more than nondepressed mothers. Finally, a "mixed" group of depressed mothers displayed a mixed pattern of intrusiveness and withdrawal. Similar observations have been made by Field (Field et al., 1990) and by Radke-Yarrow (1987) in mothers of toddlers.

Cohn and Tronick (Cohn & Tronick, 1989; Cohn et al., 1986) found important correspondences between infant behavior and maternal interactive style. Infants of intrusive mothers spent almost 70% of their time looking away from the mother but only 9% of their time looking at objects. Infants of withdrawn mothers were significantly more likely to protest and to be distressed than the infants in the other groups, suggesting that maternal withdrawal may be particularly aversive to young infants. By contrast, depressed mothers whose behavior most closely resembled the behavior of asymptomatic mothers had infants whose behavior most closely approximated the behavior of control infants. The behavior of this group of depressed mothers, however, was not identical to the behavior of control mothers, and their infants' amount of play and object attend were still reduced compared to infants of asymptomatic mothers. Finally, the infants of the mixed group of depressed mothers evidenced an inconsistent pattern of responses. They protested and attended to objects less but looked at and played with the mother more than the infants of the withdrawn mothers. In comparison to the infants of the intrusive mothers, these infants protested at similar levels, looked away less, and attended to objects and the mother at slightly higher levels.

These differential infant reactions are expectable. From the perspective of mutual regulation, infants of withdrawn mothers fail to achieve their goal for social connectedness because of the mothers' lack of response and both partners' inability to repair the interaction. Initial failures result in the infants experiencing anger, repeatedly attempting to achieve their goals, and failing. Their goal for social engagement is not achieved, and their anger is not repaired into a more positive state. Since they are unable to cope successfully on their own with this affective state, the infants become disregulated, fuss, and cry. The

predominance of negative affect compels them to devote much time to controlling their affective state. Eventually, repeated failures to change their mother's behavior and their own affective state lead to a disengaged and self-directed style of coping characterized by self-comforting, self-regulation, passivity, and withdrawal. To the extent that this coping style is successful in controlling negative affect, it becomes deployed automatically and defensively in an effort to preclude anticipated negative affect even in situations in which negative affect may not occur. When failure repeats and accumulates, these infants develop a negative affective core characterized primarily by sadness. They develop a representation of the mother as untrustworthy and unresponsive and of themselves as ineffective and helpless (Gianino & Tronick, 1988).

The infants of hostile intrusive mothers face a different regulatory problem. Because the mothers are actively disruptive of the infants' activities, reparation of the interaction does not occur. Like the infants of withdrawn mothers, these infants initially experience anger, turn away from the mother, push her away, or screen her out. Unlike the failure experience of the infants of withdrawn mothers, occasionally these coping behaviors are successful in limiting the mother's intrusiveness, and the infants' anger is not transformed into an uncontrolled disregulated state. With the reiteration and accumulation of this experience of reparation, the infants develop an affective core characterized by anger. To the extent that their coping behaviors are effective in fending off the mother, the infants eventually internalize an angry and protective style of coping that is deployed defensively in anticipation of the mother's intrusiveness. The infants become easily angry when interacting with the mother and others and frustrated when acting on objects.

Prolonged experience with withdrawn mothers might be expected to produce infants who lose self-agency and feel fragmented and depersonalized. Affectivity might be compromised to a state of anhedonia given the infants' attempts to control negative affect (Stern, 1985). This would limit the quality of the infants' interactions with people and experiences with objects. By contrast, infants of intrusive mothers may have a more intact sense of agency since their efforts are sometimes successful in limiting the mother's intrusiveness. Their sense of affectivity, however, is more likely to contain elements of rage directed at the other and at the self.

Both the intrusive and withdrawn mothers display relatively consistent interactive styles. This consistency allows for the development of stable although inappropriate infant coping strategies. Infants of mixed depressed mothers, however, are confronted with both prolonged periods of nonreparation and inconsistency in the mothers' behavior. This inconsistency may not permit these infants to develop a stable coping style and may lead to a more general form of disorganization.

Weinberg (1992) has argued that these observations need to take into account gender differences in infant regulatory and affective styles. She has hypothesized that if boys are more affectively reactive and less able to self-regulate on their own, they may be particularly susceptible to the withdrawn style of depression that denies them the regulatory dyadic support that they need. On the other hand, girls, who at 6 months of age are significantly more focused on objects than boys, may be more vulnerable to the intrusive style of depression that persistently interferes with their activities. Along with Weinberg's (1992) findings that girls show more stability of sadness than boys and boys show more stability of distancing and escape behaviors than girls, we would hypothesize that these gender differences may be the first signs presaging the differential proportion of older boys who experience behavioral problems and older girls who become withdrawn and depressed.

The research on maternal interactive styles and differential infant reactions emphasizes how critical it is to describe what the mother actually does with her infant. Knowing what a depressed mother does requires observing her interactions with her child in a number of contexts. However, to date most of the studies have taken place either in the laboratory using structured situations or in the home setting during naturalistic observations. In a unique study, Cohn and his colleagues (Cohn et al., 1986) observed mothers during structured face-to-face interactions and naturalistic observations in the home. They found a high degree of concordance between the two contexts. Nonetheless, the structured observation missed apparently important phenomena. For example, the mothers who were the most intrusive during the laboratory observation tended to avoid their infants when they were at home. Given the choice to interact or not, these mothers limited contact with the infants to comforting or caregiving activities. Preliminary data from our current research indicate that depressed mothers' style of interaction with their 3-month-old infants at home is disengaged. Compared to controls, depressed mothers were more likely to prop up a bottle so that the infant could eat alone, engaged in less spontaneous face-to-face play with the infant, expressed less positive exaggerated affect to the infant, and spent more time doing adult-focused activities such as laundry out of proximity to the infant. These findings indicate that it is important to assess depressed mothers in a variety of situations.

The caregiving of mothers of older infants and toddlers can be characterized in a similar manner to that of mothers of younger infants (Downey & Coyne, 1990). In addition, Radke-Yarrow (1987) has described stylistic differences in their caregiving that correspond to the styles of mothers of younger infants. It is not surprising, given the regulatory failures of these mothers and infants, that the infants of depressed mothers are more likely to be insecurely attached to their mother. Several researchers have noted high proportion of insecure attachments (Lyons-Ruth et al., 1986; Lyons-Ruth et al., 1990; Murray, 1992; Radke-Yarrow, Cummings, Kuczynski, & Chapman, 1985; Teti et al., 1995). From the perspective of mutual regulation, the infants of intrusive mothers might be expected to become avoidant as they elaborate an angry defensive coping style designed to limit interaction with the mother whereas infants of withdrawn mothers might be expected to become ambivalent and anxiously attached. There is some support for this hypothesis. Several researchers have suggested that infants who evidence little avoidance or resistance in the Strange Situation are likely to have a responsive mother whereas infants who show avoidance or resistance are more likely to have a hostile/intrusive or unresponsive mother (Belsky, Rovine, & Taylor, 1984; Lyons-Ruth et al., 1986). Furthermore, the infants of mixed depressed mothers, who alternate between intrusiveness and withdrawal, might be expected to be disorganized in their attachment behavior. This outcome is likely because there is no clear direction of action that would help the infants cope with the stress that they experience while interacting with their mother. Although a high proportion of disorganized behavior has been found among the infants of depressed mothers (Lyons-Ruth, 1992), further research is necessary to determine whether there is a relation between maternal social-affective style and infant attachment classification.

Around the end of the first year, infants also begin to develop an awareness of their own and their partners' intentional and affective states. Trevarthen (1979) refers to this awareness is referred as secondary intersubjectivity; Stern (1985) calls it as attunement. During this period, it is likely that the infant of a depressed mother becomes increasingly aware of the mother's affective states of sadness, anger, and hostility and of the infant's own feelings of sadness, helplessness, and anger. Awareness of these emotions may produce a great deal of anxiety in the infant, which may require an enormous effort to control. We would hypothesize that these infants become hypervigilent of their mother's affective state in order to defend themselves from the mother's affect and their own affective reactions. This defensive coping style might extend to any event that induces a highly aroused affective state, such as exciting interactions with people or intense interest in objects. Highly arousing events could disrupt the affective control the infants are attempting to maintain and reinstate the anxiety they are attempting to control. This defensive strategy might contain the anlagen of repression. There is some support for this hypothesis. Osofsky (in press) has found that infants of depressed mothers show less intense affective reactions to stressful situations and that by the first year of life they are becoming less emotionally responsive than infants of nondepressed mothers.

Maternal depression appears to have an effect on children at any developmental stage. Whether these effects are specific to the age at which the child is exposed is unclear. It is also unclear whether there are sensitive periods during the first several months of life during which infants are particularly sensitive to regulatory failures associated with maternal depression (Murray, 1992). Older children of depressed mothers show significant developmental effects, as well (Downey & Coyne, 1990). It is possible that the problems observed in older children result from earlier failures in regulation structuring the child and his

or her interactions with the mother and others in such a way that later developmental tasks are disrupted. Alternatively, maternal depression may have a compromising effect on development regardless of the child's age and that even in the absence of a history of earlier failure later exposure to maternal depression will result in developmental dysfunction. In future research, it will be critical to determine whether exposure at different ages has a differential impact on children's development.

Issues of chronicity and severity also must be considered. Teti (Teti et al., 1995) has suggested that severity and chronicity of depression may have more explanatory power than the parental diagnosis per se. Several studies demonstrate that greater severity and chronicity of maternal depression are related to greater compromise in maternal and infant functioning. Campbell (Campbell, Cohn, & Meyers, 1995) found that women whose depression lasted through 6 months postpartum were less positive with their infants during face-to-face play, feeding, and toy play than women whose depression remitted before 6 months. These women's infants also were less positive than the infants of mothers whose depression remitted. Similarly, Cohn and Campbell (1992) found that a brief depressive episode within the first 8 weeks postpartum was not related to infant insecure attachment. By contrast, longer depressive episodes lasting through the infant's first 6 months were associated with an increase of insecure attachment. Teti (Teti et al., 1995) further reports that infants and preschoolers without unitary, coherent attachment strategies tend to have mothers who are more chronically ill than children with coherent and organized attachment strategies. Finally, Frankel and Harmon (1996) found that women with double depression (i.e., both unipolar depression and dysthymia) were less emotionally available to their preschool children, showed more negative affect to the children, and had more insecurely attached children than women with major, minor, or intermittent depressions. These studies indicate that the severity/chronicity dimension is crucial to consider when evaluating the effects of maternal depression on infant and child functioning.

From the perspective of mutual regulation, diagnostic status, history, severity, and chronicity are important to the infant only to the extent that they affect the mother's behavior with her infant. If depressed mothers' behavior and affect are not compromised, the infant would have to be a mind reader or a diagnostician to experience the mother's depression. From this perspective, it is expected that women who are able to interact positively with their infants despite meeting diagnostic criteria for depression currently or in the past will have infants who show less compromise than mothers who are not able to muster the energy to engage in positive interchanges. Thus, we would hypothesize that what the mother actually does with her infant may be more important than diagnostic status per se. Furthermore, as has been suggested by Campbell (Campbell et al., 1995), the ability of mothers to pull themselves together for their infants and derive pleasure from the mother-infant relationship may be a marker of who will or will not show a chronic and severe course of depression.

It is also critical to note that the child is not exposed only to the mother. Infants and young children interact with many others—fathers, siblings, relatives, adult and child friends. The extent to which interaction with these people ameliorates or exacerbates the effects of maternal depression must be considered. Often it is implied that the effects of others will enhance the child's development. This perspective is supported by research demonstrating the importance of other relationships for children who are described as invulnerable (Garmezy & Rutter, 1983). The mutual regulation model argues that what matters is what effect, whether direct or indirect, these others have on the child's experience. For example, fathers may have a direct enhancing effect on the child's development by interacting with the child in a well-regulated manner. Fathers also may have an indirect effect on the child's functioning by enhancing the mother's regulatory capacities with her child.

Unfortunately, the literature on maternal depression suggests that fathers, relatives, and friends all too often compromise the development of the children of depressed mothers. Merikangas (Merikangas, Weissman, Prusoff, & John, 1988) has demonstrated that the partners of depressed women are likely to suffer from psychiatric illness or a family history of mental disorders, a situation that has an additive negative effect on their children's functioning. Furthermore, in families with

one depressed individual, the relations among all family members frequently are characterized by negative affect, avoidance, and poor communication (Coyne, 1976). Expanding beyond the immediate family boundaries may not change the child's situation very much. It is well established that depressed women tend to have family histories of psychopathology. For example, Campbell (Campbell et al., 1992) found that 51% of depressed women reported affective disorders in at least one parent or sibling and that the rate of psychopathology increased to 72% when other conditions were included, such as alcohol and drug abuse, anxiety disorders, and "nervous breakdowns." Furthermore, Zahn-Waxler (1992) has reported that depressed mothers have assortive friendships and that their friends are more likely to be experiencing affective disorders. This means that their children and therefore the friends of the depressed mother's child's are experiencing disregulation, as well. Thus, much of the research on the role of others suggests that the children of depressed mothers are likely to experience problematic interactions with fathers, siblings, relatives, maternal friends, and peers directly. Moreover, these people may have a disregulating effect on the mother and so further exacerbate indirectly her regulatory problems with her child. These findings suggest that the effects of maternal depression may be a social network effect in which the child's regulatory experience with the mother and others is disrupted. Nonetheless, what the mother and others do with the child and each other is still the critical pathway for effects on the child. Only detailed observational research on the nature of the child's regulatory experiences with the mother, father, family friends, relatives, and peers will permit evaluation of this social network hypothesis.

Conclusion

The research on maternal depression and its effects on children indicates that dysfunctional affective, cognitive, and interactive problems associated with depression can be transmitted to a child at a very early age. There is a heterogeneous range of outcomes in infants of depressed mothers. In comparison to the infants of nondepressed mothers, they evidence disturbances in their ability to regulate emotions, impairments in their capacity to engage objects and people, and a higher proportion of cognitive problems and insecure attachments to the mother. This diverse range of outcomes persists in older children, who evidence a variety of emotional, social, and cognitive problems and who, as they get older, begin to show psychiatric symptoms including depression (Downey & Coyne, 1990).

Many factors are associated with the effects of maternal depression on infant development. Impairment may stem from genetic, perinatal, temperamental, or environmental factors. However, while these multiple factors are critical to our understanding of the effects of maternal depression, we have argued that the process of mutual regulation is the final common pathway for the affective and regulatory problems observed in children of depressed mothers. It is our hypothesis that a chronic failure in the mutual regulation takes place between depressed mothers and their children, which results in the child reiteratively experiencing various forms of negative affect rather than the reparation of negative into positive affect. In response, the child develops coping strategies to control this negative affect, but the coping

strategies inadvertently compromise the child's development. We recognize that this hypothesis may be limited and, although there are only glimmerings of evidence, also have hypothesized that the child's regulatory experience may not be located simply with the mother but in the direct and indirect effects of the social network in which the child is embedded. Thus, the effects of maternal depression really may be the effects associated with a depressed social network that directly and indirectly disrupts the child's experience of mutual regulation.

Dysfunctional outcome is not a necessary outcome for the child of a depressed mother. The behavior of depressed individuals is heterogeneous, and protective factors may be operating. A child whose regulatory experience is characterized by successful regulation with the mother and/or others is likely to develop normally. The outcomes for children of depressed mothers, just as is the case for children of nondepressed mothers, is heterogeneous. From the perspective of mutual regulation, the pathways to normalcy and psychopathology are part of the same developmental process. While genetic, temperamental, physiological, and environmental factors play a role, the final common pathway is the slowly accumulated and eventually internalized regulatory experiences of the child.

REFERENCES

Beebe, B., Hertsman, L., Carson, B., Dolins, M., Zigman, A., Rosenweig, H., Faughey, K., & Korman, M. (1982). Rhythmic communication in the mother-infant dyad. In M. Davis (Ed.), *Interaction rhythms: Periodicity in communicative behavior* (pp. 79–100). New York: Human Sciences.

Beebe, B., & Jaffe, J. (1992). Mother-infant vocal dialogue. Paper presented in B. Beebe (Chair), *Mother-infant vocal dialogues predict infant attachment, temperament and cognition*. Symposium conducted at the International Conference on Infant Studies (ICIS), Miami, FL.

Beeghly, M., & Tronick, E. Z. (1994). Effects of prenatal exposure to cocaine in early infancy: Toxic effects on the process of mutual regulation. *Infant Mental Health Journal, 15* (2), 158–174.

Belsky, J., Rovine, M., & Taylor, D. G. (1984). The Pennsylvania Infant and Family Development: 3. The origin of individual differences in infant-mother attachment: Maternal and infant contributions. *Child Development, 55,* 718–728.

Bettes, B. A. (1988). Maternal depression and motherese: Temporal and intonational features. *Child Development, 59,* 1089–1096.

Brazelton, T. B., Koslowski, B., & Main, M. (1974). The origins of reciprocity: The early-mother infant interaction. In M. Lewis & L. Rosenblum (Eds.), *The effect of the infant on its caregiver* (pp. 49–76). New York: John Wiley & Sons.

Campbell, S. B., & Cohn, J. F. (1991). Prevalence and correlates of postpartum depression in first-time mothers. *Journal of Abnormal Psychology, 100* (4), 594–599.

Campbell, S. B., Cohn, J. F., Flanagan, C., Popper, S., & Meyers, T. (1992). Course and correlates of postpartum depression during the transition to parenthood. *Development and Psychopathology, 4,* 29–47.

Campbell, S. B., Cohn, J. F., & Meyers, T. (1995). Depression in first-time mothers: Mother-infant interaction and depression chronicity. *Developmental Psychology, 31* (3), 349–357.

Campos, J. J., Barrett, K. C., Lamb, M. E., Goldsmith,

H. H., & Stenberg, C. (1983). Socioemotional development. In M. M. Haith & J. J. Campos (Eds.), *Handbook of child psychology: Vol. 2. Infancy and developmental psychobiology* (pp. 783–915). New York: John Wiley & Sons.

Cohn, J. F., & Campbell, S. B. (1992). Influence of maternal depression on infant affect regulation. In D. Cicchetti & S. Toth (Eds.), *Developmental perspectives on depression. Rochester symposium on developmental psychopathology (Vol. 4*, pp. 103–130). Rochester, NY: University of Rochester Press.

Cohn, J. F., Campbell, S. B., Matias, R., & Hopkins, J. (1990). Face-to-face interactions of postpartum depressed and nondepressed mother-infant pairs at 2 months. *Developmental Psychology, 26* (1), 15–23.

Cohn, J. F., Matias, R., Tronick, E. Z., Connell, D., & Lyons-Ruth, K. (1986). Face-to-face interactions of depressed mothers and their infants. In E. Z. Tronick & T. Field (Eds.), *Maternal depression and infant disturbance* (New Directions for Child Development, No. 34, pp. 31–44). San Francisco: Jossey-Bass.

Cohn, J. F., & Tronick, E. Z. (1983). Three-month-old infants' reaction to simulated maternal depression. *Child Development, 54*, 185–193.

Cohn, J. F., & Tronick, E. Z. (1987). Mother-infant face-to-face interaction: The sequence of dyadic states at 3, 6, and 9 months. *Developmental Psychology, 23*, 68–77.

Cohn, J. F., & Tronick, E. Z. (1988). Mother-infant interaction: Influence is bidirectional and unrelated to periodic cycles in either partner's behavior. *Developmental Psychology, 24*, 386–392.

Cohn, J. F., & Tronick, E. Z. (1989). Specificity of infants' response to mothers' affective behavior. *Journal of the American Academy of Child and Adolescent Psychiatry, 28* (2), 242–248.

Coyne, J. C. (1976). Toward an interactional description of depression. *Psychiatry, 39*, 28–40.

Cutrona, C. E., & Troutman, B. R. (1986). Social support, infant temperament, and parenting self-efficacy: A mediational model of postpartum depression. *Child Development, 57*, 1507–1518.

Dodge, K. (1990). Developmental psychopathology in children of depressed mothers. *Developmental Psychology, 26* (1), 3–6.

Downey, G., & Coyne, J. C. (1990). Children of depressed parents: An integrative review. *Psychological Bulletin, 108* (1), 50–76.

Emde, R. N. (1983). The prerepresentational self and its affective core. *Psychoanalytic Study of the Child, 38*, 165–192.

Field, T. (1984). Early interactions between infants and their postpartum depressed mothers. *Infant Behavior and Development, 7*, 517–522.

Field, T. (1987). Affective and interactive disturbances in infants. In J. D. Osofsky (Ed.), *Handbook of infant development*, 2nd Edition, pp. 972–1005. New York: John Wiley & Sons.

Field, T. (1995). Infants of depressed mothers. *Infant Behavior and Development, 18* (1), 1–13.

Field, T., Healy, B., Goldstein, S., & Guthertz, M. (1990). Behavior-state matching and synchrony in mother-infant interactions of nondepressed versus depressed dyads. *Developmental Psychology, 26* (1), 7–14.

Field, T., Healy, B., Goldstein, S., Perry, S., Bendell, D., Schanberg, S., Zimmerman, E. A., & Kuhn, C. (1988). Infants of depressed mothers show "depressed" behavior even with nondepressed adults. *Child Development, 59*, 1569–1579.

Field, T., Sandberg, D., Garcia, R., Vega-Lahr, N., Goldstein, S., & Guy, L. (1985). Pregnancy problems, postpartum depression, and early mother-infant interactions. *Developmental Psychology, 21* (6), 1152–1156.

Fleming, A. S., Ruble, D. N., Flett, G. L., Shaul, D. L. (1988). Postpartum adjustment in first-time mothers: Relations between mood, maternal attitudes, and mother-infant interactions. *Developmental Psychology, 24* (1), 71–81.

Frankel, K. A., & Harmon, R. J. (1996). Depressed mothers: They don't always look as bad as they feel. *Journal of the American Academy of Child and Adolescent Psychiatry, 35* (3), 289–298.

Garmezy, N., & Rutter, M. (1983). *Stress, coping and development in children.* New York: McGraw-Hill.

Gelfand, D. M., & Teti, D. M. (1990). The effects of maternal depression on children. *Clinical Psychology Review, 10*, 329–353.

Gianino, A. F., & Tronick, E. Z. (1988). The mutual regulation model: The infant's self and interactive regulation, coping, and defense. In T. Field, P. McCabe, & N. Schneiderman (Eds.), *Stress and coping* (pp. 47–68). Hillsdale, NJ: Lawrence Erlbaum.

Hoffman, Y., & Drotar, D. (1991). The impact of postpartum depressed mood on mother-infant interaction: Like mother like baby? *Infant Mental Health Journal, 12* (1), 65–80.

Hopkins, J., Campbell, S. B., & Marcus, M. (1987). The role of infant-related stressors in postpartum depression. *Journal of Abnormal Psychology, 96* (3), 237–241.

Hopkins, J., Marcus, M., & Campbell, S. B. (1984). Postpartum depression: A critical review. *Psychological Bulletin, 95* (3), 498–515.

Isabella, R., & Belsky, J. (1991). Interactional synchrony and the origins of infant-mother attachment: A replication study. *Child Development, 62*, 373–384.

Kohut, H. (1971). *The analysis of the self.* New York: International Universities Press.

Kohut, H. (1977). *The restoration of the self.* New York: International Universities Press.

Livingood, A. B., Daen, P., & Smith, B. D. (1983). The depressed mother as a source of stimulation for her infant. *Journal of Clinical Psychology, 39* (3), 369–375.

Lyons-Ruth, K. (1992). From infancy to age five: Maternal depressive symptoms, family support services, and disregulated infant and child behavior among low-income families. Paper presented in R. Yando (Chair), *Longitudinal follow-up of infants of de-*

pressed mothers. Symposium conducted at the International Conference on Infant Studies (ICIS), Miami, FL.

Lyons-Ruth, K. (1995). Broadening our conceptual frameworks: Can we reintroduce relational strategies and implicit representational systems to the study of psychopathology? *Developmental Psychology, 31* (3), 432–436.

Lyons-Ruth, K., Connell, D. B., & Grunebaum, H. U. (1990). Infants at social risk: Maternal depression and family support services as mediators of infant development and security of attachment. *Child Development, 61*, 85–98.

Lyons-Ruth, K., Zoll, D., Connell, D., & Grunebaum, H. U. (1986). The depressed mother and her one-year-old infant: Environment, interaction, attachment, and infant development. In E. Z. Tronick & T. Field (Eds.), *Maternal depression and infant disturbance* (New Directions for Child Development, No. 34), pp. 61–82.

Merikangas, K., Weissman, M. M., Prusoff, B., & John, K. (1988). Assortive mating and affective disorders: Psychopathology in offspring. *Psychiatry, 51*, 48–57.

Murray, L. (1992). The impact of postnatal depression on infant development. *Journal of Child Psychology and Psychiatry, 33* (3), 543–561.

Murray, L., Kempton, C., Woolgar, M., & Hooper, R. (1993). Depressed mothers' speech to their infants and its relation to infant gender and cognitive development. *Journal of Child Psychology and Psychiatry, 34* (7), 1083–1101.

O'Hara, M. W., Zekoski, E. M., Phillips, L. H., Wright, E. J. (1990). Controlled prospective study of postpartum mood disorders: Comparison of childbearing and nonchildbearing women. *Journal of Abnormal Psychology, 99* (1), 3–15.

Osofsky, J. D. (In press). Affective development and early relationships: Clinical implications. In *Psychoanalysis and psychology* (Washington, DC: American Psychological Association).

Pelaez-Nogueras, M., Field, T., Cigales, M., Gonzalez, A., & Clasky, S. (1994). Infants of depressed mothers show less "depressed" behavior with their nursery teachers. *Infant Mental Health Journal, 15* (4), 358–367.

Radke-Yarrow, M. (1987). *A developmental study of depressed and normal parents and their children.* Paper presented at the Society of research in Child Development (SRCD), Baltimore, MD.

Radke-Yarrow, M., Cummings, E. M., Kuczynski, L., & Chapman, M. (1985). Patterns of attachment in two- and three-year-olds in normal families and families with parental depression. *Child Development, 56*, 884–893.

Rutter, M. (1990). Commentary: Some focus and process considerations regarding effects of parental depression on children. *Developmental Psychology, 26* (1), 60–67.

Sameroff, A. J., Seifer, R., & Zax, M. (1982). Early development of children at risk for emotional disorder.

Monographs of the Society for Research in Child Development, 47 (7, Serial No. 199).

Sander, L. W. (1962). Issues in mother-child interaction. *Journal of the American Academy of Child Psychiatry, 1*, 141–146.

Seifer, R. (1995). Perils and pitfalls of high-risk research. *Developmental Psychology, 31* (3), 420–424.

Stern, D. N. (1985). *The interpersonal world of the infant*. New York: Basic Books.

Teti, D. M., & Gelfand, D. M. (1991). Behavioral competence among mothers of infants in the first year: The mediational role of maternal self-efficacy. *Child Development, 62*, 918–929.

Teti, D. M., Gelfand, D. M., Messinger, D. S., & Isabella, R. (1995). Maternal depression and the quality of early attachment: An examination of infants, preschoolers, and their mothers. *Developmental Psychology, 31* (3), 364–376.

Teti, D. M., Gelfand, D. M., & Pompa, J. (1990). Depressed mothers' behavioral competence with their infants: Demographic and psychosocial correlates. *Development and Psychopathology, 2*, 259–270.

Trevarthen, C. (1979). Communication and cooperation in early infancy: A description of primary intersubjectivity. In M. M. Bullowa (Ed.), *Before speech: The beginning of interpersonal communication* (pp. 321–347). New York: Cambridge University Press.

Tronick, E. Z. (1989). Emotions and emotional communication in infants. *American Psychologist, 44* (2), 112–119.

Tronick, E. Z., & Cohn, J. F. (1989). Infant-mother face-to-face interaction: Age and gender differences in coordination and the occurrence of miscoordination. *Child Development, 60* (1), 85–92.

Tronick, E. Z., & Gianino, A. F. (1986a). Interactive mismatch and repair: Challenges to the coping infant. *Zero to Three* (Bulletin of the Center for Clinical Infant Programs), *6* (3), 1–6.

Tronick, E. Z., & Gianino, A. F. (1986b). The transmission of maternal disturbance to the infant. In E. Z. Tronick & T. Field (Eds.), *Maternal depression and infant disturbance* (New Directions for Child Development, No. 34), pp. 61–82. San Francisco: Jossey-Bass.

Weinberg, M. K. (1992). Boys and girls: Sex differences in emotional expressivity and self-regulation during early infancy. Paper presented in L. J. Bridges (Chair), *Early emotional self-regulation: New approaches to understanding developmental change and individual differences*. Symposium conducted at the International Conference on Infant Studies (ICIS), Miami, FL.

Weinberg, M. K. (1996). Gender differences in depressed mothers' interactions with their infants. Paper presented in D. M. Teti (Chair), *Maternal depression and child development: Short- and long-term sequelae for mothers, infants, and families*. Symposium presented at the 10th Biennial International Conference on Infant Studies (ICIS), Providence, RI.

Weinberg, M. K., & Tronick, E. Z. (1994). Beyond the face: An empirical study of infant affective configurations of facial, vocal, gestural, and regulatory behaviors. *Child Development, 65,* 1503–1515.

Weinberg, M. K., & Tronick, E. Z. (1996). Infant affective reactions to the resumption of maternal interaction after the still-face. *Child Development, 67,* 905–914.

Weinberg, M. K., Tronick, E. Z., Cohn, J. F., & Olson, K. (1996). Boys and girls: Gender differences in emotional expressivity and self-regulation during early infancy. (Under review.)

Weissman, M., & Paykel, E. (1974). *The depressed woman: A study of social relationships.* Chicago: University of Chicago Press.

Wolkind, S. (1981). Prenatal emotional stress: Effects on the fetus. In S. Wolkind & E. Zajicek (Eds.), *Pregnancy: A psychological and social study* (pp. 177–193) New York: Grune & Stratton.

Zahn-Waxler, C. (1992). Early antecedents of problem behaviors. Paper presented in R. Yando (Chair), *Longitudinal follow-up of infants of depressed mothers.* Symposium conducted at the International Conference on Infant Studies (ICIS), Miami, FL.

Zuckerman, B. S., Bauchner, H., Parker, S., & Cabral, H. (1990). Maternal depressive symptoms during pregnancy and newborn irritability. *Developmental and Behavioral Pediatrics, 11* (4), 190–194.

Zuckerman, B. S., & Beardslee, W. R. (1987). Maternal depression: A concern for pediatricians. *Pediatrics, 79* (1), 110–117.

22 / Psychosocial Risks for Adolescent Parents and Infants: Clinical Implications

Joy D. Osofsky

Adolescent pregnancy, which results in approximately 480,000 births each year to women under the age of 19 years, has been accompanied in the past decade by an increasing sense of hopelessness and helplessness (Ladner & Gourdine, 1985; Wright-Edelman, 1989). Many of these young women and their families feel that they have little control over their lives and few options available to them. With adolescent pregnancy comes early parenthood, forcing many young women, who are still children themselves, into the position of having to take on the responsibilities of parenthood long before most are ready or able to assume this task. In addition to medical risks, there are many psychosocial risks for adolescent mothers and their infants, including mental health concerns for the mothers and developmental problems for the infants. This chapter reviews risk factors for infants and young children of teenage mothers and discusses both the clinical implications and possibilities for intervention.

Conceptual Framework for Understanding Adolescent Mothers and Their Families

The social context for adolescent mothers and their families is frequently defined by overwhelming and often negative environmental factors including poverty, family instability, and educational and economic disadvantage. While the family context may be more positive, frequently both the individual and family must cope with social adversity including poverty and its concomitant stresses. I have found it helpful to adapt some theoretical models to aid in providing a framework for understanding the adolescent mother and her family.

The life-span developmental approach provides a perspective on intergenerational issues and how they may contribute to adolescent pregnancy. Kahn and Antonucci (1980) have suggested that social relationships be considered within a life-span developmental framework and that individuals move through life influenced, protected, and sometimes placed at risk by their social relationships. Families or, for many teenage mothers, their own single mothers try to raise their children to become competent adults within their own social group. However, mothers of teenage mothers may contribute to limiting their children's goals to those within their own views and experiences. In addition, adolescents struggle with identity and separation/individuation issues. A teenager living in a poverty environment trying to separate from her family and find her own way often is severely hampered by lack of opportunity. She may try to resolve these psychological and practical struggles by becoming pregnant, an option that confirms her femininity and identity as a woman and allows her to have a newly defined and (frequently) integrated role within the family system. Thus, the young woman resolves her identity dilemma by developing a new rapprochement (Mahler, Pine, & Bergman, 1975) with her mother and within the family. While to some this option may seem maladaptive, for many, based on traditions within the family, the solution may be viewed as a positive one (Burton & Bengston, 1985; Ladner & Gourdine, 1985).

Additional consideration from an intergenerational point of view involves the three levels of intergenerational experience that must be considered in order to understand the world of an adolescent mother and her infant and young child. Infants respond to behaviors of their mothers, which are impacted upon by past experiences of the mothers, and which also affect their interpretations of the experiences. These young mothers and children frequently are raised in very high-risk environments, which may lead to additional interpersonal struggles beyond those that accompany the usual course of development. It is extremely important to consider these intergenerational issues in attempting to understand the family environment and world of the adolescent mother and her child.

A second model uses a social ecological perspective (Bronfenbrenner, 1985, 1989; Brooks-Gunn & Chase-Lansdale, 1991; Chase-Lansdale, Brooks-Gunn, & Palkoff, 1991) to identify the context of development for the family and the individual within which teenage pregnancy occurs. The ecological perspective (Bronfenbrenner, 1989) examines interactions between the person and the environment in order to understand development and adaptation. For an adolescent mother, individual factors plus the family of origin, the network of relationships, the neighborhood, and school and work environments must be considered. The ecology of her environment in addition to her individual characteristics and prior experiences will impact strongly both on how she adjusts to the pregnancy and to young motherhood.

A third perspective, family systems theory (Hinde & Stevenson-Hinde, 1988), describes the structure of the family as an organized system made up of interdependent relationships and subsystems. Examples of the many different relationships within families that make up the subsystems have been explicated recently by Stevenson-Hinde (1990) and Emde (1991). Families of adolescent mothers, especially those of African American backgrounds, may be organized structurally quite differently from those of older mothers, including more sharing of child rearing between several individuals and generations (Holmbeck, Paikoff, & Brooks-Gunn, 1995). A focus on the family system allows assessment of the emotional quality of the family as a whole, which provides a fairly realistic understanding of the adolescent mother's family environment.

Knowledge of community-based ideologies of the context of adolescent pregnancy, including the reality of poverty, individual and family capacities to cope with the pressures and stresses, and the messages and expectations both spoken and unspoken (transmitted through behaviors and affective reactions) that are communicated is very important for an understanding of how the young woman adapts to the experience.

Psychosocial Risk Factors for Adolescent Mothers and Infants

Teenage mothers and their children suffer from both short-term and longer-term psychological, social, and economic difficulties. Poverty contributes enormously to the problems faced by teenage mothers, increasing their risk for a number of environmental difficulties including living in high-crime, high-violence areas, moving frequently, having difficulty coping with the day-to-day responsibilities and demands of raising a child, and having less social and emotional support than is usually available to older mothers. From a psychosocial perspective, adolescent mothers are less likely than older mothers to complete high school, attend college, find stable employment, marry, or be self-supporting (Chilman, 1983; Furstenberg, Brooks-Gunn, Morgan, 1987). Much evidence indicates that poverty contributes to adverse outcomes in psychological, social, emotional, and cognitive development, which places adolescent mothers as well as their children at significant risk. The stress of living in a single-parent, poverty environment can lead to higher rates of behavior problems, problems in school, and mental health risks (Kellam, Ensminger, & Turner, 1977; Spivak & Weitzman, 1987; Turner, Grindstaff, & Phillips, 1990).

Many adolescent mothers have fewer resources and are less able than older mothers to provide a positive socioemotional environment for their infants and children. Developmental conflicts specific to adolescence may interfere with their parenting ability (Fick, Peebles, Osofsky, & Hann, 1992; Peebles, Fick, Osofsky, & Hann, 1992). For example, adolescent mothers, as compared with a matched group of adolescents who were at high psychosocial risk but not pregnant, showed more identity diffusion, less autonomy, more difficulties with trust, more depression, and lower self-esteem. At times, a mismatch between the adolescent's own developmental needs and those of her infant interferes with her ability to parent (Osofsky & Eberhart-Wright, 1992).

Mental Health Risks: Maternal Depression and the Context of Poverty

The extreme risk factors in the environment of poverty within which most adolescent mothers live with their infants and children can lead not only to negative psychosocial consequences but also to significant mental health risks that may have been overlooked previously. In a recent study carried out in New Orleans on the effects of chronic community violence on 58 elementary-school children, ages 9 to 12 years (Osofsky, Wewers, Hann, & Fick, 1993), we found that almost half of the children included in the sample were born to mothers who became parents as teenagers. Further, there was a significant relationship between reported behavior problems in these children on the Child Behavior Checklist (Achenbach, 1979) and their having been parented by an adolescent mother. In addition to reported high rates of exposure to community and family violence, based on informal reports from several child abuse clinics, children of adolescent mothers are seen frequently as victims of child abuse and neglect. Informal reports from mental health clinics indicate that children of adolescent mothers are seen often with significant behavioral and personality problems. Thus, being born and raised in the family of an adolescent mother living in poverty may increase the risk of a child's being exposed to environmental and family factors that contribute to mental health risks.

Recent evidence has shown that adolescent mothers are more likely to be depressed than older mothers (Carter, Osofsky & Hann, 1991; Garrison, Schluchter, Schoenbach, & Kaplan, 1989; Hann, Castino, Jarosinski, & Britton, 1991; Osofsky, Osofsky, & Diamond, 1988). Sufficient data indicate that depressed mothers are more emotionally unavailable to their infants and children, and generally provide both a less empathic and responsive environment. Maternal depression may affect the quality of the interactive relationship between mother and child. For low-income, already-stressed dyads, maternal depression may place the infants and children at greater risk for less emotional availability and other problems in the relationship. Based on the work of my team (Carter et al., 1991; Hann et al, 1991; Osofsky et al., 1988), and that of others (Field, Healy, Goldstein, Guthertz, 1990; Radke-Yarrow, Cummings, Kuczynski, & Chapman, 1985; Tronick & Gianino, 1986; Zahn-Waxler et al., 1990), we also know that the children of depressed mothers are at higher risk for problems in affect regulation, including both increased depression or subdued affect and inappropriate aggression. According to Tronick and Gianino (1986), if the infant is able to cope with a nonresponsive environment and maintain self- and interactive regulation simultaneously, the result is likely to be positive mental health. On the other hand, if the infant cannot maintain interactive regulation, self-regulation will be the primary means of coping and the outcome is likely to be problematic. The combination of depression in the mothers and difficulty in affect regulation resulting in less emotional availability increases the risk that these infants and children will develop problematic behaviors or later psychopathology.

Parenting Risks for the Infants and Children of Adolescent Mothers

Parenting risks for adolescent mothers and infants include cognitive risks as well as socioemotional risks. Consistent evidence indicates that problems in the cognitive environment include adolescent mothers initiating less verbal interaction and being less responsive to their infants and children (Brooks-Gunn & Furstenberg, 1986; Chase-Lansdale et al., 1991; Crockenberg, 1987; Culp, Appelbaum, Osofsky, & Levy, 1988; Field, Widmayer, Stringer, & Ignatoff, 1980; Furstenberg, Brooks-Gunn, & Morgan, 1987; Holmbeck, Paikoff, & Brooks-Gunn, 1995; Osofsky, 1991; Osofsky & Eberhart-Wright, 1988, 1992). Observers of interactions between adolescent mothers and their infants frequently are struck with the quietness of the interaction. Adolescent mothers characteristically talk very little to their infants and young children, and, expectedly, the children verbalize relatively little. When these young mothers do talk, it is often to give short commands or to discipline the child rather than to elaborate responses or to make statements. Thus, many of these children grow up with impoverished cognitive environments in addition to economic and socioemotional deprivation. The increased risks and difficulties in meeting expectations when they enter the organized school environment are enormous.

In several studies, adolescent mothers as compared with adult mothers have been characterized by a lack of knowledge of developmental milestones, more punitive child-rearing attitudes, and perceptions of their own infant's temperament as more difficult (Field et al., 1980; Frodi, 1983). Both an early study (deLissovey, 1973) and a later study of teenage mothers with preterm infants (Field, 1980) reported that teenage mothers expect their children to reach developmental milestones earlier, findings that are consistent with those from our studies of teenage mothers in inner-city New Orleans (Osofsky, 1991). In their review article, Brooks-Gunn and Furstenberg (1986) conclude that even when controlling for social class, teenage mothers appear to have less knowledge about developmental milestones than do older mothers.

Adolescent mothers also exhibit less sensitive and less emotionally positive patterns of interactions with their toddlers (Hann, Osofsky, Barnard, & Leonard, 1994). When compared to the interactions observed between adult mothers and their toddlers, adolescent mother–toddler interactions were found to be less sensitive, more intrusive, less positive, and more negative. In addition, adolescent mothers and their toddlers were more likely to engage in disregulated patterns of affective interaction where either negative affects were emphasized (e.g., child cries and mother yells) or affective cues were misread by the dyad (e.g., child becomes angry and mother laughs). Participation in disregulated patterns of affect was most characteristic of adolescent mother–toddler interactions when they were compared with both socially disadvantaged and socially advantaged older mothers and toddlers (Hann, Osofsky, et al., 1994).

The developmental ramifications of the less optimal interaction patterns associated with adolescent mothers and their children may be detected early in the children's socioemotional development. Lamb, Hopps, and Elster (1987) found the distribution of infant attachment classifications to differ between infants of adolescent and adult mothers. Infants of adolescent mothers showed significantly more avoidant behavior and were more likely to be classified as avoidantly attached. More recent attachment research, including disorganized patterns of attachment in addition to secure and insecure patterns (Main & Solomon, 1990), has indicated that the infants of adolescent mothers may be at high risk for developing disorganized attachment relationships with their mothers (Hann, Castino, et al., 1991; Speiker, 1989). Some have questioned the appropriateness of measuring and interpreting attachment relationships in African American adolescent mothers according to the traditional Strange Situation procedure (Ainsworth, Blehar, Waters, & Wall, 1978) because extended family parenting patterns tend to predominate in this group (Brown, Martinez, & Radke-Yarrow, 1992). The studies based on the traditional attachment paradigm suggest that children of adolescent mothers are at higher risk for developing insecure attachment relationships. While the paradigm may not be appropriate to use with all African American groups, the insensitive, negative, and emotionally unavailable caregiving patterns that have been observed frequently with both African American and Caucasian adolescent mothers and their children are similar to those associated with both avoidant and disorganized attachment. Therefore, even if there are problems with using the attachment paradigm with adolescent mothers and their children, these dyads still appear to be at increased risk for developing patterns of interaction that appear to be less optimal. Since, in general, we see poorer social and emotional outcomes in children of adolescent mothers (Brooks-Gunn & Furstenberg, 1986; Furstenberg, Brooks-Gunn, & Chase-Landsdale, 1989; Holmbeck, Parkoft, et al., 1995; Osofsky & Eberhart-Wright, 1988; Osofsky, Eberhart-Wright, Ware, & Hann, 1992), we can question whether these poorer outcomes might result from earlier relationship difficulties. Further research is needed to establish the links between early patterns of mother-child interaction and infant attachment and later socioemotional outcomes with adolescent mothers and their children.

Resilience and Protective Factors in Adolescent Mothers and Infants

I already have noted that many adolescent mothers and their children live under conditions of chronic stress including poverty, limited educational resources, and family instability (Brooks-

Gunn & Furstenberg, 1986; Dubow & Luster, 1990; Osofsky, Osofsky, & Diamond 1988). Yet in the face of such adversities, some adolescent mothers and their children seem to do relatively well. Some young mothers go on to lead highly productive lives and are able to facilitate their children's development. The reasons explaining these successes under such difficult circumstances are not fully understood. The majority of the literature focuses on why individuals who are at risk fail. A better question to ask might be why some do not fail. What has gone right with these individuals? There is as much or more to be learned from studying the reasons for success as there is from studying failure.

When examining risk factors, it becomes apparent that some adolescent mothers show considerable resilience and that protective factors may serve as buffers against the risks. Resiliency refers to a marked ability to recover from or adjust easily to misfortune or chronic life stress; that is, adaptation despite challenging or threatening circumstances (Masten, Best, & Garmezy, 1990; Werner & Smith, 1982). By identifying protective factors, interventions can be targeted to foster the development of resilience in those individuals who are considered most vulnerable. In an earlier article (Osofsky & Eberhart-Wright, 1988), we identified protective factors in the mother, infant, and dyad that are likely to influence outcomes. Protective factors for the mother can include an ability to utilize support, goals (often with plans for a general equivalency diploma and job), consistent emotional availability, and acknowledgment of and work on difficulties in her own life. For the infant or child, protective factors can include a healthy start, which allows the child to handle crises; physical attractiveness, which lures outside adults into providing positive attention; an ability to care for and nurture the self; and an ability to use both symbolic play and others to master difficult life situations. For the dyad, protective factors can include the ability to adapt to one another's needs and unique characteristics and educational goals for both mother and child. We discuss some of these factors in more depth.

The importance of support comes up repeatedly for the young mothers, whether it is present from her family, extended family, friends, father of the child, or outside agencies. Social support generally is defined as the factors that lead individuals to believe that they are cared for, esteemed, and have people on whom they can depend in times of need (Cobb, 1976). Brooks-Gunn and Furstenberg (1986) emphasize that the availability and use of social support may buffer the individual from the possible deleterious effects of negative life events; such support may facilitate an individual's ability to handle stress. Furstenberg (1976) and Kellam et al. (1977) have reported that children of teenage mothers tend to have better developmental outcomes if there is alternative supportive child care by another person in the home. Brooks-Gunn and Furstenberg (1986) have posited several mechanisms to explain this: The person may "(1) act as a buffer, in lessening the psychological or economic impact of negative events upon the family; (2) act as a source of socioemotional support for the mother (which results in indirect benefits to the child); increased maternal well-being due to support may result in more interest in or responsivity to the child . . . ; and/or (3) act as a direct source of support for the child" (Lewis & Feiring, 1987, p. 235).

In our studies with adolescent mothers in Topeka, Kansas, and New Orleans, Louisiana, we found that both social support, particularly the young mothers' perception of support (as compared with the reported actual support) and specific support from the grandmother had significant impacts on life outcomes for both the infants and young mothers (Osofsky, 1991; Osofsky, Eberhart-Wright, Ware, & Hann 1992). Perceived support also was found to enhance the interactive relationship between the young mothers and their infants. The amount of support available to the young mother has been related to depression and self-esteem. In the New Orleans study, we found that the greater the number of people available for support to the young mother, the lower her level of reported depression and the higher her level of self-esteem. Pearson, Hunter, Ensminger, and Kellam (1990) have reported grandmothers to be a source of social support as well as socializing agents for their grandchildren. Similar findings from other studies (Kissman & Shapiro, 1990; Stevens, 1984) offer more evidence that the presence of a responsive grandmother appears to act as a buffer and as a positive influence on the child's development. These findings have strong implications for intervention, suggesting that strengthening social support systems in the mother's and infant's caregiving environment may result in reducing risk and facilitating resiliency.

In the Furstenberg, Brooks-Gunn, and Morgan (1987) follow-up study of a sample of teenage mothers and their children in Baltimore after 17 years, several factors were found to be extremely important for more successful outcomes. The young mothers' ability to continue with educational goals positively affected outcomes both for them and their children in terms of their feelings about themselves and their economic opportunities. Limiting their fertility was a second factor that positively influenced outcomes. A third major factor that seemed to impact greatly on their economic situation was whether they were married and stayed married before or after the birth of their child. Marriage provided both psychological support and a steady income to allow the family to be self-supporting. Furstenberg et al. (1987) pointed out, however, that this latter factor may have played a more significant role for a cohort growing up in the 1960s than it would today. In terms of outcomes for the children of teen mothers, "no single model described the impact of maternal career contingencies on the course of the children's development" (p. 145). However, several factors were predictive of poor outcomes, including welfare dependency, high fertility, and, at different developmental periods, unmarried status and lack of family support. The authors emphasized that the usual assumption that failure is inevitable may not be valid; they found that many of the mothers whom they studied were doing better than expected and much better than they had been doing for the first 5 years after they had the child.

In our 5-year follow-up of adolescent mothers and children in Topeka, we found that depression and self-esteem were important mediators of outcomes for both the young mothers and their infants (Osofsky & Eberhart-Wright, 1992). The relationships between child outcomes at 44 months, with particular emphasis on child behavioral conduct, and earlier indices of maternal functioning indicated that depression and self-esteem may be important mediators of outcomes, with more problematic development related to higher levels of depression and lower levels of self-esteem. At 54 months, earlier problems in maternal depression and self-esteem were found to be associated with more problematic forms of child internalizing behavior (as measured on the Child Behavior Checklist; Achenbach, 1979). In our ongoing studies of adolescent mothers and their children in New Orleans, preliminary results point in a similar direction; problems in self-esteem and depression are associated with more problematic personality issues for the adolescent mothers themselves as well as poorer outcomes for their infants in socioemotional domains. In an attempt to learn more about personality factors that may contribute to adolescent pregnancy, we are studying a sample of young mothers and a matched nonpregnant adolescent sample at high psychosocial risk. On personality measures of identity and psychosocial development based on Erikson's developmental theory, preliminary findings suggest differences between these groups. The pregnant adolescents report higher levels of identity diffusion than their nonpregnant counterparts. The nonpregnant adolescents report higher levels of identity achievement than the pregnant adolescents. On measures of psychosocial development, the pregnant group reports lower levels of trust than the nonpregnant group. This is an important area to pursue further in relation to risk factors that may contribute to early pregnancy as well as protective factors that may help an at-risk adolescent avoid early pregnancy.

Another important mediating variable is the child's dispositional attributes or temperament. Resilient children tend to have the ability, from infancy on, to gain other people's positive attention. They often possess personality characteristics, such as an appealing personality and friendliness, that elicit positive responses from family members as well as strangers (Garmezy, 1983). We have observed similar characteristics with parallel results for children of adolescent mothers (Osofsky & Eberhart-Wright, 1992). Infants who are active and socially responsive are most likely to show resilience to stress in childhood and adulthood (Werner & Smith, 1982). Lerner and East (1984) suggested that infants with easier temperaments can obtain suitable care and help with coping from their environments more readily. Cowen, Wyman, Work, and Parker (1990) found resilient outcomes in children with easy temperaments using self-report and behavioral measures of temperament. These infants were easier to manage, outgoing, and relaxed. In our work with adolescent mothers, we found several positive temperamental characteristics in infants and children that contributed to invulnerability and/or resiliency. These included a social nature apparent from birth, the ability to charm others, and a zest for living (Osofsky & Eberhart-Wright, 1992).

An examination of the relationship between risk and resiliency, including a focus on protective factors, can provide a better understanding of developmental outcomes for both adolescent mothers and their children. Knowing which individuals are at greater risk and which protective factors facilitate resiliency is crucial for the development of effective intervention programs.

Clinical Implications and Interventions for Adolescent Mothers and Infants

As part of a comprehensive approach to intervention with adolescent mothers and their infants, it is important to design programs that take into account the needs of both individuals who are going through their own developmental struggles. The intervention also should be directed both at the dyad and at the adolescent mother's broader family context. Meisels and Shonkoff (1990) provide a comprehensive review of intervention programs and strategies. Issues to be addressed in clinical intervention programs include many of the areas already discussed: support, education, personality, self-esteem, depression, match between infant and mother, and resiliency of the individual under stress.

Earlier approaches to therapeutic issues focused exclusively on the individual; however, more recent emphasis has been placed on the importance of the relationship (Sameroff & Emde, 1989) and support for individuals within a relationship context. Many adolescent mothers come from families that lack consistency and stable relationships. Therefore, first, it is important for the intervenor to build a relationship and develop trust in order to be able to provide effective interventions for the mother and child. One personality dimension that appears to discriminate between the adolescent mothers and a matched high-risk group of nonpregnant adolescents in our ongoing studies is trust, conceptualized from Erikson's developmental perspective (Erikson, 1968). Without basic trust, it is difficult to build other aspects of healthy psychological development and relationships. Thus, an intervention program for adolescent mothers should be designed to address their needs at a basic level—the level of having a trusting relationship.

Several other important tasks will be accomplished through a relationships approach to intervention. Self-esteem is an important intervening factor contributing to more positive outcomes for young mothers and their children (Furstenberg et al., 1987; Osofsky et al., 1988). For the adolescents, being able to form a meaningful trusting relationship with another person who conveys confidence in them raises their self-esteem. If the adolescents feel better about themselves, they will be able to parent their infants and children more effectively.

In developing interventions with adolescent mothers, we have found that it is most helpful to use strategies that assist the mother in empathizing with her baby. Adolescence is a developmental period during which time individuals tend to focus mainly on themselves rather than on another person. Thus, a baby or child takes away from and interferes a teenager's usual egocentric focus, when her own feelings rather than those of others predominate. For a teenager, her own feelings, not others', are crucial. Even if a young woman is already a mother, she will continue with her struggle to determine "Who am I?" Thus, helping the mother tune into her baby's feelings is difficult, but crucial, for both the baby and the relationship.

We have found that using videotaping and other techniques helps the mothers to focus playfully on their baby's feelings (Carter et al., 1991) and recognize the impact of their behaviors on the baby.

It is important to recognize that each baby and each mother is different; in fact, sometimes the most helpful information that can be imparted to the mother, either younger or older, is just that message. By recognizing the individuality of her baby, the match between baby and mother may become less important as a test of her mothering ability. This issue is particularly important for adolescent mothers and others at high psychosocial risk who may be focusing more on their own needs than on those of the baby. It is very reassuring for a mother to hear that she may not always be responsible for the difficult behaviors manifested by her baby. Encouraging the recognition and acceptance of her child's individuality may increase the mother's acceptance of her child and the patterns of interaction that will be most helpful for development.

Adolescent pregnancy and parenthood is a time of significant psychosocial risk for the young mother, her infant, and her family. This chapter has discussed factors that contribute to risk as well as protective factors that influence resiliency within individuals and dyads. While it is recognized that there are many risk factors, it is important to emphasize positive mental health; that is, to focus on what may go right rather than wrong with adolescent mothers and their infants. In this way we can plan effective preventive interventions that capitalize on the positive developmental thrust, while we work to mediate and overcome risk factors in order to optimize developmental outcome.

REFERENCES

Achenbach, T. M. (1979). The Child Behavior Profile: An empirically based system for assessing children's behavioral problems and competencies. *International Journal of Mental Health, 7,* 24–42.

Achenbach, T. M., & Edelbrock, C. S. (1981). Behavioral problem and competencies reported by parents of normal and disturbed children ages 4 through 16. *Monographs of the Society for Research in Child Development, 46,* 82.

Ainsworth, M. S., Blehar, M. C., Waters, E., & Wall, S.

(1978). *Patterns of attachment: A psychological study of the strange situation.* Hillsdale, NJ: Lawrence Erlbaum.

Baranowski, M. D., Schilmoeller, G. L., & Higgins, B. S. (1990). Parenting attitudes of adolescent and older mothers. *Adolescence, 25,* 781–790.

Belsky, J. (1984). The determinants of parenting. *Child Development, 55,* 83–96.

Benedek, T. (1970). The psychobiology of pregnancy. In E. J. Anthony & T. Benedek (Eds.). *Parenthood:*

Its psychology and psychopathology (pp. 137–152). Boston: Little, Brown.

Bibring, G. L., Dwyer, T. F., Huntington, D. S., & Valenstein, A. F. (1961). A study of the psychological processes in pregnancy and of the earliest mother-child relationship. I. Some propositions and comments. *Psychoanalytic Study of the Child, 16,* 9–24.

Broman, S. H. (1981). Long-term development of children born to teenagers. In K. Scott, T. Field, & E. G. Robertson (Eds.), *Teenage parents and their offspring* (pp. 195–224). New York: Grune & Stratton.

Bronfenbrenner, U. (1985, May). *Interacting systems in human development. Research paradigms: Present and future.* Paper presented at the Society for Research in Child Development Study Group, Cornell University, Ithaca, NY.

Bronfenbrenner, U. (1986). Ecology of the family as a context for human development. *Development Psychology, 22,* 723–742.

Bronfenbrenner, U. (1989). Ecological systems theory. *Annals of Child Development, 6,* 187–249.

Brooks-Gunn, J., & Chase-Landsdale, L. (1991). Teenage childbearing: Effects on children. In R. M. Lerner, A. C. Peterson, & J. Brooks-Gunn (Eds.), *Encyclopedia of adolescence* (pp. 103–106). New York: Garland Press.

Brooks-Gunn, J., & Furstenberg, F. F. (1986). The children of adolescent mothers: Physical, academic, and psychological outcomes. *Developmental Review, 6,* 224–251.

Brown, E., Martinez, P., & Radke-Yarrow, M. (1992). Research with diverse populations. *Newsletter of the Society for Research in Child Development.*

Burton, L. M., & Bengtson, V. L. (1985). Black grandmothers: Issues of timing and continuity of roles. In V. L. Bengtson & J. F. Robertson (Eds.), *Grandparenthood: Research and policy perspectives* (pp. 61–77). Beverly Hills, CA: Sage.

Carter, S., Osofsky, J. D., & Hann, D. M. (1991, April). *Maternal depression and affect in adolescent mothers and their infants.* Paper presented at the biennial meeting of the Society for Research in Child Development, Seattle.

Chase-Landsdale, L., Brooks-Gunn, J., & Palkoff, R. L. (1991). Research programs for adolescent mothers: Missing links and future promises. *Family Relations, 40,* 1–8.

Chilman, C. (1983). *Adolescent sexuality in a changing American society: Social and psychological perspectives for the human services professions* (2nd ed.). New York: John Wiley & Sons.

Cobb, S. (1976). Social support as a moderator of life stress. *Psychosomatic Medicine, 38,* 300–314.

Cowen, E. L., Wyman, P. A., Work, W. C., & Parker, G. R. (1990). The Rochester Child Resilence Project: Overview and summary of first year findings. *Development and Psychopathology, 2,* 193–212.

Crockenberg, S. (1987). Support for adolescent mothers during the postnatal period: Theory and research. In C. F. Z. Boukydes (Ed.), *Research on support for*

parents and infants in the postnatal period (pp. 3–24). Hillsdale, NJ: Lawrence Erlbaum.

Culp, R. E., Appelbaum, M. I., Osofsky, J. D., & Levy, J. A. (1988). Adolescent and older mothers: Comparison between prenatal maternal variables and newborn interaction measures. *Infant Behavior and Development, 11,* 353–362.

deLissovey, V. (1973). Child care by adolescent parents. *Children Today, 2,* 22–25.

Dubow, E. F., & Luster, T. (1990). Adjustment of children born to teenage mothers: The contribution of risk and protective factors. *Journal of Marriage and Family, 52,* 393–405.

Dwyer, J. (1974). Teenage pregnancy. *American Journal of Obstetrics and Gynecology, 118,* 373–376.

East, P. L., & Felice, M. E. (1990). Outcomes and parent-child relationships of former adolescent mothers and their 12-year old children. *Developmental and Behavioral Pediatrics, 11,* 175–183.

Elder, G. H., Jr., Caspi, A., & Burton, L. M. (1987). Adolescent transitions in developmental perspective: Sociological and historical insights. In M. Gunnar (Ed.), *Minnesota symposium on child development* (Vol. 21., pp. 151–179). Hillsdale, NJ: Lawrence Erlbaum.

Emde, R. N. (1991). The wonder of our complex enterprise: Steps enabled by attachment and the effects of relationships on relationships. *Infant Mental Health Journal, 12,* 164–173.

Epstein, A. S. (1979, March). *Pregnant teenagers' knowledge of infant development.* Paper presented at the Biennial Meeting of the Society for Research in Child Development, San Francisco.

Erikson, E. (1968). *Identity: Youth and crisis.* New York: W. W. Norton.

Fick, A., Peebles, C., Osofsky, J. D., & Hann, D. M. (1992). *Relationships among identity development, depression and self-esteem in pregnant and nonpregnant adolescents.* Unpublished manuscript, LSU Medical Center, New Orleans.

Field, T. (1980). Interactions of preterm and term infants with their lower and middle class teenage and adult mothers. In T. Field, S. Goldberg, D. Stern, & A. Sostek (Eds.), *High risk infants and children: Adult and peer interactions.* New York: Academic Press.

Field, T., Healy, B., Goldstein, S., & Guthertz, M. (1990). Behavior-state matching and synchrony in mother-infant interactions on nondepressed versus depressed dyads. *Developmental Psychology, 26,* 7–24.

Field, T. M., Widmayer, S. M., Stringer, S., & Ignatoff, E. (1980). Teenage, lower class, black mothers and their pre-term infants: An intervention and developmental follow-up study. *Child Development, 51,* 426–436.

Fielding, J. (1978). Adolescent pregnancy revisited. *New England Journal of Medicine, 299,* 893–896.

Frodi, A. (1983). Attachment behavior and sociability with strangers in premature and full-term infants. *Infant Mental Health Journal, 4,* 13–22.

Frodi, A., Grolnick, W., Bridges, L., & Berko, J. (1990). Infants of adolescent and adult mothers: Two indices of socioemotional development. *Adolescence, 25,* 363–374.

Furstenberg, F. F. (1976). The social consequences of teenage parenthood. *Family Planning Perspectives, 8,* 148–164.

Furstenberg, F. F., Jr., Brooks-Gunn, J., & Chase-Landsdale, L. (1989). Teenaged pregnancy and childbearing. *American Psychologist, 44,* 313–320.

Furstenberg, F. F., Jr., Brooks-Gunn, J., & Morgan, P. (1987). *Adolescent mothers in later life.* New York: Cambridge University Press.

Garcia-Coll, C. T., Hoffman, J., & Oh, W. (1987). The social ecology and early parenting of Caucasian adolescent mothers. *Child Development, 58,* 955–962.

Garmezy, N. (1983). Stressors of Childhood. In N. Garmezy & M. Rutter (Eds.), *Stress, coping and development* (pp. 43–84). New York: McGraw-Hill.

Garrison, C. Z., Schluchter, M. D., Schoenbach, & V. J., Kaplan, B. K. (1989). Epidemiology of depressive symptoms in young adolescents. *American Academy of Child and Adolescent Psychiatry, 28,* 343–351.

Geetz, C. (1973). *The interpretation of cultures.* New York: Basic Books.

Greenberg, J. R., & Mitchell, S. A. (1983). *Object relations in psychoanalytic theory.* Cambridge, MA: Harvard University Press.

Hann, D. M., Castino, R. J., Jarosinski, J., & Britton, H. (1991, April). *Relating mother-toddler negotiation patterns to infant attachment and maternal depression with an adolescent mother sample.* In J. D. Osofsky & L. Hubbs-Tait (Chairs), Consequences of adolescent parenting: Predicting behavior problems in toddlers and preschoolers. Symposium presented at the meeting of the Society for Research in Child Development, Seattle, WA.

Hann, D. M., Osofsky, J. D., Barnard, K., & Leonard, G. (1994). Dyadic affect regulation in three caregiving environments. *American Journal of Orthopsychiatry, 64,* 263–269.

Hinde, R. (1979). *Toward understanding relationships.* London: Academic Press.

Hinde, R., & Stevenson-Hinde, J. (1988). *Relationships within families: Mutual influences.* Oxford: Clarendon Press.

Hofferth, S. L., & Hayes, C. D. (Eds). (1987). *Risking the future.* Vol. 2: *Working papers.* Washington, DC: National Academy Press.

Hollingsworth, D. R., Kotchen, J. M., & Felice, M. E. (1983). Impact of gynecologic age on outcome of adolescent pregnancy. In E. R. McAnarney (Ed.), *Premature adolescent pregnancy and parenthood* (pp. 169–194). New York: Grune & Stratton.

Holmbeck, G. N., Paihoff, R. L., & Brooks-Gunn, J. (1995). Parenting adolescents. In M. Bornstein (Ed.), *Handbook of parenting* (Vol. 1, pp. 91–118). New York: John Wiley & Sons.

Kahn, R. L., & Antonuci, T. C. (1980). Convoys over the life course: Attachment, roles and social support.

In P. B. Baltes & O. G. Brim (Eds.), *Life-span development and behavior* (pp. 253–286). New York: Academic Press.

Karraker, K. H., & Lake, M. (1991). Normative stress and coping processes in infancy. In M. Cummings, A. Greene, & K. Karraker (Eds.), *Life-span developmental psychology: Perspectives on stress and coping.* (Vol. 1, pp. 85–108). Hillsdale, NJ: Lawrence Erlbaum.

Kellam, S., Adams, R., Brown, C. H., & Emsinger, M. E. (1982). The long-term evolution of the family structure of teenage and older mothers. *Journal of Marriage and the Family, 44,* 539–554.

Kellam, S. G., Ensminger, M. E., & Turner, R. J. (1977). Family structure and the mental health of children. *Archives of General Psychiatry, 34,* 1012.

Kissman, K., & Shapiro, J. (1990). The composites of social support and well-being among adolescent mothers. *International Journal of Adolescence and Youth, 2,* 165–173.

Klein, L. (1974). Early teenage pregnancy, contraception and repeat pregnancy. *American Journal of Obstetrics and Gynecology, 120,* 249.

Ladner, J., & Gourdine, R. M. (1985). Black mothers and daughters: Some preliminary findings. In V. L. Bengston & J. Robertson (Eds.), *Grandparenthood: Research and policy perspective.* Beverly Hills, CA: Sage.

Lamb, M. E., Hopps, K., & Elster, A. B. (1987). Strange situation behavior of infants with adolescent mothers. *Infant Behavior and Development, 10,* 39–48.

Lerner, R. M., & East, P. L. (1984). The role of infant temperament in stress, coping, and socioemotional functioning in early development. *Infant Mental Health Journal, 5,* 148–159.

Lewis, M., & Feiring, C. (1981). Direct and indirect interactions in social relationships. In L. Lipsitt (Ed.), *Advances in infancy research* (Vol. 1, pp. 129–161). New York: Ablex.

Lewis, M., Feiring, C., McGuffog, C., & Jaskir, J. (1984). Predicting psychopathology in six-year-olds from early social relations. *Child Development, 55,* 123–136.

Londerville, S., & Main, M. (1981). Security of attachment, compliance, and maternal training methods in the second year of life. *Developmental Psychology, 17,* 289–299.

Madge, N., & Tizard, J. (1981). Intelligence. In M. Rutter (Ed.), *Developmental psychiatry,* (pp. 245–265). Baltimore: University Park Press.

Mahler, M., Pine, F., & Bergmann, A. (1975). *The psychological birth of the human infant.* New York: Basic Books.

Main, M., & Hesse, E. (1990). Parents' unresolved traumatic experiences are related to infant disorganized attachment status: Is frighten and/or frightening parental behavior the linking mechanism? In M. Greenberg, D. Cicchetti, & E. M. Cummings (Eds.), *Attachment in the preschool years: Theory, research and intervention* (pp. 161–184). Chicago: University of Chicago Press.

Main, M., & Solomon, J. (1990). Procedures for identifying infants as disorganized-disoriented during the Ainsworth Strange Situation. In M. Greenberg, D. Cicchetti, & E. M. Cummings (Eds.), *Attachment in the preschool years: Theory, research and intervention* (pp. 121–161). Chicago: University of Chicago Press.

Maracek, J. (1985). *The effects of adolescent childbearing on children's cognitive and psychosocial development*. Unpublished manuscript.

Masten, A. S., Best, K. M., & Garmezy, N. (1990). *Developmental Psychopathology, 2*, 425–444.

McCormick, M. C. (1985). The contribution of low birth weight to infant mortality and child morbidity. *New England Journal of Medicine, 312*, 82–90.

Meisels, S. J., & Shonkoff, J. P. (1990). *Handbook of early childhood intervention*. New York: Cambridge University Press.

Osofsky, H. J., & Osofsky, J. D. (1970). Adolescents as mothers: Results of a program for low-income pregnant teenagers with some emphasis upon infants' development. *American Journal of Orthopsychiatry, 40*, 825–834.

Osofsky, J. D. (1991). *A preventive intervention program for adolescent mothers and their infants*. Final report to the Institute of Mental Hygiene, New Orleans.

Osofsky, J. D., & Eberhart-Wright, A. (1988). Affective exchanges between high risk mothers and infants. *International Journal of Psycho-Analysis, 69*, 221–231.

Osofsky, J. D., & Eberhart-Wright, A. (1992). Risk and protective factors for parents and infants. In G. Suci & S. Robertson (Eds.), *Human Development: Future Directions in Infant Psychiatry* (pp. 29–35). New York: Springer-Verlag.

Osofsky, J. D., Eberhart-Wright, A., Ware, L. M., & Hann, D. M. (1992). Children of adolescent mothers: A group at risk for psychopathology. *Infant Mental Health Journal, 13*, 119–131.

Osofsky, J. D., Osofsky, H. J., & Diamond, M. O. (1988). The transition to parenthood: Special tasks and risk factors for adolescent mothers. In G. Y. Michaels & W. A. Goldberg (Eds.), *The transition to parenthood* (pp. 209–234). New York: Cambridge University Press.

Osofsky, J. D., Wewers, S., Hann, D. M. & Fick, A. (1993). Children's exposure to chronic community violence: What are we doing to our children? *Psychiatry. 56*, 36–45.

Pearson, J. L., Hunter, A. G., Ensminger, M. E., & Kellam, S. G. (1990). Black grandmothers in multigenerational households: Diversity in family structure and parenting involvement in the Woodlawn Community. *Child Development, 61*, 434–442.

Peebles, C., Fick, A., Osofsky, J. D., & Hann, D. M. (1992). *Relationship between adolescent pregnancy, depression, self-esteem and psychosocial development*. Unpublished manuscript, LSU Medical Center, New Orleans.

Pellegrini, D. S., Mastin, A. S., Garmezy, N., & Ferrar-

ese, M. J. (1987). Correlates of social and academic competence in middle childhood. *Journal of Child Psychology and Psychiatry, 28* (5), 699–714.

Radke-Yarrow, M., Cummings, E. M., Kuczynski, L., & Chapman, M. (1985). Patterns of attachment in two and three-year-olds in normal families and families with parental depression. *Child Development, 56*, 884–893.

Ragozin, A. S., Basham, R. B., Crnic, K. A., Greenberg, M. T., & Robinson, N. M. (1982). Effects of maternal age on parenting role. *Developmental Psychology, 18*, 627–634.

Reiss, D. (1981). *The family's construction of reality* Cambridge, MA: Harvard University Press.

Reiss, D. (1989). The represented and practicing family: Contrasting visions of family continuity. In A. J. Sameroff & R. N. Emde (Eds.), *Relationship disturbances in early childhood* (pp. 191–220). New York: Basic Books.

Roosa, M. (1984). Short-term effects of teenage parenting program on knowledge and attitudes. *Adolescence, 18*, 348–360.

Sameroff, A. J. (1989). General systems and regulation of development. In M. Gunnar & E. Thelen (Eds.), *Systems and development*. Hillsdale, NJ: Lawrence Erlbaum.

Sameroff, A. J., & Chandler, M. J. (1975). Reproductive risk and continuim of caretaking casualty. In F. D. Horowitz, M. Hetherington, S. Scarr-Salapatek, & G. Siegel (Eds.), *Review of child development research* (Vol. 4, pp. 187–243). Chicago: University of Chicago Press.

Sameroff, A. J., & Emde, R. N. (Eds.), *Relationship disturbances in early childhood*. New York: Basic Books.

Spieker, S. (1989). Mothering in adolescence: factors related to infant security. (Grant No. MC-J-50535). Washington, DC: Maternal and Child Health and Crippled Children's Services.

Spieker, S. L., & Booth, C. L. (1988). Maternal antecedents of attachment quality. In J. Belsky & T. Nezworski (Eds.). *Clinical implications of attachment* (pp. 95–135). Hillsdale, NJ: Lawrence Erlbaum.

Spivak, H., & Weitzman, M. (1987). Social barriers faced by adolescent parents and their children. *Journal of the American Medical Association, 258*, 1500–1504.

Stevens, J. H., Jr. (1984). Child development knowledge and parenting skill. *Family Relations, 33*, 237–244.

Stevenson-Hinde, J. (1990). Attachment within family systems: An overview. *Infant Mental Health Journal, 11*, 218–227.

Tronick, E. Z., & Gianino, A. F., Jr. (1986). The transmission of maternal disturbance to the infant. In E. Z. Tronick & T. M. Field (Eds.), *Maternal depression and infant disturbance, New directions for child development* (No. 34, pp. 5–11) San Francisco: Jossey-Bass.

Turner, R. J., Grindstaff, C. F., & Phillips, N. (1990). Social support and outcome in teenage pregnancy. *Journal of Health and Social Behavior, 31*, 43–57.

Werner, E. E., & Smith, R. S. (1982). *Vulnerable but invincible: A study of resilient children.* New York: McGraw-Hill.

Willits, F. K. (1988). Adolescent behavior and adult success and well-being: A 37-year panel. *Youth and Society, 20,* 68–87.

Wilson, M. (1989). Child development in the context of the Black extended family. *American Psychologist, 44,* 380–385.

Wright, B. (1988). *Three generations of teenage mothers in New Orleans: Preliminary findings.* Unpublished manuscript, The Urban League of Greater New Orleans.

Wright-Edelman, M. (1989, March 27). Profile. *The New Yorker.*

Zahn-Waxler, C., Kochanska, G., Krupnick, J., & McKnew, D. (1990). Patterns of guilt in children of depressed and well mothers. *Developmental Psychology, 26,* 51–59.

Zimmerman, I. L., Steiner, V. G., & Pond, R. E. (1979). *Preschool language scale* (rev. ed.). Columbus, OH: Charles E. Merrill.

Zuckerman, B. S., Alpert, J. J., Dooling, E., Hingson, R., Kaye, H., Morelock, S., & Openheim, E. (1993). Neonatal outcome: Is adolescent pregnancy a risk factor? *Pediatrics, 71,* 489–493.

Zuravin, S. J. (1989). Severity of maternal depression and three types of mother-to-child aggression. *American Journal of Orthopsychiatry, 59,* 377–389.

23 / Vulnerability and Resilience in Young Children

Margaret O'Dougherty Wright and Ann S. Masten

Introduction

During the past 20 years, the categories of children designated "at risk" for developmental problems or psychopathology has grown exponentially. Biological, psychosocial, and environmental risk factors have been identified, and children in each of these categories have been the subject of intense investigation. In the area of biological risk there have been a series of studies of low-birthweight infants, medically vulnerable and chronically ill children, infants exposed prenatally to drugs and/or alcohol, infants and children with AIDS, and children exposed to environmental toxins (Chasnoff, 1988; Clarren & Smith, 1978; Garrison & McQuiston, 1989; Green, 1991; Horowitz, 1989; Kopp, 1983, 1987; Kopp & Kaler, 1989; O'Dougherty & Wright, 1990; Rolf & Johnson, 1990; Sameroff & Chandler, 1975; Volpe, 1992; Vorhees & Mollnow, 1987). Psychosocial and environmental risks have included the study

of children living in poverty; children of divorce; homeless children; children exposed to community violence; abused and neglected children; children whose parents are psychiatrically disturbed, alcoholic, or severely dysfunctional; children in foster care; and infants born to adolescent mothers (Cicchetti & Carlson, 1989; Emery, 1988; Garmezy & Masten, 1994; Hetherington, Cox, & Cox, 1985; Jones, Levine, & Rosenberg, 1991; Masten, Miliotis, Graham-Bermann, Ramirez, & Neemann, 1993; Osofsky, Eberhart-Wright, Ware, & Hann, in press; Richters & Martinez, 1993; Rolf, Masten, Cicchetti, Nuechterlein, & Weintraub, 1990; Rutter, 1988; Sameroff, Barocas, & Seifer, 1984; Wallerstein, Corbin, & Lewis, 1988; Werner & Smith, 1982, 1992). In addition, there has been increasing interest in examining the adaptation of children exposed to traumatic events (Eth & Pynoos, 1985; Garmezy & Rutter, 1985; Perry, Pollard, Blakley, Baker, & Vigilante, 1995; Terr, 1990; van der Kolk, 1987).

As investigators have followed the development and adjustment of children in all of these high-risk categories, it has become increasingly apparent that there is great diversity in outcomes and complexity in the developmental pathways of individual children and families (Horowitz, 1989).

Preparation of this chapter was facilitated by an Academic Challenge Grant from the state of Ohio to Dr. Wright and grants to Dr. Masten from the William T. Grant Foundation and the Minnesota Center for Research on Developmental Disabilities.

Predictions about outcome, previously focusing predominantly on vulnerability and psychopathology, have not been able to account for the high percentage of positive adaptation in these risk groups. Efforts to understand favorable developmental outcomes despite risk, vulnerability, or adversity have resulted in a search for protective processes that might further our understanding of resilience (Garmezy, 1985; Haggerty, Sherrod, Garmezy, & Rutter, 1994; Masten, 1994; Masten, in press; Masten, Best, & Garmezy, 1990, Rutter, 1990; Werner & Smith, 1982, 1992).

One of the most important tasks for developmental psychopathology is to understand the role of risk, vulnerability, and protective processes as they influence development and individual differences in the quality of adaptation (Masten & Braswell, 1991; Masten & Coatsworth, 1995). Moreover, clinicians and researchers alike have recognized the necessity of examining children *in context* in order to understand the complex factors that promote resilience (Garmezy & Masten, 1986; Rutter, 1990; Sameroff & Seifer, 1990; Sroufe & Rutter, 1984). A fundamental aspect of this orientation is an emphasis on a holistic rather than reductionistic approach to studying developmental outcome (Gunnar & Mangelsdorf, 1989; Sroufe & Rutter, 1984). Most developmental psychopathologists assume that multiple influences, both genetic and environmental, interact in the development of behavior. Bidirectional and feedback effects are anticipated, as is the need for multiple (e.g., biological, cognitive, emotional, social, environmental) levels of analysis. Given these multiple, interacting influences and transformations, a child's behavior over time can be viewed as part of a path or trajectory (Bowlby, 1988; Masten & Braswell, 1991; Masten & Wright, in press; Rutter, 1990).

This chapter examines the possible role of risk, vulnerability, and protective processes in the development of young children. First, operational definitions of the key concepts are offered to improve conceptual clarity regarding critical terms. Clinical and empirical evidence of vulnerability and resilience in young children at risk is reviewed. Resilience is explored in three different contexts: positive adaptation despite high-risk status, maintaining competence under stressful life conditions, and recovery from traumatic life experiences.

Risk Factors and Stressors

RISK FACTORS

Although many risk factors have been identified, simply listing them does not adequately define risk or clearly specify which members of the risk group are vulnerable. It is important to clarify that risk is a statistical concept and is appropriately used only for groups and not for an individual. Classifications of individuals "at risk" are based on probability estimates for experiencing a subsequent disorder or difficulty in adjustment. Thus, by their nature, risk classifications are tentative. If a child is a member of a specific risk group, it does not necessarily indicate that the child is vulnerable or that the child will develop the problem.

Consider the infant designated "at risk" due to prematurity and low birthweight as an example. Actual outcomes of infants in this risk group will vary widely depending on many factors, including the mother's health and the infant's prenatal history, the type and severity of medical complications associated with the premature birth, successfulness of medical interventions, degree of family disruption, extent of financial burden, the parents' and siblings' perception of and response to the infant, and the presence of infant and family characteristics that can moderate successful coping (e.g., socioeconomic status, marital cohesiveness, number of children in the family, family's acceptance of the condition, availability of social support, and temperament and intellectual capabilities of the infant that may affect the quality of the parent-child relationship) (O'Dougherty & Brown, 1990). The risk for problems in developmental outcome for a premature infant who suffers only mild medical complications and enters a family that is financially secure, with excellent health insurance coverage, strong social support networks, and parental confidence in their ability to cope with the additional demands of this infant differs dramatically from a premature infant of similar low birthweight with severe medical complications who is the fourth child of a single mother living in poverty with limited social support, no health insurance, and a number of additional stressors in her life.

As this example illustrates, there can be great

heterogeneity in outcome among members of a risk group identified by a single criterion. It is often the *multiplicity* of risk and the accumulation of risk factors that is clearly associated with the probability of a negative outcome (Garmezy & Masten, 1994; Masten & Wright, in press; O'Dougherty & Wright, 1990; Sameroff & Seifer, 1990). Moreover, transactional influences are important: The match and bidirectional influences between child and parent also will shape the course of development (Richters & Weintraub, 1990; Sameroff, 1983). It is also important to identify compensatory factors among high-risk children, which can include individual strengths or protective factors within the family or larger social system, as discussed in the next section. A narrow focus on a single risk variable also neglects dynamic changes in the family system over time that affect an individual child's development (Erickson, Sroufe, & Egeland, 1985; Sameroff, 1983).

Children placed in high-risk categories who demonstrate no direct evidence of either biological injury or the experience of proximal environmental stressors may not be truly "at risk" (Baldwin, Baldwin, & Cole, 1990; Rutter, 1990). Focusing more clearly on the underlying processes activated or mediated by the risk variable may allow more sensitivity and specificity in such designations (Garmezy & Masten, 1990; Rutter, 1990). As risk assessments become more refined and the impact of specific and multiple risk factors more clearly defined, the degree of certainty about who is going to experience difficulty will rise, leading to clinical predictions about prognosis rather than risk probability estimates.

STRESSORS

The word *stress* is both widely used in daily conversation and simultaneously ambiguous and imprecise. The term has come to encompass both the stressful event and the strain such stress might entail. This strain is inextricably linked to the individual's appraisal of the stressfulness of the event (Aldwin, 1994; Lazarus & Folkman, 1984). The relatively new term *stressor* is considered an event or experience that typically produces distress in people. Stressors vary along a number of dimensions: severity; acuteness of onset; duration; whether it is a normative event (experienced by virtually everyone at some time in their life—moving, changing schools, death of a parent) or a nonnormative event (such as experiencing a tornado or rape) (Masten, 1994).

Garmezy and Rutter (1983) delineate 5 categories of stressors: loss, chronically disturbed relationships, events that change the status quo, events that require social adaptation, and acute negative events. Acute stressors are often uncontrollable and/or unforeseeable, such as a tornado, flood, accident, assault, or rape. Chronic stressors, such as poverty, ongoing parental hostility, chronic illness or handicap, and chronic abuse, not only cause distress and anxiety during specific episodes but also encompass enduring adversity that can significantly disrupt and distort a child's growth and development (Garmezy & Masten, 1994; Garmezy & Rutter, 1985; Trad & Greenblatt, 1990). In some instances the event might be acute but the consequences of the event produce enduring and chronic stress, such as when a flood destroys one's community (Green et al., 1991) or a murder victim is the child's parent (Malmquist, 1984).

Stressors can affect biological systems (physiologically and/or chemically) as well as psychological systems (personal, familial, cultural). The disequilibrium following a stressful event can be reflected in a state of arousal (neurophysiological, cognitive, or emotional) that can disrupt the person's adaptation (Garmezy & Masten, 1990; Perry et al., 1995). The effects can be additive or synergistic (Arnold, 1990). For example, prenatal exposure to drugs and alcohol can directly interfere with optimal fetal brain and body growth and organ development (Volpe, 1992). Following the infant's birth, continued maternal substance abuse can have subsequent psychological effects resulting in problems in parent-infant attachment and possible neglect, child abuse, or exposure to poor environmental living conditions (Chasnoff, 1988; Singer, Farkas, & Kliegman, 1992).

Some types of stress, such as war and terrorism, comprise a number of interconnected stressors for children (separation from parents, deprivation, physical danger, anxiety about possible injury to or death of a parent). The degree to which the event is experienced directly or witnessed by the child (terrorist attack, torture) and the child's perception of his or her own degree of safety and/or control can be particularly important (Trad, 1988; Trad & Greenblatt, 1990).

Stressors producing posttraumatic stress disorder (PTSD) either are events outside the range of experience of most people or are so devastating in their impact that they would be likely to produce distress in most individuals (American Psychiatric Association, 1987). The symptoms of the disorder (nightmares, flashbacks, sleeplessness, hypervigilance, irritability, avoidance and numbing, guilt, depression, and anxiety) vary in form, duration, and severity. The degree to which preexisting vulnerabilities predispose a child to developing this disorder, and the specific factors related to different manifestations across different stressors and during different developmental periods, is currently the subject of extensive empirical and clinical investigation (Davidson & Foa, 1991a, b; Jones & Barlow, 1990; McNally, 1991, 1993; Perry et al., 1995; Pynoos, 1990; Pynoos et al., 1987; van der Kolk, 1987).

Vulnerability and Protective Factors

Vulnerabilities and protective factors moderate the effects of risk factors or stressors on adaptation. Neither is a direct effect. A vulnerability refers to a characteristic of a system (e.g., an individual, a family, or a group) that makes that system more susceptible to particular threats to development or functioning. The concept of protective factors has been used to refer to either individual or environmental characteristics that appear to facilitate better outcomes despite risk or adversity. Protective factors are presumed to reduce threats to a system's functioning or development.

Vulnerability can begin at the genetic level if an individual inherits a genetic predisposition for a metabolic, endocrinological, cardiovascular, neurological, immunologic, or psychiatric disorder. Vulnerabilities also may be acquired or exacerbated by prenatal and perinatal experiences. Early stressful experiences may create a hypersensitivity to stress, creating an increased vulnerability to fu-

ture stress (Perry et al. 1995; Rutter, 1983; Trad & Greenblatt, 1990). Psychological vulnerability evolves from a person's interactions with others and the unique biological, temperamental, and personal characteristics that influence the nature of the interaction. Taken together, these factors constitute an individual's diathesis and mediate his or her response to stress. In the diathesis-stress model (Gottesman & Shields, 1982; Meehl, 1962), an individual may inherit or acquire vulnerability to a specific medical or psychological disorder but not develop the disorder if not exposed to the eliciting stressor(s).

From a statistical/epidemiological perspective, protective factors refer to variables that appear to moderate risk. Table 23.1 presents a sampling of the most widely reported protective factors. Presumably, however, protective factors are markers of processes and actions that underlie the protective effect. *Identifying a protective factor does not tell one how it works.* Increasingly, researchers are turning from the question of what makes a difference (vulnerability and protective factors) to the processes by which resilience occurs.

For example, many studies implicate a "good parent" as the key protective factor for young children threatened by adversity (Masten et al., 1990). This is not surprising when evolutionary forces for millennia have shaped the protective role of parents in our species. Given adversity or threat, there are many ways in which a parent may function to protect a child. In some situations, a parent may actively avert a child's exposure to the adversity. In others, a parent may reassure a child, model competent behavior, or provide information. A parent may also secure additional resources when demands exceed current supplies of resources or prepare a child to face a difficult situation. Parents also contribute to the foundation of a child's confidence in self and in others by their loving and sensitive caregiving. The child responds by coming to view him- or herself as lovable and capable.

The actual behavior of an effective parent may vary in accordance with the individual development and needs of the child and the contextual circumstances. For example, parents of competent children living in dangerous urban environments have been found to be stricter and less democratic in their child-rearing practices than

TABLE 23.1

A Sampling of Protective Factors

Individual Characteristics

Good intellectual skills
Good health and physical fitness
Adaptable temperament
High self-esteem
Self-efficacy, internal locus of control
Strong sense of competence based on achievements,
    successes, special talents
Ability to persist in achieving goals
Ability to seek environments conducive to personal
    growth
Having close, trusting relationships
Religious faith
Good fortune, good luck
Attractiveness and appeal to adults
Humor

Family Characteristics and Relationships

Effective parenting
    Family warmth, cohesion, support, and good
        communication
    A good relationship with at least one parent
    Parents allow age-appropriate autonomy
    Parents are available at time of failure or distress
    Parents are able to buffer and protect child against
        excessive stress
    Parents set reasonable, consistent rules
Presence of a positive value system
Socioeconomic advantage

Extrafamilial and Community Qualities

A close relationship with a competent adult outside
    the family
Mentors and positive role models
Good schools/good day care/supportive teachers
Belonging to and participating in a group one values
    (religious, political, social, cultural)
A supportive social network
Opportunities to learn and master new skills and
    challenges

parents of children from less dangerous middle-class neighborhoods (Baldwin et al., 1990; McWhirter & Trew, 1981; Richters & Martinez, 1993). Greater parental authority and more careful monitoring may be necessary to protect children in high crime urban neighborhoods.

Effective schools may work by processes analogous to good parenting, including high expectations, positive regard for the students, good role modeling, and consistent rules (Rutter, Maughan, Mortimore, Ouston, & Smith, 1979; Wang & Gordon, 1994). Yet the precise formula that works at

one school may not work as well for a different group of children in a different time or community.

It is also important to remember that the same quality in an individual could be protective in one situation and problematic in another. Thus, for example, the child who is by nature very inhibited may be protected by this disposition from accidental injuries that arise from risk-taking behavior but may be vulnerable to internalizing symptoms or disorders (Kagan, Gibbons, Johnson, Reznick, & Snidman, 1990).

Children with High-Risk Status

CHILDREN OF MENTALLY ILL PARENTS

Children of Parents with Schizophrenia: Studies of children at risk for schizophrenia have been central to the theoretical and empirical underpinnings of developmental psychopathology (Garmezy, 1974; Garmezy & Streitman, 1974; Masten & Braswell, 1991). This work sparked the recent surge of interest in both vulnerability and resilience.

The most important model to emerge from this line of work was the diathesis-stressor framework (Gottesman & Shields, 1982). This model posited that a specific vulnerability for schizophrenia was transmitted by multiple genes but that many other biological and environmental factors contributed to the net liability for the disorder. Other genetic and environmental assets and liabilities, as well as life experiences, were hypothesized to play a role in the development of this disorder. Fundamental to this model is the idea that it is vulnerability to disorder that is inherited rather than the disorder itself. Because of differing life experiences, identical twins do not invariably develop the disorder (i.e., they are discordant) despite the same genetic vulnerability. Another important concept in this model is that net liability changes over the course of development, due to interactions between phenotype and environment and the turning off and on of genes. The concept of protective processes also is incorporated by this model. Theoretically, a very favorable environment can reduce the phenotypic manifestations of the inherent vulnerability whereas a highly stressful environment can precipitate the onset of the disorder.

The offspring of parents with schizophrenia carry an elevated risk for the disorder (approximately 10 times the population risk), and this risk appears to be specific to schizophrenia (Gottesman & Shields, 1982). Regardless of their genetic vulnerability to schizophrenia, however, many of these children live with the chronic adversities stemming from life with a mentally ill parent. In the latter case, their risk is more general and similar to risks associated with other mental illnesses in parents, such as depression (Sameroff & Seifer, 1990; Watt, Anthony, Wynne, & Rolf, 1984). Mental illness in a parent can result in ineffective parenting behavior, multiple separations and household disruptions due to hospitalizations, economic hardship, interparental conflict, and many other problems. Thus, many of the studies have found that the severity of the parent's illness and level of psychosocial disadvantage are the most powerful predictors of child adjustment (Goldstein & Tuma, 1987; Sameroff et al., 1984). Severity of parental illness and disadvantage appear to erode the quality of the caregiving environment.

Consistent with these findings is the observation that a good relationship with one parent appears to be a protective factor for the development of children with a mentally ill parent (Bleuler, 1984; Garmezy, 1985). Other protective factors observed in children living with a parent who has schizophrenia include a positive relationship with an adult outside the family, appealingness to adults, and good intellectual skills (Bleuler, 1984; Fisher, Kokes, Cole, Perkins, & Wynne, 1987).

These protective factors appear to be quite general, being found in most studies of good development in high-risk populations. They appear to be protective in general with respect to adaptation. However, it is not clear whether these general protective factors serve a specific vulnerability-reducing effect for schizophrenia. This remains to be seen. Only when the specific genetic vulnerability for this disorder can be identified accurately will it be possible to examine whether and how favorable environments or dispositions counteract the genetic vulnerability.

Children of Affectively Disordered Parents: Until recently, studies focused on the offspring of parents with depression and bipolar disorder have lagged behind the study of schizophrenia. Over the past decade, such studies have burgeoned. Results are beginning to suggest that, as with schizophrenia, there may be both general and specific risks associated with having a parent with affective disorder (Downey & Coyne, 1990; Garmezy & Masten, 1994). Genetic studies indicate an elevated risk for affective disorder in children whose biological parents have bipolar disorder or major depressive disorder. Recent studies of depressed mothers and their children also suggest that an episode of depression in one family member may increase the likelihood of an episode in another member soon after. Children and mothers have been found to have episodes of depression in close proximity to one another (Hammen, Burge, & Adrian, 1991). On the other hand, children of depressed parents also appear to have elevated problems in other spheres of behavior that are probably due to the general effects of disturbed parenting and adverse life events linked to severe mental illness in a parent (Conrad & Hammen, 1993; Downey & Coyne, 1990).

When a child's parent is severely depressed, the caregiving environment can be dramatically altered. The symptoms of depression—sad affect, emotional withdrawal, unresponsiveness, irritability, hopelessness, and lethargy—all can interfere with a parent's ability to respond to the physical and emotional needs of a children. Young children are keenly aware of changes in their parent's affective state, conveyed through facial expressions, intonation, body language, and emotional reactivity (Klinnert, Campos, Sorce, Emde, & Svejda, 1983; Osofsky & Eberhart-Wright, 1992). In a study of attachment in 2- and 3-year-olds whose mothers were depressed, Radke-Yarrow and her colleagues illustrated the relationship between expressed emotion (positive vs. negative) and patterns of attachment. Mothers of insecurely attached children expressed more negative and less positive emotion. The risk of an insecure mother-child attachment was significantly increased if the mother's affective illness was more severe (e.g., either bipolar or unipolar depression in contrast to minor depression or no affective illness). Additionally, if the depressed mother did not have a husband living with her, the prevalence of insecure attachment was significantly greater (Radke-Yarrow, Cummings, Kuczynski, & Chapman, 1985). The presence of an alternative attachment figure for the child and social support for the mother appear to be important protective factors. Overall, studies of children living with a depressed parent have pointed to later potential problems in affect regulation (sadness, anger, and aggression), self-esteem and self-worth, feelings of hopelessness, and a view of others as unpredictable, unresponsive, and/or rejecting (Beardslee, Keller, & Klerman, 1985; Osofsky et al., 1992; Radke-Yarrow et al., 1985).

Resilient children of affectively disordered parents have not yet received much research attention. One case study of 4 competent children of parents with affective disorders found familiar correlates of resilience (Radke-Yarrow & Sherman, 1990). Competence in these high-risk children was associated with better intellectual skills, social appealingness, and a particular attribute (such as being a boy) or talent valued by their parents. These children were able to garner the best of the often meager parenting resources in the family. The investigators take care to point out that these children are better described as survivors than "invulnerable." Individually they suffered inside or carried a burden of stress that concerned the investigators about the long-term costs of their positive adaptation to their parent's mental disorder. In the Beardslee and Podorefsky (1988) study of resilient young adults (mean age 19 years) whose parent or parents had experienced a severe affective disorder, all reported significant personal consequences such as economic hardship, disruption in housing, lack of parental awareness and involvement, or divorce. Their life experiences had left them with feelings of disillusionment, confusion, helplessness, and an overburdening of responsibilities. However, factors they identified as clearly helping them to achieve their own personal goals included (1) a clear ability to distinguish between their parent's illness and their own experiences; (2) an understanding that they were not the cause of the illness nor could they cure their parents; (3) an ability to talk about their parents' difficulties with sadness and empathy but without becoming overwhelmed; (4) an expectation that their future life would not be the same; and (5) pride in the active problem-solving they engaged in to help their families and themselves (Beardslee, 1990; Beardslee & Podorefsky, 1988).

Children of Adolescent Mothers: The risk for developmental problems is particularly high for infants born to adolescent mothers. The mother's young age and status as a single parent, the effect of childbearing and child rearing on her own education and subsequent employment opportunities, the constraints placed on her own resolution of age-appropriate developmental issues regarding independence, intimacy, and identity, and the greater likelihood of a problematic pregnancy and/or preterm delivery are complex and interwoven factors that potentially can disrupt the adaptation of both mother and infant (Field, Widmayer, Stringer, & Ignatoff, 1980; Osofsky & Eberhart-Wright, 1992; Osofsky et al., 1992). The multiple domains contributing to risk for developmental problems can encompass all three risk areas: poverty, heightening environmental risk, poor prenatal care and/or premature delivery, heightening biological risk (e.g., reproductive casualty), and teenage parenting, often accompanied by limited knowledge of children's development, unrealistic expectations, and ineffective child-rearing techniques (e.g., caregiving casualty) (Field et al., 1980; Osofsky, & Eberhart-Wright 1992; Sameroff & Chandler, 1975).

Several studies have begun to examine the factors that appear most influential in either derailing development or promoting positive adaptation. In the Field et al. (1980) study of poor, teenage, black mothers, the combination of a premature birth and the mother's unrealistic attitudes regarding developmental milestones and child rearing interacted to place the infant at greater risk. Term infants of teenagers matched on the other characteristics and preterm infants of adult mothers displayed better cognitive competence at 8 months of age. The preterm infants of teenage mothers who participated in an early intervention program showed more optimal growth and were perceived more positively by their mothers at both the 4- and 8-month follow-up evaluations. Family social support also emerged as a critical protective factor. For some teenagers, the greater support system at home, including grandparents, the mother's boyfriend, aunts and uncles, and cousins and friends close in age provided a range of peer and adult interaction and caregiving that was greater than that experienced by some adult married mothers who were poor (Field et al., 1980).

In addition to examining cognitive outcome, Osofsky and her colleagues have explored how the adolescent mother's responsiveness to her infant's emotional signals and reciprocal sharing of affect within the mother-infant dyad influence the infant's later prosocial behavior and development of empathy (Osofsky & Eberhart-Wright, 1992; Osofsky et al., 1992). Greater emotional availability and positive affect sharing were associated with appropriate empathic responses by the infant at 20 months of age. In contrast, negative affect sharing and nonsharing of affect by the mother was associated with fewer infant empathic responses or responses that were inappropriate (Osofsky et al., in press). This longitudinal study highlights the importance of assessing child, parent, and dyadic factors. The characteristics of a child who appeared resilient at 4½ years of age were familiar ones: good intelligence, a positive, engaging temperament, adaptability, cooperativeness, ability to turn to and availability of others to relieve distress, zest for living, compensatory factors when a weakness was present, and the ability to use symbolic play to relieve negative feelings. Mothers who appeared to be resilient were emotionally available to their children, able to protect them from crises in their own lives, willing to utilize available intervention services, able to set and reach goals that bettered their life circumstances, and willing to express negative feelings about their life while remaining generally positive in their interactions with their child. Some dyads, while vulnerable in several areas, were nonetheless particularly able to adapt to each other's needs or brought to the relationship qualities that were highly valued and subsequently nourished. Again, Osofsky et al.'s work emphasizes the importance of both reciprocity within the dyad and the strength of outside family and community factors that can facilitate the development of both mother and child (Osofsky & Eberhart-Wright, 1992; Osofsky et al., 1992).

Evidence for long-term positive adaptation is provided in Furstenberg, Brooks-Gunn, and Morgan's (1987) 17-year follow-up study of teenage mothers. Their results indicated that successful long-term outcome was associated with the mother's ability to continue her education, prevent immediate additional pregnancies, and become married. Poor outcomes were observed for mothers who were dependent on welfare, had several sub-

sequent pregnancies quickly, were unmarried, and lacked family support. These factors also were confirmed by Osofsky et al. (in press) at their 4½-year follow-up. Mothers doing well at this point had been able to obtain their General Equivalency Diploma, were employed, and displayed higher self-esteem. The importance of early preventive intervention focusing directly on the nature of the mother-infant relationship and continuing throughout the preschool period is underscored (Carter, Osofsky & Hann, 1991; Osofsky et al., 1992). These mothers' developmental struggles continue at many levels and change in nature as they engage in the effort to parent their children.

Medically Vulnerable Children: Although children born prematurely or with a chronic physical illness or handicap are at higher risk for experiencing psychosocial adjustment problems, virtually all studies have documented that there is wide variation in individual outcome (Breslau, 1985; Cadman, Boyle, Szatmari, & Offord, 1987; Kopp, 1983; Landry, Chapieski, Fletcher, & Denson, 1988; O'Dougherty, 1983; O'Dougherty & Wright, 1990; Rutter, Tizard, & Whitmore, 1970; Wallander et al., 1989, Wallander, Varni, Babani, Banis, & Wilcox, 1989). Examples of positive adaptation and maladaptation are evident within every illness group. Overall, the results of these studies suggest that adjustment cannot be predicted simply based on diagnosis, chronicity, or severity indices but is a very complex process involving the interrelationships among type of disease and personal, family, social, and medical care variables.

In discussing their findings on infants at risk due to prematurity and low birth weight, Landry and colleagues (1988) comment that "the lack of specificity about outcome is due, in part, to the practice of treating premature infants as a homogeneous group. In fact, these infants experience a variety of pre- and post-natal medical complications that might be expected to differentially effect their development" (p. 318). This observation relates equally well to studies of chronically ill or medically vulnerable children. The determinants of individual outcome are extremely complex and difficult to predict without knowledge of multiple factors. Risk, vulnerability, and effective coping must be evaluated in multiple domains, including an assessment of specific biological, psychological, and social stresses and changes in these areas over time and at different stages of the disease and the child's development (Bradley et al. 1995; Lazarus & Folkman, 1984; O'Dougherty & Brown, 1990; O'Dougherty & Wright, 1990).

Giving birth to an infant prematurely is a significant stressor that clearly portrays the complex interactions between risk and protective processes cross all three domains—biological, familial, and social. Premature birth to a socioeconomically disadvantaged mother significantly heightens the overall developmental risk for the infant (Field, 1980; Kopp, 1983, 1987; Sameroff & Chandler, 1975; Werner & Smith, 1982). Factors operative during the pregnancy that might affect fetal growth and development significantly, such as maternal undernourishment, inadequate or absent prenatal care, and delivery complications, are all correlates of poverty. Continuation of a disadvantaged economic status following the delivery can create other postnatal risk factors for the infant, including malnutrition and inadequate follow-up pediatric care.

Another striking example of the complex relationship between multiple risk factors and neurodevelopmental outcome is evident in recent research on prenatal exposure to cocaine. Infants born to mothers abusing cocaine have displayed a heightened incidence of health problems including infections, obstetric complications, prematurity, low birthweight, microcephaly, congenital abnormalities, and neonatal withdrawal and irritability (Bingol, Fuchs, Diaz, Stone, & Gromisch, 1987; Chasnoff, Burns, Schnoll, & Burns, 1985; Chasnoff, Griffith, Freier, & Murray, 1992; Madden, Payne, & Miller, 1986; Singer, Farkas, Kliegman, 1992). However, cocaine use during pregnancy is associated with a number of other maternal characteristics and health habits that are known to be independent contributors to adverse outcome, such as poor nutrition, lack of prenatal care, and polydrug use (e.g., heavy use of cigarettes, alcohol, marijuana, and other psychoactive drugs) (Chasnoff, 1988; Frank et al., 1988; Singer et al., 1992). The negative effects of the mother's nutritional status or prenatal exposure to other psychoactive drugs may be misattributed to cocaine. In addition, as Frank et al. (1988) highlight, many current samples are comprised largely of poor, inner-city minority women with little prenatal care. Cocaine use is also prevalent among upper socioeconomic status women. The risk factors and developmental outcomes of their infants have been largely unstudied. Before any conclusions can be drawn about the specific effects of cocaine use during pregnancy, and whether the severity and pattern of abuse poses an independent risk for pregnancy complications or neurobehavioral outcome, the effects of multiple risk factors and representative samples of cocaine-abusing pregnant women need to be studied (Frank, et al., 1988). In a finding similar to the results obtained in other longitudinal studies (Sameroff & Chandler, 1975; Werner & Smith, 1982, 1992), Chasnoff (1988) reports that developmental outcome at 2 years of age for infants exposed prenatally to narcotics was more directly associated with the quality of their subsequent caregiving environment than with prenatal drug exposure.

Although the long-term cognitive and behavioral effects of exposure to cocaine prenatally are still unknown, exposure to alcohol can produce a cluster of symptoms known as fetal alcohol syndrome, which includes growth deficiencies, facial abnormalities, brain and body malformations, cognitive deficits (including mental retardation), and behavioral problems, particularly hyperactivity and short attention span (Clarren & Smith, 1978; Shaywitz, Cohen, & Shaywitz, 1980; Steinhausen, Gobel, & Nestler, 1984; Streissguth et al., 1991; Streissguth et al., 1986). Not only biological but behavioral vulnerabilities can burden these children and put an added stress on the developing parent-child relationship. Infants with cognitive and/or motor deficits who are irritable, difficult to console, hyperexcitable, and highly distractible present a major challenge to stable, financially secure, effective parents. When these child problems are compounded by preexisting parental emotional and drug-related problems and lack of financial and social support, the risk for subsequent child abuse or neglect is heightened (Chasnoff, 1988; Cicchetti & Carlson, 1989).

Another consistent finding among studies of infants at medical risk has been that physical disorders or subsequent medical complications that involve documented brain damage are associated with poorer overall adaptation (Breslau, 1985; Landry et al., 1984, 1988; Seidel, Chadwick, &

Rutter, 1975). In Landry et al.'s (1984, 1988) longitudinal study of premature low-birthweight infants, problems in later (24- and 36-month follow-up) cognitive and motor development were significantly associated with the specific type and severity of medical complications that the infant experienced. Delayed development was clearly evident in infants who had experienced intraventricular hemorrhage and secondary hydrocephalus and for those who had experienced bronchopulmonary dysplasia, particularly if hospitalized for more than 16 weeks (an index of severity). Premature infants with respiratory distress syndrome or intraventricular hemorrhage alone (particularly if the intraventricular hemorrhage was not rated as severe) performed in the average range on the developmental tests, although they were significantly below their full-term control group. Continued follow-up of these infants will be particularly important in understanding the potential for recovery of function despite significant biological insult.

These and other studies of medically vulnerable infants highlight the importance of documenting the severity and nature of the biological insult. Brain imaging (computed tomography scans, ultrasound, magnetic resonance imaging) and other technological advances have allowed more accurate measurement of brain injury, which has led to a more precise identification of risk variables that do constrain adaptation (Rutter, 1990; Stewart, 1983). When "risk" is defined by a global status variable, such as perinatal complications, prematurity, low birthweight, or chronic illness, it is difficult to study resilience because the nature of the risk is unclear (Masten et al., 1990).

These issues become increasingly salient in studies focusing on multiple or cumulative risks that co-occur and on environments that have complex and interwoven risk variables (Garmezy & Masten, 1994; Masten & Wright, in press; O'Dougherty & Wright, 1990; O'Dougherty, Wright, Garmezy, Loewenson, & Torres, 1983; Richters & Weintraub, 1990; Sameroff & Seifer, 1990; Yoshikawa, 1994). One of the best-known and illustrative longitudinal projects to address these issues is the Kauai study by Werner and her colleagues (Werner, Bierman, & French, 1971; Werner & Smith, 1977, 1982, 1992). In this study 698 Polynesian and Asian children born on the

Hawaiian island of Kauai in 1955 were followed from birth to age 30. The children were studied at birth and at 1, 2, 10, 18, and 30 years of age. Over half of the sample lived in chronic poverty, and most were exposed to multiple risk factors. Key risk factors identified in this study that predicted later developmental problems included: chronic poverty, low maternal education, family conflict or instability, and moderate-to-severe perinatal stress. Approximately one third of the children experienced four or more of these risk factors, and of this "high-risk" group, approximately one third (one tenth of the total sample) were identified as resilient at the 10-, 18-, and 30-year follow-up. These resilient children were compared to a comparable high-risk subgroup who had developed problems in an effort to understand what factors might be important in fostering adaptation despite high risk. In comparing these two groups, the resilient children as infants displayed positive temperamental characteristics, were able to elicit attention from their caretakers, had a close bond with at least one caregiver, had no major separations in infancy, had no competition from a new baby in the family for at least 2 years, and had fewer congenital defects. As infants, the resilient children in this study appeared to be both less vulnerable and more protected. As preschoolers they were cheerful, responsive, self-confident, and independent. In cognitive, motor, social, and language areas they were advanced. These positive characteristics continued through the elementary school period, where they were described as good problem solvers, sociable, independent, and good communicators. As adolescents they displayed high self-esteem, an internal locus of control, an achievement orientation, social maturity, well-internalized values, and social sensitivity.

These findings raise important questions about the construct of risk (Masten et al., 1990). The child protective factors that appear to be operative (easy temperament, good intellectual abilities, positive peer relationships) also may be indicators of lower vulnerability, which may have facilitated positive parental coping and adaptation. Individual contrasts within families where there were differences in adaptational outcome among siblings would be especially useful in furthering our understanding of the interactional process between child and parent that promotes positive adaptation (Plomin & Daniels, 1987).

Children Who Experience Stressful Life Conditions

Some of the most powerful, common, and chronic adversities endured by children reflect ongoing living conditions that derive from marital conflict or change and poverty. These stressors can interfere with the care provided to children, expose them to frightening violence, and disrupt their lives by repeated changes in family structure, homes, schools, and neighborhoods.

DIVORCE AND INTERPARENTAL CONFLICT

Divorce rates gradually rose over the past century in the United States, with sharp increases in the late 1960s and 1970s and a leveling off in the 1980s (Hernandez, 1988; Norton & Moorman, 1987). From 1972 to 1982, more than 1 million children a year experienced divorce (Norton & Moorman, 1987). Approximately three quarters of divorced women remarry (Norton & Moorman, 1987), and a third of these second marriages also end in divorce (Glick, 1979). These statistics result in large numbers of children experiencing family reconfigurations.

Divorce is a complex process, involving many chronic and acute stressors. Interparental conflict, child-rearing disagreements, economic hardship, residential changes, loss of contact with one parent, and parental distress often precede, accompany, and/or follow separation and divorce (Garmezy & Masten, 1994).

The complexity of this process has made it difficult to tease apart the consequences of divorce for children. Prospective longitudinal studies have shown that some of the problems of divorced children precede the separation. One study found that the disruptive/aggressive problems of boys often attributed to the crisis of divorce may precede the separation by many years (Block, Block, & Gjerde, 1986). Examination of two epidemiological data sets, one in Great Britain and one in the United States, also has suggested that preexisting problems in children and their parents account for many of the postdivorce problems, especially in boys (Cherlin et al., 1991). On the other hand, preadolescent girls in these two data sets appeared to react to the crisis of divorce, showing increased problems in achievement and behavior.

Longitudinal studies of children following divorce suggest that gender, custody arrangements, remarriage, and ongoing conflict affect the adjustment of children (Emery, 1988). The Virginia Longitudinal Study of Divorce and Remarriage (Hetherington, 1989, 1993; Hetherington et al., 1985) has followed a sample of 4-year-old children, in which half of the parents were recently divorced and half were always married. Over the first year, considerable distress and dysfunction was observed in the children and parents. Substantial improvements occurred the second year. Girls from divorced families generally did not differ by this time from girls who had not experienced divorce. Boys who had experienced divorce continued to have more problems than boys who had not. Compared to children in conflict-ridden marriages, children of divorce were initially more distressed, but after 2 years they were better adjusted than children remaining in homes with ongoing interparenteral conflict.

Another well-known longitudinal study of divorce has followed a clinic sample of 60 divorced middle- to upper-class families for 10 years (Wallerstein & Kelly, 1980; Wallerstein et al., 1988). Although this study has methodological flaws, including no control group, it nevertheless represents the best available clinical account of age differences in the short- and long-term aftermath of divorce. Initially after divorce, preschoolers showed the most dramatic distress, expressed in such age-typical ways as crying, separation anxiety, clinginess, and loss of toileting skills. Older children expressed more anger, more worry, more antisocial behavior, declines in school achievement, and more involvement in parental disputes. After 10 years, the older children still showed intense feelings about the divorce. In contrast, children who had been younger at the time of the divorce were faring better. Despite strong initial reactions, likely related to their developmental vulnerability to disrupted parenting and to parental distress, the preschoolers appeared to be buffered for the long term by their limited ability to process and remember the events surrounding the divorce.

The level of interparental conflict has been linked to child problems before and after divorce and independent of divorce (Demo & Acock, 1988; Emery, 1982, 1988). For very young children, several processes may be involved. Experimental studies have demonstrated that preschoolers react negatively to angry interactions observed even between adult strangers (Cummings, 1987; Cummings, Iannotti, & Zahn-Waxler, 1985). Infants and preschoolers also may be quite sensitive to negative emotion expressed by a caregiver (Downey & Coyne, 1990). Distressed parents also may be less responsive to young children, less consistent as parents, and more irritable (Downey & Coyne, 1990). Younger children, because of their greater dependence on the caregivers and the amount of time they spend with caregivers, may be more vulnerable to declines in parental functioning associated with stress in the parent. Some parents who have marital problems also may have characterological problems, such as antisocial personality disorder, that are associated with poor parenting skills (Capaldi & Patterson, 1991). Similarly, alcoholism in a parent could contribute to family violence, parenting problems, and child maladjustment (Russell, Henderson, & Blume, 1985).

The most widely reported protective factor for children experiencing divorce and family discord is a familiar one: a good relationship with one parent, usually the mother (Emery, 1982; Peterson & Zill, 1986; Rutter, 1990). This relationship may function in a variety of ways. For example, a good relationship may be more likely to occur when the mother is able to contain her distress, to maintain more consistent parenting, and when the mother does not have a preexisting mental disorder, antisocial personality, or substance abuse problem. The effective parent may proactively buffer the child from observing angry interactions and prevent the child from being "caught in the middle." A parent may attempt to avoid stressors such as moving or changing schools. Better-functioning parents also may have more outside support and may depend less on their children for support.

ECONOMIC HARDSHIP AND EXPOSURE TO COMMUNITY VIOLENCE

During the 1980s in the United States, the proportion of children under 6 living in poverty rose and stayed above 20% (National Center for Children in Poverty, 1990). In large urban cities with populations of at least 100,000, childhood poverty rates exceed 40% (Children's Defense Fund, 1990). The numbers of homeless families with young children also increased, as did the proportion of homeless people who were children (Masten, 1992). Poverty in children is associated with multiple risk factors, including lower maternal education, having a single parent, inadequate prenatal and postnatal health care, lead poisoning, injuries and accidents, and maltreatment (Children's Defense Fund, 1990; National Center for Children in Poverty, 1990).

The multiplicity of risks and stressors associated with poverty often undermine development. Poor children are more likely to suffer from low birthweights, to die during their first year of life, or to have enduring physical, cognitive, and/or emotional problems. A large and growing proportion of poor children receives no immunization against major illnesses, such as polio, whooping cough, diptheria, tetanus, measles, mumps, and rubella. In some inner-city neighborhoods, 50 to 70% of preschool children are unvaccinated. Older poor children display higher rates of dropping out of school, traumatic injuries and accidents, and youth unemployment (Children's Defense Fund, 1990; National Center for Children in Poverty, 1990; Toomey & Christie, 1990).

Homeless children represent a high-risk subgroup of very poor children. The elevated rate of health problems in homeless children has been documented in a national study (Wright, 1990). Homeless children had 2 to 4 times the rates of respiratory infections, skin problems, nutritional deficiencies, gastrointestinal disorders, and chronic illnesses. Immunization delays are common, as are a wide variety of developmental delays (Masten, 1992). Many homeless mothers receive no prenatal care, and, not surprisingly, more of their babies are born prematurely and with low birthweight (Chavkin, Kristal, Seabron, & Guigli, 1987). Studies of preschoolers indicate cognitive, social, and visual-motor delays in development (Masten, 1992). Behavioral and emotional problems are also common (Holden, Horton, & Danseco; 1995).

Children and parents in areas of concentrated urban poverty also live with fear of the violence that all too frequently erupts in their neighborhoods (Christie & Toomey, 1990; Garbarino, Kostelny, & Dubrow, 1991; Kotlowitz, 1991; Pynoos & Nader, 1988; Richters & Martinez, 1993). This violence can take many forms, from murder to severe physical or sexual assault, theft, robbery or destruction of property, to verbal threats of attack, harassment, chasing, name calling, and bullying. It also can occur in any location—at home; on playgrounds; in school, parks, shopping centers, subways, and neighborhood streets (Christie & Toomey, 1990).

While news media coverage and crime statistics reports increasingly have highlighted the presence of a frightening degree of community violence, there has been little systematic study of the nature and consequences of young children's exposure to violence. Richters and Martinez's (in press) recent study of elementary school children (attending grades 1, 2, 5, and 6) in a violent neighborhood of Washington, D.C., clearly documents that a significant number of these children are either victims of or witnesses to severe violence in their community. Fourteen percent of first and second graders had witnessed someone being shot, stabbed, or raped. When violent acts such as mugging or being chased by a gang were included, the prevalence increased to 30%. The risk of witnessing severe violence increased significantly with age in this elementary school sample. Criminal victimization and exposure to violence are thought to be much higher still among secondary school students, with homicide the second leading cause of death among adolescents (Richters & Martinez, in press).

In Richters and Martinez's sample (1993), children who had been exposed to higher levels of community violence displayed more distress symptoms, such as fears, anxiety, depression, intrusive thoughts, and worries. The children's mothers, while aware of some of the events their children had witnessed, were not aware of the degree of exposure, and they significantly underestimated the degree of distress their children were experiencing. The children's underreporting and/or the parent's more limited awareness is alarming in several respects. Richters and Martinez emphasize the dual disadvantage this places on the parent(s) and child. The parent(s) who is not fully aware of the danger the child is exposed to is less likely to provide adequate supervision and to work with the child to develop effective means of preventing future victimization or exposure to violence. The children are also less likely to receive the emotional support they need from their parents to cope with their distress. Their underreporting also may reflect a growing desensitization to the violence that surrounds them as a means of shielding themselves from the frightening impact of violence. Affective blunting, emotional numbness, helplessness, a decreased ability to recognize and avoid dangerous situations, and chronic hyperarousal can be one consequence. Alternately, other children may choose defensive gang membership, chronic anger, and retaliating violence (Christie & Toomey, 1990; McDermott, 1983). Living in an environment filled with fear and violence can critically disrupt the central developmental tasks for this age—industry, achievement, and sense of confidence and self-efficacy—resulting in poor school grades, absenteeism, school failure, and diminished opportunities for employment.

In Richters and Martinez's study (1993), these young children were also exposed to high levels of violence within their homes. Thirteen percent of the mothers of fifth- and sixth-grade children reported settling arguments with their partners by threatening to use a gun or knife; 7% actually used a weapon in settling disputes. When a child witnessed a stabbing, most of the time (58%) a family member was the victim. The next section addresses the extreme distress and subsequent emotional sequelae of witnessing or experiencing family violence. However, the few available studies on young children's exposure to community violence and their distress thereafter provide compelling evidence of the immediate need for intervention programs that address the complex personal, social, and economic problems of these families.

Yet despite the considerable risk associated with poverty, not all poor children flounder. Several studies have attempted to learn how some children develop well in spite of economic hardship and dangerous neighborhoods. Although most of these studies have focused on older children and adolescents, they consistently point to a good relationship with a caregiver or surrogate parent, effective parenting, and good intellectual skills in the children (Masten, 1994; Masten et al., 1990; Werner & Smith, 1982, 1992).

Recovery from Psychosocial Trauma

CHILD MALTREATMENT

The cognitive, emotional, social, and physical development of children is intimately connected with the security and nurturance provided by their caregivers, within their environment. Certainty of the presence of a "secure base" allows for normal development and provides the foundation for exploration of new experiences and social relationships (Bowlby, 1988; Crittenden & Ainsworth, 1989). In the absence of a secure base, as in cases of child abuse and neglect, the maltreated child is at high risk for significant social, emotional, physical, and cognitive problems. Developmental theory and research about the effects of trauma in early childhood have provided a foundation for understanding possible connections among early trauma, the development of self-esteem, and later personality disorders or problems in adaptation (Masten et al., 1990). Maltreatment by a primary caregiver in early childhood can seriously jeopardize the organization and development of attachment relationships, the self, and the regulation and integration of behavior in emotional, cognitive, social, and motivational areas. Since these are the major developmental tasks of adaptation in this period of development, significant disruptions in the achievement of these developmental milestones can result in long-lasting traumatic sequelae and a high incidence of severe psychiatric disorders (Cicchetti & Carlson, 1989; Eth & Pynoos, 1985; Johnson & Cohn, 1990; McLeer, Deblinger, Atkins, Foa, & Ralphe, 1988; Putnam, 1989; van der Kolk, 1987; Widom, 1989a).

However, while many studies have indicated both short-term and long-range adaptational problems in severely maltreated children, as well as a range of psychopathological outcomes across abusive conditions, there is clearly no uniform response to childhood maltreatment (Finkelhor & Dziuba-Leatherman, 1994). Much needs to be learned about the effects of specific types of maltreatment during specific developmental phases, maltreatment varying in severity and duration, the relationship between the child and the perpetrator(s), the nature of the circumstances leading up to the abuse, and the complex interplay among vulnerability, stress, and coping skills within each child's familial context (Kendall-Tackett, Williams, & Finkelhor, 1993; Masten & Wright, in press). In addition, children can display significant sequelae at different times and in different domains—physical, cognitive, emotional, and social. Therefore, the absence of observable symptoms at one point in time does not mean that negative effects will not appear in the future. Longitudinal follow-up of children exposed to severe maltreatment is thus particularly important (Masten & Wright, in press).

Recent research on adult disorders such as borderline personality disorder, antisocial personality disorder, and multiple personality disorder has strongly suggested linkages between severe physical or sexual abuse in early childhood and later disordered functioning of the self system (Putnam, 1989; van der Kolk, 1987) or self in relation to others (Widom, 1989a, 1989b). The marked difficulty individuals with these disorders have in the organization and regulation of the self, behavior, and affect, accompanied in some individuals by symptoms of chronic posttraumatic stress disorder, have led investigators to hypothesize that severe, repeated abuse in the preschool years may be a causal factor in the development of these disorders. This hypothesis is congruent with recent developmental data documenting problems in language, cognitive development, social-emotional functioning, impulse control, frustration tolerance, and self development in severely maltreated children (Carlson, Cicchetti, Barnett, & Braunwald, 1989; Cicchetti, 1990; Crittenden & Ainsworth, 1989).

The current diagnostic formulation of posttraumatic stress disorder has been derived primarily from observations of survivors of relatively circumscribed traumatic events: combat, disaster, and rape. The posttraumatic stress disorder task force for *DSM-IV* proposed an expansion of this category to include a new category called Disorders of Extreme Stress, Not Otherwise Specified (DES-NOS) (Davidson & Foa, 1991a, 1991b). Included in this category were five groups of individuals exposed to extreme stress: sexually abused children, physically abused children, physically abused women, victims of severe crime, and victims of torture. Although this new category was not adopted in *DSM-IV*, many professionals working with these groups believe that the current posttraumatic stress disorder criteria do not adequately cover the wide-ranging symptom patterns associated with chronic victimization such as child abuse or incest and that a separate classification would be useful.

One significant concern raised in both research and public literature relates to the risk for intergenerational transmission of abuse. Widom (1989a), in her comprehensive review of literature addressing the question, concludes that empirical evidence demonstrating that abuse leads to abuse is weak. Existing studies are methodologically problematic, frequently relying on self-report data regarding prior abuse, retrospective research designs, and lack of base rate information with which to compare estimates. Although estimates range from a low 7 to a high 70%, Kaufman and Zigler (1989) estimate that approximately 30% of those abused as children subsequently will abuse their own children. However, among adults who do abuse their own children, the majority were not abused in childhood; clearly there is no simple causal relationship between the two (Widom, 1989a). Of particular importance is the finding that the majority (approximately two thirds) of abused children do not become abusive parents. While it is clearly important to look closely at factors that might facilitate "breaking the cycle of abuse" (Egeland, Jacobvitz, & Sroufe, 1988), unsubstantiated repetitions of "the cycle of violence" in popular and experimental literature can be harmful to the self-image and confidence of children who grow up in violent homes.

Several examples of resilience in maltreated children come from follow-up studies of previously abused children's effectiveness as parents later in life. Kaufman and Zigler (1989) summarized the characteristics found in a variety of studies of previously abused children who displayed later positive parenting. These included a good relationship with at least one caregiver, awareness of early abuse and a resolve not to repeat it, high IQ,

special talents, positive school experiences, physical attractiveness, a supportive spouse, physically healthy children, social support, strong religious affiliation, economic security, and effective therapy.

Widom (1991) recently reported her findings on possible mediating variables that were associated with avoiding later delinquency and criminality in a sample of 772 children with documented abuse and/or neglect. Demographic information, child and family variables, placement experiences, and type of abuse were examined. Maltreated children who later avoided arrest were significantly more likely to be female, Caucasian, and younger, probably reflecting the overall base rate patterns for arrests. They had fewer behavior problems in childhood, suggesting that whatever contributed to better outcomes may have been operating early in their lives. Females who avoided teenage pregnancy also had better outcomes, although it is not clear whether this was a matter of competence or luck, or part of an ongoing pattern of avoiding trouble. Family variables that were associated with avoidance of arrest suggested either decreased family pathology (e.g., father not an alcoholic) or severe family pathology or stressful events (e.g., mother's death) that might have resulted in direct intervention by a social service agency and placement in an improved living situation. Finally, if the mother was not employed, and by inference at home and more available to the child, the outcome also was more favorable. Factors found in other studies that have been associated with delinquency and criminality that were not replicated here included: large family size, type of abuse, and sex of perpetrator. While Widom emphasizes that these findings pertain only to avoidance of criminal arrest, and stresses that the occurrence of antisocial but not detected problems or psychological problems of either an internalizing (e.g., depression, suicide attempts) or externalizing nature were not studied, this comprehensive follow-up investigation provides additional insight into compensatory factors, if not protective processes.

Studies of abused infants and preschoolers (Crittenden, 1985; Farber & Egeland, 1987) and studies of maternal deprivation and failure to thrive (Masten & O'Connor, 1989; Rutter, 1979) also have documented that many children do recover and function adequately. This fact is particularly apparent when the caregiving environment improves. Hodges and Tizard (1989a, 1989b) found that later adjustment of adolescents reared in institutions until age 2 was best for those subsequently reared in adoptive homes rather than returned to their biological parents. Both groups, however, were less well adjusted than a comparison group of children who had experienced stable home care. Social and emotional development appears to be most disrupted by discontinuous care provided by a variety of caregivers, whereas cognitive development is most adversely affected by barren surroundings (Hodges & Tizard, 1989a, 1989b; Rutter, 1979; Tizard & Hodges, 1978; Tizard & Rees, 1974). Thus, social/emotional and cognitive domains of development may be vulnerable to disruption by different types and timing of traumatic experiences.

All of the research highlights the importance of examining the full range of adaptation/maladaptation in maltreated children Finkelhor & Dziuba-Leatherman 1993; Masten & Wright, in press). There is a need to examine abuse and neglect separately and to direct attention not only to identifying compensating factors but to begin to untangle the complex protective processes involved in order to better understand recovery and resiliency following trauma (Cicchetti, Rogosch, Lynch, & Holt, 1993; National Research Council, 1993).

Concluding Remarks

This chapter highlights the importance of viewing the descriptors *vulnerable* and *resilient* as relative and changing over time, in conjunction with changing circumstances (Masten, in press; Rutter, 1990; Werner, 1990). Neither is a fixed characteristic of an individual, a family, or a system. Werner and Smith's (1982, 1992) longitudinal study of high-risk children over a 30-year period underscores the importance of exploring and understanding both continuity and discontinuity in development within and between individuals. Reflecting on their study, Werner (1990) has written:

At each developmental stage, there is a shifting balance between stressful life events that heighten children's vulnerability and protective factors that enhance their resilience. This balance changes not only with the stages of the life cycle, but also varies with the sex of the individual and the cultural context in which he or she grows up. . . . As long as the balance between stressful life events and protective factors is favorable, successful adaptation is possible. However, when stressful life events outweigh the protective factors, even the most resilient child can develop problems. (p. 111)

The development of either competence or disorder has multifactorial determinants, and neither is static or unchanging. When these descriptors are conceptualized as traitlike, stable characteristics, often more is concealed than is actually revealed (Radke-Yarrow & Sherman, 1990). For example, assessments of competence in children who have experienced significant stress and adversity often focus on global indices of functioning in specific domains (e.g., school achievement, popularity with peers, absence of behavior problems). While this yields important information about maintaining adaptive functioning under highly stressful life circumstances, such measures do not provide an understanding of the processes that have promoted positive adaptation and often fail to assess the type and degree of personal cost and distress. Luthar's (1991) study of resilient inner-city teenagers revealed that even during apparently successful coping periods, the teens were not "trouble-free." The resilient teenagers under high stress reported more depression and anxiety than teens of comparable competence from similar backgrounds whose current life situations were less stressful. Such findings also highlight the importance of comprehensive assessment of the child in his or her environment at multiple points in time (Horowitz, 1989).

Under highly stressful circumstances, individuals with the capacity for resilience can experience a loss of adaptive functioning and distressing emotional reactions. Exploration of the factors that promote recovery following highly stressful events may provide greater insight into the compensatory and protective processes critical to recovery and a return to adaptive functioning. Again, multiple levels of analysis (biological, cognitive, social, emotional, environmental) are needed to understand individual vulnerability and resilience. In this respect, it may be useful to conceptualize both vulnerability and resilience as continuous dimensions and to examine specific triggering events or turning points that alter an individual's developmental path (Rutter, 1990).

This chapter also has provided clear documentation that children have a remarkable capacity to develop in the direction of health. Further study of the "self-righting" tendencies that facilitate normal development despite persistent adversity is greatly needed (Horowitz, 1989; Masten et al., 1990). Although severe biological insult may derail development permanently, in many instances children demonstrate the capacity for recovery and adaptive growth. Further understanding of these processes will significantly enhance our ability to intervene successfully with children who are experiencing adaptational difficulty.

REFERENCES

Achenbach, T. M. (1990). What is "developmental" about developmental psychopathology? In J. Rolf, A. S. Masten, D. Cicchetti, K. H. Nuechterlein, & S. Weintraub (Eds.), *Risk and protective factors in the development of psychopathology* (pp. 29–48). New York: Cambridge University Press.

Aldwin, C. M. (1994). *Stress, coping, and development: An integrated perspective.* New York: Guilford Press.

American Psychiatric Association. (1987). *Diagnostic and statistical manual of mental disorders* (3rd ed., rev.). Washington, DC: Author.

Arnold, L. E. (1990). Stress in children and adolescents: Introduction and summary. In L. E. Arnold (Ed.), *Childhood Stress* (pp. 1–19). New York: John Wiley & Sons.

Baldwin, A. L., Baldwin, C., & Cole, R. E. (1990). Stress-resistant families and stress-resistant children. In J. Rolf, A. S. Masten, D. Cicchetti, K. H. Nuechterlein, & S. Weintraub (Eds.), *Risk and protective factors in the development of psychopathology* (pp. 257–280). New York: Cambridge University Press.

Beardslee, W. R. (1990). Stress from parental depression: Child risk, self-understanding, and a preventive intervention. In L. E. Arnold (Ed.), *Childhood stress* (pp. 351–371). New York: John Wiley & Sons.

Beardslee, W. R., Keller, M. B., & Klerman, G. L. (1985). Children of parents with affective disorder. *International Journal of Family Psychiatry, 6,* 283–299.

Beardslee, W. R., & Podorefsky, D. (1988). Resilient adolescents whose parents have serious affective and other psychiatric disorder: The importance of self-understanding and relationships. *American Journal of Psychiatry, 145,* 63–69.

Bingol, N., Fuchs, M., Diaz, V., Stone, R. K., & Gromisch, D. S. (1987). Teratogenicity of cocaine in humans. *Journal of Pediatrics, 110,* 93–96.

Bleuler, M. (1984). Different forms of childhood stress and patterns of adult psychiatric outcome. In N. F. Watt, E. J. Anthony, & J. E. Rolf (Eds.), *Children at risk for schizophrenia* (pp. 537–542). Cambridge: Cambridge University Press.

Block, J. H., Block, J., & Gjerde, P. F. (1986). The personality of children prior to divorce: A prospective study. *Child Development, 57,* 827–840.

Bowlby, J. (1988). *A secure base: Parent-child attachment and healthy human development.* New York: Basic Books.

Bradley, R. H., Whiteside, L., Mundfrom, D. J., Blevins-Knabe, B., Casey, P. H., Caldwell, B. M., Kelleher, K. H., Pope, S., & Barrett, K. (1995). Home environment and adaptive social behavior among premature, low birth weight children: Alternative models of environmental action. *Journal of Pediatric Psychology, 20* (3), 347–362.

Breslau, N. (1985). Psychiatric disorder in children with physical disability. *Journal of the American Academy of Child Psychiatry, 24,* 87–94.

Cadman, D., Boyle, M., Szatmari, P., & Offord, D. R. (1987). Chronic illness, disability, and mental health and social well-being findings of the Ontario Child Health Study. *Pediatrics, 79,* 805–813.

Capaldi, D. M., & Patterson, G. R. (1991). Relation of parental transitions to boys' adjustment problems: I. A linear hypothesis. II. Mothers at risk for transitions and unskilled parenting. *Developmental Psychology, 27,* 489–504.

Carlson, V., Cicchetti, D., Barnett, D., & Braunwald, K. G. (1989). Finding order in disorganization: Lessons from research on maltreated infants' attachments to their caregivers. In D. Cicchetti & V. Carlson (Eds.), *Child maltreatment: Theory and research on the causes and consequences of child abuse and neglect* (pp. 494–528). New York: Cambridge University Press.

Carter, S. L., Osofsky, J. D., & Hann, D. M. (1991). Speaking for the baby: A therapeutic intervention with adolescent mothers and their infants. *Infant Mental Health Journal, 12* (4), 291–301.

Chasnoff, I. J. (1988). Drug use in pregnancy: Parameters of risk. *Pediatric Clinics of North America, 35* (6), 1408.

Chasnoff, I. J., Burns, W., Schnoll, S., & Burns, K. (1985). Cocaine use in pregnancy. *New England Journal of Medicine, 313,* 666–669.

Chasnoff, I. J., Griffith, D. R., Freier, C., & Murray, J. (1992). Cocaine/polydrug use in pregnancy: Two-year follow-up. *Pediatrics, 89,* 284–289.

Chavkin, W., Kristal, A., Seabron, C., & Guigli, P. E. (1987). The reproductive experience of women living in hotels for the homeless in New York City. *New York State Journal of Medicine, 87,* 10–13.

Cherlin, A. J., Furstenberg, F. F., Jr., Chase-Lansdale, P. L., Kiernan, E. E., Robins, P. K., Morrison, D. R., & Teitler, J. O. (1991). Longitudinal studies of divorce in children in Great Britain and the United States. *Science, 252*, 1386–1389.

Children's Defense Fund. (1990). *S.O.S. America! A children's defense budget*. Washington, DC: Author.

Christie, D. J., & Toomey, B. G. (1990). The stress of violence: School, community, and world. In L. E. Arnold (Ed.), *Childhood Stress* (pp. 297–323). New York: John Wiley & Sons.

Cicchetti, D. (1990). The organization and coherence of socioemotional, cognitive, and representational development: Illustrations through a developmental psychopathology perspective on Down syndrome and child maltreatment. In R. Thompson (Ed.), *Socioemotional development. Nebraska Symposium on Motivation* (pp. 259–366). Lincoln: University of Nebraska Press.

Cicchetti, D., & Carlson, V. (1989). *Child maltreatment: Theory and research on the causes and consequences of child abuse and neglect*. New York: Cambridge University Press.

Cicchetti, D., Rogosch, F. A., Lynch, M., & Holt, K. D. (1993). Resilience in maltreated children: Processes leading to adaptive outcome. *Development and Psychopathology, 5*, 629–647.

Clarren, S. K., & Smith, D. W. (1978). Fetal alcohol syndrome. *New England Journal of Medicine, 298* (19), 1063–1067.

Conrad, M., & Hammen, C. (1993). Protective and resource factors in high and low-risk children: A comparison of children with unipolar, bipolar, medically ill, and normal mothers. *Development and Psychopathology, 5*, 593–607.

Crittenden, P. M. (1985). Maltreated infants: Vulnerability and resilience. *Journal of Child Psychology and Psychiatry, 26*, 85–96.

Crittenden, P. M., & Ainsworth, M. D. S. (1989). Child maltreatment and attachment theory. In D. Cicchetti & V. Carlson (Eds.), *Child maltreatment: Theory and research on the causes and consequences of child abuse and neglect* (pp. 432–463). New York: Cambridge University Press.

Cummings, E. M. (1987). Coping with background anger in early childhood. *Child Development, 58*, 976–984.

Cummings, E. M., Iannotti, R. J., & Zahn-Waxler, C. (1985). Influence of conflict between adults on the emotions and aggression of young children. *Developmental Psychology, 21*, 495–507.

Davidson, J. R. T., & Foa, E. B. (1991a). Diagnostic issues in posttraumatic stress disorder: Considerations for the DSM-IV. *Journal of Abnormal Psychology, 100* (3), 346–355.

Davidson, J. R. T., & Foa, E. B. (1991b). Refining criteria for posttraumatic stress disorder. *Hospital and Community Psychiatry, 42* (3), 259–261.

Demo, D. H., & Acock, A. C. (1988). The impact of divorce on children. *Journal of Marriage and the Family, 50*, 619–648.

Downey, G., & Coyne, J. C. (1990). Children of depressed parents: An integrative review. *Psychological Bulletin, 108*, 50–76.

Egeland, B., Jacobvitz, D., & Sroufe, L. A. (1988). Breaking the cycle of abuse. *Child Development, 59*, 1080–1088.

Emery, R. E. (1982). Interparental conflict and the children of discord and divorce. *Psychological Bulletin, 92*, 310–330.

Emery, R. E. (1988). *Marriage, divorce, and children's adjustment*. Newbury Park, CA: Sage.

Erickson, M. F., Sroufe, L. A., & Egeland, B. (1985). The relationship between quality of attachment and behavior problems in preschool in a high-risk sample. In I. Bretherton & E. Waters (Eds.), *Growing points in attachment theory and research. Monographs of the Society for Research in Child Development, 50*, 147–66.

Eth, S., & Pynoos, R. S. (1985). *Post-traumatic stress disorder in children*. Washington DC: American Psychiatric Press.

Farber, E. A., & Egeland, B. (1987). Invulnerability among abused and neglected children. In E. J. Anthony & B. J. Cohler (Eds.), *The invulnerable child* (pp. 253–288). New York: Guilford Press.

Field, T. M. (Ed.). (1980). *High-risk infants and children: Adult and peer interactions*. New York: Academic Press.

Field, T. M., Widmayer, S. M., Stringer, S., & Ignatoff, E. (1980). Teenage, lower class, black mothers and their preterm infants: An intervention and developmental follow-up study. *Child Development, 51*, 426–436.

Finkelhor, D. & Dziuba-Leatherman, J. (1994). Victimization of children. *American Psychologist, 49*, 173–183.

Fisher, L., Kokes, R. F., Cole, R. E., Perkins, P. M., & Wynne, L. C. (1987). Competent children at risk: A study of well-functioning offspring of disturbed parents. In E. J. Anthony & B. J. Cohler (Eds.), *The invulnerable child* (pp. 211–228). New York: Guilford Press.

Frank, D., Zuckerman, B. S., Amaro, H., Aboagye, K., Bauchner, H., Cabral, H., Fried, L., Hingson, R., Kayne, H., Levenson, S. M., Parker, S., Reece, H., & Vinci, R. (1988). Cocaine use during pregnancy: Prevalence and correlates. *Pediatrics, 82*, 888–895.

Furstenberg, F. F., Jr., Brooks-Gunn, J., & Morgan, S. P. (1987). *Adolescent mothers in later life*. New York: Cambridge University Press.

Garbarino, J., Kostelny, K., & Dubrow, N. (1991). *No place to be a child: Growing up in a war zone*. Lexington, MA: Lexington Books.

Garmezy, N. (1974). Children at risk: The search for the antecedents of schizophrenia. Part II: Ongoing research programs, issues, and interventions. *Schizophrenia Bulletin, 9*, 55–125.

Garmezy, N. (1985). Stress-resistant children: The search for protective factors. In J. E. Stevenson (Ed.), *Recent research in developmental psychopathology. Journal of Child Psychology and Psychiatry*

Book (Suppl. No. 4, pp. 213–233). Oxford: Pergamon Press.

Garmezy, N., & Masten, A. S. (1986). Stress, competence, and resilience: Common frontiers for therapist and psychopathologist. *Behavior Therapy, 17,* 500–521.

Garmezy, N., & Masten, A. S. (1990). The adaptation of children to a stressful world: Mastery of fear. In L. E. Arnold (Ed.), *Childhood stress* (pp. 459–473). New York: John Wiley & Sons.

Garmezy, N., & Masten, A. S. (1994). Chronic adversities. In M. Rutter, L. Herzov, & E. Taylor (Eds.), *Child and adolescent psychiatry* (3rd ed., pp. 191–208). Oxford: Blackwell Scientific Publications.

Garmezy, N., & Rutter, M. (1983). *Stress, coping, and development in children.* New York: McGraw-Hill.

Garmezy, N., & Rutter, M. (1985). Acute reactions to stress. In M. Rutter & L. Hersov (Eds.), *Child psychiatry: Modern approaches* (2nd ed., pp. 152–176). Oxford: Blackwell Scientific.

Garmezy, N., & Streitman, S. (1974). Children at risk: The search for the antecedents of schizophrenia. Part I: Conceptual models and research methods. *Schizophrenia Bulletin, 8,* 14–90.

Garrison, W. T., & McQuiston, S. (1989). *Chronic illness during childhood and adolescence.* Newbury Park, CA: Sage Publications.

Glick, P. C. (1979). Children of divorced parents in demographic perspective. *Journal of Social Issues, 35,* 170–182.

Goldstein, M. J., & Tuma, A. H. (Eds.). (1987). Special section on high-risk research. *Schizophrenia Bulletin, 13* (3).

Gottesman, I. I., & Shields, J. (1982). *Schizophrenia: The epigenetic puzzle.* New York: Cambridge University Press.

Green, B. L., Korol, M., Grace, M. C., Vary, M. G., Leonard, A. C., Gleser, G. C., & Smitson-Cohen, S. (1991). Children and disaster: Age, gender, and parental effects on PTSD symptoms. *Journal of the American Academy of Child and Adolescent Psychiatry, 30,* 945–951.

Green, M. (1991). On making a difference. *Pediatrics, 87,* 712–718.

Gunnar, M. R., & Mangelsdorf, S. (1989). The dynamics of temperament-physiology relations: A comment on biological processes in temperament. In G. A. Kohnstamm, J. E. Bates, & M. K. Rothbart (Eds.), *Temperament in childhood* (pp. 145–152). New York: John Wiley & Sons.

Haggerty, R. J., Sherrod, L., Garmezy, N., & Rutter, M. (Eds.) (1994). *Stress, risk and resilience in children and adolescents: Processes, mechanisms, and intervention.* New York: Cambridge University Press.

Hammen, C., Burge, D., & Adrian, C. (1991). Timing of mother and child depression in a longitudinal study of children at risk. *Journal of Consulting and Clinical Psychology, 59,* 341–345.

Hernandez, D. J. (1988). Demographic trends and the living arrangements of children. In E. M. Hetherington & J. D. Arasteh (Eds.), *Impact of divorce, single parenting, and stepparenting on children* (pp. 3–22). Hillsdale, NJ: Lawrence Erlbaum.

Hetherington, E. M. (1989). Coping with family transitions: Winners, losers, and survivors. *Child Development, 60,* 1–14.

Hetherington, E. M. (1993). An overview of the Virginia Longitudinal Study of Divorce and Remarriage with a focus on early adolescence. Special section: Families in transition. *Journal of Family Psychology, 7,* 39–56.

Hetherington, E. M., Cox, M., & Cox, R. (1985). Long-term effects of divorce and remarriage on the adjustment of children. *Journal of the American Academy of Child Psychiatry, 24,* 518–530.

Hodges, J., & Tizard, B. (1989a). IQ and behavioral adjustment of ex-institutional adolescents. *Journal of Child Psychology and Psychiatry, 30,* 53–75.

Hodges, J., & Tizard, B. (1989b). Social and family relationships of ex-institutional adolescents. *Journal of Child Psychology and Psychiatry, 30,* 77–97.

Holden, E. W., Horton, L. A., & Danseco, E. R. (1995). The mental health of homeless children. *Clinical psychology: Science and practice, 2,* 165–178.

Horowitz, F. D. (1989, April). *The concept of risk: A reevaluation.* Invited address, Society for Research in Child Development, Kansas City, MO.

Johnson, C. F., & Cohn, D. S. (1990). The stress of child abuse and other family violence. In L. E. Arnold (Ed.), *Childhood stress* (pp. 267–295). New York: John Wiley & Sons.

Jones, J. C., & Barlow, D. H. (1990). The etiology of posttraumatic stress disorder. *Clinical Psychology Review, 10* (3), 299–328.

Jones, J. M., Levine, I. S., & Rosenberg, A. A. (1991). Special issue: Homelessness. *American Psychologist, 46* (11), 1108–1252.

Kagan, J., Gibbons, J. L., Johnson, M. O., Reznick, J. S., & Snidman, N. (1990). A temperamental disposition to the state of uncertainty. In J. Rolf, A. S. Masten, D. Cicchetti, K. H. Nuechterlein, & Weintraub, S. (Eds.), *Risk and protective factors in the development of psychopathology* (pp. 164–178). New York: Cambridge University Press.

Kaufman, J., & Zigler, E. (1989). The intergenerational transmission of child abuse. In D. Cicchetti & V. Carlson (Eds.), *Child maltreatment: Theory and research on the causes and consequences of child abuse and neglect* (pp. 129–150). Cambridge: Cambridge University Press.

Kendall-Tackett, K. A., Williams, L. M. & Finkelhor, D. (1993). Impact of sexual abuse on children: A review and synthesis of recent empirical studies. *Psychological Bulletin, 113,* 164–180.

Klinnert, M., Campos, J., Sorce, J., Emde, R., & Svejda, M. (1983). Emotions as behavior regulators: Social referencing in infancy. In R. Plutchik & H. Kellerman (Eds.), *Emotion: Theory, Research, and Experience, Vol. 2: Emotions in early development* (pp. 57–86). New York: Academic Press.

Kopp, C. B. (1983). Risk factors in development. In P. H. Mussen (Ed.), *Handbook of child psychology*

(4th ed., Vol. 2, pp. 1081–1188). New York: John Wiley & Sons.

Kopp, C. B. (1987). Developmental risk: Historical reflections. In J. D. Osofsky (Ed.), *Handbook of infant development* (2nd ed., pp. 881–912). New York: John Wiley & Sons.

Kopp, C. B., & Kaler, S. R. (1989). Risk in infancy: Origins and implications. *American Psychologist, 44* (2), 224–230.

Kotlowitz, A. (1991). *There are no children here.* New York: Doubleday.

Landry, S. H., Chapieski, L., Fletcher, J. M., & Denson, S. (1988). Three-year outcomes for low birth weight infants: Differential effects of early medical complications. *Journal of Pediatric Psychology, 13* (3), 317–327.

Landry, S., Fletcher, J., Zarling, C., Chapieski, L., Francis, D., & Denson, S. (1984). Differential outcome associated with early medical complications in premature infants. *Journal of Pediatric Psychology, 9,* 385–401.

Lazarus, R. S., & Folkman, S. (1984). *Stress, appraisal and coping.* New York: Springer.

Luthar, S. S. (1991). Vulnerability and resilience: A study of high-risk adolescents. *Child Development, 62,* 600–616.

Madden, J. D., Payne, T. F., & Miller, S. (1986). Maternal cocaine abuse and effect on the newborn. *Pediatrics, 77,* 209–211.

Malmquist, C. P. (1984). Children who witness parental murder: Post-traumatic and legal issues. *Journal of the American Academy of Child Psychiatry, 25,* 320–325.

Masten, A. S. (1992). Homeless children in the United States: Mark of a nation at risk. *Current Directions in Psychological Science.*

Masten, A. S. (1994). Resilience in individual development: Successful adaptation despite risk and adversity. In M. C. Wang & E. W. Gordon (Eds.), *Educational resilience in inner-city America: Challenges and prospects* (pp. 3–25). Hillsdale, NJ: Lawrence Erlbaum.

Masten, A. S. (in press). Resilience comes of age: Reflections on the past and outlook for the next generation of research. In M. D. Glantz, J. Johnson, & L. Huffman (Eds.), *Resilience and development: Positive life adaptations.* New York: Plenum Press.

Masten, A. S., Best, K. M., & Garmezy, N. (1990). Resilience and development: Contributions from the study of children who overcome adversity. *Development and Psychopathology, 2,* 425–444.

Masten, A. S., & Coatsworth, J. D. (1995). Competence, resilience, and psychopathology. In D. Cicchetti & D. Cohen (Eds.), *Developmental psychopathology Vol. 2: Risk, disorder, and adaptation* (pp. 715–752). New York: Wiley.

Masten, A. S. & Braswell, L. (1991). Developmental psychopathology: An integrative framework. In P. R. Martin (Ed.), *Handbook of behavior therapy and psychological science: An integrative approach* (pp. 35–56). New York: Pergamon Press.

Masten, A. S., Miliotis, D., Graham-Bermann, S., Ramirez, M., & Neemann, J. (1993). Children in homeless families: Risks to mental health and development. *Journal of Consulting and Clinical Psychology, 61,* 335–343.

Masten, A. S., & O'Connor, M. J. (1989). Vulnerability, stress, and resilience in the early development of high risk child. *Journal of the American Academy of Child and Adolescent Psychiatry, 28,* 274–278.

Masten, A. S., & Wright, M. O'D. (in press). Cumulative risk and protection models of child maltreatment. In B. B. R. Rossman, & M. S. Rosenberg (Eds.) *Multiple victimization of children: Conceptual, developmental, research and treatment issues.* Haworth.

McDermott, J. (1983). Crime in the schools and in the community: Offenders, victims, and fearful youth. *Crime and Delinquency, 29* (2), 270–282.

McLeer, S. V., Deblinger, E., Atkins, M. S., Foa, E. B., & Ralphe, D. L. (1988). Post-traumatic stress disorder in sexually abused children. *Journal of the American Academy of Child and Adolescent Psychiatry, 27* (5), 650–654.

McNally, R. J. (1991). Assessment of posttraumatic stress disorder in children. *Psychological Assessment: A Journal of Consulting and Clinical Psychology, 3* (4), 1–7.

McNally, R. J. (1993). Stressors that produce post-traumatic stress disorder in children, In J. R. T. Davidson & E. B. Foa (Eds.), *Post-traumatic stress disorder: DSM IV and Beyond* (pp. 57–74). Washington, DC: American Psychiatric Press.

McWhirter, L., & Trew, K. (1981). Children in Northern Ireland: A lost generation? In E. J. Anthony & C. Chiland (Eds.), *The child in his family. Children in turmoil: Tomorrow's children* (Vol. 7, pp. 69–82). New York: Wiley Interscience.

Meehl, P. E. (1962). Schizotaxia, schizotypy, schizophrenia. *American Psychologist, 17,* 824–838.

National Center for Children in Poverty. (1990). *Five million children: A statistical profile of our poorest young citizens.* New York: Columbia University.

National Research Council, Panel on Research on Child Abuse and Neglect, Commission on Behavioral and Social Sciences and Education. (1993). *Understanding child abuse and neglect.* Washington, DC: National Academy Press.

Norton, A. J., & Moorman, J. E. (1987). Current trends in marriage and divorce among American women. *Journal of Marriage and the Family, 49,* 3–14.

O'Dougherty, M. (1983). *Counseling the chronically ill child: Psychological impact and intervention.* New York: Viking Press.

O'Dougherty, M., & Brown, R. T. (1990). The stress of childhood illness. In L. E. Arnold (Ed.), *Childhood stress* (pp. 325–349). New York: John Wiley & Sons.

O'Dougherty, M., & Wright, F. S. (1990). Children born at medical risk: Factors affecting vulnerability and resilience. In J. Rolf, A. S. Masten, D. Cicchetti, K. H. Nuechterlein, & S. Weintraub (Eds.), *Risk and protective factors in the development of psychopa-*

thology (pp. 120–140). New York: Cambridge University Press.

O'Dougherty, M., Wright, F. S., Garmezy, N., Loewenson, R. B., & Torres, F. (1983). Later competence and adaptation in children who survive severe heart defects. *Child Development, 54,* 1129–1142.

Osofsky, J. D., & Eberhart-Wright, A. (1992). Risk and protective factors for parents and infants. In G. Suci & S. Robertson (Eds.), *Human development: Future directions in infant development research* (pp. 25–42). New York: Springer-Verlag.

Osofsky, J. D., Eberhart-Wright, A., Ware, L. M., & Hann, D. M. (1992). Children of adolescent mothers: A group at risk for psychopathology. *Infant Mental Health Journal. 13* (2), 119–131.

Perry, B. D., Pollard, R. A., Blakley, T. L., Baker, W. L., & Vigilante, D. (1995). Childhood trauma, the neurobiology of adaptation, and "use dependent" development of the brain: How "states" become "traits." *Infant Mental Health Journal, 16* (4), 271–291.

Peterson, J. L., & Zill, N. (1986). Marital disruption, parent-child relationships, and behavior problems in children. *Journal of Marriage and the Family, 48,* 295–307.

Plomin, R., & Daniels, D. (1987). Why are children in the same family so different from one another? *Behavioral and Brain Sciences, 10,* 1–6.

Putnam, F. W. (1989). *Diagnosis and treatment of multiple personality disorder.* New York: Guilford Press.

Pynoos, R. S. (1990). Post-traumatic stress disorder in children and adolescents. In B. D. Garfinkel, G. A. Carlson, & E. B. Weller (Eds.), *Psychiatric disorders in children and adolescents* (pp. 48–63). Philadelphia: W. B. Saunders.

Pynoos, R. S., Frederick, C., Nader, K., Arroyo, W., Steinberg, A., Eth, S., Nunez, F., & Fairbanks, L. (1987). Life threat and posttraumatic stress disorder in school-age children. *Archives of General Psychiatry, 44,* 1057–1063.

Pynoos, R. S., & Nader, K. (1988). Children who witness the sexual assaults of their mothers. *Journal of the American Academy of Child and Adolescent Psychiatry, 27,* 567–572.

Radke-Yarrow, M., Cummings, E. M., Kuczynski, L., & Chapman, M. (1985). Patterns of attachment in two- and three-year-olds in normal families and families with parental depression. *Child Development, 56,* 884–893.

Radke-Yarrow, M., & Sherman, T. (1990). Hard growing: Children who survive. In J. Rolf, A. S. Masten, D. Cicchetti, K. H. Nuechterlein, & S. Weintraub (Eds.), *Risk and protective factors in the development of psychopathology* (pp. 97–119). New York: Cambridge University Press.

Richters, J., & Martinez, P. (1993). The NIMH Community Violence Project: I. Children as victims of and witness to violence. *Psychiatry, 56,* 7–21.

Richters, J. E., & Weintraub, S. (1990). Beyond diathesis: Toward an understanding of high-risk environments. In J. Rolf, A. S. Masten, D. Cicchetti, K. H.

Nuechterlein, & S. Weintraub (Eds.), *Risk and protective factors in the development of psychopathology* (pp. 67–96). New York: Cambridge University Press.

Rolf, J., & Johnson, J. (1990). Protected or vulnerable: The challenge of AIDS to developmental psychopathology. In J. Rolf, A. S. Masten, D. Cicchetti, K. H. Nuechterlein, & S. Weintraub (Eds.), *Risk and protective factors in the development of psychopathology* (pp. 384–404). New York: Cambridge University Press.

Rolf, J., Masten, A. S., Cicchetti, D., Nuechterlein, K. H., & Weintraub, S. (Eds.) (1990). *Risk and protective factors in the development of psychopathology.* New York: Cambridge University Press.

Russell, M., Henderson, C., & Blume, S. B. (1985). *Children of alcoholics: A review of the literature.* New York: Children of Alcoholics Foundation.

Rutter, M. (1979). Maternal deprivation, 1972–1978: New findings, new concepts, new approaches. *Child Development, 50,* 283–305.

Rutter, M. (1983). Stress, coping, and development: Some issues and some questions. In N. Garmezy & M. Rutter (Eds.), *Stress, coping and development in children* (pp. 1–41). New York: McGraw-Hill.

Rutter, M. (Ed.). (1988). *Studies of psychosocial risk: The power of longitudinal data.* New York: Cambridge University Press.

Rutter, M. (1990). Psychosocial resilience and protective mechanisms. In J. Rolf, A. S. Masten, D. Cicchetti, K. H. Nuechterlein, & S. Weintraub (Eds.), *Risk and protective factors in the development of psychopathology* (pp. 181–214). New York: Cambridge University Press.

Rutter, M., Maughan, B., Mortimore, P., Ouston, J., & Smith, A. (1979). *Fifteen thousand hours: Secondary school and their effects on children.* Cambridge, MA: Harvard University Press.

Rutter, M., Tizard, J., & Whitmore, K. (Eds.). (1970). *Education, health, and behavior.* London: Longman.

Sameroff, A. J. (1983). Developmental systems: Contexts and evolution. In W. Kessen (Ed.), *History, theory, and methods.* Vol. 1 of P. H. Mussen (Ed.), *Handbook of child psychology* (pp. 237–294). New York: John Wiley & Sons.

Sameroff, A. J., Barocas, R., & Seifer, R. (1984). The early development of children born to mentally ill women. In N. F. Anthony, L. C. Wynne, & J. E. Rolf (Eds.), *Children at risk for schizophrenia: A longitudinal perspective* (pp. 482–514). New York: Cambridge University Press.

Sameroff, A. J., & Chandler, M. J. (1975). Reproductive risk and the continuum of caretaking casualty. In F. D. Horowitz, M. Hetherington, S. Scarr-Salapatek, & G. Siegel (Eds.), *Review of child development research* (Vol. 4, pp. 187–244). Chicago: University of Chicago Press.

Sameroff, A. J., & Seifer, R. (1990). Early contributors to developmental risk. In J. Rolf, A. S. Masten, D. Cicchetti, K. H. Nuechterlein, & S. Weintraub

(Eds.), *Risk and protective factors in the development of psychopathology* (pp. 52–66). New York: Cambridge University Press.

Seidel, U. P., Chadwick, O. F. D., & Rutter, M. (1975). Psychological disorders in crippled children: A comparative study of children with and without brain damage. *Developmental Medicine and Child Neurology, 17*, 563–573.

Shaywitz, S. E., Cohen, D. J., & Shaywitz, B. A. (1980). Behavior and learning difficulties in children of normal intelligence born to alcoholic mothers. *Journal of Pediatrics, 96* (6), 978–982.

Singer, L., Farkas, K., & Kliegman, R. (1992). Childhood medical and behavorial consequences of maternal cocaine use. *Journal of Pediatric Psychology, 17* (4), 389–406.

Sroufe, L. A., & Rutter, M. (1984). The domain of developmental psychopathology. *Child Development, 55*, 17–29.

Steinhausen, H. C., Gobel, D., & Nestler, V. (1984). Psychopathology in the offspring of alcoholic parents. *Journal of the American Academy of Child Psychiatry, 23* (4), 465–471.

Stewart, A. (1983). Severe perinatal hazards. In M. Rutter (Ed.), *Developmental neuropsychiatry* (pp. 15–31). New York: Guilford Press.

Streissguth, A. P., Aase, J. M., Clarren, S. K., Randels, S. P., LaDue, R. A., & Smith, D. F. (1991). Fetal alcohol syndrome in adolescents and adults. *Journal of the American Medical Association, 265* (15), 1961–1967.

Streissguth, A. P., Barr, H. M., Sampson, P. D., Parrish-Johnson, J. C., Kirschner, G. L., & Mortin, D. C. (1986). Attention, distraction, and reaction time at age 7 years and prenatal alcohol abuse. *Neurobehavioral Toxicology and Teratology, 8*, 77–725.

Terr, L. (1990). *Too scared to cry: Psychic trauma in childhood*. New York: Harper & Row.

Tizard, B., & Hodges, J. (1978). The effect of early institutional rearing on the development of eight year old children. *Journal of Child Psychology and Psychiatry, 19*, 99–118.

Tizard, B., & Rees, J. (1974). A comparison of the effects of adoption, restoration to the natural mother, and continued institutionalization on the cognitive development of four-year-old children. *Child Development, 45*, 92–99.

Toomey, B. G., & Christie, D. J. (1990). Social stressors in childhood: Poverty, discrimination, and catastrophic events. In L. E. Arnold (Ed.), *Childhood stress* (pp. 423–456). New York: John Wiley & Sons.

Trad, P. V. (1988). *Psychosocial scenarios for pediatrics*. New York: Springer-Verlag.

Trad, P. V., & Greenblatt, E. (1990). Psychological aspects of child stress: Development and the spectrum of coping responses. In L. E. Arnold (Ed.), *Childhood stress* (pp. 23–49). New York: John Wiley & Sons.

van der Kolk, B. A. (1987). *Psychological trauma*. Washington DC: American Psychiatric Press.

Volpe, J. J. (1992). Effect of cocaine use on the fetus. *New England Journal of Medicine, 327* (6), 399–407.

Vorhees, C. V., & Mollnow, E. (1987). Behavioral teratogeneses: Longterm influences on behavior from early exposure to environmental agents. In J. D. Osofsky (Ed.), *Handbook of infant development* (2nd ed. pp. 913–971). New York: John Wiley & Sons.

Wallender, J. L., Varni, J. W., Babani, L., Banis, H. T., DeHaan, C. B., & Wilcox, K. T. (1989). Disability parameters, chronic strain, and adaptation of physically handicapped children and their mothers. *Journal of Pediatric Psychology, 14*, 23–42.

Wallender, J. L., Varni, J. W., Babani, L., Banis, H. T., & Wilcox, K. T. (1989). Family resources as resistance factors for psychological maladjustment in chronically ill and handicapped children. *Journal of Pediatric Psychology, 14* (2), 157–173.

Wallerstein, J. S., Corbin, S. B., & Lewis, J. M. (1988). Children of divorce: A 10-year study. In E. M. Hetherington & J. D. Arasteh (Eds.), *Impact of divorce, single parenting, and stepparenting on children* (pp. 197–214). Hillsdale, NJ: Lawrence Erlbaum.

Wallerstein, J. S., & Kelly, J. B. (1980). *Surviving the break-up: How children and parents cope with divorce*. New York: Basic Books.

Wang, M. C., & Gordon, E. W. (1994). Educational resilience in inner-city America: Challenges and prospects. Hillsdale, NJ: Lawrence Erlbaum.

Watt, N. F., Anthony, E. J., Wynne, L. C., & Rolf, J. E. (Eds.). (1984). *Children at risk for schizophrenia: A longitudinal perspective*. Cambridge: Cambridge University Press.

Werner, E. E. (1990). Protective factors and individual resilience. In S. J. Meisels & M. Shonkoff (Eds.), *Handbook of early intervention* (pp. 97–116). New York: Cambridge University Press.

Werner, E. E., Bierman, J. S., & French, F. E. (1971). *The children of Kauai: A longitudinal study from the prenatal period to age ten*. Honolulu: University of Hawaii Press.

Werner, E. E., & Smith, R. S. (1977). *Kauai's children come of age*. Honolulu: University of Hawaii Press.

Werner, E. E., & Smith, R. S. (1982). *Vulnerable but invincible: A study of resilient children*. New York: McGraw-Hill.

Werner, E. E., & Smith, R. S. (1992). *Overcoming the odds: High risk children from birth to adulthood*. Ithaca, NY: Cornell University Press.

Widom, C. S. (1989a). The cycle of violence. *Science, 244* (4901), 160–166.

Widom, C. S. (1989b). Does violence beget violence? A critical examination of the literature. *Psychological Bulletin, 106* (1), 3–28.

Widom, C. S. (1991). Avoidance of criminality in abused and neglected children. *Psychiatry, 54*, 162–174.

Wright, J. D. (1990). Homelessness is not healthy for children and other living things. *Child and Youth Services, 14* (1), 65–88.

Yoshikawa, H. (1994). Prevention as cumulative protection: Effects of early family support and education on chronic delinquency and its risks. *Psychological Bulletin, 115*, 28–54.

Zahn-Waxler, C., Iannotti, R., Cummings, E. M., & Denham, S. (1990). Antecedents of problem behaviors in children of depressed mothers. *Development and Psychopathology, 2*, 271–292.

---

24 / Understanding the Social Context of Early Psychopathology

Arnold J. Sameroff

Children generally are perceived as the product of some unfolding process as they increase in size and capacity. Moving from one milestone to another, infants open their eyes and ears to the world, attend to objects in view, bring hand to eye, then hand to object to eye. Manipulating and playing with things, they come to solve problems and demonstrate an increasing understanding of the workings of their universe. This view of infants as independently developing entities belies an intimate and necessary relationship to the social world into which they are born. A linear model of child development justified a search for biological or behavioral indicators in childhood that foreshadowed later emotional or cognitive disturbances. However, longitudinal studies of child development have provided a number of surprises and offered little support for such views of direct linkages between early markers and later competencies. Research findings have led us to the following conclusions:

1. Individual differences in social and cognitive competence can be explained in large measure by differences in social environment.
2. Social contexts have substantial continuity, which may explain continuities of functioning within individuals that appear to be constitutional.
3. Theories of human development need to integrate biological, psychological, and environmental factors to make successful predictions about human development.

Sociocultural theories (Rogoff, 1990) have proposed that development is not a characteristic of the child alone but of the child in context, in a relationship to a regulatory system of parents, family, school, peers, and culture. Without examining these forces in development, we cannot understand how children follow pathways leading to competence or pathology.

For humans, the relationships of the extrauterine world are an extension of the relationships of the intrauterine one, in which there is a clear dependence on the environment for continued existence. The processes of nutrition and thermoregulation still require another person, a caregiving figure who is herself embedded in a context of caregiving relationships. Eventually infants will acquire the mobility, the manual dexterity, and the intellectual skills to regulate parts of their own growth. They will learn to go to the refrigerator to get food when hungry or to the closet to get a blanket when cold. But even at that stage, others would still have to supply the food in the refrigerator and the blankets in the closet. It is clear that, at the most basic levels of existence, other people must play a necessary role in the development of the child. What will become evident in this chapter is that the relationships with others that are necessary for physical growth are also necessary for psychological growth. Furthermore, failures in psychological growth can be attributed to failures in relationships rather than failure in the child (Sameroff & Emde, 1989).

What are the data that have forced us to move from a singular focus on individual differences in children as the major determiners of developmental outcomes to a concern with differences in their life experiences? One of the major deficiencies in research on child development has been the lack of attention to contextual factors. In the following sections we describe a research program that tried to remedy this failing and the resulting data that led us to place great importance on environmental factors in explaining childhood behavior problems.

Developmental Psychopathology

The emerging field of developmental psychopathology has begun to impact on a number of traditional problem areas in psychiatry by illuminating new possibilities for understanding the etiology, future course, and treatment of many childhood problems. Such new possibilities are contained in the dynamic models of development that are implicit in the new discipline.

One of the more articulate redefinitions of psychopathology in developmental terms has been provided by Sroufe and Rutter (1984), who saw the discipline as "the study of the origins and course of individual patterns of behavioral adaptation" (p. 18). Cicchetti (1986) enlarged this concept by rooting it in the organismic-developmental approach elaborated by Werner (1948):

. . . it is necessary to engage in a comprehensive evaluation of those factors that may influence the nature of patterns, and the different pathways by which the same developmental outcomes may be achieved. It is important to map out the processes whereby the normal course of development in the social, emotional, and/or cognitive domains, in dynamic transaction with the "inner" constitutional and "outer" environmental characteristics, may lead to outcomes that either inhibit or exacerbate early deviations or maintain or disrupt early adaptation. (Cicchetti, 1986, p. vii)

From this perspective, due to the failure of more customary models to explain how disorders arise and are maintained, a new orientation is required to interpret child behavior problems. The traditional medical model of disorder is based on the presumption that identifiable somatic entities underlie definable disease syndromes. Within traditional psychiatry, the current dominant view of disease is still strongly biomedical, with only a small role allowed for social and psychological factors in the etiology of mental illness (Engel, 1977), although these factors may have an important role in the maintenance and perhaps treatment of mental disorder. In this view, individuals are not seen as integrated systems of biological, psychological, and social functioning but rather as divided into biological and behavioral selves. If the biology changes, either through infection or cure, the behavior changes.

The developmental approach expands upon traditional models of mental disease by incorporating biological and behavioral functioning into a general systems model of developmental regulation. Within this approach, underlying entities do not exist independently of developmental organization. The expression of biological vulnerabilities can occur only in relation to the balance between coping skills and stresses in each individual's life history (Zubin & Spring, 1977). Continuities in competence or incompetence from childhood into adulthood cannot be simply related to continuities in underlying pathology or health. The relations between earlier and later behavior have to be understood in terms of the continuity of ordered or disordered experience across time interacting with an individual's unique biobehavioral characteristics. To the extent that experience becomes more organized, problems in adaptation will diminish. To the extent that experience becomes more chaotic, problems in adaptation will increase. What the developmental approach contributes is the identification of factors that influence the child's ability to organize experience and, consequently, the child's level of adaptive functioning. Obviously there is a great gap between biological models of adaptive organization and the data collected in typical empirical studies of psychiatric disorder. The Rochester Longitudinal Study (Sameroff, Seifer, & Zax, 1982) is an example of a study that was conceived as a linear analysis of the effects of parental psychopathology on children's behavior and not as a study of the interaction of complex dynamic processes. During the course of the study, however, it was found that efforts to make simple predictions about child outcome were not successful.

High-Risk Studies of Psychopathology

Mednick and Schulsinger (1968) began a movement of high-risk research projects when they initiated their study of the etiology of schizophrenia. In their paradigm, children of schizophrenic women would be examined to discover markers that were prognostic of later mental disorder. Their study was relatively unique in psychiatric research because they studied normal children, albeit those at higher than average risk for psychiatric problems.

My colleagues and I (Sameroff, Seifer, Zax, & Barocas, 1987; Sameroff & Zax, 1973) initiated a similar project using their high-risk approach to the study of schizophrenia. In our Rochester Longitudinal Study, we made a number of changes in the Mednick and Schulsinger design. Where they used school-age offspring of schizophrenic women as subjects in their Danish study, we felt that the ideal point in time to search for constitutional differences would be at birth, when the infant had not yet been subject to the social consequences of life with a schizophrenic mother. In addition, we examined parental factors other than a diagnosis of schizophrenia to determine alternate explanations for any child behavior problems we might find. Because a parent's diagnosis of schizophrenia usually is associated with chronic and severe mental disturbance, high anxiety, social incompetency, and a variety of demographic variables, and because all these factors may have an effect on the newborn condition and later development of a child, they must be adequately controlled in any study devoted to understanding the singular effect of a schizophrenic heritage. Accordingly, we began our study with pregnant schizophrenic women and planned to follow their offspring through the first 4 years of life. Our strategy was to include control populations that would allow us to assess the effects of separate aspects of psychiatric diagnosis, chronicity of disturbance, severity of disturbance, and social competency as well as the general characteristics of social class, race, educational level, and family constellation.

In addition, for our analysis of the specific effects of a woman with a diagnosis of schizophrenia on the development of her child, this group of mothers was compared with groups of mothers having diagnoses of neurotic depression, personality disorder, or no mental illness. As we expected, when the four groups were compared on mental-health criteria other than diagnosis, it was found that the schizophrenic women as a group were more chronically ill, more severe in their current symptomatology, and more socially incompetent.

During the first part of the Rochester Longitudinal Study (Sameroff et al., 1982), we assessed

children and their families at birth, and then at 4, 12, 30, and 48 months of age both in the home and in the laboratory. At each age an assessment was directed at two domains of child competence, the intellectual and the social-emotional. In our search for the roots of mental disorder, we considered three major hypotheses: (1) deviant behavior would be attributed to variables associated with a specific maternal diagnosis, for example, schizophrenia; (2) deviant behavior would be attributable to variables associated with mental illness in general, especially severity and chronicity of disorder, but no diagnostic group in particular; and (3) deviant behavior would be associated with other aspects of the family's condition, especially social status.

When we examined the results of our study, we found little support for the first hypothesis. There was no specific effect of a mother's diagnosis of schizophrenia on the behavior of her offspring during early childhood. The second hypothesis, that mental illness in general would produce substantial effects, was supported more strongly than the hypothesis regarding specific diagnosis effects. These general effects of maternal psychopathology—severity and chronicity—were ubiquitous throughout the study. Children of more severely or chronically ill mothers had poorer obstetric and newborn status. During the first year they had more difficult temperaments, lower developmental scores, and less adaptive behavior. Their mothers were less involved and more negative in affect during home observations. By 12 months of age their infants were less spontaneous and mobile when observed in the home and less responsive in the laboratory. The ill mothers remained less involved and less affectionate during home observations. When examined at 30 and 48 months of age, their children were again less responsive in the laboratory, had lower developmental test scores, and were reported by their mothers as having a variety of nonadaptive behavior patterns at home.

Our third hypothesis, that differences in family social status would produce differences in child behavior, was strongly supported. The social status effects were apparent throughout the first 4 years of life. Children from the poorest families exhibited the poorest development. Specifically, the low-socioeconomic-status (SES) children had worse obstetrical status, more difficult temperaments, and lower Bayley test scores at 4 months; less responsivity during the home and laboratory observations at 12 months; and less adaptive behavior in the home and laboratory at 30 and 48 months of age. Like their children, the low-socioeconomic-status mothers were less positive in affect and less involved with their children during our observations.

Identifying Risk Factors

When the number of differences in child behavior was compared for the diagnostic, mental illness, and social status dimensions, the highest density was found in the social status contrasts (Sameroff & Seifer, 1983). Family factors of socioeconomic status and parental factors of severity and chronicity of mental disturbance were more powerful risks than the specific psychiatric diagnoses we examined. As a study devoted to discovering the etiology of schizophrenia, the Rochester Longitudinal Study was a failure. On the other hand, as a study designed to explain why children were having behavioral problems during the preschool years, the investigation had greater success.

During the 1970s, much research attention was devoted to high-risk research targeting the offspring of schizophrenic women. As with most fads, achievements rarely match expectations, and the high-risk study of schizophrenia was no exception. The last two major conference reports of the consortium of scientists engaged in such studies contain sobering appraisals of the difficulties inherent in such research (Goldstein & Tuma, 1987; Watt, Anthony, Wynne, & Rolf, 1984). The inability of the study to find the roots of schizophrenia was not an exception in this research area.

What was learned in the Rochester Longitudinal Study was the overriding importance of attending to the context of the children in the study in order to understand their development. In the study, social status was a more powerful risk factor than any of the mental illness measures. To better understand the role of social status, more differentiated views of environmental influences needed to be taken. In order to translate this sociological economic measure into something that

would have direct impact on children, we needed to analyze the social status factor into behaviorally relevant units. We had to discover what was different about the experience of children raised in different socioeconomic environments. But first, let us review the efforts of others to find early characteristics of the child that would predict later pathology.

Perinatal Medical Condition as Developmental Risk

In an effort to determine the causes of cerebral palsy, the federal government funded a large longitudinal study. Broman, Nicholls, and Kennedy (1975) compared the effects of 169 individual biomedical and behavioral variables during infancy on 4-year intellectual performance in a sample of 26,760 children from the National Institute of Neurological and Communicative Disorders and Stroke Collaborative Perinatal Project. Although only 11 (7%) of these variables could be said to constitute social or family behavioral factors, two of these, SES and mother's education, were the most predictive of outcome of all the variables. This study demonstrated the importance of early environmental factors but did not reveal the aspects of the environment that were the most salient predictors.

Another study that contrasted the effects of early biological and social conditions on later development was the Louisville Twin Study (Wilson, 1985). The developmental status of several hundred infants was assessed from birth to 6 years of age and correlated with early biological and social factors. Although the two social factors of mother's education and SES were not correlated with developmental quotients during the first year of life, by the second year and thereafter, they became the most potent predictors of the children's intelligence.

The Kauai study of Werner and her colleagues (Werner, Bierman, & French, 1971; Werner & Smith, 1977, 1982) provides a more elaborate description of the interplay among risk factors in the child and risks in the environment. When this predominantly lower-SES sample of children was followed from birth through adolescence, more than half had learning or emotional problems by 18 years of age. However, for the most part, these developmental problems did not result from early medical conditions such as birth and pregnancy complications. Infants with severe early trauma frequently showed no later deficits unless the problems were combined with persistently poor environmental circumstances such as chronic poverty, family instability, or maternal mental health problems.

The Kauai study is in tune with others (Sameroff & Chandler, 1975) in targeting socioeconomic status and family mental health variables, such as parental attitudes, family conflict, family size, stressful life events, and the utilization of counseling and remedial assistance, as important moderators of child development. In the analyses comparing children from various groups of mothers in the Rochester Longitudinal Study, we also were able to demonstrate that both parental mental illness and social status factors were directly related to child performance (Sameroff et al., 1982). Although these analyses were helpful, they did not fully address the issue of what psychological mechanisms are responsible for the individual and group variation observed in the children's development. It was necessary to identify which factors in the family and social environment of the children in the Rochester study were associated with developmental risk.

Environmental Conditions as Developmental Risks

We subdivided the global variable of social class to see if we could identify factors that acted as environmental risks more directly connected to the children. The factors we chose ranged from proximal variables like the mother's interaction with the child, to intermediate variables such as the mother's mental health, to distal variables such as the financial resources of the family.

From the 4-year assessment of the children in the Rochester study, we chose a set of 10 environmental variables that are correlates of SES but not equivalents (Sameroff, Seifer, Barocas, Zax, & Greenspan, 1987). We then tested whether poor cognitive and social-emotional development in our preschool children was a function of low SES or the compounding of environmental risk factors found in low-SES groups. Table 24.1 presents the environmental risk variables.

To determine whether each of these factors was indeed an environmental risk condition, we compared the high-risk and low-risk group for each variable separately. For the cognitive outcomes, in all cases the low-risk group had higher scores than the high-risk group. Most of the differences were about 7 to 10 IQ points, about one-half to two-thirds of a standard deviation. Among the social-emotional competence comparisons, the low-risk group performed significantly better than the high-risk group for all but one of the comparisons. The differences between groups on these comparisons was generally about half of a standard deviation.

TABLE 24.1

Summary of Risk Variables

Risk Variables	Low Risk	High Risk
Mental illness	0–1 psychiatric contacts	More than 1 contact
Anxiety	75% least	25% most
Parental perspectives	75% highest	25% lowest
Spontaneous interaction	75% most	25% least
Education	High school	No high school
Occupation	Skilled	Semi- or unskilled
Minority status	No	Yes
Family support	Father present	Father absent
Stressful life events	75% fewest	25% most
Family size	1–3	4 or more children

NOTE: Adapted from "IQ Scores of 4-year-old Children: Social-environmental Risk Factors," by A. J. Sameroff, R. Seifer, R. Barocas, M. Zax, and S. Greenspan, 1987, *Pediatrics*, 79, pp. 343–350.

Although there were significant effects for the individual risk factors, it is clear that with only a single risk factor, most children would not end up with a major developmental problem. But what would be the result if a comparison was made between children growing up in environments with many risk factors compared to children with very few? A multiple risk score was created that was the total number of risks for each individual family. In the Rochester Longitudinal Study, the range was well distributed between scores of 0 and 8, with one family having as many as 9 risks. When these risk factors were related to children's intelligence and social competence, major differences were found between those children with few risks and those with many. On an intelligence test, children with no environmental risks scored more than 30 points higher than children with 8 or 9 risk factors, as shown in Figure 24.1. On average, each risk factor reduced the child's IQ score by 4 points.

The relation between the multiple-risk scores and the social-emotional outcome can be seen in Figure 24.2. It is clear that the effect of combining the 10 risk variables was to strongly accentuate the differences noted for the individual scores just described. As the number of risk factors increases, performance decreases for children at 4 years of age. For the social-emotional scores, the difference between the lowest and highest groups was about 2 standard deviations. Thus, the combination of risk factors resulted in a nearly threefold increase in the magnitude of differences found among groups of children relative to the effect of single variables (Sameroff et al., 1987).

These data support the view that the behavior of 4-year-old children is strongly affected by many variables in the social context, but the possibility exists that poverty may still be an overriding variable. To test for this possibility, two additional analyses were attempted. The first analysis was to determine if the relation between more risk factors and worse performance was to be found in different social classes. The families were divided into high- and low-SES groups and the effect of increased number of risks was examined

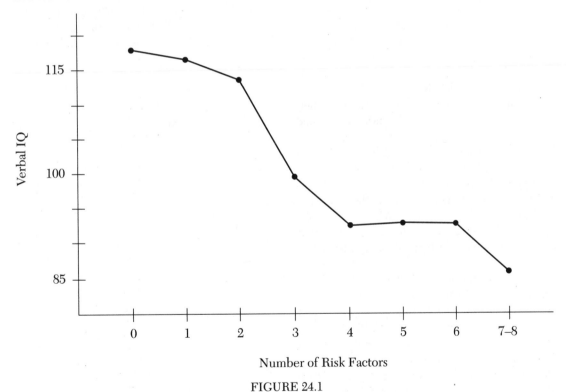

FIGURE 24.1

Effects of multiple risk sources on 4-year verbal IQ

NOTE: Adapted from "IQ Scores of 4-year-old Children: Social-environment Risk Factors," by A. J. Sameroff, R. Seifer, R. Barocas, M. Zax, & S. Greenspan, 1987, *Pediatrics, 79*, pp. 343–350.

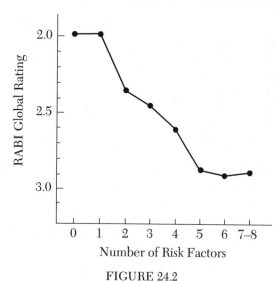

FIGURE 24.2

Effects of multiple risk scores on 4-year social-emotional competence

NOTE: Adapted from "IQ Scores of 4-year-old Children: Social-environmental Risk Factors," by A. J. Sameroff, R. Seifer, R. Barocas, M. Zax, & S. Greenspan, 1987, *Pediatrics,* 79, pp. 343–350.

within each social class group. The effects of the multiple-risk score were as clear within SES groups as well as for the population at large. The more risk factors, the worse the child outcomes for both high- and low-SES families.

The second analysis was to determine if there were consistencies in the distribution of risk factors, that is, were the same factors always present? The data from the families that had a moderate score of 3, 4, or 5 risk factors were cluster-analyzed. The families fell into 5 clusters with different sets of high-risk conditions that are listed in Table 24.2. Different combinations of factors appear in each cluster. Cluster 2 has no overlapping variables with clusters 3, 4, or 5. Minority status is a risk variable in clusters 3, 4, and 5 but does not appear in clusters 1 or 2. Despite these differences in the specific risks among families, the mean IQs were not different for children in the 5 clusters; they ranged from 92.8 to 97.7. Thus, it seems that it was not any single variable, but the combination of multiple variables, that reduced the children's intellectual performances. In every family situation, a unique set of risk or protective factors was related to children's outcome.

These analyses of the Rochester data were attempts to elaborate environmental risk factors by reducing global measures such as SES to component social and behavioral variables. We were able to identify a set of risk factors that were predominantly found in lower SES groups, but affected child outcomes in all social classes. Moreover, no single variable was determinant of outcome. Only in families with multiple risk factors was the child's competence placed in jeopardy. In the analyses of intellectual outcomes, none of the children in the low multiple-risk group had an IQ below 85, whereas 24% of the children in the high multiple-risk group did, a ratio of more than 24 to 1. Conversely, only 4% of the high-risk children had IQs above 115 whereas 55% of the low-risk children did, a ratio of 14 to 1. In families with many environmental risks (4–9 factors), 31% of children were judged to have clinical symptoms of emotional disturbance, whereas in families with few risks (0–1 factors), only 3% showed such symptoms.

The multiple pressures of environmental context in terms of amount of stress from the environment, the family's resources for coping with that stress, the number of children that must share those resources, and the parents' flexibility in understanding and dealing with their children, all

TABLE 24.2

Cluster Analysis of Families with Moderate Multiple-Risk Scores

Cluster 1	Mental Health
	Family Support
	Mother Education
	Anxiety
Cluster 2	Mother-Infant Interaction
	Mental Health
	Anxiety
Cluster 3	Family Support
	Minority Status
Cluster 4	Mother Education
	Minority Status
	Occupation
Cluster 5	Parental Perspectives
	Minority Status
	Mother Education

NOTE: Adapted from "IQ Scores of 4-year-old Children: Social-environmental Risk Factors," by A. J. Sameroff, R. Seifer, R. Barocas, M. Zax, and S. Greenspan, 1987, *Pediatrics,* 79, pp. 343–350.

play a role in the fostering or hindrance of child intellectual competencies.

Continuity of Environmental Risk

The studies that explored the effects of environmental risk factors on early development have shown major consequences for children living in multiproblem families. What are the long-term consequences of these early adverse circumstances? Will later conditions alter the course for such children, or will early experiences lock children into pathways of deviance? There is much literature on resilient characteristics of the children or protective factors in the family that may mitigate the effects of contextual risk (Masten & Garmezy, 1985; Rutter, 1987). Although we have completed such analyses (Seifer, Sameroff, Baldwin, & Baldwin, 1992), they will not be described here because this topic is reviewed in Chapter 23.

Within the Rochester Longitudinal Study, our attention has been devoted to the source of continuities and discontinuities in child performance. We recently completed a new assessment of the sample when the children were 13 years of age (Sameroff, Seifer, Baldwin, & Baldwin, 1993). Because of the potent effects of our multiple risk index at 4 years, we calculated a new multiple environmental risk score for each family based on their situation 9 years later. To our surprise, very few families showed major shifts in the number of risk factors across the 9-year intervening period. The correlation in number of risks was 0.77. The factor that showed the most improvement was maternal education, where the number of mothers who had not gotten a high school diploma or equivalent decreased from 33 to 22% of the sample. The risk factor that increased the most was single parenthood, with the number of children being raised by their mothers alone increasing from 24 to 41%.

Because of the very high stability in the number of risks experienced by these families, it was impossible to determine if the effects of early adversity were affecting the later behavior of these children. Those children who had been living in high-risk environments at 4 years of age were still living in them at 13 years of age. Moreover, these contemporary high-risk contexts were producing the same negative effects on behavior as the earlier ones had done. We found the same relationship between the number of risk factors and the child's intellectual competence; those children from families with no risk factors scored more than 30 points higher on intelligence tests than those with the most risk factors.

The typical statistic reported in longitudinal research is the correlation between early and later performance of the children. We, too, found such correlations. Intelligence at 4 years correlated 0.72 with intelligence at 13 years. The usual interpretation of such a number is that there is a continuity of competence or incompetence in the child. Such a conclusion cannot be challenged if the only assessments in the study are of the children. In the Rochester study we examined environmental as well as child factors. We were able to correlate environmental characteristics as well as child ones across time. We found that the 0.77 correlation between environmental risk scores at the two ages was as great or greater than any continuity within the child. Whatever the child's ability for achieving high levels of competence, it was severely undermined by the continuing paucity of environmental support. Whatever the capabilities provided to the child by individual factors, it was the environment that limited the opportunities for development.

Secular Trends

The thrust of a contextual analysis of developmental regulation is not that individual factors in the child are nonexistent or irrelevant, but that they must be studied in a context larger than a single child. The risk analyses discussed so far have implicated parent characteristics and the immediate social conditions of family support and life and event stressors as important moderators of healthy psychological growth in children. To this list of risks must be added changes in the historical supports for families in a given society. The importance of this added level of complexity was emphasized when we examined secular trends in the economic well-being of American families.

At 4 years of age we had divided the sample into high-, medium-, and low-risk groups based on the number of cumulative risks: 0 or 1 in the low-risk group, 2 or 3 in the medium-risk group, and 4 or more in the high-risk group. We found that 22% of the high-risk group had IQs below 85, whereas none of the low-risk sample did. Conversely, 59% of the low-risk group had IQs above 115 but only 4% of the high-risk sample did.

After the 13-year assessment, we made the same breakdown into high-, medium-, and low-risk groups and examined the distribution of IQs within risk groups. Again we found a preponderance of low IQ scores in the high-risk group and a preponderance of high IQ scores in the low-risk group, indicating the continuing negative effects of an unfavorable environment. But strikingly, the number of children in the high-risk group with IQs below 85 had increased from 22 to 46%, more than doubling. If our analysis was restricted to the level of the child and family, we would hypothesize that high-risk environments operate synergistically to further worsen the intellectual standing of these children during the period from preschool to adolescence, placing them in a downward spiral of increasing incompetence.

An alternative hypothesis was that society was changing during the 9 years between the Rochester Longitudinal Study assessments. In a study completed by the House of Representatives Ways and Means Committee (Passel, 1989), it was found that between the years 1973 and 1987, during which time we were doing this study, the average household income of the poorest fifth of Americans fell 12%, while the income of the richest fifth increased 24%.

The Regulation of Development

The purpose of this presentation has been to explore the limitations placed on understanding behavioral disorders when clinical attention is restricted to the behavior of the children taken out of their family and social context. Once the limitations are appreciated, the issue of finding an approach that provides a more complete understanding of the forces regulating development must be addressed. This approach must explain how individual characteristics and experience work together to produce patterns of adaptive or maladaptive functioning and relate how such past or present functioning influences the future.

The development of each individual is constrained by interactions with regulatory systems acting at different levels of organization. The two most prominent of these are the biological and social regulatory systems. The result of these regulatory exchanges is the expansion of each individual's ability for biological self-regulation and the development of behavioral self-regulation. Developmental advances permit children to control aspects of their environment that initially could be regulated only by caregivers. Despite this burgeoning independence, children as well as adults are never freed from a relationship to an internal biological and external social context. Should this connectedness be forgotten merely as a bout of illness or a legal transgression will remind a person of these constraints. The most important principle in a general theory of development is that individuals can never be removed from their contexts. Whether the goal is understanding causal connections, predicting outcomes, or intervention and therapy, it will not be achieved by removing the individual from the conditions that regulate development.

Most of the attention of the psychiatric community is devoted to the biological influences on behavior. Indeed, from conception to birth, interactions with the biological system are most prominent. Changes in the contemporary state of the organism's embryonic phenotype trigger the genotype to provide a series of new biochemical experiences. These experiences are regulated by the turning on and off of various gene activities directed toward the production of a viable human child. These processes continue less dramatically after birth with some exceptions, for example, the initiation of adolescence and possibly senility.

The period from birth to adulthood, however, is dominated by interactions with the social system. Again, the state of the child triggers regulatory processes, but now the regulators are in the social environment. Examples of such coded changes are the reactions of parents to their child's ability to walk or talk, and the changes in setting provided when the child reaches preschool or school age. These regulations change the experience of the child in tune with changes in his or her physical and behavioral development. The more traditional the culture, the more organized and encoded are these regulations in family and cultural socialization patterns. Indeed, the organization of experience is explicit in the great amount of attention given by educators to curriculum development and by psychologists to behavior modification plans, but the implicit organization of experience has been left to the attention of sociologists and anthropologists. The organization of a child's external experience to which a family and culture subscribes has been postulated to compose an "environtype," analogous to the biological genotype that regulates the child's internal physical experience (Sameroff, 1989).

An understanding of the developmental process requires an appreciation of the transactions between individuals, their biological inner workings, and their social outer workings. Continuities and discontinuities in competence are a joint function of these three systems, the genotype, the environtype and the phenotype (see Figure 24.3). The genotype is the system of biological regulation and organization. The environtype is the family and cultural code that regulates the developmental opportunities available to an individual. The phenotype, or in this case the individual person, transacts through development with both the genotype and environtype to determine individual status at any point in time. Individual factors are an important basis for child competence, but they

have to be recognized as only capacities until opportunities for their use arise. It is the environtype that will determine whether those opportunities are or are not available.

The Environtype

For older children, the peer groups and the school are major regulators of behavior, but for the period of early childhood, the discussion can be restricted to the hierarchical organization of environmental factors contained within the culture, the family, and the individual parent. The experience of the developing child is partially determined by the beliefs, values, and personality of the parents, partially by the family's interaction patterns and transgenerational history, and partially by the socialization beliefs, controls, and supports of the culture. Developmental regulations at each of these levels are carried within codes that direct cognitive and social-emotional development so that the child ultimately will be able to fill a role defined within society.

The ingredients of the cultural code are the complex of characteristics that organize a society's child-rearing system, incorporating elements of socialization and education. These processes are embedded in sets of social controls and social supports based on beliefs that differ in the amount of community consensus ranging from mores and norms to fads and fashions. Although the common biological characteristics of the human species have acted to produce similar developmental agendas in most cultures, there exist differences in many major features that often ignore the biological status of the individual. In most cultures, formal education begins between the ages of 6 and 8 (Rogoff, 1981), when most children have reached the cognitive ability to learn from such structured experiences. On the other hand, informal education can begin at many different ages depending on the culture's attributions to the child. The Digo and Kikuyu are two East African cultures that have different beliefs about infant capacities (deVries & Sameroff, 1984). The Digo believe that infants can learn within a few months after birth and begin socialization at that time.

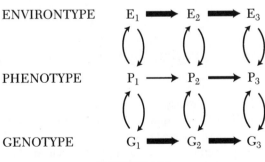

FIGURE 24.3

Regulation model of development with transactions among genotype, phenotype, and environtype.

NOTE: From *Can Development Be Continuous?* by A. J. Sameroff, Paper presented at the annual meeting of the American Psychological Association, 1985.

The Kikuyu believe serious education is possible beginning in the second year of life. Closer to home, some middle-class parents have been convinced that prenatal experiences will enhance the cognitive development of their children. Such examples demonstrate the variability of human developmental contexts.

One of the major contemporary risk conditions toward which clinical concern is directed is adolescent pregnancy. Although for certain young mothers, the pregnancy is the outcome of individual factors, for a large proportion, it is the result of a cultural code that defines maturity, family relationships, and socialization patterns with adolescent motherhood as a normative ingredient (Crockett, 1993). In such instances, focusing on the problem as one that resides wholly at the individual level would be a gross misrepresentation.

Just as cultural codes regulate the fit between individuals and the social system, family codes organize individuals within the family system. Family codes provide a source of regulation that allow a group of individuals to form a collective unit in relation to society as a whole. As the cultural code regulates development so that an individual may fill a role in society, family codes regulate development to produce members who fulfill a role within the family and ultimately are able to introduce new members into the shared system. Traditionally, new members are incorporated through birth and marriage, although more recently remarriage has taken on a more frequent role in providing new family members.

The family regulates children's development through a variety of forms that vary in their degree of explicit representation. Families have rituals that prescribe roles, stories that transmit orientations to each family member (as well as to whomever will listen), shared myths that influence individual interactions, and behavioral paradigms that change individual behavior when in the presence of other family members. Reiss (1989) has contrasted the degree to which these forms regulate family behavior through explicit prescriptions, that is, the knowledge of family rules that each member has, with the degree to which each family member's behavior is regulated by common practice, that is, the behavior of the family members when together.

There is good evidence that individual behavior is influenced by the family context. When op-erating as part of a family, the behavior of each member is altered (Parke & Tinsley, 1987), frequently without the person aware of the behavioral change (Reiss, 1981). However, there is also no doubt that each individual brings his or her own contribution to family interactions. The contribution of parents is much more complexly determined than that of young children, given the multiple levels that contribute to their behavior. Although the socializing regulations embodied in the cultural and family codes have been discussed, the individualized interpretations that each parenting figure imposes on these codes has not. To a large extent, these interpretations are conditioned by each parent's past participation in his or her own family's coded interactions, but they are captured uniquely by each member of the family. These individual influences further condition each parent's responses to his or her own child. The richness of both health and pathology embodied in these responses are well described in the clinical literature. In terms of early development, Fraiberg and her colleagues (Fraiberg, Adelson, & Shapiro, 1975) described "ghosts in the nursery" as evidence of the attributions that parents bring to their parenting from past experience. The risk factors associated with parental psychopathology have been discussed earlier as a contributor to the poor developmental status of children. It is important to recognize the parent as a major regulating agency of child development, but it is equally important to recognize that parental behavior is itself embedded in regulatory contexts.

Altering Environtypes

When children have behavioral problems, an ecological analysis requires an assessment to determine whether capacities are missing in the child or opportunities are missing in the context. The plasticity of the environtype permits compensatory regulations to be carried out in a variety of behavioral arenas. In the physical domain, wheelchairs can be provided for those who cannot walk; in the cognitive domain, sign language can be taught to deaf and retarded children; and in the social-emotional domain, parents can be trained to be more responsive to their infants. On the other hand, this same environmental plasticity can foster maladaptation through abusive parents, lack of resources for child care, and denial of education due to economic level, race, or sex.

At a historical level entire cultures can demonstrate changes in competence within generations. Flynn (1987) found massive gains in intelligence levels over the last 50 years in the United States and over the last generation in a study of 14 other nations. At a societal level, major changes can be made in the development of subpopulations at medical risk. The largest such example is the eight-center Infant Health and Development Project (The Infant Health and Development Program, 1990) in which the intelligence of low-birth weight infants was significantly increased. These studies of changes in cognitive performance have not been matched by major efforts to study societal changes in the emotional condition of children. Some social movements can be expected to have such results in young children. One is the increasing attention given to the prevention of child abuse and neglect. Another is the large federal investment in the Head Start program, which has components directed at the social-emotional as well as the cognitive development of poor children.

As an individual clinician, it is a complex enterprise to understand which environmental risks can be changed. The analysis of the deleterious effects of multiple risks on child development has a positive note. Single risk factors may have little effect on children's behavior. The mental illness of a parent, the divorce of one's mother and father, or even poverty taken alone often have been found to have minimal consequences for the social and emotional outcomes of children. It is only when these factors are compounded and multiplied that children are seriously at risk. Thus, to gain insight into a child's future progress (or lack of progress), increased attention will have to be paid to the total context of development.

REFERENCES

Broman, S. H., Nichols, P. L., & Kennedy, W. A. (1975). *Preschool IQ: Prenatal and early developmental correlates.* New York: Lawrence Erlbaum.

Cicchetti, D. (1986). Foreword in E. Zigler & M. Glick (Eds.), *A developmental approach to adult psychopathology.* New York: John Wiley & Sons.

Crockett, L. J. (1993). Early adolescent family formation. In R. M. Lerner (Ed.), *Early Adolescence: Perspectives on research, policy, and intervention.* (pp. 93–110), Hillsdale, NJ: Lawrence Erlbaum.

de Vries, M. W., & Sameroff, A. J. (1984). Culture and temperament: Influences on temperament in three East African societies. *American Journal of Orthopsychiatry 54*, 83–96.

Engel, G. L. (1977). The need for a new medical model: A challenge for biomedicine. *Science, 196*, 129–136.

Flynn, J. R. (1987). Massive IQ gains in 14 nations: What IQ tests really measure. *Psychological Bulletin, 101*, 171–191.

Fraiberg, S., Adelson, E., & Shapiro, V. (1975). Ghosts in the nursery: A psychoanalytic approach to the problems of impaired mother-infant relationships. *Journal of the American Academy of Child Psychiatry, 14*, 387–421.

Goldstein, M., & Tuma, H. (1987). High risk research: Editors' introduction. *Schizophrenia Bulletin, 13*, 369–372.

The Infant Health and Development Program (1990). Enhancing the outcomes of low birth weight, premature infants: A multisite randomized trial. *Journal of the American Medical Association, 263*, 3035–3042.

Masten, A. M., & Garmezy, N. (1985). Risk, vulnerability, and protective factors in developmental psychopathology. In B. B. Lahey & A. E. Kazdin (Eds.), *Advances in clinical child psychology* (Vol. 8, pp. 1–52). New York: Plenum Press.

Mednick, S. A., & Schulsinger, F. (1968). Some premorbid characteristics related to breakdown in children with schizophrenic mothers. *Journal of Psychiatric Research, 6*, 354–362.

Parke, R. D., & Tinsley, B. J. (1987). Family interaction in infancy. In J. Osofsky (Ed.), *Handbook of infant development* (2nd ed., pp. 579–641). New York: John Wiley & Sons.

Passel P., (1989 July 16). Forces in society and Reaganism, helped by deep hole for poor. *New York Times*, pp. 1, 20.

Reiss, D. (1981). *The family's construction of reality.* Cambridge, MA: Harvard University Press.

Reiss, D. (1989). The represented and practicing family: Contrasting visions of family continuity. In A. J. Sameroff & R. N. Emde (Eds.), *Relationship disturbances in early childhood: A developmental approach* (pp. 191–220), New York: Basic Books.

Rogoff, B. (1981). Schooling and the development of cognitive skills. In H. C. Triandis & A. Heron (Eds.), *Handbook of cross-cultural psychology: Developmental psychology* (Vol. 4, pp. 233–294). Boston:

Allyn & Bacon.

Rogoff, B. (1990). *Apprenticeship in thinking: Cognitive development in social context,* Oxford: Oxford University Press.

Rutter, M. R. (1979). Protective factors in children's responses to stress and disadvantage. In M. W. Kent & J. E. Rolf (Eds.), *Primary prevention of psychopathology. Vol. 3: Social competence in children* (pp. 117–131). Hanover, NH: University of New England Press.

Rutter, M. R. (1987). Continuities and discontinuities from infancy. In J. Osofsky (Ed.), *Handbook of infant development* (2nd ed., pp. 1256–1296). New York: John Wiley & Sons.

Sameroff, A. J. (1989). Principles of development and psychopathology. In A. J. Sameroff & R. N. Emde (Eds.), *Relationship disturbances in early childhood: A developmental approach* (pp. 17–32). New York: Basic Books.

Sameroff, A. J., & Chandler, M. J. (1975). Reproductive risk and the continuum of caretaking casualty. In F. D. Horowitz, M. Hetherington, S. Scarr-Salapatek, & G. Siegel (Eds.), *Review of child development research* (Vol. 4, pp. 187–244). Chicago: University of Chicago.

Sameroff, A. J., & Emde, R. N. (Eds.) (1989). *Relationship disturbances in early childhood: A developmental approach.* New York: Basic Books.

Sameroff, A. J., & Seifer, R. (1983). *Sources of continuity in parent-child relationships.* Paper presented at the meeting of the Society for Research in Child Development, Detroit.

Sameroff, A. J., Seifer, R., Baldwin, A. L., & Baldwin, C. A. (1993). Stability of intelligence from preschool to adolescence: The influence of social and family risk factors. *Child Development, 64,* 80–97.

Sameroff, A. J., Seifer, R., Barocas, R., Zax, M., & Greenspan, S. (1987). IQ scores of 4-year-old children: Social-environmental risk factors. *Pediatrics, 79,* 343–350.

Sameroff, A. J., Seifer, R., & Zax, M. (1982). Early development of children at risk for emotional disorder. *Monographs of the Society for Research in Child Development, 47* (7, Serial No. 199).

Sameroff, A. J., & Zax, M. (1973). Neonatal characteristics of offspring of schizophrenic and neurotically-depressed mothers. *Journal of Nervous and Mental Diseases, 157,* 191–199.

Sameroff, A. J., Seifer, R., Zax, M., & Barocas, R. (1987). Early indicators of developmental risk: Rochester longitudinal study. *Schizophrenia Bulletin, 13,* 383–394.

Seifer, R., Sameroff, A. J., Baldwin, C. P., & Baldwin, A. (1992). Child and family factors that ameliorate risk between 4 and 13 years of age. *Journal of the American Academy of Child Psychiatry, 31,* 893–903.

Sroufe, L. A., & Rutter, M. (1984). The domain of developmental psychopathology. *Child Development, 55,* 17–29.

Watt, N. F., Anthony, J., Wynne, L. C., & Rolf, J. E. (1984). *Children at risk for schizophrenia: A longitudinal perspective.* Cambridge: Cambridge University Press.

Werner, E. E., Bierman, J. M., & French, F. E. (1971). *The children of Kauai.* Honolulu: University of Hawaii Press.

Werner, E. E., & Smith, R. S. (1977). *Kauai's children come of age.* Honolulu: University of Hawaii Press.

Werner, E. E., & Smith, R. S. (1982). *Vulnerable but invincible: A longitudinal study of resilient children and youth.* New York: McGraw-Hill.

Werner, H. (1948). *Comparative psychology of mental development.* New York: International Universities Press.

Wilson, R. S. (1985). Risk and resilience in early mental development. *Developmental Psychology, 21,* 795–805.

Zubin, J., & Spring, B. (1977). Vulnerability: A new view of schizophrenia. *Journal of Abnormal Psychology, 56,* 103–126.

25 / Attachment Theory

Jude Cassidy

Attachment theory can be viewed as a comprehensive theory of personality development that provides a perspective on human development and functioning dramatically different from other theories. In fact, it was Bowlby's perceptions that existing theories did not adequately explain observed phenomena that led him to begin devising a new theory (Bowlby, 1958, 1960a, 1960b). The focus, for instance, of psychoanalytic theory on an individual's inner fantasies rather than on an individual's actual experiences was inconsistent with Bowlby's biological training, which had led him to seek to understand the interaction of organism and environment. In addition, the secondary-drive mechanisms proposed by both psychoanalytic and social-learning theorists to explain the child's relationship with the mother as derivative of her feeding the infant did not mesh with observations by Lorenz (1935) that infant geese become attached to parents who do not feed them, or with later observations by Harlow (1962) that infant rhesus monkeys, in times of stress, preferred not the wire-mesh "mother" that fed them but rather the cloth-covered "mother" that provided them contact comfort.

Dissatisfied with a variety of features of traditional theories, Bowlby sought new understanding by exposing himself to ideas and colleagues from fields such as evolutionary biology, ethology, cognitive science, and control systems theory (Bowlby, 1982). Bowlby drew upon all of these areas to formulate the innovative proposition that the infant's tie to the mother emerged as a result of evolutionary pressures. For Bowlby, this strikingly strong tie, so clearly evident particularly when disrupted, results not from an associational (secondary-drive) learning process but rather from a biologically based desire for proximity that arose through the process of natural selection.

Within contemporary developmental psychology, attachment theory is the theoretical framework within which social development is most widely examined. This is due in large part to the development of a standardized procedure for assessing individual differences in infant attachment quality, Ainsworth's Strange Situation procedure and her pioneering empirical work (e.g., Ainsworth, Blehar, Waters, & Wall, 1978). Hundreds of studies, conducted primarily in the United States but also in England, Germany, Israel, Japan, and the Netherlands, form a convergent body of research providing support for major principles of attachment theory. Recent development of systems for assessing attachment quality during childhood, adolescence, and adulthood have extended this empirical base (Cassidy & Marvin, 1992; George, Kaplan, & Main, 1985; Kobak, Cole, Ferenz-Gillies, Fleming, & Gamble 1993; Main & Cassidy, 1988; Waters & Deane, 1985). Review of this extensive literature is outside the scope of this chapter, which focuses in-

stead on theory. For reviews, see Belsky and Cassidy (1994), Bretherton (1985), and Lamb, Thompson, Gardner, and Charnov (1985).

The first section of this chapter contains a description of Bowlby's propositions related to the nature of the child's tie to the mother. The biological bases of attachment are discussed, and the developmental course of attachment in infancy and childhood is also described. In the second section, theory related to individual differences in attachment security is reviewed. Bowlby's notion of internal working models, central to understanding individual differences in security, is described, followed by theoretical discussion of what is thought to lead to secure versus insecure attachment. The final section contains a brief examination of clinical applications of attachment theory.

The Nature of the Child's Tie to the Mother

BIOLOGICAL BASES OF ATTACHMENT

The most fundamental aspect of attachment theory is its focus on the biological bases of attachment behavior (Bowlby, 1969/1982, 1973, 1980). Attachment behavior is any behavior that has the predictable outcome of increasing proximity of the child to the attachment figure (usually the mother). Some attachment behaviors (smiling, vocalizing) are signaling behaviors that signal the mother of the child's interest in social interaction and thus serve to bring her to the child for such interaction. Some (crying) are aversive and bring the mother to the child to terminate them. Some (approaching, following) are active behaviors that move the·child to the mother. Bowlby proposed that during the time in which humans were evolving, the time he called "the environment of evolutionary adaptedness," genetic selection favored attachment behaviors because they increased the likelihood of child-mother proximity.

Many predictable outcomes beneficial to the child are thought to result from the child's proximity to the parent (Bowlby, 1969/1982). These include feeding, learning about the environment, and social interaction. All of these are important. But the predictable outcome of proximity thought to give survival advantage to the child is protection from preditors. Infants who, in the environment of evolutionary adaptedness, were biologically predisposed to stay close to their mothers were less likely to be killed by predators. This is referred to as the "biological function" of attachment behavior. This is the most basic of predictable outcomes: Without protection from predators, feeding is not necessary, and learning cannot take place. Because of this biological function of protection, infants are thought to be biologically predisposed particularly to seek the parent in times of distress.

Attachment behaviors are thought to be organized into an attachment behavioral system in which the specific attachment behaviors may be less important than the internal organization of these behaviors. Bowlby (1969/1982) borrowed the concept of the behavioral system from the ethologists to describe a species-specific system of behaviors that leads to certain predictable outcomes, at least one of which offers clear survival advantage to the individual. The concept of the behavioral system involves inherent motivation. There is no need to view attachment as the by-product of any more fundamental process or "drive." This idea is supported by evidence indicating that in contrast to secondary drive theories (Freud, 1910/1957a), attachment is not a result of associations with feeding (Ainsworth, 1967; Harlow, 1962, Schaffer & Emerson, 1964). Bowlby's notion of the inherent motivation of the attachment system is compatable with Piaget's (1954) formulation of the inherent motivation of the child's interest in exploration.

Bowlby (1969/1982) adopted a control system approach to attachment behavior. Drawing on observations of ethologists who described instinctive behavior in animals as serving to maintain them in a certain relation with the environment for long periods of time, Bowlby proposed that a control systems approach also could be applied to attachment behavior. He described the workings of a thermostat as an example of a control system. When the room gets too cold, the thermostat activates the heater; when the desired temperature is reached, the thermostat turns off the heater. Bowlby described children as wanting to maintain a

certain proximity to the mother. When a separation becomes too great in distance or time, the attachment system becomes activated, and when sufficient proximity has been achieved, it is terminated. Bowlby (1969/1982; see also Bretherton, 1980) later described the attachment system as working slightly differently from a thermostat: as being continually activated (with variations of relatively more or less activation) rather than ever being completely terminated.

The child's desired degree of proximity to the parent is thought to vary at different times and in different settings, and Bowlby (1969/1982) was interested in understanding how this variation leads to relative increases and decreases in activation of the attachment system. He described three classes of causal factors: condition of the child (whether the child is sick, tired, or in pain), condition of the environment (whether it contains threatening stimuli), and the location and behavior of the mother (whether she is absent, moving away, or rejecting). Interaction among the classes of causal factors can be quite complex; sometimes only one needs to be present, and at other times several are necessary. In relation to relative deactivation of attachment behavior, Bowlby was clear that his approach has nothing in common with a model in which a behavior stops when its energy supply is depleted. For Bowlby, attachment behavior stops in the presence of a terminating stimulus. The nature of the stimulus that serves to terminate attachment behavior differs according to the degree of activation of the attachment system. If the attachment system is intensely activated, contact with the parent may be necessary to terminate it. If it is moderately activated, the presence or soothing voice of the parent or even of a familiar substitute caregiver may be sufficient.

The attachment behavioral system can be fully understood only in terms of its complex interplay with other biologically based behavioral systems. Bowlby highlighted several in relation to young children, and two, the fear and exploratory systems, will be discussed here. For Bowlby, the biological function of the fear system, like that of the attachment system, is protection. It is biologically adaptive for children to be frightened of certain stimuli. Bowlby (1973) described "natural clues to danger," stimuli that are not *inherently* dangerous but that increase the likelihood of danger. These include darkness, loud noises, aloneness, and sudden, looming movements. Because the attachment and fear systems are intertwined so that a frightened infant increases attachment behavior, infants who find these stimuli frightening are thought to be more likely to seek protection and thus survive to pass on their genes. The presence (or absence) of the attachment figure is thought to play an important role in the activation of the infant's fear system such that an available and accessible attachment figure makes the infant much less susceptible to fear.

The exploratory behavioral system is also one that is thought to be closely linked to the attachment behavioral system. The complementary yet mutually inhibiting nature of the two systems is thought to have evolved to ensure that while the child is protected by maintaining proximity to attachment figures, he or she nonetheless gradually learns about the environment through exploration. The link between these two systems is best captured within the framework of an infant's use of an attachment figure as a "secure base from which to explore," a concept first described by Ainsworth (1963) and central to attachment theory (Ainsworth et al., 1978; Bowlby, 1969/1982, 1988).

Noting the complementary activation and inhibition of these two behavioral systems, Ainsworth (Ainsworth, Bell, & Stayton, 1971) referred to an "attachment-exploration balance." Most infants balance these two behavioral systems, responding flexibly to a specific situation after assessing both the environment's characteristics and the caregiver's availability. For instance, when the attachment system is activated (perhaps by separation from the attachment figure, illness, fatigue, or by unfamiliar people and environments), infant exploration and play decline. Conversely, when the attachment system is not activated (e.g., when a healthy, well-rested infant is in a comfortable setting with an attachment figure nearby), exploration is enhanced. In terms of fostering exploration, Bowlby described as important not only the physical presence of an attachment figure but also the infant's beliefs that the attachment figure will be available if needed. A converging body of empirical work, in which maternal physical or psychological presence was experimentally manipulated, in fact has revealed support for the theoretically predicted associations between maternal availability and infant exploration (Ainsworth & Wittig, 1969; Carr, Dabbs, & Carr, 1975; Rheingold, 1969; Sorce & Emde, 1981).

It is important to clarify the distinctions among attachment behavior, the attachment behavior system, and an attachment bond (Ainsworth, 1973; Bowlby, 1982; Hinde, 1982). Attachment behavior is behavior that promotes proximity to the attachment figure. The attachment behavioral system is the organization of a variety of attachment behaviors within the individual. An attachment bond refers to a tie not between two people but rather a tie that one individual has to another individual who is perceived as stronger and wiser (e.g., the bond of an infant to the mother). Attachment behavior may or may not be present; it is situational. The attachment bond is considered to exist consistently over time, whether attachment behavior is present or not. Furthermore, the presence of attachment behavior does not necessarily indicate the existence of an attachment bond. The same behavior can serve more than one behavioral system and can have different meanings in different contexts or when directed to different people. For example, just because a baby approaches someone does not mean he or she is attached to that individual; even though approach can be an attachment behavior, it also can be an exploratory behavior.

PHASES IN THE DEVELOPMENT OF ATTACHMENT DURING INFANCY AND CHILDHOOD

Bowlby (1969/1982; see also Ainsworth, 1967) described four phases in the development of attachment during infancy and early childhood. Because development is complex and there is much individual variation in human infants, the timing of this development varies among individual infants. The four phases are as follows.

Phase 1: Undiscriminating Social Responsiveness (birth to 2 to 3 months): Several attachment behaviors are present at birth: rooting, sucking, crying, vocalizing, smiling, grasping, all of which have the predictable outcome of bringing or keeping the mother near the infant. Newborns are well adapted to respond to stimuli most likely to emanate from people. For instance, they show early preferences for listening to the human voice over other sounds and for looking at patterned over plain colored images (Fantz, 1965, 1966; Hetzer & Tudor-Hart, 1927). However, during this phase, there is very little discrimination among people. The infant will respond to nearly any stimuli, not only to a particular person: He or she will stop crying when comforted by anyone and will smile to anyone.

Phase 2: Discriminating Social Responsiveness (approximately 2 to 7 months): During this period, the infant begins to distinguish mother and other familiar people from strangers, in some modalities earlier than others. Attachment behaviors are now activated and terminated in response to specific others. Preference as well as discrimination is shown.

Phase 3: Active Initiation in Seeking Proximity and Contact (approximately 7+ months): During this phase, the infant becomes more active because of the onset of locomotion. Signaling attachment behaviors are now increasingly replaced by active attachment behaviors such as approaching and following, and there is a more coordinated use of grabbing. It is during this phase that "goal-corrected" behavior sequences emerge. Infants now can alter their behavior, continually choosing from a repertoire of attachment behaviors depending on the mother's whereabouts and the state of the environment. This is the first phase in which infants truly can be described as "attached," and it coincides with the phase that psychoanalysts call "true object relations." Nonetheless, this phase is limited by what Piaget (1926) refers to as "egocentrism."

Phase 4: The Goal-Corrected Partnership (approximately 3 years+): In order to move into this phases, the child first must be able to see things from mother's point of view, a skill facilitated by the growth of language. The child now has the ability to take into consideration the mother's plans and wishes. This phases is referred to as a "partnership" because for the first time, the child is aware of both his or her own goals and those of the mother, and can use this knowledge to negotiate a joint plan with her.

Individual Differences in Attachment

Within the context of considerable emphasis on the biologial basis of attachment, Bowlby also acknowledged the important role of learning. This was most evident in thinking related to individual differences. Despite the fact that all children, given sufficient contact with a caregiver, become attached, the *quality* of that attachment varies across relationships. In this section, I first describe Bowlby's concept of the internal working model. This notion is central to the issue of individual differences in attachment quality because it provides an explanation of the processes whereby early experience is linked with quality of attachment and later functioning. I then describe secure and insecure attachment.

INTERNAL WORKING MODELS

According to Bowlby, during the first year the child develops a set of expectancies, a set of mental representations that provide him or her with models of the workings, properties, characteristics, and behavior of attachment figures, the self, others, and the world. These working models (also called "representational models") are thought to be strongly influenced by the child's repeated daily experiences in relation to attachment, "in fact far more strongly determined by a child's actual experience throughout childhood than was formerly supposed" (1979, p. 117). (This emphasis on experience departs dramatically from Freud's focus on inner fantasies.) These models are similar to cognitive maps that permit successful navigation of an organism's environment. Unlike maps, however, working models are not static images but are flexible and adaptable representations. Bowlby relates working models to the ability to plan, and asserts that it is within the framework of these working models that the child can assess the situation and plan behavior. Thus, these models are thought to be central influences on the organization of the child's attachment behavior. The notion of working models is similar to a variety of constructs within the developmental, social, clinical, and cognitive psychology literatures: for example, to constructs such as "schema" and "relational models." (See Baldwin, 1992, for a review.)

Besides affecting behavior, working models are thought to influence feelings, attention, memory, and cognition (Bowlby, 1969/1982; Main, Kaplan, & Cassidy, 1985). They are thought to become so deeply ingrained in the individual that the ways in which they influence feelings and behavior may become automatic. This situation carries with it both advantages and disadvantages. Working models can serve a useful purpose for the child, making unnecessary the construction of a new set of expectations for each situation. This automatic use of existing models to appraise and guide behavior in new situations increases efficiency. For example, a baby who has a working model of mother as available when needed may spend less time monitoring her movements than might otherwise be the case. When models become inaccurate or outdated, however, their automatic nature may be a disadvantage because it is difficult to update them if they are not conscious.

Attachment theory emphasizes the important influence of early experience on later development, and working models are thought to be central to explaining the nature of this influence. For instance, children whose early experiences have led them to develop a working model that their needs will be attended to may be likely to wait their turn patiently for a desired toy in the preschool. In this case, the working model that others are responsive may be part of the process through which early sensitive care predicts later social competence (Sroufe, 1983). Although Bowlby viewed working models as remaining open to new input to a certain extent, he believed that with development, working models, particularly those that are unconscious, become increasingly resistant to change.

The working model of the self differs from other working models only in that its object is the self. In other ways, it is similar to working models in general: It is an active construction that, because it guides behavior, perception, and feelings,

can serve a useful purpose; yet its automatic and unconscious nature renders it resistant to change and thus potentially pathological when the model becomes outdated or inaccurate. For Bowlby (1973), there is an inextricable intertwining of the working model of the attachment figure and the working model of the self. Over time, children come to believe that their mother will behave in certain predictable ways. Based on these experiences, children simultaneously develop a complementary view of themselves. For example, if children are loved and valued, they develop a working model of the parent as accepting and responsive and a complementary model of themselves as lovable, valuable, and special. If, however, children are neglected or rejected, they come to feel worthless and of little value. Bowlby stated that this intertwining exists despite the fact that it may not be valid:

> An unwanted child is likely not only to feel unwanted by his parents but to believe that he is essentially unwantable, namely unwanted by anyone. Conversely, a much-loved child may grow up to be not only confident of his parent's affection but confident that everyone else will find him lovable too. Though logically indefensible, these crude overgeneralizations are none the less the rule. Once adapted, moreover, and woven into the fabric of working models, they are apt henceforward never to be seriously questioned. (1973, pp. 204–205)

It is important to note that even though the idea of internal working models emphasizes the behavior of the attachment figure, Bowlby (1979) acknowledges the contribution of infant characteristics. For Bowlby, as well as for other attachment researchers and theorists (e.g., Sroufe, 1985), quality of attachment represents the history of mother-child interactions and the extent to which these interactions give the baby confidence in the mother's accessibility and responsiveness. Sufficient maternal availability and responsiveness for a baby with one temperament may be insufficient for a baby with another. For Bowlby, it is the infant's confidence derived from the interplay of both maternal and infant contributions that influences attachment quality. Although Bowlby's attachment theory devotes considerable attention to the parent's contribution to the infant's working model, it does not delineate as explicitly the expected contribution of infant characteristics.

For further discussion of internal working models, see Bretherton (1985, 1990), Main et al. (1985), and Sroufe and Fleeson (1986).

INDIVIDUAL DIFFERENCES IN INTERNAL WORKING MODELS: QUALITY OF ATTACHMENT

From an ethological perspective, not only is the tendency to form attachments adaptive, but so is the ability to be flexible in the organization of the attachment system in response to environmental variation. Such tailoring of the infant's behavior to conform to environmental circumstances is described by Main and Solomon (1986) as a "strategy." The ultimate function of these strategies is thought to be protection in that they increase the likelihood of infant-parent proximity. Strategies are thought to be biologically based in that they are automatically employed and need not be in any way conscious for the individual (Main, 1990).

Secure Attachment: Most children are securely attached to their parents (Ainsworth et al., 1978; Campos, Barrett, Lamb, Goldsmith, & Stenberg, 1983). Secure attachment is thought to arise from experiences that provide the child with a working model of the parent as usually available, responsive, accepting. The parent serves the child as a secure base from which to explore, and the child develops a model of the parent as one on whom he or she can depend in times of trouble and of the self as one worthy of such care.

The strategy that secure children use to organize their attachment system is thought to be simple and direct: They use the parent as a secure base from which to explore (Ainsworth, 1984; Main & Solomon, 1986). These children are thought to have a fluid attachment-exploration balance (Ainsworth et al., 1971). They are thought to assess the condition of the environment, their own state, and the whereabouts and behavior of the mother, and then act accordingly. If the environment appears safe and is interesting and the mother is nearby, they explore. If danger appears or the mother's availability becomes threatened, they seek proximity to the mother (Main, 1990). This fluid balance reflects the belief of these children that their signals will be responded to.

Secure attachment is viewed not as incompatible with self-reliance but rather as leading to it: "an unthinking confidence in the unfailing accessibility and support of attachment figures is the bedrock on which stable and self-reliant personality is built" (Bowlby, 1973, p. 322). Both Bowlby and Ainsworth (1984) point out that contrary to some popular misconceptions of secure attachment as promoting clinging and excessive dependency, secure attachment and the certain knowledge that the parent will be available if needed is largely influential in giving the child the confidence for independent exploration. A premature attempt to push the child to independence by rebuffing attachment behavior can instead activate intense attachment behavior. The child then becomes even more concerned with the attachment figure and is therefore too preoccupied to move into independent exploration. The parental goal of promoting independence is not achieved.

Insecure Attachment: Insecure attachment is thought to result from a history of experiences with a caregiver who somehow has not provided the child with a secure base. There are many ways in which this can occur: consistent rejection, lack of availability, and extreme forms of pathological parenting (e.g., abuse, severe parental mental illness). Care of this sort is thought to lead to internal working models of others as unavailable and untrustworthy and complementary models of the self as unworthy of sensitive treatment. These experiences leave the insecure child in a more difficult position than the secure child. The secure child can count on the mother to be helpful and, therefore, has principally the environment and his or her own state to consider in relation to activation of the attachment system. The insecure child, however, has, in addition, to consider the probable way in which the mother will be unhelpful: The child must consider the environment, his or her own state, and how best to have needs met given the expected maternal behavior (Main, 1990).

The strategies that insecure children develop in response to their experiences are thought to involve manipulation of the balance between the attachment and exploratory systems such that either one or the other is emphasized. In response to a parent who is minimally or inconsistently responsive, the infant is thought to develop an understandable strategy of emphasizing attachment behavior and increasing bids for attention. Such an infant is viewed in this scheme as having a coherent strategy of exhibiting extreme dependence on the attachment figure. Main and Solomon state that "in its heightened display of emotionality and dependence upon the attachment figure, this infant successfully draws the attention of the parent" (1986, p. 112; see also Cassidy & Berlin, 1994). In response to a parent who is rejecting of an infant's attachment behavior, the infant is thought to develop a strategy of ignoring cues that might activate the attachment system and to defensively deemphasize the importance of the relation with the attachment figure (Bowlby, 1980; Main, 1981; see also Cassidy & Kobak, 1988). Correspondingly, the exploratory system may instead be emphasized. This strategy is thought to serve to permit the infant to remain in proximity to the caregiver without engaging in either angry or clingy behavior, either of which might result in further rebuff by a rejecting caregiver (Main, 1981).

Insecure attachment is thought to lead to impaired functioning in certain areas, but not all. As a result of their experiences and their internal working models, insecure children are expected to have trouble not only trusting and depending on others but also recognizing their own self-worth. These perceptions are thought to hinder the formation of supportive relationships and thus place insecure children at risk for socioemotional difficulties. However, some areas of functioning, such as work-related achievement, may be less affected.

Clinical Applications of Attachment Theory

As a clinician, Bowlby was concerned about understanding psychopathology, and such concern substantially guided his work on attachment theory. A central tenet of attachment theory is the belief that early attachment experiences have profound influences on later social and emotional functioning. Thus, many childhood and adoles-

cent psychiatric disorders are viewed as having roots in early problematic attachment relationships. Several of these disorders are discussed briefly in this section. In considering these disorders, it is important to keep in mind a crucial distinction: Although certain psychopathologies may be rooted in insecure attachment, insecure attachment itself is not to be equated with psychopathology (Sroufe, 1988). (For a discussion of the central importance of attachment theory and research to the emerging field of developmental psychopathology, see Cicchetti, Cummings, Greenberg, & Marvin, 1990; Sroufe, 1986; and Sroufe & Rutter, 1984.)

ANXIETY DISORDERS

Bowlby's (1973) theory of fear, described earlier, is central to his explanations of anxiety disorders. This theory departs radically from that of both traditional psychoanalysts and social learning theorists. Unlike Freud (1926/1959), Bowlby proposed that fears other than those of known threats from external sources can be part of healthy development and are not to be considered neurotic. Unlike social learning theorists (e.g., Sears, 1963), he did not believe a painful experience with a person or object to be necessary before one can fear it. From an ethological perspective, Bowlby viewed certain fears as biologically adaptive. For Bowlby, these are fears of situations or events that, although not dangerous in themselves, bring with them an increased risk of danger. Those who fear these are more likely to survive to pass on their genes. As mentioned, these include fears of unfamiliar objects and people, the dark, being alone, heights, loud noises, and sudden (particularly looming) movements. Thus, fears of the dark or of being alone, for instance, are understood not as neurotic but as resulting from biological predispositions emerging from natural selection. These fears are thought to be adaptive throughout the life span.

When considering individual differences in the tendency to become anxious, Bowlby (1973) recognized that infant characteristics make important contributions. He discussed the role of gender, minimal brain damage, childhood autism, and physical handicap. Based on the animal literature, he also hypothesized the existence of a genetic component in humans. During the two decades that have elapsed since the publication of Bowlby's (1973) major writings on anxiety, considerable information about the role of genetics in anxiety has emerged. Several family and twin studies have indicated that all anxiety disorders classified in the fourth edition of the *Diagnostic and Statistical Manual of Mental Disorders* (American Psychiatric Association, 1994) appear to have a substantial genetic component. (See Torgersen, 1988, for a review.) Thus, in the context of a probable genetic contribution to anxiety disorders, it is also evident that much room for environmental contribution remains: Most monozygotic twins are discordant for anxiety disorders (Torgersen, 1988). To understand the etiology of anxiety disorder, further exploration of the particular biochemical mechanisms that are inherited, of the nature of genetic and environmental interaction, and of the specific aspects of environmental experience that are influential is important. It is this last area of investigation on which Bowlby focused.

Bowlby (1973) described a variety of experiences that could lead a child to be uncertain of the availability of the attachment figure and, in turn, lead to chronic anxiety. According to Bowlby, because children have a biologically based and adaptive fear of being alone, threats of abandonment can be particularly frightening to them. Thus, parental threats of abandonment used as a means of controlling the child ("If you don't behave, I'll leave") or perhaps while exasperated ("You'll be the death of me") can lead to children's fears. Because children tend to take their parents' statements literally, such threats can be viewed as realistic experiential bases for fears of separation. Additional relevant experiences include hearing of frightening events happening to others or having experienced such events in the past. If the parent has recently been ill, or if someone close to the child has died, the child may have increased worries that something may happen to the parent.

Bowlby defined anxiety as uncertainty about the availability of the attachment figure if needed. According to clinical observations (Bowlby, 1973) and to empirical work (e.g., Ainsworth et al., 1978), most infants receive care that assures them that the caregiver will be available if needed: They have an accessible and responsive caregiver to

whom they can return as a "safe haven" should trouble arise. It is when infants do not have this certain knowledge that they can become chronically anxious.

How is this anxiety about the availability of the attachment figure manifested? According to Bowlby (1973), childhood phobias and intense separation anxiety are common results. Bowlby suggested, for instance, that what is usually called "school phobia" may in fact be a form of separation anxiety. Bowlby pointed out that children who consistently refuse to attend school are only rarely truly frightened of school, but rather much more commonly are experiencing acute separation anxiety: fear of leaving home and the attachment figure. Some children who refuse to attend school are frightened that something terrible may happen to the parent while they are away at school, and so remain home to protect the parent. Unlike the traditional psychoanalytic position (e.g., Freud, 1909/1952), which states that such a child fears his or her own aggressive impulses toward the parent, Bowlby suggested that the child's actual experiences may have led him or her to realistically fear for the well-being of the parent. Bowlby (1973) described another form of school refusal that occurs when a parent unconsciously keeps the child at home to serve as a caregiver for herself. The parent may subtly suggest that the child is too fragile or incompetent for school, and pretend that the child is staying home because he or she is unfit for the larger world. This situation often is viewed as the parent being overindulgent, when in fact the parent is placing a burden on the child by asking him or her to serve as a caregiver. These parents often did not receive care that they needed from their own parents as children and now turn to their children for such care.

Although there is as yet no empirical research examining connections between early attachment relationships and childhood anxiety disorders, there is evidence that insecurity in infancy is associated with children's fearfulness. For example, in Ainsworth's original sample, one group of insecure infants was overrepresented among the babies who showed clear-cut fear during the early free-play portion of a laboratory visit (Ainsworth, 1992). In a Japanese sample, the behavior of 7-month-olds later identified as insecure was considered more fearful than was that of infants later identified as secure (Miyake, Chen, & Campos, 1985). Inhibited exploration of the environment and shy/withdrawn behavior during peer play also have been associated with infant insecure attachment (Hazen & Durrett, 1982; Renken, Egeland, Marvinney, Mangelsdorf, & Sroufe, 1989). Finally, in a sample of British 3-year-olds, concurrent infant insecure attachment was found to be associated with a variety of forms of fearfulness in the laboratory (Stevenson-Hinde & Shouldice, 1991). (See Cassidy, 1995, for a fuller description of the connections between attachment and anxiety.)

DEPRESSION

According to Bowlby, whereas threat of loss arouses anxiety, "actual loss gives rise to sorrow" (1979, p. 130). Evidence of this connection emerged from the earliest systematic observations of children undergoing major separations from attachment figures (Robertson & Bowlby, 1952). The sequence of emotional states common to most young children was striking: Following an initial phase of protest, most children moved to a phase of despair. Once children had given up all hope of regaining the lost attachment figure, great sadness set in. This sadness is thought to be so great because of the biologically based fundamental importance of the attachment figure. Although painful, sadness is thought to be a healthy and adaptive response to loss. It permits a period of reorganization that can lead to improved adaptation to new circumstances which do not include the lost person (Bowlby, 1980).

In some cases, however, response to loss may move from sadness to depression. (Bowlby [1980] reviewed studies suggesting that children with psychiatric disorders have disproportionately experienced loss of an attachment figure.) And, according to Bowlby, early attachment experiences can influence an individual's response to loss. If the child has been made to feel incompetent and incapable of establishing satisfying relationships with others, then understandably the child fears that once the attachment figure is lost, he or she will be totally alone. If a child has been made to feel unworthy of love, he or she is likely to feel that once the attachment figure is gone,

no one will come to love the child. The child's experience-based expectations about the helpfulness of others in his or her time of distress also can play an important role in whether the response to loss becomes pathological.

Even when there is no loss, early attachment experiences are thought to play a role in childhood depression, particularly those that lead a child to "despair of ever having a secure and loving relationship with anyone" (Bowlby, 1988, p. 50). Ainsworth (Ainsworth et al., 1978), having observed that the intense cries of some infants were ignored, proposed that such repeated experiences are likely to contribute to despair. As Ainsworth pointed out, these babies learned that their signals for care would not be responded to and that they were helpless in eliciting care. Ainsworth suggested that the inability of these mothers to respond to their infants may have resulted from their own depressed preoccupations. The idea that problematic parent-child relationships may play a role in later depression characterizes much psychoanalytic and object relations theorizing (Bibring, 1953; Freud, 1917/1957b; Klein, 1932; Mahler, 1966).

Bowlby's theoretical notions about depression are also similar to theoretical viewpoints that emphasize the role of cognitive processes. For instance, Bowlby (1973) like Beck (1972), believed that depression hinges in large part on disordered cognitive beliefs about oneself, one's situation, and one's relationships. According to Bowlby, however, attachment theory goes further than Beck's theory by proposing the early experiential antecedents of these cognitive beliefs. Bowlby's notions are also highly compatible with those of Seligman (1975), who also emphasized the contribution of experiences to feelings of depression. Seligman proposed that repeated experiences with failure lead to "learned helplessness" wherein an individual loses faith in his or her abilities. According to Bowlby (1980), in most forms of depressive disorder, "the principal issue about which a person feels helpless is his ability to make and to maintain affectional relationships" (p. 247). Furthermore, as Cummings and Cicchetti (1990) have suggested, the cognitive processes thought to emerge from insecure attachment (feelings of helplessness, low self-esteem; see, e.g., Cassidy, 1988, 1990) are those that have been identified as related to depression (Kuiper & MacDonald,

1982; Peterson & Seligman, 1984). These findings strengthen the case for a link between attachment and depression and may reveal one of the processes through which this link occurs. (See also Kobak, Sudler, & Gamble, 1992.)

Recently, Cummings and Cicchetti (1990) have emphasized the importance of considering the link between attachment and depression within a transactional framework (Sameroff & Chandler, 1975). Within this scheme, the fact that insecure attachment does not lead inevitably to depression is emphasized. A model is proposed that "places attachment in the context of a large array of biological and experiential factors that affect risk for depression" (Cummings & Cicchetti, 1990, p. 356; see also Cicchetti & Aber, 1986). A variety of factors, which can be either enduring or transient in nature, are viewed as serving to either increase or decrease the likelihood of depression. It is the interplay of all these individual, familial, social, and larger environmental factors that is important. Insecure attachment is thought to increase children's vulnerability to depression by leaving them with few coping skills with which to deal with stressors and by leaving them with a decreased ability to develop relationships that could serve as a protective social support network during times of stress.

ADDITIONAL CLINICAL PERSPECTIVES

Recently there has been an upsurge in both theoretical and empirical work related to clinical issues. (See, e.g., Belsky & Nezworski, 1988; Cicchetti & Greenberg, 1992; Osofsky, 1991.) One perspective that has received increased attention examines attachment within a family systems framework (Byng-Hall, 1990; Byng-Hall & Stevenson-Hinde, 1991; Marvin & Stewart, 1990). The ways in which the quality of one relationship (e.g., the marital relationship) influences the quality of other relationships (e.g., the child-parent attachment relationship) are considered. In addition, disordered family functioning is viewed as potentially related to insecure attachments in both the current family and in the family-of-origin of the parents. Thus, increasing attention is being paid to the processes of intergenerational transmission of attachment as a means of understanding psychopathology (Jacobvitz, Morgan, Kretch-mar, & Morgan, 1992; Sroufe & Fleeson, 1986; Sroufe, Jacobvitz, Mangelsdorf, DeAngelo, & Ward, 1985). For instance, pathological role-reversal within a family may emerge when parents whose own attachment needs were unmet as children turn to their children to satisfy these needs. Or a parent may interfere with a child's independent exploration because her own lack of a secure base as a child taught her the danger of separateness and autonomy. Or a child's self-destructive behavior may be his means of keeping a disengaged parent involved in the family, thus maintaining his access to his attachment figure. This attachment perspective has proven useful in guiding intervention with troubled families (Byng-Hall, 1991; Marvin & Stewart, 1990).

Others also have recently focused attention on clinical intervention from an attachment perspective. First of all, Bowlby (1988) has described ways in which attachment theory can influence the clinician's work. This consists in large part of the therapist serving as an available and accepting attachment figure for patients, providing them with a secure base from which to explore their own feelings and behaviors. Of particular relevance is the extent to which earlier attachment relationships may be contributing to problems in current functioning and relationships. Second, a new model for treatment of children's conduct problems has been proposed (Speltz, 1990). This model, which combines traditional behavioral operant conditioning techniques with an attachment perspective, is based on the assumption that "in many cases, behaviors commonly labeled as 'conduct problems' can be viewed as strategies for gaining attention or proximity of caregivers who are unresponsive to the child's other signals" (Greenberg & Speltz, 1988, p. 206). Third, new early intervention work, aimed at reducing the incidence of insecure attachment during the first years of life, is emerging (Lieberman, Weston, & Pawl, 1991; Van den Boom, 1990).

Summary

It is clear that during the first year of life nearly all infants become attached to one or a few individuals with whom they have close contact (Ainsworth, 1967; Schaffer & Emerson, 1964). According to attachment theory, this nearly universal phenomenon is thought to result from the process of natural selection whereby infants predisposed to become attached to their caregivers survived to procreate and to contribute to the population's gene pool (Bowlby, 1969/1982). In addition to a predisposition to become attached, infants are thought to inherit the flexibility to tailor the specific organization of their attachment system to the environmental circumstances in which they are raised (Main, 1990). It is this flexibility, in combination with temperamental variation, that gives rise to individual differences in quality of attachment: security versus insecurity. Because attachment is so central to infants, the ways in which their attachment behavior is responded to is thought to have major implications for later personality development, with major traumas and disruptions contributing to psychopathology.

REFERENCES

Ainsworth, M. D. S. (1963). The development of infant-mother interaction among the Ganda. In B. Foss (Ed.), *Determinants of infant behavior* (Vol. 2, pp. 114–138). New York: John Wiley & Sons.

Ainsworth, M. D. S. (1967). *Infancy in Uganda: Infant care and the growth of attachment*. Baltimore: Johns Hopkins University Press.

Ainsworth, M. D. S. (1973). The development of infant-mother attachment. In B. M. Caldwell & H. N. Ricciuti (Eds.), *Review of child development research* (Vol. 35, pp. 1–94). Chicago: University of Chicago Press.

Ainsworth, M. D. S. (1984). Attachment. In N. S. Endler & J. McV. Hunt (Eds.), *Personality and the behavioral disorders* (Vol. 1, pp. 559–602). New York: John Wiley & Sons.

Ainsworth, M. D. S. (1989). Attachments beyond infancy. *American Psychologist, 44*, 709–716.

Ainsworth, M. D. S. (1992). A consideration of social referencing in the context of attachment theory and research. In S. Feinman (Ed.), *Social referencing and the social construction of reality* (pp. 349–367). New York: Plenum Press.

Ainsworth, M. D. S., Bell, S. M., & Stayton, D. J. (1971). Individual differences in strange-situation behavior of one-year olds. In H. R. Schaffer (Ed.), *The origins of human social relations* (pp. 17–58). New York: Academic Press.

Ainsworth, M. D. S., Blehar, M., Waters, E., & Wall, S. (1978). *Patterns of attachment*. New York: John Wiley & Sons.

Ainsworth, M. D. S., & Wittig, B. (1969). Attachment and exploratory behavior of one-year-olds in a strange situation. In B. M. Foss (Ed.), *Determinants of infant behavior* (Vol. 4, pp. 111–136). London: Methuen.

American Psychiatric Association. (1994). *Diagnostic and statistical manual of mental disorders* (4th ed.). Washington, DC: Author.

Baldwin, M. W. (1992). Relational schemes and the processing of social information. *Psychological Bulletin, 112*, 46–484.

Beck, A. T. (1972). *Depression: Causes & treatment*. Philadelphia: University of Pennsylvania Press.

Belsky, J., & Cassidy, J. (1994). Attachment: Theory and evidence. In M. Rutter, D. Hay, & S. Baron-Cohen (Eds.), *Development through life: A handbook for clinicians* (pp. 373–402). Oxford: Blackwell.

Belsky, J., & Nezworski, T. (1988). *Clinical implications of attachment*. Hillsdale, NJ: Erlbaum.

Bibring, E. (1953). The mechanisms of depression. In P. Greenacre (Ed.), *Affective disorders: Psychoanalytic contributions to their study* (pp. 13–48). New York: International Universities Press.

Bowlby, J. (1958). The child's tie to his mother. *International Journal of Psychoanalysis, 39*, 1–23.

Bowlby, J. (1960a). Grief and mourning in infancy. *Psychoanalytic Study of the Child, 15*, 3–39.

Bowlby, J. (1960b). Separation anxiety. *International Journal of Psychoanalysis, 41*, 1–25.

Bowlby, J. (1982). *Attachment and loss: Vol. 1. Attachment*. New York: Basic Books. (Original work published 1969.)

Bowlby, J. (1973). *Attachment and loss: Vol. 2. Separation*. New York: Basic Books.

Bowlby, J. (1979). *The making & breaking of affectional bonds*. London: Tavistock Publications.

Bowlby, J. (1980). *Attachment and loss: Vol. 3. Loss*. New York: Basic Books.

Bowlby, J. (1982). Attachment & loss: Retrospect & prospect. *American Journal of Orthopsychiatry, 52*, 664–678.

Bowlby, J. (1988). *A secure base*. New York: Basic Books.

Bowlby, J. (1989). Psychoanalysis as a natural science. In J. Sandler (Ed.), *Dimensions of psychoanalysis* (pp. 99–121). London: Karnac Books.

Bretherton, I. (1980). Young children in stressful situations: The supporting role of attachment figures and unfamiliar caregivers. In G. V. Coelho and P. I. Ahmed (Eds.), *Uprooting and development* (pp. 179–210). New York: Plenum Press.

Bretherton, I. (1985). Attachment theory: Retrospect and prospect. In I. Bretherton & E. Waters (Eds.), Growing points of attachment theory and research, *Monographs of the Society for Research in Child Development, 50* (1–2, Serial No. 209), 3–35.

Bretherton, I. (1990). Open communication and internal working models: Their role in the development of attachment relationships. In R. A. Thompson

(Ed.), *Socio-emotional development* (pp. 57–114). Nebraska Symposium on Motivation, 1988. Lincoln: University of Nebraska Press.

Byng-Hall, J. (1990). Attachment theory and family therapy: A clinical view. *Infant Mental Health Journal, 11*, 228–236.

Byng-Hall, J. (1991). The application of attachment theory to understanding and treatment in family therapy. In C. M. Parkes, J. Stevenson-Hinde, & P. Marris (Eds.), *Attachment across the life cycle* (pp. 199–215). London: Routledge.

Byng-Hall, J., & Stevenson-Hinde, J. (1991). Attachment relationships within a family system. *Infant Mental Health Journal, 12*, 187–200.

Campos, J. J., Barrett, K., Lamb, M. E., Goldsmith, H., & Stenberg, C. R. (1983). Socioemotional development. In M. M. Haith & J. J. Campos (Eds.), *Handbook of child psychology: Vol. 2. Infancy and developmental psychobiology* (pp. 783–915). New York: John Wiley & Sons.

Carr, S., Dabbs, J., & Carr, T. (1975). Mother-infant attachment: The importance of the mother's visual field. *Child Development, 46*, 331–338.

Cassidy, J. (1988). Child-mother attachment and the self in six-year-olds. *Child Development, 59*, 121–134.

Cassidy, J. (1990). Theoretical and methodological considerations in the study of attachment and the self in young children. In M. Greenberg, D. Cicchetti, & E. M. Cummings (Eds.), *Attachment in the preschool years: Theory, research, and intervention* (pp. 87–120). Chicago: University of Chicago Press.

Cassidy, J. (1995). Attachment and generalized anxiety disorder in adults. In D. Cicchetti & S. Toth (Eds.), *Rochester symposium on developmental psychopathology. Vol. 6: Emotion, cognition, and representation* (pp. 343–370). Rochester, NY: University of Rochester Press.

Cassidy, J., & Berlin, L. (1994). The insecure/ambivalent pattern of attachment: Theory and research. *Child Development, 65*, 971–991.

Cassidy, J., & Kobak, R. R. (1988). Ambivalence and its relation to other defensive processes. In J. Belsky & T. Nezworski (Eds.), *Clinical implications of attachment* (pp. 300–326). Hillsdale, NJ: Lawrence Erlbaum.

Cassidy, J., & Marvin, R. S., with the Attachment Working Group of the John D. and Catherine T. MacArthur Foundation Network on the Transition from Infancy to Early Childhood (1992). *Attachment organization in three- and four-year olds: Guidelines for classification.* Unpublished scoring manual. University Park: Pennsylvania State University.

Cicchetti, D., & Aber, L. (1986). Early precursors to later depression: An organizational perspective. In L. Lipsett & C. Rovee-Collier (Eds.), *Advances in infancy* (Vol. 4, pp. 87–137).

Cicchetti, D., Cummings, E. M., Greenberg, M., & Marvin, R. S. (1990). An organizational perspective on attachment beyond infancy: Implications for theory, measurement, and research. In M. Greenberg,

D. Cicchetti, & E. M. Cummings (Eds.), *Attachment in the preschool years: Theory, research, & intervention* (pp. 3–50). Chicago: University of Chicago Press.

Cicchetti, D., & Greenberg, M. (1992). The legacy of John Bowlby. *Development and Psychopathology, 3*, 347–350.

Cummings, E. M., & Cicchetti, D. (1990). Toward a transactional model of relations between attachment and depression. In M. Greenberg, D. Cicchetti, & E. M. Cummings (Eds.), *Attachment in the preschool years* (pp. 339–426). Chicago: University of Chicago Press.

Davidson, J., Schwartz, M., Storck, M., Krishnan, R. R., & Hammett, E. (1985). A diagnostic and family study of posttraumatic stress disorder. *American Journal of Psychiatry, 142*, 90–93.

Fantz, R. L. (1965). Ontogeny of perception. In A. M. Schrier, H. F. Harlow, & F. Stollnitz (Eds.), *Behavior of non-human primates* (Vol. 2, pp. 365–404). New York: Academic Press.

Fantz, R. L. (1966). Pattern discrimination and selective attention as determinants of perceptual development from birth. In A. J. Kidd & J. L. Rivoire (Eds.), *Perceptual development in children* (pp. 143–173). New York: International Universities Press.

Freud, S. (1955). Analysis of a phobia in a five-year-old boy. In J. Strochey (Ed. and Trans.), *The complete psychological works of Sigmund Freud* (hereafter *Standard edition*) (Vol. 10, pp. 5–149). London: Hogarth Press. (Original work published 1909.)

Freud, S. (1957a). Five lectures on psychoanalysis. In *Standard edition* (Vol. 11, pp. 3–56). (Original work published 1910.)

Freud, S. (1957b). Mourning and melancholia. In *Standard edition* (Vol. 14, pp. 237–258). (Original work published 1917.)

Freud, S. (1959). *Inhibitions, symptoms, and anxiety.* In *Standard edition* (Vol. 20, pp. 87–172). (Original work published 1926.)

George, C., Kaplan, N., & Main, M. (1985). *An adult attachment interview.* Unpublished manuscript, University of California, Berkeley.

Greenberg, M., & Speltz, M. (1988). Attachment and the ontogeny of conduct problems. In J. Belsky & T. Nezworski (Eds.), *Clinical implications of attachment* (pp. 177–218). Hillsdale, NJ: Lawrence Erlbaum.

Harlow, H. F. (1962). The development of affectional patterns in infant monkeys. In B. M. Foss (Ed.), *Determinants of infant behavior* (pp. 75–88). London: Methuen Press.

Hazen, N. L., & Durrett, M. E. (1982). Relationship of security of attachment to exploration and cognitive mapping abilities in two-year-olds. *Developmental Psychology, 18*, 751–759.

Hetzer, H., & Tudor-Hart, B. H. (1927). Die fruhesten Reaktionen auf die menschliche Stimme. *Quellen und Studien zur Jugendkunde, 5.*

Hinde, R. A. (1982). Attachment: Some conceptual and biological issues. In C. Murray Parkes &

J. Stevenson-Hinde (Eds.), *The place of attachment in human behavior* (pp. 60–76). New York: Basic Books.

Jacobvitz, D., Morgan, E., Kretchmar, M., & Morgan, Y. (1992). The transmission of mother-child boundary disturbances across three generations. *Developmental and Psychopathology, 3,* 513–528.

Klein, M. (1932). *The psychoanalysis of children.* London: Hogarth Press.

Kobak, R. R., Cole, H., Ferenz-Gillies, R., Fleming, W., & Gamble, W. (1993). Attachment and emotion regulation during mother-teen problem solving: A control theory analysis. *Child Development, 64,* 231–245.

Kobak, R. R., Sudler, N., & Gamble, W. (1992). Attachment and depressive symptoms during adolescence: A developmental pathway analysis. *Development and Psychopathology, 3,* 461–474.

Kuiper, N., & MacDonald, M. (1982). Self and other perception in mild depressives. *Social Cognition, 1,* 223–239.

Lamb, M., Thompson, R., Gardner, W., & Charnov, E. L. (1985). *Infant-mother attachment: The origins and developmental significance of individual differences in strange situation behavior.* Hillsdale, NJ: Lawrence Erlbaum.

Lieberman, A. F., Weston, D., & Pawl, J. (1991). Preventive intervention and outcome with anxiously attached dyads. *Child Development, 62,* 199–209.

Lorenz, K. (1935). *Instinctive behaviors.* New York: International Universities Press.

Mahler, M. (1966). Notes on the development of basic moods: The depressive affect. In R. Loewenstein, L. Newman, M. Schur, & A. Solnit (Eds.), *Psychoanalysis: A general psychology* (pp. 152–158). New York: International Universities Press.

Main, M. (1981). Avoidance in the service of attachment: A working paper. In K. Immelman, G. Barlow, M. Main, & L. Petrinovich (Eds.), *The Bielefeld interdisciplinary project* (pp. 651–693). New York: Cambridge University Press.

Main, M. (1990). Cross-cultural studies of attachment organization: Recent studies, changing methodologies, and the concept of conditional strategies. *Human Development, 33,* 48–61.

Main, M., & Cassidy, J. (1988). Categories of response with the parent at age six: Predicted from infant attachment classifications and stable over a one month period. *Developmental Psychology, 24,* 415–426.

Main, M., Kaplan, N., & Cassidy, J. (1985). Security in infancy, childhood, & adulthood: A move to the level of representation. In I. Bretherton & E. Waters (Eds.), *Growing points of attachment theory and research* (pp. 66–104). *Monographs of the Society for Research in Child Development, 50* (1–2, Serial No. 209).

Main, M., & Solomon, J. (1986). Discovery of a new, insecure-disorganized/disoriented attachment pattern. In T. B. Brazelton & M. Yogman (Eds.), *Affective development in infancy* (pp. 95–124). Norwood, NJ: Ablex.

Marvin, R. S., & Stewart, R. (1990). A family systems framework for the study of attachment. In M. Greenberg, D. Cicchetti, & E. M. Cummings (Eds.), *Attachment in the preschool years* (pp. 51–86). Chicago: University of Chicago Press.

Miyake, K., Chen, S., & Campos, J. J. (1985). Infant temperament, mother's mode of interaction, and attachment in Japan: An interim report. In I. Bretherton & E. Waters (Eds.), Growing points of attachment theory and research (pp. 276–297). *Monograph of the Society for Research in Child Development, 50* (1–2, Serial No. 209).

Osofsky, J. (Ed.) (1991). The effects of relationships on relationships: Special issue in memory of John Bowlby. *Infant Mental Health Journal, 12.*

Peterson, C., & Seligman, M. (1984). Causal explanations as a risk factor for depression: Theory and evidence. *Psychological Review, 91,* 347–374.

Piaget, J. (1926). *The language and thought of the child.* New York: Harcourt, Brace & World.

Piaget, J. (1954). *The construction of reality in the child.* New York: Basic Books.

Rapee, R. M. (1991). Generalized anxiety disorder: A review of clinical features and theoretical concepts. *Clinical Psychology Review, 11,* 419–440.

Renken, B., Egeland, B., Marvinney, D., Mangelsdorf, S., & Sroufe, L. A. (1989). Early childhood antecedents of aggression and passive-withdrawal in early elementary school. *Journal of Personality, 57,* 257–282.

Rheingold, H. L. (1969). The effect of a strange environment on the behavior of infants. In B. M. Foss, (Ed.), *Determinants of infant behavior* (Vol. 4, pp. 137–166). London: Methuen.

Robertson, J., & Bowlby, J. (1952). Responses of young children to separation from their mothers. *Courrier Centre Internationale Enfance, 2,* 131–142.

Sameroff, A., & Chandler, M. (1975). Reproductive risk and the continuum of caretaking casualty. In F. D. Horowitz, M. Hetherington, S. Scarr-Salapatek, & G. Siegel (Eds.), *Review of child development research* (Vol. 4, pp. 187–244). Chicago: University of Chicago Press.

Schaffer, H. R., & Emerson, P. E. (1964). The development of social attachments in infancy. *Monographs of the Society for Research in Child Development, 29* (3, Serial No. 94).

Sears, R. R. (1963). Dependency motivation. In M. Jones (Ed.), *Nebraska Symposium on Motivation* (Vol. 2, pp. 25–64). Lincoln: University of Nebraska Press.

Seligman, M. E. P. (1975). *Helplessness: On depression, development, & death.* San Francisco: W. H. Freeman.

Sorce, J. F., & Emde, R. N. (1981). Mother's presence is not enough: Effect of emotional availability on infant explorations. *Developmental Psychology, 17,* 737–745.

Speltz, M. (1990). The treatment of preschool conduct problems: An integration of behavioral and attachment concepts. In M. Greenberg, D. Cicchetti, &

E. M. Cummings (Eds.), *Attachment in the pre-school years* (pp. 399–426). Chicago: University of Chicago Press.

Sroufe, L. A. (1983). Infant-caregiver attachment and patterns of adaptation in the preschool: The roots of competence and maladaptation. In M. Perlmutter (Ed.), *Minnesota Symposia in Child Psychology* (Vol. 16, pp. 41–83). Hillsdale, NJ: Lawrence Erlbaum.

Sroufe, L. A. (1985). Attachment classification from the perspective of infant-caregiver relationships and infant temperament. *Child Development, 56,* 1–14.

Sroufe, L. A. (1986). Bowlby's contribution to psycho-analytic theory and developmental psychopathology. *Journal of Child Psychology and Psychiatry, 27,* 841–849.

Sroufe, L. A. (1988). The role of infant-caregiver attachment in development. In J. Belsky & T. Nezworski (Eds.), *Clinical implications of attachment* (pp. 18–38). Hillsdale, NJ: Lawrence Erlbaum.

Sroufe, L. A., & Fleeson, J. (1986). Attachment and the construction of relationships. In W. Hartup & Z. Rubin (Eds.), *Relationships and development* (pp. 51–72). Hillsdale, NJ: Lawrence Erlbaum.

Sroufe, L. A., & Jacobvitz, D., Mangelsdorf, S., DeAngelo, E., & Ward, M. J. (1985). Generational boundary dissolution between mothers and their preschool children: A relationship systems approach. *Child Development, 56,* 317–332.

Sroufe, L. A., & Rutter, M. (1984). The domain of de-velopmental psychopathology. *Child Development, 55,* 17–29.

Stevenson-Hinde, J., & Shouldice, A. (1991). Fear and attachment in 2.5-year-olds. *British Journal of Developmental Psychology, 8,* 319–333.

Torgerson, S. (1983). Genetic factors in anxiety disorders. *Archives of General Psychiatry, 40,* 1085–1089.

Torgerson, S. (1986). Childhood and family characteristics in panic and generalized anxiety disorder. *American Journal of Psychiatry, 43,* 630–632.

Torgerson, S. (1988). Genetics. In C. Last & M. Hersen (Eds.), *Handbook of anxiety disorders* (pp. 159–170). New York: Pergamon Press.

Van den Boom, D. (1990). Preventive intervention and the quality of mother-infant interaction and infant exploration in irritable infants. In W. Koops et al. (Eds.), *Developmental psychology behind the dikes* (pp. 249–270). Amsterdam: Eburon.

Waters, E., & Deane, K. E. (1985). Defining and assessing individual differences in attachment relationships: Q-methodology and the organization of behavior in infancy and early childhood. In I. Bretherton & E. Waters (Eds.), *Monographs of the Society for Research in Child Development, 50,* 41–65.

Weiss, R. S. (1982). Attachment in adult life. In C. M. Parkes & J. S. Hinde (Eds.), *The place of attachment in human behavior* (pp. 171–184). New York: Basic Books.

26 / The Psychophysiology of Temperament

Stephen W. Porges and Jane Doussard-Roosevelt

Overview

Contemporary theories of temperament have assumed that behavioral patterns are stable and are mediated by a physiological substrate. There is much debate about whether the physiological substrate represents either direct genetic influences or an interaction between genetic and environmental factors. Thus, data demonstrating physiological precursors or parallels of behavioral patterns do not confirm that the differences are genetic or immutable via environmental influences. In this chapter we present a view that various behavioral patterns are determined by the physiology of the child. However, within this presentation, we acknowledge that environmental factors (i.e., perinatal events, nutrition, illness, health care, stress, parenting style, social interactions, etc.), including impact of the child's behavior on the environment, may influence the physiology of the child and thus contribute to his or her expressed temperament.

Although theorists differ in their definitions of temperament (for a review see Seifer & Sameroff,

The preparation of this manuscript and much of the research described have been supported in part by grant HD 22628, awarded to Stephen W. Porges, from the National Institute of Child Health and Human Development. The authors would like to thank C. Sue Carter for helpful comments.

1986), there has been a shared assumption regarding biological causality. The degree to which human behavior has a constitutional basis has long been debated. Classic nature-nurture arguments have focused on the relative contribution of environmental and genetic factors in the development of various classes of behavior. The pendulum has continued to swing between the polar views of genetic versus environmental causality to where it currently rests at a midpoint appreciative of the dynamic interaction of both sources.

Most developmental scientists accept that temperament consists of biologically rooted individual differences in behavioral tendencies that are present early in life and are relatively stable across situations and time. However, researchers differ in their stated attribution of genetic causality for these biological factors. For example, Buss and Plomin (Goldsmith et al., 1987) define temperament as a set of inherited personality traits that are genetic in origin and that appear in infancy. Although interested in genetic influences, Goldsmith and Campos (Goldsmith et al., 1987) confine their definition of temperament to a behavioral level. Rothbart and Derryberry (Goldsmith et al., 1987) are less specific about the causal determinants of temperament and define temperament as "relatively stable, primarily biologically based individual differences in reactivity and self-regulation" (p. 510). Bates (1987, 1989) agrees with Buss and Plomin on the genetic origin of temperament but takes a dynamic systems perspective in which genetics serve to broadly outline the individual's responses, which are then influenced by the environment.

Temperament: A Historical Perspective

An interest in temperament is based on an appreciation that infants and children exhibit individual differences in behavioral patterns and in the development of behaviors. Galton (1869) introduced the concept of individual differences in mental development in a discussion of "individual variation" (p. 355) in his study of hereditary ge-

nius. His research focused on the study of reflexes and simple motor tasks including absolute and differential sensory thresholds and reaction time. Galton studied the families of eminent men and inferred that genetics played a major role in development. His views led to the eugenics movement, a movement intent on improving the human species through the control of hereditary factors in mating. In contrast, Watson (1930) argued that environmental factors and not inheritance served as the basis for temperament.

For Watson, heredity was responsible for the structure (e.g., stature) of the human organism, but not for psychological capacities or characteristics. In his volume entitled *Behaviorism*, Watson (1930) stated his case: ". . . there is no such thing as an inheritance of *capacity, talent, temperament, mental constitution, and characteristics.* These things again depend on training that goes on mainly in the cradle" (p. 94).

The contrasting views of Galton and Watson convey the contrasting cultures of their respective habitats of London in the late 19th century and Baltimore in the early 20th century. In London during the late 19th century, educational and professional opportunities were primarily dependent on family resources. Thus, it was difficult to observe a distinction between environmental and hereditary factors. In contrast, American cities in the beginning of the 20th century were characterized by a massive immigration from eastern Europe. In 20th-century western Europe, the intellectually disadvantaged eastern Europeans were assumed to be genetically inferior. Watson was exposed to this genetic diversity and observed that individuals who were viewed as intellectually inferior based on their country of origin were prospering when educational and professional opportunities were made available in the United States. From these observations Watson inferred that environmental factors were more important than hereditary factors. Watson's view is clearly stated in the following quotation:

Give me a dozen healthy infants, well-formed, and my own specified world to bring them up in and I'll guarantee to take any one at random and train him to become any type of specialist I might select—doctor, lawyer, artist, merchant-chief, and yes, even beggar-man and thief, regardless of his talents, penchants, tendencies, abilities, vocations, and race of his ancestors. (1930, p. 104)

Therefore, Watson advised parents to "slant" their children toward a vocation at an early age. According to him, "The vocation your child is to follow later in life is not determined from within, but from without—by you . . ." (1928, p. 39). Thus, his theory was a reflection of the American dream in which there were limitless opportunities and few constraints on success.

Watson's legacy has greatly influenced research on the psychological development of children. Other than in the case of severe mental or behavioral pathology, individual differences in behavior were assumed to be modulated by environmental factors. The behaviorist approach did not appreciate the variability in individual vulnerability to environmental factors. The research of Skinner (1958, 1968) on the treatment of behavioral problems (via behavior modification procedures) and education (via programmed instruction) shifted responsibility (control) from the child to the environment (home or school). Lack of classroom success was viewed not as a product of a temperamental characteristic but rather as the failings of the environment to identify the effective reinforcer to "control" and "optimize" behavior.

Behaviorism has been very important in the development of psychology as a science. It forced researchers to carefully identify stimulus and context conditions and to quantify response parameters with great detail. However, on the negative side, the experimental models did not allow for an understanding of the range of individual differences in behavior. Thus, behaviorism treated individual differences as a source of sampling error and neglected concepts such as temperament.

Pavlov's research (e.g., Pavlov, 1928) on the conditioned reflex, because of its quantitative reductionistic physiological measurements, furnished an enormous impetus to behaviorism. Pavlov proposed that complex behavior could be partitioned into two events—the positive and the negative conditioned reflex—which could be measured quantitatively. Pavlovian theory, although dependent on reflexes and the chaining of reflexes, evolved into a temperament typology based on the range of individual differences in establishing conditioned reflexes. Pavlov, like Galton, saw importance in individual differences and assumed that these differences were constitution-

ally determined. However, Pavlov was also similar to Watson in respecting the critical importance of environmental factors in shaping behavior.

Contemporary Research on Temperament

MATERNAL REPORTS: PHYSIOLOGICAL BASIS ASSUMED BUT NOT ASSESSED

In recent decades temperament has been "rediscovered." Research in infant temperament was stimulated by Thomas, Chess, and their colleagues in the New York Longitudinal Study (NYLS) (Thomas, Chess, Birch, Hertzig, & Korn, 1963; Thomas, Chess, & Birch, 1968; Thomas & Chess, 1977). The NYLS had as its goal the description of individual differences in infancy and the relation of these infant measures to adult personality traits. This work, and indeed all ensuing studies of infant temperament, assumes that these individual differences are stable across time and reflect underlying constitutional differences. And thus, while theorists differ in their definitions of the construct of temperament (for a review see Seifer & Sameroff, 1986), there is a shared assumption regarding causality. It is assumed that individual differences in temperament are mediated by underlying biological differences.

However, while the assumption of biological causality exists, contemporary research on infant temperament has focused less on individual differences in biological factors and more on differences in behavioral patterns. Maternal reports of infant behavior have provided the primary source of data. Maternal reports which are based on the assumption that the mother is an accurate observer of her child's behavior, have been assumed to be reliable and to reflect stable behavioral patterns.

The advantages and disadvantages of using maternal questionnaires in the study of infant/child temperament have been reviewed elsewhere (Rothbart & Mauro, 1990; Seifer & Sameroff, 1986). Both Carey (1981, 1983) and Bates (1980) have argued the relevance of maternal perceptions in temperament research. Carey notes that both parents and professionals can either make an observation of a child's behavior or have a perception of a child's behavior. While perceptions are by definition more subjective, they are not less valid than observations. Further, Bates and Bayles (1984) examined the relation between maternal perceptions and other measures of children's temperament and concluded that maternal perceptions of temperament contain both subjective and objective components. Their own dimension of "difficultness" was demonstrated to be one of the more objectively based perceptions.

In general, more global dimensions of temperament such as "difficultness" or "negative emotionality" have been found to be more stable over time than have more discrete behaviors (Belsky, Fish, & Isabella, 1991). Bates, for example, reports high stability of his Difficult dimension over time (average $r = 0.70$), accounting for almost 50% of the variance. In contrast, research with the NYLS dimensions of temperament indicates low to moderate stability of measures over time (Carey & McDevitt, 1978; McNeil & Persson-Blennow, 1988). In general, greater stability is found over shorter time periods than longer ones (McNeil & Persson-Blennow, 1988; Rothbart, 1986).

The literature on stability of temperament across various ratings sources parallels that of stability over time. The correlations are typically low to moderate in range, and are higher for dimensions of negative emotionality and difficultness than for other dimensions. Correlations between mother and father ratings are generally in the 0.3 to 0.4 range. Bates, Freeland, and Lounsbury (1979) found parental agreement in this range for three of the four factors in their Infant Characteristics Questionnaire. The strongest parental agreement was observed for difficultness ($r = 0.60$). Goldsmith and Campos (1986) assessed parental agreement on the Infant Behavior Questionnaire (Rothbart, 1981) and found low agreement on most of the scales but moderate agreement on scales tapping negative and/or highly motoric behavior.

A similar pattern is seen in studies of agreement between maternal and teacher reports. Field and Greenberg (1982) reported low to moderate corre-

lations between mothers and teachers using the Infant Temperament Questionnaire (Carey & McDevitt, 1978). The average correlations for the infant and toddler groups were $r = 0.20$ and $r = 0.35$, respectively. Goldsmith and Rieser-Danner (1986) reported moderate mother-teacher agreement for scales on the Infant Behavior Questionnaire (Rothbart, 1981) that assess negative affect and/or activity, but low agreement on all other scales.

Goldsmith and Rieser-Danner (1990) suggest that the lack of convergence of maternal ratings and the ratings of others is due to the lack of convergence in the observational base from which the raters draw their conclusions. Many of the behaviors assessed in temperament scales are very context-specific. The contexts in which teachers and other observers view the child are different from those in which the mother views the child. As Goldsmith and Rieser-Danner describe the problem, it is an "inability to provide an observer with an observational base that approximates the parent's extensive experience with the child" (p. 269).

The lack of convergence in ratings from divergent sources and the context-specific nature of many of the behaviors in question do not argue against a biological basis of temperament. They merely suggest that our means of assessing infant/child temperament are still weak and, thus, it becomes more difficult to provide a strong relationship with physiological or biological factors. The biological-behavioral relationship may be somewhat masked. Thus, any correlation between physiological and behavioral variables probably underestimates the true relationship.

GENETICS STUDIES: PHYSIOLOGICAL BASIS ESTIMATED

Behavioral Genetics: The behavioral genetics approach provides an approach to link genetic factors to temperament. The primary source of data comes from twin studies, particularly the Louisville twin study (Wilson & Matheny, 1986). Buss and Plomin (1975, 1984) presented a model of temperament that they tested with traditional behavioral genetic methods. Their theories and those of Goldsmith and Campos (1986) focus on the genetic bases of temperament. Much of the work in this area involves behavioral genetic research, and the predominant design in such research is the twin study in which monozygotic (MZ) and dizygotic (DZ) twin pairs are compared for similarity on temperament variables. Since monozygotic twin pairs are genetically identical and dizygotic twins share on average half their genes, a greater degree of similarity between MZ twins than between DZ twins is taken as evidence for the heritability of temperament traits.

Goldsmith (1983) has reviewed the twin literature and has noted the shortcomings of much of the research. Problems include small sample sizes, unsystematic subject recruitment yielding nonrepresentative samples, and poor assessment methods. In addition, in twin research there is the assumption of equal environmental influence on identical and fraternal twins. While some evidence suggests that the assumption is viable in the postnatal world (e.g., Lytton, 1977), there is evidence against the equality of prenatal environments.

There is increasing evidence that prenatal influences can have long-lasting effects on the nervous system and various aspects of behavior. For example, Clemens, Gladue, and Coniglio (1978) and vom Saal and others (vom Saal & Finch, 1988) have demonstrated in rodents that females that prenatally develop in proximity to a male littermate show alterations in genital anatomy in the male direction and as adults are more likely to show malelike patterns of sexual behavior and aggression and reduced levels of feminine sexual behavior. Thus, intrauterine events can masculinize and/or defeminize sociosexual development. Prenatal stress also affects development apparently in the opposite direction. In rats, exposure to stress during late pregnancy may both demasculinize and feminize the subsequent behavior of males (Ward, 1972). These changes represent complex interactions between fetal and maternal physiology. Steroid hormones, including those of both the adrenal and gonadal axes, are particularly potent in their capacities to have long-term effects on an organism. These systems can modulate environmental and organismic interactions, producing nongenomic changes. Thus, it is possible that even with identical genes, MZ twins may have different endocrine experiences in utero that may alter gene expression and subsequent behavior. Moreover, MZ twins often are of different sizes;

which may represent differential fetal growth patterns due to differential prenatal experiences (e.g., stress) associated with oxygenation and nutrients.

In general, twin studies have found greater evidence of heritability in subjects beyond the first year of life. The shift from primarily external control of emotions to a more internal or self-regulatory system of control is suggested as the basis for this phenomenon. Internal factors, more likely to be observed beyond the first year, are seen as more susceptible to genetic influence. In the Louisville Twin Study, Wilson, Matheny, and colleagues studied several dimensions of temperament and biological influence. Wilson and Matheny (1986) reported greater MZ versus DZ similarity on their observational and questionnaire measures of emotional tone at 18 months of age but not at 9 months of age. In a multimeasure, multioccasion twin study (Matheny, 1989), behavioral inhibition was measured by direct observation and maternal reports at 12, 18, 24, and 30 months of age in 130 twins (33 MZ pairs, 32 DZ pairs). Significant MZ-DZ differences were found for all measures at 18 and 30 months and for all but one dimension at 24 months (approach). At 9 months, two dimensions (emotional tone and fearfulness) did not reveal MZ-DZ differences. Further, the pattern of age-related changes within dimensions was more similar within MZ pairs than within DZ pairs.

Molecular Genetics: Future research with molecular genetics techniques may provide insight into temperament. Molecular genetics currently is being applied to the study of individuals with severe behavioral and psychological pathologies. Rather than treating all behavior as genetically determined, the molecular genetics model assumes that various behavioral and psychological pathologies are genetically determined (Vandenburg, Singer, & Pauls, 1986). An alternative approach is to study the behavioral patterns of individuals with confirmed genetic anomalies. Molecular genetic techniques not only identify specific anomalies but also can assess their severity. For example, with the fragile X syndrome, molecular genetic techniques can assess the degree of fragility of the X chromosome.

Recent research suggests that males with the fragile X syndrome have a temperament profile that distinguishes them from other developmentally delayed children. Goldson and Hagerman (1992) reported that fragile X males have a unique temperament characterized by poor adaptability, poor attention, high activity levels, low persistence, and resistance to approach.

A molecular genetic approach to temperament is complicated and does not necessarily assume a one-to-one correspondence between genes and the expressed temperament even with populations exhibiting severe behavioral pathologies. If temperament was determined partially or even completely by genetic factors, it still could be influenced by the environment. It is known that various genetic anomalies can respond to environmental factors. For example, dietary treatment of phenylketonuria is used to prevent severe retardation. It is possible that unique biochemical profiles underlie various temperament profiles. These biochemical conditions might be influenced by environmental factors (e.g., diet, stress, illness, drugs, pollutants, etc.). Thus, within the molecular genetics approach, individual differences in behavior still could exist that would not be genetically determined.

WESTERN PHYSIOLOGICAL APPROACHES: PHYSIOLOGICAL BASIS ASSESSED

As stated, temperament traditionally has been assessed via maternal report questionnaires while the underlying physiology has been assumed but not measured. Even behavioral genetics research of temperament is dependent on either the maternal questionnaire or other observations of behavior and uses the twin paradigm to infer genetic influences. However, these questionnaires need not be relied on. Various biological systems can be measured to provide a profile of the individual. The following sections describe other physiological systems that may influence the behavioral patterns associated with temperament.

One of the earliest attempts to link physiology and early behavioral patterns with subsequent infant and child behavioral patterns was the Fels Longitudinal Research project (Kagan & Moss, 1962). Psychophysiological studies from the Fels project attempted to identify stable psychophysiological response patterns that distinguished be-

havior along a dimension of impulsivity and reflectivity. Brief descriptions of recent studies assessing the physiology of temperament follow. (For a review, see Gunnar, 1990.)

Asymmetry of Brain Function: Two theories (Davidson & Fox, 1982; Kinsbourne & Bemporad, 1984) have posited a relationship between hemispheric laterality and temperament. Kinsbourne and Bemporad have associated the left frontotemporal cortex with activity and the right with arousal. The left region is concerned with actions on the external world while the right region is concerned with emotional reaction. Support for the theory comes from research on the effects of brain damage. Individuals with damage to the right frontal cortex exhibit emotional disinhibition. Further, Luria (1966) demonstrated an association between left-hemisphere damage and inaction or apathy and an association between right-hemisphere damage and inability to regulate emotional/social behavior. Finally, support is seen in the fact that the right hemisphere matures earlier than the left and infants exhibit chiefly emotional reactions to stimuli rather than acting upon the external world.

Davidson and Fox (1982; Fox & Davidson, 1984) also have proposed a theory relating brain laterality to temperament. The left hemisphere is associated with positive affect and approach behaviors whereas the right hemisphere is associated with negative affect and avoidance behaviors. Electroencephalogram recordings of the left and right frontal and parietal lobes in 10-month-old infants demonstrated frontal asymmetry in which greater left frontal activity was observed in response to a video of positive affect. Similarly, electroencephalogram recordings in newborns revealed greater left versus right activity accompanying an approach response to a sugar stimulus and greater right versus left activity accompanying the response to water. Recently, Fox and Davidson (1988) examined electroencephalograms in 10-month-old infants before and during episodes of stranger approach and maternal separation. Infants who cried during the stressful situations exhibited greater right frontal activation (associated with negative affect) than did noncrying infants.

Neuroregulatory Amines: Sostek, Sostek, Murphy, Martin, and Born (1981) examined monoamine oxidase and plasma amine oxidase assays on newborns in relation to their performance on the Neonatal Behavioral Assessment Scale (Brazelton, 1984). Infants with lower levels of monoamine oxidase exhibited higher arousal levels and lower consolability during testing. Infants with higher amine oxidase levels exhibited irritability earlier in the procedure than those with lower levels. Thus, monoamine oxidase and amine oxidase levels were shown to relate to the infant's alertness, arousal, and distress.

Physiological Arousal: Campos, Emde, Gaensbauer, and Henderson (1975) measured heart rate changes in infants in response to strangers. Heart rate increases were associated with high levels of arousal. Field (1981) similarly demonstrated increases in infant heart rate during face-to-face interactions when gaze aversion was present.

Adrenocortical Activity: Gunnar and colleagues (Gunnar, Connors, & Isensee, 1989; Gunnar, Connors, Isensee, & Wall, 1988) have studied negative emotionality and the adrenocortical system. Gunnar et al. (1988) measured cortisol levels in newborns following noxious and less noxious stressors. Although infants continued to exhibit behavioral distress to the less noxious stressors with repeated trials, the increase in cortisol level disappeared with repetition. The authors concluded that activation of the adrenocortical system is based on a response to the novelty or uncertainty associated with the events rather than a negative emotional response. A similar finding was obtained with 3- to 4-year-olds who received repeated blood-drawing sessions. Although children still exhibited behavioral distress to clinic visits in which blood was to be drawn, after repeated visits the cortisol level no longer was elevated. Again, it appears that the novelty aspect, not the negative emotionality, triggers the adrenocortical response.

SOVIET PHYSIOLOGICAL APPROACHES: PHYSIOLOGICAL BASIS ASSESSED

The Soviet and Western approaches to studying the physiology-temperament relationship are somewhat different (Gray, 1983). Whereas the Western approach is to study individual differences in behaviors and to then generate a theory of underlying physiology, the Soviet approach is to study individual differences in physiology and to then relate these to various personality types. For example, the Soviet (Mangan & Paisey, 1983) and Warsaw (Strelau, 1983a, 1983b) theories of temperament are based on the model that temperament can be described in terms of Pavlov's typology derived from nervous system properties.

Pavlov's initial temperament typology related the four Hippocratic temperaments—sanguine, phlegmatic, choleric, melancholic—to various combinations of the three nervous system properties of strength, balance between inhibition and excitation, and mobility or lability. A strong nervous system with an appropriate balance between central excitation and inhibition produced the normal stable temperaments (i.e., sanguine or phlegmatic). However, if the nervous system was strong and unbalanced or weak, it produced the pathological temperaments (i.e., choleric and melancholic).

Pavlov's temperament typology was based on observations of individual differences in dogs tested in the salivary conditioning experiments. However, the typology has been used to classify humans and reflects a recognition that internal differences, and not solely environmental constraints, contribute to individual differences in behavior. Thus, Pavlov departed from strict dependence on the external environment and included constitution as a determinant of behavior (Pavlov, 1928, pp. 370–378). In his latest writings, Pavlov used the terms *congenital* or *innate* rather than *inherited* types because innate properties of the nervous system may be influenced by prenatal and/or very early postnatal environmental conditions. (See Corson & Corson, 1976, p. 40.)

Neo-Pavlovian researchers have extended Pavlov's work to the study of individual differences in nervous system properties in humans. Shlyakhta and Panteleyeva (cited in Mangan & Paisey, 1983) found evidence of genetic contribution to the strength of the nervous system (i.e., MZ-DZ differences) in a reaction-time task and in an electroencephalogram-photic driving task. Two studies of the heritability of nervous system mobility found greater MZ than DZ similarity in electromyograph latencies (Panteleyeva, cited in Mangan & Paisey, 1983) and in a transformation task (Vasiletz, cited in Mangan & Paisey, 1983).

The Warsaw group's research (Strelau, 1983a, 1983b) has focused on providing "a psychological interpretation of Pavlov's notions" (1983b, p. 147). The work describes the regulative nature of Pavlov's nervous system properties and centers on the regulation of energy level in behavior, specifically activity and reactivity patterns. Their reactivity measure resembles Pavlov's measure of nervous system strength, with low reactivity relating to extreme endurance to strong stimulation (Pavlov's "strong" system) and high reactivity relating to sensory or emotional sensitivity (Pavlov's "weak" system). Strelau's work serves somewhat as a bridge between traditional Soviet typological research/theory and traditional Western behavioral research/theory.

BRIDGING THE GAP BETWEEN WESTERN AND SOVIET PHYSIOLOGICAL APPROACHES

In addition to the work of Strelau, Gray (1983) also bridges Soviet and Western approaches to the physiology-temperament relationship. Gray takes the Western approach of describing the individual differences in behavior to be explained (e.g., Eysenck's factor-analytic description of personality) but takes the Soviet approach to explaining these behaviors in physiological terms. The behavior and underlying physiology in question in Gray's work are anxiety and its neurophysiological correlates. Gray has mapped his construct of a "behavioral inhibition system" onto the septo-hippocampal system and connected structures. Much of the support for this work comes from pharmacological studies in which anti-anxiety drugs are shown to inhibit behavioral measures of anxiety as well as activity in the septo-hippocampal system (Gray, 1982). In his model, signals of punishment, signals of nonreward, and novel stimuli activate the behavioral inhibition system, which in turn produces behavioral manifestations of anxiety (operationalized as behavioral inhibition, increased arousal, and increased attention). While Gray's work has centered solely on anxiety, it represents a sophisticated and well-balanced approach to the study of the physiology-temperament relationship.

A New Physiological Model of Temperament

THE ROLE OF REFLEXES IN THE PHYSIOLOGY OF TEMPERAMENT

Historically, the literature on the biological bases of temperament consistently accepts that reflexes are dependent on the constitutional status of the nervous system. For example, both Galton (1869) and Watson (1930), who had diametrically opposed views of temperament, assumed that reflexes were innate. Galton emphasized the role of individual differences in relating reflexes and motor response speeds to variations in mental performance. In contrast, Watson did not acknowledge that individual differences in the nervous system were related to behavior (with the possible exception of severe damage of the nervous system resulting in behavioral pathology). Watson's views were shared by many researchers who thought that individual differences were due not to individual differences in nervous system organization but rather to measurement error and differences in environmentally determined motivation.

In contrast, Soviet psychology focused on the measurement of the physiological reflexes associated with orienting and classical conditioning to classify individuals. The strength and persistence of these reflexes were used to characterize individuals as having "strong" or "weak" nervous systems. The nervous system characteristics inferred from these conditioning studies were assumed to be persistent and to reflect innate characteristics. Not only were the behavioral correlates of these classifications studied, but pharmacological manipulations were attempted to change the physiological response patterns and behavior, thus emphasizing the Soviet assumption that personality and temperament were dependent on the "reflexive" nature of the nervous system.

STATEMENT OF THE MODEL

Our view of temperament merges these two approaches. Although environmental factors influence behavior, their effectiveness is dependent on constitutional factors. The nervous system in its control of physiological and behavioral responses plays a mediational role allocating resources and coordinating reflexes to deal with internal need states and external challenges. These mediational or regulatory characteristics of the nervous system are the individual differences that we view as the physiological basis of temperament. Just as Schneirla (1959) proposed that behavior could be described in terms of approach and withdrawal, we, too, use approach and withdrawal as global behavioral dimensions. The study of temperament can be capsulized into the study of the organism's pattern of approach and withdrawal to various types of stimulation. Emotion, motion, and vocal communication are the means by which the individual approaches or withdraws from animate and inanimate objects in the environment. Attention regulation, emotional regulation, and behavioral regulation are processes that underlie these responses.

We assume an "S-O-R" model to explain temperament. This model incorporates features of mechanistic (behaviorist) and organismic approaches. From a mechanistic approach, the S, or stimulus conditions of the visceral or external environment, are a determinant of behavior. In the model, behavior is denoted by the R, or response. The sequence of Rs provides observable behavioral patterns from which measures of temperament are usually derived. However, in this model, the S is not the sole determinant of behavior. Rather, the characteristics of the organism (O) expressed in nervous system function and organization mediate the impact of the environment (S) on behavior (R). The O may be assessed via the monitoring of continuously occurring visceral reflexes associated with homeostasis. Unlike other models of temperament that are based on measurement of behavior (R), this model focuses on the O as a physiological basis for temperament.

This approach was outlined initially as a hierarchical model relating physiological organization and regulation to behavior (Porges, 1983). The model has four major levels, each level being based upon the preceding level of organization and reflecting the condition of the nervous system. Level 1 represents the reflexive organization within a specific physiological system. Level 2 represents the coordination of physiological systems to maintain homeostasis and to adjust in response to both visceral and environmental challenges. Level 3 reflects the organization of overt behavior. Level 4 reflects the coordination of the social dyad.

Although most temperament models focus on the assessment of behavioral activity-reactivity levels and social behavior (i.e., Levels 3 and 4), this model suggests that these temperament dimensions may be dependent on individual differences in the physiological response systems defining Levels 1 and 2. We propose that the study of specific physiological reflexes (Level 1) and the factors that modulate these reflexes (Level 2) will provide markers for temperament. Measurable reflexes provide information regarding the nervous system because reflexes reflect the feedback characteristics of the central control of the periphery. In any reflex, an afferent (sensory) fiber conveys nerve impulses to the central nervous system, which in turn stimulates an effector (motor) fiber to produce the simple and appropriate action. Reflexes cannot operate unless the proper synaptic connections between afferent and efferent fibers are established in the central nervous system. By studying autonomic reflexes, as Pavlov did, it is possible to quantify the latency, amplitude, and recovery of reflexive behavior.

The selection of a particular reflex is critical in characterizing the nervous system organization underlying temperament. Pavlov's selection of the salivary reflex limited him to the study of event-elicited reflexes and not the spontaneous reflexes related to homeostatic regulation that we will describe. Our approach differs from Pavlov's in developing methods to evaluate the spontaneous homeostatic reflexes themselves and in examining how these reflexes change in response to a variety of sensory, emotional, and cognitive challenges. Moreover, our model provides a physiological explanation for Rothbart's temperament model (Rothbart, 1989; Rothbart & Derryberry, 1981), which emphasizes the dimensions of reactivity and self-regulation.

THE REFLEXIVE NATURE OF RESPIRATORY SINUS ARRHYTHMIA

Homeostatic processes are regulated by reflexes dependent on neural feedback. Information received at the periphery is transmitted to the central nervous system to stimulate appropriate physiological activity. Feedback loops, typical of many homeostatic processes, produce a rhythmic pattern characterized by phasic increases and decreases in neural efferent output to organs such as the heart. In many physiological systems, efficient neural control is manifested as rhythmic physiological variability. Within normal parameters the greater the amplitude of oscillation, the healthier the individual.

The autonomic nervous system, which is divided into two branches, the sympathetic and the parasympathetic, regulates homeostasis. In general, homeostatic processes are regulated primarily by the parasympathetic nervous system via the vagus nerve. The vagus is a large nerve with numerous branches communicating with many of the visceral organs. Approximately 80% of the parasympathetic nervous system is associated with the vagus and approximately 70% of the vagus is afferent. The vagus has a left and a right branch. Each branch has two source nuclei with fibers originating either in the dorsal motor nucleus (DMN) or the nucleus ambiguus (NA). The NA vagus is related to the expression of emotion, motion, and communication. The DMN vagus is related to regulation of respiratory and digestive processes. Porges (1995) has traced the evolutionary history of the NA vagus and the DMN vagus and provided a polyvagal model relating the workings of the vagal systems to behavioral responses.

Our research has focused on the quantification of respiratory sinus arrhythmia, a spontaneously occurring "reflex" in which respiratory afferents both peripherally and centrally modulate the medullary vagal efferents to the heart. Respiratory sinus arrhythmia is observed in the heart rate pattern as rhythmic variability at the frequency of respiration. Similar to other reflexes, the amplitude of respiratory sinus arrhythmia reflects a characteristic of the nervous system. The amplitude maps into the amount of efferent control of the heart via the right vagus nerve and thus serves as an index of neural regulation. The continuous reflexive nature of respiratory sinus arrhythmia provides an accurate index of cardiac vagal tone. Special statistical procedures have been developed to calculate an accurate estimate of the instantaneous cardiac vagal tone (Porges, 1985). Respiratory sinus arrhythmia is determined almost exclusively by the NA portion of the right vagus. The portion of the vagus originating in the NA regulates not only the heart but also the soft palate, pharynx, larynx, and esophagus. Changes in respiratory sinus arrhythmia in response to sensory, cognitive, and visceral challenges represent a "central command" to regulate the heart, soft palate, pharynx, larynx, and esophagus. In regulating metabolic output by shifting heart rate and by the production of vocalizations, these changes support the expression of emotion, motion, and communication.

When there are no challenging environmental demands, the autonomic nervous system, through the vagus, services the needs of the internal viscera to enhance growth and restoration. However, in response to environmental demands, homeostatic processes are compromised and the autonomic nervous system supports increased metabolic output to deal with these external challenges by vagal withdrawal and sympathetic excitation. The central nervous system, by mediating the distribution of resources, regulates the strength and latency of autonomic responses to deal with internal and external demands. Perceptions and assumed threats to survival, independent of the actual physical characteristics of the stimulation, may promote a massive withdrawal of parasympathetic tone and a reciprocal excitation of sympathetic tone. The central nervous system monitors and regulates this trade-off between internal and external needs.

SUMMARY OF THE MODEL

Our model of temperament focuses on the state of the organism by monitoring central regulation of autonomic reflexes. Specifically, the model evaluates both the "strength" of the reflex and the ability to modulate the reflex in response to definable challenges. Although the research generated by this model focuses on the measurement of heart rate patterns, the physiological and statistical approach enables strong statements regarding the central control of the reflex. First, high-amplitude respiratory sinus arrhythmia reflects a strong reflex. Second, the ability to modulate the strength of the respiratory sinus arrhythmia reflex in response to external or visceral conditions reflects the central control associated with resource allocation.

In testing our model of temperament, we have been assessing empirically whether individuals with low vagal tone and/or difficulties in regulating vagal tone will have problems with approach-withdrawal behaviors in the expression of emotion, motion, and communication. The potential to express emotion, move, and communicate enables an individual to maneuver along a continuum of approach-withdrawal with the environment. A number of behaviors are critical to this function, including dimensions of reactivity, sustained attention, and behavioral and affective self-regulation. In the following sections we present the relevant research, divided by subject age groups into neonatal research and infant research.

Vagal Tone Research

OVERVIEW

We have developed a measure of respiratory sinus arrhythmia known as the vagal tone index ($\hat{V}$). $\hat{V}$ is dependent on the amplitude of respiratory sinus arrhythmia, a spontaneous visceral reflex. However, the instantaneous amplitude or strength of the reflex is dependent on endogenous afferent-efferent feedback and the ability of central structures to regulate the visceral feedback and to dampen or amplify the reflex. In this hierarchical model of temperament, individual differences in neural regulation determine autonomic reactivity and regulation and are reflected in individual differences in behavioral reactivity and self-regulation. A number of studies have evaluated individual differences in both level and regulation of vagal tone. These studies, collectively, are providing support for our model.

NEONATAL RESEARCH

Studies using the vagal tone index have agreed that vagal tone is an index of reactivity. Porter, Porges, and Marshall (1988) showed in a sample of normal newborns that individual differences in

base-level vagal tone are correlated with heart rate reactivity to circumcision. Neonates with higher vagal tone exhibited not only larger heart rate accelerations but also lower fundamental cry frequencies to the surgical procedures. Lower fundamental cry frequencies have been hypothesized to be associated with greater vagal influences. (See Lester & Zeskind, 1982.) Consistent with these findings, Porter and Porges (1988) also demonstrated in premature infants that individual differences in vagal tone are related to heart rate response during lumbar puncture procedures.

Behavioral reactivity and irritability to environmental stimuli measured with the Neonatal Behavioral Assessment Scale (Brazelton, 1984) also are associated with vagal tone. In a sample of full-term healthy neonates, DiPietro, Larson, and Porges (1987) found that infants with higher vagal tone were more reactive and required more effort to test. When these same infants were tested at 15 months (Larson, Porges, & DiPietro, 1990), the infants who had the higher neonatal vagal tone scored higher on the Mental Development Index of the Bayley scales (Bayley, 1969) and were more motorically active and better coordinated. With heterogeneous groups of low- and high-risk preterm and full-term neonates, Fox and Porges (1985) also reported a relationship between neonatal cardiac vagal tone and the Mental Development Index at 8 and 12 months of age.

Neonatal vagal tone is related to 3-year outcome measures. Doussard-Roosevelt, Porges, Scanlon, Alemi, and Scanlon (in press) reported that the base-level vagal tone of very low birthweight infants, monitored in the neonatal intensive care unit, was related to follow-up measures in the areas of mental processing, social skills, and motor skills. Infants who had higher vagal tone performed better on the Mental Processing Composite of the Kaufman Assessment Battery for Children (Kaufman & Kaufman, 1983) at 3 years of age. Moreover, those infants who exhibited an increase in vagal tone from 33 to 35 weeks postconceptional age had better social and motor skills at 3 years of age.

In addition to base-level vagal tone, vagal tone reactivity in response to environmental demands also has been investigated. Although typically, appropriate reactivity is viewed as withdrawal of vagal tone in response to external demands, the appropriate vagal tone response is not always characterized by a suppression of vagal tone. For example, in the neonatal intensive care unit, the appropriate response to gavage feeding has been characterized as an increase in vagal tone consistent with support of digestive processes (DiPietro & Porges, 1991). Preterm neonates who demonstrated an increase in vagal tone during gavage feeding and a decrease after feeding had significantly shorter hospitalizations. Higher base-level vagal tone was associated with greater weight gain during the neonatal intensive care unit stay. Thus, healthier neonates exhibited both high vagal tone and appropriate vagal reactivity.

In summary, the neonatal research supports our model in which the organism's response to environmental challenges (e.g., circumcision, lumbar puncture procedures, the Neonatal Behavioral Assessment Scale, feeding) is mediated by the organism's physiology. Neonates with strong respiratory sinus arrhythmia reflexes (high cardiac vagal tone) exhibit appropriate autonomic, physiological, and behavioral responses (heart rate acceleration, crying, irritability, weight gain) to stimulation. The longitudinal research suggests that strong neonatal respiratory sinus arrhythmia reflexes are associated with better outcome. Further, neonates who demonstrate appropriate modulation of autonomic reflex strength in response to stimulation (vagal reactivity) are generally healthier, as demonstrated by the negative relationship between vagal reactivity and length of hospitalization in the gavage study. In general, healthier neonates exhibit higher vagal tone and appropriate vagal reactivity.

INFANT RESEARCH

Huffman, Bryan, del Carmen, Pedersen, and Porges (1992) addressed the relationship between vagal tone and temperament in 3-month old infants. The Infant Behavior Questionnaire (Rothbart, 1981) was used as well as laboratory ratings of temperament with the Garcia-Coll Behavioral Responsiveness Paradigm (B. Garcia-Coll et al., 1988). There were no significant relations between the Infant Behavior Questionnaire factors and Behavioral Responsiveness Paradigm behavioral measures, suggesting that the two measures of temperament were tapping independent processes. The vagal tone data were also consistent with this apparent independence. Base-level vagal

tone was significantly correlated with lab ratings (Behavioral Responsiveness Paradigm) of negativity and soothability. Infants with higher vagal tone were less negative and required less calming.

In contrast, the factors of the maternal reports (Infant Behavior Questionnaire) were related to vagal tone reactivity in response to the Behavioral Responsiveness Paradigm and not to base-level vagal tone. The Behavioral Responsiveness Paradigm procedure is a series of vignettes incorporating visual, auditory, and tactile stimuli. Infants who suppressed vagal tone during the paradigm were rated by their mothers as having longer duration of orienting, more frequent smiling and laughing, and greater ease of soothability as compared with infants who failed to suppress vagal tone. Thus, the Behavioral Responsiveness Paradigm was related to base-level vagal tone, and the maternal ratings on the Infant Behavior Questionnaire were sensitive to the regulatory nature of the infant's control of the autonomic nervous system. This regulatory nature should be related to a variety of behaviors, including social engagement and attention.

Stifter, Fox, and Porges (1989) have reported a relationship between vagal tone and facial expressivity. Higher base-level vagal tone is associated with greater emotional expressivity in 5-month-olds. Linnemeyer and Porges (1986) discovered that 6-month-old infants with higher base-level vagal tone were more likely to look longer at novel visual stimuli than familiar stimuli, demonstrating greater visual attention. In addition, only those infants with high vagal tone exhibited significant heart rate reactivity to the visual stimuli. Richards (1985, 1987) has offered convergent findings that infants with higher levels of respiratory sinus arrhythmia were less distractible and had larger decelerative heart rate responses to visual stimuli. Richards and Cameron (1989) reported that infants with higher levels of respiratory sinus arrhythmia were rated higher on the approach subscale of the Infant Temperament Questionnaire (Carey & McDevitt, 1978).

DiPietro, Porges, and Uhly (1992) have reported that the pattern of vagal tone reactivity to a novel stimulus at 8 months is related to developmental competence. They reported that the vagal tone response pattern to a novel stimulus was associated with the quality of play exhibited during an exploratory play session. Infants who responded to the stimulus with an increase in vagal tone more often engaged in more mature cognitive behaviors, characterized by focused examination and a greater range of exploratory play, than infants who responded with a decrease in vagal tone.

According to Greenspan (1991), infants older than 6 months of age who exhibit fussiness, irritability, poor self-calming, intolerance to change, and a hyperalert state of arousal are termed *regulatory-disordered infants*. These infants are often hyper- or hyposensitive to sensory stimuli, including auditory, tactile, visual, gustatory, and vestibular stimulation. DeGangi, DiPietro, Greenspan, and Porges (1991) evaluated differences in psychophysiological functioning between normal controls and regulatory-disordered infants who were 8 to 11 months of age. They reported a tendency for the regulatory-disordered infants to have high base-level vagal tone. More important, while the normal controls exhibited a significant relationship between base-level vagal tone and degree of vagal tone suppression during the cognitive task (i.e., higher base-level vagal tone related to greater reduction in vagal tone during the task), the regulatory-disordered infants exhibited changes in vagal tone unrelated to base-level vagal tone. The high base-level vagal tone was consistent with the high degree of behavioral reactivity observed in the regulatory-disordered infants. Moreover, the difficulties in vagal tone suppression during cognitive challenge were consistent with the defining deficits in behavioral and physiological regulation of the regulatory-disordered infant. Follow-up data at 4 years were consistent with the infant data. Difficulties in reactivity and regulation observed during infancy were exacerbated at 4 years. DeGangi, Porges, Sickel, and Greenspan (1992) reported that 8 of the 9 regulatory-disordered children had developmental, sensorimotor, and/or emotional and behavioral problems at 4 years.

Additional research has been conducted with regulatory-disordered infants. Doussard-Roosevelt, Walker, Portales, Greenspan, and Porges (1990) report findings with infants 7 to 11 months of age that are consistent with the findings of DeGangi et al. that regulatory-disordered infants have higher vagal tone than normal infants. And again, regulation of vagal tone was correlated with base-level vagal tone only for the normal control subjects. The findings support the hypothesis that the regulatory-disordered infant has specific underlying physiological characteristics consistent with the observed behaviors.

A 3-year follow-up study on this sample (Porges, Doussard-Roosevelt, Portales, & Greenspan, in press) identified the 9-month vagal tone measures as the strongest predictors of outcome behavior. Infants who at 9 months of age had higher base-level vagal tone and who exhibited greater vagal suppression during administration of the Bayley Scales of Infant Development (Bayley, 1969) had fewer behavioral problems at 3 years of age. Higher base-level vagal tone was related to fewer sleep problems (r (22) $= -0.57$) and less depressive behavior (r (22) $= -0.43, p < 0.05$) on the Child Behavior Checklist (Achenbach, 1988). Further, greater suppression of vagal tone was associated with more optimal outcomes on the three narrow-band syndrome scales associated with social behavior (Social Withdrawal, Depressed, and Aggressive behavior). Greater decreases in vagal tone were related to fewer social withdrawal problems (r (22) $= -0.42, p < 0.05$), fewer depressed behaviors (r (22) $= -0.45, p < 0.05$), and fewer aggressive behaviors, (r (22) $= -0.53, p < 0.01$). Greater decreases in vagal tone were also associated with fewer behavior problems overall as is reflected in the Child Behavior Checklist Total Score (r (22) $= -0.50, p < 0.05$). Of interest, measures of infant temperament derived from maternal reports (Infant Characteristics Questionnaire; Bates, 1984) were not related to the 3-year outcome measures. These findings suggest that the vagal tone measure provides a robust index of physiological regulation related to behavior and it may be more sensitive to developmental outcome and more characteristic of temperament than maternal reports of temperament.

In summary, the infant research provides support for our model that responses to the environment are mediated by individual differences in physiology. In general, infants with strong respiratory sinus arrhythmia reflexes (i.e., high base-level vagal tone) exhibit greater soothability, better visual attention, more approach behaviors, and greater emotional expressivity. However, a small subset of infants with strong respiratory sinus arrhythmia reflexes have regulation problems (i.e., problems related to regulation of emotion, attention, digestion, arousal, and sleep). These regulatory-disordered infants have difficulties regulating vagal tone in response to visceral and external stimulation. Poor vagal reactivity during infancy predicted behavioral problems at 3 years of age. In contrast, infants who displayed appropriate modulation of reflex strength in response to stimulation (vagal reactivity) exhibited better attention, more frequent positive affect, greater soothability, and more mature cognitive behaviors during exploratory play. Thus, low vagal tone and/or difficulties in vagal reactivity are associated with emotional and attentional problems during infancy and are risk factors for behavioral and cognitive outcomes.

Stability of Vagal Tone: We have recently evaluated the stability of the vagal tone measures (Porges, Doussard-Roosevelt, Portales, & Suess, 1994). Base-level vagal tone, suppression of vagal tone during developmental testing, and maternal perceptions of difficult temperament were assessed at 9 months and at 3 years of age. Vagal tone was stable when assessed during baseline (r (24) = 0.55) as well as developmental testing (r (24) = 0.69). Maternal perceptions of difficult temperament were also stable across this time period (r (24) = 0.71). At 9 months difficulties was correlated with higher vagal tone during baseline (r (24) = 0.43) and during testing (r (24) = 0.46). In contrast, difficultness at 3 years was related to lower baseline vagal tone. With the shared variance of 9-month vagal tone and 9-month difficultness partialed out, 9-month vagal tone remains a significant predictor of difficultness at 3 years (r (13) = −0.60).

A good measure should reflect the intra-individual variation associated with stimulus manipulations as well as have the capacity to identify stable individual differences. Vagal tone is consistent with these criteria. It has been demonstrated to be a sensitive reflection of the organism's responsivity to environmental challenges. Further, our preliminary research on the stability of the measure suggests that base-level vagal tone is stable from 9 to 36 months.

Conclusions

Vagal regulation has been cast as a primary substrate of organized behaviors to support the expression of emotion, motion, and communication. The individual can orchestrate this cluster of behaviors to either approach or withdraw from both animate and inanimate objects. This hierarchial approach assumes that individual differences in the physiological substrate will be reflected in the "higher" levels of behavior. However, behavior also can be modified by extra-physiological approaches, such as learning and conditioning. Thus, although pathology in the physiological substrate will always produce deviant behavior, deviant behavior need not always have a physiological substrate.

We have emphasized a specific biological substrate of temperament, respiratory sinus arrhythmia reflex strength and modulation. Vagal tone and vagal regulation are presented as indices of reflex strength and flexibility. While vagal regulation provides a physiological measure of temperament's constitutional basis, we have not argued that vagal regulation is genetically determined. Although genetics may play a role in the neurological function and neuroanatomical structure of the nervous system, other factors may alter the genetic expression. Our research with high-risk and preterm neonates provides a substantial data base to demonstrate that environmental constraints may contribute to individual differences in central regulation of vagal function. For example, potent environmental factors such as perinatal hypoxia can destroy the fine myelinated fibers of the vagal system and compromise vagal regulation.

The effects of pharmacological treatments on vagal tone are understood. In the healthy individual, any drug that has cholinergic influences may potentiate the strength of the vagal reflex (i.e., respiratory sinus arrhythmia), while any anticholinergic drug may attenuate reflex strength. However, the influence of drugs on regulation of vagal reflexes is not understood and has not been studied. It is possible that various drugs that enhance appropriate approach-withdrawal behavior also might enhance vagal regulation. This might explain the presumed paradoxical effects of stimulant drugs on children with attention deficit disorder. Research with heart rate variability (an estimate of vagal tone) suggests that methylphenidate (Ritalin) fostered vagal regulation in a sample of children with attention deficit disorder. Heart rate variability was suppressed during an attention-demanding task only when the children were medicated (Porges, Walter, Korb, & Sprague, 1975). Thus, although stimulant drugs are assumed not to have peripheral parasympathetic (including the vagus) effects, the drugs may influence central regulation of the vagus via complex sites of action.

Our model shares many attributes with both historical and contemporary approaches. We view specific physiological reflexes as reflecting integrative and organizational qualities of the nervous system. Both Galton and Pavlov shared this view. Galton assumed that motor response time indexed the central nervous system's processing of information. Pavlov assumed that the strength and stability of conditioned reflexes provided a similar qualitative index of the nervous system. Although we share the general approach, our model has advantages. First, by studying the strength of a spontaneously occurring reflex, we can continuously monitor the organizational and regulatory strategy of the nervous system in dealing with homeostatic demands. This provides us with the ability to assess development. Second, we can evaluate the adaptiveness and flexibility (including conditionability) of vagal reflexes by evaluating the influence of visceral and environmental factors on the strength of the vagal reflex.

The vagal regulation model is also consistent with Greenspan's view (1991) of regulation disorders. Inherent in the regulatory-disordered classification is the construct of physiological regulation. For example, the nervous system must play an important role in the infant's accommodation to varying sensory challenges and the maintenance of homeostatic processes. The infant must be able to regulate sleep states, to digest food effectively, to self-soothe in response to changing sensory stimuli, to inhibit motor and physiological activity while focusing attention, and to be capable of contingent and appropriate responses to social stimuli. All these processes require a physiological response system that is governed effectively by appropriate neural feedback. Our model provides an important, and heretofore missing, measure of the mediating physiological system.

As described, regulatory-disordered infants display high base-level vagal tone but disorganized vagal reactivity. The regulatory-disordered infant has a strong vagal reflex but the reflex is not modulated reliably by the demands of the visceral or environmental factors. Without a properly responding vagal system, the infant exhibits a variety of problems with physiological homeostasis, including digestive and sleep disorders. Moreover,

the inability to reliably modulate the reflex and inhibit physiological homeostasis via systematic vagal withdrawal to deal with environmental demands is manifested in a variety of behavioral problems. For example, the regulatory-disordered infant exhibits problems in sustaining attention, focusing interest, expressing emotion, and exhibiting socially contingent behaviors in response to pertinent social and emotional cues. Thus, the clinical definition of the regulatory-disordered infant is congruent with our physiological definition of vagal regulation difficulties.

Other researchers have approached the question of autonomic regulation and temperament. Kagan and his associates (Kagan, Reznick, & Snidman, 1987) found that children who are behaviorally inhibited in social settings tend to have higher heart rates and lower heart rate variability. Kagan speculated that these features of autonomic state reflect individual differences in sympathetic excitation. Although we share an interest in autonomic regulation, a more plausible explanation of the physiological correlates is that the high heart rate and low heart rate variability reflect low vagal tone rather than sympathetic excitation. According to our model, individuals with weak vagal reflexes would have difficulty regulating behavior along the approach-withdrawal continuum. These individuals would not respond reliably to the environment and would exhibit the "shyness" or "behavioral inhibition" described by Kagan. In contrast, individuals with strong vagal reflexes (and the potential to regulate the reflexes adaptively to environmental and internal demands) would regulate their behavior successfully along the approach-withdrawal continuum.

Research with rhesus macaques supports this interpretation. Rasmussen, Fellowes, Byrne, and Suomi (1988) reported that adolescent rhesus macaques that emigrated early from their troop had a significantly higher vagal tone than did those that remained with their natal troop. By emigrating, the monkeys with a higher vagal tone appeared to be more outgoing, less fearful, and less vulnerable to social and environmental stresses. Convergent data come from Richards and Cameron (1989), who report a significant correlation between the strength of the vagal reflex (i.e., amplitude of respiratory sinus arrhythmia) at 14, 20, and 26 weeks and the approach scale of the Infant Temperament Questionnaire (Carey & McDevitt, 1978).

We have proposed that the neurophysiological organization of the individual, reflected in the strength and regulation of autonomic reflexes, provides a physiological index of temperament. However, unlike other models (see Chapter 27), our approach to defining temperament includes bidirectional influences between the environment and the individual's nervous system. We share the view that genetics contribute to temperament. However, our view, like recent systems approaches (Cairns, 1979; Thelen, 1989), incorporates the potential for dynamic interactions between environmental factors and physiology. As Gunnar (1990) states in her review of research on physiology-temperament relations, "the psychobiologist attempts to understand the organism as a whole and not as a functioning gene machine nor as an entity shaped by external forces" (p. 387). We believe that although genetics may limit the potential range of neurophysiological and neurochemical states, it is environmental factors that are able to potentiate or restrict their function and influence behavior. Thus, environmental influences may shift behavior along the dimensions of temperament.

Historically, temperament theorists have accepted the potential shift in behavior due to severe damage to the nervous system. Consistent with these views, potent environmental influences, such as perinatal events, nutrition, injury, illness, and substance abuse, certainly can have major impact on physiological systems and potentially change nervous system organization of autonomic function and behavior. However, in contrast to most theories, we propose that more subtle environmental factors also may restructure physiological organization. For example, chronic stress via poor social interactions or inadequate emotional support by the parent might change the underlying state of neurotransmitters and produce different "set points" or "thresholds" for the regulation of autonomic function and behavior. In changing the set point, the activity and reactivity of the child might shift from being calm to being highly active and reactive. We believe that future temperament theories and research should incorporate and evaluate the dynamic relationship between the individual and the environment.

In closing, our intention in writing this chapter was to emphasize three points: first, the importance of individual differences in physiological state and organization in regulating behavior; second, the potential dynamic relationship between the individual and the environment in the organization and regulation of the central nervous system and behavior; and third, the availability of specific measurement technologies that will enable direct research assessment of the relationship between central nervous system regulation and patterns of behavior.

REFERENCES

Achenbach, T. M. (1988). *Child Behavior Checklist for Ages 2–3*. Burlington, VT: University of Vermont.

Bates, J. E. (1980). The concept of difficult temperament. *Merrill-Palmer Quarterly, 26*, 299–319.

Bates, J. E. (1984). *Infant Characteristics Questionnaire*. Bloomington: Indiana University.

Bates, J. E. (1987). Temperament in infancy. In. J. D. Osofsky (Ed.), *Handbook of infant development: Changes, continuities and challenges* (pp. 1101–1149). New York: John Wiley & Sons.

Bates, J. E. (1989). Concepts and measures of temperament. In G. A. Kohnstamm, J. E. Bates, & M. K. Rothbart (Eds.), *Temperament in childhood* (pp. 3–26). New York: John Wiley & Sons.

Bates, J. E., & Bayles, K. (1984). Objective and subjective components in mother's perceptions of their children from age 6 months to 3 years. *Merrill-Palmer Quarterly, 30*, 11–130.

Bates, J. E., Freeland, C. A. B., & Lounsbury, M. L. (1979). Measurement of infant difficultness. *Child Development, 50*, 794–803.

Bayley, N. (1969). *Bayley Scales of Infant Development*. New York: Psychological Corporation.

Belsky, J., Fish, M., & Isabella, R. (1991). Continuity and discontinuity in infant negative and positive emotionality: Family antecedents and attachment consequences. *Developmental Psychology, 27*, 421–431.

Brazelton, T. B. (1984). *Neonatal Behavioral Assessment Scale* (2nd ed.). Philadelphia: J. B. Lippincott.

Buss, A. H., & Plomin, R. (1975). *A temperament theory of personality development*. New York: John Wiley & Sons.

Buss, A. H., & Plomin, R. (1984). *Temperament: Early developing personality traits*. Hillsdale, NJ: Lawrence Erlbaum.

Cairns, R. B. (1979). *Social development: The origins and plasticity of interchanges*. San Francisco: W. H. Freeman.

Campos, J. J., Emde, R., Gaensbauer, T., & Henderson, C. (1975). Cardiac and behavioral interrelationships in the reactions of infants to strangers. *Developmental Psychology, 11,* 589–601.

Carey, W. B. (1981). The importance of temperament-environment interaction for child health and development. In M. Lewis & L. A. Rosenblum (Eds.), *The uncommon child* (pp. 31–55). New York: Plenum Press.

Carey, W. B. (1983). Some pitfalls in infant temperament research. *Infant Behavior and Development, 6,* 247–254.

Carey, W. B., & McDevitt, S. C. (1978). Revision of the Infant Temperament Questionnaire. *Pediatrics, 61,* 735–739.

Clemens, L., Gladue, B., & Coniglio, L. (1978). Prenatal endogenous androgenic influences on masculine sexual behavior and genital morphology in male and female rats. *Hormones and Behavior, 10,* 40–53.

Corson, S. A., & Corson, E. O. (1976). Philosophical and historical roots of Pavlovian psychobiology. In S. A. Corson & E. O. Corson (Eds.), *Psychiatry and psychology in the USSR* (pp. 19–58). New York: Plenum Press.

Davidson, R. J, & Fox, N. A. (1982). Asymmetrical brain activity discriminates between positive and negative affective stimuli in human infants. *Science, 218,* 1235–1237.

DeGangi, G. A., DiPietro, J. A., Greenspan, S. I., & Porges, S. W, (1991). Psychophysiological characteristics of the regulatory disordered infant. *Infant Behavior and Development, 14,* 37–50.

DeGangi, G. A., Porges, S. W., Sickel, R. Z., & Greenspan, S. I. (1992). *The longitudinal outcomes of regulatory disordered infants.* Unpublished manuscript.

DiPietro, J. A., Larson, S. K., & Porges, S. W. (1987). Behavioral and heart-rate pattern differences between breast-fed and bottle-fed neonates. *Developmental Psychology, 23,* 467–474.

DiPietro, J. A., & Porges, S. W. (1991). Vagal responsiveness to gavage feeding as an index of preterm stress. *Pediatric Research, 29,* 231–236.

DiPietro, J. A., Porges, S. W., & Uhly, B. (1992). Reactivity and developmental competence in preterm and full-term infants. *Developmental Psychology, 28,* 831–841.

Doussard-Roosevelt, J. A., Porges, S. W., Scanlon, J. W., Alemi, B., & Scanlon, K. (In press). Vagal regulation of heart rate in the prediction of outcome for very low birth weight preterm neonates. *Child Development.*

Doussard-Roosevelt, J. A., Walker, P. S., Portales, A. L., Greenspan, S. L., & Porges, S. W. (1990). Vagal tone and the fussy infant: Atypical vagal reactivity in the difficult infant. *Infant Behavior and Development, 13,* 352.

Field, T. M. (1981). Infant gaze aversion and heart rate during face-to-face interactions. *Infant Behavior and Development, 4,* 307–315.

Field, T., & Greenberg, R. (1982). Temperament ratings by parents and teachers of infants, toddlers, and preschool children. *Child Development, 53,* 160–163.

Fox, N. A., & Davidson, R. J. (1984). Hemispheric substrates of affect: A developmental model. In N. A. Fox & R. J. Davidson (Eds.), *The psychology of affective development* (pp. 353–382). Hillsdale, NJ: Lawrence Erlbaum.

Fox, N. A., & Davidson, R. J. (1988). Patterns of brain electrical activity during facial signs of emotion in 10-month-old infants. *Developmental Psychology, 24,* 230–236.

Fox, N. A., & Porges, S. W. (1985). The relationship between neonatal heart period patterns and developmental outcome. *Child Development, 56,* 28–37.

Galton, F. (1869). *Hereditary genius.* London: Macmillan.

Garcia-Coll, C. T., Emmons, L., Vohr, B. R., Ward, A. M., Brann, B. S., Shaul, P. W., Mayfield, S. R., & Oh, W. (1988). Behavioral responsiveness in preterm infants with intraventricular hemorrhage. *Pediatrics, 81,* 412–418.

Goldsmith, H. H. (1983). Genetic influence on personality from infancy to adulthood. *Child Development, 54,* 331–355.

Goldsmith, H. H., Buss, A. H., Plomin, R., Rothbart, M. K., Thomas, A., Chess, S., Hinde, R. A., & McCall, R. B. (1987). Roundtable: What is temperament?: Four approaches. *Child Development, 58,* 505–529.

Goldsmith, H. H., & Campos, J. J. (1986). Fundamental issues in the study of early temperament: The Denver Twin Temperament study. In M. E. Lamb, A. L. Brown, & B. Rogoff (Eds.), *Advances in developmental psychology* (Vol. 4, pp. 231–283). Hillsdale, NJ: Lawrence Erlbaum.

Goldsmith, H. H., & Rieser-Danner, L. A. (1986). Variation among temperament theories and validation studies of temperament assessment. In G. A. Kohnstamm (Ed.), *Temperament discussed: Temperament and development in infancy and childhood* (pp. 1–9). Lisse, The Netherlands: Swets & Zeitlinger.

Goldsmith, H. H., & Rieser-Danner, L. A. (1990). Assessing early temperament. In C. R. Reynolds & R. W. Kamphaus (Eds.), *Handbook of psychological and educational assessment of children: Personality, behavior, and context* (pp. 245–278). New York: Guilford Press.

Goldson, E., & Hagerman, R. J. (1992). *Temperament and the fragile X syndrome.* Unpublished manuscript.

Gray, J. A. (1982). *The neuropsychology of anxiety: An enquiry into the functions of the septo-hippocampal system.* New York: Oxford University Press.

Gray, J. A. (1983). Anxiety, personality and the brain. In A. Gale & J. A. Edwards (Eds.), *Physiological correlates of human behavior: Individual differences and psychopathology* (Vol. 3, pp. 31–43). New York: Academic Press.

Greenspan, S. I. (1991). *Infancy and early childhood: The practice of clinical assessment and intervention with emotional and developmental challenges.* Madison, CT: International Universities Press.

Gunnar, M. R. (1990). The psychobiology of infant temperament. In J. Colombo & J. Fagen (Eds.), *Individ-*

ual differences in infancy (pp. 387–409). Hillsdale, NJ: Lawrence Erlbaum.

Gunnar, M. R., Connors, J., & Isensee, J. (1989). Lack of stability in neonatal adrenocortical reactivity because of rapid habituation of the adrenocortical response. *Developmental Psychobiology, 22,* 221–233.

Gunnar, M. R, Connors, J., Isensee, J., & Wall, L. (1988). Adrenocortical activity and behavioral distress in human newborns. *Developmental Psychobiology, 21,* 297–310.

Huffman, L. C., Bryan, Y. E., del Carmen, R., Pedersen, F. A., & Porges, S. W. (1992). *Autonomic correlates of reactivity and self-regulation at twelve weeks of age.* Unpublished manuscript.

Kagan, J., & Moss, H. A. (1962). *Birth to maturity: A study in psychological development.* New York: John Wiley & Sons.

Kagan, J., Reznick, J. S., & Snidman, N. (1987). The physiology and psychology of behavioral inhibition in children. *Child Development, 58,* 1459–1473.

Kaufman, A. S., & Kaufman, N. L. (1983). *Kaufman Assessment Battery for Children.* Circle Pines, MN: American Guidance Service.

Kinsbourne, M., & Bemporad, B. (1984). Lateralization of emotion: A model and the evidence. In N. A. Fox & R. J. Davidson (Eds.), *The psychology of affective development* (pp. 259–292). Hillsdale, NJ: Lawrence Erlbaum.

Larson, S. K., Porges, S. W., & DiPietro, J. A. (1990). *Neonatal psychophysiological assessment and 15-month developmental outcome of healthy full-term infants.* Unpublished manuscript.

Lester, B. M., & Zeskind, P. S. (1982). A biobehavioral perspective on crying in early infancy. In H. E. Fitzgerald, B. M. Lester, & M. W. Yogman (Eds.), *Theory and research in behavioral pediatrics* (pp. 133–180). New York: Plenum Press.

Linnemeyer, S. A., & Porges, S. W. (1986). Recognition memory and cardiac vagal tone in 6-month-old infants. *Infant Behavior and Development, 8,* 43–56.

Luria, A. R. (1966). *Higher cortical functions in man.* New York: Basic Books.

Lytton, H. (1977). Do parents create, or respond to, differences in twins? *Developmental Psychology, 13,* 456–459.

Mangan, G. L., & Paisey, T. J. H. (1983). Current perspectives in neo-Pavlovian temperament theory and research: A review. *Australian Journal of Psychology, 35,* 319–347.

Matheny, A. P., Jr. (1989). Children's behavioral inhibition over age and across situations: Genetic similarity for a trait during change. *Journal of Personality, 57,* 215–235.

McNeil, T. F., & Persson-Blennow, I. (1988). Stability of temperament characteristics in childhood. *American Journal of Orthopsychiatry, 58,* 622–626.

Pavlov, I. P. (1928). *Lectures on conditioned reflexes: Twenty-five years of objective study of the higher nervous activity (behavior) of animals,* by W. H. Gantt (Trans. and Ed.). New York: International Publishers.

Porges, S. W. (1983). Heart rate patterns in neonates: A potential diagnostic window to the brain. In T. Field & A. Sostek (Eds.), *Infants born at risk: Psychological, perceptual, and cognitive processes* (pp. 3–22). New York: Grune & Stratton.

Porges, S. W. (1985, April 16). Method and apparatus for evaluating rhythmic oscillations in aperiodic physiological response systems. U.S. Patent number: 4,510,944.

Porges, S. W. (1995). Orienting in a defensive world: Mammalian modifications of our evolutionary heritage. A polyvagal theory. *Psychophysiology, 32,* 301–318.

Porges, S. W., Doussard-Roosevelt, J. A., Portales, A. L., & Greenspan, S. I. (In press). Infant regulation of the vagal brake predicts child behavior problems: A psychobiological model of social behavior. *Developmental Psychology.*

Porges, S. W., Doussard-Roosevelt, J. A., Portales, A. L., & Suess, P. E. (1994). Cardiac vagal tone: Stability and relation to difficultness in infants and 3-year-olds. *Developmental Psychobiology, 27,* 289–300.

Porges, S. W., Walter, G. F., Korb, J., & Sprague, R. L. (1975). The influence of methylphenidate on heart rate and behavioral measures of attention in hyperactive children. *Child Development, 46,* 727–733.

Portales, A. L., Doussard-Roosevelt, J. A., & Porges, S. W. (1991, November). *Nine-month cardiac vagal tone reactivity predicts three-year cognitive development and sensorimotor problems.* Paper presented at the Virginia Developmental Forum, Washington, DC.

Porter, F. L., & Porges, S. W. (1988). Neonatal cardiac responses to lumbar puncture. *Infant Behavior and Development, 11,* 261.

Porter, F. L., Porges, S. W., & Marshall, R. E. (1988). Newborn pain cries and vagal tone: Parallel changes in response to circumcision. *Child Development, 59,* 495–505.

Rasmussen, K. L. R., Fellowes, J. R., Byrne, E., & Suomi, S. J. (1988). Heart rate measures associated with early emigration in adolescent male rhesus macaques (Macaca mulatta). *American Journal of Primatology, 14,* 439.

Richards, J. E. (1985). Respiratory sinus arrhythmia predicts heart rate and visual responses during visual attention in 14 and 20 week old infants. *Psychophysiology, 22,* 101–109.

Richards, J. E. (1987). Infant visual sustained attention and respiratory sinus arrhythmia. *Child Development, 58,* 488–496.

Richards, J. E., & Cameron, D. (1989). Infant heart rate variability and behavioral developmental status. *Infant Behavior and Development, 12,* 45–58.

Rothbart, M. K. (1981). Measurement of temperament in infancy. *Child Development, 52,* 569–578.

Rothbart, M. K. (1986). Longitudinal observation of infant temperament. *Developmental Psychology, 22,* 356–365.

Rothbart, M. K. (1989). Temperament in childhood: A framework. In G. A. Kohnstamm, J. E. Bates, &

M. K. Rothbart (Eds.), *Temperament in childhood* (pp. 59–73). New York: John Wiley & Sons.

Rothbart, M. K., & Derryberry, D. (1981). Development of individual differences in temperament. In M. E. Lamb & A. L. Brown (Eds.), *Advances in developmental psychology* (Vol. 1, pp. 37–86). Hillsdale, NJ: Lawrence Erlbaum.

Rothbart, M. K., & Mauro, J. A. (1990). Questionnaire approaches to the study of infant temperament. In J. Colombo & J. Fagen (Eds.), *Individual Differences in Infancy* (pp. 411–429). Hillsdale, NJ: Lawrence Erlbaum.

Schneirla, T. C. (1959). An evolutionary and developmental theory of biphasic processes underlying approach and withdrawal. *Nebraska Symposium on Motivation, Vol. 7.* Lincoln: University of Nebraska Press.

Seifer, R., & Sameroff, A. J. (1986). The concept, measurement, and interpretation of temperament in young children: A survey of research issues. In M. Wolraich & D. K. Routh (Eds.), *Advances in developmental and behavioral pediatrics* (Vol. 7, pp. 1–43). Greenwich, CT: JAI Press.

Skinner, B. F. (1958). Teaching machines. *Science, 128,* 969–977.

Skinner, B. F. (1968). *The technology of teaching.* New York: Appleton-Century-Crofts.

Sostek, A. J., Sostek, A. M., Murphy, D. L., Martin, E. B., & Born, W. S. (1981). Cord blood amine oxidase activities relate to arousal and motor functioning in human newborns. *Life Science, 28,* 2561–2568.

Stifter, C. A., Fox, N. A., & Porges, S. W. (1989). Facial expressivity and vagal tone in five- and ten-month-old infants. *Infant Behavior and Development, 12,* 127–137.

Strelau, J. (1983a). A regulative theory of temperament. *Australian Journal of Psychology, 35,* 305–317.

Strelau, J. (1983b). Pavlov's nervous system typology and beyond. In A. Gale & J. A. Edwards (Eds.), *Physiological correlates of human behavior: Individual differences and psychopathology* (Vol. 3, pp. 139–154). New York: Academic Press.

Thelen, E. (1989). Self-organization in developmental processes: Can systems approaches work? In M. Gunnar (Ed.), *Systems in development: The Minnesota Symposium in Child Psychology,* Vol. 22. Hillsdale, NJ: Lawrence Erlbaum.

Thomas, A., & Chess, S. (1977). *Temperament and development.* New York: Brunner/Mazel.

Thomas, A., Chess, S., & Birch, H. G. (1968). *Temperament and behavior disorders in children.* New York: New York University Press.

Thomas, A., Chess, S., Birch, H., Hertzig, M., & Korn, S. (1963). *Behavioral individuality in early childhood.* New York: New York University Press.

Vandenburg, S., Singer, S. M., & Pauls, D. L. (1986). *The heredity of behavior disorder in adults and children.* New York: Plenum Press.

vom Saal, F. S., & Finch, C. E. (1988). Reproductive senescence: Phenomena and mechanisms in mammals and selected vertebrates. In E. Knobil & J. Neill (Eds.), *The physiology of reproduction* (pp. 2351–2413). New York: Raven Press.

Ward, I. L. (1972). Prenatal stress feminizes and demasculinizes the behavior of males. *Science, 175,* 82–84.

Watson, J. B. (1928). *Psychological care of infant and child.* New York: W. W. Norton.

Watson, J. B. (1930). *Behaviorism* (rev. ed.). Chicago: University of Chicago Press.

Wilson, R. S., & Matheny, A. P., Jr. (1986). Behavioral genetics research in infant temperament: The Louisville Twin Study. In R. Plomin & J. Dunn (Eds.), *The study of temperament: Changes, continuities, and challenges* (pp. 81–97). Hillsdale, NJ: Lawrence Erlbaum.

27 / Temperament

Jerome Kagan

Explanations of the stable variation in mood and behavior among children and adults have begun to acknowledge the role of inherited, physiological mechanisms, and, as a result, temperamental constructs have become popular after almost a century of exile. Two reasons for this change in view, which are complex, are dramatic advances in neurobiology and the failure of behavioristic and psychoanalytic principles to account for a substantial portion of the variance in children's behavior and psychopathology. As a result, scholars and other citizens now are more willing to acknowledge the possibility of biological contributions to psychological differences between and within sex and ethnic groups.

These historical events permitted Alexander

This research was supported in part by a grant by the John D. and Catherine T. MacArthur Foundation and the Leon Lowenstein Foundation. I thank Nancy Snidman and Doreen Arcus for their collaboration in this work.

Thomas and Stella Chess to reintroduce the idea of temperament to the psychiatric community in the early 1960s. Thomas and Chess (1977) regarded a temperamental quality as referring to a distinct style of behavior, independent of its target or the competence with which it is displayed. Interview data from 85 middle- and upper-middle-class families of infants who were rearing 138 children in the New York metropolitan area led them to posit 9 temperamental dimensions: activity, regularity, approach or withdrawal to unfamiliarity, adaptation to new situations, responsiveness, energy, a happy or irritable mood, distractibility, and attention span. Because these 9 dimensions are not independent and, in addition, were not preserved over the course of childhood, when interviews with parents and other knowledgeable adults provided the primary evidence, Thomas and Chess collapsed the findings across dimensions and posited 3 abstract categories, each defined by a profile of dimensions.

About 40% of the children were called *easy* because they were regular, approached unfamiliarity with ease, and usually had a positive mood. About 15% were classified as *slow to warm up* because they reacted to unfamiliar people or situations with an initial withdrawal and wariness. The least frequent category, about 10% of the sample, was classified as *difficult* because of frequent irritability, persistent withdrawal to novelty, and poor adaptation. This group was most likely to develop psychiatric symptoms in later childhood.

The work of Thomas and Chess motivated an empirical interest in temperament among other scholars. Some of the best known include Bates (1989), Carey and McDevitt (1978), Buss and Plomin (1984), Goldsmith and Campos (1982), and Rothbart (1989). These investigators constructed questionnaires designed to assess the stability and correlates of similar dimensions. Some investigators report modest stability from infancy through the school years and others find minimal stability; but the correlations are rarely greater than 0.4. More important, there is often a poor relation between the parents' description of their child on these questionnaires and actual observations of the child, either at home or in the laboratory. Because parents can, and often do, distort their children's characteristics and because the dimensions evaluated on the questionnaires may not be in close accord with the phenomena in nature, it is reasonable to consider an alternative strategy. If temperamental constructs are defined by inherited physiological processes and correlated behaviors and moods that emerge early in development, theoretically it should be useful to consider the behaviors that might be influenced by these biological processes. At the moment, no sturdy conceptual bridge exists between the dimensions that Thomas and Chess posited and the inherited physiology that is presumed to underlie varied temperamental styles.

A Definition of Temperament

A temperamental category, in my view, is defined by a behavioral and physiological profile that is under some genetic control. At present, most psychologists must rely primarily on a behavioral profile because scientists have not yet discovered the physiology that is part of the foundation for the behavior. This is a common historical sequence in medicine. For example, before the pathophysiology of infectious diseases was known, these diseases were defined only by their phenotypic symptoms.

The definition of a temperamental category as a changing, but coherent, profile of behavior and emotion linked to an inherited physiology acknowledges the malleability of the behavioral profile. Further, because the number of physiological profiles that might influence behavior is very large, it is likely that there will be a long list of temperamental categories. I suggest that one class of categories will rest on variation in inherited neurochemistry. A large number of different molecules and receptors monitor excitation and inhibition in the brain. It is easy to imagine that a child born with a higher than normal concentration of brain norepinephrine, for example, which can affect the excitability of limbic sites, might be excessively prone to fear. By contrast, infants born with very low levels of norepinephrine might be fearless. It is of interest that in one study, a small number of child psychiatric patients had very low concentrations of dopamine-beta-hydroxylase (DBH), an enzyme that catalyzes the conversion of dopamine to norepinephrine. Over half of these children were older boys with severe conduct disorders (Rogeness, Hernandez, Macedo,

Amyrang, & Hoppe, 1986). Because levels of DBH are under genetic control, it is possible that some extremely aggressive boys inherit a biochemistry that makes it a little more likely that they will develop this profile.

Our knowledge of the relation between variation in neurochemistry and variation in psychological characteristics is still too meager to posit the specific psychological qualities that are linked to a particular neurochemistry. Hence at this time it is necessary to rely primarily on psychological qualities in the definition of a temperamental category. However, this strategy is only temporary.

A CHOICE OF STRATEGIES

During this period of transition, when knowledge of the robust relations between physiology and behavior is fragile, two different strategies of inquiry are possible. The currently popular approach is to posit, a priori, categories that are closely related to those suggested by Thomas and Chess. One problem with this strategy is that their categories were derived from interviews with parents and, therefore, could not include concepts for which there were no easily understood English words. It is unlikely that the English language has terms for all of the significant temperamental types.

An alternative strategy, which I prefer, is to observe children's behavior and to infer the temperamental categories from these observations and associated physiological features. A child could display high levels of fear because of conditioning, modeling, or the biological preparedness that is implied by temperament. Thus, display of fear need not be the result of temperament; hence, it is important to gather information other than parental report.

ries, but conceived of the variation within each of the 9 dimensions as continua. They described the approach-withdrawal dimension, for example, as if all infants could be placed on a continuum with respect to their tendency to withdraw or to approach unfamiliar people or events. However, it is possible that children who are at the extreme on one or the other of these qualities are qualitatively different from those who are less extreme. In general, readers or listeners assume a quantitative difference between two people when they are described with words referring to particular behaviors, emotions, or talents. For example, when we say "Margaret is better at tennis than Mary," we imply a quantitative difference in ability between the two women. However, when one person is described as a member of a category and the other is not, we imply that the two differ in a set of correlated characteristics and, therefore, are qualitatively different. Thus, when we say "Mary is a member of the Olympic tennis team and Joan is not," we imply a qualitative difference in ability between the two women. Because most investigators study single features, such as activity, emotionality, or irritability, the tacit assumption is that the temperamental construct is continuous and that all irritable children belong to a homogeneous group.

I believe that temperamental categories in children are analogous to strains of animals with each type characterized by a unique profile of characteristics. Some temperamental types are common, some rare; some are obvious to observers, some are subtle; some are hard to change and some easier. When a scientific domain is immature, investigators have no choice but to invent categories that are defined primarily by surface characteristics. But when the deeper origins of the phenotypes become known, the categories often are reshuffled into new etiological groups.

Continua versus Categories

One final issue requires attention. Thomas and Chess viewed the three temperamental types—easy, difficult, and slow to warm up—as catego-

Inhibited and Uninhibited Temperamental Groups

Of the many temperamental categories that are likely to exist in nature, two are unusually obvious and represent the groups Nancy Snidman, Doreen Arcus, and I have been studying in Harvard laboratory. The group of children we call inhibited, about 15 to 20% of healthy Caucasian children, can be detected easily in the second year of life because of their consistent tendency to withdraw and to become emotionally subdued, restrained, and timid in the presence of unfamiliar situations, people, and objects. A somewhat larger group, about 30 to 35% of the same population, show the complementary profile of a relatively rapid approach to the same unfamiliar situations, often associated with a great deal of spontaneous emotion. We call these children uninhibited. About three-quarters of children originally classified as either inhibited or uninhibited in the second year of life retained their respective qualities through 7½ years of age (Kagan, Reznick, & Snidman, 1988). We presume that the children who changed their behavioral profile did so because of environmental experiences. Children with an inhibited temperaments always have the capacity to change their behavior as a result of life experiences.

PHYSIOLOGICAL DIFFERENCES

The physiological differences between the two groups implicate variation in the activity of the sympathetic nervous system as a correlate of the two types. Measurement of changes in heart rate, diastolic blood pressure, pupillary dilation, and lateral asymmetry in facial temperature reveals that the inhibited, compared with the uninhibited, children possess greater sympathetic reactivity to mild stress. They show larger magnitudes of cardiac acceleration and pupil dilation to cognitive stress and larger rises in diastolic blood pressure when their posture changes from sitting to standing. The change in posture produces a sympathetically mediated vasoconstriction in the arterial tree. Finally, thermography imaging of the face reveals that inhibited children are more likely to cool on the right side of the face to mild stress while uninhibited children are more likely to cool on the left side of the face (difference of 0.1 to 0.3° Celsius). This cooling is due to constriction of the arterioles mediated by alpha adrenergic receptors. Because the sympathetic nervous system

is more reactive on the right than on the left side of the body, these data imply greater sympathetic activity among inhibited children. However, resting baseline values for heart rate, blood pressure, and asymmetry in facial temperature are less differentiating of the two groups. This result is in accord with other investigations that also fail to find differences in baseline physiological values between or among diagnostic groups. It appears that changes in these physiological responses to an imposed stress are more differentiating of temperamental groups than are baseline values.

It is of interest that inhibited children and their first- and second-degree relatives are more likely to have or to have had allergic rhinitis and/or eczema compared with uninhibited children and their relatives (Kagan, Snidman, Julia-Sellers, & Johnson, 1991). Because the sympathetic nervous system synapses on lymphocytes that can suppress activity of certain classes of T cells, it is possible that the greater sympathetic reactivity among inhibited children and their relatives participates in the susceptibility to these atopic allergies.

Convincing support for genetic influences on these two temperamental categories comes from studies of twins at the University of Louisville (Matheny, 1989) and the Institute of Behavioral Genetics at the University of Colorado (Plomin et al., 1990). Scientists in both laboratories have found that inhibited and uninhibited behavioral styles are heritable in preschool children. The Colorado study, which currently has a sample of 100 monozygotic and 100 dizogotic pairs, has found heritabilities of 0.5 for inhibited behavior and 0.4 for uninhibited behavior.

Infant Characteristics

If inhibited and uninhibited children inherit physiologies that bias them to display their distinct behaviors, perhaps they would show prophetic signs of their style during early infancy. Research with animals implicates the importance of the amygdala and its multiple projections in mediating an organism's reaction to novelty (Dunn & Everitt, 1988). Hence, infant behaviors that are the product of high or low thresholds in the amygdala might be predictive of the two temperamental categories.

The basolateral area of the amygdala, which increases in size with phylogeny, receives information from all sensory areas (with the exception of olfaction, which synapses on the medial area). The basolateral area projects to the ventral striatum and ventral palladium, which mediate motor activity, especially flexing and extending of arms and legs to stimulation, and also sends information to the central nucleus. The central nucleus, which contains different classes of neurons, has a profound influence on emotion and the autonomic nervous system through projections to the hypothalamus and the sympathetic chain. Neurons in the central nucleus also project to the cingulate and central gray, which, in animals, mediate defensive reactions. The central gray also sends fibers to the larynx and vocal cords that mediate distress cries in puppies and kittens. Finally, the central nucleus projects to the frontal cortex, and activity in this circuit can produce desynchronization in the cortical electroencephalogram (EEG). Thus, if inhibited children have low thresholds in the amygdala and these multiple projections, we might expect high levels of motor activity, muscle spasticity, crying, cardiac acceleration, and perhaps special profiles of desynchronization in the EEG.

Longitudinal study of two independent groups of 4-month-old infants reveals that about 20% of healthy, Caucasian infants display extreme degrees of motor activity to moving mobiles, Q-tips dipped in butyl alcohol, and tape-recorded human voices. These infants extend their arms and legs in momentary spasticity, show bursts of vigorous limb activity, and, on occasion, arch their backs to the presentation of these unfamiliar events. In addition, during the periods of intense motor activity, they often fret or cry. The crying follows the rise in motor activity and appears to be a consequence of becoming aroused. We call these children *high reactive* (Kagan & Snidman, 1991).

A larger group, about one third of healthy, 4-month-old infants, shows the opposite pattern to the same stimulation. They occasionally move an arm or leg with mild vigor but rarely fuss or cry. One of their most salient characteristics is minimal motor tension in fingers, hands, legs, or trunk. We call these infants *low reactive*.

When these two temperamental groups en-

countered unfamiliar rooms, people, and toys in the laboratory at 14 and 21 months, the high-reactive infants were significantly more fearful than the relaxed ones. The evaluation of fear was based on the frequency of fretting or crying to an unfamiliar event or procedure (e.g., placement of electrodes for heart rate, placement of a blood pressure cuff, facial disapproval from an examiner or the mother, exposure to a noisy, rotating wheel, request to taste liquid from a dropper, or failure to approach a metal robot or an unfamiliar woman despite a friendly invitation to do so). At 14 months of age, 48% of the infants showed 0 or 1 fear (regarded as low fear) and 32% showed 4 or more fears (regarded as high fear). At 21 months, 34 percent showed low fear and 31 percent high fear. The typical low-reactive infant showed low fear across a 90-minute battery of various episodes; a typical high-reactive infant had 3 or 4 fears across the same battery. In addition, the low-reactive infants who showed minimal fear at 14 and 21 months, especially if they were boys, had unusually low heart rates, while the heart rate differences between the high- and low-reactive girls were minimal. This fact suggests an interaction among temperamental type, sympathetic reactivity, and gender. Although there were no major sex differences in fear at 14 months, more girls than boys in both groups showed a rise in fear between 14 and 21 months, suggesting an influence of socialization on the fearfulness of girls in the second year.

The infants who were high reactive at 4 months, compared with those who were low reactive, had higher fetal heart rates and higher heart rates at 2 weeks of age during sleep while their mother held them over the shoulder. Thus, the high sympathetic tone characteristic of older inhibited, compared with uninhibited, children is also present in high reactive infants. (See Chapter 26 for a different interpretation of this result.) As with older inhibited children, the high-reactive infants who were highly fearful in the second year were more likely to show increased cooling on the right compared with the left side of the forehead to imposed stress, while the low-reactive, low-fear children showed cooling on the left side of the forehead. In addition, Davidson (1994) and Fox, Calkins, and Bell (1994) have shown that inhibited children and high-reactive infants are more likely to show greater desynchronization of alpha activity in the right frontal area; low-reactive, uninhibited children show greater desynchronization in the left frontal area.

The high- and low-reactive infants appear to be qualitative types that cannot be placed on a continuum of arousal. Support for this statement comes from the fact that there was no relation between degree of motor activity and crying, on the one hand, and subsequent fear in the second year, on the other, within either the high- or low-reactive groups. If an infant had been classified as reactive because he or she showed extreme motor activity on 15% of the trials and crying on at least 2 episodes, that infant was as likely to be fearful in the second year as one who had a much higher motor and irritability score. This result is inconsistent with the idea of a continuum of arousal. It appears that the 4-month-old infant must pass a certain threshold in order to display vigorous motor activity and irritability. Once an infant has passed that threshold, he or she belongs to the high-reactive category.

FUTURE DEVELOPMENT

It is, of course, not possible to make firm statements about the later development of the children belonging to each of the two groups. However, some speculation is possible. The adolescent profile that will be displayed by high-reactive or low-reactive infants, who represent a little less than half of a sample of healthy Caucasian children, will depend on their home and school environments. A high-reactive infant who becomes an inhibited adolescent is likely to do well academically if raised in a home that values academic accomplishment. Because this child prefers to be alone and in control of uncertainty, rather than in frequent encounters with unfamiliar children, he or she is likely to devote a great deal of time to schoolwork and, if successful, choose an intellectual career. The same temperamental type raised in a family that does not value academic achievement cannot use school success as a compensation and may be at greater risk for personality problems.

The low-reactive, uninhibited child raised in an environment, that sets consistent standards on aggressive behavior is likely to be an extroverted child who is popular with peers. The same child raised in an environment that is unusually permissive about aggression may be at risk for a delinquent career. These expectations assume no unusual or chronic stress during the intervening years. Predictions for the remaining children who belong to neither temperamental group are much less clear.

An inhibited 3-year-old child began life with characteristics that biased that infant to react in special ways to stimulation. It is likely that the longer an inhibited child remains fearful, the more stable that behavior will be. However, some shy, fearful adolescents were neither high reactive at 4 months of age nor fearful at 1 year; their timidity was the result of a different history. These children probably acquired their shy demeanor as a result of experiences after school entrance. Thus, if all the scientist or clinician knows is that an adolescent is extremely shy, it is not possible to know the developmental route that was taken. Embryologists have argued that a cardinal rule in developmental biology is never to infer developmental mechanisms from the shape of final forms.

This warning has implications for clinicians working with children or adults who present anxiety as a primary symptom. If all that is known is that the patient is anxious, it is not possible to determine whether the person would have belonged to the high reactive-inhibited temperamental category or acquired these symptoms as a result of childhood experiences without any special, temperamental bias. In such cases it is useful to gain information on early childhood fearfulness, especially before 5 years of age. Further, physiological evidence—change in blood pressure to orthostatic challenge, heart rate acceleration to cognitive stress, blood or urine catecholamines—may help to discriminate the temperamental from the acquired syndrome. It is presumed that the former child will be less affected by changes in the environment or helped by deep dynamic interpretations than the latter but may react more positively to pharmacological treatment.

THE PROPER CONSTRUCTS

What term should we use to represent a child who showed high reactivity to stimulation at 4 months, high sympathetic tone, fear at the end of the first year, and continued timidity during later childhood? What term for the infant who began life with the same behavioral and physiological characteristics who was not unusually shy or fearful during later childhood? We propose that the terms *inhibited type* and *uninhibited type* refer to the early developmental characteristics displayed in the first year, while the terms *inhibited* and *uninhibited* refer to contemporary behavior observed during later childhood. The statement "This child is inhibited" refers to the display of shy, timid behavior by a child who presumably showed high reactivity at 4 months. The statement "This child is an inhibited type" is more hypothetical, implying that the infant inherited the genes for inhibition, as reflected in high fetal heart rate, high sleeping heart rate at 2 weeks, and high reactivity at 4 months, but this child may or may not display fearful or shy behavior during the preschool and early school years. Jung held a similar view, for he suggested that all introverted types were not necessarily shy and retiring. For some, he argued, the anima and persona were inconsistent. Many introverts develop a phenotype that is highly sociable.

We have stressed the inhibited, rather than the uninhibited, type because children in that category appear to be at greater risk for later anxiety. Nonetheless, the uninhibited type is more coherent, more stable, and, in most environments, adapts well.

Future Issues

Although there is too little evidence to permit positing other temperamental categories, some guesses are possible. At our laboratory we have been impressed with the salience and stability of a quality that most parents might call *vitality*. A small group of infants, about 10%, show unusually high levels of energy. They thrash their arms and legs but never fret or cry and vocalize and smile frequently. At later ages, they laugh with zeal. This quality is difficult to quantify for it is not captured simply by activity level. A complementary class— about 10%—displays very low energy and appears

listless. As 2-year-olds, these children often are quiet and emotionally subdued, but they do not display the frequent, intense fears to unfamiliarity characteristic of reactive infants.

Some temperamental types are rare. We have seen 1 infant from a total of almost 500 who showed a unique profile of low motor activity combined with very high irritability at 4 months. At 9 months of age, he fretted to every provocation and at 14 months maintained a sad face throughout the battery. He had frequent, uncontrolled tantrums, vocalized in short, explosive bursts, and displayed a pained facial expression without an accompanying cry or fret—a silent expression of angst. At 21 months he was willful. He resisted the placement of electrodes, ripping them off whenever they were applied, and refused almost every episode by screaming, which forced the examiner to terminate the procedure. The mother acknowledged that the boy had a tendency to bite her at home. He was not inhibited at 3½ years of age but in a peer-play situation with an unfamiliar boy of the same age, he showed an act of impulsive aggression that is rare in this context. He picked up a wooden pole and began to strike a plastic tunnel in the place where the other boy was sitting, forcing the boy to cry.

Many temperamental categories have not been discovered because they are not salient to parents and, therefore, do not emerge in questionnaire data. That is why I suggested earlier that most of the temperamental categories will have to be inferred from longitudinal observations that combine behavioral, emotional, and physiological variables.

The increased interest in temperamental constructs will generate discussion about the degree of responsibility a person has for his or her behavior. An observer's conclusion about the degree of self-conscious control an agent possesses determines the observer's evaluation of the agent, especially if the behavior violates community standards. If an observer believes that an act was deliberate, the agent is held responsible, whether that action reflects fear or aggression.

Our culture has been relatively Puritan in its commitment to the belief that *will* has preeminent power in human behavior. However, historical events during the last 30 to 40 years have eroded that view somewhat. A growing number of citizens has become willing to excuse some asocial action, including violence and fraud, because they have become persuaded that these acts are not always within an individual's deliberative sphere. Honest concern with, and guilt over, the plight of economically disadvantaged minorities has generated a reluctance to blame the victim. Moreover, advances in genetics remind us that the development of high blood pressure and cancer are not due totally to a negligent lifestyle. Many citizens are willing, therefore, to contemplate the notion that a similar rule should be applied to asocial acts or extremely timid behavior. In a recent issue of the *AARP Bulletin*, a writer excused a middle-age woman who left her older mother in a hospital, without a name or address, as an inevitable consequence of the daughter's inability to cope with her aging parent. However, it is not obvious that this new permissiveness, which minimizes will, is either healthier or more adaptive for our society than the traditional assumption that one of the many significant products of hominid evolution is our capacity to select and to control our behavior.

REFERENCES

Bates, J. E., (1989), Concepts and measures of temperament. In G. A. Kohnstamm, J. E. Bates, & M. K. Rothbart (Eds.), *Temperament in childhood* (pp. 3–26). New York: John Wiley & Sons.

Buss, A. H., & Plomin, R. (1984). *Temperament: Early developing personality traits*, Hillsdale, NJ: Erlbaum.

Carey, W. B., & McDevitt, S. C. (1978). Revision of the infant temperament questionnaire. *Pediatrics, 61,* 735–739.

Davidson, R. J. (1994). Temperament, affective style and frontal lube asymmetry. In G. P. Dawson & K. Fischer (Eds.) *Human behavior and the developing brain* (pp. 518–536). New York: Guilford Press.

Dunn, L. T., & Everitt, B. J. (1988). Double disassociations of the effects of amygdala and insular cortex lesions on conditions of taste aversion, passive avoidance, and neophobia in the rat using the excitotoxin ibotenic acid. *Behavioral Neuroscience, 102,* 3–9.

Fox, N. A., Calkins, S. D. Bell, M. A. (1994). Neural plasticity and development in the first two years of life. *Development and Psychopathology, 6,* 677–696.

Goldsmith, H. H., & Campos, J. J. (1982). Toward a theory of infant temperament. In R. N. Emde & R. J. Harmon, (Eds.), *The development of attachment and affiliative systems* (pp. 161–193). New York: Plenum Press.

Kagan, J., Reznick, J. S., & Snidman, N. (1988). Biologi-cal bases of childhood shyness. *Science, 240,* 167–171.

Kagan, J., & Snidman, N. (1991). Temperamental factors in human development. *American Psychologist, 46,* 856–862.

Kagan, J., Snidman, N., Julia-Sellers, M., & Johnson, M. O. (1991). Temperament and allergic symptoms. *Psychosomatic Medicine, 53,* 332–340.

Matheny, A. P. (1989). Children's behavioral inhibition over age and across situations. *Journal of Personality, 57,* 215–235.

Plomin, R., Campos, J., Corley, R., Emde, R. N., Fulker, D. W., Kagan, J., Reznick, J. S., Robinson, J., Zahn-Waxler, C., & DeFries, J. C. (1990). Individual differences during the second year of life: The MacArthur Longitudinal Twin Study. In J. Colombo & J. Fagen (Eds.), *Individual differences in infancy* (pp. 431–455). Hillsdale, NJ: Erlbaum.

Rogeness, G. A., Hernandez, J. M., Macedo, C. A., Amyrang, S. A., and Hoppe, S. K. (1986). Near zero plasma dopamine beta-hydroxylase and conduct disorder in emotionally disturbed boys. *American Academy of Child Psychiatry, 25,* 521–527.

Rothbart, M. K. (1989). Temperament in childhood: A framework. In G. A. Kohnstamm, J. E. Bates, & M. K. Rothbart (Eds.), *Temperament in childhood* (pp. 59–76). New York: John Wiley & Sons.

Thomas, A., & Chess, S. (1977). *Temperament and Development.* New York: Brunner/Mazel.

28 / Margaret Mahler's Theory of Separation-Individuation

Anni Bergman

Introduction

Margaret Mahler always emphasized that her original background as a pediatrician sparked her passionate interest in the human infant's early development. In her memoirs she states "For me . . . the general problem of identity, and especially the way in which one arrives at a sense of self, has always been primary. Research involving psychosis was, to my mind, always a point of departure for learning about the emerging identity and sense of self of the average child" (Stepansky, 1988, pp. 136–137). Originally she perceived that the human infant's development begins from a state of nonresponsiveness to the outside world—the "normal autistic phase"—proceeds through a phase of nondifferentiation from the mothering partner—the "symbiotic phase"—to the ultimate realization of self as separate and autonomous. In her memoirs Mahler refers to a presentation she gave together with Bert Gosliner in 1954 to the New York Psychoanalytic Society in which she described an adolescent patient, a ticquer, who was enmeshed in a symbiotic, parasitic relationship with his mother. Using this case as a pathological example, the authors then described a process by which the normal baby establishes a viable identity. In the discussion of this paper, Anna-Marie Weil suggested that this process might be named "separation-individuation." Thus, in 1954 the process of separation-individuation was first named.

A few years later Mahler decided to apply for research funds to do an observational study of the separation-individuation process in normal mothers and their infants. Mahler originally hypothesized that this process took place during the second year of life and began her research by studying a group of 1-year-olds and their mothers. Soon after the observational research began, however, she realized that by the age of 1, children were already in the midst of this process. From then on, mother-child pairs were studied beginning during the second half of the first year, which

was hypothesized to be the height of the symbiotic phase and the beginning of separation-individuation. The fact that siblings of the original subjects began to enter the project provided the researchers with the opportunity to observe infants from birth, but formal observations of the first 5 months were never made. This decision was influenced by Mahler's conviction that the infant before separation existed as part of a dual unity and that no inferences could be drawn from observational data to the internal life of the baby before the beginning of separation-individuation. Mahler was nonetheless enormously interested in and excited by the work of infant researchers and eventually had regular meetings with Daniel Stern and T. Berry Brazelton. In addition, she was an avid reader of all the early work done by infant psychiatrists, and she attended and participated in the congresses of World Association of Infant Psychiatry and Allied Disciplines. Although she also admired the new film technology that enabled infant researchers to observe mother-infant interactions not visible to the naked eye, she felt that there was an important difference between observations in the laboratory and observations in naturalistic settings.

Eventually Mahler came to realize that her earliest observations of what she had perceived to be an "autistic phase" probably were limited to the period of the first few weeks of the infant's life and that, even then, the normal infant was never completely unaware of his or her surroundings. A reformulation of what she still called the autistic phase exists as her introduction to the film *On the Phenomena Indicative of the Emergence of the Sense of Self* (Mahler, Pine, Bergman, & Smith, 1982), in which she speaks of the autistic phase as the one in which the newborn has to adjust to extrauterine existence to find a niche in the external world. The newborn has to achieve physiological homeostasis—that is, adequate inner regulation in synchrony with the vocal and gestural rhythms of the caregiver. Each infant elicits his or her own mother's caregiving, and the mother responds with coenesthetic empathy (meaning empathy through the body) to the needs of a particular infant. Although she never published such a statement in her writings, Mahler eventually gave up the idea of the "normal autistic phase" (personal communication, 1983).

In the 1950s, participating in a naturalistic observational research study was a revolutionary act for a psychoanalyst. The idea that inferences about mental life could be drawn from observing nonverbal and even early verbal interactions was not generally accepted. The research on separation-individuation, although behavioral, always had the goal of understanding an intrapsychic process. Observed behaviors were always the base for making inferences, and what allowed the observers to make inferences was comparison between subjects both simultaneously and over time. A research situation was created in which the spontaneous day-to-day relationships of mother and child could be observed in a natural playground setting. A large playroom with many attractive and colorful toys contained a small area arranged as a sitting room for mothers in which they could chat, sip coffee, or read—and from which they had a full view of and free access to their children. As soon as the children were mobile, they tended to move back and forth freely between the toy area and the mothers' sitting area. At least two participant-observers were always present to join in conversation with the mothers and play with the children.

The freedom created by this setting eventually could lead to conceptualization of the subphases of the separation-individuation process. It is important to realize that at the beginning of the study, the concept of these subphases did not exist. Instead, their conceptualization grew out of repeated observations and out of the cross-sectional methodology of the research. Psychoanalysis tends toward intensive, long-term, one-to-one observation in the psychoanalytic setting. Earlier psychoanalytic developmental research tended toward case studies rather than cross-case comparisons. What was unique about the separation-individuation research was that it combined longitudinal observations of the developmental period from 6 months to 3 years of each of the subjects with case-to-case comparison of subjects. This methodology would lead to the conceptualization of regularly occurring subphases of the

separation-individuation process. For example, at first a young toddler was observed playing contentedly at some distance from the mother. We thought that this showed particular independence on the part of this child. Only when this behavior was seen again and again in children of similar ages could a practicing subphase begin to be described and conceptualized. Similarly, when the first intense separation reactions were observed in a 15-month-old boy, it was thought that this described this specific child's relationship to his mother. Again, when separation reactions during that particular age period were observed in other children, the rapprochement subphase, with its important changes in the mother-child relationship, could begin to be conceptualized and described. Those children in whom phase-specific behaviors were somewhat exaggerated drew our attention to these behaviors and facilitated our recognition of similar patterns in other children. Only during later stages of the research, after the subphase sequences had been described, did these stages serve as a reference point for research and did an additional goal arise: to confirm or contradict the early observations and formulations.

The Separation-Individuation Process

SYMBIOSIS (4 TO 6 MONTHS)

Mahler described symbiosis based on theoretical conceptualizations of early development rather than observation. Thus, a dichotomy exists between conceptualizations of the separation-individuation process, which have a solid base in actual mother-infant observations, and descriptions of symbiosis, which are based on metapsychological formulations. Mahler states that symbiosis

describes that state of undifferentiation, of fusion with mother, in which the "I" is not yet differentiated from the "not-I" and in which inside and outside are only gradually coming to be sensed as different. Any unpleasurable perception, external or internal, is projected beyond the common boundary of the symbiotic *milieu interieur* ... which includes the mother partner's gestalt during ministrations. Only transiently ... does the young infant seem to take in stimuli from beyond the symbiotic milieu. The primordial energy reservoir that is vested in the undifferentiated "ego-id" seems to contain an undifferentiated mixture of libido and aggression. The libidinal cathexis vested in the symbiotic orbit replaces the inborn instinctual stimulus barrier and protects the rudimentary ego from premature phase-unspecific strain, from stress traumata.

The essential feature of symbiosis is hallucinatory or delusional somatopsychic *omnipotent* fusion with the representation of the mother and, in particular, the delusion of a common boundary between two physically separate individuals. (Mahler, Pine, & Bergman, 1975, pp. 44–45)

Later on Mahler states:

the infant's inner sensations form the core of the self. They seem to remain the central crystallization point of the feeling of self around which a sense of identity will become established. . . . Within this symbiotic common orbit the two partners or poles of the dyad may be regarded as polarizing the organizational and structuring processes. The structures that derived from this double frame of reference represent a framework to which all experiences have to be related before there are clear and whole representations of the self and the object world. (Mahler et al., 1975, p. 47)

After several pages of describing symbiosis in these metapsychological terms, Mahler refers to the mothering partner's holding behavior as the symbiotic organizer—"the midwife of individuation of psychological birth" (Mahler et al., 1975, p. 47). Mahler believed that vestiges of the symbiotic phase remain throughout the entire life cycle and goes on to describe different patterns of holding behaviors in different mothers showing the influence of such holding behaviors on the infant. For example, one mother appeared to breast-feed not so much because it promoted closeness but more because it was convenient and made her feel successful. Her baby's smiling response was delayed and remained unspecific well after a specific smiling response would have been expected.

We now know that symbiosis is of great importance for separation-individuation theory. Observers agree that attunement, mutual empathy, and communion between mother and infant are at their height in the period from 2 to 5 months. Thus, while Mahler sometimes described symbiosis in an abstract, metapsychological manner, she also realized the importance of the intense experience between mother and baby during that period as forming the bedrock for psychological birth.

THE FIRST SUBPHASE: DIFFERENTIATION (6 TO 9 MONTHS)

At the age of around 5 months, which is considered the height of symbiosis, the infant no longer focuses primarily on the mother's face even while nursing and being held in her arms. Once their hunger is stilled, babies now begin to look around. They may look at their hands; they may turn away from mother to look around at objects in the immediate environment. Distance perception develops, and it is typical for an infant beginning at this age to scan the environment and then look back to mother. This process of looking from mother to the outside and back, this process of increasing ability to focus on things outside of the symbiotic orbit, was named *the hatching process*. The fully hatched baby, between 8 to 10 months, has attained a new sense of alertness, can sit up freely and grasp what he or she wants. During this process of hatching several phenomena are of particular importance.

As the infant begins to hatch—to differentiate—one of the most important phenomena observed is that of *customs inspection,* a term borrowed from the work of Sylvia Brody (Brody & Axelrod, 1970). This term refers to the way an infant of that age will examine both tactilely and visually the faces of observers who are relatively unfamiliar. This examination of the nonmother's face, which is usually done in a sober and thoughtful mood, is very different from the joyful way in which the baby might squeeze or bite the mother's face. It is clear that the baby at this point is familiar with mother and reacts to her as uniquely different from the world of nonmother in which the baby begins to be intensely interested, exploring it with curiosity.

Another pattern that develops during this period is *checking back to mother.* The baby begins visually to compare mother and other, the familiar with the unfamiliar. During this process, the phenomenon of stranger anxiety develops. However, the term *stranger anxiety* was coined at a time when it was believed that until the age of about 6 months babies were not yet able to distinguish mother as unique. Recent observations have shown that the unique attachment to mother is present almost from the very beginning. The reaction to strangers that does not always lead to stranger anxiety thus is a process that is not contingent on nonrecognition of mother as different from others. Rather it is a process that results from the infant's burgeoning ability to take in the outside world, to comprehend it as being different from mother, and to react to it in a variety of different ways. The term *stranger curiosity* was coined during observations of hatching infants responding to observers and comparing these responses to their ways of being with mother. Thus, *stranger anxiety* covers a wide variety of reactions, ranging from curiosity and slight wariness to apprehension, anxiety, and distress. In *The Psychological Birth of the Human Infant,* two children of the same mother were compared with each other (Mahler et al., 1975). The older one, Peter, at 7 to 8 months, reacted to strangers briefly with curiosity and quickly with apprehension, anxiety, and crying. By contrast, Linda examined strangers with pleasure and curiosity and did not display marked stranger anxiety at any age. These comparative observations demonstrated the important differences in the specific outcome of interactions between Peter and his mother, which were often tense and unpredictable, to those of Linda, whose interactions with mother were mostly pleasurable and harmonious. From these and other observations, it was concluded that in children for whom the symbiotic phase had been characterized by pleasure, curiosity about the stranger dominated over anxiety, whereas in children in whom the symbiotic phase was less pleasurable and harmonious, wariness and anxiety predominated in the relationship to the stranger during the period of hatching.

Another important phenomenon of the differentiation subphase is the child's interest in and play with objects that belong to mother, such as her jewelry, keys, and eyeglasses. This play, initiated by the baby, usually is responded to and elaborated by the mother. These objects seem to be of special interest and value to the baby because they are perceived as being part of mother yet can be removed and thus become part of the baby and then can again be returned to mother. This back-and-forth movement between mother and baby is an important early game of interaction between them. Another mother-infant game that begins during this period of differentiation is the universal game of peek-a-boo, usually initiated at first by mother and later taken over and elaborated by the child.

During the period of differentiation, between 5 to 9 months, most babies begin some form of independent locomotion. At first they turn over and then begin to pull themselves along the floor. However, they do not yet seem quite aware that they are separating, or moving away, from mother, and mostly the preferred place for them is to be near mother, often at her feet or on her lap with face turned away from her. They also begin to be interested in making things happen, such as switching on and off lights and banging, dropping, and throwing objects.

Likely the timing of the hatching process is closely interwoven with the quality of the mother-child relationship. Thus, it was observed that in cases in which the symbiotic period of dual unity had been delayed or disturbed, the process of differentiation seems to have been delayed or premature. For example, one little girl whose mother had responded to her mechanically, without much warmth, did not seem to mold well, to become a "quasi-part of her mother" (Mahler et al., 1975). She smiled indiscriminately, and at an age when other children started to take a more active part in approach and distancing behaviors, she turned back to her own body and indulged in prolonged rocking. Thus, the differentiation process was delayed. Another child whose mother was depressed during his early infancy was late in recognizing mother as a special person. Specific smiling response was delayed, and he was late in using the visual modality, which is the first instrument to allow active distancing. Although he was late, he did not show the bland mechanical quality characteristic of the little girl. It was thought that his late hatching was adaptive. He seemed to know finally when he was ready to hatch. By contrast, a child who had a close but uncomfortable early relationship with his mother began to hatch early. He moved rapidly into the phase of differentiation, as if to extricate himself from the uncomfortable symbiosis. This child developed intense stranger anxiety, which seems to have been one of his early defensive patterns. It seemed as if the unsatisfactory symbiotic phase had prevented him from developing a reservoir of basic trust because he had to extricate himself from mother—separate early. He did so before he was truly ready and thus was easily overwhelmed by anxiety and distress.

Those children who had an unusually difficult time with separation from mother tended to have later histories of unusually early awareness of the outside world. It seems that the earliest differentiation patterns set in motion patterns of personality organization that would influence the further development of the separation-individuation process. Separation-individuation observations led to the finding that those infants whose mothers enjoyed the symbiotic phase without too much conflict seemed to start at the average time to show signs of active differentiation by beginning to distance from the mother's body. In cases in which there was ambivalence or too much intrusiveness on the mother's part, differentiation showed disturbances of various degrees and forms.

Detailed observations of the separation-individuation process allowed the observers to refine conceptualizations of stranger anxiety, showing that what had been thought of as stranger anxiety in reality encompassed a wide range of reactions vis-à-vis the stranger (Mahler et al., 1975). A similar refinement took place in the observation of separation anxiety. It was learned that separation reactions changed during the course of the subphases. They are subphase-specific, while of course they vary from child to child at any given time in development, and are closely connected to the vicissitudes of the mother-child relationship. During differentiation the child usually reacts to the mother's temporary absence not with open distress or crying but rather with a general lowering of mood. This lowering of mood was given the name *low-keyedness,* which was compared to conservation withdrawal in monkeys. It was hypothesized that this observed lowering of mood had the purpose of holding on, or conserving, the image of mother while she was not present. If a child in the state of low-keyedness was suddenly intruded upon by an observer who might be attempting to comfort or cheer him or her up, the child often broke into inconsolable crying. The intrusion of the observer forced the child to become acutely aware that mother was absent.

THE SECOND SUBPHASE: PRACTICING
(9 TO 15 MONTHS)

Early Practicing (9 to 12 months): The practicing subphase, lasting from about 10 months to about 15 months, was conceptualized in two parts: the early practicing subphase, from about 9 to 12 months, and the practicing subphase proper, from 12 to 15 months.

The practicing subphase begins with the development of independent locomotion. The ability actively to separate in space from the caregiving mother allows the baby to begin to explore the world beyond her in a much more active way. The passionate interest and investment in the mother now seems to spill over onto inanimate objects, which infants begins to explore actively, investigating their taste and texture with their mouths and hands. The maturation of locomotor and other functions brings with it an enormous expansion of the infant's world. There is more to see; there is more to touch; there is more to do. The excitement produced by the ability to propel oneself and to choose what to investigate at times seems to take precedence over the excitement in mother. However, especially during the beginning of the practicing subphase, an invisible bond seems to exist between infant and mother that unites them even when they are physically separate from one another and not in visual contact.

The child's mood during the practicing subphase is generally one of elation. There is a relative lessening of attention to mother, who during this particular period often seems to be used like an inanimate object to climb on, to step on, in order to enhance the infant's capacity for exploration. The rapidly expanding motor capacity is a special source of pleasure. Crawling, standing, coasting, and eventually walking and climbing seem to be the sources for the mood of elation. If we can think of symbiosis as the first blissful stage in human development, we can think of the practicing subphase as the second blissful period. The mastery of locomotion brings with it an enormous increment of energy and pleasure. The narcissistic investment in the body and in mastery and exploration brings about a temporary lessening in the investment in the mother, who now can be taken for granted. This slight lessening in investment in the mother also appears to protect the baby from the full realization of his or her separateness. There is a feeling of omnipotence fueled by what seems to be a silent assumption that mother always will be there when needed. The young toddler who might get tired practicing will look back to mother or go to her briefly for what has been called *emotional refueling.* Even the briefest contact with mother reenergizes the practicing child and allows him or her to continue with activities of practicing and exploring.

The advent of the ability to move independently, to practice, to explore had an especially good effect on those children who had an intense but uncomfortable symbiotic relationship. This may well have been due also to the fact that for the mother of such a child, disengagement and beginning independence comes as a relief if earlier on they were unable to relieve their infant's distress. While mothers and children had not been able to enjoy close physical contact, they could enjoy each other better now from a somewhat greater distance. As mothers became more relaxed and reassured, they also became better able to comfort and reassure their babies. On the other hand, some mothers who had enjoyed the symbiotic closeness did not take well to the transition period of practicing. Once their children left the maternal orbit, they wished for them to be grown up quickly. Interestingly, these children found it more difficult to grow up and often were demanding of closeness. In one extreme case of this sort in which a mother seemed to be able to accept her child only as a symbiotic part of herself and actively interfered with his attempts to move away, the surprising observation was made that once he could move away, he seemed to lose contact with his mother when he was at a distance from her. This is in contrast to a child whose mother enjoyed closeness but did not impede the little girl's forays into the outside world. This child was able to maintain closeness with her mother from a distance. She was reassured by looking at her mother or hearing her voice. Another girl, whose mother was not able to provide consistent emotional availability, developed normally in regard to her emerging ego functions, but it seemed that her struggle to get her mother's attention sapped her of the energy with which to invest the other-than-mother world, her own autonomous ego functions, and her own body. During the early practicing subphase she was often seen sitting at her mother's feet, apparently waiting for the bits of attention that her mother was able to provide. She could explore the outside world only briefly; the elation and enthusiasm that we saw in the other children was missing for her. Pleasure in the exercise of her autonomous functions could never take precedence over the need to stay connected to mother so that she could never ignore her mother temporarily and fully extend herself to the exploration of the world.

The optimal distance during the early practicing subphase allows the moving child freedom and opportunity for exploration at some physical distance from mother. The mother herself is needed as a stable point, a home base to fulfill the need for refueling through physical contact or even looking at mother or hearing her voice. The mother also is needed to supply enough closeness so that the child can use the mother's energies for exploration and to permit the child enough freedom from her own needs for closeness so as not to impede the child's growing ability to both be away from mother and remain in contact with her. If a mother becomes ambivalent toward the child as soon as he or she is able to move away, which interferes with the mother's ability to be empathically available, the child has difficulty functioning at a distance. It is as if the mother-child relationship during the early practicing subphase sets the tone for the further process of separation and individuation. During the early practicing subphase it is especially important that the distance be created at the child's initiative rather than the mother's. When the child leaves the mother's lap, distance modalities become important and reassuring. When the mother is not physically there, so that the child cannot use these distance modalities to stay in contact, the child's mood of elation is no longer fully present. During playroom sessions, children often stared sadly at mother's empty chair or at the door through which she left for an interview with one of the observers. Thus, relative obliviousness of mother gives way to increased awareness of separation if the mother is not present or not emotionally available.

Practicing Subphase Proper (12 to 15 months): The practicing subphase proper begins with the advent of upright locomotion. This is the beginning of "the love affair with the world" (Greenacre, 1957). "The toddler takes the greatest step in human individuation. He walks freely with upright posture. Thus the plane of his vision changes; from an entirely new vantage point he finds unexpected and changing perspectives, pleasures and frustrations" (Mahler et al., 1975, pp. 70–71). During this time, from about 12 to 16 months, libidinal cathexis shifts even more to the outside world and the growing autonomous ego functions, and the child seems at times almost intoxicated with self and the world. This period is the peak of narcissism and infantile omnipotence. Characteristically, at this time children are relatively impervious to knocks, falls, and other frustrations. Substitute familiar adults seem to be much more easily accepted than they were before. The elation characteristic of this time may be fueled with a sense of elated escape from engulfment by the mother of symbiosis. A characteristic game is running away from mother, apparently with the purpose of being swooped up by her. This is a game of mastery and reassurance that demonstrates to escaping toddlers that mother wants to catch them and swoop them up in her arms. During this period children make great strides in asserting their individuality. The first great step toward identity formation seems to occur at this time. Some mothers become poignantly aware that this is the time during which they have to begin to renounce possession of their infant's body because the infant's ability to run away dramatizes what has been happening for a while. One mother said, "When he runs away from me in the park and I have to carry that heavy little body back home, I tell myself 'You better enjoy this—it won't last long. You won't be carrying him in your arm much longer'" (Mahler et al., 1975, p. 72).

It was noticed in the separation-individuation study that frequently the first steps that the child takes without holding on are taken not toward mother but away from her, and some children take the steps in mother's absence. Often mothers seem to react to their children's first independent steps by giving them a gentle push, which seems to have a facilitating effect. If it is altogether absent, the child's ability for pleasure in individuation may suffer. This big step into the outside world often seems to create a sense of anxiety in mothers. It is as if at this point, upright locomotion almost seems to become a kind of metaphor for being able to make it in the world. At this time mothers became more interested but sometimes also more critical of their children's functioning. They began to compare notes and to worry if their child was behind. An inherent contradiction exists between the symbol of walking as the ability to make it and the reality of child who still needs, and will need for a long time, the parent's care and protection.

Some typical play activities of the practicing period proper also can be understood in terms of the toddler's need to separate and explore and the simultaneous need to remain connected to mother. For example, junior toddlers love to walk around with a pull toy behind them. We could speculate about what goes on in the children's mind at this time. Do they think, "I am Mommy with a pull toy baby who goes everywhere with me?" Or "I am Baby and have a Mommy pull toy who will go wherever I go"? Similar questions might be asked about riding on kiddie cars and tricycles, which begins to be a favorite activity at this time. Do children feel strong and powerful, like mother or father riding on his or her own car? Or do children now have a pretend parent always available on whom to ride? In the playroom observations, these riding toys were passionately coveted, and toddlers considered them to be their own, even when they temporarily dismount. In a way these toys seemed to fulfill for the children what at this point is needed from the parent, namely, to be there and support the children in their independent exploration without making demands. These toys seem to confirm the internal state of magical connection while separating that is so essential during the practicing period.

THE THIRD SUBPHASE: RAPPROCHEMENT
(15 TO 24 MONTHS)

Early Rapprochement (15 to 18 months): Around the age of 15 to 16 months, when most toddlers are quite secure in their walking, running, climbing, and ability to play happily at a distance from mother, an interesting shift was noticed in the observational nursery. Whereas earlier it had been observed that the children's locomotor capacities took them away from their mothers, now almost suddenly their directions changed and they began to move toward mother. The toddler of this age suddenly seems to rediscover the mother from whom he or she has distanced during the practicing subphase. This rediscovery of mother is joyous, and toddlers approach their mothers frequently and rarely with empty hands. They now love to bring things to mother, to bring objects from the outside world and put them into mother's lap. The size of the object brought back to mother can vary from the little crumb of cookie picked up from the floor to the big riding toy that the child can hardly carry. Interestingly, how mother receives these objects at first seems of little consequence to the toddler. If mother's lap is occupied, even possibly by a baby sibling, the object would simply be deposited near mother on a chair or on an observer's lap. Thus, it seemed that the activity itself is the driving force that is hard to discourage, just as during early practicing mother is taken for granted and the activity of moving away from her is what matters. Almost suddenly the child seems to have realized the possibility of being alone without mother, and the bringing of objects to mother's lap can be understood as a wish to share with her the discoveries in the outside world.

The relative obliviousness to mother's presence characteristic of the practicing subphase now gives way to the need to share with her and to be almost constantly concerned with her whereabouts. The toddler's awareness of separateness begins to grow, stimulated both by the ability to move away physically and by cognitive growth, the advent of representational thought. The growing awareness of separateness brings with it growing awareness and need for mother. It also brings with it the dawning realization for children of their relative smallness and lack of power and ability to do all that they wish to. In other words, their former sense of omnipotence wanes. This makes toddlers of this age much more vulnerable: No longer are they oblivious to knocks and falls and frustrations. On the contrary, they now experience these as very painful and wish the mother to undo them. Rather than being able to undo the frustrations that toddlers encounter, however, mothers often have to add to them. Toddlers now often experience routine requirements of child care, such as feeding and dressing, as an insult to their desire to be omnipotently capable and independent, and it requires utmost patience and tact on the part of the mother to help the child comply with the most necessary requirements. Toddlers of this age also give their mothers very mixed messages. They want to be close and yet they reject mother's attempt to take care of them. Mothers are also puzzled because the child, who during the practicing subphase appeared so independent, now is often demanding, sometimes clinging, requiring mother's presence and attentiveness. It is not unusual for a toddler to want to follow mother wherever she goes. This behavior was named *shadow-*

ing mother, in contrast to the equally typical tendency of toddlers to dart away suddenly and expect mother to be there to catch them and sweep them up in her arms.

Incompatibilities and misunderstandings between mother and child can be observed in normal toddlers and their mothers because these are specific to the contradictions inherent in the rapprochement subphase. Some mothers find it difficult to accept the child's demanding behaviors. Others find it difficult to tolerate gradual separation. It is not unusual for mothers at this time to separate abruptly and suddenly from their toddlers, for example, taking a new job or becoming pregnant.

Rapprochement Crisis (18 to 24 months): Individuation proceeds very rapidly during the rapprochement subphase, and the child exercises it to the limit. Yet at the same time the ever-growing awareness of separateness and vulnerability often leads the toddler to become not only demanding but coercive. The combination of the many contradictory behaviors typical of this subphase has been called the *rapprochement crisis.* It is during this time when the toddler most needs the mother's emotional availability that many mothers find it difficult to cope and become demanding of the toddler and emotionally unavailable. No matter how insistently the toddler tries to coerce the mother to act as if she were still part of him or her, the two can no longer function as a dual unit. Only slowly can the toddler begin to accept the fact that mother has separate interests and wishes. Verbal communication begins to become necessary; mutual preverbal empathy between the mother-child pair no longer suffices to create the sense of well-being in the child. At the same time, the mother can no longer make the child subservient to her own predilections and wishes. Most toddlers do not relinquish the delusion of their own grandeur and omnipotence easily. Dramatic fights and temper tantrums are characteristic of the rapprochement crisis. If, however, the mother is able to remain quietly available and share her toddler's adventures playfully, their relationship can progress and the mother's emotional participation and availability can facilitate the rich unfolding of the toddler's thought processes, language, curiosity, reality testing, and coping behaviors. Toddlers of this age often seem miraculous in what seems sudden abilities of comprehension and expressiveness. They desire, sometimes almost constantly, mother's admiration and approval and wish to show her every new skill and accomplishment. It is most important that the mother be able to mirror and admire the child's competence. These shared moments help to bridge the gap of separateness. While observing a toddler jump up and down with mastery and delight a mother looks on with admiration, and it often seems as if the child becomes filled with mother's admiration and love. Toddlers begin to imitate mothers, reflecting a powerful wish to be with and to be like her.

During this period, the beginnings of role play can be observed. Mother is asked to be fairly passive and allow herself to be used to meet the needs of the toddler's unfolding inner life. For example, a common script enacted by children of this age requires mother to cry when toddler leaves or to cry when she has been hurt. For example, a boy of 20 months bit his mother playfully and wanted her to pretend to cry. He then ran and brought her his blanket, the beloved transitional object, to comfort her. He shifted from being the playful biting or the aggressive hurtful baby to being the comforting parent. Another child told mother to cry as the girl plays that she is going to work. She quickly returns and comforts her crying mother, as she herself has been comforted. The ability to play these games, that is, to put oneself in the role of the other, reveals self and object representations on the way to object constancy as well as early identification with mother and the working through of issues and conflicts related to aggression and separation.

The rapprochement crisis is the time when conflict begins to be internalized, as can be observed in the role plays in which the internal conflict is played out with the roles reversed. Baby becomes the comforting mother, or sometimes the scolding, angry mother, while mother is supposed to be the hurt or naughty baby. Toddler likes to run away and be caught, but also wants mother to run away and pretend to catch her.

During the rapprochement subphase, many toddlers also begin to observe anatomical differences. It seems that girls become aware of anatomical difference earlier than boys, and occasionally this observation causes them great pain and anxiety. Extreme reactions to the observation of a boy's genitals seem to be connected to difficulties in the mother-child relationship. In one case the

anatomical difference was observed at a time when the father was absent for an extended period and mother became depressed. In another case mother was relatively emotionally unavailable and very preoccupied with herself. A battle around toilet training ensued, and the little girl became quite severely constipated and also showed severe separation anxieties. In this mother-child pair the child seemed to have to defend the good mother against her destructive rage. She split the object world into good and bad. The good object was always the absent one. When the mother left, the little girl had a temper tantrum and clung to her familiar observer, expressing anger toward her and kicking her while holding onto her. She found fault with everything the observer did. At the same time she was longing for her mother, but when the mother came back this child was not happy. Her first words to her mother were a demand. She did not succeed in attaining a unified object representation or in reconciling the good and bad qualities of the love object. At the same time her own self-representation and self-esteem suffered. Here we see the beginnings of internalization and character formation and the development of traits that may permanently influence further development. In other words, each child and mother have to find an individual solution of the rapprochement crisis, solutions that result in the patternings and personality characteristics with which the child enters into the fourth subphase of separation-individuation: the subphase of *beginnings of emotional object constancy and consolidation of individuality.* The role of the father during the separation-individuation process and its particular significance during the rapprochement subphase was studied by Ernest Abelin (1971, 1975, 1980).

THE FOURTH SUBPHASE: THE BEGINNINGS OF EMOTIONAL OBJECT CONSTANCY AND CONSOLIDATION OF INDIVIDUALITY (24 TO 30 MONTHS)

The achievement of affective object constancy depends on the gradual internalization of a constant positively cathected inner image of the mother. This makes it possible for the child to function separately and at a distance from mother despite moderate degrees of longing for her. The cognitive achievement of object permanence is a part of the child's ability to function separately as it enables the child to keep mother's image in mind and accept that she can be elsewhere and that knowing her whereabouts is reassuring. The slow establishment of emotional object constancy is a complex and multidetermined process that rests on trust and confidence in the love object as well as the cognitive ability to maintain a symbolic inner representation. If the ambivalence toward the mother is too great, the positive image of the mother cannot be sustained in her absence.

The development of language and symbolic play are the most important achievements that help the child master separateness as well as separation. With self and object representations more firmly established, the child is better able to enact needs, impulses, and conflicts through role play. Our ability to learn about the representational world of children through their play is dramatically increased. Role play begins to include characters from the outside world; it is no longer limited to role exchange between mother and child. This kind of play rests on a self firmly and flexibly enough established to be able to put itself in the place of the other—a hallmark in the establishment of emotional object constancy. The child is able to extend to the widening world characteristics of the self and significant others as well as aspects of their relationships. Role play reinforces connections with emotionally significant others as well as separation from them because each role enactment embodies a crucial aspect of the self and the other.

During the second half of the third year, the libidinal investment in the other helps the child to maintain emotional equilibrium in the face of absence or minor frustration. The basis for this growing stability and quality of the inner representation is the actual mother-child relationship as it unfolds in the day-to-day interaction between mother and child during the entire separation-individuation period. This relative stability, however, is not permanent and can be threatened easily by new storms arising either from the vicissitudes of further development or traumatic events in the child's life. Castration anxiety, from as early as the second part of the second year on, may threaten the development of the integration of self representations. Ongoing events can influ-

ence decisively in a negative way the consolidation of individuality and emotional object constancy. However, by the third year there is in the life of each child a particular constellation that is the result of the optimal or less than optimal empathic personality of the mother and her mothering capacities. But accidental and sometimes fateful happenings, such as sicknesses, accidents, prolonged separations, or birth of siblings, can put great strain on the developing capacity for object constancy.

Further Contributions to Separation-Individuation Theory

During the course of the study, some investigators developed special interests in one particular aspect of the separation-individuation process and its connection to psychoanalytic theory and technique. In what follows I briefly describe some of the recent research and projects directly connected with Mahler's original work.

JOHN MCDEVITT

John McDevitt was coprincipal investigator of Mahler's separation-individuation research and has contributed several papers in which he elaborates on particular issues pertaining to psychoanalytic theory and clinical practice (cf. McDevitt, 1975, 1983, 1996). In his paper entitled "Separation-Individuation and Object Constancy," McDevitt (1975) reviews object constancy as it takes place through the four subphases of the separation-individuation process, from 5 to 36 months of age. He places particular emphasis on ego development as it asserts its influence on the drives, and in particular he attends to the interrelationship of affective and cognitive structures as they contribute sometimes harmoniously and other times dissonantly to the beginning achievement of object constancy. The development of object constancy is inferred from the children observed in the separation-individuation study in which separation experiences were built into the experimental design (Mahler et al., 1975).

McDevitt begins by describing how Donna, between the age of 6 and 8 months, reacts strongly to her mother's absence and how her separation reaction is triggered by looking at the door through which mother has left sometime earlier. This indicates that she is now starting to perceive mother to some extent as separate from herself because when mother leaves the room temporarily she is not forgotten. Donna's repeated looking at the door suggests the existence of at least a rudimentary ability to remember the absent love object as well as a primitive notion of person permanence. As infants progress from differentiation to practicing (from 10 to 16 months), there begins to be more conscious awareness of the relation between mother's absence and their own distress. One-year-olds begin to search for the absent mother, try to prevent her from leaving, and indicate in her absence that they are thinking of her. By the time of rapprochement, a much greater degree of object constancy is present, but it remains subject to regression caused by moment-to-moment shifts in mood and the prevalence of anger toward the mother so that severe separation anxiety frequently occurs. Only with the resolution of the rapprochement crisis and the beginning of the fourth subphase of separation-individuation is more reliable object constancy reached.

By the time object constancy begins to be attained, the mother, whose actual presence served as a secure base from which to explore during the practicing subphase, now begins to take the form of secure and stable mental representation, which enables the toddler to engage in a variety of activities separately and independently of her. McDevitt speaks of the role of identification, which enables the child to maintain an internal tie with the mother while at the same time being able to function independently of her. Tolerance of separation is not the only sign that a greater degree of object constancy has been attained. There occurs a shift from self-centered, demanding, and clinging behaviors to more mature ego-determined object relationships. Indications that such a change has occurred include expressions of affection, trust, and confidence, regard for the interests and feelings of others, the ability to play cooperatively, sharing and taking turns, and the capacity to be concerned and make small sacrifices.

McDevitt also has been particularly interested in the emergence of internal conflict during the rapprochement subphase and has written a paper on aggression during separation-individuation (1983). In this paper he examines the emergence of hostile aggression, its precursors, and its adaptive and defensive modifications during separation-individuation. Furthermore, he demonstrates how hostile aggression contributes to the onset of intrapsychic conflict. In particular he describes the vicissitudes of the aggressive conflict in three children observed during separation-individuation and later evaluated in a follow-up study when they were 8 years old.

McDevitt cites the dictionary definition of aggression as "the forceful prosecution of one's ends." The frustration of these aims leads to anger, which he says contributes to the driving quality of hostile aggressive behavior. Although McDevitt recognizes the importance of constructive aggression, his focus is on the emergence of hostile aggression. Mother's restrictions and criticisms of her 9- to 10-month-old practicing infant become connected in the infant's mind with newly developing awareness that mother can leave and results in a crisis at this time that results in renewed clinging to mother. As a result of this crisis, infants begin to modify their angry behavior. Finally, McDevitt concludes that the aggressive potential in each child as well as the ability to modulate aggression depend on the child's endowment and on the relationship with parents. The manifestations of aggression and the ability to cope with it both influence and are influenced by the characteristics of each subphase of the separation-individuation process. Under unfavorable conditions, problems with aggression during the differentiation and practicing subphases contribute to failures during rapprochement and the fourth subphase, which in turn makes the resolution of oedipal issues more difficult. Under favorable conditions, the child's libidinal investment in the mother outweighs aggression in each subphase. Toddlers are able to reach a degree of self and object constancy that prepares them to resolve future conflicts successfully.

ANNI BERGMAN

This author, senior research associate of Mahler's separation-individuation research as well as her research on childhood psychosis (Mahler & Furer, 1968), has written case studies on 2 psychotic children in which separation-individuation theory was used to understand these children's development in therapy (Bergman, 1971, 1985). In addition, she developed a special interest in gender differences during the separation-individuation process (Bergman & Fahey, 1994) and the course of female development. She has written about the special meaning of the girl to a mother. Often a mother experiences the daughter as someone like her, which may influence her attitude toward the daughter as she separates (Bergman, 1982). She also has written about the special pleasure that the girl during early rapprochement develops and the process of sharing with mother (Bergman, 1987, 1992). In fact, it may be this closeness between mother and daughter that brings about unique difficulties in the process of separation-individuation for the girl. Another special interest is the development and significance of play during the separation-individuation process and how such play provides a window into the representational world of the infant as well as a pathway for reaching object constancy in the therapy of children with significant delays in the formation of self-object differentiation (Bergman, 1993; Bergman & Fahey, 1994).

FRED PINE

Fred Pine, consultant on research methodology during the separation-individuation research, has written extensively on the importance of separation-individuation in clinical practice and theory (Pine, 1985, 1990). In a chapter entitled "Pathology of the Separation-Individuation Process as Manifested in Later Clinical Work," Pine (1985) provides a variety of clinical vignettes in which he distinguishes pathology originating in the separation-individuation phase and indicating a not fully differentiated self from pathology in which the self is differentiated but the sense of self is disturbed in various ways originating in dynamic conflicts. He warns against accepting surface phenomena as indicators of pathology being located in the separation-individuation process. A patient may appear to have problems in that area, as indicated, for example, by a sense of being no-

body, but may in fact be well differentiated. On the other hand, a patient may have a pseudoidentity behind which is panic related to loss of self-experiences. Making the correct distinctions is of great importance because, in cases where the other is differentiated well enough, interpretation will be the main therapeutic tool. In cases where the sense of self is not differentiated sufficiently, "substantial reexperiencing of a primary object bond" is required in addition to interpretation (Pine, 1985, p. 233).

Pine (1990) also has addressed the controversies raised about Mahler's work by modern infant researchers. Pine (1992, 1994) has offered a refinement of the separation-individuation process which makes it more consistent with the findings of infant research. He has suggested a revision of the concept of the symbiotic phase, seeing symbiosis not as an ongoing state but as a series of momentary merger experiences that are affectively significant.

SELMA KRAMER

The significance of separation-individuation issues in treatment with adult patients has been examined by Selma Kramer, who has contributed to a special issue of the *Journal of the American Psychoanalytic Association* on psychoanalytic treatment technique (Kramer, 1979). With the help of clinical examples, she shows how the transference neurosis includes preoedipal conflicts that have their source in rapprochement. She shows further how the technique of the analyst helps the expression and resolution of early conflict.

OTHER RESEARCH

At this time, some investigators are carrying on further research. Anni Bergman and John McDevitt are carrying on a follow-up study of the subjects from the original separation-individuation research, who are now young adults. Patricia Nachman is the head of the Margaret S. Mahler Observational Research Nursery at The New School, where she has carried on research observations in which she compares toddlers observed in the research settings with their mothers to toddlers in the research settings with their caregivers. It is important to say that both children of working mothers and children of caregiving mothers in this sample came from reasonably intact and caring families. Subtle modifications of certain processes of the ego were observed, involving socialization, symbolization, and identification (Nachman, 1991). Calvin Settlage has been conducting a study on what he calls the "appeal cycle." He observes toddlers coping with mother's temporary emotional unavailability as she becomes involved in a discussion with the investigator, leaving the child to play on his or her own (Settlage et al., 1990).

Several other investigators have used the method of observational research done in a nursery setting. Among these are Eleanor Galenson and Herman Roiphe, who did an extensive study of gender identity (Galenson & Roiphe, 1976). Roiphe currently is studying aggression between infants (Roiphe, 1991). Wendy Olesker is the founder and director of a mother-child observa-

tional nursery at Montefiore Hospital modeled after the Mahler observational research nursery in which mothers come with their infants and toddlers and each mother pair is assigned to a resident or psychology intern for study. The main focus of her investigations has been gender difference (Olesker, 1984, 1990).

In this section I could do no more than mention the influence of Margaret Mahler's work on some of her close colleagues and coworkers. Her work is used by psychoanalysts all over the world for both its clinical and theoretical contributions. Several books of collected papers directly expand and elucidate her work (Lax, 1986; Lax, Bach, & Burland, 1980; McDevitt & Settlage, 1971), and the yearly Margaret S. Mahler Symposium in Philadelphia deals with topics that are related to separation-individuation research and theory (Akhtar & Kramer, 1996; Akhtar, Kramer, & Parens, 1995, 1996; Kramer & Akhtar, 1991, 1992, 1994; Parens & Kramer, 1993).

REFERENCES

Abelin, E. (1971). The role of the father in the separation-individuation process. In J. McDevitt & C. Settlage (Eds.), *Separation-individuation* (pp. 229–253). New York: International Universities Press.

Abelin, E. (1975). Some further observations and comments on the earliest role of the father. *International Journal of Psychoanalysis, 56*, 293–302.

Abelin, E. (1980). Triangulation: The role of the father and the origins of core gender identity during the rapprochement subphase. In R. Lax, S. Bach, & J. A. Burland (Eds.), *Rapprochement* (pp. 151–170). Hillsdale, NJ: Jason Aronson.

Akhtar, S., & Kramer, S. (Eds.). (1996). *Intimacy and infidelity: Separation-individuation perspectives.* Hillsdale, NJ: Jason Aronson.

Akhtar, S., Kramer, S., & Parens, H. (Eds.). (1995). *The birth of hatred: Developmental, clinical, and technical aspects of intense aggression.* Hillsdale, NJ: Jason Aronson.

Bergman, A. (1971). I and you. In J. McDevitt & C. Settlage (Eds.), *Separation-individuation: Festschrift in honor of Margaret Mahler* (pp. 325–355). New York: International Universities Press.

Bergman, A. (1982). Considerations about the development of the girl during the separation-individuation process. In D. Mendell (Ed.), *Early female development: Current psychoanalytic views* (pp. 61–80). New York: Spectrum.

Bergman, A. (1985). From psychological birth to motherhood: The treatment of an autistic child with follow-up into her adult life as a mother. In E.J. Anthony & G. Pollock (Eds.), *Parental influences in health and disease* (pp. 91–121). Boston: Little, Brown.

Bergman, A. (1987). On the development of female identity: Issues of mother-daughter interaction during the separation-individuation process. *Psychoanalytic Inquiry, 7*, 381–396.

Bergman, A. (1992). The mother's wish for a better self: Mutual identifications between mothers and daughters. In M. Kissen (Ed.), *Gender and psychoanalytic treatment* (pp. 38–47). New York: Brunner/Mazel.

Bergman, A. (1993). To be or not to be separate: The meaning of hide-and-seek in forming internal representations. *Psychoanalytic Review, 80*, 361–375.

Bergman, A., & Ellman, S. (1985). Margaret S. Mahler: Symbiosis and separation-individuation. In J. Reppen (Ed.), *Beyond Freud* (pp. 231–256). Hillsdale, NJ: Analytic Press.

Bergman, A., & Fahey, M. (1994). Further inquiry into negotiations of separation-individuation conflicts: A boy and a girl respond to fluctuations in mother's emotional availability. *Psychoanalytic Inquiry, 14*, 83–110.

Bergman, A., & Lefcourt, I. (1994). Self-other action play: A window into the representational world of the infant. In A. Slade & D. Wolf (Eds.), *Children at play: Clinical and developmental approaches to meaning and representation* (pp. 133–147). New York: Oxford University Press.

Brody, S., & Axelrod, S. (1970). *Anxiety and ego formation in infancy*. New York: International Universities Press.

Galenson, E., & Roiphe, H. (1976). Some suggested revisions concerning female development. *Journal of the American Psychoanalytic Association, 24,* 29–57.

Greenacre, P. (1957). The childhood of the artist: Libidinal phase development and giftedness. *Psychoanalytic Study of the Child, 12,* 27–72.

Kramer, S. (1979). The technical significance and application of Mahler's separation-individuation theory. *Journal of the American Psychoanalytic Association, 27* (Suppl.), 241–263.

Kramer, S., & Akhtar, S. (Eds.). (1991). *The trauma of transgression: psychotherapy of incest victims*. Hillsdale, NJ: Jason Aronson.

Kramer, S., & Akhtar, S. (Eds.). (1992). *When the body speaks: Psychological meanings in kinetic clues*. Hillsdale, NJ: Jason Aronson.

Kramer, S., & Akhtar, S. (Eds.) (1994). *Mahler and Kohut: Perspectives on development, psychopathology, and technique*. Hillsdale, NJ: Jason Aronson.

Lax, R., Bach, S., & Burland, J. (Eds.). (1980). *Rapprochement: The critical subphase of separation-individuation*. New York: Jason Aronson.

Lax, R. (Ed.). (1986). *Self and object constancy: Clinical and theoretical perspectives*. New York: Guilford Press.

Mahler, M., & Furer, M. (1968). *On human symbiosis and the vicissitudes of individuation: Infantile psychosis*. Westport, CT: International Universities Press.

Mahler, M., Pine, F., & Bergman, A. (1975). *The psychological birth of the human infant*. New York: Basic Books.

Mahler, M., Pine, F., Bergman, A., & Smith, J. (1976). *The psychological birth of the human infant: The separation-individuation process*. A film in three parts produced through the Margaret S. Mahler Research Foundation. (Available through the Mahler Film Library, P.O. Box 315, Franklin Lakes, NJ 07417)

Mahler, M., Pine, F., Bergman, A., & Smith, J. (1982). *On the phenomena indicative of the emergence of the sense of self*. A film produced through the Margaret S. Mahler Research Foundation. (Available through the Mahler Film Library, P.O. Box 315, Franklin Lakes, NJ 07417.)

McDevitt, J. (1975). Separation-individuation and object constancy. *Journal of the American Psychoanalytic Association, 23,* 713–742.

McDevitt, J. (1983). The emergence of hostile aggression and its defensive and adaptive modifications during the separation-individuation process. *Journal of the American Psychoanalytic Association, 31,* 273–300.

McDevitt, J. (1996). The concept of object constancy and its clinical applications. In S. Akhtar, S. Kramer, & H. Parens (Eds.), *The internal mother: Conceptual and technical aspects of intense aggression*. Hillsdale, NJ: Jason Aronson.

McDevitt, J., & Settlage, C. (Eds.). (1971). *Separation-individuation: Essays in honor of Margaret Mahler*. New York: International Universities Press.

Nachman, P. (1991). The maternal representation: A comparison of caregiver- and mother-reared toddlers. *Psychoanalytic Study of the Child, 46,* 69–90.

Olesker, W. (1984). Sex differences in 2- and 3-year-olds: Mother-child relations, peer relations, and peer play. *Psychoanalytic Psychology, 1*(4), 269–288.

Olesker, W. (1990). Sex differences during the early separation-individuation process: Implications for gender identity formation. *Journal of the American Psychoanalytic Association, 38,* 325–346.

Parens, H., & Kramer, S. (Eds.). (1993). *Prevention in mental health*. Hillsdale, NJ: Jason Aronson.

Pine, F. (1985). Pathology of the separation-individuation process. In F. Pine, *Developmental theory and clinical process* (pp. 227–247). New Haven, CT: Yale University Press.

Pine, F. (1990). Infant research, the symbiotic phase, and clinical work: A case study of a concept. In F. Pine, *Drive, ego, object & self* (pp. 232–256). New York: Basic Books.

Pine, F. (1992). Some refinements of the separation-individuation concept in light of research on infants. *Psychoanalytic Study of Child, 47,* 103–116.

Pine, F. (1994). The era of separation-individuation. *Psychoanalytic Inquiry, 14,* 4–24.

Roiphe, H. (1991). The tormentor and the victim in the nursery. *Psychoanalytic Quarter, 60,* 450–466.

Settlage, C., Rosenthal, J., Spielman, P., Gassner, S., Alterman, J., Bemesderfer, S., & Kolodny, S. (1990). An exploratory study of mother-child interaction during the second year of life. *Journal of the American Psychoanalytic Association, 38,* 705–732.

Stepansky, P. (Ed.). (1988). *The memoirs of Margaret S. Mahler*. New York: Free Press.

29 / Parent-Infant Bonding: Biologic, Psychologic, and Clinical Aspects

John H. Kennell and Marshall H. Klaus

Introduction

The process by which a mother and father become attached to their newborn infant with a love so strong that they will make great personal sacrifices for their child has been the focus of research for more than a quarter of a century. Prior to that time, however, the mother's bond to her newborn infant had been noted and commented upon by astute observers such as Donald Winnicott. A report of the effects of early and extended contact of mothers with their healthy newborn infants stimulated a wide range of research investigations of mothers, fathers, and their newborns. These studies began to provide a sketchy outline of the complex process by which parents develop an attachment to their infant as well as what enhances or distorts it. This chapter brings together information gathered from many sources and disciplines: naturalistic observations of mothering; studies of other cultures; detailed studies of maternal behavior in animals; human studies including randomized trials of mothers and fathers of premature and full-term infants using various interventions; clinical observations during medical care procedures; long-term, in-depth interviews of a small number of mothers primarily by psychoanalysts; and structured interviews. These data then are integrated into a general framework from which clinical recommendations are developed.

Definition and Measurement of the Parent-Infant Bond

This area of research has suffered from the lack of a simple tool to assess the strength and characteristics, or even the existence, of the parent-infant bond. We define a bond as a unique relationship between two people that is specific for those two and endures through time. Most studies have used an assessment of the parent's behavior primarily as evidence of interest and affectionate interaction with the baby.

The incidence and duration of breast-feeding has been used to assess the strength of the bond, but this can be criticized as not necessarily indicative, as for example, in working mothers who do not breast-feed. Possibly the most reliable measure is the parents' performance with the child over an extended period of time.

The recent avalanche of reports about young infants of cocaine-abusing mothers suffering from a lack of maternal care and attention has led to much greater awareness of the vital importance of the process by which mothers become attached to their newborn infants. Many of these women show their lack of attachment by failure to visit their sick infants, their lack of interest, and neglect. Some verbally express great love and show exemplary affection when being assessed but then thoughtlessly leave the young infant unprotected on the examining table or at home alone for hours.

Practices in Other Cultures

The process of bonding has been of special interest because it appears to touch on basic biologic principles that are significant for the survival of the infant and therefore the species. It is useful to observe practices that are still being followed in a large number of nonindustrial societies because what was chosen as a common practice in these societies may be a procedure that improves the chances of a successful outcome for both the mother and infant. Presumably those birthing, feeding, and child-rearing practices most adaptive to the life of a majority of nonindustrial societies gave the infant the best opportunity to survive and grow. If methods of providing warmth, feeding, or interaction were not adequate, the baby would not survive. Certain behavioral patterns for breast-feeding and for providing warmth by almost continuous body contact during the day and night best met the thermal as well as nutritional and immunologic needs of the infant. Practices noted almost universally then generate questions about human physiologic processes that can be tested in industrial societies. For example, in a review of geographically, linguistically, and historically representative nonindustrialized societies, "women giving birth had assistance and companionship in almost all societies" (Lozoff, Jordan, & Malone, 1988, p. 47). In 127 of 128 representative societies, a woman was present during labor and delivery. The baby was born in a familiar site with well-known attendants. When continuous emotional support for a woman during labor was systematically studied recently in the hospital, many benefits for the mother and infant were discovered. Lozoff also noted that "In 70% of the cultures ... the most common birth position was with the torso upright" (p. 47); there is now anatomical documentation for the advantages of the kneeling, squatting, or sitting positions (Russell, 1982). When pregnant women moved from the supine to the squatting and/or sitting position, it was demonstrated by radiography that the actual area of the pelvic outlet increased by 28%. Thus, the position chosen for birth by the majority of nonindustrial societies has strong support from anatomical measurements.

While studies have shown more attentive and affectionate maternal behavior when there is mother-infant contact in the first 2 or 3 hours, Lozoff and colleagues (1988) found that the bathed newborn was given to the mother in only approximately half of all nonindustrial societies; in the other half "the infant was placed in a cradle or basket ... commonly in his or her mother's sight" (p. 49).

In 7 of 9 studies in industrialized societies, women who suckled in the first hour were more likely to be breast-feeding at 2 months than mothers who started at 4 to 6 or 24 hours. However, infants were nursed at the breast in the first hour in only 48% of 81 representative agricultural societies; in 52% of these countries nursing was delayed more than 24 hours in general because colostrum was considered of no value or harmful. In spite of this delay, there was no difference in the incidence or duration of breast-feeding between the societies with early or delayed nursing. Almost all the mothers in the nonindustrial societies breast-fed successfully for many months.

This raises the question of whether mother-infant contact in privacy with protection and support over several days is more significant than what occurs in the first hour.

Actually, in 183 of 186 societies studied by Lozoff, the mother received food, support, and protection during the first days and weeks, which allowed the mother to become well acquainted with her baby and its care and establish breast-feeding. Lozoff et al. (1988) comment about the discrepancy between outcomes in nonindustrialized societies and the results of careful studies in Western societies.

The standard maternity hospital routine in industrial societies of separating mothers and babies is followed by an infant care pattern that commonly comprises frequent separations of mother and infant in the home, minimal body contact, and spaced feeding. In the context of this pattern of infant care, body contact immediately after birth may assume disproportionate significance in enhancing maternal affection. In contrast, in nonindustrial societies separation in the first hour may have less effect on the mother's later involvement with her infant because such separations are not repeated. The brief initial separation of mother and infant is universally followed by postpartum confinement of mother and baby together—a rooming-in period—which is itself followed by extensive mother-infant contact and prolonged and frequent breast feeding during the baby's early months. (p. 52)

Studies of Maternal Behavior in Animals

Studies of animal maternal behavior were in part a stimulus for the early human observations. In each species of mammals, specific ways of meeting the needs of its young have evolved to ensure survival. Detailed and careful studies in many species have described several mechanisms by which the mother develops a tie or bond to her young.

BEHAVIORAL (NONHORMONAL) EFFECTS OF CONTACT WITH YOUNG

Rosenblatt and colleagues demonstrated that when young rat pups were placed with adult males or virgin females, typical maternal behavior (nest-building and retrieving) except for breast-feeding developed over a 5- to 7-day period (Rosenblatt 1967, 1969, 1989; Rosenblatt & Siegel, 1981).

HORMONAL EFFECTS

Estradiol: A series of creative experiments revealed that in rats there is a strong early hormonal influence on maternal behavior, as well as the slower onset of a behavioral process due to association with young pups (Rosenblatt, Mayer, & Siegel, 1985; Rosenblatt & Siegel, 1981). The investigators identified the existence of a substance (presumably estradiol) present in the blood of the pregnant female for only a brief period around the time of delivery that significantly increased maternal behavior (Terkel & Rosenblatt 1972). Rosenblatt showed the importance of estradiol in the development of maternal behavior in rats. He and his associates suggested that the increase in estradiol and the rapid decline in circulating levels of progesterone that occurred 30 hours prior to delivery in the rat may facilitate the appearance of maternal behavior (Rosenblatt, Siegel, & Mayer, 1979). Researchers in France found that estrogen appeared to be the principal hormone that stimulates maternal behavior in sheep (Poindron & LeNeindre, 1980; Poindron, Levy, & Krehbiel, 1988). They noted that the onset of maternal responsiveness in sheep was related to the rise in estrogen before birth. After a 24-hour separation from their lambs, 60% of ewes treated with estrogen at the time of delivery accepted their young; only 10% of ewes not treated with estrogen accepted their lambs. Their data revealed that the effects of estrogen subsided in the early postpar-

tum period and the maintenance of maternal behavior was then related to nonhormonal factors. These results showed there was "a transition period in the shift from hormonal (internal) to nonhormonal (external stimulation) control of maternal behavior in this species" (p. 122).

A similar pattern of increase in estradiol and decrease in progesterone 3 to 5 weeks before the onset of labor in the human has also been identified (Turnbull et al., 1974).

Oxytocin: Beginning in the late 1940s, Newton and Newton emphasized the importance of oxytocin, but for several years this hormone was considered to be acting only peripherally (M. Newton & N. Newton, 1948, 1950; N. Newton 1973, 1978). However, in recent years the release of the neuropeptide oxytocin from the paraventricular nucleus and the supraoptic nucleus in the brain and the importance of its central effects in facilitating maternal behavior and the formation of social bonds has been demonstrated in animals.

Carter, Williams, and Witt (1990) demonstrated that oxytocin, working in conjunction with sex steroids, may be one component of the mechanism responsible for pair bond formation in prairie voles, a monogamous species. These investigators showed the effects of oxytocin on affiliative or attachment behavior between two adult animals of the same sex. When given oxytocin, adult voles will make a selective choice for affiliation or bonding depending on who was with them at the time. In this monogamous species, males exposed to pups become parental in less than 30 seconds and show a full range of maternal behavior. When males are exposed to pups, they have an almost immediate sharp increase in oxytocin blood levels. Sex hormones guide the number and distribution of oxytocin receptors in the brain, receptors that are necessary for the specific response to oxytocin, for example, maternal behavior. In sheep, also, the release of oxytocin in the central nervous system is involved in the mother's maternal responsiveness. Vagino-cervical stimulation, occurring during delivery, results in the intracerebral release of oxytocin and stimulates maternal behavior (Kendrick, Keverne, & Baldwin, 1987; Keverne, 1988; Keverne, Levy, Poindron & Lindsay, 1983).

Evidence is beginning to accumulate that oxytocin may have effects on the attachment behavior of the neonate in animals. Interestingly, human milk contains high levels of oxytocin. Human mothers experience a surge of oxytocin as the baby's head descends through the birth canal and repeated bursts of oxytocin ("let-down reflex") with each breast-feeding, which may explain in part the warm feelings human mothers experience when they suckle their baby. The oxytocin in the milk might enhance the nursing infant's attachment to the mother. Of course, human parents can adapt and become attached to their infants without breast-feeding. Many fail-safe processes exist to ensure the attachment of parents to infants in most circumstances. Currently a number of studies are attempting to sort out the mystery of what combinations of hormones (estradiol, progesterone, prolactin, endorphins, oxytocin) and what levels and shifts are necessary for attachment and the onset of maternal behavior is actively being studied in animals; little work is being done with humans. Opiates block the release of oxytocin, and its release decreases when mothers are stressed. In the human, does the administration of epidural anesthesia that blocks the sensory nerves carrying vagino-cervical stimulation during labor and delivery have an effect on maternal attachment? This is an important question that needs investigation.

Events Important in a Mother's Attachment to Her Infant

The infant is completely dependent on the mother or caregiver to meet all its physical and emotional needs. Thus, the strength and durability of the mother's attachment may well determine whether the baby will survive and develop optimally. Therefore, it is helpful to consider the components of the affectional bond between a mother and her infant and to determine the factors that may alter or distort its formation.

Events important to the formation of a mother's bond to her infant may occur before or during pregnancy, during labor and delivery, or after the birth of the baby in the first minutes, hours, and days.

By observing and studying mothers during these periods, it has been possible to fit together some of the interlocking pieces that lay the foundations of attachment.

BEFORE PREGNANCY

Experimental data suggest that the past experiences of the mother are major determinants in molding her caregiving role. Child development literature suggests that children are socialized by the powerful process of imitation and modeling. Long before a woman herself becomes a mother, she has learned, from the way she was mothered and through observation, whether infants are picked up when they cry, where and how much they are carried, and whether they should be chubby or thin.

Mothering Experiences: George Engel's long-term follow up of Monica, who required gastrostomy feedings for the first 2 years of her life, provides striking evidence that the way a mother cares for her baby is influenced in part by the way she was mothered herself (Engol, Reichsman, & Harvey, 1985). Due to congenital atresia of her esophagus, Monica could not be fed by mouth and was given feedings by gastrostomy tube on a strict schedule usually while lying horizontally in bed or on her mother's lap, but not in her mother's arms. (See Figure 29.1a.) Following surgical repair of the esophagus when she was 4 years old, Monica fed her doll horizontally across her knees away from her body in this same position and manner. (See Figure 29.1b.) When Monica's own four daughters were born, she fed them across her knees away from her body in a similar fashion to the way her mother had fed her. (See Figures 29.1c of Donna, her fourth baby, and 29.1d, of Adele, her first.) In spite of suggestions to hold her babies close and semivertically, the horizontal method seemed to Monica to be the easiest way to feed her babies. The babies were given one feeding at 6:00 P.M. each day in which they were held close by their father. When they became old enough to play at mothering, they fed their dolls the way Monica had fed them. However, when the girls were older, from 4 to 10 years, they began to hold their dolls easily enfolded in their arms, sometimes closely and "en face."

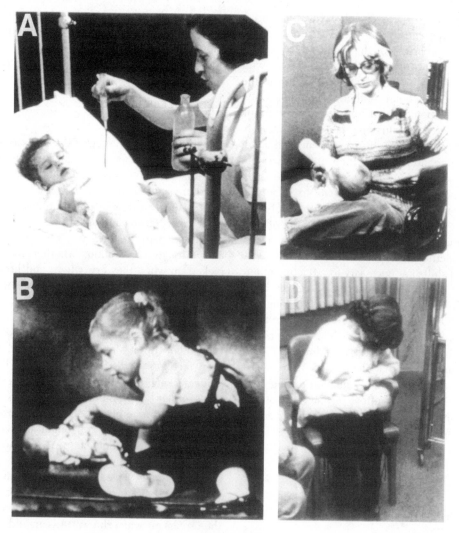

FIGURE 29.1

Monica, born with a congenital malformation, required feeding by a tube into her stomach throughout infancy. Figure 29.1a shows her being tube fed as an infant. Figure 29.1b shows her as a toddler feeding a doll without holding, in much the same position as she was fed in infancy. Figures 29.1c and 29.1d show Monica, now grown, with two of her own babies. Note that she does not hold the babies in her arms while feeding them. In contrast, her husband and sisters feed the babies by holding them in their arms in the usual face-to-face position. This long-term follow-up demonstrates the persistence of an unusual feeding pattern from one generation to another.

NOTE: Photos from *Parental Influences in Health and Disease,* edited by E. J. Anthony and G. H. Pollack, copyright 1985. Published by Little, Brown and Company. Reprinted with permission.

Cultural Practices: An unfortunate aspect of the nuclear family in the Western world is that many young women have had no exposure to the care of young infants before they have their own. This leaves them inexperienced and uncertain when their own baby arrives. In contrast, a new mother in a developing country usually has extensive experience with young infants long before she cares for her own. As a consequence she feels confident and is ready to make fine adjustments in her mothering style. The way a woman was raised, which includes the practices of her culture and the individual idiosyncrasies of her own mother's child-rearing practices, greatly influences her own behavior toward her infant (Fraiberg, Adelson, & Shapiro, 1975).

Effects of Stress: Lumley (1980) has explored the feelings and thoughts of 30 Australian mothers during their first pregnancies. In the first interview at 8 to 12 weeks' gestation, 70% of these women said they could not believe that the fetus was really there, and they never imagined or pictured the fetus as a real person. The others believed that the fetus was a real person, and they spontaneously imagined its appearance. These women were likely to describe the fetus with a feeling of concern, with anxieties about the fetus, such as the fear of miscarriage or abnormality. They predicted severe grief if they were to have a miscarriage. Those mothers who began to show early feelings of attachment came from larger families and were women whose previous work had been in nursing or teaching. Feelings of attachment were inhibited in the presence of severe physical problems in the pregnancy, when the woman's husband was not interested in the fetus, or when the husband did not provide emotional support. After the interview, mothers were asked to draw an image of the fetus. During the 8- to 12-week gestation period, the fetus was presented as shapeless and formless, but as the pregnancy progressed, the fetus developed a more human form.

The increased use of amniocentesis and ultrasound has appeared to affect parents' perceptions of their babies. Some parents have been disappointed when they discovered the sex of the baby because half of the mystery was over. Once the amniocentesis was done and the sex was known, the range of the unknown was considerably narrowed. On the other hand, these tests often have beneficial results by removing some of the anxiety about the possibility of an abnormality. Following the procedure, parents sometimes name the baby, and often they carry around an ultrasound picture of the very small fetus. The significance of these procedures to the bonding process requires further investigation.

While the creation of a normal child is a major goal of most women, most pregnant women have

hidden fears that the infant may be abnormal or reveal some of their own secret inner weaknesses.

Brazelton and Bibring have clarified in part the importance of the turmoil that occurs during pregnancy for the subsequent development of attachment to the new infant (Bibring, Dwyer, Huntington, & Valenstein, 1961; Brazelton, 1973). Reporting on the anxiety that is characteristic in prenatal interviews with mothers pregnant with their first children, Brazelton described his initial concern for whether these women would be able to adjust to mothering. What happens, Brazelton believes, is that in some way this anxiety, instead of being a destructive force, becomes "a kind of shock treatment" for reorganization. He sees the "shakeup of pregnancy as readying the circuits for new attachments, as preparation for the many choices which 'a mother' must be ready to make . . . [and] as a method of freeing her circuits for a kind of sensitivity to the infant and his individual requirements." Brazelton states that this is an example of how physicians might label a mother "anxious" or as "needing help" when her responses are more accurately described as normal anxiety.

Any stress, such as moving to a new geographic area, marital infidelity, death of a close friend or relative, previous abortion, or loss of previous children, that leaves the mother feeling unloved or unsupported or that precipitates concern for the health and survival of either her infant or herself may delay a woman's preparation for the infant and retard the attachment process. After the first trimester, behaviors that are a reaction to stress and suggest rejection of pregnancy include a preoccupation with physical appearance or negative self-perception, excessive emotional withdrawal or mood swings excessive physical complaints, absence of any response to quickening, or lack of any preparatory behavior during the last trimester.

As a result of advances in perinatal care for high-risk mothers, pregnant women with diabetes, hypertension, premature labor, or a slowly growing fetus may be hospitalized up to a month or more. Studies by Merkatz (1978) noted that mothers were primarily concerned about the baby they were carrying and only secondarily about their own health. The concerns and the loneliness of these women point up the importance of designing care for them on an individual basis that takes into account the subtleties of their changing family dynamics. It is important that a woman hospitalized on the high-risk maternity unit be visited freely by her husband or boyfriend, children, and parents. In some countries relatives are allowed to live-in.

Relations with Husband and Family: To understand better the complex events that occur during the perinatal period, attention is directed primarily to the mother-infant pair. However, it is necessary to emphasize that the father, the other siblings, and the extended family are of vital importance to this relationship. Prospective fathers go through an upheaval that is similar to that of the mothers. The social support provided by the father and family has a strong impact on the mother's attachment and care of her infant. When there is husband-wife conflict, high levels of negative affect sometimes are directed toward the infant. If one parent is insensitive in his or her handling of the infant, pacifying the baby becomes more difficult for the spouse. On the other hand, a mother's perception of her husband as supportive enhances her maternal behavior.

NEONATAL PERIOD

In the past quarter century multiple studies have focused on whether additional time for close contact of the mother and infant in the first minutes, hours, and days of life affects the quality of the mother's attachment to her infant. In three studies the extra time was added not only during the first hours of life but also during the next 3 days (Klaus & Kennell, 1982; Klaus et al., 1972). At 1 month the mothers in the group that had extra contact showed significantly more affectionate behavior toward their infants. They stood closer and watched over them more during the physical examination, soothed them more when they cried, engaged in more eye-to-eye contact and fondling during feeding, and were more reluctant to leave them with someone else.

Early Contact for Mothers with Low Levels of Social Support: One reason for undertaking the first randomized trial of the effect of early and extended contact of mothers with their full-term in-

fants was concern about the behavior of young mothers with their infants (Klaus et al., 1972). This was a low-income, minority group of primarily teenage mothers, a population in which some of the mothers seemed more eager to return to their previous activities than to nurture and attend to their new infants. The positive effects of early contact in that population and in subsequent studies has suggested that the strongest effects of early mother-infant interaction occur in poor mothers with a low level of social support.

In one study a group of mothers who had contact with their infants in the first hour after delivery showed more affectionate interaction with their newborn infant 48 hours after delivery when compared to mothers who experienced routine separation (Anisfeld & Lipper, 1983). In the analysis of their data, these investigators discovered that the effects of early contact on affectionate interaction were greatest within the group of mothers who had a low level of social support, that is, two or more of the following: women who were single, on public assistance, had not graduated from high school, and did not have the father or other family member present in the delivery room. In contrast, mothers with the same lack of social support showed the lowest level of interaction with their newborns when they experienced routine separation after delivery.

In a study involving a low-income, urban population, one group of mothers was provided with 12 additional hours of contact in the first 2 days but no contact in the first hours of life (O'Connor, Vietze, Sherrod, Sandler, & Altemier, 1980). Fifteen months later the investigators found significant differences in parenting disorders, such as child abuse, neglect, abandonment, and nonorganic failure to thrive. They found 10 of these distressing problems in the control group but only 2 among mothers who were given extended contact. They also noted that the mothers with the additional hours of contact in the first 2 days had significantly lower hospital admission rates for their infants and fewer accidents and poisonings. In contrast to this was a study of low-income mothers who had more than one pregnancy and lived in a rural area of North Carolina (Siegel, Bauman, Schaefer, Saunders, & Ingram, 1980). The aim of this investigation was to explore the effect on maternal attachment of early and extended contact as well as the effect of home visits by well-trained paraprofessionals. No significant effects resulting from the home visits were noted. However, early- and extended-contact mothers showed differences in attachment variables, such as acceptance of the infant and consoling of the crying infant, as observed in the home visit at 4 months. The infants of these mothers also showed significantly increased positive versus negative behaviors in the home at 12 months. Siegel and associates explored the differences contributed by the impact of early and extended contact on maternal attachment behavior. They calculated that 2.5 to 3% of the difference in behaviors could be explained by early and extended contact whereas between 10 and 20% of the difference was explained by background variables such as the mother's economic status, race, housing, education, parity, and age. The Siegel study emphasizes the contribution of background variables that are not easily changed.

The mother's increased physical contact with the infant throughout early infancy has impressive benefits. In a controlled trial, Anisfeld and colleagues randomly assigned low-socioeconomic-status mothers of newborn infants to an experimental group that received soft baby carriers (more physical contact) or to a control group that received infant seats (less physical contact) (Anisfeld, Casper, Nozyce, & Cunningham, 1990). At 3½ months, mothers using the soft baby carriers were more contingently responsive than control mothers to the vocalizations of their infants. The Ainsworth Strange Situation was administered when the infants were 13 months old. Significantly more experimental (more physical contact) (83%) than control infants (38%) were securely attached to their mothers. Fifteen of the 16 high users of the soft baby carriers were more securely attached.

Timing of Contact: A number of questions about the timing and duration of mother-infant contact have not been resolved, perhaps due in part to the broad range of cultural practices and environments where the baby is born and where the mother and infant spend their first days together, and in part due to the outcomes measured. Hales showed that contact in the first hour compared to 12 hours after delivery resulted in greater affectionate behavior at 36 hours (Hales, Lozoff, Sosa, & Kennell, 1977).

In a hospital where all mothers had their new-born infants on their chests for the first 45 minutes of life, Widström and associates (1990) found a significant effect on a mother's behavior with her baby when the infant touched her nipple in the first hour. After this touching of the nipple and as a result of their mother's behavior, these babies spent significantly less time in the nursery and away from their mothers compared to the other babies who had their first nipple contact an average of 9 hours after delivery. This is demonstrated in Figure 29.2, which shows the amount of time that early-nipple-contact babies and late-contact babies were in the nursery and not with their mothers.

Postpartum Effects of Doula *Support During Labor:* Two randomized controlled clinical trials of continuous emotional support by an experienced woman (*doula*) during labor in Guatemala and one in the United States have shown a decrease in labor length, in cesarean and forceps deliveries, and in use of pitocin, medication, and epidural anesthesia (Kennell, Klaus, McGrath, Robertson, & Hinkley, 1991; Klaus, Kennell, Robertson, & Sosa, 1986; Sosa, Kennell, Klaus, Robertson, & Urrutia, 1980). When routine care and *doula*-supported mothers were observed within the first hour of life with their babies after they left the delivery room in Guatemala, these mothers showed more affectionate interaction with their infants during the periods when the mothers were awake (Sosa et al., 1980).

Hofmeyr and a team of investigators in South Africa carried out a randomized *doula* study in which they obtained follow-up information 6 weeks after the delivery (Hofmeyr, Nikodem, Wolman, Chalmers, & Kramer, 1991; Wolman, 1991). They found that mothers supported by a *doula* had increased feelings of self-esteem 6 weeks later and felt they were caring for their baby better than anyone else could. Most important, the *doula*-supported mothers had a much lower score on measures of depression than women who had no *doula* during labor. Measures of anxiety also were reduced in the mothers who had received support. The mothers who had a *doula* had increased success with breast-feeding and a more positive attitude toward both their infant and their male partner. It is of interest that the infants of these mothers had significantly fewer feeding problems. When the mothers were

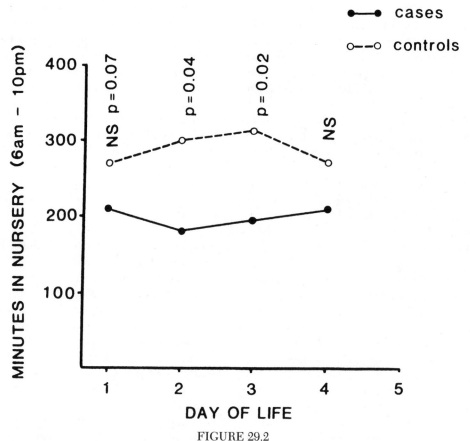

FIGURE 29.2

When the newborn infant touched the mother's nipple in the first 45 minutes of life, the baby spent significantly less time in the nursery and more time with the mother in the first 3 days of life.

asked about the amount of time they were away from their baby in a week and the number of days required to develop a relationship, there were again significant differences between the two groups. Mothers in the *doula* group said they spent 1.7 hours a week away from their baby in contrast to the no-*doula* mothers, who were away 6.6 hours. The *doula* group mothers said it took them an average of 2.9 days to develop a relationship with their baby compared to 9.8 days for the other group of mothers.

These results suggest that support during labor expedited the *doula*-group mothers' readiness to fall in love with their baby and that this attachment made them less willing to be away from their infant. These findings are with the observations of mother-infant interaction after mothers left the delivery room in the first randomized trial of *doula* support in Guatemala (Sosa et al., 1980).

There is a remarkable similarity between the results of *doula* support in the South Africa study and the behavior of mothers given early and increased contact with their newborn infants. Both groups of mothers showed or reported increased affection and attention to their baby; had an increased desire to stay home, remain with, and care for their infant in the first weeks; were more likely to pick up the baby whenever there was crying; and had an increased incidence and duration of breast-feeding. It is significant that a short intervention could produce such striking differences 6 weeks later; the period of labor and the early postpartum period are times when mothers are especially sensitive to environmental factors, and what goes on during labor and shortly thereafter may have powerful psychological consequences.

For the early development of an infant, Winnicott (1988a) emphasizes the importance of "the

298

holding environment," which includes "good-enough" maternal care that provides support, protection, and meeting physiologic needs consistently and reliably. He extended this "holding environment" concept to the needs of the mother during pregnancy, delivery, and the postpartum period (Wolman, 1991). The mother also needs a protective, supportive surrounding milieu. In a metaphorical sense, the *doula* who mothers the mother during labor and delivery provides the "holding environment" for the mother. This serves as a model for the mother to provide gentle, responsive, supportive care for her infant. Contrariwise, a mother treated roughly and left unsupported through the stressful experience of labor and delivery may follow that pattern in the care of her baby.

Winnicott (1957) stresses the father's role in the holding environment. "Fathers come into this . . . because they can help to protect the mother and baby from whatever tends to interfere with the bond between them, which is the essence and very nature of child care" (pp. 17–18).

Winnicott (1988b) describes the mother's sensitive postnatal state in this way. "The mother who is perhaps physically exhausted . . . is the one person who can properly introduce the world to the baby. She knows how to do this because she is the natural mother. But her natural instincts cannot evolve if she is scared, or if she does not see her baby when it is born, or if the baby is brought to her only at stated times (p. 78).

Fathers and Early Contact

Studies of fathers show that there are effects of early contact similar to those with mothers. When fathers were allowed to interact and establish eye-to-eye contact with their infants for 1 hour during the first hours of life, paternal caregiving greatly increased (Rödholm, 1981; Rödholm & Larsson, 1979). In another study a group of fathers given extended postpartum hospital contact with their infants, and compared to a group that had routine contact, "engaged in more en face" and vocalization with their infants during feeding 6 weeks after their baby's birth (Keller, Hildebrandt, &

Richards, 1985). They also were more involved in infant caregiving responsibilities and had higher self-esteem scores than the other group of fathers.

Criticism of Bonding Studies

Studies of early and extended mother-infant contact have been criticized because the number of differences hovered around what might be expected by chance, there were variations in the methods and timing of follow-up observations, and high-risk mothers who missed out on early contact may have felt guilty, like failures, and cheated (Lamb, 1982a,b,c). Two studies that randomly assigned middle-class mothers to receive early contact failed to replicate the results that had been found in the previous studies with poor and less educated mothers (Svejda, Campos, & Emde, 1980; Taylor & Campbell, 1979). However, there was a significant difference in the design of these two studies, since the control group of mothers did have a 5-minute period of early contact with their infants. Therefore, the studies used to criticize the previously reported bonding studies contained a significant design error. Lamb has noted that early contact may not necessarily have clear, enduring, and clinically significant benefits. However, O'Connor's (1980) well-designed and properly carried out long-term studies of 301 patients, which noted significantly decreased abuse, neglect, and nonorganic failure-to-thrive at 17 months of age, and Siegel's (1980) studies do not support Lamb's position. Nine of the investigators whose studies were challenged prepared a joint rebuttal that corrected the multiple "errors," "distortions," "inaccuracies" and "misrepresentations" in the criticisms point by point (Anisfeld et al., 1983). In another response, two respected investigators commented that "in a clinical intervention study there can be no exact replication. One cannot step in the same river twice" (Emde & Osofsky, 1983).

Studies have not clarified how much of the effect of early contact may be apportioned to the first hours and how much to the first days, but it appears that additional contact in both periods probably would be beneficial for mothers in developing a tie to their babies. Providing an opportunity for parents to be together with their baby in privacy during the first hour and throughout the hospital stay makes it possible for a mother to get to know and find her own baby. There is a need and an opportunity to conduct further studies of early contact. Sadly, research in this area came to a halt after the Lamb criticisms. Cutbacks in staff and efforts to speed up the care of patients to reduce costs have distorted or eliminated this early contact experience in some hospitals.

Other Observations that May Partly Explain Results of Early Contact Studies

INFANT APPEAL AND ABILITIES

The appearance of the healthy newborn infant, coupled with a broad array of sensory and motor abilities, pulls the mother and father to him or her and evokes responses from them. These responses result in a cascade of reciprocal parent-infant interactions that make both parties eager for further interactions and start the process of attachment. The quiet alert state of the infant during most of the first hour after delivery matches with the mother's excited ecstatic enthusiasm for interaction, particularly if she is unmedicated and has had continuous labor support and a measure of control over the events during the birth. The readiness of both members of the dyad for meeting and interacting suggests the evolutionary importance of the baby remaining with mother from birth onward because either the mother or the infant may be less responsive after the first hour. Information about infant state and the abilities of newborn infants is available in other sources (Klaus & Kennell, 1976, 1982; Klaus, Kennell, & Klaus, 1995).

HEIGHTENED SENSITIVITY OF MOTHERS

Donald Winnicott (1957) proposed that a mother goes through a period of "primary maternal preoccupation." He noted that this state of special sensitivity reached a peak at the time of delivery and then decreased in the succeeding weeks. As a result of this condition, a mother was in tune with the baby's needs and wishes so that she could respond contingently and appropriately. According to Winnicott, "Only if a mother is sensitized in the way I am describing can she feel herself into her infant's place, and so meet the infant's needs."

To develop and maintain this state, mothers need support, nurturing, and a protected environment.

UNUSUAL CAPABILITIES OF MOTHER AFTER DELIVERY

Recent studies have confirmed and extended observations of the unique capabilities of new mothers, perhaps a consequence of their being in the state of primary maternal preoccupation. Kaitz, Eidelman, and colleagues have shown that after only a few hours with their newborn infant, mothers are able to discriminate their own baby from other infants through their senses of smell, touch, vision, and hearing (Kaitz, Good, Rokem, & Eidelman, 1987, 1988, 1989). According to their studies, smell and touch appear to be the most salient sensory abilities. Sight (identifying a picture of the baby) and sound discrimination (identifying the baby's cry) take slightly longer to develop.

Clinical and Research Implications

The following changes in obstetric care suggested by research findings are recommended to enhance mother-infant attachment.

IMPROVE AND BROADEN SOCIAL SUPPORT DURING PREGNANCY

Three studies provided social support for high-risk women during pregnancy aimed at increasing the birthweight and length of gestation. These social support interventions resulted in only a significant increase in the birthweight of infants of a subgroup of teenage mothers in one study (Heins, Nance, McCarthy, & Efierd, 1990; Olds, Henderson, Tattlebaum & Chamberlin 1986).

A recent study with a high-risk group of mothers investigated the effects of comprehensive care, which included home visits by paraprofessionals, individual and group psychosocial support, practical assistance and education about self-care, and promotion of healthy behaviors during pregnancy (McLaughlin et al., 1992). This study showed a favorable effect of comprehensive care on birthweight for primiparous but not multiparous mothers.

PROVIDE POSITIVE SUPPORT DURING PREGNANCY

Positive support, praise, reassurance, and patience with the mother during the pregnancy by those who provide her care emphasize and model a pattern of behavior that the new mother is likely to show in the care of her infant. Contrariwise, rough or harsh treatment of pregnant women must be avoided, as it may result in harsh and sometimes abusive care of the new baby.

A *DOULA* FOR EVERY MOTHER AND EVERY COUPLE

Unfortunately, professionals who are harsh often do not recognize their behavior as such. A *doula* to support the mother during her labor and delivery should be provided for every mother and every couple to improve the obstetrical outcome, decrease the incidence of postpartum depression, and enhance the mother's self-esteem, her relationship with her partner, and her affectionate interaction and attachment to her baby.

EARLY AND EXTENDED PARENT-INFANT CONTACT FOR ALL PARENTS

Early and extended parent-infant contact should be an established policy for all parents if

the condition of the mother and the baby warrants. However, in the era of short stays and managed care, a recent observational study of events in the first 2 hours after delivery of a baby in a medical center showed that babies spent 24% of their time in a warmer in the delivery room out of the sight of the mother. Mothers held their babies 36% of the time and fathers only 6%. Almost two-thirds of Afro-American fathers did not hold their baby, and the times of holding were significantly shorter for teenage mothers. The entire group of 20 newborns was in the quiet alert state for the first 90 minutes, ready to interact with their mothers. Forty percent were in this state for the entire 2 hours (Mentschukoff, Kennell, & Anderson, 1995).

Powerful evidence of the importance of early and extended contact comes from a recent report from Thailand in a hospital where a disturbing number of babies were abandoned by their mothers each year. When early contact and rooming-in were provided for the mothers, there was a significant reduction in the frequency of this sad outcome, from 33 abandoned babies to only 1 per year. When early contact with breast-feeding and rooming-in have been introduced in other countries, similar marked decreases in abandonment have been reported informally. This behavior appears to be analogous to the newborn kid whose mother goat misses early contact and then refuses to feed and care for it (Buranasin 1991).

Particular emphasis should be placed on assuring early and extended parent-infant contact for all mothers who are single, teenage, from minority, and from poor, stressful households because the benefits will be greater with this group. On the other hand, if this group is deprived of well-supported, early, and extended contact with the infant in privacy, the outcome for the baby is more likely to be abusive and neglectful. If mother and baby cannot be together shortly after birth, they should be brought together as soon as possible. It is "never too late" during the hospitalization.

RANDOMIZED CONTROLLED TRIALS OF EARLY INTERVENTIONS

Early therapeutic interventions should be studied in randomized controlled trials. Studies of the effects of early discharge and a variety of recently introduced measures to provide support and education to mothers about the care of their newborn infants are necessary. This need is apparent because of the recent decrease in breast-feeding, increased maternal concerns about the care of new babies, and unanswered questions about mother-infant attachment that have arisen from clinical observations. There is special interest in effective interventions for poor mothers who come from deprived, stressful, minority households where support is lacking or inconsistent.

SOCIAL SUPPORT AT HOME AFTER DELIVERY

The almost universal provision of social support for mothers and babies during the first days and weeks in both industrialized and nonindustrialized societies stands in sharp contrast to its lack in the United States. Based on the results of randomized trials, there is now great interest in training women to be *doulas* to provide support for mothers-to-be during labor and delivery. This resulted in the formation of an organization called DONA (Doulas of North America), which has made vigorous efforts to train doulas and to encourage the provision of support after the mother goes home from the hospital are needed. By 1995 DONA had more than 1,000 members. Those who provide social support in the home after delivery require special training in assisting and encouraging mothers to breast-feed. Studies of the effects of parental leave also are needed.

EXPANDED ROLE OF THE *Doula*

For mothers-to-be with special needs, such as pregnant teenagers and single, unsupported women, it will be important to promote the so-called expanded role of the *doula*. Either paid or volunteer women with experience with their own children should be encouraged to develop a relationship with high-risk mothers as early in pregnancy as possible (the first 3 months) and to continue a close association after delivery until the child is 2 or more years. In some of the long-established programs, such as those in Traverse City, Michigan, Pontiac, Michigan, and Santa Rosa, California, volunteer women work with only one needy woman at a time, meeting with her once or twice a week during the pregnancy, going with her to the prenatal clinic visits, acting as a *doula* for her during labor, delivery, and the postpartum period, and helping her with the multiple challenges and adjustments that arise as she cares for her new baby. In Traverse City, follow-up observations on primiparous teenagers indicated that almost all mothers finished high school; only rarely did they have another baby out of wedlock, and the incidence of child abuse was extremely low. These data suggest that large controlled trials studying this type of intervention might be fruitful.

REFERENCES

Anisfeld, E., Casper, V., Nozyce, M., & Cunningham, N. (1990). Does infant carrying promote attachment? An experimental study of the effects of increased physical contact on the development of attachment. *Child Development, 61,* 1617–1627.

Anisfeld, E., Curry, M. A., Hales, D. J., Kennell, J. H., Klaus, M. H., Lipper E., O'Connor, S., Siegel, E., & Sosa, R. (1983). Maternal-infant bonding: A joint rebuttal. *Pediatrics, 72,* 569–572.

Anisfeld, E., & Lipper, E. (1983). Early contact, social support, & mother-infant bonding. *Pediatrics, 72,* 79–83.

Bibring, G. L., Dwyer, T. F., Huntington, D. S., & Valenstein, A. F. (1961). A study of the psychological processes in pregnancy and of the earliest mother-child relationship. I. Some propositions and comments. *Psychoanalytic Study of the Child, 16,* 9–27.

Brazelton, T. B. (1973). Effect of maternal expectations on early infant behavior. *Early Child Development Care, 2,* 259–273.

Buranasin, B. (1991). The effects of rooming in on the success of breastfeeding and the decline in abandonment of children. *Asia-Pacific Journal of Public Health, 5,* 217–220.

Carter, C. S., Williams, J. R., & Witt, D. M. (1990). The biology of social bonding in a monogamous mammal. In J. Balthazart (Ed.), *Hormones, brains & behavior* (Vol. 9, pp. 1–11). Basil: Karger.

Emde, R. N., & Osofsky, H. J. (1983). Bonding, humanism and science. Letter to the Editor. *Pediatrics, 72,* 749–750.

Engel, G. L., Reichsman, F., & Harvay, V. T. (1985). A 30 year longitudinal study of enduring effects in parental influences in health & diseases. In E. J. Anthony, & G. H. Pollack (Eds.), *Infant feeding behavior of a mother gastric fistula fed as an infant* (p. 29). Boston: Little, Brown.

Fraiberg, S., Adelson, E., & Shapiro, V. (1975). Ghosts in the nursery: A psychoanalytic approach to the problems of impaired infant-mother relationships. *Journal of American Academy Child Psychiatry, 14,* 387–421.

Hales, D. J., Lozoff, B., Sosa, R., & Kennell, J. H. (1977). Defining the limits of the maternal sensitive period. *Developmental Medicine and Child Neurology, 19,* 454.

Heins, H. C., Nance, N. W., McCarthy, B. J., & Efierd, C. M. (1990). A randomized trial of nurse midwifery prenatal care to reduce low birth weight. *Obstetrics & Gynecology, 75,* 341–345.

Hofmeyr, G. J., Nikodem, V. C., Wolman, W. L., Chalmers, B. E., & Kramer, T. (1991). Companionship to modify the clinical birth environment: Effects on progress and perceptions of labour and breast feeding. *British Journal of Obstetrics and Gynaecology, 98,* 756–764.

Kaitz, M., Good, A., Rokem, A. M., & Eidelman, A. I. (1987). Mothers' recognition of their olfactory cues. *Developmental Psychobiology, 20,* 587.

Kaitz, M., et al. (1988). Mothers' and fathers' recognition of their newborns' photographs during the postpartum period. *Journal of Developmental and Behavioral Pediatrics, 9,* 233.

Kaitz, M., et al. (1989). Postpartum women can recognize their infants by touch. *Pediatric Research, 25,* 14A.

Keller, W. D., Hildebrandt, K. A., & Richards, M. (1985). Effects of extended father-infant contact during the newborn period. *Infant Behavior and Development, 8,* 337–350.

Kendrick, J. M., Keverne, E. B., & Baldwin, B. A. (1987). Intracerebroventricular oxytocin stimulates maternal behaviour in the sheep. *Neuroendocrinology, 46,* 56–61.

Kennell, J. H., Klaus, M. H., McGrath, S. K., Robertson, S., & Hinkley, C. (1991). Continuous emotional support during labor in a U.S. hospital: A randomized controlled trial. *Journal of the American Medical Association, 17,* 2197–2201.

Keverne, E. B. (1988). Central mechanisms underlying the neural and neuroendocrine determinants of maternal behavior. *Psychoneuroendocrinology, 13,* 127–141.

Keverne, E. B., Levy, F., Poindron, P., & Lindsay, D. (1983). Vaginal stimulation: An important determinant of maternal bonding in sheep. *Science, 219,* 81–83.

Klaus, M. H., Jerauld, R., Kreger, N., McAlpine, W., Steffa, M., & Kennell, J. H. (1972). Maternal attachment: Importance of the first post-partum days. *New England Journal of Medicine, 286,* 460–463.

Klaus, M. H., & Kennell, J. H. (1976). *Maternal-infant bonding.* St. Louis: C. V. Mosby.

Klaus, M. H., & Kennell, J. H. (1982). *Parent-infant bonding* (2nd ed.). St. Louis: C. V. Mosby.

Klaus, M. H., Kennell, J. H., Robertson, S. S., & Sosa, R. (1986). Effects of social support during parturition on maternal and infant mortality. *British Medical Journal, 293,* 585–587.

Klaus, M. H., Kennell, J. H., Klaus, P. H. (1995). Bonding: Building the foundations of secure attachment and independence. Reading, MA: Addison-Wesley.

Lamb, M. E. (1982a). The bonding phenomenon: Misinterpretations and their implications. *Pediatrics, 101,* 555–557.

Lamb, M. E. (1982b). Early contact and maternal-infant bonding: One decade later. *Pediatrics, 70,* 763–768.

Lamb, M. E., & Hwang, C. P. (1982). Maternal attachment and mother-neonate bonding: A critical review. In M. E. Lamb & A. L. Brown (Eds.), *Advances in developmental psychology* (Vol. 2). Hillsdale, NJ: Lawrence Erlbaum.

Lozoff, B., Jordan, B., & Malone, S. (1988). Childbirth in cross-cultural perspective. *Marriage and Family Review, 12,* 35–60.

Lumley, J. (1980a). The development of maternal-foetal bonding in first pregnancy. In L. Zichellen (Ed.), *Proceedings of the 5th International Congress in Psychosomatic Medicine in Obstetrics and Gynaecology.* New York: Academic Press.

Lumley, J. (1980b). The image of the fetus in the first trimester. *Birth and the Family Journal, 7,* 5–14.

Mcclaughlin, E. J., Altemeier, W. A., Christensen, M. J., Sherrod, K. B., Dietrich, M. S., & Stern, D. T. (1992). Randomized trial of comprehensive prenatal care for low-income women: Effect on infant birth weight. *Pediatrics, 89,* 128–132.

Mentschukoff, J. D., Kennell, J. H., & Anderson, G. C. (1995). Family centered maternity care: Do we practice what we preach? *Pediatric Research* [abstract], *37,* 17A.

Merkatz, R. (1978). Prolonged hospitalization of pregnant women: the effects on the family. *Birth and the Family Journal, 5,* 204.

Newton, M., & Newton, N. (1948). The let-down reflex in human lactation. *Journal of Pediatrics, 33,* 693–704.

Newton, M., & Newton, N. (1950). Relation of the let-down reflex to the ability to breast feed. *Pediatrics, 5,* 726–733.

Newton, N. (1973). Inter-relationships between sexual responsiveness, birth and breast-feeding behavior. In J. Zubin & J. Money (Eds.), *Critical issues in contemporary sexual behavior* (pp. 77–98). Baltimore: Johns Hopkins Press.

Newton, N. (1978). The role of the oxytocin reflexes in three interpersonal reproductive acts; coitus, birth and breast-feeding. In L. Carenza, P. Pancheri, & L. Zichella (Eds.), *Clinical psychoneuroendocrinology in reproduction: Proceedings of the Serono Symposia 22.* New York: Academic Press.

O'Connor, S., Vietze, P. M., Sherrod, K. B., Sandler, H. M., & Altemeier, W. A. (1980). Reduced incidence of parenting inadequacy following rooming-in. *Pediatrics, 66,* 176–182.

Olds, D. L., Henderson, C. R., Tattlebaum, R., & Chamberlin, R. (1986). Improving the delivery of prenatal care and outcomes of pregnancy: A randomized trial of nursing home visitation. *Pediatrics, 77,* 16–28.

Poindron, P., & LeNeindre, P. (1980). Endocrine and sensory regulation of maternal behavior in the ewe. In J. S. Rosenblatt, R. A. Hinde, C. Beer, & M. C. Busnel (Eds.) *Advances in the study of behavior* (Vol. 11, pp. 75–119). New York: Academic Press.

Poindron, P., Levy, F., & Krehbiel, D. (1988). Genital, olfactory, and endocrine interactions in the development of maternal behavior in the parturient ewe. *Psychoneuroendocrinology, 13,* 99–125.

Rödholm, M. (1981). Effects of father-infant postpartum contact on their interaction 3 months after birth. *Early Human Development, 5,* 79–85.

Rödholm, M., & Larsson, K. (1979). Father-infant interaction at the first contact after delivery. *Early Human Development, 3,* 21–27.

Rosenblatt, J. S. (1967). Nonhormonal basis for maternal behavior in the rat. *Science, 156,* 1512–1514.

Rosenblatt, J. S. (1969). The development of maternal responsiveness in rats. *American Journal of Orthopsychiatry, 39,* 36–56.

Rosenblatt, J. S. (1989). The physiological and evolutionary background of maternal responsiveness. In M. H. Bornstein (Ed.), *Maternal responsiveness: Characteristics & consequences new directions for child development,* No. 43 (pp. 15–30). San Francisco: Jossey-Bass.

Rosenblatt, J. S. (1991). A psychobiological approach to maternal behaviour among the primates. In Essays in honour of R. Hinde & P. Bateson (Eds.), *The development & integration of behaviour.* Oxford: Cambridge University Press.

Rosenblatt, J. S., Mayer, A. D., & Siegel, H. I. (1985). Maternal behavior among the nonprimate mammals. In N. Adler, D. Pfaff, & R. W. Goy (Eds.), *Handbook of behavioral neurobiology* (Vol. 7, pp. 229–297). New York: Plenum Press.

Rosenblatt, J. S., & Siegel, H. I. (1981). Factors governing the onset and maintenance of maternal behavior among non primate mammals: The role of hormonal and nonhormonal factors. In D. J. Gubernick & P. H. Klopfer (Eds.), *Parental care in mammals.* New York: Plenum Press.

Rosenblatt, J. S., Siegel, H. I., & Mayer, A. D. (1979). Progress in the study of maternal behavior in the rat: hormonal, nonhormonal sensory and developmental aspects. In J. S. Rosenblatt et al. (Eds.), *Advances in*

the study of behavior (Vol. 10, pp. 226–302). New York: Academic Press.

Russell, J. G. B. (1982). The rationale of primitive delivery positions. *British Journal of Obstetrics & Gynecology, 89,* 712–715.

Siegel, E., Bauman, K. E., Schaefer, E. S., Saunders, M. M., & Ingram, D. D. (1980). Hospital & home support during infancy: Impact on maternal attachment, child abuse & neglect, & health care utilization. *Pediatrics, 66,* 183–190.

Sosa, R., Kennell, J. H., Klaus, M. H., Robertson, S. S., & Urrutia, J. (1980). The effect of a supportive companion on perinatal problems, length of labor, & mother-infant interaction. *New England Journal of Medicine, 303,* 597–600.

Spencer, B, Thomas, H., & Morris, J. (1989). A randomized controlled trial with provision of a social support service during pregnancy: The South Manchester Family Worker Project. *British Journal of Obstetrics and Gynaecology, 96,* 281–288.

Svejda, M. J., Campos, J. J., & Emde, R. N. (1980). Mother-infant bonding: Failure to generalize. *Child Development, 51,* 77.

Taylor, P. M., & Campbell, S. M. (1979). Bonding and attachment: Theoretical issues. *Seminars in Perinatology, 3,* 1.

Terkel, J., & Rosenblatt, J. S. (1972). Humoral factors underlying maternal behavior at parturition: Cross transfusion between freely moving rats. *Journal of Comparative Physiology and Psychology, 80,* 365–371.

Turnbull, A. C., Patten, P. T., Flint, A. P. F., Keirse, M. J. N. C., Jeremy, J. Y., & Anderson, A. (1974). Significant fall in progesterone & rise in oestradiol levels in human peripheral plasma before onset of labour. *Lancet, 1,* 101–103.

Widström, A. M. Wahlberg, V., Matthiesen, A. S., Enersoth, P., Uvnäs-Moberg, K., Werner, S., & Winberg, J. (1990). Short-term effects of early suckling and touch of the nipple on maternal behavior. *Early Human Development, 21,* 153–163.

Winnicott, D. W. (1957). *The child, the family and the outside world.* London: Tavistock P.

Winnicott, D. W. (1988a). Communication between infant and mother and mother and infant, compared and contrasted. In D. W. Winnicott, *Babies and their mothers.* Reading, MA: Addison-Wesley.

Winnicott, D. W. (1988b). The contribution of psychoanalysis to midwifery. *Babies and their mothers.* Reading, MA: Addison-Wesley.

Winnicott, D. W. (1988c). Dependence in child care. *Babies and their mothers* (pp. 93–94). Reading, MA: Addison-Wesley.

Wolman, W. L. (1991). *Social support during childbirth: Psychological and physiological outcomes.* Ph.D. dissertation, University of the Witwatorstrand, Johannesburg, South Africa.

30 / Early Peer Relations and Child Psychiatry

Janice Brown and Kenneth A. Dodge

This chapter provides a general overview of the role of early peer relations in psychological development. We argue that the origins of social behavior lie in the infant's interactions with adult caregivers but that very early in development peer relations take on a life of their own. Growth in peer interaction is dramatic across the first several years of life. Cooperation, negotiation, and leadership are learned during early interactions with same-age peers. We discuss the importance of peer relations in concurrent and future adjustment. The quality of a child's peer relations is a major correlate of current psychiatric adjustment and a strong marker of that child's level of risk for later psychiatric difficulties. Herein we describe empirical methods for classifying individual differences in peer relations, including classifications of adaptation to the peer group as a whole (e.g., popular, rejected, neglected, controversial, and average) as well as classifications of types of relationships (e.g., dyadic friendships). Our literature review considers: (1) the importance of peer relations, including theories of the role of peers in promoting cognitive development, the explicit role of peer relations in diagnosing psychiatric impairment, and empirical research that indicates that children with poor peer relations are at risk for later difficulties; (2) behavioral and social cognitive processes contributing to peer group status; and (3) the contribution of the peer group to the maintenance of sociometric status. The last section reviews various interventions that have attempted to improve children's peer relations so as to prevent future psychiatric impairment. For those who are interested, more complete reviews are available (e.g., Asher & Coie, 1991; Hartup, 1983).

Parental Contributions to Peer Relations

Young infants direct very little behavior toward peers. Adult caregivers play a central role in fostering the growth of peer interaction and in the quality of that interaction. Parke and Bhavnagri (1989) and Rubin and Sloman (1984) have articulated the major ways in which parents influence the development of peer relations. First, parents' interactions with infants act as a model for how interactions with other persons usually proceed. In these interactions, the infant learns expectations, such as whether another person can be trusted, is likely to respond to a smile, or is a threat. The growing child then takes this working model of relationships into interactions with peers and uses it as a template for creating peer relationships (Bowlby, 1988). The child also learns skills such as turn-taking and cooperation. MacDonald and Parke (1984) and Putallaz (1987) have observed direct correlations between the quality of parent-child play and the quality of that child's play with peers.

Parents also influence their child's development through more didactic teaching of social rules and norms. Infants as young as 12 months of age have learned to reference their parents when confronted with peer cues, especially ambiguous ones, in order to learn how to interpret the peer and how to respond (Walden, 1991). Infants who observe their parents displaying negative affect in the presence of a stranger are more likely to avoid the stranger than infants who observe their parent displaying positive affect in the same situation (Feinman & Lewis, 1983). As children grow older, their parents act as coaches to encourage their child and to direct peer interaction (Putallaz & Heflin, 1990).

Finally, parents influence their child's development of peer relations by managing that child's social environment (Parke & Bhavnagri, 1989). Parents decide whether their infant will be placed in day care and what kind of day care, how much time will be spent with other children, and what circumstances surround playtime with peers.

Early Development of Peer Play

These parental influences interact with the child's innate predilections to contribute to dramatic growth in the quality of peer play across the first 3 years of life (Eckerman, Davis, & Didow, 1989). In the first year of life, infants learn to smile at peers, to point to them, and to synchronize their looks with attempts to touch peers (Hartup, 1983). At 12 months of age, infants can imitate simple peer actions (Eckerman & Stein, 1982). Over the next 2 years, the rate of coordinated peer play triples (Eckerman et al., 1989). This play includes increased imitation but also complementary play (such as picking up a ball thrown by a peer).

During the preschool years, children learn more advanced forms of play. They move from parallel play (independent play that occurs in close proximity of a peer who is engaging in similar play), to associative play (interacting with each other using the same materials), and on to cooperative play (complex play involving different roles, rules, coordinated actions, social pretense, and joint construction) (Parten, 1932).

The Importance of Peer Relations

PEERS CONTRIBUTE TO COGNITIVE AND EMOTIONAL DEVELOPMENT

Children's relations with their peers are important for a number of reasons. Peers influence children's social, cognitive, and emotional development. Interaction with peers provides an individual child with the opportunities to learn effective communication skills (Bukowski & Hoza, 1989), to learn to control his or her aggressive behavior (Hartup, 1983), and to learn cooperative interpersonal skills (Bukowski & Hoza, 1989). Piaget (1932/1965) proposed that peer interaction contributes to the development of the cognitive skills related to perspective taking and moral reasoning. Vygotsky (1978) proposed further that the peer group provides a structure for the child's cognitive learning such that lack of sufficient exposure to normative peers could inhibit cognitive growth. Rogoff (1990) similarly has argued that some cognitive learning is not possible except in the context of a group of similarly minded peers. Peers provide a child with a sounding board for his or her ideas, a "mirror level" of cognitive sophistication against which the child can evaluate and test out ideas, and opportunities for mutual exchange that are not possible in interaction with a parent or other adult. The peer group context also has been cited as providing a secure base for emotional expression, especially during preadolescence (Bukowski & Hoza, 1989). Peers provide social support (Berndt, 1982) and contribute to the development of the concept of self (Sullivan, 1953). The nature of a child's relationships with his or her agemates thus may have an enormous impact on his or her adjustment and development. Likewise, psychiatric disorder can impair a child's ability to relate effectively with peers.

PEER MALADJUSTMENT IS A PART OF MANY PSYCHIATRIC DISORDERS

Not surprisingly, empirical studies have indicated that children who have difficulties relating to peers are highly overrepresented in referrals to child guidance clinics (Woody, 1969). Even though a child's peer interactions are not usually the focus of psychiatric inquiry, social incompetence is so closely related to psychiatric impairment that it is an explicit part of the diagnostic criteria of the fourth edition of the *Diagnostic and Statistical Manual of Mental Disorders DSM-IV* (American Psychiatric Association [APA], 1994) for at least 20 child and adult disorders and is likely to be part of the symptom cluster for at least 9 other disorders. (See Table 30.1 for a list.) Having markedly disturbed social relatedness is a symptom of attention-deficit hyperactivity disorder (from *DSM-IV:* "often interrupts or intrudes on others, e.g., butts into other children's games," p. 84), conduct disorder ("often initiates physical fights," p. 90), and autistic disorder ("failure to develop peer relationships appropriate to developmental level," p. 70) and of schizophrenia, the bipolar disorders, social phobia, and numerous personality disorders in adulthood. In addition,

TABLE 30.1

Peer Relations and Psychiatric Disorders

I. Disorders in Which Socially Incompetent Behavior Is Part of the Diagnostic Criteria

Mental Retardation (317.00 to 319.00)

Autistic Disorder (299.00)

Rett's Disorder (299.80)

Childhood Disintegrative Disorder (299.10)

Asperger's Disorder (299.80)

Attention-Deficit/Hyperactivity Disorder (314.00 to 314.9)

Conduct Disorder (312.8)

Oppositional Defiant Disorder (313.81)

Reactive Attachment Disorder of Infancy or Early Childhood (313.89)

Bipolar Disorders (296.xx, 296.89)

Social Phobia (300.23)

Paranoid Personality Disorder (301.1)

Schizoid Personality Disorder (301.20)

Schizotypal Personality Disorder (301.22)

Antisocial Personality Disorder (301.7)

Borderline Personality Disorder (301.83)

Histrionic Personality Disorder (301.50)

Narcissistic Personality Disorder (301.81)

Avoidant Personality Disorder (301.82)

Dependent Personality Disorder (301.6)

II. Disorders in Which Early Social Incompetence Probably Plays a Role

Substance Abuse Disorders (305.00 to 305.90)

Schizophrenia (295.10 to 295.90)

Delusional Disorder (297.1)

Sexual Dysfunctions and Paraphilias (302.2 to 302.9)

Impulse Control Disorders (312.30 to 312.34)

Personality Disorders (301.0 to 301.9)

III. Disorders in Which Impairment in Social Functioning May Be An Associated Feature of the Disorder

Learning Disorders (315.00 to 315.39)

Stuttering (307.00)

Tourette's Disorder (307.23)

Separation Anxiety Disorder (309.21)

Selective Mutism (313.23)

Stereotypic Movement Disorder (307.3)

Mood Disorders (296.00 to 296.90)

Anxiety Disorders (300.21 to 300.29)

Obsessive-Compulsive Personality Disorder (301.4)

---

early difficulties in relating to peers probably play a role in the development of at least 6 other categories of disorders, including substance abuse disorders and impulse control disorders. It is clear that the development of social competence is a major task of childhood, and the inability to establish peer relationships may be the single strongest indicator of psychiatric impairment.

PEER RELATIONS PREDICT LATER MALADJUSTMENT

Strong support has been found for the hypothesis that poor peer relations in childhood are predictive of later psychiatric and social impairment. (See reviews by Kupersmidt, Coie, & Dodge, 1990; Parker & Asher, 1987.) More specifically, rejection by one's peer group at the onset of elementary school has been found to predict adult schizophrenia (John, Mednick, & Schulsinger, 1982; Kohn & Clausen, 1955; Watt, 1978), psychosis (Roff, 1963), antisocial personality disorder (Robins, 1966), placement in a psychiatric register of patients at mental health clinics (Cowen, Pederson, Babigian, Izzo, & Trost, 1972), suicide (Stengel, 1971), and school dropout (Gronlund & Holmlund, 1958; Kupersmidt et al., 1990). Difficulty getting along with peers at age 8 has been found to predict bad-conduct discharges from military service 10 to 15 years later (Roff, 1961). The Cowen et al. (1972) study is particularly impressive because peer raters were contrasted directly with teacher raters of a child and found to be better predictors of long-term outcome. A patient's premorbid level of social competence also has been found to enhance the prediction of outcome among schizophrenics (Zigler & Phillips, 1961) and responsiveness to treatment among inpatients (Jacobs, Muller, Anderson, & Skinner, 1972; 1973).

Thus, the inability to relate effectively with one's peer group during early and middle childhood is a broad and nonspecific predictor of psychiatric and social morbidity. Research has not yet determined the degree to which peer rejection as an experiential phenomenon contributes to this morbidity or is merely a marker of risk. The former hypothesis is supported by the findings that peer rejection is correlated with loneliness and personal unhappiness (Asher & Wheeler, 1985) and from observational findings that peer rejection antecedes social withdrawal in some children (Dodge, Coie, Pettit, & Price, 1990). Before these issues can be explored in more detail, a description of the ways in which peer relations have been defined and the methods by which they have been studied needs to be given.

Definitions of Peer Relations

Two ways in which a child's peer relations have been defined are in terms of his or her participation in a friendship with another child and his or her sociometric status within the peer group. These definitions are very different from each other and imply an emphasis on different aspects of interpersonal functioning. Friendship applies to the interaction of a dyad. Within the context of a friendship, the child comes to establish a sense of intimacy and trust with the friend (Hartup, 1983). These tasks and the establishment of a "chumship" have been noted by Sullivan (1953) to be among the most important developmental tasks of childhood. A child who is unable to master this task may be deficient in basic interpersonal skills and subsequently is denied the opportunities of intimacy and interpersonal exploration.

A child's sociometric status is an indication of how well he or she is liked or disliked by the peer group as a whole. It is an index of how competent an individual is at getting along with a variety of other individuals. Fitting in to the peer group in childhood is a prototype for fitting in to one's employment group, community, and society as an adult. The types of skills involved in originating and maintaining a friendship are different from those involved in being accepted by one's peer group. Research on each of these aspects of peer relations therefore has focused on different types of behaviors and outcomes.

THE IMPORTANCE OF DYADIC FRIENDSHIPS

The research on children's friendships has been concerned with describing the kinds of behaviors that are displayed between children who are friends. The typical design of these studies has been to have children interact with a friend and with a nonfriend and to compare the nature of these interactions (Berndt & Ladd, 1989; Rizzo, 1989). In general, young children have been found to be more prosocial with friends than nonfriends (Masters & Furman, 1981) but also to explore differences and to allow conflicts to develop. Friends have been found to be more interactive, more affectively oriented, more concerned with being fair, and to utilize mutually directed conversational strategies (i.e., "Let's do this" versus "You do this") than nonfriends (Newcomb, Brady, & Hartup, 1979). There is mixed evidence concerning whether friends are more competitive than nonfriends (Rizzo, 1989). These differences seem to be mediated by the task conditions involved in the particular studies and are not a simple function of the nature of the relationship between the participants (Hartup, 1983).

Several recent longitudinal studies have examined the impact of dyadic friendships in early childhood on adolescent interpersonal functioning. Two competing hypotheses were examined in the context of these studies. The first was that having a mutual friend acts as a buffer against the negative impact of rejection by the peer group (Kupersmidt, Burchinal, & Patterson, 1995). Children with a mutual friend were therefore expected to demonstrate fewer internalizing and externalizing symptoms in adolescence. The second hypothesis was that forming friendships with deviant peers contributes to the development of externalizing behaviors, such as delinquency (Keenan, Loeber, Zhang, Stouthamer-Loeber, & Van Kammen, 1995; Tremblay, Masse, Vitaro, & Dobkin, 1995). In this case, children with a mutual friend were expected to demonstrate a higher rate of externalizing behaviors in adolescence.

Little evidence was found for the first hypothesis. There was no evidence that having a mutual friend either acted as a buffer against rejection by the peer group or decreased the number of externalizing symptoms displayed by children (Kupersmidt et al., 1995). However, having a mutual friend during early childhood seemed to prevent the development of internalizing symptoms and feelings of loneliness (Hoza, Molina, Bukowski, & Sippola, 1995; Parker & Asher, 1993). Mixed support was found for the second hypothesis. Aggressive and unpopular children have been found to form friendships with similar others (Cairns, Cairns, Neckerman, Gect, & Gariepy, 1988). Some support was found for the hypothesis that associating with deviant peers increases the risk of developing delinquent behavior (Keenan et al., 1995; Kupersmidt et al., 1995). Other research indicates that having deviant peer friendships does not contribute to the development of externalizing problems in adolescence over and above the influence of subjects' own history of disruptive and aggressive behavior in early childhood (Tremblay et al., 1995). Evidently more research needs to be done to clarify the relations between deviant peer friendships and externalizing outcomes.

SOCIOMETRIC STATUS INDICATES ADJUSTMENT TO THE GROUP

Sociometric status is determined by interviewing each member of the child's peer group, usually his or her classmates. In the most common form of sociometric interview, each child is asked to list the 3 classroom peers whom he or she likes the most and the 3 whom he or she likes least. Nomination scores are summed and adjusted for the size of the peer group. The difference between liking and disliking nomination scores is the child's social preference score. The sum of liking and disliking scores is a measure of social impact. Sociometric ratings by peers have proven to be reliable and valid even when collected during the preschool years (Asher, Singleton, Tinsley, & Hymel, 1979). Research has demonstrated that both liking and disliking dimensions are necessary in order to differentiate clearly the attitudes of the peer group about a particular child (Asher & Coie, 1991; Goldman, Corsini, & Urioste, 1980). From these nominations, children are divided into sociometric groups. Based on procedures developed by Coie, Dodge, and Coppotelli (1982), these groups are roughly determined as follows:

1. *Popular*—children who are often nominated as liked and seldom as disliked (about 12% of the population)
2. *Rejected*—children who are often nominated as disliked and seldom as liked (about 12%)
3. *Neglected*—children who are seldom nominated as either liked or disliked (about 8%)

4. *Controversial*—children who are often nominated as liked and as disliked (about 6%)
5. *Average*—children who do not fall in any of these categories and therefore have received an average number of liking and disliking nominations.

Children in the popular and average groups are considered to be accepted by their peer group and to have generally positive peer relations. Children who are rejected or neglected are considered to be low in peer group acceptance and therefore to have generally poor peer relations. Children who fall in the controversial group are just that; it is unclear what kind of impact these children have on their peer group.

Although this scheme is the most inclusive method of determining sociometric status, other methods have been used. In one method, only positive nominations are solicited from the peer group (i.e., each child is asked to name the 3 peers he or she likes the most). Using this method, children are classified as either popular (receiving many positive nominations) or unpopular (receiving few positive nominations). The social preference score also can be utilized as a continuous variable as opposed to a categorical variable. A high social preference score is considered to indicate high standing in the peer group. Rating scales also have been used to determine *how much* a child is liked by peers, particularly with preschool children (Asher et al., 1979). For those researchers who object on ethical grounds to soliciting negative nominations from children, rating scales can be used to substitute for negative nominations in determining status (Asher & Dodge, 1986).

Research on the Behavioral Correlates of Peer Relations

Researchers have attempted to identify the behavioral correlates of sociometric status. Methods have ranged from asking peers and teachers to describe the behaviors of specific children, to direct observation of children in classroom, playground, camp, and laboratory settings (Kupersmidt et al., 1990). The purpose of these studies is to identify the factors that are associated with, and possibly lead to, a child having poor peer relations. It is important to note that although certain behaviors have been found to be associated with different sociometric status classifications, it is very difficult to determine whether these behaviors antecede the acquisition of status or are a consequence of the experience of status. The correlational design of these studies in which children who already have achieved a particular status are observed or rated precludes any causal statements. For example, aggressive behavior is known to be the strongest behavioral correlate of peer rejection in most peer group contexts. It is not clear from the studies on behavioral correlates whether behaving in an aggressive manner leads to peer rejection or if peer rejection results in an increase of aggressive behavior, due to hurt feelings or anger at the peer group. Some researchers are getting closer to an answer to this question by observing the development of peer status over time in new peer group contexts. These studies are discussed later.

CORRELATES OF POPULAR STATUS

The behaviors associated with positive peer status are fairly consistent for children across all ages studied (Coie, Dodge, & Kupersmidt, 1990). Popular children are friendly, outgoing, cooperative, express kindness to peers, know how to make dyadic friendships, and are good sports (Hartup, 1983). Popular children often are seen as leaders by their peer group, as helpful, and as following the rules (Coie et al., 1990). Popularity also has been found to be positively associated with the tendency to defend oneself in response to peer attack (Lesser, 1959). Children who do not allow themselves to be bullied by other children are evidently viewed positively by their peer group.

CORRELATES OF REJECTED STATUS

The behaviors associated with rejected status in elementary-school children are aggressive and disruptive behaviors (Carlson, Lahey, & Neeper, 1984; Coie et al., 1982; Hartup, 1983). Rejected children are significantly more aggressive and disruptive than their average-status classmates. One study (Coie et al., 1982) found that high rates of

help-seeking at school was also strongly related to rejected status in boys. Coie et al. also found that although aggressive and disruptive behaviors are common to both rejected boys and rejected girls, cooperativeness, or the lack thereof, discriminated rejected girls from popular girls even more strongly.

Rejected status in adolescence is associated less strongly with overt aggressive behaviors, possibly because the base rate of these behaviors is lower (Coie et al., 1982). Rejected adolescents have been described by their peers as disruptive, conceited, and silly (Feinberg, Smith, & Schmidt, 1958) and as disruptive, mean, rule violators, too sensitive, and unattractive in that they were dirty or smelled badly (Elkins, 1958).

CORRELATES OF NEGLECTED STATUS

The behavioral profile of neglected children is nebulous. No overtly deviant behaviors are associated with neglected sociometric status (Coie et al., 1990). Rather, neglected children are below the mean on most of the behavior rating items associated with sociometric research (average-status children are at the mean for these items). Neglected children are below the mean on measures of sociability associated with popular status and on aggressive behavior. Although neglected children often are characterized as shy and withdrawn, the evidence on this relation is mixed. More research needs to be done on the behaviors associated with neglected status.

CORRELATES OF CONTROVERSIAL STATUS

The behaviors associated with controversial status are a combination of the behaviors associated with popular and rejected status. Controversial children demonstrate a high degree of both prosocial and aggressive behaviors (Coie et al., 1982; Dodge, 1983). They display high rates of disruptive, annoying, and aggressive behaviors, but they also demonstrate a remarkable degree of social skill and leadership ability. The proportion of controversial children in a given sample has been found to be relatively small (about 7%; Coie et al.,

1982; Dodge, 1983), and for whatever reasons, the data base on behavioral correlates of controversial status is also quite small.

BEHAVIORAL ANTECEDENTS OF PEER STATUS

The research just presented describes the types of behaviors associated with different types of sociometric status. Because sociometric status is measured concurrently with behavior, it is not possible to conclude from the research whether the behaviors contribute to sociometric status or result from it. In an attempt to determine what behaviors contribute to the acquisition of peer status, researchers have devised a method of observing sociometric status as it emerges in small play groups (Coie & Kupersmidt, 1983; Dodge, 1983). The intent of these studies is to observe children interacting with unfamiliar peers and to describe behavioral patterns that precede peer status in this new peer group. Several of these studies will be described.

Coie and Kupersmidt (1983) organized play groups consisting of 4 fourth-grade African American boys. Each boy in the group was of a different sociometric standing as assessed by their classroom peers; 1 was rejected, 1 popular, 1 neglected, and 1 average. Half the groups were comprised of boys from the same classroom, the other half were comprised of boys from different schools, in order to contrast the behavioral correlates of status in familiar versus unfamiliar groups. The groups met once a week for 6 weeks. Each play group session was videotaped, allowing the behavior of each group member to be coded at a later time. After each play group session, each group member was interviewed to determine who he liked the most in the play group. Social preference scores for each group member based on the liking scores from the play group peers were obtained.

These researchers found that, by the end of the second play group session, subjects' classroom social status was reestablished in the groups consisting of unfamiliar peers (Coie & Kupersmidt, 1983). In a related study, Dodge et al. (1990) found that in groups of 6 African American boys of either first- or third-grade age, classroom status was reestablished by the end of the third play

group session. Thus, these boys obviously carried with them certain characteristics (either behavioral or physical) that led to the acquisition of peer group status across contexts. These studies indicate that status can be conceptualized as an individual difference characteristic (in addition to being a group phenomenon). It takes just several half-hour sessions with a new group of peers before a boy replicates his standing in the peer group.

The behavior observation data of the Coie and Kupersmidt (1983) study indicated that the rejected boys were talkative, active, exhibited high rates of aversive behavior, and spent less time with the group during structured activities than did average boys. These behaviors seem to contribute both to the emergence and maintenance of rejected status for these boys because they were displayed in both familiar and unfamiliar peer group contexts (Coie & Kupersmidt, 1983). One behavior pattern exhibited by the rejected boys, solitary inappropriate play (e.g., watching aimlessly out a window, making strange noises), was found to emerge *after* status was established within the group. This behavior, therefore, seems to be a consequence of rejected status as opposed to an antecedent of rejected status. Boys who come to be rejected by peers display antisocial behaviors beginning in the first minutes of peer group interaction, but they withdraw to inappropriate solitary behaviors only after they have been rejected by peers.

Popular boys were rarely aggressive, they often reminded others of the rules, they provided suggestions and direction in ambiguous or difficult situations, and they established the norms for the group (Coie & Kupersmidt, 1983). Neglected boys were most affected by the exposure to a new peer group. Compared with those in the familiar peer groups, the neglected boys in the unfamiliar peer groups were more talkative, engaged in more prosocial behavior, and were as much involved in rough-and-tumble play as other boys. Neglected boys may therefore be able to change their sociometric status in the context of a different peer group.

Dodge (1983) studied the process of emerging peer group status in boys' play groups. Each of Dodge's groups consisted of 8 unfamiliar second-grade boys. The groups met for 8 one-hour sessions. The boys' behavior was coded live during each session by observers. The sessions were videotaped, as well, and further behavior coding was done from the videotape. Sociometric interviews were conducted with each subject after the eighth session. From these interviews, status group membership within the newly formed peer group for each subject was determined.

Dodge found a pattern of behaviors associated with the emergence of rejected status similar to the one Coie and Kupersmidt (1983) found. Boys who eventually came to be rejected by peers were those who, during the first sessions of peer play, engaged in relatively high rates of antisocial behaviors, including insults, threats, contentious statements, exclusion of peers from play, and physical aggression (Dodge, 1983). During the initial sessions of the play group, these boys displayed a high rate of trying to approach others in order to initiate play or peer group entry. Their social approaches, however, were often rebuffed by peers or led to relatively short interactions. These rejected boys became more isolated over time, perhaps in reaction to their negative reception by peers (Dodge, 1983). This pattern of reactive isolation in later sessions is similar to the finding of Coie and Kupersmidt (1983).

Rejected boys' social isolation seems to result from their rejected status as opposed to contributing to their status. Clinicians who observe an already rejected child and find that this child is socially isolated should be cautioned not to infer that the isolation causes peer rejection. Likewise, they should be cautioned that encouraging social initiations by rejected children may not necessarily lead to peer success. After all, these boys had attempted numerous social initiations during their initial encounters with peers but were unsuccessful. Their problems may be in their lack of skill at initiation rather than their lack of willingness to try. Skills training may be necessary prior to encouragement of initiation attempts that otherwise might only bring further failure.

Boys who became popular in new peer groups were those who engaged in high rates of cooperative play and social conversation and refrained from inappropriate behaviors and verbal and physical aggression (Dodge, 1983). Three of the subjects were classified as controversial. These boys engaged in even more prosocial behaviors than the popular boys did. They also displayed high frequencies of aggressive play, hostile statements, exclusions of peers, and extraneous verbalizations (e.g., making meaningless noises).

The pattern of behavior found for boys who came to be neglected by their play group peers was different from that described by Coie and Kupersmidt (1983). Dodge (1983) found that during the initial sessions of the play group, neglected children approached peers socially quite frequently. These approaches, however, often were rebuffed or of short duration, and these boys became increasingly isolated. This description is in stark contrast to the description of Coie and Kupersmidt (1983) that neglected children were more socially involved with their play group peers. This difference is probably due to the way in which neglected status is defined in each study. In the Dodge study, neglected status was defined within the play group. Thus, the behaviors observed during the play group sessions are associated with neglected status in the play group. In the Coie and Kupersmidt study, on the other hand, neglected status was defined by *classroom* peers, not play group peers. Thus, in this study, *classroom* status was associated with behavior in the play group. The Coie and Kupersmidt study does not describe the behaviors that lead to neglected status; the Dodge study does. What is demonstrated by the Coie and Kupersmidt study is that it is possible for neglected children to change their peer status when given the opportunity to interact with a different group of peers.

Social-Cognitive Correlates of Peer Status

The studies of behavioral correlates and antecedents of peer status suggest that children who come to be rejected by peers may be lacking in critical social skills, such as peer group entry and negotiation of conflict. It is hypothesized that these behavioral incompetencies are, in turn, the result of social-cognitive processing deficiencies. That is, children who are deficient or deviant in the manner in which they process social information may have a difficult time behaving competently with peers, which, in turn, may lead them to be viewed negatively by the peer group (Dodge & Feldman, 1990).

In order to test this hypothesis, researchers have constructed models of children's social information processing (Dodge, 1986; McFall, 1982; Rubin & Krasnor, 1986). These models describe the sequential steps involved in children's responding to social stimuli. Competent behavioral responding requires appropriate processing at each step. The first step involves the child's encoding of the relevant social cues (such as the peers' facial expressions, the norms for behavior in a particular context, or a peer's intention in displaying a provocative behavior). The next step consists of the child reaching an interpretation or mental representation of the meaning of these cues (e.g., making an attribution about the peer's intentions in a provocative conflict). Next, the child generates one or more behavioral responses to the situation in accordance with his or her interpretation of the cues. The child then evaluates the generated responses and chooses the one that he or she thinks will best achieve the desired outcomes. The child enacts this response and assesses its success or failure.

Researchers have found that within domains of social interaction (such as peer group entry and provocations), children's patterns or styles of processing social information are coherent and consistent and may be construed as personalitylike characteristics. Thus, some children routinely respond with hostile attributions of others' intentions, whereas others do not, and some children routinely evaluate aggression as leading to positive outcomes, whereas others do not. Next we turn to a review of the relations between each of these processing styles and a child's sociometric status.

ENCODING AND INTERPRETATION

The first steps of social information processing consist of the child encoding and interpreting a social situation. The research in this area has taken two directions. One direction has been to examine the relation between the accuracy of children's interpretations of peer intentions and their sociometric status. An example of this kind of study is one by Dodge, Murphy, and Buchsbaum (1984). These researchers showed boys and girls videotaped vignettes depicting peers behaving with one of the following intents: hostile, prosocial, accidental, and ambiguous. Subjects were presented with two tasks. For the first task, subjects were presented with three vignettes. Two vignettes depicted the same intention, whereas the

third depicted a different intention. The subjects' task was to choose the one vignette that was different from the other two. The second task presented to subjects was to ask them to identify the intention of the peer actors in a series of vignettes. The results indicated that rejected and neglected children performed more poorly than popular children on both tasks. These children were also more likely than other subjects to make specific kinds of errors. When asked to identify prosocial and accidental intentions in the second task, they made errors in the direction of a hostile attributional bias. That is, the rejected and neglected children were likely to label prosocial and accidental intentions incorrectly as hostile. Low-status children, therefore, seem to have more difficulty both discriminating among intentions and correctly labeling others' intentions.

The second direction that research on the interpretation stage of information processing has taken is to examine children's interpretations of ambiguous, or unclear, social situations. This research has demonstrated that aggressive-rejected children are more likely to attribute hostile intentions to peer provocateurs, whereas nonaggressive and nonrejected children are more likely to attribute hostile intentions to peer provocateurs, whereas nonaggressive and nonrejected children are more likely to attribute benign intentions to peer provocateurs in the identical situations (Dodge, 1980; Dodge & Newman, 1981; Guerra & Slaby, 1990; Sancilio, Plumert, & Hartup, 1989). This finding is significant because it has been found that children who attribute hostile intentions to peers are highly likely to retaliate aggressively toward them and may then become disliked by these peers (Dodge, 1980). Displaying a "hostile attributional bias" (Nasby, Hayden, & dePaulo, 1979), therefore, may contribute to children's poor peer status.

RESPONSE GENERATION

One dimension of response generation patterns that has been examined is the number of responses that children are able to generate to a hypothetical problematic social situation. Early research in this area (Spivack & Shure, 1974) found a positive correlation between the number of solutions that a child generated and his or her social adjustment. Subsequent research in this area has been mixed. Some studies have corroborated the finding that children high in peer group status generate more responses than low-status children (Asarnow & Callan, 1985; Richard & Dodge, 1982), whereas other studies have found no differences in the quantity of responses generated between high- and low-status children (Krasnor & Rubin, 1978). These mixed findings have been hypothesized to have occurred because of procedural differences among the studies and in differences in the way that subjects were selected for study (Dodge & Feldman, 1990; Gesten & Weissberg, 1979).

Another dimension of response generation that has been explored is the quality of the responses generated by children to hypothetical situations. Research in this area has consistently found that the responses generated by low-status children are more deviant and less competent than those generated by high-status children (Asher & Renshaw, 1981; Rubin & Daniels-Beirness, 1983). There is also evidence to indicate that low-status children generate more agonistic responses than high-status children (Asarnow & Callan, 1985; Rubin & Daniels-Beirness, 1983). This latter finding is not surprising given the fact that rejected children have been found to be more aggressive than their peers. Overall, then, low-status children seem deficient in the ability to generate competent responses to hypothetical social situations.

RESPONSE EVALUATION

There has not been a great deal of research conducted on the response evaluation component of social information processing. The studies that have been completed indicate that low-status children tend to evaluate socially competent responses less favorably than do high-status children and that low-status children tend to evaluate aggressive responses more favorably than do high-status children (Crick & Ladd, 1990; Dodge, Pettit, McCloskey, & Brown, 1986; Perry, Perry, & Rasmussen, 1986). Specifically, rejected children evaluate aggressive responses as leading to positive instrumental and interpersonal outcomes, and they rate these responses as "good" ones more frequently than do nonrejected children.

ENACTMENT

Skillful enactment of a response requires verbal and motor skills and a sense of timing and coordination. Again, very few studies have been done on children's enactment skills (independent of their other social information-processing skills). In general, however, low-status children have been found to be less competent at enactment of appropriate responses than are average- and high-status children (Dodge & Feldman, 1990).

THE PREDICTION OF BEHAVIOR FROM PROCESSING VARIABLES

Although deficiencies in each aspect of processing just described are associated with peer status, not every socially incompetent child displays deficits in all areas. Some socially rejected children have consistent problems at the encoding and interpretational steps (these children may have attention deficits), whereas others have problems anticipating outcomes and thinking ahead (these children may have impulsivity problems). Thus, assessing an individual's performance at all processing steps may lead to a more powerful prediction of behavior and peer status. This hypothesis was explored by Dodge et al. (1986) in two studies examining the linkages between social information processing and social behavior. These researchers assessed children's processing patterns in hypothetical peer group entry and provocation situations and behavior in actual peer group entry and response to provocation situations. These studies demonstrated that children's actual behavior in these two domains could be strongly predicted by their patterns of processing regarding hypothetical stories in the same domain. A multiple regression analysis indicated that over half of the variance in actual group entry behavior could be predicted from a child's pattern of processing hypothetical entry situations. In the domain of response to provocation, a multiple regression analysis revealed that, again, over half of the variance in aggressive behavior could be accounted for by processing patterns. Thus, specific patterns of processing can predict specific behaviors. These findings have been essentially replicated with adolescents in residential treatment (Slaby & Guerra, 1989), with elementary school students (Feldman & Dodge, 1987), and with kindergartners in a school setting (Dodge, Bates, & Pettit, 1990).

Most of the studies of processing have been cross-sectional and correlational, which precludes strong conclusions about the causal relation between processing patterns and behavior. Recently longitudinal inquiry has begun that has lent further confidence to the hypothesis that processing patterns actually *predict* later peer adjustment. Dodge et al. (1990) found that processing patterns assessed prior to the beginning of kindergarten predicted children's later peer adjustment during kindergarten, even when the prekindergarten adjustment levels were controlled statistically.

CONCLUSIONS

These studies clearly support the hypothesis that processing patterns and peer status are related. The social information processing model is intended as a description of the mental processes involved in the generation of social behaviors that determine peer status, so researchers have framed these patterns as possible antecedents of peer status. Other social cognitions have been framed as consequences of experiencing peer rejection, such as increased loneliness, personal unhappiness, and poor self-concept (Asher & Wheeler, 1985; Dodge & Feldman, 1990).

The Influence of the Peer Group on Sociometric Status

Our focus thus far has been on aspects of the individual child that contribute to his or her sociometric status. There is emerging evidence that the peer group acts in ways to maintain a child's social status, as well. In general, peers respond more favorably to the behavior of popular children than they do to that of unpopular children, presumably because of bias and reputation (Asarnow, 1983;

Dodge, 1983; Putallaz & Gottman, 1981). Even when popular children engage in negative behavior, they are perceived more positively by peers than when unpopular children behave in the same way (Asarnow, 1983; Putallaz & Gottman, 1981). Once a child has established a reputation in his or her peer group, the peer group's perception of the child's behavior seems to be based partly on his or her reputation. This reputation effect is important to keep in mind when considering how best to intervene with low-status children (Price and Dodge, 1990).

Interventions with Low-Status Children

Intervention research with low-status children has evolved over the years with respect to the targets of the intervention as well as the intervention techniques used. Early intervention studies targeted children who were socially isolated and used reinforcement and modeling techniques to increase their rate of social approach (Coie & Koeppl, 1990). Only modest success was achieved with these interventions, perhaps because, as discussed, social isolation can be a consequence rather than cause of low status. More recent interventions have targeted socially incompetent children and attempted to teach them specific skills in order to improve their peer relationships. The inclusion of peers in the intervention effort has emerged as an important component for successful behavioral and status changes, as well.

MODELING AND REINFORCEMENT INTERVENTIONS

Reinforcement by adults (Allen, Hart, Buell, Harris, & Wolf, 1964) and peers (Wahler, 1967) has been used to increase the amount of social interaction attempted by isolated children. The use of peer rewards also has been used to decrease the amount of disruptive behavior in a sixth-grade classroom (Solomon & Wahler, 1973). These interventions have been found to be effective in increasing the frequency of the subjects' interactions, but the effects have not been maintained after the reinforcement ended (Putallaz & Gottman, 1981).

Peer models have been used to increase isolated children's rates of social interaction (Furman & Gavin, 1989). After watching a film modeling prosocial interaction, isolated children significantly increased their rate of social interaction (O'Conner, 1969). Peer modeling has been found to affect children's behavior both in laboratory settings and in naturalistic environments (Abramovitch & Grusec, 1978). There is mixed evidence, however, as to whether the gains resulting from peer modeling are maintained (Putallaz & Gottman, 1981).

SOCIAL SKILLS TRAINING

Social skills training interventions have been guided by the hypothesis that children who are low in peer acceptance are prevented from establishing effective peer relationships by their own lack of social skills (Asher & Renshaw, 1981). These social skills include both social-information-processing patterns (e.g., reading peers' cues, problem solving, anticipating outcomes of behavior) and motor behaviors. The empirical basis for this work is rather strong, as reviewed earlier in this chapter. An exemplar of a social skills intervention is the coaching program developed by Oden and Asher (1977). This intervention focused on teaching four skills: participation in play; cooperation; communication by listening and talking; and validation support by looking, smiling, or offering encouragement. Children were taught the general concept underlying each skill by a coach and were then given the opportunity to practice using the skill with a peer or peers. Afterward, they received feedback and reinforcement for their performance by the coach. Oden and Asher (1977) found an improvement in sociometric ratings for the coached children immediately following the intervention as well as at a 1-year follow-up.

Some social skills training programs have demonstrated improvement in sociometric status (Bierman & Furman, 1984; Ladd, 1981), whereas others have not (Hymel & Asher, 1977). The reasons for these inconsistent outcomes is as yet unclear and need to be explored further.

PEER GROUP INTERVENTIONS

Because one's reputation in a peer group has been demonstrated to contribute to the maintenance of sociometric status, Bierman and Furman (1984) examined the effectiveness of an intervention procedure designed to improve peer attitudes toward unpopular children. Guided by the hypothesis that working toward a superordinate goal promotes group cohesiveness and reduces negative stereotyping, Bierman and Furman directed low-accepted children to work with classmates on a group task. The intervention study had 4 conditions: peer involvement in the group task; individual coaching in social skills; combined peer involvement and individual coaching; and no treatment control.

These investigators found improved sociometric ratings for children in the peer involvement and in the combined peer involvement-individual coaching conditions. These effects, however, were not maintained at a 6-week follow-up (Bierman & Furman, 1984).

In sum, promising findings have been obtained with social skills training interventions, particularly when combined with peer group interventions; however, the long-term efficacy of these interventions is still in doubt. Refinements in these interventions continue.

Conclusions

This chapter has provided an overview of the peer relations literature with regard to child psychiatry. Lack of social competence has been noted to be an integral part of numerous child and adult psychiatric disorders. Relating effectively with peers is theoretically important for normal social development and has been found empirically to predict positive adjustment outcomes in adolescence and adulthood.

The behavioral antecedents of poor peer status include aggression, disruptiveness, and lack of social skill in completing important peer tasks such as group entry and conflict negotiation. These skills deficits, in turn, appear to be related to social-information-processing patterns, such as accurately reading social cues, generating competent solutions to problems (problem solving), and anticipating outcomes of one's behavior.

These processing patterns and skill deficits have been the target of intervention efforts that have shown promising results, although long-term efficacy is still in doubt. These promising efforts have kept this field vital and are likely to lead to improved interventions in the future.

REFERENCES

Abramovitch, R., & Grusec, J. E. (1978). Peer imitation in a natural setting. *Child Development, 49,* 60–69.

Allen, E., Hart, B., Buell, J., Harris, F., & Wolf, M. (1964). Effects of social reinforcement on isolate behavior of a nursery school child. *Child Development, 35,* 511–518.

American Psychiatric Association. (1994). *Diagnostic and statistical manual of mental disorders* (4th ed.). Washington, DC: Author.

Asarnow, J. R. (1983). Children with peer adjustment problems: Sequential and nonsequential analyses of school behavior. *Journal of Consulting and Clinical Psychology, 51,* 709–717.

Asarnow, J. R., & Callan, J. W. (1985). Boys with peer adjustment problems: Social cognitive processes. *Journal of Consulting and Clinical Psychology, 53,* 80–87.

Asher, S. R., & Coie, J. D. (1991). *The rejected child.* New York: Cambridge University Press.

Asher, S. R., & Dodge, K. A. (1986). Identifying children who are rejected by their peers. *Developmental Psychology, 22,* 444–449.

Asher, S. R., & Renshaw, P. D. (1981). Children without friends: Social knowledge and social skill training. In S. R. Asher & J. M. Gottman (Eds.), *The development of children's friendships* (pp. 273–296). New York: Cambridge University Press.

Asher, S. R., Singleton, L., Tinsley, B. R., & Hymel, S. (1979). A reliable sociometric measure for preschool children. *Developmental Psychology, 15,* 443–444.

Asher, S. R., & Wheeler, V. (1985). Children's loneliness: A comparison of rejected and neglected peer status. *Journal of Consulting and Clinical Psychology, 53,* 500–505.

Berndt, T. J. (1982). The features and effects of friendship in early adolescence. *Child Development, 53,* 1447–1460.

Berndt, T. J., & Ladd, G. W. (Eds.) (1989). *Peer relationships in child development.* New York: John Wiley & Sons.

Bierman, K. L., & Furman, W. (1984). The effects of social skills training and peer involvement on the social adjustment of preadolescents. *Child Development, 57,* 151–162.

Bowlby, J. (1988). *A secure base: Parent-child attachment and healthy human development.* New York: Basic Books.

Bukowski, W. M., & Hoza, B. (1989). Popularity and friendship: Issues in theory, measurement, and outcome. In T. J. Berndt & G. W. Ladd (Eds.), *Peer relationships in child development* (pp. 15–45). New York: John Wiley & Sons.

Cairns, R. B., Cairns, B. D., Neckerman, H. J., Gect, S. D., & Gariepy, J. L. (1988). Social networks and aggressive behavior: Peer support or peer rejection. *Developmental Psychology, 24,* 815–823.

Carlson, C. L., Lahey, B. B., & Neeper, R. (1984). Peer assessment of the social behavior of accepted, rejected, and neglected children. *Journal of Abnormal Child Psychology, 12,* 189–198.

Coie, J. D., Dodge, K. A., & Copottelli, H. (1982). Dimensions and types of social status: A cross-age perspective. *Developmental Psychology, 18,* 557–571.

Coie, J. D., Dodge, K. A., & Kupersmidt, J. B. (1990). Peer group behavior and social status. In S. R. Asher & J. D. Coie (Eds.), *Peer rejection in childhood* (pp. 17–59). New York: Cambridge University Press.

Coie, J. D., & Koeppl, G. K. (1990). Adapting intervention to the problems of aggressive and disruptive rejected children. In S. R. Asher & J. D. Coie (Eds.), *Peer rejection in childhood* (pp. 309–337). New York: Cambridge University Press.

Coie, J. D., & Kupersmidt, J. B. (1983). A behavioral analysis of emerging social status in boys' groups. *Child Development, 54,* 1400–1416.

Cowen, E. L., Pederson, A., Babigian, H., Izzo, L. D., & Trost, M. A. (1972). Long-term follow-up of early detected vulnerable children. *Journal of Consulting and Clinical Psychology, 41,* 438–446.

Crick, N. R., & Ladd, G. W. (1990). Children's perceptions of the outcomes of social strategies: Do the ends justify being mean? *Developmental Psychology, 26,* 612–620.

Dodge, K. A. (1980). Social cognition and children's aggressive behavior. *Child Development, 51,* 162–170.

Dodge, K. A. (1983). Behavioral antecedents of peer social status. *Child Development, 54,* 1386–1399.

Dodge, K. A. (1986). A social information processing model of social competence in children. In M. Perlmutter (Ed.), *Minnesota symposia on child psychology* (Vol. 18, pp. 75–127). Hillsdale, NJ: Lawrence Erlbaum.

Dodge, K. A., Bates, J. E., & Pettit, G. S. (1990). Mechanisms in the cycle of violence. *Science, 250,* 1678–1683.

Dodge, K. A., Coie, J. D., Pettit, G. S., & Price, J. M. (1990). Peer status and aggression in boys' groups: Developmental and contextual analyses. *Child Development, 61,* 1289–1309.

Dodge, K. A., & Feldman, E. (1990). Issues in social cognition and sociometric status. In S. R. Asher & J. D. Coie (Eds.), *Peer rejection in childhood* (pp. 119–155). New York: Cambridge University Press.

Dodge, K. A., Murphy, R. M., & Bushsbaum, K. (1984). The assessment of intention-cue detection skills in children: Implications for developmental psychopathology. *Child Development, 55,* 163–173.

Dodge, K. A., & Newman, J. P. (1981). Biased decision-making processes in aggressive boys. *Journal of Abnormal Psychology, 4,* 375–379.

Dodge, K. A., Pettit, G. S., McClaskey, C. L., & Brown, M. (1986). Social competence in children. *Monographs of the Society for Research in Child Development, 51* (2, Serial No. 213).

Eckerman, C. O., Davis, C. C., & Didow, S. M. (1989). Toddlers' emerging ways of achieving social coordinations with a peer. *Child Development, 60,* 440–453.

Eckerman, C. O., & Stein, M. R. (1982). The toddlers' emerging interactive skills. In K. H. Rubin & H. S. Ross (Eds.), *Peer relationships and social skills in childhood* (pp. 41–71). New York: Springer-Verlag.

Elkins, D. (1958). Some factors related to the choice status of ninety eighth-grade children in a school society. *Genetic Psychology Monographs, 58,* 207–272.

Feinberg, M. R., Smith, M., & Schmidt, R. (1958). An analysis of expressions used by adolescents at varying economic levels to describe accepted and rejected peers. *Journal of Genetic Psychology, 93,* 133–148.

Feinman, S., & Lewis, M. (1983). Social referencing at ten months: A second-order effect on infants' responses to strangers. *Child Development, 54,* 878–887.

Feldman, E., & Dodge, K. A. (1987). Social information processing and sociometric status: Sex, age, and situational effects. *Journal of Abnormal Child Psychology, 15,* 211–227.

Furman, W., & Gavin, L. A. (1989). Peers' influence on adjustment and development: A view from the intervention literature. In T. J. Berndt & G. W. Ladd (Eds.), *Peer relationships in child development* (pp. 319–340). New York: John Wiley & Sons.

Gesten, E., & Weissberg, R. (1979, September). *Social problem-solving training and prevention: Some good news and some bad news.* Paper presented at the annual meeting of the American Psychological Association, New York.

Goldman, J. A., Corsini, D. A., & de Urioste, R. (1980). Implications of positive and negative sociometric status for assessing the social competence of young children. *Journal of Applied Developmental Psychology, 1,* 209–220.

Gronlund, N. E., & Holmlund, W. S. (1958). The value of elementary school sociometric status scores for predicting pupils' adjustment in high school. *Educational Administration and Supervision, 44,* 225–260.

Guerra, N., & Slaby, R. (1990). Cognitive mediators of aggression in adolescent offenders: II. Intervention. *Developmental Psychology, 26,* 269–277.

Hartup, W. (1983). Peer relations. In P. Mussen (Ed.), *Handbook of child psychology* (Vol. 4, pp. 103–196). New York: John Wiley & Sons.

Hoza, B., Molina, B. S. G., Bukowski, W. M., & Sippola, L. K. (1995). Peer variables as predictors of later childhood adjustment. *Development and Psychopathology, 7,* 787–802.

Hymel, S., & Asher, S. R. (1977). *Assessment and training of isolated children's social skills.* Paper presented at the biennial meeting of the Society for Research in Child Development, New Orleans.

Jacobs, M. A., Muller, J. J., Anderson, J., & Skinner, J. R. (1972). Therapeutic expectations, premorbid adjustment, and manifest distress levels as predictors of improvement in hospitalized patients. *Journal of Consulting and Clinical Psychology, 39,* 455–461.

Jacobs, M. A., Muller, J. J., Anderson, J., & Skinner, J. R. (1973). Prediction of improvement in coping with pathology in hospitalized psychiatric patients: A replication study. *Journal of Consulting and Clinical Psychology, 40,* 343–349.

John, R. S., Mednick, S. A., & Schulsinger, F. (1982). Teachers' reports as predictors of schizophrenia and borderline schizophrenia: A Bayesian decision analysis. *Journal of Abnormal Psychology, 91,* 399–413.

Keenan, K., Loeber, R., Zhang, Q., Stouthamer-Loeber, M., & Van Kammen, W. B. (1995). The influence of deviant peers on the development of boys' disruptive and delinquent behavior: A temporal analysis. *Development and Psychopathology, 7,* 715–726.

Kohn, M., & Clausen, J. (1955). Social isolation and schizophrenia. *American Sociological Review, 20,* 265–273.

Krasnor, L., & Rubin, K. H. (1978, June). *Preschoolers' verbal and behavioral solutions to social problems.* Paper presented at the annual meeting of the Canadian Psychological Association, Ottawa.

Kupersmidt, J. B., Burchinal, M., & Patterson, C. J. (1995). Developmental patterns of childhood peer relations as predictors of externalizing behavior problems. *Development and Psychopathology, 7,* 825–843.

Kupersmidt, J. B., Coie, J. D., & Dodge, K. A. (1990). The role of poor peer relationships in the development of disorder. In S. R. Asher & J. D. Coie (Eds.), *Peer rejection in childhood* (pp. 274–305). New York: Cambridge University Press.

Ladd, G. (1981). Effectiveness of a social learning method for enhancing children's social interaction and peer acceptance. *Child Development, 52,* 171–178.

Lesser, G. S. (1959). The relationship between various forms of aggression and popularity among lower-class children. *Journal of Educational Psychology, 50,* 20–25.

MacDonald, K., & Parke, R. D. (1984). Bridging the gap: Parent-child play interaction and peer interactive competence. *Child Development, 55,* 1265–1277.

Masters, J. C., & Furman, W. (1981). Popularity, individual friendship selections, and specific peer interaction among children. *Developmental Psychology, 17,* 344–350.

McFall, R. M. (1982). A review and reformulation of the concept of social skills. *Behavioral Assessment, 4,* 1–35.

Nasby, W., Hayden, B., & dePaulo, B. M. (1979). Attributional bias among aggressive boys to interpret unambiguous social stimuli as displays of hostility. *Journal of Abnormal Psychology, 89,* 459–468.

Newcomb, A. F., Brady, J. E., & Hartup, W. W. (1979). Friendship and incentive condition as determinants of children's task-oriented social behavior. *Child Development, 50,* 878–881.

O'Conner, R. D. (1969). Modification of social withdrawal through symbolic modeling. *Journal of Applied Behavioral Analysis, 2,* 15–22.

Oden, S., & Asher, S. R. (1977). Coaching children in social skills for friendship making. *Child Development, 48,* 495–506.

Parke, R. D., & Bhavnagri, N. P. (1989). Parents as managers of children's peer relationships. In D. Belle (Ed.), *Children's social networks and social supports* (pp. 241–259). New York: John Wiley & Sons.

Parker, J. G., & Asher, S. R. (1987). Peer relations and later personal adjustment: Are low-accepted children at risk? *Psychological Bulletin, 102,* 357–389.

Parker, J. G., & Asher, S. R. (1993). Friendship and friendship quality in middle childhood: Links with peer group acceptance and feelings of loneliness and social dissatisfaction. *Developmental Psychology, 29,* 611–621.

Parten, M. (1932). Social participation among preschool children. *Journal of Abnormal and Social Psychology, 27,* 243–269.

Peery, J. C. (1979). Popular, amiable, isolated, rejected: A reconceptualization of sociometric status in preschool children. *Child Development, 50,* 1231–1234.

Perry, D. G., Perry, L. C., & Rasmussen, P. R. (1986). Aggressive children believe that aggression is easy to perform and leads to rewards. *Child Development, 57,* 700–711.

Piaget, J. (1965). *The moral judgment of the child.* New York: Free Press. (Originally published 1932.)

Price, J. M., & Dodge, K. A. (1990). Peers' contributions to children's social maladjustment. In T. J. Berndt & G. W. Ladd (Eds.), *Peer relationships in child development* (pp. 341–370). New York: Wiley-Interscience.

Putallaz, M. (1987). Maternal behavior and children's sociometric status. *Child Development, 58,* 324–340.

Putallaz, M., & Gottman, J. M. (1981). Social skills and group acceptance. In S. R. Asher & J. M. Gottman (Eds.), *The development of children's friendships* (pp. 116–149). New York: Cambridge University Press.

Putallaz, M., & Heflin, A. H. (1990). Parent-child interaction. In S. R. Asher & J. D. Coie (Eds.), *Peer rejection in childhood* (pp. 189–216). New York: Cambridge University Press.

Richard, B. A., & Dodge, K. A. (1982). Social maladjustment and problem solving in school-aged children. *Journal of Consulting and Clinical Psychology, 50,* 226–233.

Rizzo, T. A. (1989). *Friendship development among children in school.* Norwood, NJ: Ablex.

Robins, L. N. (1966). *Deviant children grown up.* Baltimore: Williams & Wilkins.

Roff, M. (1961). Childhood social interactions and young adult bad conduct. *Journal of Abnormal Social Psychology, 63,* 333–337.

Roff, M. (1963). Childhood social interactions and young adult psychosis. *Journal of Clinical Psychology, 19,* 152–157.

Rogoff, B. (1990). *Apprenticeship in thinking: Cognitive development in social context.* New York: Oxford University Press.

Rubin, K. H., & Daniels-Beirness, T. (1983). Concurrent and predictive correlates of sociometric status in kindergarten and grade one children. *Merrill-Palmer Quarterly, 29,* 337–352.

Rubin, K. H., & Krasnor, L. R. (1986). Social-cognitive and social behavioral perspectives on problem solving. In M. Perlmutter (Ed.), *Minnesota symposia on child psychology* (Vol. 18, pp. 1–68). Hillsdale, NJ: Lawrence Erlbaum.

Rubin, Z., & Sloman, J. (1984). How parents influence their children's friendships. In M. Lewis (Ed.), *Beyond the dyad* (pp. 223–250). New York: Plenum Press.

Sancilio, M. F. M., Plumert, J. M., & Hartup, W. W. (1989). Friendship and aggressiveness as determinants of conflict outcomes in middle childhood. *Developmental Psychology, 25,* 812–819.

Slaby, R. G., & Guerra, N. G. (1989). Cognitive mediators in adolescent offenders: I. Assessment. *Developmental Psychology, 24* (4), 580–588.

Solomon, R. W., & Wahler, R. G. (1973). Peer reinforcement of classroom problem behavior. *Journal of Applied Behavioral Analysis, 6,* 49–55.

Spivack, G., & Shure, M. B. (1974). *The problem solving approach to adjustment.* Washington, DC: Jossey-Bass.

Stengel, E. (1971). *Suicide and attempted suicide.* Harmondsworth, England: Penguin.

Sullivan, H. S. (1953). *The interpersonal theory of psychiatry.* New York: W. W. Norton.

Tremblay, R. E., Masse, L. C., Vitaro, F., & Dobkin, P. L. (1995). The impact of friends' deviant behavior on early onset of delinquency: Longitudinal data from 6 to 13 years of age. *Development and Psychopathology, 7,* 649–667.

Vygotsky, L. S. (1978). *Mind in society: The development of higher psychological processes.* Cambridge, MA: Harvard University Press.

Wahler, R. G. (1967). Child-child interactions in five field settings: Some experimental analyses. *Journal of Experimental Child Psychology, 5,* 278–293.

Walden, T. A. (1991). Inant social referencing. In J. Garber & K. A. Dodge (Eds.), *The development of emotion regulation and dysregulation* (pp. 69–88). New York: Cambridge University Press.

Watt, N. E. (1978). Patterns of childhood social development in adult schizophrenics. *Archives of General Psychiatry, 35,* 160–165.

Woody, R. (1969). Behavioral problem children in the schools: Recognition, diagnosis, and modification. New York: Appleton-Century-Crofts.

Zigler, E., & Phillips, L. (1961). Social competence and outcome in psychiatric disorder. *Journal of Abnormal and Social Psychology, 63,* 264–271.

31 / "We Hold These Truths to Be Self-Evident": The Origins of Moral Motives in Individual Activity and Shared Experience

Robert N. Emde and Robert B. Clyman

This chapter sets forth our model of the development of moral motives during the first 4 years of life. In reviewing relevant research on moral development, we discover multiple paradoxes and surprises. Consider the paradox implicit in Jefferson's historic words: "We hold these truths to be self-evident, that all men are endowed by their creator with certain inalienable rights; that among these are life, liberty, and the pursuit of happiness."

Why did Jefferson proclaim democratic ideals that are already "self-evident" to all? In part, the answer may lie in a phenomenon we consider central to understanding moral behavior: Many "self-evident," closely held values are often not criticized, assumed, and may not be conscious. Jefferson's pronouncement makes explicit what has been implicit; these are the values he poses to be at the core of democratic ideals.

This chapter reviews how infants and young children may develop moral motives, expectations, and rules without consciously reflecting on those rules. At later ages, inclinations formed earlier may be so "self-evident" that the individual may act morally in accordance with internalized rules without first consciously thinking about them. We do not need to recall the Golden Rule

("Do unto others as you would have them do unto you") in order to act in accordance with it. Jefferson's words point to another important observation that we include in our model. The words contain another contradiction that has been made poignant by our historical perspective. There is an unspoken limitation on a quality because it implies only to men of one race. The task of articulating implicit assumptions, and of attending to cultural variations in ideals and practices, continues to be an urgent task for us.

Last, our title suggests still another paradox: The young child develops moral motives as a result of activity that is uniquely individual yet is also a result of experience that is shared with caregivers. Taking account of such paradoxes, we believe, will lead us to a more integrative perspective on the vicissitudes of moral behavior as we understand it in particular infants and young children.

Early Development of Self from a Moral Perspective

Our view of self-experience is that it is, from the beginning, shared. The development of a sense of self occurs along with the development of the sense of others who are evaluated as being important. Self-experience is as much affective as it

Dr. Emde's work is supported by the National Institute of Mental Health project grant MH22803 and Research Scientist Award 5 K02 MH36808. The work reviewed in this chapter was also supported by the John D. and Catherine T. MacArthur Foundation Research Network on Early Childhood Transitions.

is cognitive, and, beginning in early infancy, our model proposes that the internalizations of self contain important moral aspects.

A surprising feature of the model concerns the nature of morality itself. Not only do we see it earlier in development, we also see it more broadly than many. Morality often involves struggles and dilemmas, but it is also positive and freely flowing, and it involves the young child's activation of internalized rules about "dos" as well as about "don'ts."

A BASIS FOR SELF AND MORAL MOTIVES PRIOR TO AWARENESS

Our model's perspective about consciousness may be the most paradoxical and surprising of all. We have come to the view that most moral motivation and action is not conscious. Psychoanalysts, however, will be surprised that the domain of nonconscious mental activity that we deem of most importance for early moral motives and activity is one that Freud had not envisioned. In addition to *preconscious* mental activity (what is not in any moment's consciousness but can be brought into awareness with effort, such as remembering one's address) and in addition to *dynamically unconscious* mental activity (what is warded off because of associations with a painful past or expectations of pain in the future, such as anger at a loved one who has died), there is the area of procedural *nonconscious* mental activity. The latter kind of mental activity has come into the purview of the cognitive sciences and the artificial intelligence community only recently and, since it is used throughout our model, it deserves further comment.

Procedural knowledge refers to information that underlies a skill but need not be represented in consciousness in order for an individual to manifest the skill (Cohen & Squire, 1980). Declarative knowledge, in contrast to procedural knowledge, refers to information that can be brought into consciousness through recognition or recall. Procedural knowledge is demonstrated when a child speaks grammatically without conscious knowledge of grammatical rules or when a skillful psychotherapist intervenes with a patient without first consciously planning the intervention. To paraphrase Ryle (1949), we do not have to think before we act in order to act intelligently. Rules that govern complex behavior need not be represented consciously for the behavior to be rule-governed. Indeed, typically we are conscious of the outcome of information processing but unaware of the processing itself. Recently these ideas have been implemented in a new form of artificial intelligence, referred to as parallel distributive processing, where neuronlike units interact to yield complex rule-governed behavior, although the rule is never explicitly learned or represented (Rummelhart, McClelland, & the PDP Research Group, 1986). Similarly, we believe infants can acquire complex behaviors without consciously learning rules. This capacity for procedural knowledge develops by the end of the first year of life, more than 1 year before the development of recall (Mandler, 1983; Piaget, 1952), with the beginning of expressive language as indicated by personal pronouns or 2-word speech (Bates, Bretherton, & Snyder, 1988), or with the development of reflective self-awareness (Lewis & Brooks-Gunn, 1979) at the end of the second year of life.

We might consider, as an example of procedural knowledge, how young infants demonstrate skillful regularities in their face-to-face turn-taking behavior with their caregivers. Such procedural knowledge emerges from the children's biologically prepared capacities interacting with emotionally sensitive caregivers. Complex rules that regulate reciprocity are acquired, yet we need not postulate that an infant must first think about reciprocity prior to manifesting it. In such a fashion, we believe that early moral motives develop in a self that operates procedurally (Clyman, 1991; Emde, Biringen, Clyman, & Oppenheim, 1991). Such a perspective on important behaviors developing in action, prior to representation, is also consistent with the foundations of Piagetian theory wherein such sequences are emphasized in cognitive development (Piaget, 1952).

A wide variety of early moral behaviors operate procedurally. In addition to early reciprocity, infants and young children demonstrate empathy, prosocial behavior, compliance with parental directives, and avoidance of prohibitive actions, without there being any evidence that they first recall explicit rules prior to acting on them. Rather, they demonstrate procedural knowledge of implicit rules. Empirically, young children's knowledge of implicit rules can be inferred not only from observing their rule-governed behavior but also by observing their responses when assumed rules are violated. Kagan (1981), in such a fashion, demonstrated that infants show anxiety in response to flawed objects, indicating their implicit knowledge of internalized standards.

One important class of procedurally governed actions that plays a prominent role in moral behavior is emotional signaling. The organized expression of emotion in the face or voice, as well as the reception of emotional signals from important others, provides a background of coherence for both self- and moral regulation. This has been conceptualized as the affective core of self (Emde, 1983), and it indicates, from our point of view, the operation of emotional procedures (Clyman, 1991). The young infant in a playroom who monitors parents in order to detect indications of emotional availability or unavailability (Sorce & Emde, 1982) or the infant who perceives parental emotional signals and modifies behavior accordingly (Klinnert, Campos, Sorce, Emde, & Svedja, 1983) demonstrates the operation of nonconscious, automatic emotional procedures. Thus, social referencing is based on procedural knowledge about the consistency of emotions in self and others. The infant can use parental emotional signals without thinking about the consistency in emotional expression, thereby demonstrating procedural knowledge concerning the meaning of such interactions (Emde et al., 1991).

With development, interindividual emotional signaling becomes intraindividual emotional signaling, a phenomenon psychoanalysts since Freud (1926/1959) have referred to in terms of the construct of signal affect systems (also see Emde, 1980). The experience of moral emotions such as shame or guilt can alert us not only to the fact that we have violated a norm but also to the possibility that we are contemplating an action that will do so. As such, emotional signaling acts procedurally to organize our attention, motivation, and, subsequently, our behavior.

The construct of procedural knowledge should not be used without certain caveats. The limits of the construct are not yet known, and the best way to characterize different types of nonconscious information processing is the subject of intense current interest. (For a review, see Richardson-

Klavehn & Bjork, 1988.) The idea of procedural knowledge, however, provides a new and important frame in which to theorize and test hypotheses about moral development.

SELF DEVELOPMENT: INDIVIDUAL ACTIVITY AND SHARED EXPERIENCE

It always seems a bit awkward to use the word "self" as a noun, because it may lead to a tendency to think of self as an entity rather than a construct of convenience. Even from a functionalist orientation, this usage may lead to a tendency to think of an organization that is static rather than changing over time. But perhaps most awkward of all, the noun "self," even from a developmental orientation, may lead us to think of individual development in an isolated fashion. The construct of self, instead, refers to a dynamic organization of regulatory functions that serves to characterize an individual in relation to others. Let us take up the points about self as individual activity and then as shared experience.

We think of self as an organizing mental process and a regulator of experience—where this includes an individual's sense of continuity, confidence, mastery, and, at a later age, esteem. Regulation of experience, according to these dimensions, is based on knowledge of one's active, purposeful existence. It involves knowing what is one's own body and what is not one's own body and, similarly, what is one's own activity and what is not one's own activity. A sense of coherence and agency are cardinal features of the self system along with a sense of control (i.e., ownership of body and action). Elsewhere (Emde et al., 1991) we have spoken of the paradox in that coherence and sense of agency are maintained across time in the midst of developmental change, new events, and accommodations to increasing complexity. Self can be thought of as a regulator of stability in the midst of active exploration and perturbation—perhaps as a regulatory "constant" for the dynamic equilibria of adaptation, wherein the regulatory constant itself undergoes replenishment and change.[1]

And now to shared experience. Self is a relational construct. Self development can be thought of only as self-in-relation-to-other development.

Thus, the psychological development of the sense of self necessarily involves and coincides with the psychological development of the sense of the other and, more particularly, with the development of the sense of self in relation to significant others (Lazarus, 1991; Lewis & Brooks-Gunn, 1979; Stern, 1985). The case can be made that self-recognition and the maintenance of integrity are two biological functions that permeate all of life. As such, they serve to define individuality at levels involving a variety of systems within the organism in relation to each other, and they also serve to define individually at levels involving the organism in relation to the external environment. At all levels, whether one is considering molecular genetics, immune functions, or organismic functioning in a group, self is a relational construct; self exists only in relation to others. Thus, early self not only has to do with the sense of agency but of recognition and of the maintenance of integrity along the developmental course of increasing complexity. Species, gender, family, and group are all involved in self- and other recognition and in integrity maintenance at successive levels of organization. Some personality theorists have preferred terms such as *identity* and *ego-integrity* over self as being more relational (cf. Erikson, 1950; Lazarus, 1991). Such terms necessarily take into account self-development in relation to others at particular times in one's life and in relation to cultural values. They highlight the fact that one's identity grows out of experience with others who share one's culture. Shared information from everyday activities often is acquired and stored procedurally, removed from consciousness, and therefore recalcitrant to modification. Information of this sort often is brought into consciousness only when others who do not share the same assumptions notice the discrepancy between two views, as happens, for example, when academic papers are debated or when anthropologists conduct field work.[2]

Moral Motives in Early Infancy

Having situated moral development within a broader framework of self-development and the different types of information and emotion processing in infancy, we turn our attention to a description of basic motives. We find that moral motives, derived from basic motives, are linked to what feels right in action. They develop transactionally from the interplay of biological capacities and environmental exigencies, and come to involve the establishment of procedures, expectations, and shared goals.

BASIC MOTIVES AND AFFECTIVE CORE

This developmental period lasts from birth to approximately 1½ years of age. Our theory, based on recent interdisciplinary research (Emde, 1988), suggests that early moral motives grow from a set of basic motives. Basic motives are regarded as inborn tendencies built into our species by evolution and present in earliest infancy. They are necessary for development, are activated in the context of the caregiving relationship, and persist throughout life. Because they underlie the development of moral motives in this age period, it is necessary to review them in summary fashion.

Activity, the first basic motive, is presupposed by all contemporary theories of development, although usually it is not made explicit (Bertalanffy, 1968; Piaget, 1952). It includes formulations about basic tendencies for exploration, intrinsic motivation, and mastery (Berlyne, 1960; Deci, 1975; Harlow, 1953; Hendrick, 1939; Hunt, 1965; Izard, 1977; Morgan & Harmon, 1984; White, 1963), and it also includes more recent research formulations about inborn developmental agendas and expectancies (Haith, 1980, 1985).

Self-regulation, a second basic motive, refers to an inborn tendency for regulation of behavior as well as physiology. Such regulation includes state cycles of sleep and wakefulness and cycles of infant attentiveness, as well as the regulation of vital developmental functions that are goal-oriented. There are multiple ways of reaching developmental goals, as Bertalanffy (1968) pointed out. Accordingly, with respect to developmental functions, there is a strong self-regulatory tendency to return to the developmental pathway after deficit, deviance, or perturbation (Clarke & Clarke, 1976; Sameroff & Chandler, 1976; Waddington, 1962).

Social fittedness, a third basic motive, results from research that has shown that infants come into the world preadapted for initiating, maintaining, and terminating human interactions. The infant has a propensity for participating in eye-to-eye contact, for showing prolonged alert attentiveness to the stimulus features contained in the human voice and face, and for integrative capacities that must be considered remarkable preadaptations for the dynamic complexities of human interaction (e.g., processing sequential information, cross-modal perception, early forms of social imitation and orienting; Meltzoff, 1985; Papousek, 1981; Stern, 1985). Social fittedness is also a strong, probably inborn, propensity in parents, as well, as demonstrated by Papousek and Papousek (1979) in their studies of "intuitive" or automatic parenting behaviors. These behaviors are species-wide, nonconscious, and do not seem to result from individual experience, according to the Papouseks; they include the way a baby is held, the quality of gesturing, and an automatic tendency for baby talk. (See also Snow, 1972.) Research on behavioral synchrony between infants and caregivers also illustrates this point about social fittedness (Brazelton & Als, 1979; Condon & Sander, 1974; Haith, 1977; Meltzoff, 1985; Stern, 1977; Tronick & Glanino, 1986) as does joint visual referencing later in the first year that has been taken to indicate an inborn potential for a "shared visual reality" (Butterworth & Jarrett, 1980; Scaife & Bruner, 1975).

Affective monitoring is a fourth basic motive of our theory. The infant has a propensity from the start to monitor experience according to what is pleasurable and unpleasurable. From the mother's point of view, infant affective expressions guide caregiving. A newborn infant's cry communicates a demand message of "come, change something"; later, an infant's smile communicates a message of "keep it up—I like it." From the infant's point of view, emotional communications become increasingly prominent with development. During the middle of the first year, the infant begins to engage in social referencing, a phenomenon we have studied in our research group wherein there is a searching out of emotional expressions of significant others during situations of uncertainty in order to guide behavior.

A fifth basic motive is that of *cognitive assimilation.* From the start, the infant explores the environment, seeking what is new in order to make it familiar. Cognitive assimilation overlaps with the first motive we have designated as activity, but we believe it deserves separate emphasis so that we can label a more directed tendency to "get it right" about the environment. This motive comes directly from the theorizing of Piaget (1952), who referred to cognitive assimilation as "a basic fact of life." Recent research has shown the power of this fundamental organizing activity as well as its relative stability as an individual characteristic from infancy to early childhood (Bornstein & Sigman, 1986).

It is important to point out that these basic motives are listed separately for theoretical convenience. They are overlapping and inseparable in their functioning. Moreover, although we attribute them to the individual, it is in the caregiver/infant relationship experience that the basic motives become activated, acquire meaning, and develop into more complex motivational structures. Thus, it is in the context of the relationship experience where we see the integration of what we have referred to as the affective core of self and our early moral motives.

Our theory of an affective core providing a sense of continuity for self stems from our newer organizational perspectives about affects (Emde, 1980; Sroufe, 1979). Affects are seen as active, ongoing, and adaptive features of our lives that serve both motivational and evaluative functions. In addition to mobilizing action according to built-in goals (Campos, Butterfield, & Klinnert, 1985; Lazarus, 1991), affects at any given time allow us to monitor our own states of being and our engagement with the world. They also allow us to monitor others and their needs, intentions, and states of well-being. The theory of affective self adds still another dimension to these adaptive functions—namely, that because of a basic biological organization, a patterned affective core of responsiveness gives us a sense of consistency. Our affective core allows us to know we are the same in spite of the many ways we change. Our affective core also gives us a sense of consistency of others' and our own humanness. Thus, it can be regarded as a core for intersubjectivity as well as for self.

The evidence for the theory of affective core of self is summarized in Emde (1983). Our theory proposes that the affective core gives meaning and consistency, individuality, and a sense of uniqueness to experience. It is also important to emphasize that although we theorize that, from earliest infancy, emotions provide a sense of coherence for self-regulatory experience, this can occur only if there is a "self-regulating other" (Sander, 1985; Stern, 1985). The coherence of experience results from an emotionally available caregiver who is continually responsive to a particular active, self-regulating, socially interactive, emotional infant—an infant who is "getting it right" in the midst of a particular developmental world that is expanding socially. It can be said that the infant develops particular emotional procedures for monitoring the caregiver's emotional availability (Clyman, 1991). After the middle of the first year, emotional communication with others becomes more complex. By 7 months, the infant engages in social referencing, seeking out emotional signals of others in order to guide behavior when there is uncertainty (Feinman & Lewis, 1983; Klinnert et al., 1983). It is through social referencing that a host of emotional procedures and guidelines for action become internalized with respect to particular social contexts. Emotions become shared and guide action.

Before moving into our direct discussion of early moral motives, we would point out that our theoretical perspective has a strong background in the thinking of a number of psychoanalytic theorists. These include notions of caregiving interactions being conceptualized as affective "dialogues" (Spitz, 1965) in terms of "good enough mothering" (Winnicott, 1965) and in terms of the parents' sensitivity and attunement to the infant's emotional cues and needs (Bowlby, 1973; Brazelton & Cramer, 1990; Mahler, Pine & Bergman, 1975; Osofsky & Eberhart-Wright, 1988; Stern, 1985). Similarly, the caregiver's regulatory role in structuring the continuity of early experience is reminiscent of the concept of the parent's acting as a "container" (Bion, 1962) or as a "holding environment" (Winnicott, 1965). The concepts of Margaret Mahler and her colleagues concerning the toddler's need for "emotional refueling" with the caregiver in the midst of exploratory initiatives (Mahler et al., 1975) are perhaps best known. The school of psychoanalysis that has recently come to be known as "self psychology" has been particularly explicit in these matters. The caregiver's available responsiveness for the child's affective states ("mirroring") has been considered

necessary for coherence to develop; self-fragmentation and forms of narcissistic pathology may be outcomes when there is a deficit of such experience (Kohut, 1971, 1977; Stolorow, Brandchaft, & Atwood, 1987).

MORAL MOTIVES: INTERNALIZING THE "DOS"

Our developmental observations have led us to highlight an obvious point that has not received sufficient attention in theories of morality; namely, that all systems of morality have "dos" alongside of "don'ts." In the second year of life, the toddler becomes willful and acquires the use of negation, and parents become preoccupied with issues of discipline and of "don'ts" in addition to nurturing (Biringen, Emde, Campos, & Appelbaum, 1995; Maccoby & Martin, 1983). The child's internalization of dos begins earlier, however, and we have come to believe that this process becomes structuralized as a core aspect of moral development. Our theory seeks to portray how experience becomes internalized in such a way that the child gains extensive procedural knowledge concerning reciprocity as well as prototypic rules for what should be and what should not be.

The infant learns a great variety of "rules" as a shared aspect of the caregiving experience, before there is conflict and as a positive aspect of the early moral self. Along the lines of our theme, internalized rules may be thought of as having a dual origin—both in inborn propensity and in expectable caregiver relationship experiences. Rules involving "reciprocity," for example, can be thought of as developing quite naturally from the basic motive of social fittedness. Early face-to-face turn-taking interactions with mother provide well studied examples of internalized rules about reciprocity that become particularized in the course of infants/caregiver relationship experiences (Brazelton & Als, 1979; Stern, 1977; Trevarthen, 1979; Tronick, 1980). Research has clearly shown that rules about how to communicate—about how to engage, maintain, and terminate social interaction—are operative well before language (Bruner, 1982; Kaye, 1982). They are internalized as a result of caregiving experiences (often highly pleasurable experiences in games) and—

important for the theme of this chapter—they come to form early motives and coherent procedures for social turn-taking. The reader may ask: Is this a basic form of morality? We believe it is. Systems of morality typically emphasize a sense of human reciprocity with some version of the Golden Rule: "Do unto others as you would have them do unto you."

The infant's learning about rules of social interaction involves repeated experiences of "affect attunement," as Stern (1985) has conceptualized it, and caregiving interactions increasingly involve shared intentions as well as assumptions about others' mental states (Kaye, 1982; Trevarthen, 1979). What has been called "intersubjectivity" is based on consistent caregiving interactions that generate expectations that are cognitively coherent as well as procedural memories that our theory proposes become constituent in a consolidated affective core of self. This perspective brings us to one other point. Early moral motives are strongly positive on one condition: that adequate support is provided from consistent caregiving. Our theory proposes that the fundamental modes of development become differentiated so that a basic positive morality occurs through internalizing the dos of everyday interactions. This morality includes elements of a sense of reciprocity, an internalized sense of everyday rules (e.g., about what to do, when, and what belongs where), empathy, and some internalized standards. Affect plays a major role as pleasure in "getting it right" and is confirmed by the caregiver's expression of pride in the child's accomplishments. That the emotional availability of the caregiver is central is also emphasized by our consideration of the importance of negative emotions and "internalizing the don'ts."

MORAL MOTIVES: INTERNALIZING THE DON'TS

Repeated interactions with caregivers also provide the vehicle for the infant's internalization of "don'ts." Social referencing and negotiation are two processes that we have come to give major emphasis as a result of our observations. Both of these processes involve dynamic, affective communications that come to mediate internalized

procedures for self-regulation of what is prohibited and should be restrained.

Social referencing begins sometime after the middle of the first year and becomes prominent in the latter quarter of the child's first year as well as in the second year of life. As we mentioned earlier, infants who encounter a situation of uncertainty tend to seek emotional information from a caregiver (or significant other person) in order to resolve the uncertainty and regulate behavior. For example, an infant who sees a toy robot enter a room will look to mother. If mother smiles or expresses interest, the infant is encouraged to approach and touch the robot; if mother expresses fear or anger, the infant will avoid the robot. In our longitudinal observations, we have found that a similar searching for emotional signals and use of these signals occurs during prohibitions. At the beginning of the child's second year, a toddler typically looks back and forth to mother or father and makes use of perceived emotional expressions (in face and voice), testing the parents' authority and clarity of prohibition messages. Repeated looking occurs either after or before a prohibited act, with the child seeking resolution of uncertainty or confirmation for a decision about acting in the emotional signal of the parent. Elsewhere (Emde, Johnson, & Easterbrooks, 1988), we have described our longitudinal research observations that suggested developmental steps in the early internalization of prohibitions, steps that we conceptualized as occurring normatively under the watchful eyes of the caregiver. By the middle of the second year the child gives some evidence of having internalized some prohibitions and rules for don'ts, so long as the parent is physically present, emotionally available, and can be referenced.

Our longitudinal observations concerning the internalization of don'ts also reveal that social referencing was embedded in a larger process of negotiation that characterize interactions between infant and caregiver. In our longitudinal study of prohibitions mentioned earlier, parents repeatedly came with their infants to our playroom laboratory that had a variety of interesting toys, objects, and potential "prohibitables" in the room. We did not instruct parents to prohibit the child from touching any objects but left such emotional communications to vary according to family style and shared meaning. Under these circumstances, a toddler's movement toward a prohibited object rarely began with a clear emotional message of prohibition from the parent. Typically, parents offered initial emotional messages that expressed a mixture of interest, curiosity, and pleasure, along with mild prohibitions; these messages were then "tested" by a toddler who continued moving toward the tempting object. It was only toward the end of a sequence of communications, when the toddler was about to touch a tape recorder, for example, that a parent might decide to be clear and unequivocal, with a stern, glaring, message of "No, don't touch!" Toddlers experienced many variations of prohibition sequences in response to their initiations, and they often charmed their parents with positive message exchanges in the course of "getting their way" or "resisting temptation." What seemed to be internalized in these kinds of experiences were not prohibitions in any simple way but, instead, strategies of negotiation in the midst of emotional communication and the consequences of these strategies. Negotiation, even though it involves the don'ts of early moral development, also can be thought of as a positive principle of morality, as having its roots in repeated attempts to "get it right" in social interactions. Shared meaning is negotiated in the course of back and forth exchanges with a significant other (including during social referencing).

As a result of our findings, we are tempted to say that the internalization of early relationship experiences is largely the internalization of negotiated interactions. What the young child internalizes are strategies of action with particular others in varying contexts. Thus, again, we come to the view that development is an extraordinarily dynamic and creative process in its use of individual activity and shared experience. Development not only involves processes of construction and coconstruction, it also involves the internalization of dynamic procedures of negotiation.

Moral Motives in Late Infancy

Moral motives in late infancy involve what feels right that one can change. They involve the beginnings of moral emotions, willfulness, responsibility, and the consciousness of self in the presence of another.

The approximate age of this developmental period is from 1½ to 3 years. Its onset is marked by a momentous developmental transition that can be designated as the demarcation between early and late infancy. Piaget (1952) marked this transition as that from sensorimotor to representational intelligence, wherein there is a new degree of the child's understanding of things and people in their absence and a beginning understanding of causal relationships such that means and ends can be separated. Transformational changes in cognitive development at this age have been reviewed by McCall (1979). Those focusing on language emphasize still another developmental transition at this time. The infant moves from 1-word to multiword speech and the beginnings of grammar (Bates et al., 1988). We emphasize still another feature of this transition that demarcates it as the watershed between early and late infancy: the onset of reflective self-awareness (Emde, 1983; Kagan, 1981; Lewis & Brooks-Gunn, 1979). The infant now recognizes (as has been shown experimentally) when his or her facial image has been altered by a rouge mark in a mirror reflection; moreover, the child begins to use personal pronouns, and there are frequent references to "me" and "mine."

DEVELOPMENTAL PATHWAYS

Let us trace the developmental progression of the moral motives we have portrayed in early infancy after the onset of this developmental transition.

We have just described the beginnings of internalization of don'ts, of parental prohibitions. Our longitudinal observations compelled us to realize that the process of internalization involved repeated experiences of negotiations of plans and actions in relation to back-and-forth emotional communications in particular contexts. Following the developmental watershed we have described, such internalizations become more complex and active in the midst of the infant's experiencing increasing willfulness and intentions that are separate from others. Alternate possibilities for actions and experiences of negotiating with significant others become internalized. A broader array of conflicting intentions between self and significant others are experienced, and their consequences increasingly appreciated. Thus, during this developmental period, moral motives for restraint in the midst of conflicts around "don'ts" with significant others show increasingly complex development. Our observations have pointed to the fact, long appreciated by psychoanalytic observers (e.g., Ferenczi, 1927) that such internalized restraint involving prohibitions initially is limited in its impact to conditions in which the prohibiting significant other is present. Our research model emphasizes the role of social referencing in this process; thus we have described the normative regularity of restraint developing "under the watchful eyes of the other" (Emde, Johnson, & Easterbrooks, 1988).

When we consider our basic motives of infancy, additional pathways of development become apparent, leading to new phenomena with more complex moral motivations at this age. Toward the end of the second year, the tendency for cognitive assimilation, for "getting it right," shows itself in a new affective way. In some contexts the child shows anxiety when internal standards are violated. When faced with a familiar object that is dirty or otherwise flawed, the child may evidence distress, along with an urge to correct what is viewed as a discrepancy from what was expected (Dunn, 1988; Kagan, 1981). Is this a form of morality? Again, we believe it is. Kagan, who deserves credit for linking this developmental milestone to the onset of reflective self-awareness, has highlighted that all systems of morality require internalized standards along with a sense of uneasiness when prototypic standards are violated. It is no small matter, therefore, that, by the end of the second year, the child's early moral self has internalized and developed moral procedures that guide such a process.

Still another pathway that shows transformation involves the development of basic motives for turn-taking, communication, and social cooperation. The new positive feature of early morality that develops at this age concerns empathy. Research has shown that toward the end of the child's second year, toddlers come to feel distress at another's expressed discomfort and begin to show tendencies of wanting to help or comfort (Radke-Yarrow, Zahn-Waxler, & Chapman, 1983; Zahn-Waxler & Radke-Yarrow, 1982). The emergence of empathy appears to have a number of

components with maturational and genetic contributions (Zahn-Waxler, Robinson, & Emde, 1992). Some researchers have suggested that the empathy may have evolved in the course of our biology as a natural countertendency to aggression against others (Hoffman, 1977; Kagan, 1984). Clinical and other evidence suggests also that empathy and its corresponding tendency for helping are influenced by the quality of repeated, empathically attuned experiences with caregivers. As Stern (1985), Trevarthen, (1979), and Kaye (1982) have pointed out, caregiving interactions in early infancy increasingly involve shared intentions and assumptions about others' mental states. Consistent caregiving interactions and what has been called "intersubjectivity" depend not only on expectations that are cognitively coherent but also on procedural memories that are coherently modeled in what we refer to as a consolidated affective core of self.

CHARACTERISTICS OF MORAL EMOTIONS

Moral motives, as they develop from basic motives, necessarily involve emotions. The emotional signaling with respect to the moral motives of late infancy, however, is of a different quality from what has occurred earlier. By the end of the second year, a new set of patterned emotions begins to emerge, which we refer to as "moral emotions." These emotions, which include pride, shame, and the forerunners of guilt, have a different kind of organization from the basic discrete emotions (of joy, surprise, anger, fear, sadness, interest, and disgust). Recently Zahn-Waxler and Kochanska (1990) have argued that early forms of guilt develop from the affective arousal connected with tendencies to reparation in connection with experiences of empathy. Like all emotions, they build upon previously acquired developmental accomplishments, but they also have a number of new qualities. They are predominantly internal, are more complex than the discrete emotions, and do not have any simple correspondence to emotional expression in the face, voice, or posture. They are based on relationships—on a past history of experience with particular individuals in particular contexts. Thus, they presuppose a developed sense of shared meaning. They are based on some sense of struggle, dilemma, or conflict; further-more, they are linked to moral rules and moral motives.

Perhaps most important, moral emotions are anticipatory; that is, they often are "signal affects" in the psychoanalytic sense (Freud, 1926/1959). They portend, or represent, the consequences of an intended (or undesired) outcome. As such, they organize our attention to the possibility that a rule violation has occurred, or the possibility of hurting another, or the possibility of helping or "doing right." Thus, from the point of view of our considerations about consciousness, they have the function of making implicit or preconscious moral goals conscious. Moral emotions compel us to focus on moral rules and ideals, thereby organizing and motivating our behavior. With development, moral emotions typically involve multiple appraisals of self in relation to one or more meaningful others (including, presumably, the "generalized other" of Mead, 1934). Along these lines, such emotions may include the perception that other(s) will appraise our action as positive or negative, whether the other perceives of us as in control of our behavior, and whether we are seen as responsible for our actions (Lazarus, 1991).

The complex coordination of multiple appraisals suggests an emerging taxonomy of moral emotions. An initial dichotomy in moral emotions may be whether the emotion is elicited in response to one's own actions or in response to another's actions. Let us address the former group first. When an appraisal of our own action (or our appraisal of how the other appraises our action) is positive, pride or hubris may result. When such an appraisal is negative, shame, guilt, or embarrassment may result. Lewis (1991) has suggested that hubris is differentiated from pride, and shame from guilt or regret, by the presence of global versus specific attributions, respectively.

Moral emotions that are elicited by others' actions call for additional appraisals. We judge if the individual who is acting feels positively or negatively and whether this state of affairs makes us feel positively or negatively. The result is classifiable as a 2 × 2 matrix. The emotion that results when we appraise has no term in English but may be an important component in friendships and love. When we feel negatively that the other feels negatively, we may feel empathy or sympathy. When we feel badly that the other feels positively,

it may result in envy or jealousy (depending on whether the situation is dyadic or triadic). If we feel positively when the other feels negatively, the emotion may be hostile pleasure, or pleasure over another's misfortune—an emotion deserving further investigation in both normative and at-risk children. Much later in development, individuals can have empathy for themselves as well as take pleasure in their own misfortune, the latter being traditionally termed masochism. The last point to note emerges from our interest in shared meaning. When the valence of our appraisal is shared with the other (where we both feel positively, or both feel negatively), we are likely to consider the emotion to be a *moral* emotion (in the positively evaluated sense). When our appraisals are discrepant (as in envy, jealousy, and hostile pleasure, where one feels positively and the other feels negatively), the valence of the emotions are not shared and these emotions have more negative connotations.

Our model presupposes shared meaning—a common sense of past, current context, and future possibilities. But we are also mindful that not all "moral behavior," even with signaling moral emotions, requires awareness or judgment. We have taken this point of view with respect to early infancy, namely, that young infants manifest moral motives and behavior in internalized reciprocal functioning and "getting it right" about internalized family rules. We suspect that in this age period, most everyday "moral" actions involve procedures that are relatively automatic; they do not require awareness or reflective judgment. Only when there is a change or perturbation of some kind is consciousness required for moral behavior, we suspect, and this involves particular frustrations and interpersonal conflicts that vary with the particular child's temperament and family style as well as circumstances.

The moral emotions, with their internal signaling functions, organize tendencies to action. Thus, as they become patterned in early development, they become important features of moral motives. The emotions we discussed earlier as part of the moral motives of this age period can be thought of as early prototypic moral emotions. Both empathic arousal and distress about perceived violation of internalized standards carry with them an experienced desire for repair of the situation. They result from the activation in particular contexts of expectations and schemes that have been built up from earlier experience.

Emotions that begin to emerge during this period are more patterned and often are experienced as longer-lasting than discrete emotions. As such, they can enter into configurations of mood (and, later, as aspects of character and personality). *Pride* is the earliest appearing, and, we believe, normatively the most pervasive of these complex moral emotions. Pride is developmentally continuous with earlier mastery pleasure and pleasure from assimilation and "getting it right." The more patterned emotion of pride carries with it a "puffed-up" feeling and often a "puffed-up" posture in the presence of a significant other. As this moral emotion develops during this age period, it becomes internalized such that there is pleasure experienced from "getting it right" with an imagined significant other who may not be present.

The counterpoint of pride is shame. Shame is a moral emotion that also arises interpersonally and increasingly becomes internalized as a guide for moral action. Earlier psychoanalytic theorists linked shame to the experience of toilet training during this age period (Fenichel, 1945), and Erikson (1950) linked it to broader experiences of autonomy. Although we and others (e.g., Lewis, 1991) have observed patterned shame with an averting of gaze and a shrinking-away posture (the opposite of puffed up postures of pride as Darwin noted in 1877), we believe its beginnings show extensive variation during the child's second and third years. In some family cultures, shaming experiences are salient during this age; in others they are not. The internalized experience of shame always contains an image of one or more significant others, along with a devastating feeling of wanting to shrink out of sight. According to our model, this patterned internalized moral regulating emotion typically becomes more prominent at three years and after.

Shame has its origins in early face-to-face interactions with significant others. Although it becomes internalized and continues to develop as a moral emotion throughout life, shame keeps as a core feature the vivid imaging of significant others. Thus, in our view, it involves a special form of social referencing. The role of social referencing in the developmental process by which shame experiences are transformed from the interpersonal-intersubjective to the intra-individual level of experience is described elsewhere (Emde & Oppenheim, 1995). As social referencing becomes internalized, we envision that it has two components of shared meaning. One component can be thought of as related to pride and the dos of early moral development. This component involves the seeking of guidance from internalized referents with whom one has a dialogue in situations of uncertainty. The experience of internalized dialogue results in a feeling of encouragement, of joint interest, of expansion, and of a shared sense of "we-ness" that we have characterized elsewhere as an executive sense of we or "we-go" (Emde, 1988). In contrast, the other component of internalized social referencing can be thought of as relevant to the don'ts of early moral development. Internalized significant others are experienced as being vigilant and as seeing one as not "measuring up" (i.e., inadequate). The feeling is one of deflation, of shrinking, and of shame. There is a feeling of smallness and aloneness rather than of "we-go."

The developmental forerunners of guilt also may appear during this age period but, according to our theoretical model, patterned guilt appears even later. Zahn-Waxler and Kochanska (1990) have argued, based on their research observations, that an early internalized sense of responsibility and what may be a forerunner of guilt may accompany sympathetic arousal and lead to prosocial and reparative behaviors. (See also Kochanska, 1993.) Child observers have noted a "hurt-feelings look" during this age period when the child presumably has a sense of having caused a problem or hurt another or engaged in a transgression. It is debatable, however, whether guilt is common, even in an early form, during this age. Observers have noted that reparative behaviors (such as might indicate early conscience) are less likely when the child of this age is the cause of distress to others (such as a sibling) and that early reparative behaviors in such contexts often involve conflict and ambivalence (Zahn-Waxler, 1995).

In contrast to shame, which involves visual imaging, our model proposes that guilt as an internalized moral emotion principally involves auditory channels of emotional communication. Thus, a form of social referencing mediating guilt would involve internalized dialogues with dos and don'ts having inner voices in conversations supplementing imagined visual scenarios. Support for such an idea is provided from observations of toddlers' and preschoolers' monologues before bedtime (e.g., see Dore, 1989) and during solitary play, both of which sometimes seem to be "reenvoicements" of disciplinary parental actions (e.g., the child utters "no!" as she looks at a desired but prohibited object). Whether more complex internalized social referencing processes involving guilt have dialogues with inner voices and whether those involving shame have dialogues with imagined faces is an area that calls for additional research. Certainly the linkage of guilt with internalized voices draws our attention to the role of language acquisition in moral development.

At the end of the second year, the child is typically entering into multiword speech. Along with what has been referred to as the "vocabulary burst," the child develops the use of language not only for reference but for predication and for propositional declarations (Bates, 1992; Bates et al., 1988). Toward the end of the third year, the child also develops the capacity for emotionally coherent narrative speech and discourse (Wolf, 1990). By 3 years of age, the child typically comes to have what many have regarded as a "narrative self" (Buchsbaum & Emde, 1990; Stern, 1985). The child is now able to hold two or more possibilities in mind and engage in internal representations that may be connected with moral emotions. Such a capacity forms a background for when the internalized voices of guilt may become structured in scenarios of self-criticism. This brings us to moral motives in the preschooler.

Moral Motives in the Preschooler

Moral motives in the preschooler involve what feels right in a world that has possibilities. They involve making coherent meaning by establishing narratives and the use of imagination as well as play.

By 3 years of age, the child has developed a coherent narrative sense and has a capacity for discourse, for telling a significant other about events that have happened, even when the other was not present at the event. The narrative world is one in which there is a storylike flow of events with scenarios, high points, and multiple possible outcomes and resolutions. As Bruner (1986) has put it, there is increasing appreciation of other possible minds and other possible worlds. The preschooler increasingly becomes fascinated by the world of possibilities in fantasy and play. Indeed it is at this age that fantasy and trial action become prominent, not earlier. The prominence of imagination, fantasy, and play during this period has been reviewed from the standpoint of recent research by Harris (1989) and by Singer and Singer (1990). The child is now able to deal with competing alternative outcomes, to bear them in mind, and to distinguish between reality, pretense, and the appearance of reality (Flavell, Green, & Flavell, 1986; Wolf & Grollman, 1982; Wolf, Rygh, & Altshuler, 1984). From the standpoint of moral development, it can be shown that the child can struggle with simple forms of "moral dilemmas" (Emde & Buchsbaum, 1989).

Thus, moral motives in the preschooler involve a major set of developmental transformations. Anticipated alternative outcomes now involve the child's expanded social world that is reflected in internalized representation. The child moves beyond twosomes and enters into the "family drama," or the Oedipus complex, as Freud described it. The child may experience a shifting set of loyalties between parents (increased affection and erotic feelings toward the parent of the opposite sex and rivalry toward the parent of the same sex) and becomes aware of a sense of exclusion from parental intimacy in a new way. In addition to forming narrative representations of the family drama and its variations, the child comes to "narrativize" sibling experiences and scenarios involving rivalry, envy, and caring. Similarly, toward the end of this period the child comes to narrativize peer experiences and begins to expand socially referencing processing to peers (cf. the process of establishing "reference groups" as written about by sociologists; Feinman, 1992).

From the perspective of social cognition, the child comes to understand the complementarities, boundaries, and eventually the intersections of family roles (Watson & Fischer, 1980). Correspondingly, moral emotions of shame, guilt, and anxiety begin to color the dramatic patterns of narrative flow in the experienced world. As this happens, the child increasingly tries out possibilities of action in the context of his or her developing understandings either in play or in fantasy.

Moral Motives and Consciousness Reconsidered

Our model has portrayed the origins of moral motives during three developmental phases of the child's increasingly complex activity and shared experience. In each of these developmental phases, the child's emotional organization and its embeddedness in emotional communication systems with significant others is central. Thus, in early infancy, a basis for moral motives was portrayed as what feels right with another; in late infancy what feels right in a world where one can change things; and in the preschooler what feels right in a world of narrative possibilities. Emotions are basic motivational processes. They are linked not only to direct actions on the dimension of approach-withdrawal as Darwin pointed out long ago (Darwin 1872; see Frijda, 1986, for a contemporary statement), but they also are linked to goals and thinking (see Barrett & Campos, 1987; Lazarus 1991). Our discussion presupposes the development we have portrayed through the preschooler phase. In early development, we believe that a great deal of moral development is internalized without consciousness and reflective self-awareness; we also have suggested that once reflective self-awareness develops, considerable moral activity continues that is nonconscious. Next we consider further the role of nonconscious and conscious activity with respect to moral emotions and motives.

PSYCHODYNAMIC AND PROCEDURAL INFLUENCES ON EMOTIONAL REGULATION

Psychodynamically oriented psychologists are not accustomed to thinking about nonconscious procedural knowledge influencing moral regulation. But we can now appreciate than an individual's "preferences" and inclinations reflect a variety of stored moral procedures. Many of these procedures are mutually defined, shared, and implicit goals that feel good as they regulate behavior. Others may be used in defensive or protective ways. "Signal affects" may operate on the basis of procedural knowledge. According to psychoanalytic theory, small doses of anxiety or guilt that trigger defense mechanisms, other emotions, or overt behavior are activated automatically under specific circumstances that are perceived as dangerous (Brenner, 1975; Engel, 1962; Freud 1926/1959). Debates exist in the psychoanalytic literature about whether it is useful or not to portray such signal affects as unconscious; we consider it likely, however, that components of an organized emotional experience can be warded off or disconnected from that experience, whether it be perceptions, goals, or actions in relation to feeling states. Components of signal affects therefore can be organized procedurally without conscious awareness. But what about the relations between psychodynamic processes and other nonconscious processes? We are just beginning to frame appropriate questions. Do moral emotions forecast in a *procedural way* the consequences of an intended outcome? To what extent do we have procedural knowledge with respect to psychodynamic organizations of experience and make use of such knowledge?

The following anecdote from a 5-year-old severely abused child studied by Dr. Jill Hodges of the Anna Freud Centre in London illustrates why these questions may be fruitful to ask. In collaborative research with our MacArthur program, Hodges used story stem narratives (see Buchsbaum, Toth, Clyman, Emde, & Cicchetti, 1993; Emde & Buchsbaum, 1989) to probe for themes dealing with family conflict and early moral development. The child was in a foster home, which was going well, but he was fearful of being removed (a realistic concern on the child's part because of external circumstances). The child had suffered extensive physical and emotional trauma in the first 3 years and was very much concerned about being a good boy and in control. During the first series of play narratives in response to standard story stems, the child's responses seemed to be characterized by "keeping the lid on" and making things turn out well without much difficulty. The following transcript is in response to the story stem in which the tester portrays a parental argument in doll play between mother and father. Mother doll says to father doll, "You lost my car keys—you always do!" Father doll says, "I did not." The tester then says, "Show me and tell me what happens now" and, as is characteristic in our story stem narratives, two additional child dolls are present of the same sex as the child.

TESTER: (finishes story stem)
CHILD: So . . . Dad says, they're in my pocket! And Mommy says . . . Oh, well give them back then. . . . So George (shows Mommy and Daddy approaching each other) . . . "thank you . . ." . . . So George went to bed . . . (Lies George doll down) . . . Dreaming . . . He had the shark.
TESTER: He had the shark, when he was dreaming?
CHILD: Yes, so he had . . . a lot of dreams. . . . And was . . . scared . . . (voice trails off)

In discussing this narrative, we marveled at the child's seeming implicit knowledge of the fact that if you keep the lid on, you will have bad frightening dreams with the shark. The child seemed to sense an aspect of psychodynamic dream theory. We wondered: To what extent do children during the preschool years have procedural knowledge about the consequences of dynamic configurations? Even though we, as psychodynamic clinicians, have not thought this way before, the fact that children might have such knowledge makes considerable sense. The historical origins of psychodynamic discoveries are instructive. Freud gave explicit credit for many of his central formulations about unconscious motivation not only to his clinical observations but also to what he learned from authors and dramatists. Well-known examples include the structural theory of id, ego, and superego conflicts as seen in Dostoevsky's *The Brothers Karamazov* and the Oedipus complex as revealed by Sophocles' *Oedipus Rex*. From our current perspective, we could say that Dostoevsky and Sophocles did not make explicit a psychodynamic theory, but instead had procedural knowledge of the consequences of central dynamic configurations and made this knowledge manifest in literary form.

Is there a quality of "self-evident" mentation that keeps it out of consciousness? At this point, we might return to Jefferson's paradox. He bolstered his argument by claiming that the ideas he propounded were "self-evident" and therefore

known to all. Yet it was because these ideas were not conscious for everyone, but instead were implicit, that he felt the need to articulate them. Furthermore, there were unarticulated assumptions about the limitations concerning those who were considered to be endowed with the inalienable rights—only men of a certain race—and Jefferson could assume that other Caucasian men, like him, shared these assumptions and that, therefore, they did not come to be articulated. Recent critiques of Kohlberg's (1982) theory of moral development have pointed out assumptions related to a male-oriented research program (Gilligan, 1982) and these remind us of the need to be vigilant to other cultural and time-bound hidden assumptions, which may be so "self-evident" to us as to be nonconscious while they influence our theoretical and empirical work.

Such considerations suggest that moral behavior often may involve nonconscious mental processes. A host of questions are evoked. Are certain components and scenarios of moral motives procedurally organized, automatic, and not accessible to consciousness? Do moral emotions regulate and maintain behavior in accordance with internal standards, without requiring that one think about a rule that one has violated or obeyed, or might obey? And to what extent are there imagined nonconscious scenarios involving others? To what extent are there multiple alternative scenarios that are nonconscious, with moral emotions regulating behavior despite the dimmest glimpses of feeling states or awareness of the scenarios? To what extent are such alternative nonconscious scenarios, acting in parallel processing modes, involved in producing our sense of a "generalized other" (Mead, 1934) that increasingly provides an additional source of moral regulation?

INDIVIDUAL GOALS, ACTIONS, AND SHARED
EXPERIENCE: MORAL EMOTIONS AS
INTEGRATING INFLUENCES

Our view of morality has been a broad one, including the individual's internalized propensities about what to do as well as what not to do. Regulation has been a central idea. We deal with the development of morality in ways similar to that proposed by Hoffman (1983), who has defined moral internalization as the process whereby individuals increasingly come to regulate inevitable conflicts between personal needs and social obligations. We believe that emotions contribute to such regulation. Emotions are both individually existentially felt—organizing our orientations, evaluations, and goals—and socially constructed and shared. At all ages, moral emotions are significant, integrating influences, whether we see ourselves as being more individually oriented or more communally oriented in our democratic society (cf "self-contained individualism" versus "self in relation"—Hermans, Kempen, & van Loon, 1992; Sampson, 1988). Moral emotions also can be negative emotions throughout life—constricting, disruptive, and nonregulatory instead of regulatory. From a developmental point of view, moral emotions can lead to increased exploration, information gathering, and higher organized levels of functioning. They can lead to the appreciation of more complexity and to engaging such complexity as well as a "resetting" of one's perspectives. Moral emotions, however, also can be constrictive, entropic, and painfully discombobulating. This fact is indicated not only in much psychoanalytic literature where the consequences of guilt, moral anxiety, and shame are apparent in symptom formation, but it also is seen in broader aspects of everyday life, where self-righteous indignation leads to a narrowing of view and motives that are often hateful.

A balance of moral emotions as integrating influences is needed. More research is called for, we believe, concerning the early development of such regulatory balances if we are to promote the healthy development of individuals as well as our shared democratic values of citizenship.

Summary and Conclusion: Risky Opportunities and Establishing Commitment

We have reviewed a model for the development of moral motives during the child's earliest years. The early self is a moral one and has dual origins in a set of biologically prepared motives and interactions with emotionally available caregivers. The model, based on recent research, contains many surprising elements that are not apparent, and we have evoked Jefferson's historic phrase from the Declaration of Independence to highlight some aspects of truths that come to be regarded as self-evident. Early moral motives arise both from individual activities and from shared experience and, in our view, are stored as procedural knowledge. As such, they contain the opportunities and limitations of a person's historical time and culture. Early moral motives reflect skills, emotional communication, and internal emotional signaling, and they result from the internalization of a multiplicity of rules—including those about what to do and what not to do in familiar environments and about reciprocity and turn-taking in social encounters. Typically moral emotions develop as integrating and regulatory influences, but they also can be disruptive or constricting. Empathy, wanting to repair standards that are violated, and mastery/pride are all positive moral emotions that typically develop in the child's first 2 years. Similarly, ways of dealing with conflict and getting "one's way" by negotiation involves skillful procedures that develop in the early years considerably before developmental theorists had appreciated heretofore. Variations in these procedures under stress and less-than-optimal circumstances are deserving of more clinical and research attention, as are the developmental circumstances that lead to shame and guilt.

We look now to further implications. In the course of development, the child faces increasing challenges and establishes commitment to a coherent line of possibilities among alternatives. Such alternatives include choices among competing personal needs, prosocial inclinations, social obligations, and a variety of needs of others. We have portrayed how many of these challenges are processed at the level of procedural knowledge and are regulated by moral emotions, probably known to the individual only by a sense of "what feels right." We also have portrayed how the bulk of early moral development occurs in a positive, nonconflictual manner, as a conjoint influence of self-development involving both individual activity and shared experience. We close our chapter with two additional reflections.

First, we need to remind ourselves that interpersonal conflicts become more prominent beyond the child's early years. Observations of preschool children in Minnesota in the 1930s showed that aggression and selfish behaviors among peers vastly outnumbered kind and shared interactions (Murphy, 1937) and similar findings resulted from more recent observations in California (Bronson, 1981). Home observations have emphasized the high incidence of teasing and hurting in early sibling relationships, and among 3-year-olds, hurting incidents were observed to be as common as comforting on occasions when a younger sibling was in distress (Dunn, 1988; Dunn & Kendrick, 1982). What we have reviewed in our model are positive factors offsetting the child's selfish and fighting tendencies seen later with peers. Our model has portrayed that such offsetting factors may be basic in the sense of being derived from fundamental modes of development. Thus, the infant monitors his or her own experience and that of significant others according to what feels right in the surroundings and according to goals that are increasingly complex and shared. It is a task for the future to understand more about family, situational, and cultural variation with respect to positive features of moral development in order to enhance offsetting factors to the development of harsh negative and aggressively violent features of morality and development.

A second reflection is related to the first. It is not only the child who faces increasing challenges in committing to alternatives. So do we as developmental researchers and citizens. We believe there is an urgent need for us all to commit to understanding more about moral motives amid variations in the context for early development. Because most of the research we have reviewed has been conducted with advantaged Caucasian families in the United States, we do not know which aspects of our model will be generalizable and which aspects will require cultural specification. The impact of different environments, particularly amid variations in family and community violence, deserve increased attention (Osofsky, 1993). Additional, important questions remain about gender differences in the ontogeny of early moral motives. The strength of our society today is increasingly acknowledged to be found in its particulars of ethnic and cultural diversity. Both as citizens and as developmentalists, we need to study the inculcation of values for citizenship in our democracy. We must examine variations in values, whether coherent or disrupted. A revitalized developmental social psychology could well have a new emphasis that examines values in the context of early motives, that examines the crucial relation between emotions and moral behavior, and that appreciates the diverse contexts within which we live.

We hope that our model provides one useful guide for such an approach.

NOTES

1. These ideas are based on the regulatory principles of adaptation both for general systems theory (Bertalanffy, 1968) and for Piagetian cognitive-developmental theory (see the maintenance of equilibria between assimilation and accommodation; Piaget, 1952).

2. Terms such as *ego integrity* also reflect a manifestation of a central developmental process involving individual activity; namely, integration that takes place along with differentiation. Developmental biology also brings us to what is a dual meaning of the word *integrity*. For example, Gottlieb (1992) cogently demonstrates that differentiation, as well as integration, requires co-actions of genetic and environmental influences at increasingly complex levels of organization.

REFERENCES

Barrett, K. C., & Campos, J. J. (1987). Perspectives on emotional development II: A functionalist approach to emotions. In J. D. Osofsky (Ed.), *Handbook of infant development* (2nd ed., pp. 555–578). New York: John Wiley & Sons.

Bates, E. (1992). Language development. In E. Kandell & L. Squire (Eds.), *Current Opinion in Neurobiology, 2,* 180–185 (special issue on cognitive neuroscience).

Bates, E., Bretherton, I., & Snyder, L. (1988). *From first words to grammar—individual differences and dissociable mechanisms.* New York: Cambridge University Press.

Berlyne, D. E. (1960). *Conflict, arousal, and curiosity.* New York: McGraw-Hill.

Bertalanffy, L. von (1968). *General system theory foundation, development, application.* New York: Braziller.

Bion, W. R. (1962). *Learning from Experience.* New York: Basic Books.

Biringen, Z., Emde, R. N., Campos, J. J., & Appelbaum, M. I. (1995). Affective reorganization in the infant, the mother, and the dyad: The role of upright locomotion and its timing. *Child Development, 66* (2), 499–514.

Bornstein, M. H., & Sigman, M. (1986). Continuity in mental development from infancy. *Child Development, 57,* 251–274.

Bowlby, J. (1973). *Attachment and Loss: Vol. 2, Separation.* New York: Basic Books.

Brazelton, T. B., & Als, H. (1979). Four early stages in the development of mother-infant interaction. *Psychoanalytic Study of the Child, 34,* 349–369.

Brazelton, T. B., & Cramer, B. G. (1990). *The earliest relationship.* Reading, MA: Addison-Wesley.

Brenner, C. (1975). Affects and psychic conflict. *Psychoanalytic Quarterly, 44,* 5–28.

Bronson, W. C. (1981). *Toddler's behavior with age-mates: Issues of interaction, cognition, and affect.* Norwood, NJ: Ablex.

Bruner, J. (1982). *Child's talk: Learning to use language.* New York: W. W. Norton.

Bruner, J. S. (1986). *Actual minds, possible worlds.* Cambridge, MA: Harvard University Press.

Buchsbaum, H. K., & Emde, R. N. (1990). Play narratives in thirty-six-month-old children: Early moral development and family relationships. *Psychoanalytic Study of the Child, 40,* 129–155.

Buchsbaum, H. K., Toth, S. L., Clyman, R. B., Cicchetti, D., & Emde, R. N. (1993). The use of a narrative story stem technique with maltreated children: Implications for theory and practice. *Development and Psychopathology, 4* (4), 603–625.

Butterworth, G., & Jarrett, N. (1980, September). *The geometry of pre-verbal communication.* Paper presented to the annual conference of the developmental psychology section of the British Psychological Society, Edinburgh.

Campos, J. J., Butterfield, P. M., & Klinnert, M. D. (1985, April). *Cardiac and behavioral differences of negative emotion signals: an individual differences perspective.* Poster presented at the meetings of the Society for Research in Child Development.

Clarke, A. M., & Clarke, A. D. B. (1976). *Early experience: Myth and evidence.* London: Open Books.

Clyman, R. B. (1991). The procedural organization of emotions: A contribution from cognitive science to the psychoanalytic theory of therapeutic action. *Journal of the American Psychoanalytic Association* (Supple.).

Cohen, N. J., & Squire, L. R. (1980). Preserved learning and retention of pattern-analyzing skill in amnesia: Dissociation of knowing how and knowing that. *Science, 221,* 207–210.

Condon, W. S., & Sander, L. W. (1974). Synchrony demonstrated between movements of the neonate and adult speech. *Child Development, 45,* 456–462.

Darwin, C. (1872). *The expression of the emotions in man and animals* (2nd ed.). New York: D. Appleton.

Darwin, C. (1877). A biological sketch of an infant. *Mind, 2,* 285–294.

Deci, E. (1975). *Intrinsic motivation.* New York: Plenum Press.

Dore, J. (1989). Monologue as reenvoicement of dialogue. In K. Nelson (Ed.), *Narratives from the crib* (pp. 231–260). Cambridge, MA: Harvard University Press.

Dunn, J. (1988). *The beginnings of social understanding.* Cambridge, MA: Harvard University Press.

Dunn, J., & Kendrick, C. (1982). *Siblings.* Cambridge, MA: Harvard University Press.

Emde, R. N. (1980). A developmental orientation in psychoanalysis: Ways of thinking about new knowledge and further research. *Psychoanalysis and Contemporary Thought, 3* (2), 213–235.

Emde, R. N. (1983). The prerepresentational self and its affective core. *Psychoanalytic Study of the Child, 38,* 165–192.

Emde, R. N. (1988). Development terminable and interminable: I. Innate and motivational factors from infancy. *International Journal of Psycho-Analysis, 69,* 23–42.

Emde, R. N., Biringen, Z., Clyman, R. B., & Oppenheim, D. (1991). The moral self of infancy: Affective core and procedural knowledge. *Developmental Review, 11,* 251–270.

Emde, R. N., & Buchsbaum, H. K. (1989). Toward a psychoanalytic theory of affect: II. Emotional development and signaling in infancy. In S. I. Greenspan & G. H. Pollock (Eds.), *The course of life: Vol 1. Infancy* (rev. ed.). Madison, CT: International Universities Press. (Previously published as *The course of life: Psychoanalytic contributions toward understanding personality development.*)

Emde, R. N., Johnson, W. F., & Easterbrooks, M. A. (1988). The do's and don'ts of early moral development: Psychoanalytic tradition and current research. In J. Kagan & S. Lamb (Eds.), *The emergence of morality* (pp. 245–277). Chicago: University of Chicago Press.

Emde, R. N., & Oppenheim, D. (1995). Shame, guilt, and the oedipal drama: Developmental considerations concerning morality and the referencing of critical others. In J. P. Tangney & K. W. Fischer (Eds.), *Self-conscious emotions: The psychology of shame, guilt, embarrassment and pride* (pp. 413–436). New York: Guilford Press.

Engel, G. (1962). Anxiety and depression-withdrawal: The primary affects of unpleasure. *International Journal of Psycho-Analysis, 43,* 89–97.

Erikson, E. (1950). *Childhood and society.* New York: W. W. Norton.

Feinman, S. (Ed.) (1992). Social referencing and the social construction of reality in infancy. New York: Plenum Press.

Feinman, S., & Lewis, M. (1983). Social referencing at ten months: A second-order effect on infant's responses to strangers. *Child Development, 54* (4), 878–887.

Fenichel, O. (1945). *The psychoanalytic theory of neurosis*. New York: W. W. Norton.

Ferenczi, S. (1927). Psycho-analysis of sexual habits. In *Further contributions to the theory and technique of psycho-analysis* (E. Glover, Trans.) (pp. 259–297). London: Hogarth Press.

Flavell, J. H., Green, F. L., & Flavell, E. R. (1986). Development of knowledge about the appearance-reality distinction. With commentaries by M. W. Watson and J. C. Campione. *Monographs of the Society for Research in Child Development, 51* (1 Serial No. 212).

Freud, S. (1959). Inhibitions, symptoms and anxiety. In J. Strachey (Ed. and Trans.), *The standard edition of the complete psychological Works of Sigmund Freud* (Vol. 20, pp. 87–175). London: Hogarth Press. (Originally published 1926.)

Frijda, N. J. (1986). *The emotions*. Cambridge: Cambridge University Press.

Gilligan, C. (1982). *In a different voice: Psychological theory and women's development*. Cambridge, MA: Harvard University Press.

Gottlieb, G. (1992). *Individual development & evolution*. New York: Oxford University Press.

Haith, M. M. (1977). Eye contact and face scanning in early infancy. *Science, 198,* 853–855.

Haith, M. M. (1980). *Rules that babies look by*. Hillsdale, NJ: Lawrence Erlbaum.

Haith, M. M. (1985). *Today's baby: Technology's product or nature's accomplishment?* Lecture presented at the University of Denver.

Harlow, H. F. (1953). Motivation as a factor in the acquisition of new responses. *Nebraska Symposium on Motivation, I,* 24–29.

Harris, P. L. (1989). *Children and emotion. The development of psychological understanding*. New York: Basil Blackwell.

Hendrick, I. (1939). *Facts and theories of psychoanalysis* (2nd ed.). New York: Alfred A. Knopf. (Originally published 1934.)

Hermans, H. J. M., Kempen, H. J. G., & van Loon, R. J. P. (1992). The dialogical self. *American Psychologist, 47* (1), 23–33.

Hoffman, M. L. (1977). Moral internalization: Current theory and research. In L. Berkowitz (Ed.), *Advances in experimental social psychology* (Vol. 10, pp. 86–133). New York: Academic Press.

Hoffman, M. L. (1983). Affective and cognitive processes in moral internalization. In E. T. Higgins, D. N. Ruble, & W. W. Hartup (Eds.), *Social cognition and social development: A sociocultural perspective* (pp. 236–274). New York: Cambridge University Press.

Hunt, J. McV. (1965). Intrinsic motivation and its role in psychological development. In D. Levine (Ed.), *Nebraska symposium on motivation* (pp. 189–282) Lincoln: University of Nebraska Press.

Izard, C. E. (1977). *Human emotions*. New York: Plenum Press.

Kagan, J. (1981). *The second year: The emergence of self-awareness*. Cambridge, MA: Harvard University Press.

Kagan, J. (1984). *The nature of the child*. New York: Basic Books.

Kaye, K. (1982). *The mental and social life of babies: How parents create persons*. Chicago: University of Chicago Press.

Klinnert, M. D., Campos, J. J., Sorce, F. J., Emde, R. N., & Svedja, M. J. (1983). Social referencing: Emotional expressions as behavior regulators. In R. Plutchik & H. Kellerman (Eds.), *Emotion: Theory, research and experience, Vol. 2: Emotions in early development* (pp. 57–86). Orlando, FL: Academic Press.

Kochanska, G. (1993). Toward a synthesis of parental socialization and child temperament in early development of conscience. *Child Development, 64,* 325–347.

Kohlberg, L. (1982). *The philosophy of moral development*. San Francisco: Harper & Row.

Kohut, H. (1971). *The analysis of the self*. New York: International Universities Press.

Kohut, H. (1977). *The restoration of the self*. New York: International Universities Press.

Lazarus, R. S. (1991). *Emotion and Adaptation*. New York: Oxford University Press.

Lewis, M. (1991). *Shame. The exposed self*. New York: Free Press.

Lewis, M., & Brooks-Gunn, J. (1979). *Social cognition and the acquisition of self*. New York: Plenum Press.

Maccoby, E., & Martin, J. (1983). Socialization in the context of the family: Parent-child interaction. In W. M. Hetherington (Ed.), *Socialization, personality and social development* (Vol. 4, pp. 1–101). New York: John Wiley & Sons.

Mahler, M. S., Pine, F., & Bergman, A. (1975). *The psychological birth of the human infant: Symbiosis and individuation*. New York: Basic Books.

Mandler, J. (1983). Representation. In J. H. Flavell & E. M. Markman (Eds.), *Handbook of child psychology: (Vol. 3); Cognitive development* (pp. 420–494). New York: John Wiley & Sons.

McCall, R. B. (1979). The development of intellectual functioning in infancy and the prediction of later I.Q. In J. D. Osofsky (Ed.), *Handbook of infant development* (pp. 707–741). New York: John Wiley & Sons.

Mead, G. H. (1934). *Mind, self and society*. C. Morris (Ed.), Chicago: University of Chicago Press.

Meltzoff, A. N. (1985). The roots of social and cognitive development: models of man's original nature. In T. M. Field & N. A. Fox (Eds.), *Social perception in infants* (pp. 1–30). Norwood, NJ: Ablex.

Morgan, G. A., & Harmon, R. J. (1984). Developmental transformations and mastery motivation: Measurement and validation. In R. N. Emde & R. J. Harmon (Eds.), *Continuities and discontinuities in development* (pp. 263–291). New York: Plenum Press.

Murphy, L. (1937). *Social behaviour and child personality.* New York: Columbia University Press.

Osofsky, J. D. (1993, June). Violence in the lives of young children. Position paper prepared for the Task Force on the needs of young children, Carnegie Corporation of New York.

Osofsky, J. D., & Eberhart-Wright, A. (1988). Affective exchanges between high risk mothers and infants. *International Journal of Psycho-Analysis, 69,* 221–232.

Papousek, H. (1981). The common in the uncommon child. In M. Lewis & L. Rosenblum (Eds.), *The uncommon child* (pp. 317–328). New York: Plenum Press.

Papousek, H., & Papousek, M. (1979). Early ontogeny of human social interaction: Its biological roots and social dimensions. In K. Foppa, W. Lepenies, & D. Ploog (Eds.), *Human ethology: Claims and limits of a new discipline* (pp. 456–489). Cambridge: Cambridge University Press.

Piaget, J. (1952). *The origins of intelligence in children,* Margaret Cook (Trans.). New York: International Universities Press. (Originally published 1936.)

Radke-Yarrow, M., Zahn-Waxler, C., & Chapman, M. (1983). Children's prosocial dispositions and behavior. In E. M. Hetherington & P. H. Mussen (Eds.), *Handbook of child psychology; Vol. 4; Socialization, personality, and social development* (4th ed., pp. 469–545). New York: John Wiley & Sons.

Richardson-Klavehn, A., & Bjork, R. A. (1988). Measures of memory. *Annual Review of Psychology, 39,* 475–543.

Rumelhart, D. E., McClelland, J. L., and the PDP Research Group. (1986). *Parallel distributed processing: Explorations in the microstructure of cognition. Vol. 1: Foundations.* Cambridge, MA: MIT Press.

Ryle, G. (1949). *The concept of mind.* New York: Barnes and Noble.

Sameroff, A. J., & Chandler, M. (1976). Reproductive risk and the continuum of caretaking casualty. In F. D. Horowitz (Ed.), *Review of the Child Development Research.* (Vol. 4, pp. 187–244). Chicago: University of Chicago Press.

Sampson, E. E. (1988). The debate on individuality. *American Psychologist, 43* (1), 15–22.

Sander, L. (1985). Toward a logic of organization in psychobiological development. In K. Klar & L. Siever (Eds.), *Biologic response styles: Clinical implication* [Monograph] (pp. 20–36). Washington, DC: American Psychiatric Press.

Scaife, M., & Bruner, J. S. (1975). The capacity for joint visual attention in the infant. *Nature, 253,* 265–266.

Singer, D. G., & Singer, J. L. (1990). *The house of make-believe. Children's play and the developing imagination.* Cambridge, MA: Harvard University Press.

Snow, C. E. (1972). Mother's speech to children learning language. *Child Development, 43,* 549–565.

Sorce, J. F., & Emde, R. N. (1982). The meaning of infant emotional expressions: Regularities in caregiving responses in normal and Down's syndrome infants. *Journal of the Child Psychology and Psychiatry, 23* (2), 145–158.

Spitz, R. (1965). The evolution of dialogue. In M. Schur (Ed.), *Drives, affects, behavior* (Vol. 2, pp. 170–190). New York: International Universities Press.

Sroufe, L. A. (1979). Socioemotional development. In J. D. Osofsky (Ed.), *Handbook of infant development* (pp. 462–516). New York: John Wiley & Sons.

Stern, D. N. (1977). *The first relationship: Mother and infant.* Cambridge, MA: Harvard University Press.

Stern, D. N. (1985). *The interpersonal world of the infant.* New York: Basic Books.

Stolorow, R., Brandchaft, B., & Atwood, G. E. (1987). *Psychoanalytic treatment: An intersubjective approach.* Hillsdale, NJ: Analytic Press.

Trevarthen, C. (1979). Communication and cooperation in early infancy: A description of primary intersubjectivity. In M. Bullowa (Ed.), *Before speech: The beginning of interpersonal communication* (pp. 321–347). Cambridge: Cambridge University Press.

Tronick, E. (1980). The primacy of social skills in infancy. In D. B. Sawin, R. C. Hawkins, L. O. Walker, & J. H. Penticuff (Eds.), *Exceptional infant* (Vol. 4, pp. 144–158). New York: Brunner/Mazel.

Tronick, E., & Gianino, A. (1986). The transmission of maternal disturbance to the infant. In E. Tronick & T. Field (Eds.), *Maternal depression and infant disturbances* (pp. 5–11). San Francisco: Jossey-Bass.

Waddington, C. H. (1962). *New patterns in genetics and development, Vol. 21.* New York: Columbia University Press. (Columbia Biological Series.)

Watson, M. W., & Fischer, K. W. (1980). Development of social roles in elicited and spontaneous behavior during the preschool years. *Developmental Psychology, 16,* 483–494.

Wellman, H. M., Cross, D., & Bartsch, K. (1986). Infant search and object permanence: A meta-analysis of the A-not-B error. *Monographs of the Society for Research in Child Development, 51* (3, Serial No. 214).

White, R. W. (1963). Ego and reality in psychoanalytic theory. *Psychological Issues, Monograph No. 11.* New York: International Universities Press.

Winnicott, D. O. (1965). Ego distortion in terms of true and false self. In *The maturational processes and the facilitating environment* (pp. 140–152). New York: International Universities Press.

Wolf, D. (1990). Being of several minds: Voices and versions for a heterogeneous self. In D. Cicchetti & M. Beeghly (Eds.), *The self in transition: Infancy to childhood* (pp. 183–212). Chicago: University of Chicago Press.

Wolf, D., & Grollman, S. (1982). Ways of playing: Individual differences in imaginative play. In K. Rubin & D. Pepler (Eds.), *The play of children: Current theory and research* (pp. 1–19). New York: Karger.

Wolf, D., Rygh, J., & Altshuler, J. (1984). Agency and experience: Actions and states in play narratives. In I. Bretherton (Ed.), *Symbolic play* (pp. 195–217). Orlando, FL: Academic Press.

Zahn-Waxler, C., & Kochanska, G. (1990). The origins of guilt. In R. Thompson (Ed.), *Nebraska symposium*

338

on motivation, 1988: Socioemotional development (pp. 183–258). Lincoln: University of Nebraska Press.

Zahn-Waxler, C., & Radke-Yarrow, M. (1982). The development of altruism: Alternative research strategies. In N. Eisenberg (Ed.), *The development of prosocial behavior.* New York: Academic Press.

Zahn-Waxler, C., & Robinson, J. (1995). Empathy and guilt: Early origins of feelings of responsibility. In *Self-conscious emotions: The psychology of shame, guilt, embarrassment, and pride* (pp. 143–173). New York: Guilford Press.

Zahn-Waxler, C., Robinson, J., & Emde, R. N. (1992). The development of empathy in twins. *Developmental Psychology, 28* (6), 1038–1047.

32 / **Infant-Parent Psychotherapy**

Jeree H. Pawl and Alicia F. Lieberman

People always have taken an interest in the nature of the relationship between parents and children. From whatever perspective, how children are "raised" has seemed significant. Whether the hand that is rocking the cradle is ruling the world or parents are being admonished that sparing the rod is spoiling the child, the view that how parents treat their children has an outcome of some interest has long been held. "How-to" advice to parents also has a long history, albeit one in which the advice shifts dramatically over the years.

Psychoanalytic theory has held that individual experience shapes significant aspects of individual personality functioning. A true developmental history consists not only of the vicissitudes of "stages of development" but also of the actual experiences that children have with people, particularly within their primary relationships. Harry Stack Sullivan's (1938, 1953) emphasis on the vital importance of the "interpersonal" relationship added significantly to this climate. At the most extreme nurture end of the nature-nurture spectrum, Watson (1928) maintained that social conditioning made it possible simply to create individuals tailored to demand. The dissemination of this perspective stemming from both psychoanalytic and behavioral theories in scholarly and popular materials during the first third of the 20th century placed a clear emphasis on the salience of interactive experience to individual development. During the next 30 years, Burlingame and Freud (1942, 1944), Provence and Lipton (1962), Spitz (1965), Bowlby (1969), and many others demonstrated with dramatic intensity the effects of maternal deprivation and loss on the well-being of infants. Levy (1943) and others focused on how maternal characteristics affected young children. Milton Senn (1954) edited a book on the problems of infancy and childhood whose focus was on early emotional development and also the effects of experience. And within these contexts there gradually emerged an interest in and conceptualization of something called preventive psychiatry. Gerald Caplan was one of its most vigorous and imaginative proponents.

At the International Institute of Child Psychiatry in August of 1954, a "prevention" movement began to take a very clear shape. *Emotional Problems of Early Childhood* (Caplan, 1955), a book that resulted from the conference, became a leading textbook in child psychiatry and clinical psychology and included an entire section on preventive psychiatry containing descriptions of interventions with parent and infant dyads ranging from the most direct to the most indirect. In his own chapter, "Recent Trends in Preventive Child Psychiatry," Caplan outlined and discussed in great detail the justifications for and the kinds of interventions with parents and their infants and toddlers that might be undertaken. He described a need to ameliorate the "pathogenic parent-child relationship" through methods described as "child-centered therapy" (with the parent) or "focused case work." Further, he emphasized providing service through well-baby clinics and on consulting to and training nurses, pediatricians, and other front-line contacts so that they could offer some aspects of mental health support to young families in order to prevent later difficulties. Caplan had outlined this approach in an earlier paper (1951).

By the early 1970s, Selma Fraiberg (1980) was directing an infant-parent psychotherapy demonstration project focusing on early parent-child relationships and incorporating a home-visiting model. Until then home visits had been used only briefly or intermittently as a mode of delivering psychotherapy. Her use of the phrase "ghosts in the nursery" captured in a vivid and compelling way the recognition of the role of parental histories as shapers of parents' perceptions of and relationships with their infants and hence the infants themselves. Fraiberg's primary focus was on the interferences created by those "malignant ghosts," and her intent, like Caplan's, was to "free" the baby from the parents' internal conflicts.

Perhaps most important was Fraiberg's sophisticated integration of social work principles and techniques with psychoanalytic understanding of dynamics and psychoanalytic techniques. This blend contributed a flexibility and freedom when working with parents and their infants that was crucial to the development of the work.

Basic Considerations

One of the primary questions in infant-parent psychotherapy and a question that renews itself in each treatment is: Who is the patient? An accurate but less than adequate answer is "both." The parent and the baby create a relationship, and each makes potent contributions to it. In a sense, it is this relationship we are treating, and the relationship involves both parent and child. Sameroff and Emde (1989) embraced this conceptual focus on relationship as a way of developing an appropriate developmental model for looking at the disturbances in infancy.

Conceptually, this goal is rather obvious and easy. Practically, it is a difficult stance to maintain. It is particularly difficult when a parent is signifi-

cantly disturbed and the baby is seemingly quite ordinary in the most positive sense—neither particularly active nor passive, neither overly sensitive nor unresponsive, unstable or poorly regulated. The infant may, however, bear a striking resemblance to the biological father who abandoned both child and mother, and, as a result, the baby's very existence may carry a constant negative valence for the mother.

Although such provoking and disturbing effects may involve the baby, they are not really contributions stemming from any of his or her actual, unique qualities. The mother provides the *meaning* of the baby. Likewise, the mother's own feelings and expectations may perceive ordinary characteristics of the child in such a way that they are rendered aggravating or aggressive. All the qualities of the baby, including parental perception of him or her, do produce an effect. Equally important, each baby registers events uniquely, as only he or she can.

Fraiberg's original intervention population involved blind babies and their parents, a fortuitous circumstance that ensured that the baby's contribution could not be overlooked. It also ensured that the idiosyncratic, singularly personal, and unique responses of each parent to each baby also would be highlighted.

Today, practitioners are more alert to the infant's contribution to the interaction due to a similar dramatic effect. They are aware that babies may be markedly affected by exposure to drugs in utero. This creates an awareness of the salient influences of the unique qualities of each individual infant. The work of Thomas and Chess (1977) on temperament, Escalona (1976) and Colombo and Fagan (1990) on individual differences, and Brazelton (1979) on joint regulation argue for the need for a relationship framework in order to understand the importance of mutual child and parent influence. Current stresses and difficulties of all kinds facing many parents also guarantee that *their* unique perceptions and contributions are not ignored. Thus, researchers and practitioners are increasingly aware that appreciating the contribution of only the parent or only the infant is insufficient. While in an individual dyad, one partner may have more influence than the other, the person who intervenes—the therapist—must recognize the uniqueness and relevance to the relationship of both parent and child. Often the therapist must maintain this perspective in the face of great odds.

Who Is Referred: The Evaluation Process

The range and kinds of difficulties for which parent and child are referred are remarkably varied. Referrals not initiated by the parents themselves tend to reflect the most serious of concerns regarding the baby's safety and well-being. Also, in the last 10 years, more of the families referred are in more serious trouble than ever before. Because of the complexity of the situations prompting the referrals, the process of evaluation is increasingly important. The therapist must gather information in order to decide whether infant-parent psychotherapy is the treatment of choice and whether forming a working alliance with the parent(s) seems possible.

Motivation and Expectations

Parents may be referred by an authority figure with whom they feel they must comply, or they may be mandated to treatment by a court. They may be reluctant, reluctant but curious, or desperate for help. These differences in parental motivation markedly influence how the work with the therapist will begin and unfold. If the parent is also a current or former user of illegal drugs or alcohol, is raising a child alone, is new to the mainstream culture, or has a history of serious rejection or abuse, these conditions too will powerfully influence what can happen in treatment or if it can happen at all. Who the parents are and how they and the therapist come to be meeting with one another are the most important factors shaping the initial evaluation. The following case example is taken from clinical notes by Jeree Pawl.

CASE EXAMPLE

It took several minutes for Mrs. W. to answer the therapist's knock on her door. When she did, she barely acknowledged my introduction but nonetheless opened the door wide and stepped back to let me into a cluttered and grubby kitchen, smelling of cigarettes and fried fish. A baby was asleep in a car bed on the floor and there was a beaten up easy chair in the corner by a door leading to another room. Mrs. W. nodded toward the chair and sat down at a table in a straight chair. She looked very tired and certainly disinterested. I decided to introduce myself again. This time she heard Sara B.'s name (the pediatric nurse practitioner) and she said, with greater liveliness, "Oh—Sara!" I said I guess she hadn't heard me say Sara's name at the door so she really didn't know who I was. Her face suggested that she was not sure if I was criticizing her or not so I said, "I get the idea there are a lot of people parading through here. What is it like for you?" "Well," she said, "I don't mind so very much but I don't really know what the different ones do—but I guess they're supposed to come and . . ." She drifted off. We then began a conversation about how many people there were and tried to identify them. With a little encouragement, she began describing them in terms of size, shape, and personality and began to become more animated—even slightly amused by her own characterizations. I joined her by lightheartedly describing myself in the same way, and she laughed. I remarked that she was certainly very observant even if she didn't know who came from where or for what. By this time we were able to begin to talk a bit about how it really felt to her to have all these visitors.

This kind of awareness of where we as therapists may fit in the institutional involvements people are experiencing is crucial. This process of "beginning at the beginning" is paramount to ensure that consideration and respect characterize the therapeutic treatment of the parent.

Therapist-Parent Relationship

If treatment is to develop effectively, the therapist's attitude and behavior must, from the beginning, reflect the fact that parents are full partners in the relationship. Parents must be engaged as full partners during the evaluation and in the course of whatever type of treatment eventually evolves. While it is too simple to say that the therapist is doing something *with* the parents rather than *to* them, nonetheless this is an accurate description. This attitude of respect must pervade the therapeutic relationship, both because it is an agent of change in itself and because it makes it possible for other aspects of treatment to occur.

The therapist's attitude toward the parent must parallel aspects of the relationship that he or she is striving to create between parent and child. Although the therapist does not deny various areas of expertise, the way that expertise is delivered is an essential part of the therapeutic relationship and hence of the treatment. Recognizing this is, in fact, another aspect of the therapist's expertise.

The quality of the relationship between therapist and parent is crucial in infant-parent psychotherapy because it is an important mutative factor. Eventually we hope to see changes in the parent expressed in the parent-child relationship. Although these positive qualities of experience provided within the therapist/patient relationship are not a sufficient factor, they are necessary ones if change is to occur. The parameters of respect, concern, accommodation, and steady basic positive regard are crucial aspects of the therapeutic relationship and are central aspects of the process of treatment. The more disturbed the parent, the more crucial this becomes. Only in the positive context of this kind of relationship can the parent's negative transference to child and therapist be experienced and discussed usefully.

Some aspects of this positive regard have been called a corrective emotional experience (Alexander, 1948, 1956); sometimes they been viewed negatively as an artificial manipulation of the parent's experience by the therapist with only the most temporary effect, if any. But, in fact, those positive parameters that do characterize parent/therapist relationships must exist to provide a necessary contrast to the parents' conscious and unconscious negative expectations of what relationships can be. In this sense, the therapist's empathic attunement serves as the background against which the parental negative expectations can be experienced and understood. There must be a contrast in this figure-ground relationship, or they will merge irretrievably. People whose experiences have been uniformly harsh and bleak find it difficult to perceive any significant divergence from those experiences. Their expectations and defenses are organized to protect them from disappointment and offer an efficient though costly way to be the least vulnerable and the most prepared.

When any of the essential parameters of the transactions between therapist and parent match the parent's negative expectations, no useful progress can be made. It is easy to imagine therapeutic relationships that are permeated with sexism, racism, authoritarianism, classism, and disrespect, attitudes that may match the early or current experience and expectations of parents so perfectly that their expectations are either confirmed very consciously or they are never even perceived or the focus of discussion at all.

It is also true that very subtle "matches" occur that can obscure the existence of problem areas that the parent should experience clearly and both parent and therapist should understand. The effectiveness of the therapeutic encounter will be undermined totally if the expectations engendered in parents by basic and pervasive flaws in their early relationships are matched by the therapist. Consider the case of patients with serious deprivations who nevertheless have a general sense of faith in "therapy" who enter a relationship with an authoritarian or sexist therapist. While the relationship may be engaging and useful to some degree, the patient will never come to grips with problems obscured by the "match" between their unconscious expectations and the therapist's biases. Even though these matches may be paramount in the patient's psychopathology, they are an unnoted, unaddressed parameter of the patient-therapist relationship, and as such they deter therapeutic progress, even though the patient's "belief" in therapy may sustain the treatment. In contrast, unmotivated patients who are coerced into entering a therapeutic relationship will not develop any truly useful therapeutic alliance at all if the relationship is not free of such undermining matches. All therapists should be aware of the specific negative expectations they may be confirming with their patients and what cost this is having; a failure to do so with severely deprived patients to whom the efficacy of treatment itself must be demonstrated—will render treatment impossible. The quality of the relationship and what it conveys is central. The following case example is taken from Jeree Pawl's notes 6 months into treatment.

CASE EXAMPLE

Mrs. S. lay on the floor, reaching for a toy for her daughter, Tiffany, that had rolled far under the couch. "You know," she said, "I don't sing that song anymore." "You mean the one from that TV show you were always singing?" I asked. "Yeah," she said, still reaching under the couch, "the one that goes 'I want to go somewhere where everybody knows my name.' *You* know my name. Dr. *Lopez* knows my name. I don't have to sing it anymore."

This statement is a clear but shyly delivered reference to her sense of connectedness and of being seen—an experience stemming from the qualities of the two therapeutic relationships she has been experiencing, qualities absent in her earliest experiences in her family.

A week later Mrs. S. said (this time looking at me), "You know, nobody in my house ever said good morning to anybody. I like it that it's the first thing Tiffany says to me in the morning—even when she's not really ready to get up—she says "good morning, Mommy." I asked what that felt like to her—why it mattered? Mrs. S. said, "'Cause then I know I am in the world. I'm real. I exist."

Winnicott (1971), in speaking of the mirror role of mother and family in child development, has said "... I am seen, so I exist" (p. 114). Feeling "seen" had a significant effect on Mrs. S., a very disturbed patient. The effect stemmed from the qualities shared in the two relationships she cites. She gradually has experienced the qualities of genuine concern, respect, consideration, and accommodation as a sense of existing for someone. She can discern her impact on someone else, and she comprehends that she is in continual existence for them. Elsewhere Pawl (1995) has described this as the experience of being "held in someone's mind" and noted the crucial effect of its absence or presence in infancy and toddlerhood. Providing this experience for a patient for whom it was missing can be signally important in treatment.

Therapist-Child Relationship

The relationships between therapists and the children involved are as varied as those between therapists and the parents. Although the intent is to influence the parent-child relationship through the parent-therapist relationship and the work of therapy, other routes of influence are also available, as the child is present during treatment. Not only does the child's presence provide rich observational opportunities that can be exploited fruitfully, but as the child grows older, direct interaction inevitably occurs. Sometimes the parent may thrust an infant on the therapist, or, more naturally, the baby may need to be appropriately admired. How the therapist does this influences parental perception and sometimes direct handling. The following case example is from Jeree Pawl's notes.

CASE EXAMPLE

I was unsure whether Deborah [the mother] wanted me to ask to hold Armand or not—whether I was seeming not interested enough. I watched her carefully and came closer to where they sat. She turned Armand so I could see him better and I squatted down. I said, "Hi, Armand," and smiled at him. Deborah then asked, rather shyly, if I would like to hold him, with what I felt was a clear hope that I would. I thanked her, sat down next to her, and held him. When I held him I spoke to him and commented that to me, he looked not so sure of "this new face." I said for him when she took him back, "There—now that's the face I know and like." Deborah smiled happily and said, "Hi, Armand— you're back." This was not her typical style but she seemed to enjoy trying it on.

In this brief moment, the therapist has interacted with the baby (age 3 months) directly, but it is an interaction different from that which happens between Armand and his mother. The therapist spoke to the baby and hypothesized about his preferences. Importantly, the mother seemed to like the therapist's actions; this fact suggests that in her case, her *not* talking to her baby was due to her depression and that the potential for more verbal interaction between mother and baby exists as treatment becomes more effective. This example also illustrates how what happens between therapist and child may influence the parent in a variety of ways.

Still, the 2- or 3-month-old will neither need nor demand a separate relationship with the therapist as will a more mobile older infant. The therapist's responsibility throughout is to understand the effect that his or her relationship with the child has on the parent as well as the effect that his or her relationship with the parent has on the child. This is a rich field of exploration, containing as it does the potential for envy, jealousy, competition, cooperation, consideration, and a balancing of needs. The presence of both baby and parent creates a texture of interlocking transferences, countertransferences, and other possibilities that are wonderfully complex, splendidly useful, and highly demanding. The therapist must monitor these processes continually to ensure that they continue to contribute usefully and positively to the treatment.

The Experience of the Therapist

Many parents who are referred to community agencies for infant-parent psychotherapy are ones who suffered extreme deprivation as children. Their needs are enormous and their expectations often are very negative. The therapist somehow must bridge this chasm without tumbling into it. The therapist must gratify some needs of these parents in such a way that they can feel, both emotionally and concretely. Other parents may take a concerned and considerate attitude for granted. They expect such treatment much of the time and may even perceive it when it is not there. But the most troubled parents will need to struggle very hard in order to perceive concern at all even when it is there. Their special needs call for specific kinds of therapist responses. Initially, concrete assistance in response to a concrete need may be the only way to convey any sense of concern, respect, or consideration. If so, this concrete assistance (with transportation, transactions with agencies, grocery shopping, and so on) constitutes a necessary beginning.

As a result of the need to be especially forthcoming and responsive to the parent, the therapist must determine his or her own level of tolerance to the parent's need. In order to respond to and manage a sometimes desperate level of need in a parent, the therapist must learn his or her own limits, know quickly where actions are leading, what unkeepable promises may be made inadvertently, and how flexible he or she can be. The therapist must not only predict what parents may need or want but also his or her capacity to respond to those needs. For the most part, the actual capacity of the therapist matters less than his or her own awareness of what that capacity is and will continue to be over time. Generous responses turn to cruelties if they cannot be sustained. Responding is not the danger. The danger is responding at first and then failing to respond.

In working with severely deprived parents, therapists probably need a somewhat higher threshold of willing availability and tolerance for inconvenience than that required for working with patients with less negative expectations. The requirements of office visits and home visits are very different. A therapist's reaction to a parent failing to keep an appointment is rather different when being pondered in the comfort of a cozy office chair as opposed to while standing on a stoop in the rain in front of a closed door.

Another source of therapist stress is the complex feelings aroused when working directly with the parent and infant in a troubled relationship. The therapist's ability to remain empathic to the "abusive" parent is sorely tested when a child is treated in ways that seem damaging or dangerous. While reportable abuse presents its own set of complicated problems, therapist toleration of other painful treatment of children—the joyless silence of the depressed mother's interactions, the abrupt and harsh admonishments of an extremely enraged mother—which will take time to ameliorate, presents a tremendous challenge. Any response that is not clinically sound in relation to the parent could readily disrupt treatment, and then there is no hope to alleviate the situation for child or parent.

In addition, the area of parent-child relationships evokes in all practitioners complex feelings about their own early history, feelings that may or may not be quite recognized or understood and that present an ever-present danger that therapists will act out in ways harmful to those whom they aim to help.

Awareness of the ready arousal of such conflictual feelings, good supervision while in training, and the ready availability of collegial or more formal consultation is a necessary and fruitful safeguard against these ready provocations.

Gathering Information

A main goal of the evaluation is to achieve some mutual agreement with the parent about the agenda for treatment if, in fact, treatment is to occur. Parent or therapist or both may find that proceeding from evaluation to treatment is not desirable.

Given that many referred patients in the public sector are not seeking treatment on their own, therapists should gather necessary information through a relatively natural conversation and must respect the fact that many parents believe that they do not need any help with their children. As good social work instructs, therapists begin where the person is and build a relationship from there. During the initial evaluation, the primary consideration is to establish a relationship. As the parents guide the discussion, choosing the topics and shifting from one to the other or watching TV (in a home visit), therapists can learn readily what the basic background affects are, what the habitual coping and defense mechanisms are, and, most important, how the parents want to be seen and understood. The parents always know they are being seen "because of the baby," but they rarely understand why. Often they are insulted and angry about the referral; while these emotions must be dealt with first, the therapists should, simultaneously and throughout the interview, observe how the parents appear to experience the child and how the child is functioning developmentally and affectively. It is also crucial to hear parents' experience of and understanding of their child directly.

Developmental testing often is a very useful component of the evaluation process. In addition to providing information about the child's predilections, talents, and areas of difficulty, testing presents a microcosm of the parent/child relationship. It also offers an immediate opportunity to discuss the child's style and capacities as well as strengths and vulnerabilities. Most parents are very anxious concerning tests of their children,

even if the evaluation is presented as an opportunity to "see the things in a short time that we would naturally see if we followed the child around all day." Another useful way to present testing is as a way to see how children like to learn, what is interesting to them and what is not, and how they respond to things that are hard and things that are easy.

Watching a videotape of the testing with parents also offers a good opportunity to gather their impressions and reflections and begin the process of further work. Often a parent who is consumed by the personal trials in life will manage to use the opportunity for bringing his or her child into focus that the evaluation process affords. This can provide the parent and the therapist a way of investing the child with a clearer personhood than the child currently has, one less distorted by parental need. It is very important, however, to make a clinical judgment as to whether this focus on the child at the beginning of treatment will, for whatever reason, interfere with the creation of a working alliance and positive relationship with the parent. Too much anxiety, competition, and unwelcomed direct focus on the child may totally alienate a parent. The evaluation may prove more useful at a later time.

The Role and Usefulness of Diagnosis

The diagnosis of parents both shapes and is shaped by the course of evaluation and treatment. The relationship between diagnostic classification and predicting the probable course and outcome of treatment is complex. Parents with only relatively severe disorders may respond less well to infant-parent psychotherapy than those with more serious disorders. This finding is consonant with research findings that psychiatric diagnosis is not a good predictor of disturbances in the ability to be an adequate parent (Sameroff, Seiffer, & Zax, 1982).

It also seems that parents' emotional investment in their infant affects their ability to make use of treatment on behalf of their child. This parental investment in the child makes it possible to utilize infant-parent psychotherapy with patients who might be unlikely candidates for more conventional insight-oriented psychotherapy as it is traditionally delivered. Other factors ordinarily seen to argue against successful involvement in individual therapy, such as low educational level, social marginality, and inability to be introspective, also do not seem to interfere so as to preclude infant-parent psychotherapy. In fact, many of the parents do gradually become introspective, insightful, and highly articulate. Clearly, this has much to do with the flexible, relationship-oriented nature of the treatment plus the leverage provided by the investment parents have in the well-being of their child.

Making diagnoses with confidence and usefulness decreases as the objective difficulties of the parents' daily lives increase. Sureness in diagnostic accuracy decreases when the conditions are less stable or significantly affected by poverty, especially increasingly violent urban poverty. Situations of homelessness also confound therapists' ability to diagnose with confidence. Is this young new mother suffering from postpartum depression, or is her current external situation the major contributor to her depression? Considerations of these kinds must be weighed continually.

In addition, both the referral context and the wish to achieve a balanced, more egalitarian relationship with the parent preclude a more formal psychiatric interview. If such an interview is deemed necessary for any reason, it is done by referral elsewhere. Thus, the role of psychiatric diagnosis has a different place in infant-parent functions and psychotherapy. It is merely one of the ways in which one tries to understand how someone views herself and her world.

In the course of the evaluation, therapists want to formulate a sufficient diagnostic impression to be able to assign a diagnosis from the fourth edition of the *Diagnostic and Statistical Manual of Mental Disorders* (American Psychiatric Association, 1994). There is no question that such a diagnosis and the process of determining it are useful in various kinds of decision making. They may help, for example, in deciding whether to refer a parent for individual treatment in conjunction with infant-parent psychotherapy, and if so, how such a referral should be made. Additionally, the discipline involved in thinking systematically about the strengths and vulnerabilities of a parent in an objective framework aids in anticipating

likely difficulties in treatment and suggests likely idiosyncracies of a parent's perception of the infant.

The process of arriving at a diagnosis also informs the clinical decisions made about focus and timing. Very often mothers with serious narcissistic disorders are intolerant of the ordinary demands of their baby and of the therapist paying any direct attention to the baby during a session. Both situations interfere with the fulfillment of their wish to be the exclusive focus of the therapist's attention, and they experience an acute sense of loss as a result. In these cases, the focus initially must be primarily on the mother and only eventually on the discomfort such shifts in attention produce within her.

Narcissistically injured mothers also are likely to experience any comment about child rearing or any observations of the baby as somehow critical of them as mothers. Often these women take even questions regarding their opinions or feelings as hurtful, infuriating, critical comments. Until these women can experience other comments uncritically, therapists may need to avoid any comment on the baby's experience. The women's sense of themselves and of the therapeutic relationship may need considerable strengthening before they can assume a more reflective stance. The internal changes that will allow this stance stem from a therapist's unfailing, empathic, and responsive availability.

As mentioned previously, parents whose styles of thinking are relatively concrete and whose experiences in relationships have been chronically impoverished may perceive expressions of concern and understanding only if the therapist's actions make them totally explicit, and even concrete expressions may be discerned only after some period of time. Initially, direct intervention on these parents' behalf—driving them somewhere or going with them to an inconvenient or anxiety-provoking appointment, responding with information and/or help so they can obtain needed free food, or straightening out their agreement with a landlord—may be the only way that these parents can begin to experience being cared about. It also may be the only way they can experience the therapist as useful, which a therapist should indeed be perceived to be. Patients who think they should be in therapy because they need it and believe it will help them find their therapist "useful." In such cases, the therapist is joining the patient in doing what the patient thinks needs to be done. Patients who lack a belief in the need for or efficacy of therapy find a therapist useful if they experience being with and talking to the therapist as emotionally supportive or even clarifying. But some patients cannot "feel" this sense of meaningful usefulness unless it produces a product or a literal, concrete reduction in externally produced stress. With these patients (and most of our parents are), such concrete changes are needed before they can experience a relationship as helpful and rewarding rather than burdensome and disappointing. Such seriously deprived parents feel unworthy of care and attention even as they also may feel enormous rage. Gradually, however, whatever sheer glee they feel (and they often do) in exploiting someone who is essentially a stranger—the therapist—for their own ends is transformed. Instead, the parents come to sense that they are not exploiting the therapist but that he or she is genuinely willing to accomodate and be useful because he or she finds it natural that the parents are worth the effort of investment time and energy. This recognition enhances the parents' sense of worth and often allows them to feel more invested in and concerned for their babies. The psychological growth that accompanies the gradual evolution of this process is often astounding. As one patient put it: "First I didn't even believe there was a candy store—then I thought I could at least press my nose to the window. Now I'm inside and I can't quite believe it." The discussion in which this comment occurred was very complex, but the metaphor captures one important aspect of her sense of moving from disbelief that a relationship could provide anything, to being somewhat overwhelmed and amazed by the possibilities.

Parents who have antisocial personality disorders and engage in criminal and/or dangerous activities need to have wholly realistic responses from the therapist in regard to those activities. The therapist needs to express clear concern regarding the safety of both parent and baby. This firm and serious tone often creates the necessary climate for encouraging real exploration of the reasons for the dangerous behavior. Similarly, parents who endanger their children in other ways need to hear that "This won't do" in very clear terms. Often these parents experience not being allowed to act out in dangerous ways with considerable relief.

Less deprived patients and those with sturdier senses of self-will need less concrete demonstration of concern although they may need more emotional availability and candor than is traditional. Therapy with parents most resembles the more familiar psychodynamic model when the parents are willing and eager to explore the past in the context of current experiences with the baby.

Nonetheless, whatever type of approach is needed, from the most concrete to the least, it is the quality of the relationship between therapist and parent that is paramount. The linking of early and shaping parental experiences with current disturbances in the parents' relationship with their child always rests on the therapist's painstaking and unswerving appreciation of the parents' subjective experience and on the need for the therapist's genuine concern and respect.

The Treatment Process

In its early days, infant-parent psychotherapy was described as comprising four major therapeutic modalities: concrete assistance, emotional support, developmental guidance, and psychotherapy (Fraiberg, 1980). One or another modality might predominate, depending on the individual circumstances of the case and the stage of treatment, but all four could be called upon as an integral part of the therapist's repertoire, and all four were integrated seamlessly, whenever needed, and were equally important components of the therapeutic process.

From our current perspective, it is more accurate to describe emotional support not as a separate modality but rather as the overarching attitude the therapist brings to the work. This view is inherent in our earlier emphasis on the quality of the therapeutic relationship as an important mutative factor in treatment. At its best, emotional support incorporates genuine respect, empathy, and reciprocity as qualities that are experienced and then internalized gradually by the parent and ultimately become stable characteristics of the relationship with the child.

As we stressed earlier, treatment begins during the first assessment session. In this sense, there is no basic difference in the therapeutic approaches employed during assessment and during treatment. The difference is rather one of degree: Once the parents accept the offer of treatment and an explicit agreement to continue the work is made, the therapist has greater parental permission to explore, question, raise issues, and suggest clarifications or interpretations.

The issue of timing is crucial. An offer of concrete assistance may be just right for a parent who is daunted by the task at hand or who needs a concrete demonstration that a therapist means what he or she says when talking about "finding ways to make things better" for the family. Yet the same parent may perceive a similar offer as infantilizing or demonstrating a lack of trust when he or she is in a different state of mind or at a later stage of treatment. Similar considerations of timing and appropriateness apply to developmental guidance and psychological interpretations as well.

It is useful to think of developmental guidance and psychological interpretation as points along a continuum rather than as discrete categories. Formally, of course, their definitions make them appear as separate forms of intervention. Developmental guidance involves providing information about age-appropriate behaviors, interests, concerns and conflicts, and suggesting appropriate and possible parental responses based on their developing understanding of their child. Psychological interpretations, on the other hand, involve understanding a parent's reactions to the child in the context of his or her early experience, current circumstances, or intrapsychic conflicts.

These formal definitions obscure an important link between developmental guidance and interpretation. To be most useful, the content of both forms of intervention needs to emerge from a process of exploration where a parent's subjective experience is actively sought out and incorporated into the work. Didactic teaching has had a very limited role in infant-parent psychotherapy. Information is always embedded in a broader understanding of the strengths and conflicts in the parent-child relationship and how these relate to the impediments in the parent toward a more empathic and reciprocal interaction with the child.

Often parents begin a session asking for the therapist's advice about how to solve a specific problem: clinginess, refusal to be toilet trained, temper tantrums, or many of the myriad challenges of infancy and toddlerhood. The therapist may already understand clearly the source of the difficulty and can perhaps, give immediate, thoughtful advice about the appropriate course of action. The temptation to impart "wisdom" is great in these circumstances, but therapists who yield to this temptation may soon experience a seemingly inexplicable change in the emotional tone of the exchange. The parents' eyes may glaze over, or the expressions of interest may acquire a decidedly phoney tone, or they may protest that that is exactly what has been done all along, and it has not worked. Although therapists might feel frustrated in such situations, the message is clear: The parents are not ready to listen.

In such cases, the outcome might be more rewarding for all involved if the therapist refrains from offering information right away and answers a question with another question that says basically: "What have you tried, and what happens when you do it?" While listening to the response, the therapist can gain invaluable information that can be incorporated later while working with the parent toward an effective course of action. As the parent describes the situation in detail, or (more effectively still) when the therapist observes the child's problematic behavior unfold during the session, the many components of the situation and the existing obstacles to an easy solution become clear. These challenges include such things as the child's constitutional vulnerabilities, temperamental proclivities and emerging defensive style, parental child-rearing values (which may be culturally determined, idiosyncratically personal, or a bit of both), and parental fears and misperceptions. Included as well are the parallels between the current situation and the parents' own childhood experiences and perhaps even their unconscious resistances to a solution. All of these factors need to be woven into an approach to the problem that parents and child will experience as consistent with who they are rather than simply reflecting an "expert's" view of how children should be raised.

As mentioned earlier, infant-parent psychotherapy is commonly identified as a "ghosts in the nursery" approach to treatment. This expression has great value in conveying the active influences of the results of the parents' experiences and conflicts on their relationship with the child. This conceptualization has given a distinctly psychodynamic stamp to infant-parent psychotherapy. By enabling parents to understand the relationship of their current feelings toward a child to their own childhood experiences, therapists can help them experience their child for who he or she is rather than as the child appears through the distorting lens of parental projection and conflict.

It is important to underline, however, that most often there is no one-to-one correspondence between well-delineated parental conflicts and a set of negatively colored attitudes toward or perceptions of the child. When parents suffer from pervasive characterological disorders, when the day-to-day circumstances are crushing to their sense of personal dignity and hope in the future, or when both conditions operate at the same time—all these circumstances, intrapsychic problems, and conflicts about the child seem to unite because they reflect the parents' deepest levels of self-experience rather than circumscribed areas of psychological distress. In these circumstances the therapeutic relationship can become the most immediate and most potent vehicle to eventual change.

Treatment Formats

The hallmark of infant-parent psychotherapy is the infant's presence during the therapeutic sessions. This presence allows the therapist to observe, understand, and intervene in the immediacy of the moment as the emotions between parent and child are expressed spontaneously and with full intensity rather than recalled (and edited) by the parent in the relative detachment of an individual session.

Yet in certain situations, the child's presence inhibits therapeutic progress. For example, a parent may need to delve into painful personal experiences in a setting where the needs and demands of a young child do not constantly divert his or her attention. A couple may need a protected setting where they can speak freely to each other about their marital difficulties and how these spill over onto the ways they interact with their child. The child him- or herself, once receptive language is acquired, may need to be protected from listening to disturbing parental accounts. Situations such as

these call for a modification of the joint parent(s)-child-therapist session format. In addition, when the target child is a toddler, the element of competition, whether between parent and child for the therapist's attention or between parent and therapist for the child's, may indicate a strong need for a different format. It is wholly possible to do infant-parent psychotherapy in the absence of the child if the therapist holds the child firmly in his or her mind. This psychological presence allows the therapist to associate freely the content of the parent's material, both verbal and behavioral, to meanings for the child and the parent-child relationship. This is only a step beyond the therapist's need to represent and hold the child in mind even when the child is present but is essentially ignored or rejected by the parent. Although the process is clinically challenging, through comments and questions the therapist makes judicious decisions as to when the child can be made effectively and productively present. Frequently it is most effective for the therapist and parents to search together for a flexible form where individual and/or couple sessions may be interspersed or primary with those in which the child is present. Stern (1995) has commented on the importance of this kind of flexible approach to successful treatment.

Home visits also have been an unusual yet typical feature in the format of infant-parent psychotherapy. Visiting families in their own homes allows therapists to appreciate with unmatched vividness the day-to-day experience of the baby and the parents. Clinical considerations as well as parental choice are the basis of what treatment choice is decided upon: a home visit format, a more traditional program-centered approach, or some mix thereof. In setting, composition of the sessions, and focus of the work, flexibility and attunement to the unique needs of each case are the most reliable ingredients of infant-parent psychotherapy and in fact the most reliable hallmark.

Training

The training of infant-parent psychotherapists has important parallels to the clinical work. Working

349

with the troubled infants of troubled parents is often extremely emotionally draining. Supervisors must pay close attention to student experiences to prevent serious clinical mistakes based on countertransference reactions. These reactions may run the range from a total identification with the maltreated infant at the expense of empathy for the parents, to collusion with the parents in the maltreatment of the baby, to unrealistic rescue fantasies involving the parent, the baby, or both.

In addition to presenting emotional challenges to the beginning practitioner, infant-parent psychotherapy calls for expertise in several fields simultaneously. The therapist needs to be conversant in normal and deviant development in infancy and toddlerhood as well as being skilled in assessing adult psychopathology and in clinical observation and intervention.

As a result of the need for expertise in several areas, infant-parent psychotherapy is essentially a multidisciplinary undertaking. It can be practiced successfully by psychologists, psychiatrists, behavioral pediatricians, social workers, nurses, learning disabilities specialists, and practitioners of other professions concerned with infants and their families. Each profession brings its own core of specific knowledge. Infant-parent psychotherapy contributes a unique focus on the parent-child relationship and its psychological underpinings.

Close and sustained supervision is key in training infant-parent psychotherapists. One hour of supervision for each clinical contact with a family is indicated at least for the first year of training and perhaps also for the second year, depending on the severity of the problems posed by the case and the advancing skills of the clinician.

The emotional tone of the supervision needs to parallel the parameters the supervisor seeks to foster in the therapeutic relationship. A supervisor's attitude needs to be one of openness, warmth, and respect for the student's experience. Information should be conveyed in a context of dialogue and the opportunity to elicit and elucidate doubts and disagreements. The supervisor needs to monitor continuously his or her own attitude of empathy for the student's uncertainties, emotional reactions, and even therapeutic mistakes. Only in this context will the student feel supported enough to truly dare to engage flexibly and thoughtfully with the troubled families with whom he or she must work.

Weekly case reviews attended by faculty and trainees are a valuable training forum. They allow the trainees to partake of each other's experience and promote a lively exchange of opinion that makes it clear that infant-parent psychotherapy is not monolithic and that equally experienced therapists may disagree strongly about the optimal clinical direction in a particular case.

Seminars in infant and toddler development, psychoanalytic, object relations, and attachment theory, as well as clinical technique are also important in providing a cohesive theoretical and clinical background that brings together the multiplicity of disciplines represented by the trainees. It is this melding of perspectives that continues to enrich the work that therapists do with infants, toddlers, and their parents.

REFERENCES

Alexander, F. (1948). *Fundamentals of psychoanalysis.* New York: W. W. Norton.

Alexander, F. (1956). *Psychoanalysis and psychotherapy.* New York: W. W. Norton.

American Psychiatric Association. (1994). *Diagnostic and statistical manual of mental disorders* (4th ed.). Washington, DC: Author.

Bowlby, J. (1969). *Attachment and loss. Vol. 1: Attachment.* New York: Basic Books.

Brazelton, T. B. (1979). Joint regulation of neonate-parent behaviors. In E. Tronick (Ed.), *Social interchange in infancy* (pp. 7–22). Baltimore: University Park Press.

Burlingame, D. T., & Freud, A. (1942). *Young children in war-time.* London: Allen & Unwin.

Burlingame, D. T., & Freud, A. (1944). *Infants without families: The case for and against residential nurseries.* London: Allen & Unwin.

Caplan, G. (1951). A public health approach to child psychiatry. *Mental Hygiene, 25,* 2.

Caplan, G. (1955). Recent trends in preventive child psychiatry. In G. Caplan (Ed.), *Emotional problems of early childhood* (pp. 153–163). New York: Basic Books.

Columbo, J., & Fagan, J. (Eds.) (1990). *Individual differences in infancy: Reliability stability and prediction.* Hillsdale, NJ: Lawrence Erlbaum.

Escalona, S. (1968). *The roots of individuality.* Chicago: Aldine.

Fraiberg, S. (Ed.) (1980). *Clinical studies in infant mental health.* New York: Basic Books.

Levy, D. (1943). *Maternal overprotection.* New York: Columbia University Press.

Pawl, J. (1995). The therapeutic relationship as human connectedness: Being held in another's mind. *Bulletin of Zero to Three/NCCIP, 15,* 4.

Provence, S., & Lipton, R. C. (1962). *Infants in institutions.* New York: International Universities Press.

Sameroff, A., Seiffer, R., & Zax, M. (1982). Early development of children at risk for emotional disorders. *Monographs of the Society for Research in Child Development, 47* (7, Serial No. 199).

Sameroff, A., & Emde, R. (Eds.) (1989). *Relationship disturbances.* New York: Basic Books.

Senn, M. E. (Ed.) (1954). *Problems of infancy and childhood.* New York: Jewish Foundation.

Spitz, R. A. (1965). *The first year of life.* New York: International Universities Press.

Stern, D. (1995). *The motherhood constellation.* New York: Basic Books.

Sullivan, H. (1938). Psychiatry: Introduction to the study of interpersonal relations. *Psychiatry, 1,* 121–134.

Sullivan, H. (1953). *The interpersonal theory of psychiatry.* New York: W. W. Norton.

Thomas, A., & Chess, S. (1977). *Temperament and development.* New York: Basic Books.

Watson, J. B. (1928). *Psychological care of infant and child.* New York: W. W. Norton.

Winnicott, D. W. (1971). *Playing and reality.* New York: Tavistock Publications.

33 / The Developmental Structuralist Model of Early Personality Development

Stanley I. Greenspan

The diagnosis and treatment of emotional and developmental disorders in infants and young children requires the clinician to take into account all facets of a child's experience. It is necessary, therefore, to have a model with which to look at how constitutional-maturational (i.e., regulatory), family, and interactive factors work together as children progress through each developmental phase.

The developmental model formulated in this chapter (Greenspan, 1979, 1989, 1992) can be visualized with the infant's constitutional-maturational patterns on one side and the infant's environment, including caregivers, family, community, and culture, on the other side. Both of these sets of factors operate through the infant-caregiver relationship, which can be pictured in the middle. These factors and the infant-caregiver relationship, in turn, contribute to the organization of experience at each of six different developmental levels, which may be pictured just beneath the infant-caregiver relationship. (See Figure 33.1.)

Each developmental level involves different tasks or goals. The relative effect of the constitutional-maturational, environmental, or interactive variables will therefore depend on and can be understood only in the context of the developmental level they relate to. The influencing variables are best understood not as they might be traditionally, as general influences on development or behavior, but as distinct and different influences on the six distinct developmental and experiential levels. For example, as a child is negotiating the formation of a relationship (engaging), his mother's tendency to be very intellectual and prefer talking over holding may make it relatively harder for him to become deeply engaged in emotional terms. If, constitutionally, he has slightly lower than average motor tone and is hyposensitive with regard to touch and sound, his mother's intellectual and slightly aloof style may be doubly difficult for him, as neither she nor the child is able to take the initiative in engaging the other.

Let us assume, however, that he more or less negotiates this early phase of development (grandmother, who lives with him, as well as his father are very "wooing" caregivers). At age 3, when the developmental phase and task is different, he may have an easier time, even though his mother has not changed. His intellectual mother is highly creative and enjoys pretend play as well as give-and-take logical discussions. No longer

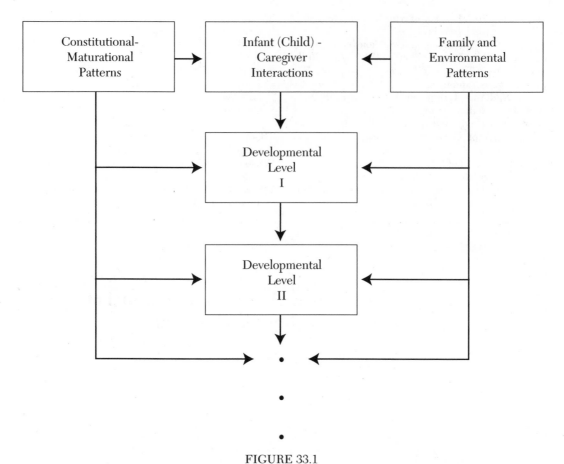

FIGURE 33.1

The functional emotional assessment scale for infancy and early childhood

anxious about her son's dependency needs, she is more relaxed and available for play and chit-chat. The task is no longer simply one of forming a relationship but of learning to represent (or symbolize) experience and form categories and connections between these units of experience. Mother's verbal style is now quite helpful to him, especially given his need for a lot of verbal interaction. In other words, the same caregiving pattern can have a very different impact, depending on the tasks of the particular developmental level. Each developmental level of experience is therefore a reference point for the factors that influence development.

What is potentially unique about this particular clinical and research model (Greenspan, 1989) is the ability it gives us to look at the back-and-forth influence of highly specific and verifiable, constitutional-maturational factors on interactive and family patterns and vice versa, in relationship to specific developmental processes (and to relate these processes to later developmental and psy-

chopathologic disorders). Very useful intervention models focus on specific influences such as the caregiver's feelings, fantasies, or support system, or on certain phases of early development (Brazelton & Cremer, 1990; Fraiberg, 1980; Provence, 1983; Provence & Naylor, 1983). The goal of this model is to look at all the major influences throughout the different stages of development. Each of these factors is discussed individually, followed by a brief case example and discussion of how they work together.

Developmental Levels

This model contains six developmental levels, which include the infant-child's ability to accomplish the following:

1. Attend to multisensory affective experience, while at the same time, organize a calm, regulated state and experience pleasure.
2. Engage with and evidence affective preference and pleasure for a caregiver.
3. Initiate and respond to two-way presymbolic gestural communication.
4. Organize chains of two-way communication (opening and closing many circles of communication in a row), maintain communication across space, integrate affective polarities, and synthesize an emerging prerepresentational organization of self and other.
5. Represent (symbolize) affective experience (e.g., pretend play, functional use of language). This ability calls for higher level auditory and verbal sequencing ability.
6. Create representational (symbolic) categories and gradually build conceptual bridges between these categories. This ability creates the foundation for such basic personality functions as reality testing, impulse control, self-other representational differentiation, affect labeling and discrimination, stable mood, and a sense of time and space that allows for logical planning. This ability rests not only on complex auditory and verbal processing abilities but on visual-spatial abstracting capacities as well. The theoretical, clinical, and empirical rationale for these developmental levels is discussed in *The Development of the Ego* (Greenspan, 1989).

At each of these levels, the clinician looks at the range of emotional themes organized (e.g., can the child play out only dependency themes and not aggressive ones; is aggression "behaved" out?). The clinician also looks at the stability of each level. Does a minor stress lead a child to lose her ability to represent, interact, engage, or attend?

In regard to their use in day-to-day clinical work, the six developmental levels can be collapsed into four essential processes that characterize development in infants and young children. These processes have to do with how an infant and parents or caregivers negotiate the various phases of their early interactions. It is necessary to understand how these four processes serve as a basis for diagnosis and treatment.

SHARED ATTENTION AND ENGAGEMENT

Usually in the first 4 months of life, a baby learns to look, listen, attend, and also to experience pleasure and comfort, dependency, and warmth with the caregiver. But it is important to look for this core process in 2- and 3-year-old children as well. Is the problem the youngster is having (whether it be a sleep problem or a behavioral problem, such as hitting another child), related to difficulties with proper negotiation of this core process of attention and engagement?

TWO-WAY COMMUNICATION

Normally, between 4 and 8 months, babies are learning how to go beyond a simple state of connectedness and shared attention into a state of cause-and-effect interaction. At this point, there should be an emotional, social, and intellectual dialogue going on, in addition to a motor dialogue and a sensory dialogue, between the caregiver and the baby. This is the root of two-way communication.

One way to think about two-way communication is the process of opening and closing circles of communication. When the mother, father, or therapist takes an interest in a child, the first circle of communication is opened. When she responds, the child is closing the circle, and when the parent responds in turn, he or she is opening another circle. When the child responds again, she has closed a second circle. A circle of communication involves following a child's lead with interest, responding in some way, and the child then responding to the parental initiative. The child's response closes the circle. In very simple communications, such as with a 4- to 6-month-old, a parent may get just 1 or 2 circles. By 15 or 16 months, it should be possible to get 20 or 30 closed circles in a row, as the baby takes a parent by the hand, walks to the refrigerator, and points to the door, or tries on a hat and has fun imitating a caregiver's or therapist's gesture.

A difficulty in two-way communication processes in older children may show up as a problem in controlling aggression. The core problem may be that gestural communication was never negotiated. For example, most children learn to comprehend limits from gestures, not from words. By 16 or 17 months, the look on Daddy's face or a pointing finger will tell most babies whether they are safe or in danger. Toddlers can gauge approval or disapproval based on this, because they possess a more complex version than the 4- to 12-month level of two-way communication. Two-way communication establishes very important behavioral parameters.

SHARED MEANINGS

The third core process involves the level of shared meanings, when, by 18 to 24 months, a baby is learning to use representations (symbols or emotional ideas) to comprehend his or her world. In pretend play, children use phrases such as "Me mad," "Me sad," "Give me that." Any time words convey intentionality or play involves representations or symbols that have emotional themes or content, the child has moved into this third level of shared meanings. A child who does well at the early level of engagement and has two-way gestural communication may have a problem at this higher level. The problem could be fantasy related. A child who is withdrawn and seems to be unattached could be fearful that if he gets close to people they will bite him. A 3½-year-old who has a fantasy of being bitten will pull away from people. Therapists cannot immediately assume that what they see in front of them is necessarily the essence of the problem. A complete diagnostic workup is needed to discern what is happening at the level of shared meanings and symbols.

EMOTIONAL THINKING

The fourth process is representational differentiation, or emotional thinking. From about ages 2½ or 3 to about 4½ to 5 years, children learn to categorize shared meanings. They categorize units of thought or ideas into different configurations. They see connections between images or representations or symbols. They can categorize in dimensions of time—what is now; what is in the future; what is in the immediate past. This ability is critical for limit-setting and impulse control—"Something I do now is going to impact on you later," or "If I do this, I'll be punished later." They also begin to categorize in terms of space—"what is immediately in front me; what is in the next room; what is around the corner?" This capacity is critical, because knowing that mother is in the next room and not in California makes a child feel much more secure. To be able to conceptualize a sense of space and distance and to define what is "me" and what is "not-me," what is inside me and what is outside me (a child's basic boundary), what is reality and what is fantasy, all relates to what is self and what is nonself. Emotional thinking also includes the ability to categorize different emotional themes: What is dependency? What is aggressiveness? What is assertiveness? What is the difference between healthy assertiveness and destructive aggressiveness? Children at this age are learning to make these kinds of distinctions and categorize these sorts of experiences.

In addition, children are learning to integrate feeling and thought. A younger child can talk sadly yet look happy, and the therapist may not think anything is wrong. The 2-year-old may be gleeful while saying "Die, die." But if a 4-year-old behaves the same way, the therapist should wonder, "Hey, what isn't working here?" The 4-year-old should have an integration of the idea and the emotion.

In a number of areas, categorizations of units of intrapsychic life allow a child to begin to make connections and to reason between them. The 4½-year-old can figure out, "I hit Johnny because yesterday he hit me." The reasoning incorporates both time and feelings—a piece of anger in one time interval relates to a piece of anger in another time interval. Or, "I didn't get what I wanted, therefore, I'm mad." As development continues into latency and adolescence, it is this fourth process, the ability to categorize and make connections and various permutations of these connections, that gets more sophisticated and evolves into the ability to deal with the peer group and form an identity.

It is important to note that each of these new organizational levels puts demands on the infant to organize new types of experience. For example, engaging the animate world or caregivers and becoming emotionally involved and dependent on human relationships demands that the infant adjust to the unpredictable behaviors, mood shifts, and frustrations of a real person. While children can bang a block on the kitchen floor and reliably hear a sound, they may not get back a vocalization or receive a hug every time they vocalize or reach out invitingly with the arms. When infants learn to use words and can form an internal picture of the mother, they now rely on their word and their picture to convey certain internal feeling states, such as security. The language and symbolic mechanisms underlying this representational ability initially may not be as reliable as mother's continuing physical (and tactile) presence. Auditory or verbal sequencing difficulties or sensory hyper- or hyporeactivity in any modality can easily compromise such emerging symbolic capacities. Yet at the same time, the ability to engage as well as the ability to represent or symbolize experience provides enormous flexibility and new adaptive range for the growing infant. In this respect, and new level of organization is, indeed, a double-edged sword.

CASE EXAMPLE

Observing the Four Developmental Levels in a 3-Year-Old: A 3-year-old girl would hardly look at, and would not talk to, the therapist. However, she was clearly warmly engaged with her father and held onto him as if he were a security blanket. She came along readily with him into the playroom, and when he invited her to play, she said, "Play with me," and indicated her desire to get down on the floor and play with him. She was attentive to her toys and held several dolls very tightly. She was also very attentive to her father and made sure he was in view. If anyone else came near her, she would both hug her dolls and want to either touch her father or be near him. As the therapist tried to talk to her or show her toys, she tended to tune in only to what she was most interested in—her daddy and her dolls. With great effort, she could pay attention to another person; she could listen to a voice or exchange gestures. She was attentive and could focus for a few minutes on what she wanted to, but she was unable to move around and take in, visually and auditorily, the room, all the people in the room, or the toys in the room; nor could she move smoothly and easily from one attentional realm to another.

She engaged her father very warmly and used him as her security whenever something intruded or made her feel scared. However, she hardly spoke a word; if other people in the room talked or moved around, she gave her father mostly looks or smiles, or tentative and frightened glances.

She related warmly to the dolls, but had a difficult time engaging new people; she tended to look at them fleetingly but would not talk to them. She would place the dolls inside or outside the doll house; she answered questions with "yes" or "no." When her father started to play with her, he had to do all the talking. He also had to carry out all the action for her; she would say only "yes," "no," or just nod.

While she slowly warmed up, she kept herself less than fully engaged with the interviewer. She did smile and giggle, but a sense of reserve constrained her range of warm, pleasurable feelings. In contrast, there was a sense of involvement and connection between the girl and her father, although he, too, was rather constricted in his range of affect and did not show a lot of exuberance or pleasure.

In terms of two-way communication, she was initially quite passive: She let her father initiate the dialogue. For example, he would say, "Do you want to play with this doll or that doll?" She would nod or shake her head or occasionally say "yes" or "no." Communication even with him was limited to closing one or two circles. She would respond to his questions with some circle-closing answers but would not elaborate or show any inclination to continue the dialogue. Even though she tended to be passive and cautious, there was a sense that she was aware of what she wanted to do. Her verbal responses were quite deliberate, and from her passive position she orchestrated the drama that her father played out around her. She behaved similarly with the clinician about 15 minutes into the session. She was gradually becoming more relaxed.

As the clinician exchanged simple gestures with her, he sought to expand the range of the gestures to include different themes, such as exploration, conflict, aggression, and warmth. She was able to engage cautiously in each. In her drama that dealt with aggression, for example, she stomped on "the monster" with her foot and had her doll attack the monster, but she closed only 2, 3, or 4 circles in a row, instead of 10 or 20, as one would expect at her age. She abruptly switched themes, which suggested that aggression made her anxious. She was able to mobilize a verbal component to her gestural signals, however, by responding to "why" questions with low-level answers, such as responding to "Why does the boy want to be in the house?" with "he wants to eat dinner." When she played out a theme of dependency, she fed the dolls repetitively, but she did not develop the theme further. She evidenced a constriction in her range of affect at the gestural level and was unable to close many circles in a row.

She showed the ability for both representational elaboration and differentiation (i.e., the ability to connect ideas). When asked who gets angry at her, she was able to say "Mommy and Daddy"; when her father asked her "Why?" she said, "Because I wouldn't share my ice cream." She had a few instances of elaborate representational play, when, for example, she wanted the doll to go to sleep in the house and wanted to put various other animals into the house. She seemed to have a plan in mind. But she did not spontaneously elaborate on any related themes. Either her father or the clinician constantly had to engage her and help her be representational.

Therefore, she was capable of shared attention, very gradual engagement, two-way gestural communication, representational elaboration, and the early stages of representational differentiation. At each stage, however, she evidenced a significant constriction in the range of affect and depth and elaboration of the drama or dialogue. She often depended on the other person to move her from one theme to another. She was more comfortable with themes of dependency than themes of aggression. While she was able to stomp joyfully on the monster, she changed themes quickly afterward. She continued and developed the dependency themes more easily. Her father seemed similarly tense and constricted. Mother was not present in this session, but she, too, tended to avoid assertiveness and tended to be anxious and overprotective.

Through this case example, we can see how, in a relatively short period of time, the clinician can observe how a child does or does not evidence the capacities associated with each stage of development. We also see how the clinician can look at the depth and range of theme dealt with at each level as well as the degree to which they are elaborated (number of circles opened and closed in a row). The child just described was consistent in behavior over a number of sessions. These patterns were also consistent with her history. Not surprisingly, she was having difficulty interacting, talking, and playing with peers in her preschool program. A plan was developed for her parents to help her become more elaborate at each stage and to become more comfortable with aggression and assertiveness.

Different factors influence the four processes described earlier and illustrated in this case example. These factors determine whether an infant and his or her family successfully negotiate these levels of development. As indicated earlier, these factors include constitutional-maturational and family patterns.

Constitutional-Maturational Patterns

The clinician should observe the following constitutional-maturational characteristics during assessment.

1. Sensory reactivity, including hypo- and hyperreactivity in each sensory modality (tactile, auditory, visual, vestibular, olfactory)
2. Sensory processing in each sensory modality (e.g., the capacity to decode sequences, configurations, or abstract patterns)
3. Sensory affective reactivity and processing each modality (e.g., the ability to process and react to degrees of affective intensity in a stable manner)
4. Motor tone
5. Motor planning

An instrument to clinically assess aspects of sensory functions in a reliable manner has been developed and is available (DeGangi & Greenspan, 1988, 1989a, b).

Sensory reactivity (hypo- or hyperreactivity) and sensory processing can be observed clinically. Is the child hyper- or hyposensitive to touch or sound? The same question must be asked in terms of vision and movement in space. In each sensory modality, does the 4-month-old "process" a complicated pattern of information input or only a simple one? Does the 4½-year-old have a receptive language problem and is, therefore, unable to sequence words he hears together or follow complex directions? Is the 3-year-old an early comprehender and talker, but slower in visual-spatial processing? If spatial patterns are poorly comprehended, a child may be facile with words, sensitive to every emotional nuance, but have no context, never see the big picture (the proverbial "forest"); such children get lost in the "trees." In the clinician's office, they may forget where the door is, or have a hard time picturing that mother is only a few feet away in the waiting room.

In addition to straightforward "pictures" of spatial relationships (i.e., how to get to the playground), they also may have difficulty with seeing the emotional "big picture." If the mother is angry, the youngster may think the earth is opening up and he is falling in, because he cannot comprehend that she was nice before, and she will probably be nice again. Such a child may be strong on the auditory processing side but weak on the visual-spatial processing side.

Children with a lag in the visual-spatial area can become overwhelmed by the affect of the moment. Precocious auditory-verbal skills often intensify the situation. These children, in a sense, overload themselves and do not have the ability to see how it all fits together. Thus, at a minimum, the clinician needs a sense of how the child reacts in each sensory modality, how she processes information in each modality, and particularly, as she gets older, a sense of her auditory-verbal processing skills in comparison to visual-spatial processing skills.

It is also necessary to look at the motor system, including motor tone, motor planning (fine and gross), and postural control. Observing how a child sits, crawls, or runs; maintains posture; holds a crayon; hops, scribbles, or draws; and makes rapid alternating movements will provide a picture of the child's motor system. His security in regulating and controlling his body plays an important role in how he uses gestures to communicate his ability to regulate dependency (being close or far away), his confidence in regulating aggression ("Can I control my hand that wants to hit?"), and his overall physical sense of self.

Other constitutional and maturational variables have to do with movement in space, attention, and dealing with transitions. Further research with the role of these individual differences in an infant's regulatory capacities will pinpoint the processing, reactivity, and motor style that leads to attentional and behavioral problems (DeGangi & Greenspan, 1989a).

As can be seen, the constitutional and maturational variables are one set of influences on children's ability to regulate behavior, affect, and later on, thought. These variables may therefore also be thought of as "regulatory factors" when they are a prominent feature of a disorder of behavior, affect, or thought. Such a disorder may be considered a "regulatory disorder."

Family Contributions

In addition to constitutional and maturational factors, it is important to describe the family contribution with regard to each of the four core processes. If a family system is aloof, it may not negotiate engagement well; if a family system is intrusive, it may overwhelm or overstimulate a baby. Obviously, if a baby is already overly sensitive to touch or sound, the caregiver's intrusiveness will be all the more difficult for the child to handle. Thus we see the interaction between the maturational pattern and the family pattern.

A family system may throw so many meanings at a child that he or she is unable to organize a sense of reality. Categories of me/not-me may become confused, because one day a feeling is yours, the next day it is the mother's, next day it is the father's, the day after it is little brother's; anger may turn into dependency, and vice versa. If meanings shift too quickly, a child may be unable to reach the fourth level—emotional thinking. A child with difficulties in auditory-verbal sequencing will have an especially difficult time (Greenspan, 1989).

The couple is a unit in itself. How do husband and wife operate, not only with each other, but how do they negotiate on behalf of the children, in terms of the four processes? A couple with marital problems still could successfully negotiate shared attention, engagement, two-way communication, shared meanings, and emotional thinking with their children. But marital difficulties could disrupt any one or a number of these developmental processes.

Each parent is also an individual. How does each personality operate vis-à-vis these four processes? While it may be desirable to have a general mental health diagnosis for each caregiver, the clinician also needs to functionally observe which of these levels each caregiver can naturally and easily support. Is the parent engaged, warm, and interactive (a good reader of cues)? Is he or she oriented toward symbolic meanings (verbalizing meanings) and engaging in pretend play, and can the caregiver organize feelings and thoughts, or does one or the other get lost between reality and fantasy? Are there limitations, in terms of these four levels, and if so, what are they?

Each parent also has specific fantasies that may be projected onto the children and interfere with any of the four levels. Does a mother see her motorically active, distractible, labile baby as a menace and therefore overcontrol, overintrude, or withdraw? Her fantasy may govern her behavior. Does a father, whose son has low motor tone, see his boy as passive and inept, and therefore pull away from him or impatiently "rev" him up?

In working only with the parent-child interaction, and not the parent's fantasy, a clinician may be dealing with only the tip of the iceberg. The father may be worried that he has a homosexual son, or the mother may be worried that she has a monster for a daughter (one who reminds her of her retarded sister). All these feelings may be stewing, and they can drive parent-child interactions.

In the first session of a diagnostic workup, I let parents talk about their child; I do not interrupt very much. I listen for their associations. When, for example, they finish telling me what the symptoms are, I say, "Tell me more about Billy." Often elements of their fantasies spontaneously emerge in that first session. In the second meeting I have with a family, I go through the developmental history. I try to learn about their wishes for their baby and how they felt about the baby at each stage and age. I take the parents through the four processes: finding out how they negotiated shared attention and engagement, two-way communication, shared meanings, and emotional thinking. For example, was the child a self-starter who initiated activities and pulled them in, or was the child passive so that they initiated the communication? What was going on in their lives, in terms of what they were thinking and feeling? What was going on in their marriage? Often, fantasies will develop further during this second meeting.

Then I have a third meeting with the parents, which is devoted to them as individuals and as a couple and to the family as a system. I want to know their backgrounds, their emotional makeup, and what they were like as children growing up. In this session, if it hasn't come up before (we now know each other better), they often will talk about their worries; for example, about a brother who was hyperactive and destructive or about a sister who was a show-off or about the way their mothers aggressively criticized them, and how they worry about being too like their mothers. A governing fantasy may emerge that explains why a parent shies away from a baby's aggressiveness (e.g., the parent does not want to be too controlling like his or her own mother). Or, perhaps, a parent is trying not to be as aloof as his or her mother was and is, instead, overly bossy with their 18-month-old. In a similar way, I try to discover, as a part of the family's overall fantasy about itself, the couple's and family's collective fantasies about the new baby.

Infant-Caregiver Relationship Patterns

We have discussed the developmental levels; the constitutional-maturational variables; and the family, couple, and parental characteristics, including the organizing fantasies the parents have about their child, and how this all plays out in the four developmental levels.

Next, we focus on the caregiver-infant relationship. As indicated earlier, it is this relationship that mediates these other variables and, in addition, determines how each of the four developmental processes is successfully or unsuccessfully negotiated.

Often, parents come in with their baby, and I watch the parent-infant interaction in the first session, while I am listening to their concerns. With an older child, a 4-year-old, for example, I have them wait to bring the child in, because I want them to talk freely at the outset.

Usually, I ask each parent to play with their child for at least 15 or 20 minutes, and then I play with the child for about the same amount of time. I look for a pattern of interaction in the context of the four core processes. I also look for the range of emotional themes in each of the four core processes and the stability of these processes. For example, a 4-year-old may be playing out wonderful fantasies of fairy princesses going off to a castle and being tied up by an evil witch and then being saved by the hero. While I am interested in the content, I first keep an eye on how the child is relating with his or her caregiver (and later on with me) as well as the breadth of emotion and the stability of the relatedness.

How are they negotiating shared attention? Is the child attending well until the parent intrudes; then does the child pull away and become distracted? Or is the child only attentive to the toys, marching to his or her own drummer and not attending to the parent? Is the parent laid back and slow to make overtures? Depressed caregivers often talk to their child in slow rhythm with much longer pauses than expected. Sometimes children who are potentially good attenders begin to get preoccupied and distracted because the parent's rhythm is not compelling enough to keep them involved. I may be able to confirm these children's skill when I interact with them myself. Therapists must observe the baby or child with caregivers and with the therapists and then reach a conclusion about the baby, the parent, and how they negotiate each developmental process together.

After observing the quality of shared attention (actually, all the developmental processes are being observed simultaneously), I observe how the child and the parent are engaging. I look at the depth and warmth and the richness of their sense of connectedness, the chemistry between the two of them. Therapists must train themselves to look simultaneously at a multiplicity of issues.

Next, I observe two-way communication, focusing initially on gestural issues. What is the quality of child and parent's eye-to-eye contact, smile-to-smile, affect-to-affect? What is the frown-smile interaction like? Are their motor gestures interactive? Are they opening and closing gestural circles together, or, gesturally, are they each marching to different drummers? In looking at gestures, size and complexity of the pattern also must be observed. Are basic emotions of acceptance, approval, and pride; or rejection, hostility, danger, and bossiness communicated via this system; or is the communication system so constructed that only one of these is being dealt with? In looking at the two-way communication, I am looking at the baby's side, the mother's or father's side, and the interactive pattern.

Next, I look at shared meanings. For example, with a 2-year-old or older, is there pretend play? If so, what is the theme of the play? But before I get to the content of the theme, I look at how elaborate the drama is. Is it a shallow drama of simple dependency, with the dolls hugging—and nothing else happening—or is it a rich drama that is flexible and encompasses a broad range of themes? How deep is the drama, in terms of the complexity of each theme? Is the drama constricted or wide-ranging in terms of affects? Then I look at the content. Is the child predominantly concerned with separation, dependency, aggression, neediness, sexual curiosity, or all of the above, and what happens in the drama? Is the scared child helped or left alone to fend off the tiger or the evil witch?

Last, I look at the level of emotional thinking, the categorization of meanings, and how the child connects different ideas. Is he using "buts" and "becauses"; is he connecting subplots with a larger plot?

At both levels of "ideas," I look at whether the parent supports the symbolic activity or not. Does the parent, when the child is playing out themes of aggression, say, "Oh, you must be tired . . . you must be hungry," thereby changing the theme and distracting the child? Or, when the child is playing out dependency, does the mother pick her up and hug her as opposed to letting her play it out with the dolls? In this instance, the mother may subconsciously be saying to the child "Go back to an earlier level of concreteness and behaving. Don't stay at the symbolic level because symbols are more scary to me than behavior." For some parents, the symbol is more anxiety provoking than the behavior, and they would rather return to a lower level.

Even when a parent stays with the representational or symbolic level, he or she can be more or less reflective. The child says, "Get me my juice now." The unreflective concrete parent says "yes" or "no," indirectly supporting the child's sense of urgency. Even a "no" supports the urgency because the child's demand is taken literally. The reflective parent says "Boy, you sure sound like you need it immediately," thereby helping the child reflect or symbolize the sense of urgency. After a brief discussion, and depending on the circumstances, the parent may get the juice or help the child get it for himself, or let the child accept a delay and wait. The key is the parent's tendency to take his or her child literally or to help the child symbolize. In areas of their own anxieties, parents tend to be more concrete.

While most parents may respond to their child's demanding attitude with a concrete "no," some parents will be concrete in all areas of a child's affects, including sexual curiosity, dependency wishes, interest in assertiveness, and so forth. For example, a child says to a parent, "I want to see your bottom!" An anxious, concrete parent might say, "No! Don't talk that way!" A reflective parent might be concerned with where such a wish has originated and reflectively ask, "Where does that idea or wish come from?" (The parent will be wondering if a brother or sister or friend said something, etc.) After the wish is reflected on, the parent might explain to the child why his or her goal will not be implemented. Interestingly, in looking at degrees of concreteness or degrees of reflectiveness, the clinician can look at which of the child's themes brings forth a reflective or concrete attitude. Average parents would be concrete if their child is too demanding but would deal with sexual curiosity in a reflective way. Very concrete parents would deal with both in a concrete manner.

I next look at how well parents deal with logic and reality. Does the parent give accurate feedback to his or her child and encourage her to elaborate her ideas in a logical way? Or does the parent get avoidant or so mixed up, confused, and lost in the daughter's world that emotional thinking is compromised? Does the parent support the use of "but" and "because" to connect ideas?

Putting the Pieces Together

For each of the four levels, or core processes, it is necessary to look at a child's constitutional and maturational status, the family and parent and couple patterns, and the actual caregiver/parent-child interaction. For each of the four levels, the clinician must look at what is influencing the successful or compromised negotiation at that level. For children 3 years and older, the therapist should reach a conclusion about their processes on all four levels. Children less than age 3, should be assessed on however many levels they should have attained (e.g., 2½-year-olds should have reached the first three levels; 14-month-olds should have attained the first two levels).

Looking at all the variables for each developmental level may seem very complex. However, not every system always contributes equally. In some cases, the maturational system may be the major contributor, and the family may be playing a minor role. In other cases, the parent's projections may be playing the major part, and while there are some unique maturational patterns, they are a minor theme, perhaps setting the stage for some of the parental distortions but not in itself the controlling variable.

Nevertheless, the clinician needs to have a con-

ceptual framework that touches on all these points in order to avoid, for example, dealing with the maturational system and ignoring the family and interactions, or vice versa. If the therapist focuses on just one developmental level (e.g., the current one) and fails to look at others (e.g., the earlier levels), he or she may be missing the predominant issues. If the child is "spacey" and not engaged, and the therapist is dealing with meanings, he or she may be missing the boat. The therapist may play and talk with a child who needs instead to be wooed into a relationship. A distracted, unengaged child's main problem may be conflict at the level of meaning. Successfully engaging the child may not deal with his fear of aggression, being "eaten up."

Therefore, our model looks at the constitutional-maturational, family, and interactive factors, as they influence a series of developmental processes. This model can accommodate and further elaborate many of the currently and historically important research trends in infancy.

For example, there is an important and valuable literature on "temperament" as a way of capturing the infant's innate tendencies. Our focus on specific constitutional and maturational variables attempts to build on what we know about temperament in a new and, we hope, promising manner. Most of temperament research relies on parental reports of the infant's capacities rather than "hands-on" assessment of the infant. In addition, most temperament constructs tend to assume that there is a general tendency within the infant toward such global behaviors as introversion or extraversion. In this model, these global behavioral tendencies are hypothesized to be secondary to highly specific "hands-on" verifiable infant tendencies, such as tactile or auditory sensitivity or motor tone and motor planning difficulties. Furthermore, we seek to relate each maturational tendency to specific developmental processes, which are influenced also by family variables.

In addition, there is a growing literature on attachment difficulties using an experimental paradigm focusing on the infant's reaction to a Strange Situation (Ainsworth, Bell, & Stayton, 1974). This important body of work not only helps categorize caregiver-infant interaction patterns, it relates problems in later childhood to qualities of the infant-caregiver attachment pattern at 1 year of age (which also can be related to earlier caregiver patterns). In our model, we attempt to examine interaction patterns at each of the 6 developmental stages and also relate them not only to caregiver patterns but to the infant's individual variations in terms of physical and maturational differences (an important component of the infant's adaptive capacities).

The goal of the model presented here is to understand how all the relevant factors influence a child's behavior. Behavior is viewed not simply as what a child does, but how he or she organizes experience. As a child's capacity to organize experience changes, new relationships between various family, constitutional-maturational, and interactional factors influence this capacity.

CASE EXAMPLE

Regulatory Problem: A 7½-month-old infant's mother worried that "He cries any time I try to leave him, even for a second. If I'm not standing right next to him when he is sitting on the floor, he cries and I have to pick him up. He's a tyrant. He's waking up four times at night and is a fussy eater. He eats for short bursts [breast-feeding] and then stops eating. I'm feeding him all the time."

The mother was feeling cornered, controlled, manipulated, and bossed around. Her baby was like a *fearful dictator* (therapist's term). She said, "That's the perfect way to describe him." The father was impatient with the mother; he felt that she indulged the baby too much. He was getting "fed up," because she had no time for him.

Mother was frightened of aggression and was very dependent on her own mother. She was very fearful of any discomfort that her baby might experience; she wanted the baby to be happy (meaning no crying). It made her "shake" to think that her baby could be uncomfortable. The father, an angry sort of person, took the opposite approach—a "John Wayne," tough-it-out strategy. In interactions with the baby, each showed his or her characteristic pattern.

The baby was very interactive and sensitive to every emotional nuance. As he came into the room, he immediately caught my eye. We exchanged smiles and motor gestures. He interacted with his parents with smiles, coos, and motor movements. Father intruded somewhat. He would roughhouse until the baby would cry, put the baby down, and then roughhouse again. Mother, in contrast, was very gentle, but she had long

silences between her vocalizations. During her long silences, the baby would rev up, get more irritable, and start whining. This became a pattern—whining with the mother and fearful crying with the father. Even before he could finish his motor gestures or vocalizations, his mother moved in and picked him up, gave him a rattle, or spoke to him. In this way, she undermined his initiative. Even while whining, however, he was interactive and contingent.

Upon physical examination, this baby was sensitive to loud noises as well as light touch on the arms, legs, abdomen, and back. He had a mild degree of low motor tone and was posturally insecure. He was not yet ready to crawl.

From a regulatory perspective, babies who are constitutionally most worrisome are those who are oversensitive to the environment, to normal sounds and sensations, and, at the same time, have poor control over their motor system. Because of their motor immaturity, they are unable to do much to correct their sensitivities themselves. They are passive victims of their own sensory and motor systems.

Mother, terribly frightened of her own and her infant's potential assertiveness, was unable to help her baby learn assertive coping because she was so overprotective. At the same time, however, she was *undernurturing*, evidenced most notably in the empty spaces in the rhythm of her speech. She was not silent consciously. She wanted to do everything possible for her baby, but her own depression and anxiety kept her from having a securing and soothing vocal or gestural rhythm. The spaces in her vocal pattern conveyed a sense of emotional emptiness. At the same time, father was impatient and moved in too quickly. The baby was receiving challenges from all sides.

Related to the mother's patterns were worrisome fantasies that her baby would get sick and not survive. These were related to anger at her own very ambivalent mother. Behind father's John Wayne approach was his relationship to his own austere, strict father. Father had been taught to "control" his needs and longings very early in life.

In terms of mastering the first developmental challenge of shared attention and engagement, the infant's constitutional and maturational patterns did not compromise development. This was an attentive, engaged baby. But at the second developmental stage, intentional communication and assertiveness, he was a passive reactor. He was not learning to initiate two-way communication, to be assertive and take charge of his interactions. His low motor tone was compromising his ability to control his motor movements. His sensory hyperreactivity was compromising his ability to regulate sensation. He was frequently overloaded by just the basic sensations of touch and sound. At the same time, he was not receiving support from his mother through the nurturing and rhythmic caregiving that would foster self-initiative. Father obviously was not supporting assertive communication either.

This family required therapeutic work on a number of fronts simultaneously. We went over the infant's special constitutional-maturational patterns. Hands-on practice helped the parents help their baby be attentive and calm. We worked on how to play with the baby; how to get in front of him and help him to take more initiative. We also worked on how to help mother to be more patient and wait for the baby to finish what he started, and how to support his initiative (e.g., putting something in front of him while he was on his tummy in order to motivate him to crawl and reach). We worked on getting mother to put more affect into her voice and to increase the rhythm and speed of her vocalizations; we worked on getting the father to be more gentle. We explored the parents' own feelings about the interactions—the father's tough upbringing and the mother's fear of her own assertiveness, of her baby being injured, and their own associated family patterns.

Gradually, the baby began to sleep through the night and became more assertive and less clinging and fearful. He also became happier. He was slow to reach his motor milestones, so an occupational therapist began to work with him and to give the parents advice on motor development and normalizing his sensory overreactivity. In 4 months, this infant was functioning in an age-appropriate manner with a tendency toward a cautious but happy and assertive approach to developmental challenges.

Children with Severe Regulatory Problems

A number of children come in with severe communication problems, sensory under- and overreactivity, processing difficulties, motor delays, and "autistic" features, with the diagnosis of per-

vasive developmental disorder or atypical development. Such children often have problems at all of the developmental levels described earlier: attention, engagement, two-way gestural communication, and the symbolization of emotions.

At each developmental level there are problems on all fronts: familial, maturational, and interactional. The constitutional problems with sensory reactivity and processing (of a severe nature, especially auditory-verbal processing), motor tone and motor planning, family system problems, parent-child interaction problems, as well as problems with the parents' own reactions and fantasies about the child, undermine attending, forming relationships, being intentional, and using words or complex symbols and gestures to convey needs or desires. Treatment involves a comprehensive approach. With these children, however, professionals often may try to work with splinter skills at the symbolic level and not enough with the regulatory difficulties and the early levels of engagement, shared attention, and gestural interactions. Four-times-a-week play therapy that focuses on all developmental levels, occupational therapy twice a week (for some children), speech therapy twice a week, parent counseling once or twice a week, and a psychoeducational program 5 half-days a week are elements of a comprehensive program. With such a program, many children we have treated in the last few years have done remarkably well. Within 6 months, for example, withdrawn preschoolers have become comfortable with dependency and closeness, seeking out their parents and learning to be intentional. Within 1 year, they have begun to symbolize affect and become comfortable with peers. Over time, specific severe learning disabilities become the focus of treatment as the pervasive emotional difficulties improve. Compared to children where the focus is on controlling behavior and splinter skills, working comprehensively on the underlying regulatory difficulties and their associated emotional patterns leads to children having greater warmth and spontaneity.

For each case, the clinician must pinpoint the family system dynamics, the parents' fantasies, the baby's constitutional-maturational contributions, and the caregiver-child interactions for each developmental level: attention and engagement, two-way communication, shared meanings, and emotional thinking.

Conclusion

The infant and child's ability can be viewed in the context of sensory, motor, interactive, and family patterns. Each of these variables can, in turn, be viewed in the context of a number of developmental-emotional levels of functioning. This model provides a construct that is sensitive to an infant's individual differences; to family and environmental patterns on the one hand and to the infants' emerging adaptive and psychopathological patterns on the other hand. It provides a bridging construct between genetic, prenatal, perinatal, or early developmental variables and later developmental outcomes. This type of construct may be particularly useful for understanding the developmental course of conditions where multiple etiological factors interact with one another or where the impact of certain etiological factors is part of a dynamic system. It also has implications for constructing a comprehensive treatment approach that can work with the multiple intervening variables that influence the course of development.

REFERENCES

Ainsworth, M., Bell, S. M., & Stayton, D. (1974). Infant-mother attachment and social development: Socialization as a product of reciprocal responsiveness to signals. In M. Richards (Ed.), *The integration of the child into a social world* (pp. 99–135). Cambridge: Cambridge University Press.

Brazelton, T. B., & Cramer, B. G. (Eds.). (1990). *The earliest relationship*. Reading, MA: Addison-Wesley.

DeGangi, G., & Greenspan, S. I. (1988). The development of sensory functioning in infants. *Journal of Physical and Occupational Therapy in Pediatrics, 8*, 3.

DeGangi, G., & Greenspan, S. I. (1989a). The assessment of sensory functioning in infants. *Journal of Physical and Occupational Therapy in Pediatrics, 9*, 21–33.

DeGangi, G., & Greenspan, S. I. (1989b). *Test of sensory functions in infants*. Los Angeles: Western Psychology Services.

Fraiberg. S. (1980). *Clinical studies in infant mental health: The first year of life*. New York: Basic Books.

Greenspan, S. I. (1979). Intelligence and adaptation: An integration of psychoanalytic and Piagetian developmental psychology. *Psychological Issues, 12* (3/4, Monograph 47/48). New York: International Universities Press.

Greenspan, S. I. (1989). *The development of the ego: Implications for personality theory, psychopathology, and the psychotherapeutic process*. Madison, CT: International Universities Press.

Greenspan, S. I. (1992). *Infancy and early childhood: The practice of clinical assessment and intervention with emotional and developmental challenges*. Madison, CT: International Universities Press.

Provence, S. (1983). *Infants and parents: Clinical case reports* (Vol. 2). New York: International Universities Press.

Provence, S., & Naylor, A. (1983). *Working with disadvantaged parents and their children: Scientific and practical issues*. New Haven, CT: Yale University Press.

SECTION III

Clinical Syndromes of Infancy and Early Childhood

34 / Feeding Disorders of Infants and Toddlers

Irene Chatoor

Feeding is an early and significant form of interaction between mothers and infants. Their interactions during feeding have been identified as essential in the understanding of infant development in general (Ainsworth & Bell, 1969; Brody & Axelrod, 1970; Field, 1978) and failure to thrive in particular (Casey, Bradley, & Wortham, 1984).

Failure to thrive is a common and often serious problem in pediatrics. The term describes infants and young children who demonstrate failure in physical growth, often with delay of social and cognitive development. Between 1 and 5% of pediatric hospital admissions in the United States have been reported to exhibit failure to thrive (Berwick, Levy, & Kleinenman, 1982; English, 1978). The diagnosis is made when the child's decelerated or arrested growth results in weight and height measurements that fall below the third percentile on the Boston Growth Standards, or when infants demonstrate a persistent deviation below the established growth curve across 2 major percentiles over time (Woolston, 1985).

In the past, feeding disorders and failure to thrive have been used as separate diagnostic entities. Whereas failure to thrive has been used primarily by pediatricians to describe inadequate growth and development in infants and young children, behaviorists have focused on the treatment of feeding problems. Failure to thrive has a long history as a diagnostic label. Since the beginning of this century, when Chapin (1908) first described it in institutionalized infants, there has been an increasing awareness that organic as well as psychosocial factors can lead to growth failure in infants and young children. This led to a dichotomous approach to failure to thrive: organic and nonorganic FTT. During the last two decades several authors (Budd et al., 1992; Casey, Bradley, & Wortham, 1984; Homer & Ludwig, 1981), have pointed to a third mixed category of failure to thrive that combines organic and nonorganic factors.

The observation of feeding has been of primary importance in understanding how psychosocial factors contribute to feeding problems that lead to growth failure. Various approaches have been proposed to integrate the assessment of feeding with the diagnostic approach to failure to thrive (Linscheid & Rasnake, 1985; Woolston, 1985). Some authors (Chatoor, Schaefer, Dickson, & Egan 1984; Chatoor, Dickson, Schaefer, & Egan, 1985; Lieberman & Birch, 1985) have proposed a developmental line to understand feeding disorders that can be the sequela of, be associated with, or lead to failure to thrive.

Failure to thrive describes a symptom rather than a disorder and is thus analogous to fever, which can be the presenting symptom of various underlying disorders. In order to gain a better understanding of the failure of physical, emotional, and cognitive development in infants and young children, focusing on feeding appears more meaningful. Infants and young children cannot regulate their food intake independently of a caregiver; hence, feeding assumes an important role in the relationship of infants and young children with their primary caregivers, usually mothers. Herein I propose classification of feeding disorders based on the suggestions for diagnostic criteria for psychiatric disorders by Wing (1973, 1979): (1) a limited syndrome can be reliably agreed upon; (2) possible links to etiology, pathophysiology, and underlying processes of normal functioning can be hypothesized; (3) uses of pharmacologic and social treatments depend on proper diagnosis; and (4) diagnosis is linked to prognosis. In addition, most feeding disorders meet criteria for relationship disorders proposed by Anders (1989): (1) symptoms may be expressed by one individual but reflect the relationship and are expressed in relationship tasks; (2) symptoms are problematic and disruptive to the routines of daily living for one or both partners; (3) interactions are assessed as inflexible or insensitive; and (4) the relationship has stagnated or failed to progress along the expected developmental course. Anders points out that a relationship disorder does not preclude that individual psychopathology in one or both partners may coexist.

In keeping with the diagnostic criteria suggested by Wing and Anders, I differentiate three developmental feeding disorders associated with failure to thrive, (1) feeding disorder of homeostasis, (2) feeding disorder of attachment, and (3) feeding disorder of separation (infantile anorexia); and the posttraumatic feeding disorder, which can occur at any stage of feeding development.

Recently, the *DSM-IV* introduced Feeding Disorder of Infancy or Early Childhood as a new diagnostic category. The diagnostic criteria require that the feeding disturbance is manifested by persistent failure to eat adequately with significant failure to gain weight or significant loss of weight over at least 1 month, that the feeding disturbance is not due to an associated gastrointestinal or other general medical condition, and that the onset of the feeding disorder is before age 6 years. These criteria serve as a very useful umbrella diagnosis for the specific feeding disorders I propose.

ing, play, and the regulation of sleep. In a number of studies, Chatoor and associate have used the direct observation of feeding and play to diagnose specific interactional patterns of mothers and infants (Chatoor, Egan, Getson, Menvielle, & O'Donnell, 1988; Chatoor, Getson, Menvielle, & Egan, 1990; Chatoor & Menvielle, 1987). These patterns differentiate feeding-disordered infants from healthy ones and various types of feeding-disordered infants from each other (Chatoor, 1991). Dyadic reciprocity versus dyadic conflict can be observed during feeding as well as during play. It is important to address whether dysfunctional patterns of interaction are observed only during feeding or are evident during play, as well, and whether the regulation of sleep or toilet training is an additional area of conflict.

All these areas of the infant's functioning involve patterns of regulation to which both the infant and the caregiver contribute. Anders (1989) designated six patterns of regulation and regulatory dysfunction: appropriate regulation, overregulation, underregulation, inappropriate regulation, irregular regulation, and chaotic regulation.

Assessment of Feeding Disorders

Each of the feeding disorders should be assessed within the primary relationships of the infant or toddler. It is important to begin the evaluation with an assessment of the current relationship between the infant and his or her primary caregiver including an exploration of the history of that relationship. Then, as Anders (1989) suggested, each of the partners as individuals, including the caregivers' past histories, needs to be evaluated. Finally, the family's socioeconomic background, stresses, and the social support system should be considered.

INFANT-CAREGIVER RELATIONSHIP

The current and past relationship of the infant and his or her caregivers should be evaluated across several areas of interaction, including feed-

INFANT AND CAREGIVERS AS INDIVIDUALS

Next, the assessment has to focus on each of the individuals, the infant and his or her caregivers.

The infant's temperament can be assessed through direct observation and through caregivers' descriptions of him or her. Infants vary greatly in their expression of hunger and satiety and in their ability to self-regulate. Several authors (Plomin, Loehlin, & Fries, 1985) have pointed to the interaction of the genotype and the environment. These authors found "a positive relationship between the Restriction/Punishment factor in the home environment and difficult temperament at 12 months of age, suggesting the possibility of feed back based relationships involving the child's genetic propensities" (p. 398). Scarr and McCartney (1983) have proposed an interesting theory that asserts that people make their own environment. They hypothesize that genotypic differences affect phenotypic differences in three ways: a passive kind provided by biologically related parents, an evocative kind through responses elicited from others, and an active kind through the selection of different environments by different people.

In addition to the infant's temperament, the presence of any organic problems that might interfere with feeding or contribute to the feeding difficulties needs to be assessed. Infants with respiratory or cardiac disease tire out quickly during feeding and impose special demands on the caregivers to regulate their food intake. Infants with anatomic abnormalities of the oropharyngeal and gastrointestinal tract or those with neurologic, metabolic, or renal disease frequently display special feeding problems. Toddlers with autism frequently exhibit extreme food selectivity and impose special demands on their caregivers.

The primary caregivers' psychosocial functioning and their prior relationship history are an important part of the assessment. A depressed mother will be emotionally less available to her infant; an anxious and overwhelmed mother may overreact or misinterpret the infant's cues. A mother caught up in substance abuse may be greatly impaired in her ability to care for her infant.

In addition to assessing the mother's present state of psychosocial functioning, her experience of past relationships with her parents or with other significant people in her life also needs to be explored. Fraiberg, Anderson, and Shapiro (1975) have pointed to the lack of nurturing in the mother's own infancy and childhood and the lack of a satisfying relationship with another emotionally supportive person as contributors to the mother's inability to nurture her infant. A more recent study by Main and Goldwyn (1984) systematically explored the mother's attachment behaviors from her childhood into adult life, revealing that the mother's experience of her own mother as rejecting was related to specific distortions in her cognitive processes, to rejection of her infant, and to the infant's avoidant insecure attachment as observed in the laboratory.

FAMILY SUPPORTS AND STRESSORS

Finally, the family's psychosocial functioning along with its support system and standing within the culture need to be considered. Family problems or socioeconomic stressors may both limit support for maternal caregiving and interfere with the allocation of proper attention and nutrition to the infant. Drotar and Eckerle (1989) reported that families with infants with nonorganic failure to thrive had more problematic relationships and showed lower cohesion and expressiveness than did the families of physically healthy infants. In addition, these families showed less cultural involvement. Altemeier, O'Connor, Sherrod, & Vietze (1985) reported that family stressors differentiated families whose infants were not thriving from those whose infants were developing well. The most common stressor involved the relationship between the infant's mother and father. Other studies have indicated that families of infants with nonorganic failure to thrive (FTT) had lower socioeconomic levels and demonstrated greater social isolation with less help and support for child rearing than was true for families of well-thriving infants (Bithony & Newberger, 1987). Although the exact mechanisms by which the family affects the mother-infant relationship are not known, these studies indicate that, whether directly or indirectly, the problems in family relations and the lack of a social and cultural support system can contribute to dysfunction in the mother-infant relationship.

Developmental Feeding Disorders

Anna Freud (1946) first described a developmental line for eating, which she called "from suckling to rational eating." During this developmental process, the infant and toddler depend greatly on the caregiver for the regulation of food intake. The regulation of eating is internally controlled by cues of hunger and fullness; externally it is influenced by the availability of food, the taste and texture of food, and the emotional experiences during the presentation of food. Any one of these factors can interfere with the healthy regulation of eating. The infant may not perceive signals of hunger because of illness or because of other competing external stimuli. The mother may lack the financial resources to provide the infant with adequate food, she may be too depressed to remember to feed her infant, or the infant may reject the taste or texture of the food presented. The emotional experiences of the infant during feeding may be so stimulating and distracting that he or she cannot focus on feeding, or so low in stimulation that the infant falls asleep and stops feeding.

Because of the multiplicity and diversity of the factors that can contribute to feeding problems at various stages of development, Chatoor et al. (Chatoor, Schaefer, et al., 1984; Chatoor et al., 1985) suggested a developmental classification of feeding disorders associated with failure to thrive. This classification incorporates a multifactorial etiology including various organic as well as psychosocial factors that can create, exacerbate, or be a sequela to the infant's feeding and growth problem. This developmental classification of feeding disorders draws from Greenspan and Lourie's (1981) stages of early infant development and Mahler's (Mahler, Pine, & Bergman, 1975) concept of separation and individuation. Chatoor et al. classify three stages of feeding development in which adaptive and maladaptive behaviors in both the infant and the mother can be identified: homeostasis, attachment, and separation.

FEEDING DISORDER OF HOMEOSTASIS

In the first 2 or 3 months of life, the infant begins to establish regular patterns of sleep arousal, hunger satiation, and elimination. The mother helps to modulate the infant's physiological and affective states by creating an environment responsive to the infant's individual characteristics. By reading and interpreting the infant's cues correctly, the mother helps the infant to reach and maintain the state of quiet alertness necessary for feeding.

Infants with difficult temperamental traits, central nervous system immaturity, or medical illnesses are especially at risk for failing to develop adequate feeding behaviors during this stage. Mothers who are anxious, depressed, or otherwise impaired have difficulty interpreting the infant's cues correctly. Frequently the combination of infant vulnerability and maternal difficulty lead to the severe feeding problems seen at this stage of development. Table 34.1 presents criteria that can diagnose this developmental feeding disorder.

Mother-Infant Interaction: Chatoor, Getson, et al. (1990) studied 74 feeding-disordered infants and toddlers referred for psychiatric evaluation. Of these 8 infants met the just-described criteria for feeding disorder of homeostasis. Their average age was 3 months. These infants were matched by age, sex, and race with 8 infants who were feeding and thriving well. All infants and toddlers were offered 20-minute feeding period followed by a 10-minute play period during which they were videotaped from behind a one-way mirror in two adjacent hospital offices.

Observations were rated on the Feeding and Play Scales developed by Chatoor et al. (1990); these in turn were subjected to discriminant function analysis for the two groups, conducted for each of the 5 subscales of the Feeding Scale and the 4 subscales of the Play Scale. The feeding-disordered group differed significantly from the control group on the first subscale on both scales, a subscale called Dyadic Reciprocity that describes the mutual engagement and positive affect of mother and infant. The feeding-disordered infants appeared less responsive and less connected to their mothers.

Treatment of Infants with Feeding Disorder of Homeostasis: Treatment must be individualized, taking into consideration both the maternal as well as the infant factors that have interfered with feeding. Treatment must be directed toward the infant, toward the mother, and toward the mother-infant interaction. The interventions might range from treating the mother's depression, to introducing nasogastric tube feedings to substitute for oral feedings in an infant who tires easily because of cardiac problems while simultaneously offering a pacifier during these gavage feedings. Bernbaum, Pereira, Watkins, and Peckhom (1983) have shown that regular offering of a pacifier during gavage feedings facilitated the infant's learning to suck and swallow. Later these infants learned to feed more quickly and gained weight faster than did a control group. Furthermore, although both groups of infants were taking in the same amount of milk through gavage feedings, the infants who were stimulated to suck a pacifier seemed to absorb their feedings more effectively.

A second intervention directed toward the infant is the use of sham feedings during gastros-

TABLE 34.1

Feeding Disorder of Homeostasis

Feedings are characterized by poor reciprocity between mother and infant and inadequate food intake.

1. Onset between birth and 3 months of age

2. Irregular feeding pattern and poor food intake:
   a. Intake varies in quantity
   b. Feeding varies in timing

3. Infant shows poor regulation of state:
   a. Irritability or easy fatiguability
   b. Poor sleep or excessive sleepiness
   c. Irregular sleep pattern

4. Parental anxiety; depression; parental psychopathology and/or psychosocial stressors that lead, individually or collectively, to an inability to read the infant's cues

5. Failure to thrive

6. Frequently associated organic problems:
   a. Prematurity, dysmaturity
   b. Cardiac or pulmonary disease
   c. Functional or structural abnormalities of the oropharynx or gastrointestinal tract (cleft palate, gastroesophageal reflux, esophageal atresia, etc.)

tomy feeding in infants with esophageal atresia. In a study of 7 such infants, Dowling (1977) noticed that those who had only gastrostomy feedings for the first months of life had severe difficulties learning how to suck, chew, and swallow. Moreover, these infants seemed to have no awareness of hunger or satiety. Dowling demonstrated that, by introducing sham oral feedings, he could prevent these feeding problems and developmental delays with a second group of infants born with esophageal atresia. During gastrostomy feedings, the mothers were instructed to hold their infants and to have them suck from a bottle with milk that was then collected from an esophageal fistula at the neck. Children who had been fed this way quickly learned to signal their hunger and satiety. The mothers could read these cues and feed the infants accordingly. Once the esophagus was surgically corrected, the infants learned to feed orally without much difficulty.

Mother-infant interactional problems observed during the assessment can be addressed by working with the mother. The therapist and the mother can watch together a videotape of the mother and infant during feeding, at which time the therapist shares observations and helps the mother to become a better self-observer. The therapist serves as an interpreter between mother and infant by reinforcing mutual cueing and helping the mother read her infant's signals more effectively. In the work with the mother, it is important that the therapist focus on positive and contingent maternal reactions to the infant rather than on maladaptive responses. Maternal self-esteem can be undermined all too easily if the mother experiences the therapist as critical.

Early regulation of feeding has a significant impact on the infant's overall motivation and drive (Dowling, 1977). Successful self-regulation of the infant lays the foundation for the next stage of development, whereas feeding difficulties early in life frequently leave infant and mother vulnerable to problems during later stages of development.

FEEDING DISORDER OF ATTACHMENT

From 2 to 6 months of age, social exchanges between mother and infant become more prominent. The infant distinguishes the mother more clearly from other adults and is more likely to actively engage and to elicit social responses from her. During this developmental stage, if the mother is unavailable, depressed, noncontingent in her responses to the infant, or unable to provide an adequate social experience, the infant is at risk for being fed inadequately and for the development of failure to thrive.

The literature on nonorganic failure to thrive has concerned itself primarily with exploring this particular type of disturbance. Much has been written about mothers whose infants suffer from this type of growth disorder. Fishhoff, Whitten, and Petit (1971) found that 10 of 12 mothers with failure-to-thrive infants demonstrated character disorders, whereas only 2 were considered psychoneurotic. Evans, Reinhart, and Succop (1972) have distinguished three groups of parents with failure to thrive infants and classified them along a continuous spectrum of psychopathology.

Fraiberg (Fraiberg et al., 1975) has pointed out how the lack of nurturing in the mother's own infancy and childhood and the lack of a satisfying relationship with another emotionally supportive person together lead to the mother's inability to nurture her infant. Gordon and Jamieson (1979) studied attachment in 12 infants 12 to 19 months old who had been hospitalized during the first year of life with a diagnosis of nonorganic failure to thrive and compared these attachment patterns to those of matched controls. Six of the 12 nonorganic FTT infants and two of the 12 controls were classified as insecurely attached. In addition, nonorganic FTT infants showed marked inhibition of affect during separation from the mother. Powell and Low (1983) described distinct target behaviors that characterized infants with nonorganic FTT: inactivity, irritability, posturing, lack of affect, lack of or decreased vocalizations, poor eye contact, crying when approached, lack of response to human stimuli, and indifference to separation. These behaviors are indicative of the infant's difficulty in mutual engagement. Although these studies do not answer questions of etiology regarding the infant's difficulty in attachment, hospitalization and the affectionate and consistent care by a primary care nurse frequently show that these infants can be engaged successfully.

Table 34.2 presents criteria that can diagnose this developmental feeding disorder.

Mother-Infant Interaction: Twenty infants with failure to thrive classified as attachment disorders who averaged 8 months of age and 20 infants matched by age, sex, and race who were feeding and thriving well were observed with their mothers during 20 minutes of feeding and 10 minutes of play. In both situations the clinical group showed less mother-infant reciprocity as evidenced in less visual and vocal engagement, less physical closeness, and lack of pleasure in their interactions. During the feeding, the mothers of the failure-to-thrive infants were less contingent to the infant's cues, and during the play, they were more oblivious to the infant's activities.

Treatment of Infants with Feeding Disorder of Attachment: Treatment needs to be individualized and should address their physical and developmental needs. Because of the complexity of the issues involved, a multidisciplinary team comprised of a pediatrician, nutritionist, physical or occupational therapist, social worker, and child psychiatrist is generally required. Because of the large number of personnel involved, the seriousness of the disorder, and the degree of malnutrition, hospitalization frequently is necessary. This allows for both a thorough assessment and initiation of nutritional rehabilitation.

During the hospitalization, a number of specialized interventions can be carried out that focus on the infant, including nutritional rehabilitation, development stimulation, and emotional nurturance. It is important to assign a primary care nurse and to limit the number of alternative caregivers as much as possible. The goal is to facilitate a special relationship between the primary caregiver and the infant.

Improvement in the infant's health and affective availability then can be used to capture the mother's interest and engage her more actively in the treatment process in order to form an alliance for treatment after discharge. Because mothers of these infants frequently present with a variety of social and psychological disturbances, their problems need to be explored while work goes on with the infant. Many of these mothers experienced deprivation or losses during their own childhood and, to protect themselves from further hurts, they avoid engaging in any therapeutic relationship. Some mothers are too impaired to move beyond their distrust and avoidance of those who want to help. However, nurturance of the mother is a first and critical step in the treatment in order to facilitate her potential to nurture the infant (Fraiberg et al., 1975). The infant's hospitalization provides a critical time to assess whether the mother can be

TABLE 34.2

Feeding Disorder of Attachment

Feedings are characterized by lack of mutual engagement and pleasure in the relationship.

1. Onset between 2 and 8 months

2. The infant shows lack of age-appropriate social responsivity:
   a. Lack of visual engagement:
      hypervigilance when people are at a distance
      avoidance of eye contact when approached closely
   b. Lack of smiling response
   c. Lack of vocal reciprocity
   d. Lack of anticipatory reaching when picked up (when infant is more than 5 months old)
   e. Lack of molding and cuddling when held

3. Parental depression or personality disorder; high psychosocial stress; drug or alcohol abuse leading (individually or collectively) to lack of affectionate care and feeding of the infant

4. Failure to thrive

5. Development
   a. Delay in motor milestones
   b. Poor muscle tone evidenced by:
      hyperextension when picked up
      surrender posture when held
   c. Delayed cognitive development

engaged in a therapeutic relationship or whether the infant needs to be placed in alternative care.

DISORDER OF SEPARATION (INFANTILE ANOREXIA)

From 6 to 36 months, coinciding with the rapid gains in locomotion, fine motor skills, language acquisition, and capacity for symbolic representation, the infant becomes more aware of him- or herself as a separate individual. With the development of this emerging aspect of the infant's sense of self, and the new demands he or she places on the environment, mother and infant must negotiate in general issues of autonomy and parental control. While the infant is transitioned to self-feeding, mother and infant need to negotiate in particular who is going to put the spoon in the infant's mouth.

In 1983, Chatoor and Egan published a clinical report on the diagnosis and treatment of an eating disorder that starts during the developmental period of separation and individuation and is characterized by food refusal or extreme food selectivity and undereating. They called it a separation disor-

der and later, because of its similarities to anorexia nervosa, infantile anorexia nervosa (Chatoor, 1989; Chatoor, Egan, Getson, Menvielle, & O'Donnell, 1988). Later Chatoor called it infantile anorexia (Chatoor et al., 1992). The onset of this disorder is usually between 6 months and 3 years, with a peak onset around 9 months of age. The parents report a history of the infant's food refusal or extreme food selectivity and undereating in spite of all efforts to increase food intake. The feeding difficulties stem from the infant's thrust for autonomy. Mother and infant become embroiled in conflicts over autonomy and control, which manifest primarily during the feeding situation. This leads to a battle of wills over the infant's food intake. Characteristically, parents mention that they have tried "everything" to get the infant to eat—usually coaxing, cajoling, bargaining, distracting, or forcing food into the infant's mouth. This separation-related conflict interferes with the infant's development of somatopsychological differentiation as described by Greenspan and Lieberman (1980). The process of learning to distinguish somatic sensations, such as hunger and satiety, from emotional feelings, such as affection, anger, or frustration, is clouded by noncontingent responses by the parent to cues coming from the infant. As a result of this confusion of somatic and psychological feeling states, the infant's eating is controlled by his or her emotional experiences with the caregiver instead of by his or her physiological needs. This situation leads to primarily external regulation of eating.

Table 34.3 presents criteria that can diagnose this developmental feeding disorder.

Mother-Infant Interaction: The study of 42 infants with infantile anorexia nervosa who averaged 20 months of age and 30 control subjects matched by age, sex, and race revealed significant differences in mother-infant interactions between the two groups (Chatoor, 1991; Chatoor, Egan, et al., 1988). The feeding-disorder group demonstrated less dyadic reciprocity, less maternal contingency, more dyadic conflict and struggle for control. This group's play also was characterized by less dyadic reciprocity, more dyadic conflict, less maternal responsiveness to the infant's needs, and more maternal intrusiveness.

Parental Characteristics: The clinical assessment revealed two major groups of mothers who seemed unable to negotiate issues of autonomy versus dependency successfully with their infants during this developmental phase of separation and individuation. One group of mothers seemed to be more comfortable with the infant's autonomy during play but had developed a "blind spot" when dealing with the infant during feeding. These dyads usually had experienced some transient feeding difficulties when the infant was ill, which seemed to have "sensitized" the mother to worry excessively about the child's growth. These mothers seemed to feel insecure in their parental role and measured their competence by how well the infant ate. Because of high anxiety during feeding, these mothers were unable to read the infant's cues correctly. Feeding became an increasingly frustrating task as the youngster refused to eat in an effort to assert more autonomy and control.

Another group of mothers reported intense conflicts and/or lack of appropriate limit setting by their own parents during their growing years, which frequently had continued into their adult years. They had been informed of poor childhood eating behaviors by their mothers or remembered their own battles over food during childhood. They did not want to be harsh and punitive like their own parents, but they lacked the emotional experience of alternative role models. These un-

TABLE 34.3

Feeding Disorder of Separation (Infantile Anorexia)

Feeding is characterized by food refusal by the infant and by lack of appropriate limit-setting by the caregiver. This leads to conflict, struggle for control, or bargaining.

1. Onset between 6 months and 3 years, during infant's transition to self-feeding

2. Food refusal by infant:
    a. Varies from meal to meal
    b. Varies among different caregivers

3. Parent's anxiety about infant's food refusal expressed by:
    a. Coaxing infant to eat more
    b. Distracting infant with toys or by playing games to induce infant to eat
    c. Feeding infant around the clock, including at night
    d. Trying different types of food if infant does not eat
    e. Force-feeding infant

4. Failure to thrive:
    a. Initially loss of weight or lack of weight gain
    d. Gradually stunting of linear growth resulting in dwarfism

5. Development:
    a. Delay in motor development in severe cases secondary to malnutrition
    b. Delay in expressive speech in some infants who appear to refuse to talk as they refuse to eat
    c. Cognitive development progresses well

resolved conflicts over control interfered with these mothers' ability to set appropriate limits with their youngsters. In addition, these mothers had difficulty reading their own cues of hunger and fullness and tended to regulate their eating externally. Likewise, they had difficulty reading their infants' cues and felt responsible for their food intake.

Infant Characteristics: Many infants with this disorder were observed to show intense interpersonal sensitivity and reactivity to social exchanges with their caregivers. They appear so involved in the external world that they seem oblivious to internal cues of hunger. Many mothers report that from early on, these infants showed little interest in feeding. In addition to this interpersonal sensitivity, these infants are characterized by persistence and stubbornness. They pose a great challenge to their caregivers, particularly in the second year of life, when they become assertive in general and during feeding in particular.

Treatment of Youngsters with Feeding Disorder of Separation: Treatment is focused on helping the parents negotiate issues of autonomy and control with their toddlers in order to facilitate internal regulation of eating.

The intervention consists of six stages:

1. Form a therapeutic alliance with the mother.
2. Reframe the infant's difficult temperament.
3. Reassure parents about the infant's cognitive development.
4. Discuss developmental conflicts of the infant.
5. Advise parents on how to change the infant's feeding behavior.
6. Discuss limit-setting for inappropriate behaviors of the infant.

It is evident that many of these mothers reexperienced with their infants feelings of ineffectiveness and helplessness they had suffered during their childhood with their parents; accordingly, the therapeutic process begins in the initial interview with the parents. As Bromwich (1990) outlined in describing treatment of parent-infant interactions, the first stage should be support of parental self-confidence, because high self-esteem and self-confidence in the role of parent decreases tension and increases the mother's sensitivity to other's cues. From the first contact of

the therapist with the infant and his or her parents, the primary goal is empowerment of the parents (Chatoor et al., 1992). An empathic approach is necessary to allow these mothers to open up to the therapist, to share their struggles with the infant, and to admit to their difficulty around limit setting. Only after this groundwork has been done can direct psychoeducational intervention begin.

The second stage occurs at the end of the evaluation, when the therapist meets with both parents to share the results of the assessment. The therapist compares the mother's description of the infant's temperament with his or her own observations of the infant in the office or laboratory. The infant's interpersonal sensitivity is discussed as an asset but also as a vulnerability. The therapist explains how the infant becomes so caught up in interpersonal interactions that it appears difficult for him or her to focus on his or her internal state of hunger or fullness. Consequently the parents have to work extra hard not to engage in distracting interactions during feeding, in order to allow the infant to become more internally focused. Then the therapist discusses the infant's "stubbornness" in a similar way, as both an asset and a challenge to the parents because the infant wants to be in control at all times. The "little executive" is discussed as somebody who needs firm limit setting in order to allow this characteristic to become a positive drive instead of the driving force of an oppositional disorder.

After this discussion of the infant's specialness, the infant's developmental level is addressed. Many parents of FTT infants are highly educated and have heard or read about the developmental delays in infants with failure to thrive. Interestingly, there has been no correlation between malnutrition and developmental deficits in infants with this disorder. The child's developmental level is discussed, and if appropriate, the parents are reassured that in this type of failure to thrive, the malnutrition does not appear to affect the infant's cognitive development. This is a critical part of the intervention. The fear of developmental deficits secondary to the infant's poor food intake is a driving force behind the parents' efforts to get the infant to eat through noncontingent behaviors, such as distracting, bargaining, cajoling, or even force-feeding.

After discussion of the infant's temperament and developmental level, the therapist explores the conflict in the mother-infant relationship from a developmental point of view. The therapist helps the parents understand the conflicts between autonomy and dependency during this developmental period—the wish of the infant to self-feed but still have mother's attention. The parents are helped to understand how the food refusal serves both sides of this conflict. By refusing to accept the food offered by the mother, the infant feels independent and in control, and by getting the mother anxiously engaged in all kinds of distractions and bargaining, the infant has all the attention he or she wants. Consequently, the infant will not give up the food refusal.

Following the explanation of the infant's developmental conflicts, parents are provided with behavioral techniques that allow the infant more autonomy during feeding, while setting limits on inappropriate, maladaptive behaviors. They are given general "food rules": (1) facilitate self-feeding by offering finger food, a second spoon, or a little dish with food while feeding the infant; (2) feed the infant at regular times and do not offer milk and snacks between these regular meal and snack times in order to allow the infant to experience hunger; and (3) limit mealtimes to 30 minutes and terminate the meal earlier if the infant refuses to eat, plays with the food without eating, throws food or eating utensils in anger, or does so in order to provoke the parents. To facilitate somatopsychological differentiation, to help the infant distinguish physiologic hunger for food from emotional hunger for attention, the parents are encouraged to separate mealtimes from playtimes. They are asked to deal with the infant's intake in a neutral matter, neither playing games to distract the infant in order to sneak a bite into the infant's mouth nor exaggerating their approval for every mouthful swallowed. Parents also are requested to withhold expressions of disapproval and frustration if the infant eats little or nothing. They are reassured that experiencing hunger is the only means of inducing the infant to eat. In this way, the infant's attention can be focused on his or her inner state of hunger or satiety rather than on interactions with the parents. Parents are encouraged to introduce a playtime after the meal to provide the attention they had previously showered on the infant when trying to induce him or her to eat.

Each of the food rules is discussed to give the parents a chance to see whether they are comfortable with it and can implement it at home. Frequently, mothers anticipate intense protest and provocative behaviors by their toddler. Discipline in the form of "time out" has to be discussed in detail with most parents to help them deal with their toddler more effectively. At the end, the parents are asked how much time they want to practice the new rules before they check in with the therapist again. Working through these six stages can take from 2 to 8 sessions.

Parents who are able to support one another can apply this approach, and usually, within a few days or weeks, they succeed in changing the infant's eating pattern. However, parents who are in conflict with one another, or mothers who continue to struggle with unresolved issues of control stemming from their own childhood, cannot follow through with these behavioral instructions. In these cases, the second phase of treatment can involve couples' therapy to address these unresolved marital conflicts or individual psychotherapy for the mother to deal with her struggle over control by bringing out the "ghosts" from her childhood, as Fraiberg et al. (1975) described so pointedly. Some parents are resistent to therapy and change. Long-term follow-up of these infants is not available at this time.

Rumination Disorder

Rumination is a syndrome characterized by the regurgitation of food, which then may be partially or completely rechewed, reswallowed, or expelled. Frequently the infant inserts a hand in the mouth to initiate the process. Later he or she may be able to bring up the food by arching the back, sucking the tongue, or contracting the abdominal muscles. The syndrome is observed most commonly in infants. Although rumination is much more prevalent among the mentally retarded, it also has been described in children and adults of normal intelligence. More recently, rumination has been reported in adults in association with bulimia nervosa (Fairburn & Cooper, 1984; Larocca, 1988). In infants rumination can lead to electrolyte imbalance, weight loss, dehydration, and death. In older children and adults the condition is usually of a more chronic nature.

The term *rumination* was introduced by Freund in 1903, who considered it a form of pylorospasm. Since then there has been much controversy in the literature regarding both the etiology and the treatment of this syndrome. When Grulee did the first review of the world literature on rumination in 1917, he was able to identify only 6 cases. He concluded that the condition was due to hyperexcitability of the involuntary muscles and that treatment should consider the psychic needs of the child. Cameron (1925) illuminated the condition by his descriptions of the ruminating infant and his conceptualization of the ruminating behavior as "learned." He recognized that rumination does not spring full-blown and that before the infant achieves dexterity, rumination differs little from vomiting. A review of the world literature by Williams (1955) demonstrated a wide variety of hypotheses about rumination. By then, some researchers considered it to be an anatomical problem causing reflux, a condition to be treated by thickening of the formula and positioning the child erect. At that time rumination was treated with mechanical restraints such as arm splints, jaw stabilizers, tight head bonnets, or chair straps. Some used local anesthetics to the throat, esophagus, and stomach. Williams himself suggested treating the "spastic hyperkinetic infant" with antispasmodics and sedation. Since then four major approaches to the understanding of rumination and its treatment have emerged: organic, physiological, psychodynamic, and behavioral.

ORGANIC APPROACH

Herbst, Friedland, and Zboraliski (1971) propose that rumination can be one of the symptoms of gastroesophageal reflux. They reported 3 cases of rumination that showed no signs of maternal deprivation but radiographically demonstrated a sliding hiatal hernia with reflux. Through special radiographic techniques such as cinefluorography, they were able to observe that the classic sucking movements of the tongue and mouth occurred after the entire esophagus was markedly distended with refluxed barium. They concluded that these oral maneuvers appeared to result in opening of the superior esophageal sphincter, allowing some barium to enter the mouth, and that subsequent deglutition initiated a peristaltic wave that emptied the esophagus of refluxed barium. They also concluded that the oral movements could have been performed by the patient in an attempt to empty the esophagus of refluxed gastric contents or reflexively, as a response to retrograde esophageal dilation.

PHYSIOLOGICAL APPROACH

Based on their experience with two adult women, a 33-year-old with a lifetime rumination history and a 23-year-old with rumination and bulimia, Blinder, Bain, and Simpson (1986) postulated that opiate receptor insensitivity or reduced endorphinergic transmission may be implicated in rumination. In both women, paregoric, an opiate agonist, totally inhibited postingestive rumination, whereas naltrexone administered intravenously inhibited this opiate agonist effect. Premeal administration of both intravenous metochlopramide and oral haloperidol (Haldol) also abolished rumination. This effect was also blocked by intravenous naloxone.

PSYCHODYNAMIC APPROACH

Within a psychodynamic formulation as described by Stein (Stein, Rausen, & Blau, 1959), rumination is seen as a somatic symptom of an unsatisfactory mother-infant relationship. It develops when the infant, who has limited ability to express psychic disturbance, uses the somatic pathway to relieve tension. In his paper on psychosomatic problems in infants, Lourie (1955) described the "pleasurable, voluntary and habitual act of rumination as the infant's recoil from the environment and the people in it." He was the first to point out that overstimulation as well as understimulation, and too much environmental tension as well as too little environmental satisfaction "make it unsafe for the infant to maintain investment in the love object"; thus, of necessity, the infant turns to his or her own body for satisfaction.

When a poor mother-infant attachment relationship exists, a mother may either not be able to meet her infant's needs for stimulation or may be unable to screen out excess stimulation. An infant who is unable to evoke appropriate responses from mother may well turn to rumination as a tension-releasing and self-soothing activity. Rumination in infants has been described in connection with poor attachment of the infant to the mother or as a consequence of the partial or total unavailability, of the primary caregiver (Chatoor, Dickson, & Einhorn, 1984).

BEHAVIORAL APPROACH

Advocates of the behavioral approach believe that rumination is a learned behavior. Learning theory focuses on the consequences of behavior. The concept of reinforcement is used to explain the strengthening or maintenance of desirable as well as undesirable behavior. If other more positive attention is lacking, then the attention that follows rumination, even in the form of disapproval, can be a powerful reinforcer (Winton & Singh, 1983).

A number of treatment methods have been developed based on the assumption that rumination is a learned habit, that is, an operant that is maintained by a consequence and that has to be unlearned by counterconditioning (Lavigne & Burns, 1981).

AN INTEGRATED BIOPSYCHOSOCIAL MODEL
FOR RUMINATION

Rumination is a disorder that can be seen along a continuum. At one end of the spectrum, a patient might have gastrointestinal pathophysiology, such as a hiatal hernia and reflux, and little psychopathology. At the other end of the spectrum would be the converse, where a patient might have no organic gastrointestinal pathology and severe psychopathology in the relationship with the primary caregiver. In infants, an organic illness not necessarily related to the gastrointestinal tract, such as otitis media, might lead to vomiting. At some point the infant seems to learn to initiate

the vomiting him- or herself and turns it into rumination in an effort to achieve self-regulation.

The primary caregiver, usually the mother, plays an important role in the infant's self-regulation. A perceptive mother will adjust the infant's environment to provide adequate stimulation, while protecting the infant from overstimulation and helping the baby to relieve tension. If something interferes with the development of a mutually gratifying relationship between mother and child or if something interrupts their relationship, the infant turns to rumination as a way of self-regulation. At times, the pathology may lie in the mother, stemming from deprivation in her own background; at other times, the tension of the parents' marital relationship, the loss of an important relative, or the social circumstances with which the mother struggles may not allow her to be as sensitive to the infant's needs as is required at that time. On the other hand, some infants have innate difficulties in achieving self-regulation. Infants with a labile autonomic nervous system may present with problems of disregulation of the respiratory and gastrointestinal tract; infants with reflux or with autism require extraordinary care to facilitate better regulation. Apparently, when infants either fail to elicit or lose loving attention or tension-relieving responses from the caregiver, they resort to rumination as a means of self-soothing and relief of tension.

Once infants discover rumination as a means of self-regulation, it may develop into a habit that is difficult to break. Like other symptoms, such as body rocking, head banging, or hair pulling, rumination can take on the form of a habit disorder.

The following hypothesis is proposed:

Rumination stimulates the endogenous opioid system and leads to relief of tension and self-soothing. The infant, child, or adult resorts to rumination as a means of self-regulation when the external world is not able to gratify vital needs. Once established, rumination becomes addictive and takes the form of a habit disorder.

This hypothesis gains support from the study by Blinder et al. (1986), and from animal studies by Herman and Panksepp (1978) on the role of opioids in the mediation of social attachments. "Opioids" (also called endorphins) are endogenous peptides that act like morphine or heroin in the central nervous system. Experiments with guinea pigs demonstrated that morphine, an opiate agonist, produced powerful dose-dependent decreases in separation distress vocalizations emitted by both infant and juvenile guinea pigs tested in social isolation; on the other hand, naloxone, an antagonist, increased separation distress. They also found that morphine decreased the amount of time a juvenile guinea pig chose to remain in close proximity with its mother, suggesting that agonists may be capable of replacing a function normally served by endorphins in the maintenance of social attachments. Panksepp, Herman, and Conner (1978) postulate that endorphins mediate social attachment and that an infant becomes physiologically dependent on its mother for endorphin stimulation. Separation triggers endogenous endorphins withdrawal. Administration of morphine, an opiate agonist, may act as a physiological substitute for the caregiver, whereas naloxone may simulate the separation from mother by stimulating endogenous endorphin withdrawal. The history of ruminating infants frequently reveals either a lack of attachment or a disruption of the attachment between mother and infant.

In the context of Herman and Panksepp's hypothesis of the mother's important role in endorphin stimulation in the infant, it can be assumed that these infants either fail to develop endorphins or suffer from endorphin withdrawal when the mother-infant relationship is disrupted. Rumination can be understood as a self-initiated activity by the infant to stimulate endorphin production and achieve self-regulation. Once rumination has been learned, the endorphin hypothesis helps explain its addictive quality.

TREATMENT

Proposed methods of treating rumination have been as diverse as theories concerning its etiology. Besides the surgical interventions and the early use of mechanical restraints, treatment has been primarily psychodynamic, behavioral, or a combination of both.

A number of treatment methods have been based on the assumption that rumination is a learned habit—that is, an operant maintained by a consequence, and one that therefore has to be

unlearned by counter conditioning. Lang and Melamed (1969) reported using electric shock with a 9-month-old infant, after extensive treatment involving dietary changes, restraints, and considerable nurturance by the nursing staff had failed to stop the rumination. Others have reported successful treatment by electric shock (Bright & Whaley, 1968; Linscheid, Thomas, & Cunningham, 1977). Since the shock treatment introduces a punishment procedure that may cause resistance in the parents and in the hospital staff, a number of alternative behavioral treatment approaches have been developed over the last few years. Aversive taste stimuli (lemon juice or hot sauce) have been put on the infant's tongue during rumination to serve as a negative conditioner for this maladaptive behavior (Becker, Turner, & Sajwaj, 1978; Sajwaj & Agras, 1974). Others have addressed rumination by combining aversive and reward stimuli. Upon initiation of rumination, they placed two drops of hot sauce on the infant's tongue and set the infant down in the crib. The positive reward comes (Murray, Keele, & McCarver, 1976) as soon as the tongue movements stop; at that point they attend to the infant and pick him up again.

Lavigne and Burns (1981) point to difficulties inherent in using aversive taste stimuli as punishment. Since the rumination frequently occurs when the infant is out of the caregiver's reach, the infant is not getting a consistent response; indeed, he or she is on a variable ratio schedule that can delay learning. They also found that some infants become adapted to these aversive taste stimuli. These authors suggest programs of both social rewards and punishments. Immediately upon rumination, the procedure combines scolding and time out, shouting "no," placing the infant down, and leaving the room for 2 minutes. If the infant is not ruminating upon the caregiver's return, he or she is picked up, washed, and played with as a reward. After the baby is hospitalized briefly, the authors report that this treatment could be carried out by the parents on an outpatient basis.

Richmond, Eddy, and Green (1958) were early proponents of a psychodynamic approach based on the assumption that rumination is symptomatic of a disturbance in the mother-child relationship. They found that mothers of ruminating infants often had marital conflicts or personality problems that interfered with their ability to relate appropriately to their babies. Others (Stein et al., 1959) who have followed this approach have suggested that the infant be cared for by a nurturing mother substitute while mother is being helped through psychotherapy to deal with her own problems.

Before any one treatment is considered, Chatoor, Dickson, and Einhorn (1984) point to the importance of looking at each child individually. The observation of mother and infant during feeding and during play can provide valuable information as to how much pleasure mother and infant derive from each other, and how effectively the mother responds to signs of distress or tension in the infant. The diagnostic evaluation needs to determine whether the infant has learned to expect little gratification from caregivers and has turned to rumination as a means for self-regulation in the service of relief of tension, or, whether the infant uses rumination for self-stimulation, or both. It is also important to look at organic factors, such as reflux, that might contribute in a major way to the development and maintenance of this pattern. As Chatoor and Dickson (1984) demonstrated, treatment needs to be individualized according to the meaning of the infant's symptom and the dynamics of the parent-infant relationship.

Posttraumatic Feeding Disorder

In severe cases, this feeding disorder is characterized by total food refusal; in milder cases, by the refusal to accept or swallow textured food. It is seen most commonly in infants who have been medically ill, such as those who have undergone painful manipulation of the oral cavity by insertion of tubes or vigorous suctioning, who have experienced pain during feeding because of refluxesophagitis, or who have had episodes of gagging and choking during feedings. Infants who have undergone such adverse experiences appear to associate anything related to feeding with pain, and they show fear in anticipation of feedings. Some show distress when approached with a bottle or become fearful when touched in the perioral area. In some infants, the anticipatory fear of being fed is so severe that they cry or vomit at the sight of the bottle or the high chair. On the other hand, some parents report that when these infants are drowsy and unaware of what they are doing, they are able to drink from the bottle.

From a study of 5 latency-age children, Chatoor, Conley, and Dickson (1988) observed that one incident of choking was enough to lead to severe fear of eating and choking and resulted in food refusal. Although the parents did not consider the choking event as very serious or life threatening, these children developed many of the symptoms of a posttraumatic stress disorder: They were preoccupied with the fear of choking and dying; they dreamed of choking or dying; and they avoided any activity that could be associated with choking. Some were afraid to go to sleep out of fear of choking to death. One girl would sit up in bed propped up by several pillows and refuse to lie down to sleep out of fear that her loose tooth would come out during her sleep and choke her.

It is difficult to say what the inner experience of a young nonverbal infant may be. However, the affective expressions of infants provide a window to their inner life. These infants' behavior clearly indicates that they are frightened and that the fear seems to be aroused by the anticipation of eating. Since this fearful refusal to eat frequently follows traumatic oral experiences, this author has called it a posttraumatic feeding disorder (Chatoor et al., 1992). In severe cases it is characterized by refusal to have anything put in the mouth, and in milder or in partially treated cases by refusal to chew or swallow solid food. If such infants are forced to open their mouth and if they then are fed forcefully, severe distress is triggered and they become even more fearful the next time around. Their fear seems to override any awareness of hunger; in severe cases, infants will become so dehydrated as to threaten life unless fed via a nasogastric or gastrostomy tube. In cases where infants refuse solids but takes liquids, nutrition might not be a problem.

Table 34.4 presents proposed diagnostic criteria for posttraumatic feeding disorder.

In time, secondary complications of this feeding disorder develop. If infants refuse to put anything in their mouth over weeks, months, or years, they do not get any practice in sucking, chewing, and swallowing. They do not learn how to move their tongue in the side of the mouth and move

TABLE 34.4

Posttraumatic Feeding Disorder

Feedings are characterized by total food refusal or refusal to eat or swallow textured food. The infant shows distress if pressured into feeding, but otherwise mother and infant show good reciprocity.

1. Rather sudden onset
   a. After an episode of choking
   b. After medical illness or after medical procedures associated with pain of the oropharynx or esophagus, such as gastroesophageal reflux, insertion of feeding or endotracheal tubes, or suctioning of the oropharynx

2. Infant appears to associate feeding with pain leading to:
   a. Total food refusal (severe cases)
   b. Anticipatory anxiety about putting bottle or food in mouth (infant cries at sight of high chair, bottle, or spoon)
   c. Crying, gagging, choking or vomiting when force-fed

3. Infant appears to associate swallowing textured food with pain (milder or partially treated cases) expressed by:
   a. Drinking liquids but refusing textured food
   b. Accepting textured food but holding it in cheecks and spitting it out later
   c. Crying, gagging and chocking when force-fed

4. Parental anxiety secondary to food refusal by infant

5. Dehydration and acute weight loss in severe cases

6. Delay in oral motor development secondary to lack of practice in feeding

7. Secondary behavioral feeding problems

---

food effectively to the pharynx to be swallowed. When infants finally relax enough and put food in the mouth, they frequently choke and gag. This evokes old fears, and again they refuse to accept food in the mouth.

In addition, as these infants mature cognitively, they become more aware of cause and effect in their interactions with caregivers. They learn to anticipate certain emotional responses and behaviors in caregivers, whether the children refuse to eat or whether they put some food in the mouth. The food refusal usually arouses such intense feelings of anxiety, anger, or frustration in the parents that they try anything to get these infants to eat, including coaxing, cajoling, bargaining, pleading, distracting, or forcing food down an infant's throat. Since nothing seems to work, the parents become inconsistent, trying one method after another, and feeding time becomes a highly emotional experience for infant and parent. The infant learns to exercise control over the parents' emotions and behaviors by opening or closing the mouth. This severely interferes with an infant's development of somatopsychological differentiation (the ability to differentiate somatic sensations such as hunger or satiety from emotional feeling states, such as need for affection, feelings of anger

and frustration). Earlier this was described as an important developmental milestone during the transition to self-feeding, which occurs during the developmental phase of separation. The secondary complications of the lack of development of oropharyngeal coordination and of somatopsychological differentiation perpetuate the feeding disorder.

In some cases the picture becomes mixed, particularly in toddlers or young children, where symptoms of a posttraumatic feeding disorder are combined with infantile anorexia. In these cases, a child initially may refuse to eat textured food out of fear of choking but then become engaged in a battle of wills over eating with a parent who is unable to deal with the child's food selectivity (Chatoor et al., 1992).

TREATMENT

All the complicating factors just described must be considered if treatment is to be effective. As a first step, it is important to help the parents understand the dynamics of a posttraumatic feeding disorder, and to become active participants in the treatment. Treatment of the infant involves three steps: desensitization, introduction of food, and regulation of food intake.

Desensitization: The infant needs to be desensitized to the fear of eating. This is best done after thorough exploration of what seems to trigger anticipatory anxiety about eating. Frequently the sight of the bottle or placement in the high chair are enough to distress the infant. In these cases, these objects should be presented without being associated to feeding until the infant is comfortable and can tolerate being exposed to them. If the infant is frightened to be touched around the mouth, the mother should engage in pleasurable touching until the infant is comfortable opening the mouth, mouthing a toy, or can take a spoon without fear. Since mothers are frequently so upset by their child's problem that it is hard for them to break out of old patterns, a professional may have to initiate the desensitization process and model for the mother. Once the infant is able to mouth toys without fear, food can be introduced.

Introduction of Food: It is important to begin with water so the child does not associate feeding with milk. Also, the infant might have difficulty with oropharyngeal coordination and might gag or choke; this is less likely and less harmful when drinking water. Once the infant is comfortable with drinking water, juices and then milk can be introduced. Some infants respond better to smooth semisolids such as yogurt, pudding or ice cream. Infants or toddlers who can participate in the feedings are less anxious if they are given a spoon and a dish, and when they are encouraged to self-feed. It is very important that a professional assess the infant's oromotor coordination and work with the infant directly on chewing and swallowing semisolids that dissolve in the mouth, before any type of textured food is introduced that can lead to choking. Again, a hierarchy of solid food should be followed. Meats should be kept until last in order to avoid frightening choking experiences. During this stage the emphasis is on teaching the infant oromotor skills. Since many infants like to imitate, modeling the placing of food in the mouth and how to chew and swallow is very helpful. As long as the infant works on desensitization and oromotor coordination, there should be no emphasis on the amount of food taken in, and positive reinforcement should be given liberally to newly acquired skills; for example, "You opened your mouth nicely, that was good chewing, good swallowing."

Regulation of Food Intake: Once the infant has fairly good feeding skills, the experience of hunger becomes an important new goal. This is the time to work on the regulation of tube feedings. Continuous infusion at night and fewer bolus feedings during the day need to be considered to make the infant hungry at feeding time. During this time it is also important to cut down on the volume of the tube feedings in order to stimulate hunger. This is best done at regularly planned 2- to 4-week intervals. During this transition the infant might lose some weight; however, it is important that parents do not exert pressure on the infant to eat more; rather they must allow him or her to learn how to regulate intake according to physiological needs. Usually this step requires time and patience.

In summary, posttraumatic feeding disorder has become a new challenge in the treatment of severely ill infants. Many intertwining factors contribute to this severe feeding disorder, and successful intervention generally requires an integrated multidisciplinary team approach.

Pica

Pica is defined as the persistent eating of a nonnutritive substance. Infants and toddlers with this disorder typically eat plaster, paint, paper, clothing, hair, animal droppings, sand, or pebbles. The onset of pica is usually during the toddler age, between 12 and 24 months. Since young infants mouth objects quite commonly, it is difficult to make the diagnosis of pica in the first year of life. Millican et al. (1962), who surveyed the prevalence of pica in three groups of children age 1 to 6 years, reported that pica occurred in 32% of a black low-income group, in 10% of a white middle- and upper-income population, and was the highest, 55%, in a group of children hospitalized for accidental poisoning. The prevalence of pica dropped sharply in both high- and low-income groups after the age of 3 years. Wortis et al. (1962) reported that out of 272 premature infants they followed, at the age of 30 to 33 months 22% had pica. Millican et al. (1968) postulated that the higher incidence of pica in the black low-income group was due partially to the cultural acceptance of pica. They observed that 63% of mothers with children with pica had pica themselves. Gutelius, Millican, Layman, Cohen, and Dublin (1962) reported that 87% of children with pica had either mothers and/or siblings with pica.

The most common complication of pica is lead poisoning from the ingestion of paint or paint-soaked plaster. Neurologic complications of chronic lead poisoning may present with hyperactivity, short attention span, mental retardation, and convulsive disorder. Other complications are the development of a bezoar, a ball of hair, plant, or undigestible chemical substances that can lead to intestinal obstruction (Barnhard & Mittleman, 1986). One study (Marchi & Cohen, 1990) suggested that a history of pica in early childhood increases the risk for subsequent eating disorders (anorexia nervosa and bulimia nervosa) in adolescence.

Various hypotheses have been proposed to explain the phenomenon of pica. Organic, psychodynamic, socioeconomic, and cultural factors have been implicated in the etiology of this disorder. There are reports of pica induced in rats by iron deficiency (Woods & Weisinger, 1970) or by a low-calcium diet (Jacobson & Snowdon, 1976). Some clinical studies confirm the association between iron deficiency and pica (Ghaziudin & McDonald, 1985; Reynolds, Binder, Miller, Chang, & Horan, 1968), whereas Gutelius et al. (1962) concluded in a double-blind study, that intramuscular iron was no more effective than saline injection in reducing pica. In young children pica has been associated with relative environmental deprivation (Madden, Russo, & Cataldo, 1980) or parental psychopathology (Lourie, 1977). Singhi, Singhi, and Adwani (1981) have reported on the role of psychosocial stress in the families of children with pica and found a strong association with maternal deprivation, parental neglect and child beating, impoverished parent-child interactions and disorganized family structure. Vermeer and Frate (1979) have pointed to the cultural acceptance of pica, especially in rural families of African lineage. Millican, Dublin, and Lourie (1979) propose a

multifactorial etiology where constitutional, developmental, emotional, socioeconomic, and cultural factors interact with each other. They observed that young children with pica showed a high degree of other oral activities, such as thumb sucking and nail biting. They interpreted the ingestion of inedible substances as a distorted form of instinctual seeking of gratification and as a defense against the loss of security caused by lack of parental availability and nurture. They report that these children experienced frequent separations from one or both parents, followed by replacement by inadequate or rapidly changing caregivers. In addition, the investigators observed that the mothers seemed to encourage oral gratification in response to the child's expression of anxiety or distress. In response to the infant's distress, the mothers would offer the pacifier or the bottle with milk as substitute for their personal involvement in helping the infant cope.

Millican, Dublin, and Lourie (1979) also stress the seriousness of this disorder. The younger children were, as a group, somewhat retarded in their use of speech and showed conflicts about their dependency needs and aggressive feelings. Half of the adolescents evidenced some degree of depression, and several had personality disorders, primarily of passive dependent borderline or type. Many continued to engage in other forms of oral activity such as thumb sucking, nail biting, aberrant food habits, and tobacco, alcohol, and drug abuse.

TREATMENT

Treatment must reflect the various factors that appear to contribute to this disorder. Lourie (1977) proposed a psychoeducational treatment approach. Mothers need to be taught the dangers of pica and helped to become more available to their children. This requires social support for the mothers, who may be economically deprived and socially isolated. The mother's depression or other psychopathology need to be addressed before she will be able to nurture and supervise her infant or toddler more adequately. The child's nutritional state needs to be monitored, and any iron deficiency or lead poisoning needs to be treated.

REFERENCES

Ainsworth, M. D., & Bell, S. M. (1969). Some contemporary patterns of mother-infant interactions. In A. Ambrose (Ed.), *Stimulation in early infancy.* New York: Academic Press.

Altemeier, W. A., O'Connor, S. M., Sherrod, K. B., & Vietze, P. M. (1985). Prospective study of antecedents for nonorganic failure to thrive. *Journal of Pediatrics, 106,* 360–365.

Anders, T. F. (1989). Clinical syndromes, relationship disturbances and their assessment. In A. J. Sameroff & R. N. Emde (Eds.), *Relationship disturbances in early childhood* (pp. 125–144). New York: Basic Books.

Barnhard, J. S., & Mittleman, R. E. (1986). Unusual deaths associated with polyphagia. *American Journal of Forensic Medical Pathology, 7,* 30–34.

Becker, J., Turner, S., & Sajwaj, T. (1978). Multiple behavioral effects of the use of lemon juice with a ruminating toddler age child. *Behavior Modification, 2,* 267–272.

Bernbaum, J. D., Pereira, G. R., Watkins, J. B., & Peckham, G. J. (1983). Nonnutritive sucking during gavage feeding enhances growth and maturation in premature infants. *Pediatrics, 71,* 41–45.

Berwick, D. M., Levy, J. C., & Kleinerman, R. (1982). Failure to thrive: Diagnostic yield of hospitalization. *Archives of Diseases of Childhood, 57,* 347–351.

Bithony, W. G. & Newberger, E. H. (1987). Child and family attributes of failure to thrive. *Journal of Developmental and Behavioral Pediatrics, 8,* 32–36.

Blinder, B. J., Bain, N., & Simpson, R. (1986). Evidence for an opiod neurotransmission mechanism in adult rumination. *American Journal of Psychiatry, 143,* 225.

Bright, G. O., & Whaley, D. L. (1968). Suppression of regurgitation and rumination with aversive agents. *Michigan Mental Health Bulletin, 2,* 17–21.

Brody, S., & Axelrod, S. (1970). *Anxiety and ego formation in infancy.* New York: International Universities Press.

Bromwich, R. M. (1990). The interaction approach to early intervention. *Infant Mental Health Journal, 11,* 66–79.

Budd, K. S., McGraw, T. E., Farbisz, R., Murphy, T. B., Hawkins, D., Heilman, N., & Werle, M. (1992). Psychosocial concommitants of children's feeding disorders. *Journal of Pediatric Psychology, 17,* (1), 81–94.

Cameron, H. C. (1925). Forms of vomiting in infancy. *British Medical Journal, 1,* 872–876.

Casey, P. H., Bradley, R., & Wortham, B. (1984). Social and nonsocial home environments and infants with nonorganic failure to thrive. *Pediatrics, 73,* 348–353.

Chapin, H. D. (1908). A plan of dealing with atrophic infants and children. *Archives of Pediatrics, 25,* 491–496.

Chatoor, I. (1989). Infantile anorexia nervosa: A developmental disorder of separation and individuation. *Journal of the American Academy of Psychoanalysis, 17,* 43–64.

Chatoor, I. (1991). Diagnosis, mother-infant interaction, and treatment of three developmental feeding disorders associated with failure to thrive. Institute II: A Developmental Perspective on Eating Disorders from Infancy to Adulthood. Presented at the annual meeting of the Academy of Child and Adolescent Psychiatry.

Chatoor, I., Conley, C., & Dickson, L. (1988). Food refusal after an incident of choking: A posttraumatic eating disorder. *Journal of the American Academy of Child and Adolescent Psychiatry, 27,* 105–110.

Chatoor, I., & Dickson, L. (1984). Rumination: A maladaptive attempt at self-regulation in infants and children. *Clinical Proceedings Children's Hospital, 40,* 107–116.

Chatoor, I., Dickson, L., & Einhorn, A. (1984). Rumination: Etiology and treatment. *Pediatric Annals, 13,* 924–929.

Chatoor, I., Dickson, L., Schaefer, S. & Egan, J. (1985). A developmental classification of feeding disorders associated with failure to thrive: Diagnosis and treatment. In D. Drotar (Ed.), *New directions in failure to thrive: Research and clinical practice* (pp. 235–258). New York: Plenum Press.

Chatoor, I., & Egan, J. (1983). Nonorganic failure to thrive and dwarfism due to food refusal: A separation disorder. *Journal of the American Academy of Child Psychiatry, 33,* 294–301.

Chatoor, I., Egan, J., Getson, P., Menvielle, E., & O'Donnell, R. (1988). Mother-infant interactions in infantile anorexia nervosa. *Journal of the American Academy of Child and Adolescent Psychiatry, 27,* 535–540.

Chatoor, I., Getson, P., O'Donnell, R., Menvielle, E., & Egan, J. (1990). *The development of observational scales for mother-infant interactions.* Scientific Proceedings of the annual meeting of the American Academy of Child and Adolescent Psychiatry, 56.

Chatoor, I., Kerzner, B., Zorc, L., Persinger, M., Simenson, R., & Mrazek, D. (1992). Two-year old twins refuse to eat: A multidisciplinary approach to diagnosis and treatment. *Infant Mental Health, 13,* 252–268.

Chatoor, I., & Menvielle, E. (1987). *The assessment of feeding and play behaviors of infants and young children under the age of three.* Scientific Proceedings of the Annual Meeting of the American Academy of Child and Adolescent Psychiatry, 18.

Chatoor, I., Schaefer, S., Dickson, L., & Egan, J. (1984). Nonorganic failure to thrive: A developmental perspective. *Pediatric Annals, 13,* 829–843.

Chatoor, I., Schaefer, S., Dickson, L., Egan, J., Conners, C. K., & Leong, N. (1984). Pediatric assessment of nonorganic failure-to-thrive. *Pediatric Annals, 13,* 844–850.

Dowling, S. (1977). Seven infants with esophageal atresia: A developmental study. *Psychoanalytic Study of the Child, 32,* 215–256.

Drotar, D., & Eckerle, D. (1989). The family environment in nonorganic failure to thrive: A controlled study. *Journal of Pediatric Psychology, 14,* 245–257.

English, P. C. (1978). Failure to thrive without organic reason. *Pediatric Annals, 7,* 774–781.

Evans, S. L., Reinhart, J. B., & Succop, R. A. (1972). Failure to thrive: A study of 45 children and their families. *Journal of the American Academy of Child Psychiatry, 11,* 440–457.

Fairburn, C. G., & Cooper, P. J. (1984). Rumination in bulimia nervosa. *British Medical Journal, 288,* 826–827.

Field, T. (1978). The three R's of infant-adult interactions: Rhythms, repertoires and responsivity. *Journal of Pediatric Psychology, 3,* 131–136.

Fishhoff, J., Whitten, C. F., & Petit, M. G. (1971). A psychiatric study of mothers of infants with growth failure secondary to maternal deprivation. *Journal of Pediatrics, 79,* 209–215.

Fraiberg, S., Anderson, E., & Shapiro, V. (1975). Ghosts in the nursery. *Journal of the American Academy of Child Psychiatry, 14,* 387–421.

Freud, A. (1946). The psychoanalytic study of infantile feeding disturbances. *Psychoanalytic Study of the Child, 2,* 119–132.

Freund, W. (1903). Uber Pylorusstenose im Sauglingsalter. *Mitteilungen Grenzoebiet Medicine Chirturgie, 11,* 309–326.

Ghaziuddin, N., & McDonald, C. (1985). A clinical study of adult coprophagics. *British Journal of Psychiatry, 147,* 312–313.

Gordon, A. H., & Jamieson, J. C. (1979). Infant-mother attachment in patients with non-organic failure to thrive syndrome. *Journal of the American Academy of Child Psychiatry, 18,* 251–259.

Greenspan, S. I., & Lieberman, A. F. (1980). Infants, mothers and their interaction: A quantitative clinical approach to developmental assessment. In S. I. Greenspan & G. H. Pollock (Eds.), *The course of life, Vol. 1: Infancy and early childhood* (pp. 271–312). Bethesda, MD: National Institute of Mental Health.

Greenspan, S. I., & Lourie, R. S. (1981). Developmental structuralist approach to classification of adaptive and pathologic personality organizations: Infancy and early childhood. *American Journal of Psychiatry, 138,* 725–735.

Grulee, C. G. (1917). Rumination in the first year of life. *American Journal of Diseases of Children, 14,* 210–218.

Gutelius, M. F., Millican, F. K., Layman, E. H., Cohen, G. J., & Dublin, C. C. (1962). Children with pica: Treatment of pica with iron given intramuscularly. *Pediatrics, 29,* 1012–1023.

Herbst, J., Friedland, G. W., & Zboraliski, F. F. (1971). Hiatal hernia and rumination in infants and children. *Journal of Pediatrics, 78,* 261–273.

Herman, B. H., & Panksepp, J. (1978). Effects of morphine and naloxone on separation distress and approach attachment: Evidence for opiate mediation of social effect. *Pharmacology, Biochemistry, and Behavior, 9,* 213–220.

Homer, C., & Ludwig, S. (1981). Categorization of etiology of failure to thrive. *American Journal of Diseases of Children, 135,* 848–851.

Jacobson, J. L., & Snowdon, C. T. (1976). Increased lead ingestion in calcium deficient monkeys. *Nature, 162,* 51–52.

Lang, P. J., & Melamed, B. G. (1969). Avoidance conditioning therapy in an infant with chronic ruminative vomiting. *Journal of Abnormal Psychology, 74,* 1–8.

Larocca, F. E. (1988). Rumination in patients with eating disorders. *American Journal of Psychiatry, 145,* 1610.

Lavigne, J. V., & Burns, W. J. (1981). Rumination in infancy: Recent behavioral approaches. *International Journal of Eating Disorders, 1,* 70–82.

Lieberman, A., & Birch, M. (1985). The etiology of failure to thrive: An interactional developmental approach. In D. Drotar (Ed.), *New directions in failure to thrive* (pp. 250–277). New York: Plenum Press.

Linscheid, T. R., & Rasnake, L. K. (1985). Behavioral approaches to the treatment of failure to thrive. In D. Drotar (Ed.), *New directions in failure to thrive* (pp. 279–294). New York: Plenum Press.

Linscheid, T. R., Thomas, R., & Cunningham, C. E. (1977). A controlled demonstration of the effectiveness of electric shock in the elimination of chronic rumination. *Journal of Applied Behavior Analysis, 10,* 500–563.

Lourie, R. S. (1955). Treatment of psychosomatic problems in infants. *Clinical Proceedings Children's Hospital, 2,* 142–151.

Lourie, R. S. (1977). Pica and lead poisoning. *American Journal of Orthopsychiatry, 41,* 697–699.

Madden, N. A., Russo, D. C., & Cataldo, M. F. (1980). Environmental influences on mouthing in children with lead intoxication. *Journal of Pediatric Psychology, 5,* 207–216.

Mahler, M. S., Pine, F., & Berman, A. (1975). *The psychological birth of the human infant.* New York: Basic Books.

Main, M., & Goldwyn, R. (1984). Predicting rejection of her infant from mother's representation of her own experiences: Implications for the abused abusing interactional cycle. *Child Abuse & Neglect, 8,* 203–217.

Marchi, M., & Cohen, P. (1990). Early childhood eating behaviors and adolescent eating behavior. *Journal of the American Academy of Child and Adolescent Psychiatry, 29,* 112–117.

Millican, F. K., Dublin, C. C., & Lourie, R. S. (1979). Pica. In J. D. Noshpitz (Ed.), *Basic handbook of child psychiatry, Vol. 2: Disturbances in development* (pp. 660–666). New York: Basic Books.

Millican, F. K., et al. (1968). Study of an oral fixation: Pica. *Journal of the American Academy of Child Psychiatry, 7,* 79.

Millican, F. K., et al. (1962). The prevalence of ingestion and mouthing of nonedible substances by children. *Clinical Proceedings Children's Hospital, 18,* 207–214.

Murray, M. E., Keele, D. K., & McCarver, J. W. (1976). Behavioral treatment of rumination: A case study. *Clinical Pediatrics, 15,* 591–596.

Panksepp, J., Herman, B., & Conner, R. (1978). The

biology of social attachments: Opiates alleviate separation distress. *Biological Psychiatry, 13*, 607–617.

Plomin, R., Loehlin, J. C., & Fries, J. C. (1985). Components of "environmental" influences. *Genetic and Environmental Psychology, 21*, 391–402.

Powell, G. F., & Low, J. (1983). Behavior in nonorganic failure to thrive. *Journal of Developmental and Behavioral Pediatrics, 4*, 26–33.

Reynolds, R. D., Binder, H. J., Miller, M. B., Chong W. W., & Horan, S. (1968). Pagophagia and iron deficiency anemia. *Annals of Internal Medicine, 69*, 435–440.

Richmond, J. B., Eddy, E., & Green, M. (1958). Rumination. *Pediatrics, 22*, 49–55.

Sajwaj, J. L., & Agras, S. L. (1974). Lemon juice therapy: The control of life threatening rumination in a six month old infant. *Journal of Applied Behavior Analysis, 7*, 551–563.

Scarr, S., & McCartney, K. (1983). How people make their own environments: A theory of genotype-environmental effects. *Child Development, 54*, 424–435.

Singhi, S., Singhi, P., & Adwani, G. B. (1981). Role of psychosocial stress in the cause of pica. *Clinical Pediatrics, 20*, 783–785.

Stein, M. L., Rausen, A. R., & Blau, A. (1959). Psychotherapy with an infant with rumination. *Journal of the American Medical Association, 171*, 2309–2316.

Vermeer, D. E., & Frate, D. A. (1979). Geophagia in rural Mississippi: Environmental and cultural contexts and nutritional implications. *American Journal of Clinical Nutrition, 32*, 2129–2135.

Williams, C. G. (1955). Rumination in a Bantu baby. *South African Medical Journal, 29*, 692–695.

Wing, J. K. (1973). International variations in psychiatric diagnosis. *Triangle, 12*, 31–36.

Wing, J. K. (1979). The concept of disease in psychiatry. *Journal of the Royal Society of Medicine, 72*, 316–321.

Woods, S. C., & Weisinger, R. S. (1970). Pagophagia in the albino rat. *Science, 169*, 1334–1336.

Woolston, J. (1985). Diagnostic classification: The current challenge in failure to thrive research. In D. Drotar (Ed.), *Research and clinical practice* (pp. 225–233). New York: Plenum Press.

Wortis, H., Rue, R., Heimer, C., Braine, M., Redlo, M., & Freedman, A. M. (1962). Children who eat noxious substances. *Journal of the American Academy of Child Psychiatry, 1*, 537–547.

35 / Disorders of Affect in Infancy and Early Childhood

Leon Cytryn and Donald H. McKnew, Jr.

Theoretical Framework

Comprehensive studies have now confirmed the high prevalence of anxiety and depressive disorders in the general adult population (Robins & Regier, 1991; Weissman, Leaf, & Tischler, 1988; Weissman, Leckman, Merikangas, Jammon, & Prusoff, 1984). Furthermore, most of these adults follow a chronic and intermittent course, despite improved psychotherapeutic and psychopharmacological efforts. These medical conditions cause not only untold emotional suffering to the patients and their families but also great financial loss to the families and society in general. These facts have stimulated interest in primary prevention as a fruitful approach to diminishing the prevalence of these disorders.

This approach has led to the investigation of ever younger children who might have either full-blown mood disorders or identifiable precursors. Several factors have encouraged such investigations. First, we have discovered that many adults with depressive or anxiety disorders can date the early signs or the full clinical picture of their illness to prepubertal and in some cases preschool years. Second, the children of parents with depressive and anxiety disorders have been found to have a significantly higher incidence of such disorders than the general population (Weissman et al., 1984). Conversely, in studying young children with depressive or anxiety disorders, often the same or similar disorders are found in their parents and other first-degree relatives.

Depression in young children most commonly presents as a dysthymic disorder, but it also can appear as a major depressive disorder. Only rarely do we see young children with bipolar disorder.

In the same way, anxiety in young children most commonly presents as school phobias or other variants of separation anxiety, agoraphobia, avoidant disorder, and overanxious disorder. In studying and treating affectively disturbed young children, investigators have found that their parents report significant signs or symptoms of such disorders dating back to toddlerhood and even infancy. Such findings were among several developments that have led to the now-burgeoning field of infant and toddler psychiatry, which in turn has given rise to the field of developmental psychopathology. This discipline concerns itself with integrating the vast body of knowledge about the interaction of human development with the natural course of mental illness. This new approach provides the theoretical framework for this chapter on affective disorders.

We must clarify our use of the term *affective disorder.* This term often is used as a synonym for depression or mood disorders. In this chapter, however, the term *affective* is used to cover anxiety as well as depressive phenomena, both of which involve disorders of affect. This approach seems justified because in infants, anxious and depressive affects often cannot be differentiated. Also, as is discussed in other chapters, there is a strong linkage (comorbidity) of anxiety and depressive disorders in childhood.

Developmental Issues

AFFECTIVE DEVELOPMENT

Many of the factors that determine future emotional development are already present at birth. According to the differentiation hypothesis of emotional expression, only two basic emotions are present at birth: undifferentiated distress and excitement (Bridges, 1932). All the remaining emotions gradually evolve from these two, based on the maturation of the central nervous system and life experiences. In contrast, the discrete-emotions view holds that the neural substrate for all emotions is already present at birth, and many of their characteristics (primarily facial expres-

sions) can be elicited and observed even in early infancy (Izard, 1978). Proponents of both these theories agree that with the passage of time, emotions become more differentiated and more complex as they become connected to cognitive growth and language development and become increasingly internalized. Already in the first 7 to 9 months of life, observable emotions include anger, sadness, interest, fear, joy, and surprise. Obviously, the whole gamut of affects is crucial to both normal and abnormal personality development and functioning. We choose, however, to focus our attention on fear and sadness, which are the basis of affective disorders.

These same potentially pathological emotions serve crucial adaptive functions and are indispensable to the personality development of infants and toddlers—even to their very survival. The same fear that underlies all anxiety disorders in later life has a crucial survival role of signaling to the mother (or caregiver) that her child is in danger. In the same way, sadness, which underlies all depressive disorders in later life, elicits a positive emotional response in the form of nurturing, which may be crucial in maintaining an empathic bond between parent and child.

In the second year, cognitive growth promotes the first appearance of the additional emotions of guilt, shame, contempt, and shyness. These emotions also have adaptive functions; further, they are crucial to moral development and vital to the survival of society. In early infancy these emotional states largely serve as signaling functions, and their expression is dependent on external events (Lazarus, Canner, & Folkman, 1980). They become, however, gradually internalized by the growing child, largely because of cognitive growth that enables the process of self-object differentiation.

During this gradual process of elaboration and internalization of affects, several milestones herald specific stages of development. Somewhere around the eighth month of life, both separation anxiety and fear of strangers appear in most infants. These phenomena represent expectable developmental processes, which grow out of the child's ability to differentiate between self, parents, and other people. As a rule, these processess may last until the third or even the fourth year of life, proceeding alongside infant socialization.

While childhood depression generally has been recognized as a separate disorder for only about 25 to 30 years, over the past century several child psychoanalysts have studied in great detail the development of depressive states in infants and young toddlers.

OBJECT RELATIONS

According to object relations theorists, there is little differentiation between the mother and the child in the first 3 months, even though it is recognized that an infant can recognize his or her mother already in the first week of life (Brazelton, Koslowski, & Main, 1974). In the following months the infant becomes increasingly aware of distinct differences between self and mother (Spitz, 1962). This process of differentiation culminates at about 8 months of age, when the previously mentioned phenomena of separation and stranger anxiety appear. In the ensuing months, the baby continues to move away from mother visually and literally in an effort to learn about the world around him or her, while still maintaining a strong tie to mother, who continues to function as a safe harbor (Mahler, Pine, & Bergman, 1975). In addition to attaining their own identity, infants begin to view the mother as a whole person, who contains both "good" nurturing qualities as well as "bad" punitive qualities. A process called object constancy is attained at about 1 year of age (Solnit, 1982).

During the second year of life, the phase of so-called separation-individuation continues, with the infant making increasingly bold forays to explore the environment while returning periodically to the safety of the mother. If the mother rebuffs the child's periodic returns to her (rapprochement), mistaking it for a sign of excessive dependency, the child may feel rejected; such rejection, if repeated, may sow the seeds of a future depressive predisposition (Mahler, 1972).

Margaret Mahler (1972) and her associates described two sisters, Ann and Susan, as good examples of the mother's special importance during the period when the child is becoming an individual. Toward the end of the first year of life, when children are beginning to realize that there is more to the world than themselves and their mothers, Ann often sat at her mother's feet and patiently begged for attention. Most often she begged in vain. The investigators say that, as a result, she had little psychic energy for the next period of her development, the *practicing phase*. During this period, Mahler found, the normal child takes delight in trying out new skills, particularly the ability to get around by him- or herself. The child crawls or walks farther and farther from mother's feet and often becomes so absorbed in activities that for long periods of time he or she seems oblivious to the mother's presence. But Ann would make only brief excursions away from her mother. This period, in which the usual child is exuberant, lasted only a relatively short while for her, and she acted subdued during most of it.

Later, Ann was plainly an unhappy little girl who could not easily endure separation from her mother, did not get along well with other adults and children, and showed little joy when her mother returned after short, everyday absences. In one camera-recorded scene she has a tantrum when her mother starts to leave the room. At first she insists on going along but then gives up and just stands there. Finally, when she retires to the play area for the youngest babies, she turns her back on the others and is clearly hurt and angry.

Ann is described as already vulnerable—already in trouble. Unless through further experience the girl is amply compensated for the rejections and other disappointments of her earliest years, the investigators believe she may well develop emotional problems.

By the time Ann's younger sister, Susan, entered the study, the mother was still somewhat aloof and self-centered, but she had mellowed. Every so often she would put the baby down and bury herself in the newspaper. But Susan was by nature more outward-going and determined than Ann. When she wanted her mother's attention, she knew how to go about getting it. In one photographed scene, she tugs at her mother's dress, looks beseechingly at her, and finally starts to pull herself up to her mother's knee. The viewer can almost hear the mother say, "Oh, the heck with it," as she lays down the paper and picks up the baby. Sometime later Susan looks distressed when her mother leaves the room, but—unlike Ann—soon turns happily to playing with others in the room. She is joyful when her mother returns. Mahler emphasizes that a child who has a good relationship with her mother shows relatively little tendency toward depression in early life and is better prepared emotionally than other children to handle what life offers.

Most people, while accepting the general concept of maternal rejection as one causative factor in the etiology of later depressive states, do not accept such a rigid timetable for this or any one stage of emotional development because of the plasticity and adaptability of the human psyche.

The foregoing issues of separation and individuation are also tied to the beginning development of shame and guilt, well established in third year of life, which play a crucial role in depression (Lewis, 1979). Shame is tied to the development of self-esteem requiring reasonably completed individuation, while guilt is more dependent on the strength of the mother-child bond. Both shame and guilt are crucial to the development of depressive feelings. It may be for that reason that the first reported cases of childhood depression were detected in children nearing the end of the third year of life.

Another pioneer in this field was psychiatrist René Spitz. He had been interested in child development when in the 1940s he came upon 123 young children being raised in a South American nursery. He found that a number of them tended to withdraw from social contact, lose weight, have trouble sleeping, and become ill—behavior much like that being noticed by doctors nowadays in many older children who have suffered a loss and become depressed. Spitz called this behavior *anaclitic* (leaning upon) *depression* (Spitz & Wolf, 1946). It lasted up to 3 months, after which some patients assumed a rigid, frozen posture.

Spitz searched for a common cause of such behavior. He found that all the children who developed the symptoms just cited had been separated from their mothers somewhere between the sixth and eighth month of life for an unbroken period of at least 3 months. They had had no mother or good mother-substitute to lean upon, hence the term *anaclitic*. When the separation ended in less than 6 months, Spitz found, usually the children suddenly turned "friendly, gay, approachable, and the withdrawal, disinterest, and rejection of the outside world, the sadness disappeared as if by magic" (p. 328).

How about the children whose mothers did not come back and who lacked a good substitute?

Sptiz was able to study that question in a foundling home, where the lost mothers had not been restored. Here the picture of depression was as clear-cut as in the nursery but continued to a more advanced stage. In the worst cases, the children became stuporous, agitated, or retarded. It appeared that most could not be brought back to normal. In fact, 24 of the 91 children who were studied died as a result of their condition, after reaching a stage of physical deterioration called marasmus.

ATTACHMENT

More than any other person, psychoanalyst John Bowlby (1969) laid the groundwork for the theory of attachment. According to this theory, during the first year of life the child forms a strong bond to the mother through a series of predictable developmental stages, such as recognition of mother, smiling, separation anxiety, and fear of strangers. Normally this mother-child bond is firmly established by 1 year of age. Where Bowlby differs from the traditional analytic view is in his belief that the child is born with a set of innate mechanisms designed to evoke the maternal tie to the child. Prominent among these are smiling, crying, sucking, clinging, and following. Bowlby and his collaborators noticed that children separated from their mothers, such as when hospitalized, went through a predictable sequence of emotional states. They named these protest, despair, and detachment. During the phase of protest, the baby is restless, angry, and vocal. Several days later, when the period of despair appears, the child becomes withdrawn, visibly sad, often refusing food and any contact with substitute caregivers. Finally, the period of detachment is characterized by more normal behavior, which includes a positive response to the caregiver. However, when, during this period, the mother returns, the child appears indifferent to her presence, indicating a still-existing disturbance of the mother-child bond.

One of Bowlby's collaborators, Mary Ainsworth, provided the first reliable method to assess the attachment behavior, classify the quality of such attachment, and describe deviant forms of attachment (Ainsworth, Blehar, & Waters, 1978). The method she devised is called the Strange Situation. This involves a series of graded separations between infant and mother. The child's behavior is assessed each time he or she is reunited with his mother. A coding system has been devised that includes three major groupings: Group A infants, labeled *avoidant,* are characterized by resisting contact with the mother upon reunion; Group B infants, labeled *securely attached,* approach the mother looking for proximity and contact; Group C infants, called *ambivalently attached,* are characterized by passivity, minimal exploration, and ambivalent reunion behavior with mother, marked by clinging or pushing the mother away. Each of these groups is divided into several subgroups representing variants of the above-mentioned behaviors. Attachment behavior has been linked to the earliest forms of both anxiety and depression.

Shaeffer and Callender (1959) also continued Bowlby's studies. They found that if infants *under* 6 months were separated from their mother by hospitalization, the previously mentioned three stages of disturbance did not occur. However, when the hospitalization occurred after 6 months, which usually coincided with the appearance of separation anxiety and stranger anxiety, the stages of protest, despair, and detachment would invariably occur. This study indicates that the attachment bond between infant and mother must be well established before its interruption causes psychic distress in the child.

TEMPERAMENT

Current interest in the study of temperament dates from the beginning of the New York Longitudinal Studies of Thomas, Chess, and their co-workers in the mid-1950s (1977). They defined temperament as "the behavioral style of the individual child," incorporating the child's "characteristic tempo, rhythmicity, adaptability, energy expenditure, mood and focus of attention" (Thomas & Chess, 1977, p. 24). They established the following categories of temperament by using a content analysis of structured parent and teacher interviews: activity level, rhythmicity, approach or withdrawal after being exposed to a

new stimulus, adaptability, threshold of responsiveness, intensity of reaction, quality of mood, distractibility, attention span, and persistence.

These investigators defined three basic temperamental clusters:

1. "Easy children" are characterized by regularity, positive approach responses to new stimuli, high adaptability to change, and mild or moderate intensity of mood that is predominantly positive.
2. "Difficult children" are characterized by irregularity in biological functions, negativity, withdrawal responses to new stimuli, slow adaptability to change, and intense, mostly negative mood responses.
3. "Slow-to-warm-up children" are marked by a combination of negative responses of mild intensity to new stimuli with gradual adaptability after repeated contact. Their reactions are less intense, and, with repeated experiences and without pressure, such children gradually come to show quiet and positive interest and involvement.

Chess and Thomas view temperament as in constant interaction with the environment. Within this interactional framework, they introduced the concept of *goodness and poorness of fit.* At any age, if the individual's temperament, abilities, and motivations are consonant with the environmental expectations and demands, a goodness of fit will exist and good personality adjustment and functioning would be expected. If, however, the environmental demands and expectations are dissonant with the individual's temperament and abilities, poorness of fit will result, unfavorably influencing the individual's adjustment, functioning, and course of psychological development.

Such an interactive approach implies that neither the child's temperamental and other characteristics nor the environmental demands are in themselves accurate predictors of future adaptation and functioning. Rather, the interaction between the growing child and its environment holds the key to future psychological development (Lerner, 1984). No formal data support a strictly genetic or environmental etiology of temperament. Chess and Thomas followed 133 children from early infancy to adult life and found an impressive continuity of temperamental characteristics over time in many, but not all, of their subjects.

These investigators have reported that the children who belonged to the difficult child temperamental category were more likely to develop behavior disorders in early and middle childhood. They stressed, however, that behavioral disturbances can develop with any temperamental constellation, even that of the "easy child" (Chess & Thomas 1984), if there exists a poorness of fit or dissonance between the child's capacities and the environmental demands and expectations.

BEHAVIORAL INHIBITIONS IN CHILDREN: A POSSIBLE PRECURSOR TO ANXIETY DISORDERS

It is possible that precursors of anxiety disorders may manifest in infancy and toddlerhood as specific behaviors related to temperament. Children who are shy and inhibited withdraw, and, when confronted with a novel situation, "They typically stop their ongoing behavior, cease vocalizing, seek comfort from a familiar figure" (Kagan, Reznick, Clarke, Sidman, & Garcia-Coll, 1984, p. 2212). Some investigators associate these early temperamental traits with a risk for development of overanxious or avoidant disorder in childhood (Kagan et al., 1986). Jerome Kagan and his colleagues at Harvard found that approximately 10 to 15% of children "appear predisposed to be irritable as infants, shy and fearful as toddlers and cautious and introverted when they reach school age" (Biederman et al., 1990, p. 21). Their study also indicates that the tendency to approach or withdraw from a novel situation is a relatively enduring temperamental trait (Kagan, 1984; Resnick et al., 1986).

Kagan and his colleagues have ingeniously and extensively studied the role of this "behavioral inhibition to the unfamiliar" as a possible early precursor of anxiety disorders in childhood and adult anxiety disorders such as panic disorder and agoraphobia. To this end they studied children of parents with panic disorders and agoraphobia and those of parents with other psychiatric disorders (Rosenbaum et al., 1988). The rates of behavioral inhibition in children of parents with panic disorder and agoraphobia were significantly higher than for the comparison group.

Next the correlation between behavioral inhibition and childhood anxiety disorders was investigated in the previously mentioned children of parents with panic disorders and agoraphobia and an existing nonclinical sample of children followed by Kagan and associates identified at 21 months as either inhibited or uninhibited (Biederman et al., 1990). The investigators found that inhibited children had increased risk for multiple anxiety and phobic disorders, suggesting that behavioral inhibition may be associated with risk for anxiety disorders in children.

Studies of Infants and Toddlers of Bipolar (Manic-Depressive) Parents

Our first study included seven male children with a bipolar parent studied longitudinally, beginning at age 1. Each boy was matched with a boy of the same age but with healthy parents (Cytryn et al., 1984). In 4 of the index families the mother was bipolar; the father was bipolar in the remaining 3 families. All of the bipolar parents were on lithium and considered to be in remission at the time of the study.

The goal of the study was to evaluate attachment behavior as well as the nature of affiliative expression and quality of social relationships in the infants as they grew. A modified Ainsworth paradigm was used at 12, 15, and 18 months of age (Gaensbauer & Harmon, 1981). The ratings of attachment were based on traditional measures developed by Ainsworth and her colleagues (1978). Ratings of emotional expression were measured by the methods developed by Harmon and Culp (1981).

Results of the study most relevant to a developmental perspective are: (1) over time, from 12 to 18 months, insecure, ambivalent attachment increased in the infants with a bipolar parent; (2) these infants had less capacity for self-regulation of their emotional equilibrium, especially in handling fear and anger; and (3) only 1 of these infants showed a predominantly depressive mood at times.

Problem behaviors in the two groups of children were examined. Beginning when the boys were 1 year old, a staff member visited the home each month. Based on their cumulative observations and mothers' reports, the home visitors identified various psychological symptoms in the child. These included phobias, sleep disturbances, eating problems, excessive shyness, passivity, hyperactivity, poor impulse control, self-punitive behaviors (e.g., head banging), excessive dependency, social language problems, disturbances in regulation of affect, temper tantrums, echolalia, and resistance to physical contact. Children with a bipolar parent were rated as having both significantly more problems and more severe problems than children from control families.

Peer interactions were investigated at age 2½ years. At this time the control group was enlarged to 12 children. Each boy in the study group came to the laboratory for two sessions with his mother and a same-age playmate and his mother (Zahn-Waxler, McKnew, Cummings, Davenport, & Radke-Yarrow, 1984). Children from bipolar families showed more inappropriate aggression, hurting their friends with greater frequency than controls did. They also showed substantially less altruism toward their peers, most noticeably reflected in less sharing.

The same children were used to investigate the development of object relations. Children from bipolar and normal families performed similarly on tests of object permanence and self-recognition. However, children from bipolar families were more frequently judged insecure in their attachment relationship to the mother at age 26 months (86% in bipolar families vs. 30% in controls). Early impairments in object relations were manifested in tasks that involved interactions with people.

The same 7 sons of bipolar parents and their controls were given a psychiatric evaluation at age 6 (Zahn-Waxler et al., 1988). On the basis of these assessments, diagnoses were made using criteria from the third edition of the *Diagnostic and Statistical Manual of Mental Disorders* (*DSM-III*; American Psychiatric Association [APA], 1980). In the group with bipolar parents, 3 had a unipolar depressive disorder, 3 had a conduct disorder, 3 had an overanxious disorder, and 3 had a separation anxiety disorder. All 7 children had at least one *DSM-III* diagnosis, and the majority had two or more diagnoses. Of the control children, 3 had separation anxiety disorder and 2 had simple phobia; none had depressive or conduct disorder diagnoses.

The authors also participated in a study of toddlers of 120 families in which mothers either had no history of psychiatric illness or suffered from a major or minor affective disorder. All parents were given a psychiatric interview and were diagnosed according to the Research Diagnostic Criteria of Robert Spitzer, Jean Endicott, and Lee A. Robins (1972). The children ranged in age from 15 months to 54 months and the sexes were evenly distributed.

To be considered at high risk for the later development of psychopathology, a child must have been rated as dysfunctional in each of these four areas: (1) the quality of the child's relationship with his or her mother; (2) the child's dominant mood; (3) the child's ability to regulate mood; and (4) the child's mastery in play both when observed with mother and when observed with the psychiatrist. Of the 120 children, 16 were considered dysfunctional in both settings. These 16 children, considered to be the most disturbed in the entire sample (Cytryn, McKnew, & Sherman, 1987), presented the following four patterns or syndromes of maladaptation.

SYNDROME 1 (SOCIALLY AND EMOTIONALLY ISOLATED CHILDREN)

Only 1 child fit the group called Syndrome 1, and he displayed a detached style of relating to mother. In most scenes he initiated almost no interaction with his mother and often ignored her presence. There seemed to be little warmth, empathy, or caring between them. The child's style of mood regulation was overcontrolled. His affect was blunted even when he appeared annoyed with his mother. The boy never lost control of his moods with the psychiatrist; rather, for 30 minutes he was entirely mute. His pattern of mastery in play was characterized by minimal play activity. He functioned best when playing on his own in the presence of his mother. This child worried us the most. His lack of emotional expression and of social relatedness suggested a schizoid quality to his evolving personality. Neither parent of this child had a psychiatric diagnosis.

SYNDROME 2 (DYSPHORIC CHILDREN)

Three girls displayed this pattern, relating to their mother in an emotionally isolated yet physically close style. These children initiated very little interaction with their mother, and their dominant mood was one of sadness or apathy. Often they were simply very still, doing and saying little. They were easily frustrated and revealed few resources for coping, often becoming whiny or clingy. One of the girls began head banging when her mother lay down for a nap. None of these children could be separated from her mother for the psychiatric interview. Since each of the girls cried bitterly, the mothers had to be allowed to stay for the entire interview. All displayed anhedonia (lack of pleasure in activities that would be expected to be pleasurable), showing little interest in play materials, almost no exploration in the laboratory apartment, withdrawal from the psychiatrist and from the novel play materials he presented. These children appeared clinically depressed. Each of them had a mother with a unipolar major depressive disorder. In addition, 1 of the fathers had a recurrent major depression and 1 was absent from the home; 1 father had no psychiatric diagnosis.

SYNDROME 3 (ANGRY AND ANXIOUS CHILDREN)

This pattern was observed in 8 cases (4 boys, 4 girls). The children's dominant mood was anger, alternating with anxiety. These children demonstrated little ability to regulate their moods, often expressing their anger by throwing temper tantrums, acting aggressively toward their mothers, and smashing toys. During the psychiatric interview, many of these children appeared very fearful and lost control completely, weeping excessively and clinging to mother. They showed one of two patterns of poor coping with play materials. One group showed some curiosity and appropriate play with toys; however, when they were faced with frustration or adult limit setting, their play became dysfunctional. They fell apart and often became aggressive toward either the toy or the adult. The other play pattern was seen in children who appeared so angry that they were out of control.

These children showed minimal interest in play materials and spent most of their time in disorganized activity, temper tantrums, or aimless wandering. Two of the mothers in this group had major depression and 2 had minor depression, while 4 had no psychiatric diagnosis. Among the fathers, 4 had major depression, 3 had no psychiatric diagnosis, and 1 was absent.

SYNDROME 4 (STRUCTURE-DEPENDENT CHILDREN)

Four boys were classified as Syndrome 4. These children showed the best relationship to their mothers of all the high-risk children and at times were able to behave warmly and empathically. They also showed a wide range of emotions, including pleasure and joy. However, when the mother withdrew her attention, these boys had difficulty maintaining control; they often became angry, uncooperative, and verbally or physically aggressive toward the mother. Without structure, they became oppositional, belligerent, and excessively angry. Play was good when supervised. With toys enabling aggression, there were problems with impulse control, and without adult attention, these children became angry and even destructive of play materials.

At times they were able to show joy and pleasure and to play competently with adult supervision. However, they appeared to have little, if any, ability to maintain self-control without an adult structuring the situation. All mothers in this group had a mood disorder: 1 had major depression, 1 was bipolar, and 2 had minor depression. Among the fathers, 2 had major depression, 1 was alcoholic, and 1 had no psychiatric diagnosis.

Radke-Yarrow and her colleagues studied these same families using a somewhat different methodology (Radke-Yarrow, Nottleman, Martinez, Fox, & Belman, 1992). In addition to the psychiatric interviews of the children, the maternal report on the Child Behavior Checklist (CBC) was used; also, while our study focused on the most disturbed children, Radke-Yarrow chose to cast a much wider net, including much less disturbed children.

The psychiatric assessment of the same toddlers just reported on yielded the following results. Fifty-four percent of children of unipolar mothers, 43% of children of normal mothers, and only 18% of children of bipolar mothers had a "problem status," which included such areas of concern as separation anxiety, generalized anxiety, disruptive behavior, and depressive symptoms. When the psychiatric assessment of the children was combined with the mothers' reports, the following results were obtained: 66% of the children of unipolar mothers, 46% of those of normal mothers, and only 25% of those of bipolar mothers had a "problem status."

Three of the five components of this "problem status" are of special interest. Depressive symptoms were found in 7% of the toddlers of unipolar mothers; none were found in the children of either normal or bipolar mothers. Symptoms of anxiety were present in 34% of the toddlers with unipolar mothers, 30% of those with normal mothers, and only 9% of those with bipolar mothers. The "disruptive-aggressive" symptoms cluster was found in 34% of toddlers with unipolar mothers but in only 14% of those with both normal and bipolar mothers.

While the results of our and Radke-Yarrow's approaches to this study of 120 toddlers differ somewhat, probably due to different methodology, they agree on two fundamental issues: First, serious depressive disorder is very rare in toddlers and occurs predominantly in the offspring of unipolar parents, and second, the frequency of serious psychopathology in toddlers of bipolar parents does not differ from that in children of normal controls.

In the first family study (Cytryn et al., 1984) described earlier, the children of bipolar parents showed serious disturbances from at least the second year of life. In contrast, the children of bipolar parents in the second family study did not differ from normal controls in the rate of psychopathology. This disparity may be related to the fact that the bipolar parents in the first study were severely ill, had all been on medication, and had experienced one or more psychiatric hospitalizations. The children's home environment was extremely disturbed and marked by disorganization, conflict, chaos, unpredictability, and alienation. The bipolar parents in the second study, on the other hand, had much less severe illness. None had been hospitalized, few were on medication, and their family life was not marked by the extremes noted in the first study.

These studies indicate that the risk of psychopathology in offspring of mood-disordered parents parallels the severity of parental psychopathology.

Clinical Issues

Anxiety disorders of early childhood are outgrowths of two normal developmental milestones characterized by anxiety, namely separation anxiety and stranger anxiety. Behavioral inhibition occurring in infancy is often a precursor of future anxiety disorder. Anxiety disorders in infancy and toddlerhood are worrisome if they present in an exaggerated form but would rarely be diagnosed as a pathological state before the age of 3.

In contrast, most clinicians, with some notable exceptions, including Margaret Mahler, do not view depression as a part of normal psychological development in infants and toddlers. However, we do recognize depressivelike states in this age group that are environmentally caused and labeled by *DSM-IV* (APA, 1994) as reactive attachment disorder of infancy or childhood. This condition was called anaclitic depression by Spitz (1962), hospitalism by Bakwin (1949), and despair by Bowlby (1969).

Reactive attachment disorder is characterized by persistent failure to initiate or respond to most social interactions. Infants with this disorder exhibit a lack of visual tracking, reciprocal play, and vocal imitation or playfulness; apathy; and little or no spontaneity. Later they lack curiosity or social interest. This condition is always brought on by grossly pathogenic care, as evidenced by one of the following: (1) persistent disregard of the child's basic emotional needs for comfort, stimulation, and affection; (2) persistent disregard for the child's basic physical needs, including nutrition, housing, and protection from outside danger; or (3) repeated changes of primary caregiver so that stable attachments are not possible.

Even though depressive states are not seen as normal developmental stages in infancy, unlike separation anxiety and fear of strangers, which have a strong survival value for navigation in a hostile world, Bowlby (1969) and Engel (1962) have argued that depressive mood states in infants and toddlers also have survival value in that they evoke sympathy, primary caregiving, and lead to reuniting the child with his or her mother or providing adequate substitute mothering and improved care.

Summary

This chapter deals with the development of normal and abnormal affect in infants and toddlers, in an effort to trace the origin of depressive and anxiety disorders in younger children. Fear and sadness, which underlie all such disorders, already develop in the first few months. They serve crucial adaptive functions and are indispensable to the personality development of the infant and toddler, even to the child's very survival.

Pathological distortions of these emotions evolve and become increasingly more complex as the child ages. The incidence and intensity of such distortions depend on many factors, including: the inborn temperamental propensities of the child and its cognitive growth, parent-child interaction, and family psychopathology. As a rule, severe affective disorders manifest themselves during infancy and early childhood only under the impact of overwhelming environmental stress.

REFERENCES

Ainsworth, M., Blehar, M. C., & Waters, E. (1978). *Patterns of attachment: A psychological study of the strange situation.* Hillsdale, NJ: Lawrence Erlbaum.

American Psychiatric Association. (1980). *Diagnostic and statistical manual of mental disorders* (3rd ed.). Washington, DC: Author.

American Psychiatric Association. (1994). *Diagnostic and statistical manual of mental disorders* (4th ed.). Washington, DC: Author.

Bakwin, H. (1949). Emotional deprivation in infants. *Journal of Pediatrics, 35*, 512–521.

Biederman, J., Rosenbaum, J. F., Hirshfeld, D. R., Faraone, S. V., Bolduc, E. A., Gerston, M., Meninger, S. R., Kagan, J., Snidman, N., & Resnick, J. S. (1990). Psychiatric correlates of behavioral inhibitions in young children of parents with and without psychiatric disorders. *Archives of General Psychiatry, 47*, 21–26.

Bowlby, J. (1969). *Attachment Vol. 1.* New York: Basic Books.

Brazelton, T. B., Koslowski, B., & Main, M. (1974). The origin of reciprocity: the early mother-infant interaction. In M. Lewis & L. A. Rosenbloom (Eds.), *The effect of the infant on its caregiver* (pp. 49–74). New York: John Wiley & Sons.

Bridges, K. N. B. (1932). Emotional development in early infancy. *Child Development, 3*, 324–341.

Chess, S., & Thomas, A. (1984). *Origins and development of behavioral disorders.* New York: Brunner/Mazel.

Cytryn, L., McKnew, D. H., & Sherman, T. (1987). *Psychopathological syndromes in toddlers.* Paper presented at the 140th annual meeting of the American Psychiatric Association, Chicago, IL.

Cytryn, L., McKnew, D. H., Zahn-Waxler, C., Radke-Yarrow, M., Gaensbauer, T. J., Harmon, R. J., & Lamour, M. (1984). Affective disturbances in the offspring of affectively ill patients—a development view. *American Journal of Psychiatry, 141*, 219–222.

Engel, G. L. (1962). Anxiety and depression withdrawal: The primary affects of unpleasure. *International Journal of Psycho-analysis, 43*, 89.

Gaensbauer, T. J., & Harmon, R. J. (1981). Clinical assessment in infancy utilizing structured playroom situations. *Journal of the American Academy of Child Psychiatry, 20*, 264–280.

Harmon, R. J., & Culp, A. M. (1981). The effect of premature birth on family functioning and infant development. In I. Berlin (Ed.), *Children in our future.* Albuquerque: University of New Mexico Press.

Izard, C. E. (1978). On the development of emotions and emotion-cognition relationships in infancy. In M. Lewis and L. A. Rosenbloom (Eds.), *The development of affect* (pp. 389–413). New York: Plenum Press.

Kagan, J. (1984). *The nature of the child.* New York: Basic Books.

Kagan, J., Reznick, J. S., Clarke, C., Sidman, N., & Garcia-Coll, C. (1984). Behavior inhibition to the unfamiliar. *Child Development, 55*, 2212–2225.

Lazarus, R. S., Canner, A. D., & Folkman, S. (1980). Emotions: A cognitive-phenomenological analysis. In R. Plutchik & H. Kellerman (Eds.), *Theories of emotion* (Vol. 1, pp. 189–217). New York: Academic Press.

Lerner, J. A. (1984). The import of temperament for psychosocial functioning: Tests of goodness of fit model. *Merrill-Palmer Quarterly, 30*, 177–188.

Lewis, H. B. (1979). Shame in depression and hysteria. In C. Izard (Ed.), *Emotions in personality and psychopathology* (pp. 369–396). New York: Plenum Press.

Mahler, M. S. (1972). Rapprochment subphase of

the separation-individuation process. *Psychoanalytic Quarterly, 41,* 487–506.

Mahler, M. S., Pine, F., & Bergman, A. (Eds.) (1975). *The psychological birth of the human infant.* New York: Basic Books.

Radke-Yarrow, M., Nottleman, E., Martinez, P., Fox, M. B., & Belman, B. (1992). Young children of affectively ill parents: A longitudinal study of psychosocial development. *Journal of the American Academy of Child and Adolescent Psychiatry, 31,* 68–77.

Resnick, G. S., Kagan, J., Snidman, N., Gosten, M., Baak, K., & Rosenberg, A. (1986). Inhibited and uninhibited children: A follow-up study. *Child Development, 57,* 660–680.

Robins, L. N., & Regier, D. A. (1991). *Psychiatric disorders in America: The Epidemiological Catchment Area study.* New York: Free Press.

Rosenbaum, J. F., Biederman, J., Gerston, M., Hirshfeld, D. R., Meninger, S. R., Herman, J. B., Kagan, J., Reznick, J. S., & Snidman, N. (1988). Behavioral inhibition in children of parents with panic disorder and agoraphobia. *Archives of General Psychiatry, 45,* 463–470.

Schaeffer, H. R., & Callender, W. M. (1959). Psychological effects of hospitalization in infancy. *Pediatrics, 24,* 528–539.

Solnit, A. J. (1982). Developmental perspectives on self and object constancy. *Psychoanalytic Study of the Child, 32,* 201–217.

Spitz, R. A. (1962). Autoerotism examined: The role of

early sexual behavior patterns in personality formation. *Psychoanalytic Study of the Child, 17,* 283–315.

Spitz, R. A., & Wolf, K. M. (1946). Anaclitic depression: An inquiry into the genesis of psychiatric conditions in early childhood. *Psychoanalytic Study of the Child, 24,* 313–342.

Spitzer, L., Endocott, J., & Robins, E. (1972). Research Diagnostic Criteria. *Archives of General Psychiatry, 35,* 773–782.

Thomas, A., & Chess, S. (1977). *Temperament and development.* New York: Brunner/Mazel.

Weissman, M. M., Leaf, P. J., & Tischler, M. (1988). Affective disorders in five United States communities. *Psychological Medicine, 18,* 141–153.

Weissman, M. M., Leckman, J. R., Merikangas, K. R., Jammon, G. D., & Prusoff, B. A. (1984). Depression and anxiety disorder in parents and children: Results from the Yale Family Study. *Archives of General Psychiatry, 41,* 845–852.

Zahn-Waxler, C., Mayfield, A., Radke-Yarrow, M., McKnew, D. H., Cytryn, L., & Davenport, Y. B. (1988). A follow-up investigation of offspring of parents with bipolar disorder. *American Journal of Psychiatry, 145,* 506–509.

Zahn-Waxler, C., McKnew, D. H., Cummings, E. M., Davenport, Y. B., & Radke-Yarrow, M. (1984). Problem behaviors and peer interactions of young children with a manic-depressive parent. *American Journal of Psychiatry, 141,* 236–240.

36 / Substance Abuse, Fetal Alcohol Syndrome, and Related Neonatal Disorders

Judy Howard and Leila Beckwith

Mental health professionals play a key role in addressing the complex issues surrounding family substance abuse. An infant born to an alcoholic and/or addicted parent enters a family system where a range of biological and environmental events may influence normal social and emotional development. Further, the interplay among these events is also significant. Genetic and congenital factors, for instance, can result in greater vulnerability to environmental adversities. However, even in the absence of other risk factors, environmental stresses alone—many of which are commonly elements of the substance-abusing "lifestyle" (e.g.,

conflict, domestic violence, family breakup)—have been related to future conduct disorders in children (Offord, 1989).

As long as alcohol and/or other drug abuse remains a factor within a family system, specialized clinical services are critical to foster the physical and mental health of all family members. In order to be effective, these interventions must be based on professionals' understanding of addiction and how the addict's craving for alcohol and/or other drugs preempts other life concerns, including family welfare. Further, it is important that professionals understand the impact of alcohol and other drugs upon the user him- or herself as well as upon fetal development in cases of prenatal substance abuse.

This chapter provides a brief overview of the incidence of parental substance abuse, the impact of prenatal alcohol and other drug exposure on the developing fetus, parenting problems commonly associated with substance abuse, and clinical implications for the mental health practitioner.

Background

The prevalence of alcohol and other drug use by men and women between the ages of 18 and 45 is very difficult to determine with any real accuracy. However, some statistics have been put forth. In a 21-state study conducted between 1985 and 1988, regarding alcohol consumption by women of childbearing age, approximately 25% of pregnant women and 55% of nonpregnant women reported some use of alcohol, with an average of 4.2 drinks per month for pregnant women and 8.7 for non-pregnant women (Serdula, Williamson, Kendrick, Anda, & Byers, 1991). This study showed that women who were smokers, single, less educated, and younger reported the heaviest consumption of alcohol. However, in considering these statistics, it is important to bear in mind the fact that these estimates were based on maternal self-report, and self-reports, as compared with actual sales data, have consistently been shown to underestimate consumption (Midanik, 1982; Smith, Remington, Williamson, & Anda, 1990).

With respect to illicit substances, in 1990 it was estimated that 5 million women of childbearing age within the United States used illicit drugs (General Accounting Office, 1990). Again, however, exact figures are not easily obtained. One complicating factor is the fact that most individuals who abuse drugs are polysubstance abusers (i.e., they use more than one drug), and most include alcohol among their "repertoire." Further, an individual's report of using only alcohol or a single drug may be unreliable, in part due to his or her inaccuracy in recalling actual drinking or drug use during periods of intoxication.

Finally, figures regarding the number of alcohol- and other drug-affected infants who are born annually have been even more difficult to ascertain. One study estimated that over 7,000 children are born with fetal alcohol syndrome each year (Abel & Sokol, 1987). However, this report did not address the number of infants born with fetal alcohol effects, which are also a consequence of maternal alcohol consumption during pregnancy. Reports of the annual number of infants born prenatally exposed to cocaine have ranged from 91,500 to 240,000 (Besharov, 1989; General Accounting Office, 1990; Gomby & Shiono, 1991). However, these figures do not address prenatal exposure to heroin, methamphetamine, phencyclidine (PCP), and other substances of abuse.

Over the years, the realization that alcohol and other drug abuse by women of childbearing age is linked to adverse effects on children has shifted the primary focus of much research from the adult user to the substance-abusing family as a whole. One example of this changing focus has been the publication of a long-term study of adults with fetal alcohol syndrome (Streissguth et al., 1991) and their deviant developmental course. Other researchers are gathering longitudinal data regarding children who were exposed to illicit substances in utero as well as information regarding substance-abusing parents' own family backgrounds, personality disorders among chronic substance abusers, caregiving patterns within the home setting, attachment behaviors between substance-abusing mothers and their toddlers, and treatment approaches for serving these complex families.

The Impact of Alcohol and Other Drugs on the Developing Fetus and Child

An entire spectrum of substances used by women during pregnancy—including alcohol, cocaine, heroin, marijuana, methadone, and nicotine—have been reported consistently to hinder fetal growth and development. Further, a number of maternal health, nutritional, and other lifestyle factors that are associated with substance abuse also can interfere with these processes in utero. Researchers have reported a broad continuum of interferences, ranging from fetal demise, to preterm delivery, to intrauterine growth retardation—that is, lower birthweight, shorter length, and/or smaller head circumference—in full-term infants, to an increased incidence of mental retardation, decreased IQ, and/or attention deficits even in children with normal intelligence.

Any use of alcohol or other drugs by a pregnant woman has the potential to affect fetal health and well-being. However, most of our knowledge in this area is based on studies of chronic substance abusers. Little is known regarding the effects of experimental or sporadic alcohol and/or other drug use during pregnancy, in part because the identification of occasional users is much more difficult. Even with respect to chronic use, subject selection presents challenges—as noted, self-report is not always a reliable indicator of alcohol and/or other drug consumption, and many patients who deny use may be eliminated from research projects.

Research in this field is further complicated by the fact that it is not always possible to ascertain the trimester during which use occurred. Additionally, researchers often are unable to tease out the effects of specific substances of abuse. This is the case primarily because polysubstance abuse is the most characteristic pattern among users, but it also is due to the fact that drugs sold on the street commonly are adulterated with other substances. In other cases the market may shift, and this, too, can complicate research findings. For example, while clients may enter a study at a point in time when they are abusing one primary substance (e.g., cocaine), by the time the study is underway, another substance may have gained predominance in the marketplace, and clients may have shifted to this entirely different drug (e.g., heroin). Even urine toxicology screens, often performed at delivery as an objective means of identifying maternal substance abuse, reflect drug use only during a brief, 72-hour window of time.

Further, at this time we are unable to address the effects of paternal abuse of alcohol and/or other drugs on the developing fetus. In this new field of research, only very limited data are available. Reports from animal studies have shown that the offspring of males who have been given morphine, methadone, or marijuana prior to mating have been affected, even when drugs have not been administered to the females (Dalterio & De Rooji, 1986; Joffee et al., 1976; Sonderegger, O'Shea, & Zimmerman, 1979). Furthermore, researchers using human subjects have demonstrated that the children of alcoholic fathers are more likely to have lower birthweights, and sons are more likely to perform less well in school than their sisters or children of nonalcoholics (Little & Sing, 1988; Tarter, Jacob, & Bremer, 1990).

Additional confounding factors that make research in this field especially challenging include the multiplicity of environmental influences that contribute to infant outcomes. Substance-affected children may be placed with multiple caregivers as child protective services agencies and the juvenile courts make decisions regarding child placement. The most common reason for out-of-home placement is potential harm to young children due to parental intoxication, but such decisions also may be based on parents' enrollment in residential drug treatment facilities that exclude children or parental incarceration related to activities such as prostitution or drug sales.

Finally, many of the standardized measures currently used to evaluate the development of infants and children of substance-abusing mothers are not sufficiently sensitive to identify more subtle behavioral and cognitive deficits that may have implications for future functioning. Thus, more sophisticated research measures and the involvement of a well-informed and interdisciplinary team are critical in this field.

FETAL ALCOHOL SYNDROME AND FETAL ALCOHOL EFFECTS

Alcohol is a known teratogen (i.e., an agent that causes developmental malformations) that is related to an entire range of birth defects, including death, malformation, growth retardation, and functional impairment. Fetal alcohol syndrome (FAS) was first described as a specific pattern of malformation by Jones, Smith, Ulleland, and Streissguth in 1973. It has been called one of the leading known teratogenic causes of mental retardation in the Western world (Clarren & Smith,

1978) and is estimated to occur in approximately 1.9 of 1,000 births (Abel & Sokol, 1987). FAS is a medical diagnosis that is characterized by intra-uterine as well as postnatal growth retardation and/or microcephaly, a pattern of physical anomalies (including characteristic minor facial abnormalities), and a range of central nervous system dysfunction that may include developmental delay, hyperactivity, problems with attention or learning, intellectual deficits, and/or seizures (Olson, Burgess, & Streissguth, 1992; Smith, 1979). Children with FAS also may have cardiac defects and/or minor abnormalities of joints and limbs (Streissguth, Herman, & Smith, 1978).

However, not all children who were exposed to alcohol in utero develop FAS. Many exhibit less severe consequences related to maternal alcohol use during pregnancy, or what is known as fetal alcohol effects (FAE). This determination generally is based on a maternal history of alcohol consumption during pregnancy, the presence of one or two facial characteristics associated with FAS, moderate growth deficiency, and developmental disability with no other known etiology. Although children with FAE may function within the normal range intellectually, they often exhibit various maladaptive behaviors and less easily recognizable central nervous system effects. These may include learning disabilities, hyperactivity, and problems with speech and language and/or attention span (Streissguth & LaDue, 1985). FAE has been estimated to be as much as 3 times as common as FAS (Olson et al., 1992).

Still other children who were exposed to alcohol in utero appear to be unaffected. These diverse outcomes may be related to the complex interplay of a variety of complicating factors, including the amount of alcohol consumed, the circumstances and timing of exposure, and differences in individual health and sensitivity (Streissguth & LaDue, 1985).

Infancy: In a landmark 1981 study on alcohol and pregnancy (Streissguth, Martin, Martin, & Barr, 1981), after adjusting for a variety of confounding variables, children of alcohol-using mothers were shown to have a greater incidence of impaired growth (with respect to birthweight, length, and head circumference), increased tremulousness, lower Apgar scores, decreased habituation (i.e., a measure of how quickly an infant stops

responding to repeated stimuli), weak suck, decrease in the vigor of body activity, and an increased incidence of minor dysmorphic characteristics associated with FAS (including low birthweight and microcephaly). At 8 months of age, these children also had significantly lower mental and motor scores.

A 1986 study of middle-class alcohol-using mothers over 30 years of age (O'Connor, Brill, & Sigman, 1986) showed a strong relationship between the mothers' drinking prior to pregnancy and infant mental development. In this study, maternal self-report of alcohol use prior to pregnancy, as opposed to maternal report of consumption during pregnancy, was the factor that correlated to the infants' later mental development. Infants whose mothers reported that they drank more before becoming pregnant had lower mental scores than infants whose mothers reported consuming smaller amounts of alcohol, although the deficits were not as pronounced as those found in children with FAS.

Preschool Years: Preschool-age children with FAS or FAE often have been observed to be hyperactive, oversensitive to touch and other stimulation, and inattentive; some have demonstrated fine motor problems as well as severe temper tantrums and difficulty with transitions (Olson et al., 1992). However, mental disabilities are the most debilitating aspect of fetal alcohol exposure (Streissguth & LaDue, 1985), and, even with adjustment for confounding variables, maternal alcohol use during early pregnancy has been significantly related to lower IQ scores in offspring at 4 years of age (Streissguth, Barr, Sampson, Darby, & Martin, 1989).

Middle Childhood: In older children with FAS and FAE, hyperactivity, distractibility, impulsivity, and memory difficulties also have been observed. Further, although these children generally appear to be affectionate and interested in other persons, they also have been noted to lack the social skills to develop friendships and the judgment to keep away from strangers. In school, they may exhibit a tendency toward concrete thinking that can interfere with their comprehension of more abstract concepts, causing particular difficulty with mathematics (Olson et al., 1992).

Adolescence and Adulthood: One report on adolescents and adults with FAS or FAE noted that these research subjects tended to "plateau" in learning at school (Olson et al., 1992). This fact alone would not necessarily indicate to a professional that these individuals were at serious risk for future problems with independence or inappropriate social growth. However, study participants' ongoing problems with poor judgment, impulsivity, and attention deficit interfered with successful employment and their ability to establish stable living arrangements. From a mental health perspective, a person's awareness of a difficulty making and keeping friends, securing and/or maintaining employment, and achieving financial independence and responsibility can place a him or her at risk for future problems, such as depression and alcohol abuse, that require intervention.

Another recent clinical report focusing on adolescents and adults with FAS indicated that the facial anomalies characteristic of this syndrome gradually became less noticeable as the children grew into adolescence and adulthood (Streissguth et al., 1991). However, their physical stature was noted to be short, and head circumferences remained in the microcephalic range. Further, the developmental and cognitive disabilities that had been observed in these individuals as children persisted into later life. As has been observed in younger children with FAS or FAE, problems with abstractions such as time, space, cause and effect, and a decreased ability to generalize from one situation to another were evident. This commonly resulted in academic difficulty with arithmetic as well as problems in the more general interpersonal realm. The average IQ score for the subjects in this study was just into the mentally retarded range, extending from as low as 20 (severely retarded) to 105 (normal). Although most of the patients had required some remedial help in school and on the average functioned academically at the early grade-school level, 42% had an IQ score above 70 and for this reason could not qualify easily for special community services after leaving school. The 58% percent whose IQ scores were 70 or below could be classified as disabled more readily and thus had been eligible to receive special community services.

The overall level of adaptive functioning observed among all participants in this study was also of great concern. The most common behavioral problems included poor concentration and attention deficit. Research subjects also demonstrated difficulty perceiving social cues, dependency, stubbornness or sullenness, social withdrawal, teasing and bullying, crying or laughing too easily, impulsivity, periods of high anxiety, and problems with judgment, comprehension, and abstraction. Conduct problems (e.g., lying and defiance) also were observed in some study participants.

Compounding the biological risks noted in this study (i.e., microcephaly and facial dysmorphism), the environmental situations surrounding these individuals also were noted to be multiproblem. Subjects had lived, on the average, in 5 different principal homes during their lifetimes. ("Receiving homes" and temporary shelters were not included in these calculations.) Among patients for whom accurate data could be collected, a significant percentage (69%) of their biologic mothers were known to be dead, either due to alcohol-related illnesses or alcohol-related causes (e.g., homicide, suicide, falls, automobile accidents). Further, almost one third of these individuals were never raised by their biologic mothers—they had been given up for adoption at birth or abandoned in the hospital.

PRENATAL EXPOSURE TO ILLICIT DRUGS

Unlike cases of prenatal alcohol exposure, where some longitudinal studies have been conducted over an extended period of time, prenatal exposure to illicit substances remains an area where we have only limited knowledge; furthermore, what we do know has been assembled over a relatively short period of time. During the 1970s researchers began to look at the effects of prenatal heroin abuse, focusing on the child from the newborn period until 2 years of age. Methadone, a synthetic opiate, was introduced as a treatment for pregnant heroin addicts during the 1970s, and it was determined that this drug did not cause congenital malformations or interfere significantly with fetal growth. Babies of methadone-maintained mothers tended to have higher birthweights than infants of heroin-abusing women, and, furthermore, the overall developmental scores of methadone-exposed children at

24 months of age fell within the normal range. Based on these observations, many members of the drug treatment community sighed with relief, believing that a safe medical treatment for pregnant heroin addicts had been found. Thus, longitudinal investigation of more subtle biological effects (e.g., fine motor incoordination, delayed speech and language, increased activity levels) related to prenatal heroin and methadone exposure was put on a back burner. In time, however, some worrisome reports of adverse effects in young children who had been prenatally exposed to methadone did begin to appear (Rosen & Johnson, 1982; Wilson, Desmond, & Wait, 1981).

Though substance-abusing mothers usually have one or two preferred drugs of abuse, as noted earlier, the most common form of drug abuse is polysubstance abuse; thus, research subjects generally admit to using alcohol, nicotine, and marijuana along with their preferred primary substance(s). The bulk of the research on maternal substance abuse that has been conducted to date has focused on the effects of in utero exposure to heroin, methadone, cocaine, methamphetamine, and phencyclidine. It has been difficult to tease out the individual effects related to these specific drugs; however, researchers have noted a characteristic constellation of signs and symptoms among infants of addicted women, regardless of the reported substances of abuse.

Infancy: Where there is a maternal history of prenatal abuse of illicit substances, studies have reported an increased incidence of fetal demise, preterm delivery, and intrauterine growth retardation. Preterm delivery (i.e., birth at less than 37 weeks' gestational age), for instance, generally is estimated to occur in less than 10% of the newborn population; however, about one third of prenatally substance-exposed children are born preterm. Drug-exposed infants also show an increased risk of intrauterine growth retardation as compared with the general population. Thus, there is evidence that prenatal substance abuse can negatively affect fetal growth and interrupt the normal 9-month gestation that constitutes term delivery.

Even when there has been no prenatal drug exposure, fetal growth impairment, as shown by subnormal head size and/or intrauterine growth retardation, has been associated with an increased incidence of later speech and language problems, attention deficits, and difficulties in school. A link between fetal growth impairment and behavioral development also has been identified in children who were exposed to drugs in utero. One study of children who were prenatally exposed to cocaine and/or marijuana, alcohol, and nicotine found that cocaine exposure was the single best predictor of small head circumference in children from birth through age 2, and that small head circumference, in turn, was associated with poorer developmental scores at 2 years of age (Chasnoff, Griffith, Freier, & Murray, 1992).

Health concerns for infants who were prenatally exposed to drugs include an array of disorders. For example, there is a reported increased incidence of sudden infant death syndrome (SIDS) among such children (Chavez, Ostrea, Stryker, & Smialek, 1979; Davidson Ward et al., 1990; Householder, Hatcher, Burns, & Chasnoff, 1982; Kandall, Gaines, Habel, Davidson, & Jessop, 1993). More commonly known as "crib death," SIDS is defined as the sudden death of an infant under 1 year of age that remains unexplained after autopsy, investigation of the death scene, and review of the case history. Children who die from SIDS commonly exhibit no other sign of illness immediately prior to their death.

These infants also are more frequently exposed to infectious diseases, either prenatally or at the time of delivery. It is not uncommon for addicted women to resort to a lifestyle that involves multiple sexual partners or prostitution. They may engage in such activities for many reasons, not the least of which is to obtain drugs to sustain their drug habit. This lifestyle, as well as any history of intravenous (IV) drug use, can place an individual at increased risk for acquiring a variety of infectious diseases. Because many infectious agents cross the placenta, an infant may then acquire his or her mother's infections during pregnancy and delivery. The infectious diseases most commonly seen in infants of substance abusers include gonorrhea, syphilis, herpes, chlamydia, hepatitis B, and AIDS.

An additional health risk that seems to be increased in full-term newborns who were prenatally exposed to cocaine and methamphetamine is the occurrence of hemorrhagic infarctions in the central nervous system. Among one group of such infants who had uncomplicated deliveries and who had been exposed prenatally to cocaine and methamphetamine, one-third were noted to have small central nervous system bleeds or infarctions that were apparent upon cranial ultrasound examination (Dixon & Bejar, 1989). In addition to vascular changes in the central nervous system, electroencephalogram abnormalities also have been noted, particularly in the temporal and frontal lobes (Dixon & Bejar, 1989; Doberczak, Shanzer, Senie, & Kandall, 1988; Hoyme et al., 1990). There have been reports of interferences in other organ systems, as well, including limb development and kidney structure (Bingol, Fuchs, Diaz, Stone, & Gromisch, 1987).

In addition to these health concerns, many prenatally drug-exposed infants have been reported to demonstrate neurobehavioral symptoms that indicate difficulty with state regulation during the first year of life. Caregivers frequently report that these infants are unable to organize normal sleep-wake cycles. Although most infants develop predictable sleeping patterns by 4 to 6 months of age, some prenatally drug-exposed infants continue to demonstrate sleeping patterns more typical of a newborn through the first year (or even, although more infrequently, throughout early childhood). It is not uncommon for some of these infants to sleep only for brief periods of time, which can be extremely exhausting for caregivers.

Among some prenatally drug-exposed infants, feeding patterns are also deviant. For instance, infants exposed prenatally to heroin and/or methadone may suffer ongoing vomiting and ineffectual sucking motions that contribute to poor growth and weight gain during the first 6 months. More recently, it has been noted that infants exposed prenatally to cocaine and methamphetamine demonstrate a different pattern of feeding difficulties and insufficient weight gain. They frequently have hyperphagia (i.e., excessive sucking and swallowing as if from extreme hunger) and uncoordinated sucking.

Substance-exposed infants also run an elevated risk of failure to thrive, a syndrome of disordered growth and development characterized by a marked deceleration in weight gain and a slowing in acquisition of developmental milestones (Rudolph, 1991). In prenatally drug-exposed infants, failure to thrive may be due to both biological and environmental factors. The pattern of poor sucking, swallowing difficulties, and distractibility that

has been observed in many of these infants can contribute to this syndrome. Further, children who live in dysfunctional, substance-abusing families are at increased risk for receiving inadequate nutrition on a consistent basis. In addition, emotional neglect can contribute to insufficient weight gain; thus, drug-exposed infants often do not receive adequate nurturing and actually may turn away when food is offered.

With respect to the influence of specific drugs of abuse on a young infant's muscle tone and movements, there has been extensive documentation of the early withdrawal syndrome among newborns who were prenatally exposed to heroin and methadone. These infants typically are tremulous, irritable, and hypertonic (Finnegan, 1975; Wilson, Desmond, & Verniaud, 1973). They have poor motor control, attend less well to visual stimuli, and may have increased responses to auditory stimuli (Hans, Marcus, Jeremy, & Auerbach, 1984).

Cocaine and methamphetamine also have been demonstrated to have worrisome effects on infants exposed to these substances in utero. Unlike hyperirritable newborns suffering heroin or methadone withdrawal, during early infancy many cocaine-exposed infants may appear lethargic and poorly responsive, and display fluctuating muscle tone ranging from hypotonia to hypertonia with mild tremors (Oro & Dixon, 1987). While awake and alert, these infants often are easily overstimulated and may experience rapid emotional state changes that can fluctuate from quiet sleep to irritable crying within an extremely brief span of time. Further, as time passes infants who were lethargic during the immediate postnatal period sometimes have been noted to become more irritable and difficult to console.

One study of neonatal infant cries also found that prenatal cocaine exposure potentiated both an excitable and a depressed syndrome. Infants who had been prenatally exposed to cocaine had cries of longer duration, higher fundamental frequency, and a more variable format frequency than control infants. The controls were born to mothers who were similar demographically as well as with respect to cigarette, alcohol, and marijuana use during pregnancy. Further, intrauterine growth retardation was associated with cocaine exposure, and affected children had cries that were fewer in frequency, with longer latency, lower amplitude, and more dysphonation (Lester et al., 1991). These data have served to substantiate clinical observations regarding the difficulty caregivers often experience in reading cocaine-exposed infants' cues as well as in soothing these often irritable young infants.

Finally, studies have been conducted with infants prenatally exposed to the synthetic anesthetic and hallucinogen phencyclidine (PCP). The investigators have documented irritability, tremors, darting eye movements, and increased sensitivity to environmental stimuli (Howard, Kropenske, & Tyler, 1986; Strauss, Modanlou, & Bosu, 1981). PCP-exposed infants also commonly demonstrate difficulty in organizing sleep-wake cycles, a phenomenon observed in infants prenatally exposed to other substances of abuse.

In addition to the symptoms just described, children who were exposed to cocaine and PCP in utero may show altered visual attention. In one study, exposed 6-month-old infants were compared to control infants with respect to their preference for novelty tasks and in spontaneous play with a block and a ball. On the first trial, it was found that the drug-exposed children exhibited no preference for the novel stimulus, whereas the control children did. Further, the control children gazed at the toys more frequently while manipulating them and looked at toys more frequently after dropping them than did children in the drug-exposed group. This study indicates that subtle alterations in gaze behavior may be associated with prenatal drug exposure (Beckwith & Howard, 1991).

Early Childhood: As substance-exposed children leave infancy and toddlerhood, the majority have organized their sleep-wake cycles, are eating successfully, have become less irritable, attend visually to their caregivers, and may look as if they no longer experience any negative effects related to their prenatal drug exposure. When standardized developmental evaluations are administered to assess motor, cognitive, language, and personal-social areas of behavior, most studies report that these young children as a group (whether exposed to heroin, methadone, cocaine, methamphetamine, and/or PCP) tend to score within the low-normal range as compared with non-drug-exposed groups, who score within the median normal range (Johnson, Diano, & Rosen, 1984; Kal-

tenbach & Finnegan, 1984; Rosen & Johnson, 1982; Sowder & Burt, 1980; Wilson et al., 1973).

However, as these children enter the early childhood period, the battery of available testing measures becomes more abundant, enabling professionals to assess subtler developmental behaviors. Using these more sensitive tools, substance-exposed children frequently do, in fact, demonstrate behavioral patterns that may indicate an increased risk for problems with socialization and learning, and several studies have described behaviors that may be viewed as precursors to future learning and emotional difficulties.

As one developmental pediatrician noted many years ago, the quality of methadone-exposed children's interactions with toys and with persons in the environment is different from that of children who were not prenatally exposed to drugs (Wilson, 1976). More specifically, another publication during that same year noted that toddlers who had been prenatally exposed to heroin and methadone were behaviorally observed to be highly energetic, active, talkative, and very reactive to sensory stimulation. At the same time, they had overall developmental scores within the normal range. Further, although these youngsters appeared to be genuinely interested in toys and objects as well as in people, their overall persistence, goal-directedness, and attention spans appeared to be somewhat brief. While engaged in play activities, the children seemed immature, frequently mouthing and banging the toys rather than demonstrating more complex manipulations and constructive play (Lodge, 1976).

Again in 1979 a report describing preschoolers who had been heroin-exposed prenatally stated that the children's overall performance with respect to intellectual functioning was within the normal range. However, the parents rated these youngsters as having difficulty with physical, social, and self-adjustment. Areas of significant concern included uncontrollable temper, impulsiveness, aggressiveness, low levels of self-confidence, and difficulty in making and keeping friends (Wilson, McCreary, Kean, & Baxter, 1979).

A 1985 study examining the long-term effects of prenatal methadone and polysubstance exposure reported that 24-month-old children seemed to have difficulty with highly structured tasks or tasks involving verbal instructions. Between 37 and 84 months of age, youngsters who had been exposed prenatally to methadone and other drugs were described as having a higher incidence of problems with fine and gross motor coordination, poor balance, increased activity levels, decreased attention span, and speech and language delays as compared with children in the control group (Rosen & Johnson, 1985).

Although these reports referred primarily to children who were prenatally exposed to heroin and/or methadone, more recent research has shown that youngsters who were exposed to a variety of substances often demonstrate poorer language skills, shorter attention span, increased distractibility, hyperactivity, a less organized approach to activities, and greater impulsivity. One recent longitudinal study, for instance, reported that 30 to 40% of preschool children who had been prenatally exposed to cocaine demonstrated learning and language difficulties (as assessed by standardized developmental measures) (D. Griffith, personal communication, 1990). With respect to poor interpersonal skills, additional studies have reported aggressive behaviors, emotional lability, and difficulties with social interactions (Young, Wallace, & Garcia, 1992).

At the University of California at Los Angeles (UCLA), we have described the organization of unstructured play behavior in toddlers whose mothers had used a range of substances that included heroin, methadone, cocaine, methamphetamine, and PCP. These children had not experienced perinatal complications and had normal developmental scores. Over time, however, they demonstrated a significantly decreased ability to structure play that required focused attention, sequencing of activities, and persistence with any single scheme of play (e.g., feeding a baby doll or putting the baby to bed), as compared with a group of preterm children who had been respirator-dependent following birth but who also had normal developmental scores. With respect to environmental factors, those prenatally drug-exposed children who had secure relationships with their caregivers demonstrated better organization in play and better attention spans than those who had insecure attachments (Rodning, Beckwith, & Howard, 1989).

Another study at UCLA compared full-term children who had been prenatally exposed to PCP

and cocaine with full-term children born to non–substance-abusing mothers who lived in the same geographic area and were of similar ethnicity and socioeconomic status. At 24 months of age, the prenatally drug-exposed children demonstrated significantly more immature play strategies, less sustained attention, and fewer positive social interactions with their caregivers. There was substantial variability, however, within the drug-exposed group, with a significant minority indistinguishable in play from the control children. When these children were compared with other drug-exposed children, as well as with children in the control group, protective factors within the child and environmental mitigation of the adverse effects of prenatal substance exposure became evident. The drug-exposed children whose play was similar to that of the control children were born to mothers who had more years of education, and the youngsters themselves had higher developmental quotients and experienced more sensitive and responsive caregiving during the first year of life (Beckwith et al., 1994).

Within a preschool setting, prenatally drug-exposed children from 3 to 5 years of age have been reported to have problems with hypersensitivity to environmental stimuli compounded by an inability to self-regulate (e.g., they may be impulsive and have difficulty attending to the task at hand). Further, many exhibit sporadic mastery of tasks (e.g., a child may be able to complete a puzzle one day, but the following day seems unable to organize him- or herself in order to complete the task). Fine as well as gross motor difficulties may make some of these children appear awkward and clumsy, while others may have speech and language delays (Johnson & Cole, 1992).

Middle Childhood, Adolescence, and Adulthood: Very little longitudinal research has evaluated the impact of prenatal drug exposure into middle childhood, adolescence, and adulthood. One study of older children living with addicted parents found that 57% of the children between 3 and 7 years of age performed more poorly on tests measuring IQ and perceptual motor performance (Sowder & Burt, 1980). These children also had greater anxiety, more insecurity, and shorter attention spans. A few studies examining the behaviors of prenatally drug-exposed children placed in out-of-home care reported that the children demonstrated learning difficulties in school, poor school adjustment, and problems in their relationships with adults as well as peers (Fanshel, 1975; Nichtern, 1973; Sowder, Carnes, & Sherman, 1981). Additionally, mental health problems were more frequent in these populations.

Additional reports describing older children and teenagers being raised by parents who were in drug treatment have reported that these children also demonstrated behavioral and school adjustment problems, although it was not ascertained whether the children had in fact been prenatally exposed to drugs (Herjanic, Barredo, Herjanic, & Tomelleri, 1979; Sowder & Burt, 1980). Further, researchers looking at the school performance of 8- to 17-year-old children of addicted parents found that teachers reported more behavior problems, repeated grades, and absences (Sowder & Burt, 1980). Children of addicts also have been noted to exhibit an increased number of delinquent acts, and these acts were considered more serious than those of children in the control group. Finally, these youngsters were more likely to abuse drugs and be in drug treatment programs themselves.

SUMMARY

Based on the preceding review of characteristics that have been described among children who were prenatally exposed to alcohol and/or other drugs, the reader now should have a beginning understanding of the physical growth and observed patterns of behavior in children with known prenatal exposure to alcohol and/or other drugs of abuse. It is important to bear in mind, however, that all of the researchers just cited have noted that the behaviors described are no doubt the result of a combination of biological as well as environmental factors. The following discussion of parental behaviors and lifestyle provides a more inclusive perspective on these complex family systems. Without this additional information, mental health professionals will be unable to develop meaningful treatment strategies to meet the needs of so many of these family members.

The Impact of Alcohol and Other Drug Abuse on Parenting

Parental alcohol and/or other drug abuse generally can be characterized by a theme of overriding need: The alcoholism or addiction supersedes everything else in the addicted individual's life. Alcohol dependency, for example, has been described as compulsion, loss of control, and continued consumption of alcohol despite adverse consequences (Smith, Milkman, & Sunderwirth, 1985). A key feature of the disorder of addiction is denial. As a result, personal health, financial security, safety, and relationships with others all may be neglected as the substance abuser focuses on sustaining his or her habit.

The following discussion is based primarily on what is known about only one member of the parenting dyad: the pregnant woman who is chemically dependent. More extensive empirical data addressing the addicted father's contribution to the lifestyle of the spouse or significant other as well as to the developing fetus and child are not available yet.

IDENTIFICATION OF PARENTAL ALCOHOL AND/OR OTHER DRUG ABUSE

Because of the risks associated with prenatal abuse of alcohol and/or other drugs, it is critical that professionals learn to identify pregnant substance-abusing clients as early as possible in order to address the complex medical, social, financial, and other needs of this population more effectively. However, the identification of these parents presents a number of challenges. For example, a young parent who is a heavy drinker or who abuses cocaine and/or marijuana commonly does not exhibit obvious physical findings related to chronic substance abuse (i.e., a dissipated appearance, liver disease, evidence of chronic brain syndrome).

Further, many substance abusers, especially those who are young parents, may not be open about their use of alcohol and/or other drugs. They may be embarrassed or in denial regarding the extent of their problem. However, using clinical intuition, a professional may be alerted to potential substance abuse by a client on the basis of a variety of indicators (Jessup & Green, 1987). These may include historical factors (e.g., clinical depression, multiple emergency room visits, incidents involving domestic violence, older children who are in out-of-home placement or who have learning disabilities of hyperactivity), medical conditions (e.g., poor nutritional status, sexually transmitted diseases, delivery of a child with intrauterine growth retardation), and/or observable behaviors (e.g., alcohol on the breath, inappropriateness, slurred speech, staggering gait, mood swings).

COMPLICATING FACTORS OFTEN ASSOCIATED WITH SUBSTANCE ABUSE

The majority of parents who abuse alcohol and/or other drugs come from difficult family backgrounds. Once again, however, the bulk of knowledge regarding the family histories of adult substance abusers who are parents pertains more to women's negative experiences during childhood than to men's. A large number of substance-abusing women, for instance, report that their own parents also abused alcohol and/or other drugs (Cuskey & Wathey, 1982), and many also report that they endured physical, sexual, and/or emotional abuse as children (Howard, Beckwith, Rodning, & Kropenske, 1989; Ryan, Ehrlich, & Finnegan, 1987). Unfortunately, we have only limited information regarding the incidence of physical and sexual abuse within the male alcoholic/addict population (Friedrich, Beilke, & Urquiza, 1988). In any event, even without the complicating factor of addiction, individuals who come from such traumatic backgrounds may find it difficult to be nurturing parents themselves.

Persons who come from abusive backgrounds also often have problems with low self-esteem, and this, in turn, can influence their educational achievements and social support networks. Studies have shown that substance-abusing women report having fewer friends and more intense feelings of loneliness than non–drug-abusing women (Tucker, 1982). Further, most adult women who are current substance abusers and who grew up in homes where parents also used alcohol and/or other drugs report problems with attending to educational tasks as well as low motivation to seek high school diplomas or college degrees. Based on clinical experience, the authors of this chapter have found that it is not uncommon for substance-abusing women to question whether their past learning difficulties in school may have been related to their own parents' use of alcohol and/or other drugs at the time of conception or during pregnancy.

Additionally, in an ongoing project at UCLA in which researchers are making a concentrated effort to interview pregnant addicts individually prior to their initiation into treatment programs, we have learned that most of these women report serious psychiatric disorders, including paranoid ideation, thought disorder, depression, and anxiety, in addition to alcohol and/or other drug abuse. Other investigators also have found a significant association between drug use and psychiatric disorder. For example, in one report describing 533 opiate-dependent men and women in treatment, 70% of study participants had had a psychiatric disorder at some time during their lives, and 87% currently met the criteria for at least one psychiatric disorder other than substance abuse (Regan, Ehrlich, & Finnegan, 1987). Although it is not clear whether psychiatric disorder is an antecedent or a consequence of drug use, it is likely that it is both a potentiator of substance abuse as well as a condition that is exacerbated by the neurotoxic effects of drugs.

EFFECTS OF SUBSTANCE ABUSE ON CURRENT MENTAL STATUS

In addition to the background experiences that chemically dependent parents bring into the family environment, professionals need to acquaint themselves with the specific impact of various substances of abuse on the user's mental state. Next we provide a brief overview of these effects.

Alcohol: Alcohol is a depressant that interferes with thinking and motor control. The user may experience a lack of inhibition, which in turn may result in aggression.

Stimulants: Stimulant compounds, such as cocaine (including crack) and methamphetamine, produce feelings of alertness and elevated energy levels with decreased anxiety and social inhibitions. When the acute drug effect comes to an end, a "crash" ensues. Users commonly become unable to experience pleasure, take limited interest in their environments, and have very low energy levels (Gold, Washton, & Dackis, 1985). Individuals who experience sleep disturbances may turn to sedatives, opiates, marijuana, or alcohol to ease agitation and induce slumber.

Opiates: Opiates, such as heroin, are depressants that produce a feeling of well-being in the user, along with episodes of drowsiness. Heroin withdrawal symptoms are more violent physiologically than those associated with the stimulants. They may include strong muscle contractions, intense perspiration, writhing, and nausea (Finnegan & Wapner, 1987). The classic opiate withdrawal is a continuing state during which the user experiences an ongoing desire to alleviate the symptoms through repeated administration of the drug.

Phencyclidine (PCP): Another substance of abuse, PCP (or "angel dust"), is an inexpensive synthetic drug, originally developed as an anesthetic, that may produce a wide spectrum of behaviors, ranging from delirium tremens and acute psychiatric illness to sedation, superhuman strength, violent acts, aggression, or a heightened state of euphoria (Fauman & Fauman, 1980; Pradhan, 1984; Rawson, Tennant, & McCann, 1981).

Marijuana: In low doses, marijuana can cause restlessness and a dreamy relaxed state, while stronger doses can induce rapidly fluctuating emotions and hallucinations or image distortions. Some users experience physical effects that include red or bloodshot eyes, dryness of the mouth and throat, increased appetite, and impaired muscular coordination. Reduced reactions, intensified concentration on surroundings, decreased ability to concentrate on tasks, an altered sense of time, impaired short-term memory, meaningless giggly conversation, anxiety, and psychological dependency are additional effects.

Given the behavioral effects of the various substances just described, it is clear that abuse of any of these drugs must have a profound impact on an individual's interactions with others as well as on parenting ability. The complexities of day-to-day responsive parenting are incongruent with altered mental status as seen in chronic addicts. Such people have difficulty meeting the ongoing life-supporting and emotional needs of a newborn infant and dependent child.

RELATIONSHIPS AND PARENTING SKILLS

The often-heard phrase "the lifestyle of the addict" evokes an image of an individual whose daily experiences revolve around the procurement and use of drugs. However, when the addict happens to be a pregnant woman or a father-to-be, that image becomes more complex. The focus shifts to the unborn child and how those parents will manage the responsibilities of caring for their offspring. A combination of circumstances that we often take for granted needs to be present in order to foster the growth of a baby. The mother-to-be, for instance, has a responsibility to seek prenatal care and ensure adequate nutrition. The father-to-be has a responsibility to support the mother's care of herself and the unborn child. Together, they need to secure housing, dependable income, preparations for the baby's arrival, and, if the parents are addicts, drug treatment for themselves.

In one longitudinal study examining the parenting behaviors of 47 amphetamine users, the environmental experiences of children of mothers who continued to use after pregnancy were disturbing (Billing, Eriksson, Larsson, & Zetterström, 1979). This Swedish research project showed that young children who were discharged home with mothers who had used amphetamine throughout pregnancy suffered the most adverse infancies during the 12 months of follow-up, as compared with infants whose mothers had discontinued drug use upon becoming aware of pregnancy and infants who were placed in institutions or foster homes following birth. One-third were removed from the care of their mothers because of parental neglect, approximately 40% were hospitalized one or more times, and over 50% had developmental and/or emotional problems.

Another longitudinal project followed the neurobehavioral development of children born to women on methadone maintenance and children born to women in a drug-free comparison group (Johnson, Glassman, Fiks, & Rosen, 1987). The relative impact of maternal drug abuse and postnatal family functioning on children's intellectual functioning at age 3 could then be evaluated. Maternal drinking, cigarette smoking, and, especially, illicit drug abuse had a clear influence on developmental outcome, mediated by both medical and environmental factors. Medically, substance abuse was related to complications during labor, delivery, and early neonatal course that, in turn, were associated with less adequate development in the children at 36 months. Environmentally, substance abuse was associated with a lower level of maternal education, more sporadic employment, and increased history of mental illness. These factors, in turn, were associated with more chaotic living conditions involving more frequent moves, more crowding, and an increased incidence of family violence; these directly and adversely affected the children's functioning at 36 months of age. Whereas maternal drug abuse was a significant prenatal risk factor, its effects were amplified by adverse postnatal family functioning. Still, despite the recognized significance of environmental influences on developmental outcome, little research has been conducted in this area.

MOTHER-CHILD INTERACTION AND ATTACHMENT

Past research has shown that even when there is no evidence of gross abuse or neglect, insecure attachment may be a precursor to future emotional disturbances in children (Ainsworth, Blehar, Waters, & Wall, 1978). Because this is such a crucial area of behavior, the actual quality of relationships and social interactions that prenatally drug-exposed infants experience with their caregivers has become a new area of focus for professionals in the field of perinatal alcohol and other drug abuse.

In one study, researchers videotaped methadone-maintained women and comparison group women as these mothers fed, diapered, and played with their 4-month-old infants in the laboratory (Jeremy & Bernstein, 1984). There was no simple difference between the groups. On the other hand, the methadone-maintained women tended to have lower IQ scores, fewer years of education, and less stable, satisfying relationships with their babies' fathers; and it was these poor maternal resources that correlated to deficiencies in interaction. In sum, methadone use was embedded within a matrix of risk factors that adversely affected mother-infant interaction.

To our knowledge, only one study to date has examined the home environments of children born to substance-abusing families (Rodning, Beckwith, & Howard, 1991). This study assessed the quality of attachment in the laboratory at 15 months of age and also systematically observed the rearing environments and caregiving behaviors provided at home by biologic, extended family, and foster caregivers to prenatally drug-exposed infants in their care during the first year of life. The substance-exposed infants and their caregivers were compared with infants of similar minority ethnic and low socioeconomic status who had been born to non–substance-abusing mothers residing in the same geographic area. Measures of the caregiving environments by both the HOME Inventory and the Ainsworth Rating Scales of Maternal-Care Behavior showed the biologic substance-abusing mothers to be significantly more rejecting, ignoring, neglecting, and interfering, and less sensitive to their infants than the comparison mothers. Extended family caregivers, foster parents, and comparison group mothers did not differ. The majority of drug-exposed infants were insecurely attached to their caregivers, whereas the majority of non–substance-exposed comparison infants were securely attached. Changes in caregivers during the first year of life did not explain the increase in insecure attachment. Moreover, poverty—a condition affecting both the drug-exposed and the control group— also was not the reason for the insecurity, nor was it necessarily associated with unresponsive or insensitive caregiving.

Research findings point to a similar situation with prenatal exposure to alcohol, which also has been linked to an increased occurrence of insecure attachment between mothers and infants in an economically advantaged sample. A path analysis has suggested that prenatal alcohol exposure was associated with increased infant irritability and that infant irritability increased the likelihood of insecure attachment (O'Connor, Sigman, & Kasari, 1992).

Implications for Mental Health Practice

In families where parents have problems with alcohol and/or other drug abuse, it is crucial for clinicians to consider the needs and dynamics of the family as a whole. The biological risks that have been reported in children prenatally exposed to alcohol and/or other drugs can make many of these youngsters particularly vulnerable to developing problems with learning and low self-esteem. These biological factors, coupled with the negative environmental influences that so often are associated with parental substance abuse (e.g., family discord, domestic violence, multiple caregivers), also can place these children at increased risk for future personality disorders. Thus, treatment efforts need to focus on the parents as well as on the children and must be comprehensive in scope.

Such comprehensive intervention requires an interdisciplinary approach that is critical for addressing the multiple needs of families affected by parental substance abuse. For example, a social worker can help a family with issues related to stabilizing income and housing. This is often a critical area for these families, as substance abusers commonly have problems with ongoing employment and frequently expend funds that are needed for rent and other basic costs of living on alcohol and/or other drugs. Issues related to ongoing family health and nutrition lie within the domain of the health care team. Families affected by parental substance abuse often have needs related to treatment of sexually transmitted diseases, dental care, family planning, and prenatal care (including nutritional counseling and information about the effects of alcohol and other drugs on the developing fetus). Pediatricians and child development specialists are essential in focusing on children's issues, such as infant care, early intervention, age-appropriate activities that can be im-

plemented within the family home, and later school placements that foster children's learning. Additionally, when parents are willing to engage in treatment, substance abuse treatment counselors need to become involved in order to address the complex issues related to addiction, including peer pressure, relapse, types of treatment programs (e.g., residential outpatient, transitional), and treatment options (e.g., methadone maintenance). In collaboration with these other disciplines, the mental health professional is in a better position to help family members deal more effectively with issues related to their mental health. These issues may be related to parental histories of child abuse, family violence, addiction and/or alcoholism, and school failure as well as problems related to codependency among other family members and parent-child interactions.

It also is important to bear in mind the intergenerational nature of family dysfunction and parental substance abuse. Thus, mental health efforts need to involve treatment for the mental health disorders of alcoholic or addicted parents among the interventions designed to prevent later psychiatric problems in their children. In order to plan effective treatment strategies for substance-abusing families, the professional needs to take into account what is known about the causes of mental health disorders in adults, over and above the problem of substance abuse, as well as the effects of parental mental health problems on children.

It has been found that a variety of community and socioeconomic factors, such as residence in an inner-city and low socioeconomic status, as well as involvement with an antisocial peer group, are risk factors associated with mental health problems (Langner, Herson, Greene, Jameson, & Goff, 1970; Rutter, Cox, Tupling, Berger, & Yule, 1975). However, even more important, parental and family factors such as poor parenting, marital discord, large family size, discordant mother-child relationships, and parents with psychiatric impairment have been shown to contribute significantly to future psychiatric disturbances in children. In fact, if such adverse family influences are taken into account, the risk to these children for future mental disorders drops to the same level as that which has been attributed to children in the general population (Rutter & Quinton, 1984). Further, research has shown that children not living with their mentally ill parents did not evidence any increase in later psychiatric disorders if they were raised in alternative family settings and not in institutions (Feldman, Stiffman, & Jung, 1987).

The effects of addiction per se have not been isolated as a potential factor in most research that has been conducted with parents who have personality disorders. However, as we have learned more about substance-abusing parents of young children, it has become clear that many have an underlying personality disorder that exists along with the addiction. Further, alcoholic or addicted parents of young children frequently demonstrate many of the same behaviors that have been reported in parents who have mental disorders—an increased incidence of marital and family discord, negative feelings toward children, impairment of parenting ability. Thus, much research related to the effects of parental mental disorder on children also may be useful in developing treatment strategies for substance-abusing families.

The association between parental personality disorders and children's future personality disturbances is most clear when family dysfunction results in children's exposure to hostile or aggressive behavior (Rutter, 1989). Evidence suggests that even very young children may be affected by such domestic tension—toddlers appear to be very quick to perceive negative feelings among family members (Zahn-Waxler, McKnew, Cummings, Davenport, & Radke-Yarrow, 1984)—and this often interferes with the young child's sense of security in the parent-child dyad. Further, children's behaviors do not necessarily coincide chronologically with those of their parents—that is, a child may not exhibit increased negative behavior at the height of a parental outburst or decreased negative behaviors while a parent is in control (Hobbs, 1982; Rutter & Quinton, 1984). Thus, the mental health professional needs to recognize the potential for a "delayed reaction" and not conclude that a child's risk is diminished if he or she does not show an immediate response to parental hostility. Research has shown that the psychiatric risk to children can continue until well after the remission of the parental disorder, although the risk is greater if it persists (Billings & Moos, 1986; Rutter & Quinton, 1984).

A factor that is unique to substance-abusing families that can further complicate the parent-child relationship is the "revolving door" cycle

(i.e., parental loss and regaining of child custody) that often ensues following the identification of a parental substance abuse problem and concerns about child safety. One of the deleterious effects of this situation upon parental self-perception may be a "learned helplessness" whereby parents may not take the initiative to improve their situations. For instance, a few parents may abandon their infants, while others may appear to take little interest in their children who are placed outside the parental home. Still others may have repeat pregnancies in order to "replace" children who have been removed from their custody. The impact of multiple placements with multiple caregivers upon a child's social-emotional and cognitive development may be even more profound. Unfortunately, no studies have been conducted with this population to determine the negative impact of this type of experience upon parents and children. However, one study of children whose parents had psychiatric disorders did indicate that youngsters who were placed in stable foster care settings or for whom family harmony was restored tended to be at decreased risk (Rutter, 1989).

Although it is important to consider potential risk factors such as those just listed, individual differences do exist in all families, and it is helpful also to focus on the specific problems that are present within the family setting and on how individual family members actually respond to one another. Only as we begin to examine family members' individual histories and the circumstances that they identify as significant (both negatively and positively) in their experience can we begin to sort out family strengths. In addition to the many vulnerabilities we encounter in substance-abusing families, families do exhibit strengths. For example, a good relationship with a parent or with a teacher or clergy member may be a protective factor. By incrementally building on these strengths, we can help decrease environmental adversities for all family members.

In summary, treatment of the substance-abusing family needs to focus on decreasing biological risk to future children by curtailing alcohol and/or other drug abuse during pregnancy as well as on improving environmental factors. Because alcoholism and drug addiction are chronic health disorders that commonly involve multiple relapses and remissions, intervention with substance-abusing families must be an ongoing effort provided by an interdisciplinary team. Although we recognize that prenatal drug exposure acts both biologically and environmentally through the addicted parent and poorer family functioning, the implications for treating these families lie in changing behaviors. Professionals need to work with parents to help them become sober and/or drug-free, improve self-esteem, and become self-reliant; with families as a whole to improve family health, nurturing, and functioning, and to decrease discord; and with children to foster learning and to develop trust in meaningful relationships with adult caregivers.

REFERENCES

Abel, E. L., & Sokol, R. J. (1987). Incidence of fetal alcohol syndrome and economic impact of FAS related anomalies. *Drug and Alcohol Dependency, 19,* 51–70.

Ainsworth, M. D. S., Blehar, M. C., Waters, E., & Wall, S. (1978). *Patterns of attachment.* Hillsdale, NJ: Lawrence Erlbaum.

Backwith, L., & Howard, J. (1991, April). *Development of toddlers exposed prenatally to PCP and cocaine.* Paper presented at the biennial conference of the Society for Research in Child Development, Seattle, WA.

Beckwith, L., Rodning, C., Norris, D., Phillipsen, L., Khandabi, P., & Howard, J. (1994). Spontaneous play in two-year-olds born to substance-abusing mothers. *Infant Mental Health Journal 15* (2), 189–201.

Besharov, D. J. (1989, Fall). The children of crack: Will we protect them? *Public Welfare,* 7–11.

Billing, L., Eriksson, M., Larsson, G., & Zetterström, R. (1979). Occurrence of abuse and neglect of children born to amphetamine addicted mothers. *Child Abuse and Neglect, 3,* 205–211.

Billings, A. G., & Moos, R. H. (1986). Children of parents with unipolar depression: A controlled 1-year follow-up. *Journal of Abnormal Child Psychology, 14,* 149–166.

Bingol, N., Fuchs, M., Diaz, V., Stone, R. K., & Gromisch, D. S. (1987). Teratogenicity of cocaine in humans. *Journal of Pediatrics, 110* (1), 93–96.

Chasnoff, I. J., Griffith, D. R., Freier, C., & Murray, J. (1992). Cocaine/polydrug use in pregnancy: Two-year follow-up. *Pediatrics, 89,* 284–289.

Chavez, C. J., Ostrea, E. M., Jr., Stryker, J. C., & Smialek, Z. (1979). Sudden infant death syndrome among infants of drug-dependent mothers. *Journal of Pediatrics, 95* (3), 407–409.

Clarren, S. K., & Smith, D. (1978). The fetal alcohol syndrome. *New England Journal of Medicine, 298,* 1063–1067.

Cuskey, W. R., & Wathey, B. (1982). *Female addiction.* Lexington, MA: Lexington Books.

Dalterio, S. L., & De Rooji, D. C. (1986). Maternal cannabinoid exposure: Effects on spermatogenesis in male offspring. *International Journal of Andrology, 9,* 250–258.

Davidson Ward, S. L., Bautista, D., Chan, L., Derry, M., Lisbin, A., Durfee, M. J., Mills, K. S. C., &

Keens, T. G. (1990). Sudden infant death syndrome in infants of substance-abusing mothers. *Journal of Pediatrics, 117* (6), 876–881.

Dixon, S. D., & Bejar, R. (1989). Echoencephalographic findings in neonates associated with maternal cocaine and methamphetamine use: Incidence and clinical correlates. *Journal of Pediatrics, 115* (5), 770–778.

Doberczak, T. M., Shanzer, S., Senie, R. T., & Kandall, S. R. (1988). Neonatal neurologic and electroencephalographic effects of intrauterine cocaine exposure. *Journal of Pediatrics, 113* (2), 354–358.

Fanshel, D. (1975). Parental failure and consequences for children: The drug-abusing mother whose children are in foster care. *American Journal of Public Health, 65* (6), 604–612.

Fauman, M. A., & Fauman, B. J. (1980). Chronic phencyclidine (PCP) abuse: A psychiatric perspective. *Journal of Psychedelic Drugs, 12* (3–4), 307–315.

Feldman, R. A., Stiffman, A. R., & Jung, K. G. (1987). *Children at risk: In the web of parental mental illness.* New Brunswick, NJ: Rutgers University Press.

Finnegan, L. P. (1975). Narcotics dependence in pregnancy. *Journal of Psychedelic Drugs, 7* (3), 299–311.

Finnegan, L. P., & Wapner, R. (1987). Narcotic addiction in pregnancy. In J. R. Neibyl (Ed.), *Drug use in pregnancy* (pp. 203–222). Philadelphia: Lea and Febiger.

Friedrich, W. N., Beilke, R., & Urquiza, A. (1988). Behavior problems in young sexually abused boys. *Journal of Interpersonal Violence, 3,* 21–27.

General Accounting Office (1990, June). *Drug-exposed infants: A generation at risk* (Publication GAO/HRD-90–138). Washington, DC: Author, Human Resources Division.

Gold, M. S., Washton, A. M., & Dackis, C. A. (1985). Cocaine abuse: Neurochemistry, phenomenology and treatment. In N.J. Kozel & E. H. Adams (Eds.), *Cocaine use in America: Epidemiological and clinical perspectives* (NIDA Research Monograph 61) (pp. 130–150). Rockville, MA: National Institute on Drug Abuse.

Gomby, A., & Shiono, P. H. (1991). Estimating the number of substance-exposed infants. *Future Child, 1,* 17–25.

Hans, S. L., Marcus, J., Jeremy, R. J., & Auerbach, J. G. (1984). Neurobehavioral development of children exposed in utero to opioid drugs. *Neurobehavioral Teratology*, 249–273.

Herjanic, B. M., Barredo, V. H., Herjanic, M., & Tomelleri, C. J. (1979). Children of heroin addicts. *International Journal of the Addictions, 14*, 919–931.

Hobbs, P. (1982). The relative timing of psychiatric disorder in parents and children. *British Journal of Psychiatry, 140*, 37–43.

Householder, J., Hatcher, R., Burns, W., & Chasnoff, I. (1982). Infants born to narcotic-addicted mothers. *Psychological Bulletin, 92*, 453–468.

Howard, J., Beckwith, L., Rodning, C., & Kropenske, V. (1989). The development of young children of substance-abusing parents: Insights from seven years of intervention and research. *Zero to Three, 9* (5), 8–12.

Howard, J., Kropenske, V., & Tyler, R. (1986). The long-term effects on neurodevelopment in infants exposed prenatally to PCP. In D. H. Clouet (Ed.), *Phencyclidine: An update* (National Institute on Drug Abuse Research Monograph Series 64, pp. 237–251). Rockville, MD: National Institute on Drug Abuse.

Hoyme, H. E., Jones, K. L., Dixon, S. D., Jewett, T., Hanson, J. W., Robinson, L. K., Msall, M. E., & Allanson, J. E. (1990). Prenatal cocaine exposure and fetal vascular disruption. *Pediatrics, 85* (5), 743–747.

Jeremy, R. J., & Bernstein, V. J. (1984). Dyads at risk: Methadone-maintained women and their four-month-old infants. *Child Development, 55*, 1141–1154.

Jessup, M., & Green, J. R. (1987). Treatment of the pregnant alcohol-dependent woman. *Journal of Psychoactive Drugs, 19* (2), 193–203.

Joffe, T. J., Peterson, J. M., Smith, D. J., & Soyka, L. F. (1976). Sub-lethal effects in offspring of male rats treated with methadone before mating. *Research Communications in Chemistry, Pathology and Pharmacology, 13*, 611–621.

Johnson, D. J., & Cole, C. K. (1992, Winter). Extraordinary care for extraordinary children. *School Safety*, 7–9.

Johnson, H. L., Diano, A., & Rosen, T. S. (1984). 24-month neurobehavioral follow-up of children of methadone-maintained mothers. *Infant Behavior and Development, 7*, 115–123.

Johnson, H., Glassman, M. B., Fiks, K. B., & Rosen, T. S. (1987). Path analysis of variables affecting 36-month outcome in a population of multi-risk children. *Infant Behavior and Development, 10*, 451–465.

Jones, K. L., Smith, D. W., Ulleland, C. N., & Streissguth, A. P. (1973). Pattern of malformation in offspring of chronic alcoholic mothers. *Lancet, 1*, 1267–1271.

Kaltenbach, K., & Finnegan, L. P. (1984). Developmental outcome of children born to methadone maintained women: A review of longitudinal studies. *Neurobehavioral Toxicology and Teratology, 6*, 271–275.

Kandall, S. R., Gaines, J., Habel, L., Davidson, G., & Jessop, D. (1993). Relationship of maternal substance abuse to subsequent sudden infant death syndrome in offspring. *Journal of Pediatrics, 123* (1), 120–126.

Langner, T. S., Herson, J. H., Greene, E. L., Jameson, J. D., & Goff, J. A. (1970). Children of the city: Affluence, poverty and mental health. In V. L. Allen (Ed.), *Psychological factors in poverty* (pp. 185–202). Chicago: Markham.

Lester, B. M., Corwin, M. J., Sepkoski, C., Seifer, R., Peucker, M., McLaughlin, S., & Golub, H. L. (1991). Neurobehavioral syndromes in cocaine-exposed newborn infants. *Child Development, 62*, 694–705.

Little, R. E., & Sing, S. F. (1988, June). High proof paternity: Dads who drink conceive low birth weight infants. *Health*, 20.

Lodge, A. (1976). Developmental findings with infants born to mothers on methadone maintenance: A preliminary report. In G. Beschner & R. Brotman (Eds.), *National Institute on Drug Abuse symposium on comprehensive health care for addicted families and their children* (Services Research Report 017-024-00598-3, pp. 79–85). Washington, DC: U.S. Government Printing Office.

Midanik, L. (1982). The validity of self-reported alcohol consumption and alcohol problems: Literature review. *British Journal of Addiction to Alcohol and Drugs, 77*, 357–382.

Nichtern, S. (1973). The children of drug users. *Journal of the American Academy of Child Psychiatry, 12* (24), 24–31.

O'Connor, M. J., Brill, N.J., & Sigman, M. (1986). Alcohol use in primiparous women older than 30 years of age: Relation to infant development. *Pediatrics, 78* (3), 444–450.

O'Connor, M. J., Sigman, M., & Kasari, C. (1992). Attachment behavior of infants exposed prenatally to alcohol: Mediating effects of infant affect and mother-infant interaction. *Development and Psychopathology, 4*, 243–256.

Offord, D. R. (1989). Conduct disorder: Risk factors and prevention. In D. Shaffer, I. Philips, & N. B. Enzer (Eds.), *Prevention of mental disorders, alcohol and other drug use in children and adolescents* (OSAP Prevention Monograph 2, DHHS Publication No. [ADM] 89-1646, pp. 275–307). Rockville, MD: Office for Substance Abuse Prevention.

Olson, H. C., Burgess, D. M., & Streissguth, A. P. (1992). Fetal alcohol syndrome (FAS) and fetal alcohol effects (FAE): A life-span view, with implications for early intervention. *Zero to Three, 13* (1), 24–29.

Oro, A. S., & Dixon, S. D. (1987). Perinatal cocaine and methamphetamine exposure: Maternal and neonatal correlates. *Journal of Pediatrics, 111* (4), 571–578.

Pradhan, S. N. (1984). Phencyclidine (PCP): Some human studies. *Neuroscience and Biobehavioral Reviews, 8*, 493–501.

Rawson, R. A., Tennant, F., & McCann, M. A. (1981). Characteristics of 68 chronic phencyclidine abusers who sought treatment. *Drug and Alcohol Dependency, 8*, 223–227.

Regan, D. O., Ehrlich, S. M., & Finnegan, L. P. (1987). Infants of drug addicts: At risk for child abuse, neglect, and placement in foster care. *Neurotoxicology and Teratology, 9,* 315–319.

Rodning, C., Beckwith, L., & Howard, J. (1989). Characteristics of attachment organization and play organization in prenatally drug-exposed toddlers. *Development and Psychopathology, 1,* 277–289.

Rodning, C., Beckwith, L., & Howard, J. (1991). Quality of attachment and home environments in children prenatally exposed to PCP and cocaine. *Development and Psychopathology, 3,* 351–366.

Rosen, T. S., & Johnson, H. L. (1982). Children of methadone-maintained mothers: Follow-up to 18 months of age. *Journal of Pediatrics, 101* (2), 192–196.

Rosen, T. S., & Johnson, H. L. (1985). Long-term effects of prenatal methadone maintenance. In T. M. Pinkert (Ed.), *Current research on the consequences of maternal drug abuse* (NIDA Research Monograph 59, pp. 73–83). Rockville, MD: National Institute on Drug Abuse.

Rudolph, A. M. (1991). Neglect: Failure to provide essentials. In *Rudolph's Pediatrics* (19th ed., pp. 844–845). San Mateo, CA: Appleton and Lange.

Rutter, M. (1989). Psychiatric disorder in parents as a risk factor for children. In D. Shaffer, I. Philips, & N. B. Enzer (Eds.), *Prevention of mental disorders, alcohol and other drug use in children and adolescents* (OSAP Prevention Monograph 2, DHHS Publication No. [ADM] 89-1646, pp. 159–189). Rockville, MD: Office for Substance Abuse Prevention.

Rutter, M., Cox, A., Tupling, C., Berger, M., & Yule, W. (1975). Attainment and adjustment in two geographical areas: 1. The prevalence of psychiatric disorder. *British Journal of Psychiatry, 126,* 493–509.

Rutter, M., & Quinton, D. (1984). Parental psychiatric disorder: Effects on children. *Psychological Medicine, 14,* 853–880.

Ryan, L., Ehrlich, S., & Finnegan, L. (1987). Cocaine abuse in pregnancy: Effects on the fetus and the newborn. *Neurotoxicology and Teratology, 9,* 295–299.

Serdula, M., Williamson, D. F., Kendrick, J. S., Anda, R. F., & Byers, T. (1991). Trends in alcohol consumption by pregnant women 1985 through 1988. *Journal of the American Medical Association, 265* (7), 876–879.

Smith, D. E., Milkman, H. B., & Sunderwirth, S. G. (1985). Addictive disease: Concept and controversy. In H. B. Milkman & H. J. Shaffer (Eds.), *The addictions: Multidisciplinary perspectives and treatments* (pp. 145–159). Lexington, MA: Lexington Books.

Smith, D. W. (1979, October). The fetal alcohol syndrome. *Hospital Practice,* 121–128.

Smith, P. F., Remington, P. L., Williamson, D. F., & Anda, R. F. (1990). Alcohol consumption and problem drinking: Comparison of sales data with surveys of self-reported alcohol use in 21 states. *American Journal of Public Health, 80,* 309–312.

Sonderegger, T. B., O'Shea, S., & Zimmerman, E. (1979). Progeny of male rats treated neonatally with morphine pellets. *Proceedings of the Western Pharmacology Society, 11,* 137–139.

Sowder, B. J., & Burt, M. R. (1980). Children of addicts and nonaddicts: A comparative investigation in five urban sites. In *Heroin-addicted parents and their children: Two reports* (DHHS publication [ADM] 81–1028, pp. 19–35). Rockville, MD: National Institute on Drug Abuse.

Sowder, B. J., Carnes, Y. M., & Sherman, S. N. (1981). *Children of addicts in surrogate care.* Unpublished manuscript prepared for the Services Research Branch, National Institute on Drug Abuse, Institute for Human Resources Research.

Strauss, A. A., Modanlou, H. D., & Bosu, S. K. (1981). Neonatal manifestations of maternal phencyclidine (PCP) abuse. *Pediatrics, 68* (4), 550–552.

Streissguth, A. P., Aase, J. M., Clarren, S. K., Randels, S. P., LaDue, R. A., & Smith, D. F. (1991). Fetal alcohol syndrome in adolescents and adults. *Journal of the American Medical Association, 265* (15), 1961–1967.

Streissguth, A. P., Barr, H. M., Sampson, P. D., Darby, B. L., & Martin, D. C. (1989). IQ at age 4 in relation to maternal alcohol use and smoking during pregnancy. *Developmental Psychology, 25* (1), 3–11.

Streissguth, A. P., Herman, C. S., & Smith, D. W. (1978). Intelligence, behavior, and dysmorphogenesis in the fetal alcohol syndrome: A report on 20 patients. *Journal of Pediatrics, 92* (3), 363–367.

Streissguth, A. P., & LaDue, R. A. (1985). Psychological and behavioral effects in children exposed to alcohol. *Alcohol Health and Research World, 10* (1), 6–12.

Streissguth, A. P., Martin, D. C., Martin J. C., & Barr, H. M. (1981). The Seattle longitudinal prospective study on alcohol and pregnancy. *Neurobehavioral Toxicology and Teratology, 3* (2), 223–233.

Tarter, R. F., Jacob, T., & Bremer, D. L. (1990). Specific cognitive impairment in sons of early onset alcoholics. *Alcoholism: Clinical and Experimental Research, 13,* 786–789.

Tucker, M. B. (1982). Social support and coping: Applications for the study of female drug abuse. *Journal of Social Issues, 38* (2), 117–137.

Wilson, G. (1976). Management of pediatric medical problems in the addicted household. In G. Beschner, & R. Brotman, (Eds.), *National Institute on Drug Abuse symposium on comprehensive health care for addicted families and their children, 20–21 May 1976* (Services Research Report 017-024-00598-3, p. 74). Washington, DC: U.S. Government Printing Office.

Wilson, G., Desmond, M. M., & Verniaud, W. M. (1973). Early development of infants of heroin-addicted mothers. *American Journal of Diseases in Children, 126,* 457–462.

Wilson, G. S., Desmond, M. M., & Wait, R. B. (1981). Follow-up of methadone-treated and untreated narcotic-dependent women and their infants: Health, developmental, and social implications. *Journal of Pediatrics, 98* (5), 716–722.

Wilson, G. S., McCreary, R., Kean, J., & Baxter, J. C. (1979). The development of preschool children of heroin-addicted mothers: A controlled study. *Pediatrics, 63* (1), 135–141.

Young, N. K., Wallace, V. R., & Garcia, T. (1992). Developmental status of three- to five-year-old children who were prenatally exposed to alcohol and other drugs. *School Social Work Journal, 16,* 1–15.

Zahn-Waxler, C., McKnew, D. H., Cummings, M., Davenport, Y. B., & Radke-Yarrow, M. (1984). Problem behaviors and peer interactions of young children with a manic-depressive parent. *American Journal of Psychiatry, 141,* 236–240.

37 / The Child with Mental Retardation

Robert M. Hodapp and Connie Kasari

The field of mental retardation has recently witnessed a series of findings and controversies that make it particularly interesting to child psychiatrists. These issues include difficult definitional questions; new types of retardation; peculiar developmental findings; new perspectives on families; and new approaches to dual diagnosis, early intervention, and the role of the psychiatrist and other professionals. Indeed, the number and complexity of issues in mental retardation cut across a variety of different disciplines, including but not limited to child psychiatry.

Classification, Assessment, and Prevalence

The first of these controversial areas is the problem of definition. For the past decade, the main professional organization in mental retardation, the American Association on Mental Retardation (AAMR), has defined mental retardation as follows: "Mental retardation refers to significantly subaverage intellectual functioning resulting in or associated with impairments in adaptive behavior and manifested during the developmental period" (Grossman, 1983, p. 11).

This definition essentially involves three factors: (1) *subaverage intellectual functioning,* which usually is defined as a score on an IQ test that is two or more standard deviations below the mean of the population (usually, an IQ less than 70);

(2) *impairments in adaptive behavior,* usually assessed with the AAMR, Vineland, or other scales of adaptive behavior; and (3) *manifested during the developmental period* (i.e., first occurring before 18 years of age).

While not perfect, this three-factor definition has held up reasonably well over the past decade. Recently, however, the AAMR has published a revised classification manual (AAMR, 1992). While retaining the three-factor format, this manual emphasizes the importance of adaptive behavior and divides this construct into a number of domains. These include: communication, self-care, home living, social skills, community use, self-direction, health and safety, functional academics, leisure, and work. Deficiencies in any two or more of these areas are considered impairments in adaptive behavior. In addition, the IQ cut-off has been changed to a range, from 70 to 75, as opposed to the prior cut-off of 2 standard deviations below the population mean (Grossman, 1983; American Psychiatric Association [APA], 1987).

As might be expected, heated controversy has accompanied this new AAMR manual. Even prior to its formal publication, Jacobson and Mulick (1992) decried the unwieldiness of the new definition. They noted that the criterion of deficits in any two adaptive subdomains—some of which now have no standardized assessments—makes the assessment of deficits in adaptive behavior almost impossible. These authors also criticize the "floating" nature of the IQ criterion: With an IQ cut-off at IQ 70 or 75, the diagnosis of mental retardation becomes increasingly subjective.

The ultimate outcome of the new AAMR definition remains unknown. In commenting on the

414

change in the IQ criterion, MacMillan, Gresham, and Siperstein (1993) note that *"Twice as many people are eligible* [to be diagnosed with mental retardation] when the cutoff is 'IQ 75 and below' as when it is 'IQ 70 and below'" (p. 327; emphasis in original). Similarly, Hodapp (1995a) has noted the unwieldiness of the new definition, particularly its adaptive component (see also Gresham, MacMillan & Siperstein, 1995).

Faced with such competing definitions, the American Psychiatric Association (1994) adopted some features from the original definition, others from the 1992 AAMR definition. Specifically, *DSM-IV* criteria include IQ scores of 70 or below (from the Grossman 1983 definition) and deficits in 2 areas of adaptive behavior (as in the AAMR 1994 definition). For a review of this controversy, see Hodapp and Dykens (1996).

Although open to criticism, the 1992 AAMR definition highlights trends arising within the mental retardation field. For example, while the vagueness of the IQ cut-off (i.e., IQ 70 to 75) is regrettable, the decision reflects the recent deemphasis placed on psychometric measurements of intelligence. The *Larry P.* case (MacMillan, Hendrick, & Watkins, 1988)—and its resultant prohibition on the use of IQ tests to diagnose children with retardation in California—is the most well-known example of this trend; other states and systems (e.g., schools), are also giving IQ tests lesser weighting than previously. The concerns about the possible racial and ethnic biases of IQ tests provide one source of disenchantment with such tests, although no good alternatives have yet been proposed.

A related trend involves the growing recognition of the importance of adaptive behavior in individual functioning. In fact, particularly among children with mild impairments, IQ scores poorly predict real-world adaptation. The lack of a relationship between IQ and adaptation extends into adulthood as well: In several studies of adults with retardation, individuals with IQs of approximately 50 to 85 (or "borderline" levels of intellectual functioning) were found to vary widely in their everyday performances. Some of these adults held jobs, were married, and lived independent lives, whereas others at equivalent IQ levels were totally or partially dependent on others (Ross, Begab, Dondis, Giampiccolo, & Meyers, 1985). From a sample of Scandinavian young men with IQs from

50 to 70, Granat and Granat (1973, 1978) demonstrated that the best predictors of *not* being identified as mentally retarded were being punctual and hardworking, getting along with others, and not being depressed.

Along with the deemphasis on IQ tests and the increased attention to adaptive behavior, the AAMR definition attempts to highlight the contextual nature of individual functioning. That is, all individuals function better given the presence of certain social, financial, educational, or other supports.

Still, even allowing for these understandable trends, the new AAMR definition seems problematic. Adaptive behavior, for example, is composed of areas (e.g., self-direction, leisure, health and safety) for which no standardized measures currently exist, and the IQ cut-off of 70 to 75 introduces a degree of uncertainty that exacerbates already-existing problems.

Besides being unwieldy, the new definition also complicates the issue of establishing the prevalence of mental retardation. Until now, mental retardation has been thought to affect some 3% of the population. Beginning during the 1970s, however, Mercer (1973) criticized the 3% figure, arguing that only about 1% of the population should be so classified. Mercer asserted that the 3% figure is based on four invalid assumptions: (1) that IQ is the sole criterion of mental retardation (or that IQ and adaptive behavior are perfectly correlated); (2) that equal percentages of persons will be diagnosed as retarded at every age; (3) that IQ is stable; and (4) that the death rates of persons with mental retardation are identical to those of the nonretarded population.

Each of the four assumptions is problematic. Regarding the relationship between IQ and adaptive behavior, this relationship differs due to the individual's level of impairment. At lower levels of intelligence (e.g., below IQ 40 to 50), IQ and adaptive behavior quotients are highly correlated; such correlations are seen in both children (Kahn, 1992) and adults (Ross et al., 1985). Above IQ 50, however, the relationships are more variable, and the extent to which the two are *not* related lowers the 3% figure, although to what extent remains unclear.

In the same way, prevalence rates of mental retardation change at different ages. Although prevalence rates of children with below 50 IQs are steady at 0.4% throughout childhood (Abramowicz & Richardson, 1975), children with lesser degrees of impairment are most often diagnosed during the school-age years. Thus, higher percentages of children ages 6 to 16 are diagnosed with mental retardation, with lesser numbers identified both before and after this time (c.f. MacMillan, 1982). Indeed, professionals often talk of a "decertification" of mental retardation that occurs during the postschool years, as young adults who had previously been considered to be mentally retarded are no longer so diagnosed. In the same way, the degree to which school and academic performance intricately involved in diagnosis has led some to propose the presence of a "six-hour retarded child," the child who is considered to be retarded only within the school context. Again, as with the assumption of IQ as the sole diagnostic criterion, the degree to which prevalence rates of non–school-age children are below 3% will lessen the prevalence of mental retardation.

A third problematic assumption concerns the stability of IQ. While reasonably stable after age 4 (Vernon, 1979), any individual child's IQ score will fluctuate slightly. To some extent, the AAMR's (1992) IQ cut-off of 70 to 75 acknowledges this fact. Also, as children scoring below IQ 70 will tend to perform slightly higher on a subsequent IQ test (due to regression effects), uncertain prevalence rates of mental retardation result.

A fourth assumption concerns death rates. In contrast to a life expectancy of 75 or so years for the person without mental retardation, persons with mental retardation die at earlier ages. Such shorter life spans most often occur in individuals who are nonambulatory, are profoundly impaired intellectually, and have associated physical disabilities. In addition, several specific types of mental retardation have associated health problems that make these individuals at high risk for earlier deaths. Thus, although the life span of children with Down syndrome has risen from 9 years in 1912 (c.f. Penrose, 1963) to 50 or so years during the 1980s (Dupont, Vaeth, & Videbech, 1986), heart defects, respiratory diseases, and the onset of premature Alzheimer's after the age of 35 years (Zigman, Schupf, Lubin, & Silverman, 1987) continue to plague such persons. Similarly, the obesity and weight fluctuations of persons with Prader-Willi syndrome shorten their life spans

(Cassidy, 1992; Dykens & Cassidy, in press). As with the first three assumptions, the shorter life expectancies of persons with retardation lead to prevalence rates below 3% of the general population.

How many persons are mentally retarded? Given that IQ is not the sole diagnostic criterion, prevalence rates are not stable with age, IQ fluctuates, and persons with retardation have higher death rates, it seems unlikely that 3% of the population is mentally retarded. At the same time, a 1% rate may also be too low. The actual prevalence rate may never be agreed upon, especially given definitional debates that continue to characterize the professional fields interested in mental retardation.

Levels and Types of Mental Retardation

Since all persons with retardation are not alike, efforts continue as to the best ways of categorizing such persons. Two different approaches are generally used, one focusing on degree of intellectual deficit, the other on the type of mental retardation.

LEVEL OF IMPAIRMENT

In differentiating by level of impairment, the degree to which the child is impaired is compared to same-age peers. Four categories are generally used: mild, moderate, severe, and profound.

The category of *mild mental retardation* (IQs from 55 to 69) includes the majority of persons with retardation. Individuals with mild retardation vary widely in their adaptive abilities. As children, individuals at this level of retardation are often mainstreamed into classes with nonretarded children; as adults, many live independent or semiindependent lives. As noted earlier, many of the most difficult definitional issues concern this group.

Comprising the second largest category of mental retardation, persons with *moderate men-*

tal retardation (IQs from 40 to 54) are more affected—intellectually and adaptively—than are
persons with mild retardation. Although some will
live independent lives, the majority require at
least some supervision in school, work, and living
settings. In addition, whereas many persons with
mild mental retardation show no obvious cause of
their retardation, most persons with moderate retardation show a clear organic etiology.

With the help of educational and training advances, persons with *severe mental retardation*
(IQs from 25 to 39) are generally able to achieve
basic self-help and communication skills. Still, virtually all persons with severe mental retardation
require some supervision throughout life. As
adults, many such individuals perform well in supervised workshops and group homes, and most
show a clear organic cause of their retardation.

Individuals with *profound mental retardation*
(IQs below 20 or 25) are the most impaired intellectually and adaptively, achieving only the most
basic communication and self-help skills. In addition, individuals with profound mental retardation
often suffer from physical deformities and associated health problems.

THE TWO-GROUP APPROACH AND
RECENT EXTENSIONS

A second approach to classification relates to
the cause of the child's retardation. Zigler's (1967)
"two-group approach" to mental retardation began this differentiation process, with more recent work refining and extending this approach.
Briefly, the two-group approach hypothesizes that
there are two types of individuals with mental retardation. The first group is composed of individuals showing no clear organic etiology to their retardation. Called by a variety of names, familial or
cultural-familial retarded individuals often come
from lower socioeconomic backgrounds. Persons
with familial retardation are generally mildly retarded and often have one or more relatives who
are themselves mentally retarded.

The second group is comprised of individuals
who show one of the approximately 300 organic
causes of mental retardation. These include *prenatal causes* such as fetal alcohol syndrome, accidents in utero, and all of the genetic disorders;

perinatal causes such as anoxia and prematurity;
and *postnatal* causes such as meningitis and head
trauma. This group accounts for somewhat less
than half of all cases of mental retardation
(Zigler & Hodapp, 1986).

The two-group approach has recently been extended to examine more closely the different
types of organic retardation (Burack, Hodapp, &
Zigler, 1988). Particularly as concerns individual
genetic disorders (Dykens, 1995; Hodapp & Dykens, 1994), specific etiologies lead to different
behavioral profiles and initial indications as to
gene-behavior relationships. Among the most
interesting disorders in this regard are fragile X
syndrome and Prader-Willi and Angelman's syndromes.

Fragile X Syndrome: After Down syndrome,
fragile X syndrome is the second most common
genetic—and most common hereditary—cause
of mental retardation. Unlike most X-linked disorders, fragile X syndrome does not follow the
"classic" pattern of affected males and unaffected
female carriers. Twenty percent of genetically
affected males are impaired intellectually; conversely, about one-third of female carriers are
themselves affected with the disorder. (See Dykens, Hodapp, & Leckman, 1994, for a review.)

First described in a family study by Martin and
Bell (1943), the genetics of this peculiar disorder
are only now beginning to be understood. Herbert
Lubs first noticed the pinched, constricted "fragile" site on the long arm of the X chromosome in
1969. But for several years, Lubs's discovery could
not be replicated. Only in 1977 did it become
clear that the fragile site in fragile X syndrome
only shows itself when karyotypes are performed
in the absence of folate. In 1991, the actual gene
for fragile X syndrome (the FMR-1 gene) was discovered at a particular portion of the X chromosome (Xq27). Even more recently, two other features of the disorder have become apparent:
Fragile X syndrome has been shown to consist of
an overly large number of cytosine-guanine-
guanine (CGG) repeats at the FMR-1 site and the
overabundance of CGG repeats combines with a
chemical process called methylation to decrease
production of a particular protein, thereby leading
to fragile X's characteristic physical and behavioral features.

As a result of these genetic anomalies, males

with fragile X syndrome display a long, thin face and large, prominent ears. After puberty, these males show enlarged testes. Females with fragile X show some of these physical features, but to a lesser extent.

Behaviorally, too, individuals with fragile X syndrome show particular, etiology-specific characteristics. Their abilities to process sequential, step-by-step information is particularly impaired relative to simultaneous (or holistic) processing (Dykens, Hodapp, & Leckman, 1987). In addition, these males slow in development at or near the pubertal years; such plateauing occurs in both intellectual (Dykens et al., 1989; Hodapp et al., 1990) and adaptive development (Dykens, Hodapp, Ort, & Leckman, 1993).

Prader-Willi Syndrome and Angelman's Syndrome: In a similar way to fragile X syndrome, the "twin syndromes" of Prader-Willi syndrome and Angelman's syndrome inform us about the nature of genetic disorders and hereditary in general.

Prader-Willi syndrome is a genetic disorder in which the affected individuals are mildly retarded. After a period of hypotonia and failure to thrive in infancy, as children and adults these individuals are almost always extremely obese (Cassidy, 1992). Along with their obesity, individuals with Prader-Willi syndrome suffer from obsessions with food, hoarding, pica, and other maladaptive behaviors (Dykens, Hodapp, Walsh, & Nash, 1992; Dykens, Leckman, & Cassidy, in press).

In contrast, individuals with Angelman's syndrome are generally severely to profoundly retarded. Their most salient physical characteristic is an awkward "puppetlike" gait; indeed, children with this disorder have often been referred to as having the "happy puppet" disorder. As implied by the name, these children, although nonverbal, appear jovial most of the time.

At first glance, Prader-Willi syndrome and Angelman's syndrome would seem distinct both physically and behaviorally. Recent studies have found, however, that both groups suffer from a similar genetic disorder, a deletion of material from the same portion of the 15th chromosome (c.f. Cassidy, 1992). More recently still, molecular analyses have found that, when the deleted material comes from the mother, the child has Angelman's syndrome; when the deletion comes from the father, Prader-Willi syndrome results.

These two disorders indicate for the first time the importance of both the nature of the genetic anomaly *and* the parent from whom that anomaly came.

The cases of fragile X syndrome and Prader-Willi and Angelman's syndromes, then, tell us much about the relationships between genetic disorders and subsequent behavior. Such knowledge, most of which has emerged in the past few years, should continue to grow through the study of these and other mental retardation disorders in the years to come.

Developmental Issues

In addition to definitional, classificatory, and genetic issues, important new findings are accruing as to the development of children with retardation. These findings extend and update a perspective that has historically been called the developmental approach to mental retardation.

From the 1920s on, developmentalists such as Piaget, Werner, and Vygotsky have been interested in the development of children with retardation (Hodapp & Zigler, 1995). But only in the past 25 years have more sustained developmental analyses occurred. Much of this sustained analysis has resulted from Zigler's developmental approach to mental retardation. In a series of papers beginning in the late 1960s, Edward Zigler (1967, 1969) formulated this approach with three major hypotheses: similar sequence, similar structure, and similar reactions.

The *similar sequence hypothesis* predicts that children with retardation develop in identical order through Piagetian, early language, or other universal sequences of development. The *similar structure hypothesis* predicts that, when matched to nonretarded children on overall levels of cognitive functioning (e.g., on mental age, or MA), children with retardation will show no particular defects or areas of weakness beyond their overall, general delays; and the *similar reactions hypothesis* predicts that children with retardation will react to the external environment as do nonretarded children. In contrast to the first two hypotheses, however, children with retardation do suffer from more failure experiences and therefore develop a set of personality-motivational characteristics that differ from nonretarded children.

Especially regarding the similar sequence and structure hypotheses, Zigler was careful to apply these ideas only to children with familial retardation; these developmental principles do not necessarily cover children with organic retardation. As Zigler (1969) noted, "If the etiology of the phenotypic intelligence (as measured by an IQ) of two groups differs, it is far from logical to assert that the course of development is the same, or that even similar contents in their behaviors are mediated by exactly the same cognitive process" (p. 533).

In contrast to this limitation to children with familial retardation, various developmentalists have recently attempted to examine a wider, more "liberal" developmental approach (e.g., Cicchetti & Pogge-Hesse, 1982; Hodapp, Burack, & Zigler, 1990). This more liberal approach extends developmental principles to children with Down syndrome (Cicchetti & Beeghly, 1990), fragile X syndrome (Dykens, Hodapp, & Leckman, 1994), and other organic forms of mental retardation. In addition, this modified approach incorporates the wider sense of "development" as currently used in developmental psychology. As a result, the developmental approach to mental retardation now features an emphasis on mother-child interaction, families, and other social systems in which children with retardation develop (Hodapp & Zigler, 1995). Thus, the developmental approach has been modified over the past two decades, both in how it is defined and to whom it is applied (Hodapp, in press). The following review therefore focuses on children with all types of retardation and includes updates on a variety of developmental topics.

SEQUENTIAL DEVELOPMENT

The hallmark of any developmental approach involves an orderly sequence of stages, or the prediction that children with retardation go through these stages in the same order as do nonretarded children. Across different tasks using different methodologies, Weisz and Zigler (1979) found that, almost without exception, children with retardation traverse similar sequences as do nonretarded children. In addition, this sequence holds

for all children with retardation, including those with various organic forms.

The identification of such similar sequences is by now well established and has a variety of theoretical and practical implications. Theoretically, the presence of such sequential development— even in the face of different organic impairments—shows the robust nature of many (particularly earlier-occurring) sequences in development (Hodapp, 1990). Practically, such sequences provide both an ordered curriculum for intervention (Hodapp & Dykens, 1991) and a way to assess children with diverse forms of mental retardation (Dunst, 1980).

STRUCTURES AND CROSS-DOMAIN RELATIONS

In contrast to the similar sequence hypothesis, findings of similar structures have been more complicated. These findings do, however, promise to tell us much about the way that developments in various areas do or do not go together.

Compared to children of the same mental ages, children with familial mental retardation do not show particular deficits in their cognitive functioning, especially when examined using Piagetian tasks (Weisz & Yeates, 1981). However, some deficits in information processing may be present, and these deficits may be due either to the less-interesting nature of these tasks (Weisz, 1990) or to some deficit this group has in performing information processing (but not on Piagetian) tasks (Mundy & Kasari, 1990). The finding of information-processing deficits and the reason for such deficits need to be explored further.

In contrast to familial retarded children, children with different forms of organic retardation are clearly deficient compared to MA-matches, with the deficits often specific to the child's type of mental retardation. For example, children with Down syndrome are particularly weak in linguistic grammar (Fowler, 1990) and in nonverbal requesting (Mundy, Sigman, Kasari, & Yirmiya, 1988) but are better at pragmatics or the communicative uses of language (Beeghly & Cicchetti, 1987). Males with fragile X syndrome perform poorly on tasks of sequential abilities relative to their levels on simultaneous processing and achievement (Dykens et al., 1987).

The most startling findings on cross-domain

functioning come from the study of Williams syndrome, a rare, presumably genetic disorder. Williams syndrome involves a micro-deletion on chromosome 7 involved in the production of elastin. As a result, these children show a characteristic, "pixielike" appearance along with their moderate levels of retardation (Pober & Dykens, in press). These children also show relatively spared levels in vocabulary and in other linguistic skills (Bellugi, Wang, & Jernigan, 1994). Compare, for example, the story narratives of two children—one with Down syndrome and one with Williams syndrome—as they describe a story about a boy and dog's pet frog and how, during the night, the frog gets away. The two children are matched on IQ, overall mental age, and chronological age.

Child with Down syndrome:
He looks in the bowl. He . . . sleep. Then the frog got away. He looked in the bowl . . . and it empty.
Child with Williams syndrome:
Once upon a time there was this boy who had a dog and a frog. And it was night time. And there was a . . . bowl. And the boy and the dog looked in the . . . looked in the bowl. Then, it was nighttime and time for the boy to go to bed. But, as the boy and the dog were sleeping the frog climbed out. And, when it was morning [whispers] "The frog was gone." (Reilly, Klima, & Bellugi, 1991, p. 377)

As these vignettes demonstrate, Williams syndrome children are particularly adept at several aspects of language. They produce long and complicated sentences, and also seem able to skillfully narrate a story, using linkages, time clauses ("And then . . ."), and the extralinguistic devices (whispering, sound effects) that help build interest. The stories of identical-level children with Down syndrome are not nearly so advanced. Indeed, as children with Williams syndrome appear to be performing language that is above their level of cognition they help us to understand how achievements in various domains do (or do not) go together.

FAMILY FUNCTIONING

Research on family functioning has been influenced by the expanded developmental perspective that also examines mothers, fathers, siblings, and the family unit as a whole, both at one time

and as the child develops. Most of this work has occurred within the past decade. Although a full review of such work is beyond the scope of this chapter (see Krauss, Simeonnson & Ramey, 1989; Minnes, 1989 for reviews), several themes are noteworthy.

Stress-Coping Perspective: Research on families of children with disabilities has moved from what might be called a "pathology" perspective to one that emphasizes factors that lead to successful coping. Early work on mothers of children with disabilities emphasized the ways in which mothers "mourn"—as in a death—the loss of the idealized perfect infant (Solnit & Stark, 1961). Later workers noted that mothers also experience strong emotional reactions at other times, particularly during periods of increased stress, as when the child enters adolescence (Wikler, 1986).

In an attempt to understand what helps families of children with disabilities, various workers have identified stressors on the family. For example, two-parent families cope better than single-parent families (Beckman, 1983), and women in better marriages cope better than those in less harmonious marriages (Friedrich, 1979). Similarly, higher socioeconomic status families do better than poorer families, and the support of the mother's close personal friends seems particularly important (Crnic, 1990). Although many of these findings are intuitively obvious, they remain important nonetheless.

Recent work has also emphasized the nature of social network support for mothers of children with disabilities. Kazak and Marvin (1984) have noted that mothers of children with disabilities often have smaller but more intense social networks. These networks, often including only the mother's own mother and a few extended family members or close friends, can simultaneously be supportive and claustraphobic. In addition, Suelzle and Keenan (1981) find that, as children get older, mothers use social supports less often, even as they simultaneously experience a "pile-up" of stressors (Minnes, 1989). Mothers of older children with disabilities would seem, then, to require more attention from social service professionals (Wikler, Wasow, & Hatfield, 1981).

Differences among Families: All families of children with disabilities are not identical. In studies of families of children with severe retardation, Mink, Nihira, and Meyers (1983; also Mink, Meyers, & Nihira, 1984) identify five family "types" for children with severe mental retardation: (1) cohesive, harmonious families; (2) control-oriented, somewhat unharmonious families; (3) low-disclosure, unharmonious families; (4) child-oriented, expressive families; and (5) disadvantaged, low-morale families. Surprisingly, families of children with Down syndrome were most often of the first, or cohesive-harmonious, type, leading to suggestions about effects of the child's type of disability on family functioning (Hodapp, 1995b).

Such differences in families may be partially attributable to the meaning of the child and the child's disability to the family. Using more anthropological, cross-cultural perspectives of child development, Gallimore, Weisner, Kaufman, and Bernheimer (1989) note that all children (disabled and nondisabled) develop within families that have particular views of children and child rearing. As a result of these views, parents set up a series of activities to foster certain goals for the children and families. In families with a child with retardation, these "activity settings" vary enormously. Some families emphasize cognitive interventions for the child, others focus on the social development of the child with disability, whereas still others value activities for the other, nonhandicapped children in the family. Although this type of "ecological" family work is just beginning, it promises to tell us much about how families of children with retardation differ one from another.

Sophisticated Models of Family Functioning: Many different models of family functioning are currently being used to examine families of children with retardation. To date the most frequently employed has been the so-called Double ABCX model (Minnes, 1989). The Double ABCX model stipulates that the nature of the initial crisis reaction (X) is a function of specific characteristics of the child (A), mediated by the family's internal and external resources (B) and by the family's perceptions of the child (C). Furthermore, child characteristics, family resources, and family perceptions of the child can all change and evolve as the child gets older. This model, while general, helps to organize many of the findings just described. It also emphasizes that families show no single familial reaction to all children with disabilities, or at all points during the child's development.

Dual Diagnosis

Compared to even a decade or two ago, mental health researchers and clinicians now realize that children with mental retardation can suffer from the complete range of psychiatric symptoms and disorders. Research on the so-called dually diagnosed child—the child with both retardation and psychiatric disorder—has become an important new area of mental retardation, albeit one in which much more work is needed. Clinically, the child who is dually diagnosed often presents the clinician with some of the most complex diagnostic and therapeutic dilemmas in the field. The following review highlights several of the important issues in this growing area.

EPIDEMIOLOGY

Although virtually all epidemiologic studies of persons who are dually diagnosed have weaknesses, many have begun to suggest that mental illness in mentally retarded populations is both common and linked to several different factors. Most striking has been the sheer percentage of persons with both mental retardation and psychiatric conditions. In the Isle of Wight study, Rutter, Tizard, and Whitmore (1970) found that, among 10- to 11-year-old children with retardation, 30 to 42% met criteria for psychiatric disturbance; in contrast, only 6 to 7% of nonretarded 10- to 11-year-olds were psychiatrically impaired. Equally high prevalence rates among people with retardation have been found in other studies of both children (Koller, Richardson, Katz, & McLaren, 1982) and adults (Gostason, 1985). Taken together, roughly one third to two thirds of individuals with retardation are reported to have some form of psychopathology. In contrast to earlier thinking, then, individuals with mental retardation seem to be at particularly increased risk for psychiatric illnesses of many types.

In addition to the increased risk of psychopathology per se, risks for particular disorders may vary by the child's degree of retardation. For example, schizophrenia is estimated to occur in 2 to 3% of individuals with retardation (as compared to 1% of nonretarded persons), but most cases are found among persons who are more severely retarded. Corbett (1985) emphasized that those with mild retardation show increased rates of externalizing disorders as well as increases in other nonpsychotic disorders, whereas individuals with more severe retardation are more likely to show childhood psychosis, hyperkinetic disorders, and severe stereotypies. Curiously, some reports note higher rates of psychopathology in persons who are *less* severely retarded (Gostason, 1985; Iverson & Fox, 1989); such findings run directly contrary to the clinical axom that the presence of psychopathology is roughly proportional to the degree of retardation. Clearly, more research is needed.

Besides the child's degree of retardation, a host of other factors also affect the prevalence of psychiatric disorders in retarded populations. These risk factors include language disorders, school failure, brain injury, seizures, low socioeconomic status, family strain, and physical disabilities. (See Corbett, 1985, for a review.) The presence of each increases the likelihood of psychopathology in the child with retardation.

A final risk factor—for both more and specific types of psychopathology—is the child's syndrome of retardation (Dykens, in press). For example, boys affected with fragile X syndrome commonly (up to 75% of cases) exhibit inattention, distractibility, and hyperactive behavior (Bregman, Leckman, & Ort, 1988). Fragile X syndrome and autism can also co-occur, although this association is probably weaker than originally thought, with approximately 3 to 5% of autistic individuals showing evidence of the fragile site (Einfield, 1989; Fisch, 1992; Rutter et al., 1990). Other disorders may be even more prone to autism: For example, recent reports suggest that approximately 30% of children with tuberous sclerosis also meet criteria for autism (Smalley, Smith, Guttierrez, & Tanguay, 1992).

Although a booming area, the delineation of the prevalence, types, and correlates of psychopathology in retarded populations all must be considered preliminary. Studies are often performed using small and nonrepresentative samples, with little attention given to the child's level of retardation or to the age of the samples studied. Similarly, studies often employ differing definitions of specific psychopathological conditions; the varying criteria used to diagnose autism in studies examining males with fragile X syndrome is but an extreme example in this regard. (See Dykens et al., 1994, for a review.) Still, even given these caveats, children with retardation can clearly suffer from additional psychiatric conditions.

ASSESSMENT

Along with the sampling and definitional problems just described, the major stumbling block in dual-diagnosis research involves the measurement of psychopathology per se. Specifically, most diagnostic measures and procedures are designed for nonretarded samples who are in their middle childhood through adolescent years. At issue is whether it is appropriate to use these instruments (e.g., Schedule for Affective Disorders and Schizophrenia for School Age Children [Kiddie-SADS], behavioral rating scales) with children of limited cognitive abilities. Given that many types of psychopathology involve reporting one's feelings and thinking, measurement issues are of obvious importance. To the extent possible, self-report should be used for verbal retarded persons. Recent data support the use of measures such as the Beck Depression Inventory (Beck, Carlson, Russell, & Brownfield, 1987) with adolescents with mild mental retardation. Caregiver reports should also be used to assess changes over time, specific behavioral manifestations of disorders, and patterns of symptoms.

Related to the issue of measurement is the possible presence of "diagnostic overshadowing" in mental retardation. Led by Reiss and Szysko (1983), many researchers argue that the fact that a child is mentally retarded often leads clinicians to feel that the child cannot also suffer from other psychopathology. In this sense, mental retardation may "overshadow" other conditions. Although just how often such overshadowing occurs remains unclear, it is nevertheless an important reminder that, in the case of clients with retardation, clinicians may be more prone to diagnostic errors of omission rather than of comission.

Although diagnostic overshadowing and measurement of psychopathology in general remain important issues, several attempts are being made to modify or create psychopathology measures for use with persons with retardation. One such scale is the Psychopathology Instrument for Mentally Retarded Adults (Senatore, Matson, & Kazdin, 1985), and other instruments will soon be forthcoming. At present, clinicians should treat all measures cautiously, and employ multimethod and multiinformant approaches as much as possible. Such assessments might include observational measures of the child, more traditional assessments of both categories of disorder (e.g., structured or semistructured diagnostic interviews with the caregiver), and important dimensions of behavior (e.g., rating scales for inattentive and hyperactive behaviors by teachers or caregivers). To date, no specific clinical or laboratory tests are of proven validity for psychiatric diagnoses among children with mental retardation.

TREATMENT

Combined with the recent focus on psychopathology has come an interest in treating dually diagnosed individuals. So far, such attempts have mirrored efforts to treat identical conditions in the general population. For example, stimulant medications have proven effective in treating the hyperactivity and attention problems in boys with fragile X syndrome (Hagerman, Murphy, & Wittenberger, 1988), just as behavioral modification techniques are of demonstrated utility in stopping the self-abusive behavior of many children with mental retardation (Cipani, 1989).

But as Bregman (1991) notes, medications and behavior modification are only a few of the many psychotherapeutic techniques currently being tried with dually diagnosed populations. Over the past few years, almost every technique used with nonretarded children has been attempted with children with retardation: These techniques include ecological and educational interventions, psychotherapy by verbal and nonverbal (e.g., play therapy, drawing, etc.) means, all sorts of behavioral and cognitive behavioral techniques, and psychopharmacological interventions. In addition, specific interventions have recently been proposed for children and adults with different genetic forms of mental retardation (Dykens & Ho-

dapp, 1996). Although future research will tell us how effective each technique is with children of various etiologies or levels of impairment, the entire gamut of clinical approaches is currently being tried with psychiatrically impaired retarded populations.

Early Intervention

Early intervention is a widespread and commonly accepted service for retarded and at-risk children and their families. These services have recently evolved in several ways. First, infants and young children themselves are now the recipients of services throughout the United States. As an outgrowth of Public Law 94-142 (the Education for All Handicapped Children Act of 1975), services have recently been extended to the 0- to 3-year period. The main law in this regard, Public Law 99–457, provides strong federal incentives to intervene during these early years.

Second, more sophisticated developmental, behavioral, and other models are currently being used with young children with retardation (Guralnick, 1991). Such services capitalize on the latest developmental information concerning sequences, cross-domain relations, and mother-child interactions. In addition, recommendations have been made to tailor interventions differently to young children who have different types of handicaps; even in the earliest years, then, the child with Down syndrome (Gibson, 1991) may differ from the child with fragile X syndrome or other types of retardation (Hodapp & Dykens, 1991).

Third, a major emphasis on the family has arisen in early intervention work (Krauss & Hauser-Cram, 1992). Some of this family-focus arises from the law itself; indeed, PL 99-457 requires that early intervention specialists develop a "Family Intervention Plan" as well as the more usual IEP (or Individualized Educational Plan). This legal requirement reflects—and makes even more pronounced—the importance of including the family in early intervention services.

Finally, early intervention services are now performed by professionals from a host of different disciplines. These professionals include early childhood special education teachers, clinical and developmental psychologists, social workers, physical therapists, occupational therapists, speech-language pathologists, pediatricians, and child psychiatrists. Furthermore, many of these disciplines have recently developed particular subspecialties to address specific needs during the early childhood years. For example, the entire field of infant psychiatry (and organizations such as World Association of Infant Psychiatry and Allied Disciplines) is directly focused on psychiatric issues during infancy, albeit not on children with retardation per se. In the same way, a variety of professions now have either specialized organizations or journals dealing with young children: journals such as *Zero to Three, Topics in Early Childhood Special Education, Infant Mental Health Journal*, and the *Journal of the Division of Early Childhood* (of the Council for Exceptional Children) all attest to the growing and cross-disciplinary interest in early intervention.

The Role of the Psychiatrist

Given mental retardation's range of definitional, developmental, genetic, and psychiatric issues, the child psychiatrist is ideally situated to serve many roles when caring for children with retardation and their families. For younger patients, the psychiatrist may serve as the coordinator of a comprehensive diagnostic assessment. Such assessments involve aspects of the child's development, of the functioning and coping of each family member, and of the family as a whole.

Child psychiatrists can also help disentangle for families the difficult genetic and medical issues arising from mental retardation. Families, for example, may have difficulties understanding what fragile X syndrome means for the child who has the disorder; for the mother, father, and/or sibling who may carry it; for unaffected siblings; and for extended family members. Schools and other service agencies also require the latest information concerning these and other disorders. In the same way, therapies with dually diagnosed persons will increasingly utilize the entire armamentarium of therapies currently used with any child and family, including but not limited to medication and psychotherapeutic services.

Like many conditions, then, mental retardation is simultaneously a problem in development, (often) a medical condition, a family issue, and a societal concern. Furthermore, new controversies and information have arisen in each of these areas. It is therefore more important than ever that child psychiatrists and other mental health personnel have a clear and up-to-date understanding of children with mental retardation and their families.

REFERENCES

Abramowicz, H. K., & Richardson, S. (1975). Epidemiology of severe mental retardation in children: Community studies. *American Journal of Mental Deficiency, 80,* 18–39.

American Association on Mental Retardation. (1992). *Mental retardation: Definition, classification, and systems of supports.* Washington, DC: Author.

American Psychiatric Association. (1987). *Diagnostic and statistical manual of mental disorders* (3rd ed., rev.). Washington, DC: Author.

American Psychiatric Association. (1994). *Diagnostic and statistical manual of mental disorders* (4th ed.). Washington, DC: Author.

Beck, D. C., Carlson, G., Russell, A., & Brownfield, F. (1987). Use of depression rating instruments in developmentally and educationally delayed adolescents. *Journal of the American Academy of Child and Adolescent Psychiatry, 26,* 97–100.

Beckman, P. J. (1983). Influence of selected child characteristics on stress in families of handicapped infants. *American Journal of Mental Deficiency, 88,* 150–156.

Beeghly, M., & Cicchetti, D. (1987). An organizational approach to symbolic development in children with Down syndrome. In D. Cicchetti & M. Beeghly (Eds.), *Symbolic development in atypical children. New directions for child development* (pp. 5–29). San Francisco: Jossey-Bass.

Bellugi, U., Marks, S., Bihrle, A. M., & Sabo, H. (1988). Dissociation between language and cognitive functions in Williams Syndrome. In D. Bishop & K. Mogford (Eds.), *Language development in exceptional circumstances* (pp. 177–189). London: Churchill Livingstone.

Bellugi, U., Wang, P., & Jernigan, T. (1994). Williams syndrome: An unusual neuropsychological profile. In

S. H. Broman & J. Grafman (Eds.), *Atypical cognitive deficits in developmental disorders* (pp. 23–56). Hillsdale, NJ: Lawrence Erlbaum.

Bregman, J. (1991). Current developments in the understanding of mental retardation. II. Psychopathology. *Journal of the American Academy of Child and Adolescent Psychiatry, 30,* 861–872.

Bregman, J. D., Leckman, J. F., & Ort, S. I. (1988). Fragile X syndrome: Genetic predisposition to psychopathology. *Journal of Autism and Developmental Disorders, 18,* 343–354.

Burack, J. A., Hodapp, R. M., & Zigler, E. (1988). Issues in the classification of mental retardation: Differentiating among organic etiologies. *Journal of Child Psychology and Psychiatry, 29,* 765–779.

Cassidy, S. B. (1992). Introduction and overview of Prader-Willi Syndrome. In S. B. Cassidy (Ed.), *Prader-Willi syndrome and other chromosome 15q deletion disorders.* New York: Springer-Verlag.

Cicchetti, D., & Beeghly, M. (Eds.). (1990). *Children with Down Syndrome: A developmental perspective.* New York: Cambridge University Press.

Cicchetti, D., & Pogge-Hesse, P. (1982). Possible contributions of the study of organically retarded persons to developmental theory. In E. Zigler & D. Balla (Eds.), *Mental retardation: The developmental-difference controversy* (pp. 277–318). Hillsdale, NJ: Erlbaum.

Cipani, E. (Ed.). (1989). *The treatment of severe behavior disorders: Behavior analysis approaches.* Washington, DC: American Association on Mental Retardation.

Corbett, J. A. (1985). Mental retardation: Psychiatric aspects. In M. Rutter & L. Hersov (Eds.), *Child and adolescent psychiatry: Modern approaches* (2nd ed., pp. 661–678). Oxford: Blackwell Scientific Publications.

Crnic, K. (1990). Families of children with Down syndrome: Ecological contexts and characteristics. In D. Cicchetti & M. Beeghly (Eds.), *Children with Down syndrome: A developmental approach* (pp. 399–423). New York: Cambridge University Press.

Dunst, C. J. (1980). *A clinical and educational manual for use with the Uzgiris-Hunt Scales for infant development.* Baltimore: University Park Press.

Dupont, A., Vaeth, M., & Videbech, P. (1986). Mortality and life expectancy of Down's Syndrome in Denmark. *Journal of Mental Deficiency Research, 30,* 111–120.

Dykens, E. M. (1995). Measuring behavioral phenotypes: Provocations from the "new genetics." *American Journal on Mental Retardation, 99,* 522–532.

Dykens, E. M. (In press). DSM meets DNA: Genetic syndromes' growing importance in dual diagnosis. *Mental Retardation.*

Dykens, E. M., & Cassidy, S. B. (In press). Prader-Willi syndrome: Genetic, behavioral, and placement issues. *Child and Adolescent Psychiatry Clinics of North America.*

Dykens, E. M., & Hodapp, R. M. (1996). *Treatment is-*

sues in genetic mental retardation syndromes. Manuscript submitted for publication.

Dykens, E. M., Hodapp, R. M., & Leckman, J. F. (1987). Strengths and weaknesses in the intellectual profiles of males with fragile X syndrome. *American Journal of Mental Deficiency, 92,* 234–236.

Dykens, E. M., Hodapp, R. M., & Leckman, J. F. (1994). *Development and psychopathology in fragile X syndrome.* Newbury Park, CA: Sage.

Dykens, E. M., Hodapp, R. M., Ort, S. I., Finucane, B., Shapiro, L., & Leckman, J. F. (1989). The trajectory of cognitive development in males with fragile X syndrome. *Journal of the American Academy of Child and Adolescent Psychiatry, 28,* 422–426.

Dykens, E. M., Hodapp, R. M., Ort, S. I., & Leckman, J. F. (1993). Trajectory of adaptive behavior in males with fragile X syndrome. *Journal of Autism and Developmental Disorders, 23,* 135–145.

Dykens, E. M., Hodapp, R. M., Walsh, K., & Nash, L. (1992). Adaptive and maladaptive behavior in Prader-Willi syndrome. *Journal of the American Academy of Child and Adolescent Psychiatry, 31,* 1131–1136.

Dykens, E. M., Leckman, J. F., & Cassidy, S. L. (In press). Obsessions and compulsions in individuals with Prader-Willi syndrome. *Journal of Child Psychology and Psychiatry.*

Einfield, S. L., Molony, H., & Hall, W. (1989). Autism is not associated with the fragile X syndrome. *American Journal of Medical Genetics, 34,* 187–193.

Fisch, G. (1992). Is autism associated with the fragile X syndrome? *American Journal of Medical Genetics, 43,* 47–55.

Fowler, A. (1990). The development of language structure in children with Down syndrome. In D. Cicchetti & M. Beeghly (Eds.), *Children with Down syndrome: A developmental perspective* (pp. 302–328). New York: Cambridge University Press.

Friedrich, W. N. (1979). Predictors of coping behavior of mothers of handicapped children. *Journal of Consulting and Clinical Psychology, 47,* 1140–1141.

Gallimore, R., Weisner, T., Kaufman, S., & Bernheimer, L. (1989). The social construction of ecocultural niches: Family accommodation of developmentally delayed children. *American Journal of Mental Retardation, 94,* 216–230.

Gibson, D. (1991). Down syndrome and cognitive enhancement: Not like the others. In K. Marfo (Ed.), *Early intervention in transition: Current perspectives on programs for handicapped children* (pp. 61–90). New York: Praeger.

Gostason, R. (1985). Psychiatric illness among the mentally retarded: A Swedish population study. *Acta Psychiatrica Scandinavia, 71* (Suppl. 318), 1–117.

Granat, K., & Granat, S. (1973). Below-average intelligence and mental retardation. *American Journal of Mental Deficiency, 78,* 27–32.

Granat, K., & Granat, S. (1978). Adjustment of intellectually below-average men not identified as mentally retarded. *Scandinavian Journal of Psychology, 19,* 41–51.

Gresham, F. M., MacMillan, D. L., & Siperstein, G. M. (1995). Critical analyses of the 1992 AAMR definition: Implications for school psychology. *School Psychology Quarterly, 10,* 1–9.

Grossman, H. J. (Ed.) (1983). *Manual on terminology and classification in mental retardation* (3rd rev.). Washington, DC: American Association on Mental Deficiency.

Guralnick, M. (1991). The next decade of research on the effectiveness of early intervention. *Exceptional Children, 58,* 174–183.

Hagerman, R., Murphy, M., & Wittenberger, M. (1988). A controlled trial of stimulant medication in children with fragile X syndrome. *American Journal of Medical Genetics, 30,* 377–392.

Hodapp, R. M. (1990). One road or many? Issues in the similar sequence hypothesis. In R. M. Hodapp, J. A. Burack, & E. Zigler (Eds.), *Issues in the developmental approach to mental retardation* (pp. 49–70). New York: Cambridge University Press.

Hodapp, R. M. (1995a). Definitions in mental retardation: Effects on research, practice, and perceptions. *School Psychology Quarterly, 10,* 24–28.

Hodapp, R. M. (1995b). Parenting children with Down syndrome and other types of mental retardation. In M. Bornstein (Ed.), *Handbook of parenting. Vol. 1. How children influence parents* (pp. 233–253). Hillsdale, NJ: Lawrence Erlbaum.

Hodapp, R. M. (In press). Developmental approaches to children with disabilities: New perspectives, populations, prospects. In S. S. Luthar, J. A. Burack, D. Cicchetti, & J. R. Weisz (Eds.), *Developmental psychopathology: Perspectives on risk and disorder.* New York: Cambridge University Press.

Hodapp, R. M., Burack, J. A., & Zigler, E. (Eds.) (1990). *Issues in the developmental approach to mental retardation.* New York: Cambridge University Press.

Hodapp, R. M., & Dykens, E. M. (1991). Toward an etiology-specific strategy of early intervention with handicapped children. In K. Marfo (Ed.), *Early intervention in transition: Current perspectives on programs for handicapped children* (pp. 41–60). New York: Praeger.

Hodapp, R. M., & Dykens, E. M. (1994). Mental retardation's two cultures of behavioral research. *American Journal on Mental Retardation, 98,* 675–687.

Hodapp, R. M., & Dykens, E. M. (1996). Mental retardation. In E. Mash & R. Barkley (Eds.), *Child psychopathology* (pp. 362–389). New York: Guilford Press.

Hodapp, R. M., Dykens, E. M., Hagerman, R., Schreiner, R., Lachiewicz, A., & Leckman, J. (1990). Developmental implications of changing trajectories of IQ in males with fragile X syndrome. *Journal of the American Academy of Child and Adolescent Psychiatry, 29,* 214–219.

Hodapp, R. M., & Zigler, E. (1995). Past, present, and future issues in the developmental approach to mental retardation. In D. Cicchetti & D. Cohen (Eds.), *Manual of developmental psychopathology* (Vol. 2, pp. 299–331). New York: John Wiley & Sons.

Iverson, J. C., & Fox, R. A. (1989). Prevalence of psychopathology among mentally retarded adults. *Research in Developmental Disabilities, 10,* 77–83.

Jacobson, J. W., & Mulick, J. A. (1992). A new definition of mental retardation or a new definition of practice? *Psychology in Mental Retardation and Developmental Disabilities, 18,* 9–14.

Kahn, J. V. (1992). Predicting adaptive behavior of severely and profoundly mentally retarded children with early cognitive measures. *Journal of Intellectual Disability Research, 36,* 101–114.

Kazak, A., & Marvin, R. (1984). Differences, difficulties, and adaptation: Stress and social networks in families of handicapped children. *Family Relations, 33,* 67–77.

Koller, H., Richardson, S., Katz, M., & McLaren, J. (1982). Behavior disturbance in childhood and the early adult years in populations who were and were not mentally retarded. *Journal of Preventive Psychiatry, 1,* 453–468.

Krauss, M. W., & Hauser-Cram, P. (1992). Policy and program development for infants and toddlers with disabilities. In L. Rowitz (Ed.), *Mental retardation in the year 2000* (pp. 184–196). New York: Springer-Verlag.

Krauss, M. W., Simeonsson, R., & Ramey, S. L. (Eds.) (1989). Special issue on research on families. *American Journal on Mental Retardation, 94* (No. 3).

Lubs, H. (1969). A marker X chromosome. *American Journal of Human Genetics, 21,* 231–244.

Luckasson, R. (Ed.) (1992). *Classification in mental retardation.* Washington, DC: American Association on Mental Retardation.

MacMillan, D. L. (1982). *Mental retardation in school and society* (2nd ed.). Boston: Little, Brown.

MacMillan, D. L., Gresham, F. M., & Siperstein, G. L. (1993). Conceptual and psychometric concerns about the 1992 AAMR definition of mental retardation. *American Journal on Mental Retardation, 98,* 325–335.

MacMillan, D. L., Hendrick, I. G., & Watkins, A. V. (1988). Impact of *Diana, Larry P.,* and P. L. 94–142 on minority students. *Exceptional Children, 54,* 24–30.

Martin, J. P., & Bell, J. A. (1943). A pedigree of mental defect showing sex-linkage. *Journal of Neurological Psychiatry, 6,* 154–157.

Mercer, J. (1973). The myth of three percent prevalence. In C. E. Meyers (Ed.), *Socio-behavioral studies in mental retardation. Monographs of the American Association on Mental Deficiency, 1.*

Miller, J. (1987). Language and communication characteristics of children with Down syndrome. In S. M. Pueschel, G. Tingey, J. Rynders, A. Crocker, & D. Crutcher (Eds.), *New perspectives on Down Syndrome* (pp. 233–262). Baltimore: Brookes.

Mink, I., Meyers, C., & Nihira, K. (1984). Taxonomy of family life styles: II. Homes with slow-learning children. *American Journal of Mental Deficiency, 89,* 111–123.

Mink, I., Nihira, K., & Meyers, C. (1983). Taxonomy of family life styles: I. Homes with TMR children. *American Journal of Mental Deficiency, 87,* 484–497.

Minnes, P. M. (1989). Family stress associated with a developmentally handicapped child. *International Review of Research in Mental Retardation, 15,* 195–226.

Mundy, P., & Kasari, C. (1990). The similar structure hypothesis and differential rate of development in mental retardation. In R. M. Hodapp, J. A. Burack, & E. Zigler (Eds.), *Issues in the developmental approach to mental retardation* (pp. 71–92). New York: Cambridge University Press.

Mundy, P., Sigman, M., Kasari, C., & Yirmiya, N. (1988). Non-verbal communication in Down syndrome children. *Child Development, 59,* 235–249.

Penrose, L. S. (1963). *The biology of mental defect.* London: Sidgwick & Jackson.

Pober, B., & Dykens, E. M. (In press). Williams syndrome: An overview of medical, cognitive, and behavioral features. *Child and Adolescent Psychiatry Clinics of North America.*

Reilly, M., Klima, E., & Bellugi, U. (1991). Once more with feeling: Affect and language in atypical populations. *Development and Psychopathology, 2,* 367–391.

Reiss, S., & Szysko, J. (1983). Diagnostic overshadowing and professional experience with mentally retarded persons. *American Journal of Mental Deficiency, 87,* 396–402.

Ross, R. T., Begab, M. J., Dondis, E. H., Giampiccolo, J. S., & Meyers, C. E. (1985). *Lives of the retarded: A forty-year follow-up study.* Stanford, CA: Stanford University Press.

Rutter, M., Macdonald, H., Le Couteur, A., Harrington, R., Bolton, P., & Bailey, A. (1990). Genetic factors in child psychiatric disorders. II. Empirical findings. *Journal of Child Psychology and Psychiatry, 31,* 39–83.

Rutter, M., Tizard, J., & Whitmore, K. (Eds.) (1970). *Education, health, and behavior.* London: Longmans.

Senatore, V., Matson, J., & Kazdin, A. (1985). An inventory to assess psychopathology of mentally retarded adults. *American Journal of Mental Deficiency, 89,* 459–466.

Smalley, S., Smith, M., Gutierrez, G., & Tanguay, P. (1992). Autism and tuberous sclerosis. *Journal of Autism and Developmental Disorders, 22,* 339–355.

Solnit, A., & Stark, M. (1961). Mourning and the birth of a defective child. *Psychoanalytic Study of the Child, 16,* 523–537.

Suelzle, M., & Keenan, V. (1981). Changes in family support networks over the life cycle of mentally retarded persons. *American Journal of Mental Deficiency, 86,* 267–274.

Vernon, P. (1979). *Intelligence: Heredity and environment.* San Francisco: W. H. Freeman.

Weisz, J. (1990). Cultural-familial mental retardation: A developmental perspective on cognitive performance and "helpless" behavior. In R. M. Hodapp, J. A. Burack, & E. Zigler (Eds.), *Issues in the developmental approach to mental retardation* (pp. 137–168). New York: Cambridge University Press.

Weisz, J., & Yeates, K. (1981). Cognitive development in retarded and nonretarded persons: Piagetian tests of the similar structure hypothesis. *Psychological Bulletin, 90,* 153–178.

Weisz, J., & Zigler, E. (1979). Cognitive development in retarded and nonretarded persons: Piagetian tests of the similar structure hypothesis. *Psychological Bulletin, 86,* 831–851.

Wikler, L. (1986). Periodic stresses of families of older mentally retarded children: An exploratory study. *American Journal of Mental Deficiency, 90,* 703–706.

Wikler, L., Wasow, M., & Hatfield, E. (1981). Chronic sorrow revisited: Parent versus professional depiction of the adjustment of parents of mentally retarded children. *American Journal of Orthopsychiatry, 51,* 63–70.

Zigler, E. (1967). Familial mental retardation: A continuing dilemma. *Science, 155,* 292–298.

Zigler, E. (1969). Developmental versus difference theories of mental retardation and the problem of motivation. *American Journal of Mental Deficiency, 73,* 536–556.

Zigler, E., & Hodapp, R. M. (1986). *Understanding mental retardation.* New York: Cambridge University Press.

Zigman, W. B., Schupf, N., Lubin, R. A., & Silverman, W. P. (1987). Premature regression of adults with Down syndrome. *American Journal of Mental Deficiency, 92,* 161–168.

38 / Infants and Toddlers with Medical Conditions and Their Parents: Reactions to Illness and Hospitalization and Models for Intervention

Susan K. Theut and David A. Mrazek

Introduction

New research findings and innovative approaches have focused attention on the importance of the early years of development for physically ill children. Medical illnesses and hospitalizations can disturb a child's developmental course and affect the nature of the child-parent relationship. The extent of this interference depends on a host of interacting factors. One of the most important determinants for the child is the parents' ability to cope with their own anxieties regarding the child's illness (Prugh, Staub, Sands, Kirschbaum & Lenihan, 1953). This ability subsequently affects the parents' capacity both to provide emotional security for the child facing a critical situation and to help modulate the experience. Other important factors influencing the child's adaptation include the nature of the illness, the hospital experience, the child's developmental phase and cognitive understanding, and the child's constitutional endowment and resilience. Important factors that influence the parents' coping include their ability to negotiate the medical care system, the strength of the parents' relationship with one another, the responsiveness of the medical care system, and the parents' receptiveness to psychological intervention.

This chapter describes the reactions of infants and toddlers to hospitalization. It also discusses how parents differentially adapt to acute and chronic illnesses. The process of mourning a loss and the concept of anticipatory grief are of central importance. A general approach to the process of intervention is presented with a specific clinical example.

Infants' and Toddlers' Reactions to Hospitalization

Most children show some reaction to hospitalization (Prugh et al., 1953). In some measure, this reaction is a function of their developmental phase (Zetterstrom, 1984). All hospitalizations require some transfer of care from the mother to maternal substitutes; as a result, there is always a degree of separation from mother. For certain infants and toddlers, this separation can be the most distressing aspect of hospitalization.

Schaffer and Callender (1959) observed the reactions of hospitalized infants less than 1 year of age. They reported the classic signs of protest, despair, and detachment (Bowlby, 1961) for infants between 7 months and 12 months of age. Attachment theory (Ainsworth, Blehar, Waters, & Wall, 1978; Bowlby, 1973) highlights the potentially disorganizing consequence of poorly modulated separation of the infant from the mother.

Several studies suggest that the reaction to hospitalization is most marked between the ages of 1 and 4 years (Illingworth & Holt, 1955; Mrazek, Anderson & Strunk, 1984; Prugh et al., 1953). In 1953 Prugh et al. reported that children 2 to 4 years old showed the most intense reaction to separation from parents. This reaction included continual crying, apprehensive behavior, and screaming when approached by an adult. Somatic aspects of anxiety including urinary frequency, diarrhea, and vomiting also were observed, as was the affective withdrawal characteristic of anaclitic depression (Spitz & Wolfe, 1946). Other common reactions were disturbances in feeding behavior (anorexia, overeating, refusal to chew food), demand to return to the bottle, regressive loss of control of bladder or bowel function, fear of the dark, and sleep disturbances (insomnia, nightmares, restlessness). Hyperactivity, irritability, and an increase in aggressive behavior were seen in some infants, while others displayed self-soothing behavior, such as thumb sucking and rocking.

These reactions should be placed within the context of toddlers who are transitioning from the sensorimotor to the preoperational stage of cognitive development (Piaget, 1926; Piaget & Inhelder, 1969). Since these children cannot understand cause-and-effect relationships, they may attach irrational interpretations to illnesses, such as punishment for misbehavior. Preoperational children do not yet understand such concepts as conservation or reversibility (Burbach & Peterson, 1986), and may accordingly be particularly frightened by the removal of body fluids because they may fear they cannot be replaced. Children in this age group have a very limited capacity to understand and test reality; in the face of stress, they tend to exhibit what has been described as magical thinking.

It therefore may be difficult to distinguish children's reactions to the illness from reactions to hospitalization. For example, as a direct physiological result of the illness, children may exhibit a combination of fatigue, irritability, anorexia, and sleep disturbances that resembles the symptoms of an emotional reaction to overwhelming stressors.

Parental Reaction to Hospitalization

Parents who learn that their child is seriously ill and must be hospitalized exhibit three general phases of reaction, as described by Richmond (1958). The initial phase of denial and disbelief occurs in reaction to the immediate shock of the news and may last from hours to weeks. The second phase, fear and frustration, occurs if the child does not begin to improve or if it appears that the child has developed a chronic or handicapping condition. Parents can show anxiety, depression, anger, and guilt as they wonder if they "caused" the illness or failed to prevent serious sequelae by ignoring early symptoms. Such parents will be quick to feel criticized by medical staff. In an effort to cope with this guilt, parents may unconsciously blame each other or join together to blame the child's part-time caregiver, prior medical care, or the current hospital staff.

If the parents are able to work through the denial and fear, they may enter the third phase, which is intelligent inquiry and planning. In this stage the parents begin to accept the help of the staff to learn about the illness. As a result, they become more prepared to participate in the medical decision process and eventually can begin to make long-term plans. In this phase, parents learn both to cope with the uncertainties associated with their child's prognosis and to support their child effectively. During this phase there is a danger that parents may become overprotective and overcontrolling, particularly if their child does not recover quickly. The parents' reaction to a life-threatening illness may result in long-term psychosocial development problems for the child, which Green and Solnit (1964) have described as the vulnerable child syndrome.

The Impact of the Hospital Setting on Parents

The hospital setting and medical caregivers represent a foreign environment for parents and children. Large hospitals rely on multidisciplinary teams, with rotating staff (daily and monthly), and are hierarchically organized, often with interns, residents, and fellows. They are thus innately confusing and can be an overwhelming situation for parents. The frequent questions parents raise about how decisions of care are made illustrate their lack of comprehension of the system.

While technological sophistication has increased, the medical staff frequently are unable to predict the course and outcome of a child's illness. This fact can lead parents to believe that the staff is withholding information from them. Parents may feel isolated from the decision-making process, which often occurs during staff meetings. In addition, parents understandably are confused by medical terminology. They may feel threatened in their role as parents by hospital staff because, on a temporary basis, the medical team make the decisions and spend more time with the child. One parent described this feeling by saying "Whose baby is this anyway?"

Medical units function in a fashion that is foreign to most parents. For most families, the medical staff hierarchy, the importance of orders, and the scheduling arrangements for special tests or procedures are new concepts. Parents can experience new medical technology in a variety of ways. The complexity of the machines in the hospital may reassure some parents, who feel that they have chosen a state-of-the-art center for their child's care. Others may feel isolated and overwhelmed by technology they do not understand and experience as threatening.

Medical teams should strive to make decisions with the parents and to deliver care while keeping the family informed. In critical situations the staff's primary responsibility is to stabilize the patient. At these times parents often feel isolated and helpless. One of the functions of a liaison child psychiatrist is to facilitate communication between the team and the parents so that the parents understand the process. Young children cannot voice dissatisfaction about their care to their parents. Parents need conscientiously to elicit feedback about the course of the child's treatment decisions and serve as advocates for their child. At the same time, highly sensitive parents may become unrealistic about their child's needs and be perceived as demanding and irrational by the staff. The psychiatric consultant often must serve as a systems analyst who can define interpersonal problems and negotiate solutions.

Parental visits to the hospital and their degree of involvement with the child are important issues. Some parents may view a severely ill baby as "damaged" and feel that visiting is hopeless. Some parents have competing responsibilities outside the hospital, such as the needs of other children and the demands of their own work, which make it difficult to be at the hospital every day. This is particularly true of tertiary care centers where a child may be referred from a long distance away and the parents find it difficult to make arrangements to stay with the child. Every effort should be made to facilitate at least one parent staying with a hospitalized child. If this proves to be impossible, the liaison child psychiatrist can share the realities of the parents' situation with the hospital staff. It is hoped that they will then be less critical of parents who do not stay with their child.

While modern hospitals either encourage "rooming in" or have liberal visiting privileges, many parents still feel that their role is unclear and that they are in the way. Special units, such as the neonatal intensive care unit and burn unit, may seem particularly alien given their special restrictions and requirements, such as sterile dress.

The Process of Intervention for the Parents of Medically Ill Children

The clinician working with the parents of an ill infant or toddler has six basic tasks. These include:

1. Forming an alliance and assessing the parents' reactions to the ill child, the nature of the illness, and the hospitalization.
2. Clarifying information and helping the parents process their reactions.
3. Helping the parents understand their child's reaction to illness and hospitalization within a developmental framework.
4. Assisting the parents in defining their roles on the medical unit.
5. Maintaining an ongoing therapeutic relationship with the parents.
6. Facilitating communication between the staff and the parents.

One of the most important aspects of the child's adaptation depends on the parents' ability to cope with their own anxieties and subsequently support their child. The clinician's immediate and ongoing goal is to form an alliance with the parents in order to facilitate the intervention. In the initial meeting, a history of the child's illness and hospitalization should be obtained, including how the parents were told of the child's illness. In order to be able to assess the parental ability to understand the illness, it is important to explore several areas, namely: the parental perception of the illness, the treatment, the prognosis and the long-term outcome. An important aspect of this process is to evaluate the parents' coping skills.

A developmental history of the infant or toddler is crucial to assess the child's reaction to the illness. It is also important to understand how the parents experienced previous pediatric illnesses and hospitalizations. Both difficult or helpful experiences with the hospital staff in the past should be elicited. A social history should include knowledge of divorce, parental illness, other children at home, employment demands, financial pressures, and support from family and friends. This information will shape practical interactions between the family and staff. For example, divorced parents who have been granted joint custody will not only require equal information before medical decisions can be made, but they must be in agreement about such decisions. The medical staff may have missed pertinent information about the family in their rush to provide care.

One of the most important aspects of an intervention with the parents of a physically ill child is to provide accurate information about the child's medical treatment and course. Some parents will seek reassurance about outcome that cannot be given. Furthermore, it is always important to balance the reality of the illness and a grave prognosis with the need to maintain hope. Because of their denial of the child's illness at the outset, many parents cannot cope with the knowledge of a guarded prognosis. Other functions include monitoring issues that need to be discussed by the team and identifying areas of conflict between the staff and the parents that impede the care. It is important to talk with the parents about how the nature of the illness and treatment may affect the child's behavior, and how these changes may influence family patterns of interaction. For example, children with overwhelming infections often are too ill to respond to parents in their usual way. Such anticipatory guidance can make a child's regressive behavior more comprehensible to parents, who would otherwise be confused by the onset of more immature behavior during a hospital stay.

All parents need an orientation to the staff, the hospital, and the restrictions of the particular unit. Parents who are staying with their child need to know where they can sleep. If an orientation is not provided, it is little wonder that parents may feel that their needs have been minimized.

One function of the liaison psychiatrist is to help the parents become involved with the child on the medical unit (Cleary et al., 1986). This function includes communicating to and helping the staff appreciate the nature of the parents' situation. Increasing the frequency and quality of communication often avoids schisms between the team and the parents. Parents may have specific needs that can be met by a referral to someone to help them with financial problems, insurance problems, or with their quest for local housing. Some parents may need help to define what their role as a parent is while they are in the hospital and what they can do to help care for their child. This is especially important in regard to procedures and to postsurgical restrictions. Parents may need special coaching on how to relate to a child who is severely ill and unable to respond to them. Parents are usually eager to bring favorite toys or a picture of the family to help the child feel more at home in the hospital. The parents need to know how to handle the child physically, or what activity is allowed and what is restricted. For example, parents often need direction about whether they can help feed the child, take the child for a ride in the unit wagon, or whether they need to restrict the child's intake of fluids.

Seeing the child with the parents usually helps in assessing the parents' interactions with the child, especially after surgery. If the child's appearance will be affected by surgery, parents should be warned, so that they can be prepared when they first see their child. Many parents are frightened to see their child immobilized or surrounded by machinery. Empathetic statements to the parents about their feelings and fears upon seeing their child in this situation can be helpful, particularly if linked to truthful updates about the child's progress and the immediate medical plans.

Optimally intervention should continue throughout the hospital stay. As the hospitalization proceeds and more serious problems emerge, parents often encounter inconsistencies and disagreements among the medical team members. The liaison psychiatrist can facilitate communication between the staff and the parents by convening and chairing a meeting to discuss concerns and reach a resolution.

The Structure of Intervention

Ideally, all hospitalized children should be screened to assess the need for a psychiatric consultation. The nursing staff caring for the child is often the first to recognize and request such a consultation. Any member of the medical team can suggest such an assessment.

Intervention can occur at a number of levels and with varying degrees of intensity, depending on the nature of the illness and the needs of the parents. It is becoming increasingly common for the infant mental health specialist to be part of the pediatric team and to serve as a pediatric liaison (Horner, Theut, & Murdoch, 1984). This usually occurs in situations where there is a frequent need for intensive intervention services, such as on a neonatal intensive care unit. In this liaison role, the infant psychiatrist makes rounds with the medical team and attends their team meetings. As a result, the clinician has ongoing knowledge of the child's condition and the staff reactions to the child and parents. With such ongoing contact, the liaison clinician can facilitate communication between the staff and family, address specific parental concerns, and serve as a ongoing resource to the family. This model is especially important for children in critical condition.

The advantage of this arrangement is that it allows for early identification and immediate intervention: There is a high level of utilization of services because the liaison psychiatrist becomes identified with and perceived as a valued part of the team. As a result, the medical staff is more likely to enlist the help of the liaison psychiatrist.

On a general medical floor, such as an infectious disease or postsurgical unit, the intervention model may be less intense, but it still offers a continuing presence. Often an infant mental health specialist meets with the staff once or twice per week to consult about specific children and families who are of current concern. There is a risk that marginal families who are barely coping may not be readily recognized. Nurses and child life personnel often serve as the initial contact by recognizing those parents who are angry, isolated, unresponsive, or overly involved. The initial contact person has to assess what services he or she will be able to deliver directly, when a situation will require consultation from the infant mental

health specialist, and when the family needs referral to another clinician. For example, a mother with a postpartum depression whose premature baby is in the neonatal intensive care unit for several weeks may best be served by a referral to an outside psychiatrist who will remain in contact with the mental health specialist on the unit. In this instance, the liaison role with the treating psychiatrist and the medical staff becomes pivotal to the child's care.

At times the mental health specialist may need to explain to the medical team that their expectations for the parents may be unrealistic. For example, if the parents have not shown a high degree of investment in the baby, the intensive care staff may have concerns about relinquishing the baby at discharge. Medical staff may judge the parents by how often they have visited the child. This may not be a fair assessment if the staff is not aware of other circumstances that have prevented the parents from being more available to the child. The liaison person also needs to help the team understand the needs of the parents. The staff may need assistance in teaching the parents how to care for a baby whom the parents perceive as fragile.

Intervention with the Young Child

It is essential to help toddlers understand the illness, the hospitalization, and the medical procedures that they are encountering; such intervention needs to be performed in ways that are consistent with children's cognitive level (Rasnake & Linscheid, 1989). Children in the preoperational period should be prepared for a procedure or an operation; details of what the actual experience is like should be explained to them. For example, toddlers should be given basic facts about the procedure, with the emphasis on who will be there at the start, where they will go, what the anesthesia will be like, and who will be there when they awaken. Children can be helped to understand medical procedures through drawings, doll play, and puppet presentations (Schulz, Raschke, Dedrick, & Thompson, 1981). Younger children who are awaiting kidney transplants can be prepared for the operation by the doctor, nurse, or child life specialist (Anderson et al., 1985) showing them where the new kidney will be placed by means of a simple drawing or a doll. In subsequent play settings, children often act out what they have been told and express their worries. The child's nurse or child life specialist can provide ongoing help to the child as the youngster presents the anticipatory feelings and fantasies about what will take place.

Infants and Toddlers with Acute Illnesses

The birth of a baby who is unexpectedly ill presents a major challenge to parents. During pregnancy parents create fantasies about and expectations for their baby (Leifer, 1977; Pines, 1972). The image of the expected baby represents a composite of both parents and their families and extends to the child's physical appearance, temperament, and development. The psychological preparation for the new baby involves the wish for a perfect child and the fear of a child who is defective (Solnit & Stark, 1961).

The birth of a seriously ill baby represents a significant deviation from the expected perfect child. In these situations the parents grieve the loss of the expected baby and struggle to change their expectations to conform to the present baby. Parents may view the child as damaged, which may in turn lead to its rejection. Five stages of parental reactions have been described: shock, denial, sadness and anger, adaptation, and reorganization (Drotar, Baskiewicz, Irvin, Kennell, & Klaus, 1975). Early intervention contributes to a more optimal parental attachment and adjustment. Parents of an ill neonate struggle with the complicated tasks of getting to know their baby at the same time as they are trying to come to terms with the ultimate implications of the illness. Thus, holding and touching the baby are the common ways that new parents relate to an infant. In this case, however, the child's medical condition may prohibit such interactions. The mother's physical status after a difficult delivery or cesarean can inhibit the pro-

cess. The baby may be surrounded by monitors and intravenous bottles such that the parents may be too frightened or timid to touch their baby. Other parents become so involved with the child's care that they never leave the hospital.

Infants and Toddlers with Chronic Illnesses

When a child is diagnosed with a chronic illness, the parents' view of a healthy child must change. Parental reactions form a continuum from a perception that the illness will present a new set of challenges, but that the child will be able to master them, to the belief that the child is now "damaged" and life will be difficult at best. With some chronic illnesses, parents must change their perception of the child continually as the illness evolves and presents new situations. These new perceptions influence the parents' relationship with the child. Parents who view the child as vulnerable and fragile may become overly protective and have difficulty helping the child resume normal development.

Children and families who face a chronic illness are confronted with the need for an ongoing series of adaptations (Pless & Pinkerton, 1975). The child's final status will depend on a number of factors, including the time of onset of the illness, the nature of its etiology, the certainty of the diagnosis, the degree of physical deformity and disability, the projected prognosis and outcome, and the parents' ability to help the child (Mrazek, 1991). The parents face numerous stressors, including financial pressures, the need for frequent doctor visits, and hospitalizations. The child's developmental stages are affected as the normal milestones are delayed. The unpredictability and uncertainty of the exacerbations and their outcome create their own stress.

The interventions for these children and families need to be long term. Comprehensive programs that provide medical care and support services are best. Their goal should include the normalization of the experience for the parents. Although some parents may not require intensive services after the child is stabilized, their care also needs to be long term.

Impact of Chronic Illness on the Development of Young Children

The first 4 years of life encompass a time of rapid development and pose the child a variety of physical, social, and emotional tasks. Children struggle to master such areas as cooperative play with peers, a developing body image, a sense of autonomy, a sense of self, physical independence, and separation from parents. All this occurs in parallel with an expanding cognitive development. A chronic illness that isolates the child from both interaction with peers and the stimulation of preschool clearly delays the child's progress (Travis, 1976). For example, the child with hemophilia who requires repeated blood samples may have problems developing a consolidated body image. The treatment of almost all chronic illnesses necessitates immobilization for some time (e.g., children on dialysis or children with leukemia undergoing chemotherapy); this in turn interferes with their developing sense of autonomy and physical independence. Children who previously had mastered an appropriate degree of separation from their parents frequently regress as they continue to experience the anxiety and pain of a chronic medical illness. In all cases, the extent of the impact depends on the child's developmental level and the severity of the interference from both the medical illness and the level of treatment.

Impact of the Child's Chronic Illness on Relationships with Peers and Siblings

Young children develop social competence through their interaction with siblings and peers.

As children mature, they move from independent and parallel play to cooperative play. Chronic illness, with its frequent medical appointments, hospitalizations, and treatments, often interferes with children's opportunities for social experience. Siblings and peers may express fear of children who appear fragile or physically different and may accordingly interact with them less or in a stilted manner. Fearful that they will develop the same illness, the peers may ignore a child with a chronic illness. Some parents are reluctant to enroll their ill child in activities, because they feel the youngster cannot be consistent in attendance; often the parents do not want to explain to yet another party their child's problems or special needs.

The chronically ill child in a medical setting may become accustomed to interacting primarily with adults and to having most needs met very quickly. If placed in a class with peers, the sick youngsters may gravitate to the adults because they are most comfortable in these relationships. The give and take in cooperative play may be the most difficult area for these children to master.

The team members must help the parents understand the importance of peer relationships and the variety of opportunities available to assist their child in developing social relationships (play groups, preschools, church nurseries). Parents will need assistance in how to help the teachers understand their child's needs. The emphasis should be on the rich experience this will provide for the child's social development.

ASTHMA IN THE TODDLER AS AN EXAMPLE OF A CHILD WITH A CHRONIC ILLNESS

For very young children, a severe asthmatic attack can be a particularly frightening emotional experience. Toddlers cannot understand their sudden inability to breathe. The panic induced by not being able to get air into their lungs can lead to further bronchoconstriction and thus exacerbate their respiratory symptoms. When such an attack is precipitated by an emotional confrontation with a parent, the situation becomes more complicated because the child's source of security is also a central part of the conflict.

One of the normal tasks of parenting a 2-year-old child is to set adequate limits and gradually obtain an appropriate level of behavioral compliance. Temper tantrums during the second year of life can be challenging, but most parents learn that they are a normal developmental phase that all children experience. However, when a severely asthmatic child has a violent tantrum, the emotional distress can lead to bronchoconstriction, sudden dyspnea, and a frightening trip to the emergency room. Some parents decide that giving in to their child's demands is preferable to running the risk of precipitating a violent attack. This conflict-avoidant pattern of parenting was documented in a sample of preschool children with severe asthma. These children were studied systematically using an observational paradigm that could be coded to reveal the nature of the mother-child interactions. These asthmatic children were not only more frequently oppositional, but, in approximately 75% of the oppositional sequences, their parents gave in to their child's willfulness. In contrast, a control sample of healthy preschoolers were studied and found to be noncompliant with their parents' instructions in only one-third of their somewhat less frequent oppositional sequences (Mrazek et al., 1984).

Given that intense emotional distress can lead to an overt asthma attack, there has long been an interest in the role of emotional stressors in the initial onset of the illness. Given that asthma is clearly a genetic illness, the children of asthmatic parents are at increased risk for developing the disease. If one parent is asthmatic, the odds are about 1 in 5 that the child will develop asthma. If both parents have the illness, the risk of developing the disease increases to 50%. In these children, biological risk factors such as early respiratory infections and high levels of serum immunoglobulin E are associated with the expression of asthma (Mrazek, Klinnert, Brower, & Harbeck, 1990). Furthermore, early problems in parenting have been shown independently to be associated with an increased likelihood of developing the illness (Mrazek, Klinnert, Mrazek, & Macey, 1991). Currently studies are under way that have been designed to help parents understand the potential role of emotional factors in disease expression. The ultimate objective of these interventions is to demonstrate that by modification of these risk factors the onset of asthma can be delayed or prevented.

Anticipatory Grief

Loss is an ongoing issue for all parents of a chronically ill infant or toddler. Parents must alter their image of the child at each developmental stage. The optimal intervention is to allow the parents to grieve the loss of the expected child, while helping them adjust to their child's current level of adaptation.

Anticipatory grief is the process of experiencing the phases of normal postdeath grief in the face of a potential loss of a significant person (Fulton & Gottesman, 1980; Rando, 1986). Some of the components of anticipatory grief are anger, guilt, sadness, feelings of loss, and decreased ability to function at usual tasks. Anticipatory grief is especially significant and pertinent for parents whose child has a chronic illness. It is a particularly useful concept to invoke when working with parents whose child is coping with a protracted and deteriorating illness or suffering from a disease with no known cure such as AIDS.

Intervention with Parents and the Dying Child

Despite the best efforts of the medical staff, there will be occasions when the infant's or toddler's condition deteriorates and the staff is unable to prevent death. Delivering the news that a child has a fatal illness is a complicated task. The first step is to supply the parents with honest and complete information about the diagnosis and prognosis, which allows ongoing communication both to help the parents express their sadness and begin to say good-bye to the child and to help the family cope with the aftermath. A dying child may cause the parents to question the quality of the child's life and the necessity to continue treatment. Occasionally there are disagreements within the team or between the team and the parents regarding the degree of medical support. The liaison consultant's role is vital in helping the parents and staff communicate and discuss the parents' wishes. If no agreement can be reached, the consultant may then request an ethics consultation to help the parents and staff review the child's course, prognosis, and quality of life. Someone outside the treatment unit may offer a novel perspective and help all concerned to explore their feelings and options.

Mourning consists of preoccupation with the lost object along with the affective burdens of anger, sadness, and guilt (Freud, 1917, 1957; Lindemann, 1944; Osterweis, Solomon, & Green, 1984; Parkes, 1985). Parents can be assisted by an explanation that mourning is a normal experience, and that each may grieve differently and may not be experiencing the same feelings at a given time. Supportive therapy can be helpful immediately after the child's death. The staff members who helped the family at the time of the death become important for the parents. A phone call a month after the child's death provides the parents with a sense of caring and connectedness. Referral to a therapist who understands issues of mourning may be needed.

Prevention of Adverse Effects of Hospitalization

The prevention of adverse effects from hospitalization for infants and toddlers involves three major efforts: (1) preparation for hospitalization by providing the children and parents with information about what will occur; (2) maintaining the child's contact with the parents during hospitalization; (3) reducing the amount of time spent in the hospital (Byrne & Cadman, 1987).

Parents serve as the secure base for infants and toddlers who are hospitalized. The parents' preparation for hospitalization greatly determines the effect on the child. Parents need to understand the reasons for the hospitalization and the nature of the surgery or procedure; they are then better able to anticipate what will happen and better prepared to assist their child. With proper management, their anxiety level decreases, and they are able to provide comfort and reassurance to the child. This preparation can involve films,

books, visits to the hospital, or visits from a nurse to the home. Parents also need to know how children developmentally respond to illness, surgery, and hospitalization so that they can be prepared for the variety of reactions they may encounter.

One of the most important concepts to communicate to parents is the impact of separation on infants and toddlers. Parents should be told that despite the presence of the medical and nursing staff, contact with the parents will greatly reduce child's separation fears. It is important for the parents to be present on the unit during painful procedures, although perhaps not in the same room. Hence, it is important for the parents either to visit frequently or to room in.

The third part of decreasing adverse effects is to reduce the time children are hospitalized. The change in insurance benefits, with the associated decrease in allowances for hospitalization, has resulted in many day-surgery programs in which children enter the hospital in the morning and go home that night.

Since young children cannot understand the concept of time, it is not useful to tell them of impending hospitalization or procedures until shortly before the event. For example, a child should be prepared for a lumbar puncture immediately before the procedure, not a day in advance.

Caregivers Other than the Parents

Although this chapter has focused on intervention with the biological parents, at times the primary caregivers are grandparents, older siblings, extended relatives, or foster parents. In these situations, the clinician will need to consider the nature of the relationship and commitment to the child. At times the court will select a guardian or appoint a family member as guardian. The medical team often can make recommendations to the court regarding these appointments in the best interests of infants and toddlers based on their observations of interaction during hospitalization.

Effect on Siblings

Parents frequently request help in explaining their child's medical illness to siblings. It is important that the parents prepare the siblings appropriately with simple explanations aimed at the child's developmental level. Parents should be told that siblings often worry that they might have contributed to the condition, or that they will develop the same illness. Often parents request to have the siblings visit the ill child. Such requests should be considered on an individual basis and weighed on the basis of various factors. Thus, if the ill child is surrounded by high-technology machinery and cannot in any case respond to the sibling, it is best to discourage such visits. Alternatively, for certain children, not visiting a sibling may generate disturbing fantasies.

Discharge Planning

Even after parents adapt adequately to the child's medical illness and hospitalization, discharge planning may arouse new anxieties and a different set of concerns. Parents may question whether they will be able to care for the child at home, away from the support of the hospital and staff. Parents often have to learn new skills in caring for the child, such as sterile dressings changes or how to respond to the alarm on the monitor; they may feel criticized by the staff in the face of their initial blunders. Some parents fear a crisis and a return to the hospital. Many parents will be concerned that the illness will reoccur and that the long-term outcome will be problematic. Helping parents to work through these concerns and to make appropriate plans for discharge is a central role of the infant psychiatrist. New parents may feel overwhelmed by the challenge of caring for their child for the first time, independent from the hospital. Parents also need help in allowing the child to resume normal activities. A follow-up phone call a week later can provide continuity after discharge, assess how the family has made the transition, and direct future attempts to help the family find a therapist.

Summary

This chapter has discussed the impact of acute and chronic medical illness and hospitalization on infants and young children and their parents. It highlights the need for members of the medical team to work closely with the family in order to help parents understand both their child's and their own reactions to these experiences. The parents benefit by having these explanations delivered in terms of their child's developmental stage.

The mental health members of the team have a special role in fostering the relationship between the parents and the medical team. One of the most important aspects of their work is in helping the parents and medical team prevent adverse effects of the medical illness and hospitalization.

REFERENCES

Ainsworth, M. D. S., Blehar, M. C., Waters, E., & Wall, S. (1978). *Patterns of attachment: A psychological study of the strange situation.* Hillsdale, NJ: Lawrence Erlbaum.

Anderson, A. S., Bergeson, P. S., Bushore, M., Cravens, J. H., Dudgeon, D. L., Evans, H. E., Gold, H. R., & Shattuck, G. B. (1985). Child life programs for hospitalized children. *Pediatrics, 76* (3), 467–470.

Bowlby, J. (1961). Childhood mourning and its implications for psychiatry. *American Journal of Psychiatry, 118,* 481–498.

Bowlby, J. (1973). *Attachment and loss: Vol. 2. Separation.* New York: Basic Books.

Burbach, D. J., & Peterson, L. (1986). Children's concepts of physical illness: A review and critique of the cognitive—developmental literature. *Health Psychology, 5* (3), 307–325.

Byrne, C. M., & Cadman, D. (1987). Prevention of the adverse effects of hospitalization in children. *Journal of Preventive Psychiatry, 3* (2), 167–190.

Cleary, J., Gray, O. P., Hall, D. J., Rowlandson, P. H., Sainsbury, C. P. Q., & Davies, M. M. (1986). Parental involvement in the lives of children in hospital. *Archives of Disease in Childhood, 61,* 779–787.

Drotar, D., Baskiewicz, A., Irvin, N., Kennell, J., & Klaus, M. (1975). The adaptation of parents to the birth of an infant with a congenital malformation: A hypothetical model. *Pediatrics, 56,* 710–717.

Eiser, C. (1984). Communicating with sick and hospitalized children. *Journal of Child Psychology and Psychiatry, 25* (2), 181–189.

Freud, S. (1957). *Mourning and melancholia.* In J. Strachey (Ed. and Trans.), *The standard edition of the complete psychological works of Sigmund Freud* (Vol. 14, pp. 243–258). London: Hogarth Press. (Originally published 1917.)

Fulton, R., & Gottesman, D. J. (1980). Anticipatory grief: A psychosocial concept reconsidered. *British Journal of Psychiatry, 137,* 45–54.

Green, M., & Solnit, A. J. (1964). Reactions to the threatened loss of a child: A vulnerable child syndrome. *Pediatrics, 34,* 58–66.

Horner, T. W., Theut, S. K., & Murdoch, W. G. (1984). Discharge planning for the high-risk neonate: A consultation-liaison role for the infant mental health specialist. *American Journal of Orthopsychiatry, 54* (4), 637–647.

Illingworth, R. S., & Holt, K. S. (1955). Children in hospital: Some observations on their reactions with special reference to daily visiting. *Lancet, 271* (2), 1257–1262.

Leifer, M. (1977). Psychological changes accompanying pregnancy and motherhood. *Genetic Psychology Monographs, 95,* 55–96.

Lindemann, E. (1944). Symptomatology and management of acute grief. *American Journal of Psychiatry, 101,* 141–148.

Mrazek, D. A. (1991). Chronic pediatric illness and multiple hospitalizations. In M. Lewis (Ed.), *Child and adolescent psychiatry* (pp. 1041–1050). Baltimore: Williams & Wilkins.

Mrazek, D. A., Anderson, I. S., & Strunk, R. C. (1984). Disturbed emotional development of severely asthmatic preschool children. *Journal of Child Psychology and Psychiatry, 26* (Suppl. 4), 81–94.

Mrazek, D. A., Klinnert, M. D., Brower, A., & Harbeck, R. J. (1990). Predictive capacity of elevated serum IgE for early asthma onset. *Journal of Clinical Immunology, 85,* 194.

Mrazek, D. A., Klinnert, M., Mrazek, P., & Macey, T. (1991). Early asthma onset: Consideration of parenting issues. *Journal of the American Academy of Child and Adolescent Psychiatry, 30,* 277–282.

Osterweis, M., Solomon, F., & Green, M. (1984). *Bereavement: Reactions, consequences & care.* Washington, DC: National Academy Press.

Parkes, C. M. (1985). Bereavement. *British Journal of Psychiatry, 146,* 11–17.

Piaget, J. (1926). *The language and thought of the child.* London: Routledge and Kegan Paul.

Piaget, J., & Inhelder, B. (1969). *The psychology of the child.* New York: Basic Books.

Pines, D. (1972). Pregnancy and motherhood: Interaction between fantasy and reality. *British Journal of Medical Psychology, 45,* 333–343.

Pless, I. B., & Pinkerton, P. (1975). *Chronic childhood disorder—Promoting patterns of adjustment.* Chicago: Henry Kimpton.

Prugh, D. G., Staub, E. M., Sands, H. H., Kirschbaum, R. M., & Lenihan, E. A. (1953). A study of the emotional reactions of children and families to hospitalization and illness. *American Journal of Orthopsychiatry, 23,* 70–106.

Rando, T. A. (1986). Understanding and facilitating anticipatory grief in the loved ones of the dying. In T. A. Rando (Ed.), *Loss and Anticipatory Grief* (pp. 97–130). Lexington, MA: Lexington Books.

Rasnake, L. K., & Linscheid, T. R. (1989). Anxiety reduction in children receiving medical care: Developmental considerations. *Developmental and Behavioral Pediatrics, 10,* 169–175.

Richmond, J. B. (1958). The pediatric patient in illness. In M. H. Hollender (Ed.), *The psychology of medical practice* (pp. 195–211). Philadelphia: W. B. Saunders.

Schaffer, H. R., & Callender, W. M. (1959). Psychologic effects of hospitalization in infancy. *Pediatrics, 24,* 528–539.

Schulz, J. B., Raschke, D., Dedrick, C., & Thompson, M. (1981). The effects of a preoperational puppet show on anxiety levels of hospitalized children. *Children's Health Care, 9,* 118–121.

Solnit, A. J., & Stark, M. H. (1961). Mourning and the birth of a defective child. *Psychoanalytic Study of the Child, 16,* 523–537.

Spitz, R. A., & Wolfe, K. M. (1946). Anaclitic depression. In A. Freud, H. Hartmann, & E. Kris (Eds.), *The psychoanalytic study of the child, 2,* 313–342.

Travis, G. (1976). *Chronic illness in children.* Stanford; CA: Stanford University Press

Zetterstrom, R. (1984). Responses of children to hospitalization. *Acta Paediatrica Scandinavia, 73,* 289–295.

39 / Coping and Young Children with Motor Deficits

G. Gordon Williamson

What type of early intervention makes a significant difference in a child's life: teaching specific skills or the functional application of those skills to manage the requirements of daily living? Certainly achievement of object permanence, a pincer grasp, or any other skill is very important. However, positive meaning is not generated by a developmental skill per se but by its contribution to the child's ability to cope with self and the environment.

This chapter focuses on the adaptive behavior of infants, toddlers, and preschool children with motor deficits. These children may be motorically challenged due to a physical disability (e.g., cerebral palsy, spina bifida), general developmental delay, or secondary motor dysfunction associated with certain conditions (e.g., Down syndrome, prematurity, drug exposure, regulatory disorder). For maximal benefit, therapeutic and educational intervention needs to enhance simultaneously their motor control—the capacity to plan and coordinate movements—(Replacement clarifying "motor control") and their coping competence. By emphasizing the child's transactions with the environment, physical movement becomes a means of supporting his or her adaptive functioning. Intervention that helps make this linkage inclines the child to develop a belief that the world is a safe and satisfying place in which he or she can be successful.

The chapter first describes the coping process of young children and the internal and external resources that influence it. To validate the importance of coping as a focus of intervention, a study is summarized that compares the coping characteristics of children with and without disabilities who are under 3 years of age. Given this clinical foundation, the discussion then addresses motor

This chapter is adapted from *Coping in young children: Early intervention practices to enhance adaptive behavior and resilience,* by S. Zeitlin and G. G. Williamson, 1994, Baltimore: Paul H. Brookes, P.O. Box 10624, Baltimore, MD 21285-0624. Copyright 1994 by Paul H. Brookes Publishing Company. Adapted with permission.

control and how it contributes to an infant's emerging adaptive ability. The development of coordinated movement during infancy is described, as is the vulnerability generated by the atypical movement patterns observed in infants with disabilities. Next, intervention options are presented that are based on the transactional coping process. These options serve as a guide for designing services to foster motor control and coping. Special attention is placed on direct and indirect intervention strategies that regulate sensory experiences, facilitate physical positioning and mobility, and encourage the therapeutic use of play.

Coping in Young Children

Coping refers to how the child manages situations perceived as threatening or challenging. It is the process of making adaptations to meet personal needs and to respond to the demands of the environment (Williamson, Zeitlin, & Szczepanski, 1989). The child's coping style is influenced by his or her developmental skills, temperament, prior experience, areas of vulnerability, and the demands of the environment (Murphy & Moriarty, 1976). By drawing on coping resources, the infant attempts to maintain or enhance feelings of well-being.

For intervention purposes, the process of coping is described by a theoretically sound, 4-step model (See Figure 39.1). Generally speaking, in young children coping is predominately emotionally driven and reflects rudimentary cognitive processing. However, it is useful to consider the several interrelated steps: first, determine the meaning of an event, then develop an action plan, next implement a coping effort, and finally evaluate the outcome (Zeitlin & Williamson, 1994). The coping process may be initiated by an event occurring in the environment (e.g., a demand by

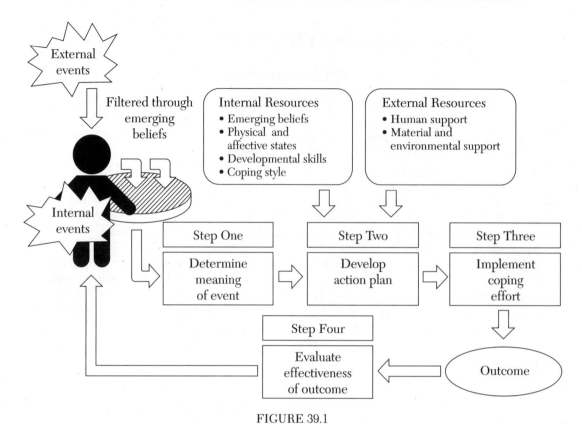

FIGURE 39.1

The coping process of young children.

the caregiver) or within the child (e.g., a need for food, comfort, or to express preferences). Ultimately, it is the child who gives meaning to the event based on his or her perception of it as harmful, threatening, or challenging to his or her sense of well-being (Lazarus & Folkman, 1984).

Given this interpretation, the child then decides what to do. The child's internal and external resources influence this decision. Key internal resources are the child's emerging beliefs, physical and affective states, developmental skills, and coping style. The essential external resources involve both human and material/environmental supports. As a consequence of this decision making, the child implements a coping effort to deal with the situation. The child then evaluates the result of this effort to determine whether it was successful or not.

A child with adequate coping resources is better able to manage the demands of daily living, master new learning, and generate positive feelings of self-esteem. It is important for the prac-

titioner to evaluate the status of each of these resources because of their impact on the child's perception and management of life events (Greenspan, 1992; Werner, 1989; Williamson & Zeitlin, 1990). In this chapter the emphasis is on motor development and coping style. However, the following discussion provides an overview of each of the internal and external coping resources.

INTERNAL RESOURCES

From birth an infant's experiences shape *emerging beliefs* about self and the environment (Stern, 1985). Beliefs are a doubly used resource in coping. They provide the screen through which all perceptions of events are filtered, and they influence decision making by forming expectations for the outcome of an action. That is, beliefs provide a continuity of perception that organizes experience and serves as a motivator for the initiation or avoidance of specific actions (Bandura, 1986). In young children, emerging beliefs relevant to coping are related to an evolving sense of efficacy—the power to produce an effect, control events, and trust others to be responsive to needs.

Another internal resource, *physical and affective states,* may be considered at the time of a specific coping transaction or in the context of their general status over a period of time. Physical state refers to the child's health and bodily condition. For example, the coping capacity of a toddler with cerebral palsy may be undermined due to upper respiratory infections related to impaired breathing patterns or to the fatigue induced by the high energy requirements of moving with spastic muscles. Affective state refers to a child's characteristic mood and feelings (e.g., happy, anxious, depressed).

The child's repertoire of *developmental skills* is also a significant internal resource. Although children acquire increasingly complex skills as they mature, each child has a unique pattern of development influenced by his or her constitution and transactions with the environment. Skills in all areas of development—motor, cognitive, communicative, social, and emotional—are the building blocks for function. They are integrated and applied in specific situations as part of coping efforts.

Coping style is the typical behavioral pattern a child uses to manage the routines, opportunities, challenges, and frustrations encountered in daily living. The authors (Zeitlin, Williamson, & Szczepanski, 1988) developed the Early Coping Inventory to assess the behavioral characteristics documented in the research literature, or identified by expert clinical judgment, as critical to coping in infants and toddlers. The instrument evaluates a child's coping style according to three descriptive categories—sensorimotor organization, reactive behavior, and self-initiated behavior.

Sensorimotor organization refers to the child's regulation of psychophysiological functions and the ability to integrate the sensory and motor systems. These sensorimotor behaviors involve such factors as the organization of state and arousal, self-comforting behaviors, managing the intensity and variety of sensory stimuli, and the quality of motor control.

Reactive behaviors are used to respond to external demands of the physical and social environment. Among these are: the ability to adapt to daily routines and limits set by the caregiver, to accept warmth and support from familiar persons, and to respond to vocal and gestural direction.

Self-initiated behaviors are autonomously generated behaviors used to meet personal needs and to interact with objects and people. Whereas reactive behaviors are closely contingent on environmental cues, self-initiated behaviors are more spontaneous and intrinsically motivated. They include, for example, the ability to initiate action to communicate a need, to demonstrate persistence during activities, and to apply previously learned behaviors to new situations.

EXTERNAL RESOURCES

Human supports are a primary external resource influencing the child's coping competence. In addition to meeting basic care needs, parents are instrumental in fostering the attachment and trust required for emotional development. Thus, the infant's subjective experience with the caregiver helps shape an emerging sense of self. This relationship provides a source of comfort when distressed and serves as a secure base from which the child can venture into the world. Thus, in the provision of early intervention services (Brazelton & Cramer, 1990), the quality of the parent-child relationship and the degree of mutually rewarding interaction are fundamental areas of concern. Likewise, the support provided to family members influences their availability to the child.

The other external coping resource involves *material and environmental supports.* Material supports refer to such resources as adequate food, clothing, shelter, and toys. Environmental supports are the conditions of the physical surroundings that can facilitate or interfere with coping efforts, such as space, air, temperature, noise, and light. Physical environments that are chaotic, disorganized, overstimulating, or lacking in stimulation increase the risk for maladaptive outcomes in young children.

So far the discussion has highlighted the nature of the coping process and emphasized the major internal and external resources that influence the ability of young children to cope. We now shift our

TABLE 39.1

Most and Least Adaptive Coping Behaviors of the Disabled Children

Most Adaptive (Situationally Effective)	Least Adaptive (Minimally Effective)
Accepts warmth and support from familiar persons	Unable to change behavior when necessary to solve a problem or achieve a goal
Responds to a variety of sounds	Fails to find a way of handling a new or difficult situation
Reacts to a variety of visual stimuli	Does not enter new situations easily or cautiously as the situation demands
Completes self-initiated activity	
Expresses likes and dislikes	Cannot balance independent behavior with necessary dependence on adults
	Often uses behavior inappropriate to the situation

focus to address the adaptive functioning of young children who are developmentally delayed and disabled.

Coping Behaviors of Children with Special Needs

Infants and toddlers with special needs frequently have fewer resources to support adaptive coping efforts. For example, a disability may limit the acquisition of developmental skills and thereby restrict the variety and sophistication of available coping strategies. Parents may be less accessible as a supportive external resource if they are experiencing psychological distress or exhaustion from the requirements of daily caregiving (Turnbull & Turnbull, 1990). Also, children with disabilities often have to manage additional stressors such as treatment regimes, hospitalization, restrictions in activity, and disruptions in daily routines (Williamson, Szczepanski, & Zeitlin, 1993). Thus, they frequently face a greater number of stressors with a limited repertoire of coping resources.

We conducted a study that investigated the coping characteristics of children between 4 and 36 months of age using the Early Coping Inventory (Zeitlin & Williamson, 1990). The study examined the coping behaviors of 1,035 children with developmental delays or disabilities and 405 children with typical development. Seventy-three

day care and early intervention programs participated in the study from 22 states and Canada.

Heretofore, clinical impressions and previous research had suggested that differences exist between the coping abilities of young children with and without disabilities (Barrera & Vella, 1987; Carlton, 1988; Meisels & Shonkoff, 1990); the results of this investigation supported these views. In this study, the disabled group was significantly less skilled in coping competence. As a group, their coping behaviors tended to be situationally effective. That is, behaviors used successfully in one type of situation were not generalized to other types of situations. In contrast, the coping behaviors of the nondisabled group were effective. The least adaptive behaviors of the disabled group were minimally effective—often erratic, rigid, or limited in expression. Table 39.1 provides a list of the most and least adaptive behaviors of this group. The greatest difference between the two groups lay in the character of their self-initiation. The coping patterns of the children with disabilities tended to be less autonomous and more passive.

It is important to note, however, that in this study, both sets of children included some individuals with consistently effective coping behaviors and others with minimally effective behaviors. This finding suggests that the presence of a disability as such does not mean that a particular child will have ineffective coping. Rather, it suggests a greater vulnerability to the stress of daily living.

Now we shift our attention to focus on the acquisition of motor control in infancy in order to understand its importance as a resource for adaptive functioning. From this perspective the discussion then targets the impact of atypical motor development on coping and provides suggestions for intervention with children who have physical disabilities.

Acquisition of Motor Control in Infancy

One of the infant's most crucial achievements during the first year of life is learning to deal with gravity. At birth, an infant is already capable of the basic movements. The young child can extend (straighten), flex (bend), move laterally (side to side), and rotate (twist or turn). However, two important elements are missing: the postural control necessary to assume increasingly advanced developmental positions against gravity and the coordination necessary to bring together a wide variety of movement patterns in order to accomplish a task (Gilfoyle, Grady, & Moore, 1990). Thus, every baby is challenged to develop the control of posture and movement that will enable him or her to discover the world and manage it successfully.

The development of postural control against gravity proceeds in a cephalo to caudal direction (i.e., from the head toward the feet). In the course of achieving such control, the infant acquires coordination of movement in a predictable sequence—extension, flexion, lateral movement, and rotation (Williamson, 1987). The acquisition of this control expands the child's repertoire of available coping strategies. The infant's development of control of extension against gravity is quickly counterbalanced with emerging control of the opposite movement pattern of flexion. Only when extensor and flexor movements are coordinated does the infant demonstrate organization of lateral movements that allow weight-shifting of the body side to side. Rotation is the most sophisticated of the movement patterns and is therefore the last to be mastered.

During play, the infant practices these movements and learns to organize them for functional use. During the first year of life, when the infant is in the prone-lying position, the head-to-foot development of controlled extension can be seen readily. At 1 month of age, the child rests in a curled posture when lying on the abdomen and has the arms tucked under the body. By 2 to 3 months of age, however, control of extension progresses to the midback, enabling the infant to lift the head and chest off the mat and bring the arms out to the side of the body. Gradually extension progresses to the low back, allowing the infant to use extensor muscles to raise the buttocks off the mat (the playful "bottom-lifting" of the 4-month-old child). Around 5 to 6 months, extensor control crosses the hips so that the legs come into alignment with the body and are no longer in a flexed posture to the side (the "frog-legged" position). The infant celebrates this achievement by joyous rocking on the belly for countless hours. At approximately 7 months of age, the infant has conquered gravity in the prone position and displays controlled extension throughout the body (the Landau reaction).

Concurrent with the development of extension, the infant is acquiring control of flexion. It can best be seen when the child is supine. When resting on the back, the 2-month-old infant assumes an asymmetrical posture with the head usually to one side. During the next month, the infant learns to maintain the head in the body's midline due to developing coordination of the flexor muscles of the neck. This emerging flexor control becomes dramatically expressed in the symmetrical, midline-oriented play of the 4-month-old infant. The child enjoys bringing the arms together in order to pluck on clothing, mouth objects, and touch the bottle or breast during feeding. All of these activities contribute to sensory, cognitive, and emotional development and rely on the infant's expanding flexor skills. By 5 months of age, the infant engages in more body-oriented play by bringing the hands to the knees and lifting the head off the mat to look at the body. Greater control of flexion in the trunk (torso) and legs allows the infant of 6 to 7 months to grasp the feet, suck on the toes, and rock with delight in this flexed posture. Thus, the child has mastered gravity in the supine position and has an enhanced sensorimotor foundation for exploring the world.

When movements of extension and flexion are counterbalanced, lateral control appears. Around 4 months, the infant begins to right the head laterally in space when the body is tilted to one side during caregiving activities such as bathing or dressing. At this time, the child has adequate lateral control of the trunk to play in a side-lying position and not fall onto the abdomen or back. During the next few months, the infant learns to shift weight side to side when propping on the forearms or extended arms in the prone position. This ability to weight-shift laterally allows the child to free one hand to reach for objects. It also facilitates social interaction since the infant can attend more directly to the surroundings. By 7 months of age, the infant has sufficient control of lateral movements to "pivot on the belly" in a circle during play.

The emergence of controlled rotation of the head, trunk, and extremities is founded on the development of extension, flexion, and lateral movement. Therefore, it is the most difficult movement pattern for the infant to coordinate. In the early months, rotation usually is associated with reaching or kicking. As the infant reaches for an object, the upper trunk tends to twist in order to support the movement of the arm. Likewise, kicking of the legs often elicits rotation in the lower trunk. These activities generally introduce early rolling. The infant reaches across the body when on the back, loses balance, and flips over. With practice, the child learns to roll with controlled rotation (i.e., the head turns, the shoulders follow, then the trunk, and finally the pelvis).

In large part, it is trunk rotation that enables an infant to assume new positions such as sitting, crawling, or standing and to move with balance from one position to another. In every new position, the infant must learn to coordinate extension, flexion, lateral movement, and rotation in order to be mobile in that posture (e.g., reciprocal crawling, walking). The acquisition of motor skills is based on the infant's ability to organize the movements available at birth into increasingly sophisticated adaptive movement strategies.

Atypical Motor Development

Motor control does not develop in a vacuum; it emerges within the context of a child learning to cope with daily activities. Movement becomes relevant when used to meet personal needs and to respond adaptively to the demands of the environment. Many infants who are developmentally delayed or disabled have difficulty organizing the sensory and motor systems in a way that allows for successful interaction with objects and people. This vulnerability strongly influences their coping efforts. Frequently they are born with low muscle tone and may have an additional dysfunction in sensory processing. As a result, their development of functional movement is blocked (Zeitlin & Williamson, 1994). Generally, these infants start to develop extension but fail to counterbalance it with quality control of flexion. As a consequence, the more sophisticated lateral movements and those of rotation do not develop adequately (Scherzer & Tscharnuter, 1990; Williamson, 1987). Thus, these infants have limited movement patterns available for exploration, learning, and interpersonal engagement.

For instance, an infant with low muscle tone characteristically develops a predominance of extensor movement. There may be a tendency to pull the head and shoulders back with too much force. At the same time, the opposing flexor movements, such as reaching forward with the arms, are slow to develop. With repetition, the atypical patterns of extension may become habitual and hinder further development. These extensor movements make it difficult for the infant to acquire head control, to suck appropriately on a nipple, to assume a good prone-on-elbows position, or to play with the hands together in sitting. Since balanced control of extension and flexion is not attained, lateral movements and rotation often fail to develop properly. Therefore, postural control and coordination may be insufficient for the achievement of motor milestones. In addition, this clinical picture may interfere with the infant's capacity to elicit attention, nurturance, and care from the parents. As a result, parent-child interaction may be strained—which places at risk their ability to establish a positive attachment and sense of relatedness.

Infants with an athetotic type of cerebral palsy serve as an illustration. These infants are initially "floppy" and demonstrate increasingly erratic movement patterns over time. To compensate for the low muscle tone and disorganization, they

444

learn to stiffen (tense) their muscles in order to achieve some level of control. For example, they may elevate the shoulder girdle to stabilize the head ("shrug" the shoulders up), arch the trunk into extension, and stiffen the arms and legs at the extremes of range. Since the infants are typically more involved on one side of the body than the other, the head tends to turn asymmetrically to a preferred side. Consequently, they may turn and pull away from the parents when being held. Similarly, their attempt to coordinate movement results in general stiffening, which prevents them from molding to the adult's body and cuddling in the arms. Parents may interpret such postural responses as rejection by the infant and feel incompetent in their caregiving skills.

Interactive demands are further exacerbated by the following problems that may interfere with communication: (1) marked fluctuations in attention and arousal by the infant with athetosis, (2) facial expressions that vary from a flat affect to grimacing due to altering muscle tone, (3) difficulty in maintaining eye contact related to positioning of the head, (4) incoordinated vocalizations that are hard to understand, and (5) deficits in the use of manual gestures (e.g., giving and showing behaviors with objects, pointing). Hence, reading the child's cues is often confusing and exacting. As a consequence, there tends to be an interactive mismatch and breakdown in communication due to missed emotional signals or the misreading of signals.

Intervention with these families must focus on the primacy of the parent-child relationship. Parents need to learn how to interpret with accuracy the subtle communicative signs of the infant with athetosis and to act accordingly. Such an understanding often leads to a decompression of emotional tension and an appreciation that both partners are trying to interact as best they can. The parents also must acquire skills in ways to handle and position the child, so that the influence of aberrant movement patterns is decreased and the child is provided with adequate proximal stability of the head and trunk. The emphasis should fall on enhancing mutual self-esteem and efficacy within the context of daily activities. These issues are addressed in greater detail in our discussion of options for educational and therapeutic intervention.

Intervention Options

Intervention is directed toward increasing the effectiveness of the child's transactions with the environment. Children cope most adaptively when there is a congruence between their coping resources and environmental demands and expectations (Sameroff & Fiese, 1990). A goal of intervention is to encourage a "goodness-of-fit" between resources and demands, so that the infant can manage daily living with a sense of well-being. In the course of this process, the child modifies previously learned coping strategies and develops new ones.

Three primary intervention options address the components of this transactional process. Each option is designed to establish a better fit between the child and the environment. One can change demands to be congruent with the child's capabilities, enhance the child's internal and external coping resources, and provide accurate contingent feedback regarding the child's efforts. Due to the transactional nature of the coping process, all three intervention options are frequently applied at the same time.

The first option, changing demands, requires active collaboration of parents and practitioners to ensure they have an adequate understanding of the child. This knowledge enables them to set expectations that match the child's ability to meet them. Specific intervention strategies include establishing appropriate therapeutic goals, modifying demands when necessary, and grading environmental stressors. For example, it is helpful to introduce early the concept that functional independence for the child with major physical involvement may best be achieved by a combination of wheelchair use and ambulation with braces. One mode of locomotion may be preferred over the other, depending on the circumstances. The wheelchair may be more practical in a crowded shopping mall, whereas ambulation with crutches may be more efficient in the home. By establishing realistic and shared goals for intervention, parents, professionals, and the child can place ambulation training in proper perspective and avoid the narrow attitude that walking is always the desired means of mobility.

The second option, enhancing coping resources, increases the child's ability to produce effective coping efforts. In the context of fostering developmental skills, for example, the infant is helped to learn more adaptive ways of coping. This approach requires that intervention goals and objectives link skill acquisition to functional coping outcomes. For instance, an objective to improve coordination of the arms may be connected to enhancing the child's ability to engage in dramatic play, to demonstrate self-reliance in feeding or dressing activities, or to express emotions (e.g., use of gestures for emotional signaling such as raising the arms for a hug).

The third option, providing contingent feedback, involves parents and professionals responding appropriately to the child's efforts. Through this feedback, the child learns the impact of his or her behavior on the environment. When an effective coping effort receives positive and accurate feedback, both the infant and adult feel successful and experience pleasure in the interaction. Such reinforcement of effective coping leads to a sense of mastery that usually is reflected in subsequent coping efforts.

These intervention options may be implemented through direct and indirect intervention strategies. For children with physical limitations, these strategies need to highlight four particular areas of concern: grading sensorimotor experiences, utilizing proper positioning, providing a means of mobility, and using play within the context of intervention.

Direct and Indirect Strategies

Adapting the initial work of Hildebrand (1975), it is helpful to classify intervention strategies according to whether the environment is being managed or the child is being interacted with directly. Indirect strategies influence a child's behavior by modifying the environment to encourage exploration and discovery. They involve management of the surrounding space, materials, and equipment. Common indirect strategies include: eliminating distractions and providing structure for the impulsive child, establishing a balanced routine of active and quiet activities for the child who is prone to fatigue, using adapted seating equipment and power-operated toys for the child with physical disabilities, and providing novel play materials with familiar toys for the child who has difficulty adjusting to new experiences. Through these indirect strategies the adult "sets the stage" for the child to be productive and successful.

Direct intervention strategies focus on influencing the child's behavior through specific interaction with the adult. Familiar direct strategies involve: modeling appropriate behaviors for the child to imitate (including risk taking and coping with failure), prompting or cueing to facilitate generalization of skills across situations, giving accurate feedback for coping efforts, labeling emotions to help the child handle diverse feelings, and providing physical handling procedures to enable the child to produce coordinated movement. Timing is important when using direct strategies. If guidance is implemented too soon, the child receives a message of doubt and incompetence. In contrast, intervention that is delivered too late may allow the child to experience excessive frustration and revert to ineffective coping behaviors, such as the habitual use of temper tantrums.

In most cases, some combination of direct and indirect strategies are used to support adaptive functioning. Indirect approaches are particularly helpful in promoting the child's self-initiation. Sometimes very slight modification of an environmental factor can result in self-generated, purposeful behavior. A caution in the use of direct strategies is that they tend to place the child in a respondent role. Adults often assume a rather dominant, lead-taking posture when interacting with young children who are motorically disabled (Hanzlik, 1989; Rosenberg & Robinson, 1988). Their actions often are geared to eliciting responses from the infant, which they then reinforce. Overuse of this interactional pattern can result in passivity, inattention, or defensive reactions by the child.

Parents and professionals may need to alter their interactional style to achieve greater reciprocity. Coping and development are enriched when adults encourage and extend rather than prescribe and control the child's activity. Mahoney and his associates (1986) offer the following recommendations for helping adults become more contingent in their interactions: respond to the behaviors initiated by the child, achieve balanced turn-taking by each partner, and provide equal opportunities for control. Thus, the infant learns that intrinsically motivated behavior can generate mutually satisfying transactions.

The use of direct and indirect strategies to implement the intervention options is illustrated by the case of Jackie. She was a 20-month-old child with ataxic, disorganized movements who had difficulty completing self-initiated activities. At home, Jackie could not be left alone to play since she required adult direction to choose and complete activities. Her play consisted of frenetically pulling toys off the shelf in her room for brief visual inspection before throwing them on the floor to explore the next one. An observation of Jackie's home environment indicated that she was overwhelmed by the demand to choose a play object from an extensive array. The setting was modified to provide a more limited selection of three toys. At times her mother augmented this indirect approach by modeling different ways to play with a chosen toy. When appropriate, her mother complimented Jackie on playing with a specific toy for an extended period of time.

such an emotional state, spasticity is increased, undesired movement patterns are reinforced, and skilled performance is impeded. Likewise, the child's trust of the adult is undermined. The challenge is to grade the choice, intensity, and variety of environmental demands based on the child's changing ability to process and organize sensory information for an adaptive response (Greenspan & Greenspan, 1989).

Managing the infant who is intolerant of movement illustrates this point. Intervention involves the introduction of slow, carefully monitored movement experiences. In grading the intervention, it is generally easiest for the child to tolerate movement while being held in a maximally supported position as the adult moves (e.g., held in the arms as the adult gently steps in various directions). The next progression is to move the child while supported on the adult's lap (e.g., shifting the infant side to side by raising and lowering the adult's legs). Motion therefore is translated through the adult's body to the infant. Over time, the child may be able to accept direct facilitation of movement on a stable surface such as the floor or a tabletop. For the toddler, self-initiated movements may be tolerated more readily than those superimposed by an adult's handling.

Personalizing Sensory Experiences

Therapeutic and educational experiences need to be graded systematically to assure that the infant is not bombarded with sensory stimulation. Infants vary greatly in their capacity to control states of arousal, habituate to disturbing events, and organize their movements in response to the surroundings (Brazelton & Cramer, 1990; Greenspan, 1992). Some infants are hyporeactive and require rather active stimulation to become engaged. However, most infants with motor deficits are hyperreactive and readily overload with multisensory stimulation.

The child may respond to overstimulation by active withdrawal (arching, running away), turning off (staring into space, yawning), rejection (pushing away with the hands or feet), or signaling distress (crying, verbalizing). When a child is in

Proper Positioning

In the course of normal development, young children spontaneously and frequently move from one position to another as they change play activities, explore their surroundings, and interact with others. In contrast, children with motor deficits tend to maintain rather static postures for prolonged periods of time (e.g., supine lying or propped-up sitting). This restricted physical activity not only limits opportunities for participation in family life but also can undermine emotional growth. For instance, a child may be unduly frightened by a loud noise, because she is unable to turn to the sound for assurance that she is not personally threatened.

It is essential that parents and professionals identify together a variety of alternative positions that can be provided throughout the day and that are appropriate to the task at hand. Of particular concern is the need for positions that allow the child to be involved in social interactions with the family. It is helpful to review the progression of family and caregiving routines within a typical day and then determine how the child can be physically handled and positioned for optimal participation. What are safe and appropriate positions in the kitchen, dining room, bathroom, living area, or bedroom? Are any modifications or adapted equipment required to ensure proper positioning? Are there options that enable the child to play in an independent, self-initiated manner? What are the best alternatives for fostering parent-child communication and motorically vigorous play such as roughhousing?

The ability of the child with a motor deficit to be engaged can vary, depending on his or her physical position. Some children may regress in their behaviors when in a position requiring greater postural control. For example, a developmentally delayed infant who has poor balance may be able to demonstrate only primitive play schemes in a sitting position (e.g., holding, mouthing, and looking at objects). When lying supine, however, the same child may have adequate control of the arms for shaking, waving, and banging toys together. A baby may play best when lying supine, in an infant seat, or on the adult's lap. An older child may be most functional in supported or independent sitting. At any rate, the child should be well positioned before engaging in activity in order to attend, feel emotionally secure, and have the hands free. If balance is poor, the child may tend to tense the trunk and arms for stability, use the arms for support in a propping fashion, or resist reaching away from the body for fear of falling.

Depending on the child's age and physical status, various positions can be considered: supine lying, prone lying, side lying, floor sitting, short sitting (the typical posture in a chair), standing, and carrying positions. Keep in mind that during caregiving and intervention, positioning should not be static. Instead, the child and adult should move together in a dynamic fashion. When the infant is on the adult's lap, for instance, the child should be encouraged to move between these positions (and their innumerable combinations) during interaction. The professional literature describes in detail principles for physical handling and positioning as well as adaptations that may be required (Campbell, 1989; Scherzer & Tscharnuter, 1990; Williamson, 1987). We next present a few positions for illustrative purposes.

Playing on the floor is a natural aspect of parent-child interaction and early intervention activities. The child needs to have a number of floor sitting positions that allow for optimal functioning and social exchange. In general, postures such as ring sitting or cross-legged sitting, which are symmetrical and provide a wide base of support, are easiest to maintain. If necessary, external support can be provided by having the child use a floor seat or lean against a wall. In this manner the child is made posturally secure and is thus able to cope more effectively.

The child also needs to be well positioned in a regular chair, high chair, stroller, or wheelchair. This requires sitting equally on both buttocks with the hips well back into the chair. With the pelvis properly placed, the trunk is usually in erect alignment and the legs are positioned to provide a wide base of support. The feet should rest firmly on the floor or on a footrest; in this way a right angle (90 degrees of flexion) is maintained at the hip, knee, and ankle joints. Some modifications of this position and specially adapted equipment may be required for children with abnormal muscle tone or an imbalance of muscle action in the trunk.

Mobility

Independent mobility contributes both to the social and emotional well-being of children and to their physical development. The capacity to roll, crawl, and later walk expands their ability to explore the physical surroundings, to get needs met, to control the level of personal involvement in situations, and to release physical energy and psychological tension. Poor locomotor skills can restrict these coping-related functions.

A therapeutic priority is to teach the child a means of functional mobility as early as possible. For example, for many infants with spina bifida, physical therapy initially focuses on teaching a modified crawling pattern and the ability to scoot on the buttocks by use of the arms. Standing and ambulation with braces are then introduced at 12 to 18 months of age (Williamson, 1987). Special equipment may be purchased or adapted to supplement these efforts. In the prone position, the child may propel a scooter board by use of the arms. Tricycles may be modified with trunk supports and footstraps. In addition, various types of riding toys are available that can be activated by either the hands or the feet.

Mobility is an important factor that helps young children achieve separation and later individuation in their psychosocial development. Parents are used as a safe base from which the infant moves out into the world. Through varying means of locomotion, the young child experiments with autonomy by practicing leave-taking and reunion.

For children with physical disabilities, this natural process may be disrupted. The infant may not have mobility skills that allow practice in controlling experiences of separation. Therefore, parents must adapt caregiving so that the motor deficit does not unnecessarily interfere with emotional development. This is a particular challenge for parents who are highly protective or ambivalent in regard to their child's emerging independence. The child can be taught compensatory strategies such as visually checking-in with the parent. Another way to facilitate autonomy is to encourage the child to play independently in the presence of the caregiver. If the child is unable to follow the mother around the house while she is performing daily chores, the use of transitional objects may assist the child to manage the short periods of being alone (e.g., accepting a favorite teddy bear as a comforting substitute).

Play

Play is an essential area of concern for two primary reasons. Most significantly, it provides an opportunity for the child to organize thoughts, feelings, and skills within the context of discovering the new and making sense of the familiar. Play integrates the child's internal and external worlds. It is a spontaneous, voluntary involvement that is initiated and regulated by the child. The acts of play are performed for their own intrinsic reward. Since the child is in command, the contraints of reality can be ignored for free expression of emotions, fantasy, and imagination (Fewell & Kaminski, 1988).

Second, within professional practice, play can serve as a medium for remediation of specific physical, mental, or psychosocial deficits. The practitioner can create a play milieu that facilitates the acquisition of developmentally appropriate skills in an emotionally rich environment. Therapeutic and educational intervention that fails to appreciate this natural drive to play can result in distress, resistance, or boredom by the child. The incorporation of play activities into professional practice with children who are motorically challenged usually involves: adapting the size and type of play materials, modifying the position of the child and the placement of toys, adjusting handling procedures in a dynamic manner to enable the child to be engaged, and controlling the nature and degree of interpersonal interaction (Anderson, Hinojosa, & Strauch, 1987).

A key to facilitating motor control is for the child to be motivated through play experiences that build on emerging cognitive, social, and communicative skills. By providing activities that promote active engagement, the child can practice purposeful movement patterns within a personally gratifying context. The following brief vignettes illustrates ways that play was employed to expand the motor and coping competence of specific children with physical limitations.

• To encourage side-to-side rolling, the teacher sang to an 8-month-old infant with a motor delay while he was lying on his back. When the boy was attending to her voice and face, she leaned in one direction, which led him to turn his head and roll onto his side. She continued the singing as she leaned in the opposite direction and elicited a head turn and partial roll onto the other side. Thus, by building on the child's social and attending skills, the teacher sought to foster his motor development.
• Intervention was personalized for a toddler with poor sitting balance and a rather passive cop-

ing style. The little girl was prepositioned in a stable, floor-sitting position and encouraged to swipe overhead to pop bubbles or bat a balloon. These playful activities provided immediate contingent feedback regarding the success of her reaching efforts. As a result she demonstrated an unusual degree of persistence during the session. At the same time the activities stimulated the combined action of the abdominal and extensor muscles of the trunk, which is necessary for an erect sitting posture.

• To enhance imaginary play and rotation of the trunk, the therapist placed a preschool child with spastic diplegia astride a bolster in the sitting position. She initially invited him to reach down to the side with both hands to pick up large stuffed animals from the floor. (Reaching bilaterally to the side encourages rotation of the trunk rather than lateral bending, which is easier.) He would identify and pet each animal before placing it in the "zoo" on the other side. The therapist then commented that the animals may be hungry. This suggestion elicited a play sequence in which the child lifted imaginary vegetables from one side and reached across his body to feed the animals on the other side. Therefore, he experienced controlled rotation of the trunk toward both directions. If the child started to become physically tight during the session, the therapist gently rocked the bolster in order to decrease spasticity of the trunk and limbs.

• A girl, who had been prenatally exposed to drugs, disliked crawling and preferred to scoot on her buttocks in sitting. The parents were taught simple crawling games that the child found highly motivating. They would play hide-and-seek or "I'm going to catch you" to great squeals of delight. Thus, the child was learning to master a challenging motor skill while expanding her reciprocal social interaction.

The development of symbolic or dramatic play is particularly crucial for children with limited physical capabilities. It provides them with an opportunity to manifest thoughts and emotions that are more typically expressed through gross motor activities. Symbolic play provides a natural outlet for the expression of themes related to control, fear, anxiety, dependency, aggression, and loss. Some children with disabilities tend to stay at a rather concrete level of play, such as combining common objects together (e.g., putting cups on saucers, using a brush to comb the hair). Through modeling and elaboration, the practitioner or parent can extend the play content to a more representational and dramatic level. Initially intervention should emphasize helping the child pretend actions that involve the self and, later, to pretend with a doll or the adult. Over time, the child is assisted to use one object to represent another.

Imaginative play situations may incorporate the use of stuffed animals, puppets, and miniature people, with accompanying environments that represent the home, gas station, or school. Likewise, pretend play episodes may entail dressing up, going to the store, having a tea party, and playing house. The therapeutic benefit of play is demonstrated by the case of Max, a bright 4-year-old child with spina bifida, who was scheduled to have hip surgery. He was helped to prepare for the operation by playing "doctor and nurse" with his preschool peers during the preceding weeks. They dressed up in uniforms and surgical gowns, played with a toy doctor's kit, and gave each other "pills" and physical therapy. Gradually, as he rehearsed the coming event and practiced coping strategies, Max's fears seemed to diminish.

James was a child with spastic cerebral palsy who was having great difficulty adjusting to the arrival of a baby sister. His anger and resentment were demonstrated through irritability and a marked increase in muscle tone throughout his body. He was emotionally and physically becoming "tied up in knots." Occupational therapy during this period involved procedures to reduce his spasticity followed by opportunities to play in a doll corner. Through her handling and positioning, the therapist provided dynamic external support; this allowed James to express freely a diverse range of emotions and actions. His ambivalence regarding how to manage his current situation was dramatically evidenced by his play sequences. At times a baby doll would be smashed by He Man, eaten by a monster, and left in a trash can. At other times the doll would be hugged, comforted, and "made okay." It was very critical that the therapist avoid the tendency to tell James to "be nice" to the baby. Instead she provided an opportunity for him to learn to cope with his inner self (i.e., his mixed feelings).

450

Summary

This chapter has emphasized the importance of facilitating the motor control of young children within the context of expanding their adaptive behavior. Intervention options based on the coping process allows parents and practitioners to foster more effective transactions by changing demands, enhancing coping resources, and providing contingent feedback. Of particular relevance for children with motor deficits is the use of direct and indirect intervention strategies. These serve to personalize their sensory experiences, provide proper positioning and mobility, and capitalize on their love of play. In this way improvements in postural control and coordination are closely linked to meaningful functional outcomes.

REFERENCES

Anderson, J., Hinojosa, J., & Strauch, C. (1987). Integrating play in neurodevelopmental treatment. *American Journal of Occupational Therapy, 41,* 421–426.

Bandura, A. (1986). *Social foundations of thought and action: A social cognitive theory.* Englewood Cliffs, NJ: Prentice-Hall.

Barrera, M. E., & Vella, D. M. (1987). Disabled and nondisabled infants' interactions with their mothers. *American Journal of Occupational Therapy, 41,* 168–172.

Brazelton, T. B., & Cramer, B. G. (1990). *The earliest relationship: Parents, infants, and the drama of early attachment.* Reading, MA: Addison-Wesley.

Campbell, P. H. (1989). Posture and movement. In C. Tingey (Ed.), *Implementing early intervention* (pp. 189–208). Baltimore: Paul H. Brookes.

Carlton, S. B. (1988). *The relationship between temperament and coping in handicapped and nonhandicapped infants and young children.* Unpublished doctoral dissertation, Rutgers, The State University of New Jersey, New Brunswick.

Fewell, R. R., & Kaminski, R. (1988). Play skills development and instruction for young children with handicaps. In S. L. Odom & M. B. Karnes (Eds.), *Early intervention for infants and children with handicaps: An empirical base* (pp. 145–158). Baltimore: Paul H. Brookes.

Gilfoyle, E. M., Grady, A. P., & Moore, J. D. (1990). *Children adapt.* Thorofare, NJ: Charles B. Slack.

Greenspan, S. I. (1992). *Infancy and early childhood: The practice of clinical assessment and intervention with emotional and developmental challenges.* Madison, CT: International Universities Press.

Greenspan, S., & Greenspan, N. T. (1989). *The essential partnership.* New York: Viking Press.

Hanzlik, J. R. (1989). Interactions between mothers and their infants with developmental disabilities: Analysis and review. *Physical and Occupational Therapy in Pediatrics, 9,* 33–47.

Hildebrand, V. (1975). *Guiding young children.* New York: Macmillan.

Lazarus, R., & Folkman, S. (1984). *Stress, appraisal, and coping.* New York: Springer.

Mahoney, G., Powell, A., Finnegan, C., Fors, S., & Wood, S. (1986). The transactional intervention program. In D. Gentry, J. Olson, & M. Veltman (Eds.), *Individualizing for families.* Moscow: University of Idaho Press.

Meisels, S. J., & Shonkoff, J. P. (Eds.). (1990). *Handbook of early childhood intervention.* Cambridge: Cambridge University Press.

Murphy, L. B., & Moriarty, A. (1976). *Vulnerability, coping and growth.* New Haven, CT: Yale University Press.

Rosenberg, S. A., & Robinson, C. C. (1988). Interactions of parents with their young handicapped children. In S. L. Odom & M. B. Karnes (Eds.), *Early intervention for infants and children with handicaps* (pp. 159–177). Baltimore: Paul H. Brookes.

Sameroff, A. J., & Fiese, B. H. (1990). Transactional regulation and early intervention. In S. J. Meisels & J. P. Shonkoff (Eds.), *Handbook of early childhood intervention* (pp. 119–149). Cambridge: Cambridge University Press.

Scherzer, A. L., & Tscharnuter, I. (1990). *Early diagnosis and therapy in cerebral palsy.* New York: Marcel Dekker.

Stern, D. N. (1985). *The interpersonal world of the infant.* New York: Basic Books.

Turnbull, A. P., & Turnbull, H. R. (1990). *Families, professionals, and exceptionality: A special partnership* (2nd ed.). Columbus, OH: Merrill.

Werner, E. E. (1989). Children of the garden island. *Scientific American, 260,* 106–111.

Williamson, G. G. (Ed.). (1987). *Children with spina bifida: Early intervention and preschool programming.* Baltimore: Paul H. Brookes.

Williamson, G. G., Szczepanski, M., & Zeitlin, S. (1993). Coping frame of reference. In P. Kramer & J. Hinojosa (Eds.), *Frames of reference for pediatric occupational therapy* (pp. 395–436). Philadelphia: Williams & Wilkins.

Williamson, G. G., & Zeitlin, S. (1990). Assessment of coping and temperament: Contributions to adaptive functioning. In E. D. Gibbs & D. M. Teti (Eds.), *Interdisciplinary assessment of infants* (pp. 215–226). Baltimore: Paul H. Brookes.

Williamson, G. G., Zeitlin, S., & Szczepanski, M. (1989). Coping behavior: Implications for disabled infants and toddlers. *Infant Mental Health Journal, 10*, 3–13.

Zeitlin, S., & Williamson, G. G. (1990). Coping characteristics of disabled and nondisabled young children. *American Journal of Orthopsychiatry, 60*, 404–411.

Zeitlin, S., & Williamson, G. G. (1994). *Coping in young children: Early intervention practices to enhance adaptive behavior and resilience.* Baltimore: Paul H. Brookes.

Zeitlin, S., Williamson, G. G., & Szczepanski, M. (1988). *Early Coping Inventory.* Bensenville, IL: Scholastic Testing Service.

40 / Gender Identity Disorders of Childhood

Susan Coates and Sabrina Wolfe

Diagnostic Criteria

At present, gender identity disorder (GID) of childhood is one of a number of syndromes classified according to the content of the symptom without any consideration of etiology. As with eating disorders, a case could be made that GID should be reclassified among disorders of attachment in childhood that result in chronic anxiety reactions.

Table 40.1 presents the criteria for gender identity disorder from the fourth edition of the *Diagnostic and Statistical Manual of Mental Disorders* are (*DSM-IV* American Psychiatric Association [APA], 1994)

No reliable estimate exists for the incidence of gender identity disorder in the general population. Clinical experience indicates that it is an extremely rare syndrome. Boys are referred for evaluation more often than girls, with a ratio of observed cases of approximately 5 to 1 (Zucker & Green, 1992). We do not know whether this is the true prevalence of the disorder or whether it reflects greater social tolerance of cross-gender behavior in girls. No data exists suggesting variation in the frequency of the disorder by ethnicity or socioeconomic class.

Boys with GID have been studied far more extensively than girls; as a result the primary focus of this chapter, particularly around issues of etiology and treatment, will be on boys.

In the first extensive longitudinal study of boys with gender identity problems, Green (1987) found that by adolescence, roughly three quarters of 44 boys appeared to be developing a homosexual and/or bisexual sexual orientation and approximately one quarter of them were developing a heterosexual sexual orientation. Zucker (see Zucker & Bradley, 1995) combined the results for several other outcome studies and found that of 41 boys studied, 66% had an atypical outcome; 51% were homosexual, 12% were transsexual, 2% were transvestitic, and 34% were heterosexual. More recently, Zucker and Bradley (1995) have reported that in a follow-up study of a sample of 45 boys, roughly 30 to 40% appeared to be on a bisexual or homosexual course while roughly 60% appeared to be on a heterosexual courses; in addition, 20% were intensely gender dysphoric and appeared to be on a transsexual course.

At our current stage of knowledge we are unable to predict future sexual orientation in any individual child. The pathways to both heterosexuality and to homosexuality are likely to be very complex, involving multiple biological and experiential factors interacting at many levels of development.

Adult transsexual men retrospectively report acute gender dysphoria dating back as far as they can remember; nonetheless, it has yet to be established how many of these men would have merited a true diagnosis of the childhood disorder. A majority of adult homosexual men report a sig-

TABLE 40.1

Diagnostic Criteria for Gender Identity Disorder

A. A strong and persistent cross-gender identification (not merely a desire for any perceived cultural advantages of being the other sex).

In children, the disturbance is manifested by four (or more) of the following:

(1)   repeatedly stated desire to be, or insistence that he or she is, the other sex

(2)   in boys, preference for cross-dressing or simulating female attire; in girls, insistence on wearing only stereotypical masculine clothing

(3)   strong and persistent preferences for cross-sex roles in make-believe play or persistent fantasies of being the other sex

(4)   intense desire to participate in the stereotypical games and pastimes of the other sex

(5)   strong preference for playmates of the other sex. . . .

B. Persistent discomfort with his or her sex or sense of inappropriateness in the gender role of that sex.

In children, manifested by any of the following: in boys, assertion that his penis or testes are disgusting or will disappear or assertion that it would be better not to have a penis, or aversion toward rough-and-tumble play and rejection of male stereotypical toys, games, and activities; in girls, rejection of urinating in a sitting position, assertion that she has or will grow a penis, or assertion that she does not want to grow breasts or menstruate, or marked aversion toward normative feminine clothing. . . .

C. The disturbance is not concurrent with a physical intersex condition.

D. The disturbance causes clinically significant distress or impairment in social, occupational, or other important areas of functioning.

NOTE: From the *Diagnostic and Statistical Manual of Mental Disorders* (4th ed., pp. 537–538), American Psychiatric Association, 1994, Washington, DC: Author. Copyright 1994 by American Psychiatric Association. Reprinted with permission.

nificant degree of gender nonconforming interests and behavior in childhood, particularly the avoidance of rough-and-tumble play and an interest in solitary activities and in artistic pursuits (Bell, Weinberg, & Hammersmith, 1981; Saghir & Robins, 1973). Based on currently available data, only a very small minority (the upper limit is about 15%) would have met the criteria for childhood GID.

The long-range social adaptation of boys with GID has not been systematically studied yet. Clinical studies of adolescents with extremely "feminine behavior" have found a high incidence of peer relation difficulties, depression, and suicidal behavior (Bradley et al., 1984). In a study of suicidal behavior in adults, Harry (1983) found that among men, high levels of cross-gender behavior in their childhood was associated with suicidal behavior in adulthood. This obtained whether the adults were homosexual or heterosexual. This area of study has received very little attention; it is important that it become a focus of future research.

Neither prospective nor retrospective studies have yet to be conducted on girls with childhood gender identity problems.

Clinical Presentation

GID is a readily recognized syndrome characterized by persistent cross-gender fantasies and behavior. The child intensely dislikes being the gender he or she is and actively wishes to be the opposite gender. The disorder is deeply rooted in the child's early attachment relationships; usually it is first observed between the ages of 2 to 3 when the child begins to develop an autonomous sense of self as separate from the mother.

Once established, the cross-gender fantasies and behavior become embedded in the child's coping strategies and self-image. It is not uncommon for young children without clinical problems to display passing cross-gender fantasies and behavior (Linday, 1994; Sandberg, Meyer-Bahlburg, Ehrhardt, & Yager, 1993). The issue is one of degree and the role that this complex of factors comes to play in the child's adaptive functioning. What is notable about the cross-gender fantasy and behavior in GID is their *pervasiveness, persistence, and duration;* often they take on a compulsivelike quality. Once established, these elements will evolve and develop as the child does, becoming progressively more autonomous from the forces that set them in motion and moving inexorably to become an internalized psychological structure.

The manifestations of the disorder will vary depending on the child's age. The 2- to 3-year-old boy will show a prolonged and marked preference for his mother's clothing; he will lack the flexible interest seen in typical 2-year-olds who enjoy dressing up in everyone's clothes, Mommy's as well as Daddy's, sister's as well as brother's. The cross-gender fantasy also will incorporate the mother's activities, and the boy will engage in such behaviors as pretending to put on jewelry and makeup like Mommy. Moreover, his cross-gender interest will have an urgent and pressing quality to it that lacks the joy and and easy spontaneity typical of children's play. In addition, he will have a strong preference for playing with girls rather than boys. He will prefer activities such as doll play, often with a special interest in Barbie, and his favorite stories are likely to be ones with female heroines, such as "Cinderella," "The Little Mermaid," "Snow White," or Dorothy from *The Wizard of Oz.* By the time the boy is 3, he is likely to imitate heroines while watching videotapes and will often demand to watch them over and over again. In time, the capacity to imitate feminine gestures, attitudes, and voices may well become remarkable. A majority of boys with GID will at some time express anatomical dysphoria, voicing a wish to be rid of their penis, attempting to hide it between their legs, or, in extreme cases, even threatening to mutilate themselves.

In girls, the manifestations of GID are generally the mirror opposite of those that appear in boys. That is, the little girl will prefer to imitate Daddy or big brother. She will insist on wearing pants on all occasions. She may say that she has a penis or will grow one when she gets older, and she will have a marked preference for the company and activities of boys rather than girls. Some girls with GID will urinate only standing up; they may further insist that they be allowed to use the boy's bathroom in school. Indeed if they are not permitted to do so they may refuse to go to the bathroom until they return home. Some girls demand that they be addressed with a boy's name or adopt a gender-neutral name, such as using their initials only.

In evaluating girls, it is critical to distinguish girls with GID from tomboys. Girls with GID are, by definition, intensely unhappy that they are girls. Although tomboys prefer to wear pants and are usually athletic, they do not show extreme rigidity in this preference and do not have the dysphoria and intense dislike of being a girl that is characteristic of girls with GID (Green, Williams, & Goodman, 1982). Girls with GID, by contrast, have an extreme aversion to wearing culturally defined feminine clothing in any situation whatsoever, and, if required to wear a dress on a special occasion often will react with panic and refuse to attend the function at all. In addition, they either act out or verbalize intense discomfort with their sexual anatomy.

Cognitive Developmental Level

Between the ages of 2 and 4, experience, and peer socialization as well as cognitive level will all affect the presentation of the disorder. It is not uncommon, for example, for a 2-year-old boy with the disorder to twine a scarf around his neck, use a towel to pretend he is wearing a skirt, and announce: "Look at me, Mommy, I'm a girl." At this age, fantasy and reality are not well differentiated, and the child may truly believe that he has changed his gender by changing his clothes and/or activities. By the age of 4, the child will almost never believe he really is a girl; instead, the cross-gender fantasy is expressed in terms of wishing to be a girl or pretending that he is a girl.

The evolution of the clinical presentation during these years can be viewed against a backdrop of the developing general cognitive capacity to understand the concept of gender. By 12 months, infants have tacit categories for gender. By 16 to 20 months, as language emerges, they have labels for adult males and females. By 28 months, they have labels both for male and female peers and for themselves (Fagot, 1993). It is at this age, when the child can label self and peers correctly, that gender first becomes a salient characteristic for children—and it immediately becomes an important part of their self-concept as well as a primary organizer of their behavior. Once children can label their own gender and that of their peers, they show a marked increase in their preference for play with same-sex peers and for stereotypically same-sex activities (Fagot, Leinbach, & Hagan, 1986). In girls there is also a marked decrease in aggression (Fagot, 1993). Children typically experience their own gender as an integral part of their self-concept (with all the narcissistic investment that this implies). In cases of GID, this process of consolidating a basic, positive, affectively charged sense of gender identity is derailed, and the child is unable to consolidate a positive sense of his or her gender identity.

Moreover, even by age 4 or 5, the further cognitive capacities needed to understand that gender is unchanging are not necessarily in place. Many children may exhibit confusion when asked whether a change of activities will lead to a change of gender (gender constancy) or whether they will always be or have always been the same gender (gender stability). This confusion appears to arise from several sources, in part because the children have not yet acquired the general cognitive developmental structures needed for this understanding and in part because they do not yet have the domain-specific knowledge that genitals are the defining characteristic of gender categorization. Indeed, by age 5, less than half of all children understand the defining role of the genitals in establishing one's gender (Bem, 1989). There is a degree of normal variation in the age at which children come to understand gender constancy, gender stability, and the fact that the genitals are definers of gender. Not until about age 6 do most children understand this categorization with any constancy and depth. The issue for GID is that the child's immature cognitive development can be brought into the service of solving pressing psychodynamic needs. Zucker et al. (1993) have found that children referred for problems with gender identity have significantly more cognitive confusion about gender than either normal children or clinical controls.

The period during which cognitive understanding of gender develops overlaps with another important developmental period, when children's newly established locomotive capacity thrusts them into new challenges around issues of separation and attachment. How best to conceptualize this phase is a matter of current debate. From the perspective of traditional psychoanalytic theory,

newly acquired locomotive capacity triggers the onset of the rapprochement crisis, a stormy but putatively necessary substage of separation individuation (Mahler, Pine & Bergman, 1975). In this conception, outwardly observable ambitendency both toward and away from the mother is said to reflect a developmentally inevitable ambivalence on the part of children about experiencing themselves as separate. Recent research by Lyons-Ruth (1991) has shown that at this stage, ambivalent behavior toward the mother is not a universal phenomenon. Moreover, she argues that "longitudinal evidence unequivocally supports the position that the unambivalent seeking of comfort or contact associated with secure attachment during the rapprochement period is related to more adaptive social behaviors as a toddler" (p. 11) and not the reverse, as separation-individuation theory implies. However we ultimately conceptualize this period, it seems to be a time of increased vulnerability for self-development in a relational context. The nature of the vulnerability is under active investigation and is important for an increasing understanding of why childhood gender identity disorders emerge primarily in this limited time frame.

By the time children are referred for evaluation, the clinical presentation of the disorder may be further complicated by their discerning that their cross-gender fantasies have become upsetting to parents. Accordingly, children may deny such wishes on direct questioning. However, when asked indirectly about interests, or about why it is better to be one gender or another, the children will readily give evidence of the depth of their preoccupation and of their dysphoria with the gender they actually are.

Onset of GID in Boys

In some cases the disorder appears to have a gradual onset; in others, most often between the ages of 2 to 3, the onset is rapid with the cross-gender behavior and patterns becoming consolidated in a period of weeks to a few months. Most cases, however, do not present for evaluation until the child is about 4 or 5. Often the parent has been told by a teacher or pediatrician that this is a passing phase that the child will grow out of. It may take a year or two for the parent to realize that this is by no means a passing phase and that the child is not going to grow out of it. Clinical observation also suggests that the disorder typically emerges in the context of severe family stress; it often involves trauma to the mother that results in her becoming depressed, anxious, and emotionally inaccessible to the child. In some instances the mother remembers (or, at any rate, reports) the traumatic event only after intervention has begun and not during the initial evaluation.

In very rare instances, usually involving pathological mourning, a mother will deliberately cross-dress a son, give him a girl's name, and treat him as if he were a girl. An example from literature is the poet Rainer Maria Rilke, whose mother had lost a daughter before he was born. She repeatedly played games with him in which she gave him a girl's name, and she dressed him as a girl until the age of 5 when he was sent off to school (Kleinbard, 1993; Rilke, 1949).

PRODROMAL PHASES OF GID

When dealing with very young toddlers, it is important to be sensitive to the prodromal stages of GID. A precocious 1½-year-old may already have a persistent fascination with his mother's clothes and with female heroines in books and videos and may already be persistently imitating them in his play. Even at this very early age, a careful diagnostic interview can uncover the child's use of cross-gender fantasies to manage anxiety. These early manifestations of the disorder usually occur in the context of serious marital difficulties or in situations of serious direct trauma to the child, such as a life-threatening illness and/or major surgery. In the former instances, the child often will actively rebuff the father's attempts to play and to make social contact. In these situations, the child is either expressing mother's rage at the father or believes that contact with the father will result in loss of mother's emotional availability.

No hard and fast rules can be given for evaluating the prodromal phases of the disorder at the earliest ages, since the behavior will vary according to the child's precocity and the prevailing family climate. Indeed, prior to the age of 2, a child may be well on his or her way along the path to a GID yet not meet the full diagnostic criteria. The clinician must proceed on the basis of assessing the intensity of the child's cross-gender fantasy and, of equal importance, the dynamic and defensive uses to which it is being put. All this, moreover, in the context of simultaneously assessing family dynamics. Even at this early age, the need for prompt intervention is great.

Differential Diagnosis

THE WISH TO BE BOTH GENDERS

As the developmental summary given earlier suggests, prior to roughly 2½ to 3½, when children learn to categorize correctly by gender, all children experience themselves as able to do and be all things male and female. Thus, little boys may believe that they can give birth and still be boys, little girls that they may grow a penis while yet remaining girls. Once the child gives up this illusion, there is a loss involved. Some toddlers whose narcissism is especially brittle may have trouble negotiating this period and will show behavioral signs that they still harbor some of the old hopes of being both genders; indeed, they may well express rage and envy at whichever parent or sibling seems to them to have dashed their hopes. (See Fast, 1984, for further discussion.) This is not GID—in GID the child wants to be the opposite gender, not both. If, however, the child's distress at making this developmental transition is excessive, further evaluation is warranted.

GENDER NONCONFORMITY

A different phenomenon involving cross-gender interests sometimes is observed in children who have a well-established and positive sense of their own gender identity. A little boy may take up an interest in cooking, in growing flowers, or in play-acting and may not enjoy rough-and-tumble play. A little girl may discover that she is a better athlete than most of the boys her age and begin to enjoy exercising her skills accordingly. This kind of behavior constitutes gender nonconformity and is not accompanied by a dislike of one's gender. It is not a pathological phenomenon and, indeed, may well be indicative of a greater degree of ego flexibility and health.

TRANSIENT CROSS-GENDER WISHES AND INTERESTS

Occasionally, transitory reactions of this kind may be seen in children whose gender identity is reasonably well established but who show a sudden upsurge in cross-gender interests and behavior in response to a familial crisis. Although these behaviors may be intense, they rarely meet the full criteria for GID. Typically, in boys, the nature of the stress involves some catastrophic loss that has had a significant emotional impact on the mother, making her emotionally inaccessible. The loss may be the death of a family member, or a loss of status or health suffered by the mother or the father. This may arise in the face of severe physical illness or severe financial loss that seriously troubles the mother and the entire family system. Or the mother may have a traumatic experience such as being mugged or raped that makes her particularly fearful of and/or furious at men. In effect, the boy is indicating that he has either been cued by the mother or else has developed the fantasy on his own that his maleness might be dangerous or emotionally unacceptable either to the mother or to himself, and he responds by switching to being a girl. In these cases, when the family crisis subsides, the behavior usually disappears and does not alter the child's basic gender identity. Were the behavior to continue for more than a few months (usually 3 months is a marker of outside limits), family intervention is almost always warranted.

CHILDREN WITH INTERSEX CONDITIONS

Where a true intersex condition exists—that is, where there is genital ambiguity—it may give rise to confusion about gender but rarely to GID (Meyer-Bahlburg, 1991). This is a different syndrome. However, intersex children who have significant confusion about their gender should receive help.

Predisposing Factors

Despite extensive investigation, to date no direct evidence has been found that either genetic or hormonal influences are at work in GID. Accordingly, unless a genital abnormality such as a hypospadias is present, no endocrine or other physical workup is warranted. Indirect evidence has arisen from animal research and from spontaneously occurring endocrine disorders that suggests that genes and hormones do not directly affect gender identity but do affect aspects of stereotypical gender role behavior, such as rough-and-tumble play (Ehrhardt & Meyer-Bahlburg, 1981).

Boys with GID avoid rough-and-tumble play, are typically shy and inhibited in new environments, and are slow to warm up in strange situations. Once they do make a connection to people, their attachments are often intense. That any or all of these and other temperamental characteristics might be etiologically related to specific, identifiable prenatal hormonal influences, with their attendant impact on brain structuralization, must, for the moment, remain an intriguing theoretical possibility.

From a behavioral standpoint, boys with GID appear to be a subgroup of what Kagan (1989) has identified as "inhibited" children. Such children, who constitute approximately 15% of the normal population, are characterized by very high reactivity and high rates of central nervous system arousal. Behavioral inhibition can be seen as a way of coping with this physical endowment; where other boys will be bold and aggressive, these "inhibited" children tend to hold back and to be anxious until they acclimatize themselves to new situations. Such children also may have difficulty managing their own aggression, which can escalate quickly past the threshold where they can tolerate it and/or express it in socially acceptable ways. Such children need support from adults in managing their anxiety, particularly in the face of transitions. They are unusually reliant on caregivers to provide them with clues as to whether a situation is safe or not and to help them to regulate their anxiety. In our experience, the majority of boys with GID display this reactive inhibited temperamental style (Coates, Hahn-Burke, & Wolfe, 1994).

A different way of conceptualizing the contribution of temperament is in terms of an affective diathesis (Bradley, 1985, 1990). The high rates of anxiety disorders and depression in their parents suggest that these children may be especially vulnerable to separation anxiety and depression. Over half of all children with GID have sufficient symptoms to warrant a separate diagnosis of separation anxiety disorder (Coates & Person, 1985; Lowry & Zucker, 1991), and over half have symptoms of depression as well (Coates & Person, 1985).

These two alternative conceptualizations of the nature of temperamental predisposition are essentially complementary rather than mutually exclusive. On both bases, moreover, it can be expected that children so endowed would show greater than average need for an attachment relationship. And, indeed, this is what is seen clinically. Albeit concerned about separation and slow to warm up, these children tend to form especially intense though often anxious connections to available adults (Coates & Wolfe, 1995). They will scan the interviewer's face intently and pick up the slightest emotional cues readily. In a study using the Ainsworth separation paradigm, 73% of boys with GID were insecurely attached to their mothers (Goldberg, in press).

Beyond the need for, and readiness to engage in, an attachment bond, these boys also seem to have special sensory sensitivities generally (Coates et al., 1994; Stoller, 1968). They are unusually reactive to odors and color and are sometimes responsive to sound and texture. Not only do these boys appear more alive to the sensory world, but they are also more vulnerable to it. Thus, one child will gag if the family car passes a garbage truck, and another will refuse to wear a shirt unless the tag is taken out. Such a boy's typical aversion to rough-and-tumble play may be accounted for in part by his inhibited and reactive temperament, special sensory sensitivities, and strong empathic attunement to others, which can in turn interfere with the normal aggressiveness.

As with their specific behavioral characteristics, far less is known about any constitutional predispositions to GID in girls. Like boys, girls with GID tend to have sensitive, reactive temperaments, but unlike boys with GID, who tend to be behaviorally inhibited, girls with GID are often oppositional and aggressive. They often appear to be bold and are often highly invested in athletic activities. Zucker and Bradley (reported in Zucker & Green, 1993) found that girls with GID had a higher activity level and overall indicators of extroversion than did both siblings and clinical and normal controls. Despite their extroversion, our clinical impression is that these girls have as high an anxiety level as do the boys, but, because of their temperaments, they manage their anxiety with different coping strategies. Since girls with GID are only now beginning to be studied systematically, the mechanisms whereby constitution and early experience interact to produce the disorder are not yet fully known. Clinical experience suggests, however, that theirs is a different pathway to the disorder from that of boys.

Parental Psychopathology and Parental Tolerance in Boys with GID

Research has shown that in addition to constitutional predisposition, two additional risk factors are almost invariably at work: inadvertent parental reinforcement for the cross-gender behavior and significant parental psychopathology.

In his original study, Green (1974) identified a lack of discouragement of cross-gender behavior by the primary caregiver as a necessary factor for the disorder to develop. Since that time, all observers who have studied the syndrome agree that initial parental encouragement of the child's cross-gender behavior is almost always present. Not infrequently, mothers will smile at or at least be more attentive to the child when he is involved in cross-gender behavior. Often mothers will view the behavior as an indicator that the child is unusually sensitive, or artistically gifted, or as evidence that the child is not destructive, as they typically believe rough-and-tumble boys to be.

Fathers, as well, often view their son's behavior as an indicator of artistic giftedness.

Parents are usually unaware of the significance of the symptoms or of the anxiety that the child is binding with cross-gender behaviors, because in many cases the child's suffering is going on silently and is being hidden from them. Even for clinicians, children's presentation can be very confusing, because these children often are using manic defenses to manage underlying feelings of being unheard or unreal or of being anxious and depressed. When first evaluated, the children are often "on," and are intense and entertaining, although this presentation often lacks real vitality and authenticity. In many cases, either through the use of projective testing early in the assessment process or in direct discussions treatment when children feel that it is safe to show their underlying feelings, the anxiety and depression become more obvious. In play therapy and often during the assessment, a lack of vitality can be observed directly in the joyless, repetitive, unelaborated play of many boys with GID.

By age 4, in addition to a psychiatric interview, projective testing is almost always useful in understanding the children's inner experience. Projective testing that focuses on a sequence analysis of content can bring into relief the associations that trigger cross-gender fantasies, thus highlighting the conflicts that are most central in fueling these fantasies. Typically, in boys with GID, these associations involve issues of loss, annihilation, and aggression.

Mothers and fathers often see the child's cross-gender behavior as simply an indicator of his creativity. Indeed many of these boys are extremely talented and have considerable potential for creativity (Coates, Freedman & Wolfe, 1991; Stoller, 1968). What actually is observed clinically, however, is that before the child and family have received psychological help, the boy's creativity is being exhausted and constricted in an enactment that is essentially anxiety-driven and joyless. Indeed, one of the major goals of psychotherapy is to restore the child's creativity.

The fact of universal initial parental encouragement by both mothers and fathers for the cross-gender behavior has led some researchers to intervene with behavioral techniques. Both positive and negative reinforcement strategies have been tried. Research indicates, however, that such intervention only reduces the specific target behaviors, and clinical experience suggests strongly that the net effect is to drive the cross-gender fantasy underground. Beyond this, such interventions of necessity do not address the child's underlying anxiety or the ongoing parental psychopathology. Nor do they address the derailment of the child-mother and child-father attachment bonds that were involved in the onset of the disorder and that usually are making their own contribution to perpetuating it, or the important dynamic and psychic-structural uses in the service of which the child currently may be employing the behavior.

Parental psychopathology is an extremely important risk factor in this disorder. Studies of the families of boys have revealed a very high incidence of long-standing psychopathology in the parents, including, most notably, depression, anxiety disorder, and problems with substance abuse (Bradley, 1985; Marantz & Coates, 1991; Mitchell, 1991; Wolfe, 1990). Indeed, in every systematic study to date and regardless of the kind of depression inventory used, maternal depression has emerged as a major and consistent factor. Furthermore, lately evidence has emerged (Zucker & Bradley, 1995) that maternal depression, anxiety, and hostility were particularly high during the child's first 3 years of life. Significant paternal psychopathology also has emerged as a prominent risk factor (Wolfe, 1990); substance abuse and difficulties with impulse control are frequently encountered, as are depression and anxiety.

Operating between long-standing psychopathology and witting or unwitting encouragement of the cross-gender behavior are a host of other parental attitudes also found associated with the disorder. Mothers of boys with gender identity disorder are more prone than mothers of boys who have not been referred for psychiatric difficulties (clinically unreferred) to exhibit attitudes and child-rearing patterns that interfere with the child's capacity to function as separate person in his own right. By their own self-report, many of these mothers are more dependent on and less differentiated from their sons; likewise, they have greater difficulty in separating from their sons and are more likely to be disapproving of their sons' relationships with others (Marantz & Coates, 1991). In addition, again by their own self-report, they are more likely to employ authoritarian and intrusive forms of control as compared to mothers of clinically unreferred boys (Marantz & Coates, 1991; Mitchell, 1991).

Clinical experience suggests, in addition, that mothers of boys with GID interfere with the developing autonomy of these youngsters by failing to foster and empower their emotional tie to the father. Research has demonstrated that the degree to which a father is involved with his children is determined primarily by the mother's influence. (See Lamb & Oppenheim, 1989, for a review.) A mother who talks to a child about his father when he is away and enjoys the time that the father and son spend together communicates to her son that he can have a relationship with his father without jeopardizing his emotional tie to her. In effect, this "vitalizes" the son's relationship to the father (Atkins, 1981, 1984). The majority of mothers of boys with GID have significant difficulty in supporting this essential part of the child's development. The child often interprets the failure to foster this development as "Mommy does not like men or is not interested in men; if I like one or become like one, I will lose Mommy."

The fathers of boys with GID contribute to the difficulty in developing a relationship with their sons by being overly sensitive to rejection. If their initial attempt to engage their son is not successful, they readily give up and withdraw rather than persevere until they can find a means of emotionally connecting to their son. This in turn makes them unavailable as a model for identification. Since fathers play a major role in the socialization of aggression in boys (Herzog, 1982), the father's inaccessibility can interfere with the boy developing strategies for coping with aggression.

Maternal anxiety often focuses on typical masculine assertiveness and love of rough-and-tumble activities. Mothers of boys with GID are often fearful that their sons will get hurt and may prohibit all forms of roughhousing (Coates & Zucker, 1988; Green, 1987). They overreact to minor physical illnesses. Many are proud that their boy is a sensitive, well-behaved "mother's helper," that he is "gentle" and "angelic," not aggressive or "bullying like other boys" (Coates, 1990). Mothers of boys with GID are often on a hair trigger about aggression and confuse and conflate healthy rough-and-tumble play with destructiveness (Coates, 1990).

Clinical experience indicates that the fathers consistently fail to provide a counterbalance to the maternal prohibitions and injunctions. Sometimes the failure is due to straightforward emotional inaccessibility; other times explosive, aggressive behavior on the part of the father makes the child fear for his own and his mother's safety and makes him fearful that by becoming male, he will become a person who is out of control and destructive, and who thereby could jeopardize his tie to his mother, his primary caregiver.

In short, in these families, long-standing parental psychopathology, most especially in the regulation of affect, gives rise to and becomes embedded in attitudes and practices that operate to discourage stereotypically assertive masculine play and to reward stereotypically feminine play. Clinically, these attitudes are inextricably linked to parental psychopathology; which, in turn, often is linked to the parent's previous life experiences as they are represented and intertwined with current fantasies relating to gender categories, although the specifics vary from case to case. The mothers of boys with GID, and most often the fathers, as well, have reorganized and embedded into the domain of gender categorization their own unresolved lifelong conflicts about abandonment, loss, autonomy, and the management of aggression.

Intercurrent Trauma and the Derailment of Attachment

It might seem from the foregoing discussion that the intersection of parental psychopathology and tolerance for the cross-gender behaviors together with the boy's temperamental predisposition might be sufficient to produce the disorder. Both clinical experience and systematic research indicates, however, that it is rarely this simple. The child's cross-gender fantasy is not simply a passive response to the parental milieu; on the contrary, it represents an active attempt by the child to forge a creative solution to what would otherwise be experienced as a catastrophic and massively disorganizing situation.

Clinical experience suggests that the context in which GID arises most often is the loss of the emotional availability of the mother. This is usually due to depression, a situation that is otherwise known to have deep and far-reaching impact on the child's development (Emde, 1980, 1983). In most cases, when it occurs, this loss represents a change from what had previously been a tolerable or, in some cases even a satisfactory mother-infant relationship. Most often mothers of boys with GID report that the first 6 to 8 months of infancy went relatively smoothly and, indeed, constituted an especially rewarding period from the mother's point of view. It seems that at this early age, the child's high capacity for bonding typically offsets whatever difficulties an unusually low threshold for arousal might create, and the child's behavior falls within the range that the mother finds acceptable in terms of her own fantasies and wishes connected to the child. Despite the temperamental vulnerabilities of these children, the majority of mothers seems to adapt to their sensitivities in the first 6 months of life and describe them as easy babies.

Sooner or later the child begins to separate from the mother by losing interest in breast-feeding, for example, or by beginning to walk and becoming able to explore the environment on his own. Once this happens, matters often become more problematic. Clinical observation suggests that many mothers of boys with GID have difficulty remaining affectively available to their child during this phase; where this situation does not precipitate the onset of a separation anxiety disorder outright, it makes the vulnerable child anxiously attached. In about three quarters of the cases, traumatic events within the family further significantly complicate the situation. These events precipitate massive anxiety and clinically significant depression in the mother, rendering her suddenly and profoundly emotionally inaccessible to her child. This in turn derails that mother-son attachment bond. Clinical observation suggests that in a majority of cases, the consolidation of the cross-gender behavior occurs in the immediate wake of this traumatic experience.

The effect of the trauma on the mother is almost invariably compounded both by her own preexisting psychopathology and by the father's inability and/or unwillingness to intervene effective either in helping her to cope or in taking over her function as the primary caregiver. The effect on a boy who is temperamentally sensitive to loss is overwhelming. The abrupt loss of the primary caregiver to her own depression may be likened psychologically to a confrontation with what A. Green (1986) describes as the "dead mother," a mother who is present but "not there" and who is therefore gone but cannot be mourned. The son of a depressed mother loses not only the mother's emotional availability but also her reliability, her capacity to comfort him, her affect attunement, and her availability to help him make meaning out of his moment-to-moment experience. In young children, such a loss is catastrophic and threatens to destablize not only the children's sense of security but also their developing sense of self. The children will search for any means within their capacity to restore this emotional tie if at all possible.

In assessing etiology, the clinician should keep in mind that a multitude of risk factors operating together are necessary to produce this disorder. It is important to be on the alert for additional contributing causes, since some of these may emerge only during the course of a prolonged assessment or well after treatment has begun. In general, cascading anxiety, depression, and trauma in the family will intersect with the child's temperament, which is itself perhaps exacerbated by the trauma, at a specific developmental period before the disorder emerges. However, there are multiple pathways to childhood GID, and not all of them have been detailed in the literature. While we can distinguish nonspecific factors, such as maternal depression, which serve to increase the child's anxiety and desperation, and specific factors, such as maternal encouragement of the cross-gender behavior, which orient the child toward the specific "solution" of GID, a comprehensive, fully integrated etiological model adequate to the description of all cases has yet to be achieved.

Psychopathology in Children

About 60% of boys with GID meet the criteria for a *DSM-III-R* separation anxiety disorder, and most of the remaining third have significant symptoms of separation anxiety (Coates & Person, 1985; Zucker, Bradley & Sullivan, in press). In addition, over 50% score in the clinical range on the depression scale of the Child Behavior Checklist (Achenbach & Edelbrock, 1983), and one third have suicidal ideation (Coates & Person, 1985). Boys with GID have greater overall psychopathology than boys who have not been referred for psychiatric evaluation, and their overall degree of psychopathology is similar to other psychiatrically referred children (Bates, Skilbeck, Smith, & Bentler, 1974, 1975; Bradley, Doering, Zucker, Finegan, & Gonda, 1980; Coates & Person, 1985; Zucker, 1985, 1990b). Using Achenbach and Edelbrock's (1983) two factor analysis of qualitative difference in the kinds of psychopathology assessed by the Child Behavior Checklist, Zucker (1990b) has shown that boys with GID fall into the overcontrolled and internalizing subgroup as opposed to the externalizing subgroup.

Although systematic studies of psychological functioning in girls have not yet been published, Zucker (Zucker & Bradley, 1995) using the Child Behavior Checklist finds comparable levels of psychopathology in girls with GID to that of boys with GID. In contrast to boys, girls show a mixture of internalizing and externalizing behavioral problems.

Psychodynamics in Boys with GID

Although it is impossible to get a perfectly clear window on the mind of a 2-/3-year-old, what appears to happen in essence is that, triggered by the mother's emotional inaccessibility, the boy experiences severe separation anxiety. He attempts to manage this anxiety via a fantasy solution in which he imagines himself as "being Mommy" rather than "being with Mommy." In effect, he substitutes an identification for a relationship. Imitation of a lost or absent person is a familiar psychological mechanism. We have speculated that at this young developmental age, where imitation is a major mode of thought, it is all the more apt to be used defensively where the child encounters circumstances requiring an extreme solution. And to restate, these children, have a constitutionally heightened need for attachment, which already may have been heightened further by previous

trauma, these children truly do experience the loss of the mother to her own depression as a catastrophe.

Individual talents at mimicry frequently are found in these children. Many mothers describe their sons as having had unusual imitative capacities before the onset of the cross-gender symptoms. The child may use this capacity in part in an attempt to understand an experience that he cannot assimilate or otherwise metabolize. As Emch (1944) suggests, acting like a person or "becoming" the person allows a child to predict what the person will do, so as not to be taken off guard and hurt by that person.

The child's cross-gender behavior serves multiple functions, both intrapsychic and interpersonal. On an interpersonal level, the child altruistically sacrifices his authentic development by transforming himself into an "other" that he imagines will help restore his mother. We have speculated that one of the important perpetuating factors in boyhood GID is that the boy's cross-gender behavior succeeds, at least momentarily, in engaging and enlivening the "dead mother"—she may find it cute or funny—which the boy may experience as partly restoring the lost mother-child emotional relationship (Coates & Wolfe, 1995). In this psychological situation, the mother's positive response would serve as a particularly powerful external reinforcer to the boy's cross-gender behavior.

The child's cross-gender fantasy often interlocks with the mother's internal world in various and very precise ways. By becoming a girl, he may, for example, be offering himself as a replacement for a lost female child or other deceased relative who had not been adequately mourned. Or he may be reassuring her that he is not aggressive, abusive, or abandoning, an array of qualities that he intuits his mother equates with maleness. Clinical experience repeatedly has shown that the child's cross-gender fantasy most often constitutes a "solution," one that works for the mother as well as for the child.

No matter how creative and reparative a solution the cross-gender fantasy may be, it still does not successfully bind the child's anxiety. The continuing dysphoria is often poignantly expressed. One 3-year-old boy said: "I hate myself. I don't want to be me. I want to be someone else. I want to be a girl." In some cases, the profound dysphoria may be manifest in self-destructiveness, including preoccupations with suicide and, in rare instances, attempts to mutilate one's own genitals.

The boy's suffering can be obscured by a maniclike presentation that initially can be confusing to the clinician. For example, during his evaluation, one little boy drew a very elaborate and colorful picture of a lady that included a brightly colored rainbow. After he had entered therapy and continued to draw similar pictures, he was asked what was at the end of his rainbow. He responded, "A big black pit filled with dead bodies and bones." It is not uncommon for boys with GID to use manic defenses to cover dysphoric affect.

Some children express a sense of loneliness and intense psychological suffering directly. They may volunteer that "Nobody likes me" or "I wish I was dead" or "Why did God make me a boy?" As treatment proceeds, and some of their creativity is freed up, the children often are capable of producing remarkably moving and detailed accounts of their suffering. One boy, reported elsewhere (Coates, Friedman, & Wolfe, 1991) marshaled his artistic talents to produce a series of drawings entitled "My Story." Utilizing *Guernica*-like figures, he portrayed the terror and psychological pain of being transformed into a woman against one's will. Another boy told a story in which a boy is informed by a monster that the only way to make contact with what he described as his "dead" mother was to turn into her.

Once the cross-gender fantasy is established, it may successfully reduce traumatic levels of anxiety. With this, it becomes readily available for use in less traumatic situations where the child has not yet developed effective coping strategies. These include brief periods of maternal loss (such as a hospitalization) and maternal emotional unavailability, separations and transitions, and occasions that evoke the child's aggression. The use of the fantasy to manage separation, for example, can be seen readily in therapy at the end of individual sessions. Often when we announce that the session will soon be over, the child will begin expressing or dramatizing cross-gender fantasies. Over the course of therapy, one little boy had begun to spend sessions making models of boys out of clay; at the end of a session, however, he would smash up the boys and make a girl before he would leave.

Once the child invents his "solution," the increasing autonomy that it gives him from his family also serves to perpetuate the defense. Moreover, the family dynamics and the additional complication of increasing social ostracism by male peers (preventing normative peer socialization of gender) will all interact and further lock in this solution.

The cost to the child is that he continues to develop an inauthentic self, a self based primarily on the needs of others (Winnicott, 1954). This impairs his capacity to feel real and to feel recognized, known, and nurtured by others. The failure to restore an authentic self in turn leads to further alienation, often resulting in depression and sometimes suicidal preoccupations. The poet Rilke, whose mother wanted him to be a girl, suffered lifelong from a false self and had feelings that he was unreal, lifeless, and that his center was unheard and unknown (Kleinbard, 1993). In his notebooks, which were largely autobiographical, he uses images such as living behind a mask and being a vacant spot (Rilke, 1949).

In girls, the constellation of dynamic factors appears to be different, as does the intersection with temperament. (Where a girl of a sensitive, inhibited temperament is traumatized by sudden maternal withdrawal, clinical experience suggests that unless other factors come into play, she will respond not with cross-gender fantasies but with the development of a separation anxiety disorder or an exaggerated hyperfemininity.)

Systematic research on girls with GID is only just beginning, but clinical experience suggests that the combination of predisposing familial factors that are found clinically most often in girls appears to be somewhat different. Girls with GID perceive the female role as devalued and disidentify with their mothers while identifying with males whom they alternately perceive as aggressive and as nurturant. In general, girls with GID appear to equate changing their gender with their emotional, and sometimes even physical, survival. By the school-age years, girls with GID will manifest significant levels of psychopathology and behavioral disturbance.

The extremely low incidence of GID in both girls and in boys indicates that a multiplicity of risk factors must be present simultaneously and operate with a rare severity to produce the disorder. In attempting to understand the disorder in both boys and girls, it must be borne constantly in mind that no matter how readily GID may fit in with prevailing family dynamics and interpersonal realities, it still represents an intrapsychic solution indicative of severe anxiety about separation, aggression, and annihilation in the child.

Initial Assessment

Assessment of childhood GID must focus on evaluating the symptom in the context of the family. This must include an understanding of the meaning and function of the cross-gender disorder for the child intrapsychically as well as an appreciation of the role that it plays in maintaining his attachment relationships. No single set of psychodynamic factors has yet been identified for the families of these boys, nor it is likely that any ever will be. Accordingly, the clinician has to assess the family from the point of view of several systems, while keeping in mind the potentially variable role the child will play in each, depending on his age, developmental needs, and psychodynamics. In addition to the two primary parental relationships—each parent with the child—the clinician also must assess the relationship between the father and the mother. In many cases it is critical to have the nanny be a part of the evaluation because, in our experience, nannies often have a surprisingly significant role in perpetuating the GID. Teacher consultation is often critical, as well. Many nursery school teachers have been found to encourage a child's cross-gender behavior.

In the course of an interview with the parents, it is relatively easy to establish the diagnosis of GID on the basis of symptoms. From a therapeutic perspective, the critical task is to understand the function of the symptom in the family context and its role in the child's intrapsychic organization. The clinician must take a careful developmental history that focuses on the family context, the parental relationship at the time of the emergence of the cross-gender behavior, and the child's temperament. An evaluation of the sense of self, gender identity, and cognitive understanding of

gender are essential components of a comprehensive psychiatric interview with the child.

The following questions can be integrated into either a semistructured interview or a play therapy interview with children referred for gender identity problems. Weissman et al. (1987) have found that, in general, children are far more able to report the details of their disorders than their parents. Our clinical observations suggest that this too is the case with children with GID; usually they are able to express their confusion and dysphoria about their gender identity either directly or in the metaphor of play. Despite the fact that parents have brought their child to be evaluated for GID, they are often unaware of the full extent of the child's preoccupations and dysphoria.

Gender identity is a subdivision of self-concept and overall identity and, as such, its assessment should be included in any comprehensive evaluation of a child presenting with significant emotional difficulties. Gender identity is evaluated most effectively in the context of an exploration of the self-concept and of overall identifications. The following are suggested questions for a semistructured interview. The wording of the questions is geared to the cognitive developmental level of children ages 3 to 6. Clinicians may find it appropriate to alter wording to match the developmental level or family background of a particular child. Also, clinicians should select questions that are most appropriate for the case they are evaluating; given a particular family structure, some questions may not be indicated.

The questions under self-concept and identifications are useful in comprehensive psychiatric evaluations of any child. Those under cognitive understanding of gender and feelings about one's gender are useful when the general interview suggests that the child may have problems in the domain of gender identification.

SELF-CONCEPT

1. Tell me some things that you like about yourself.
2. Do you like yourself just the way you are?
3. Do other kids like you?
4. What are some of the things that other kids like about you?
5. What kinds of things do you sometimes do that get other kids a little mad at you?

6. If you could change anything you wanted to about yourself, what would you change?
7. If you could be anybody else in the world for a day who would you like to be?
8. What would you like to be when you grow up?

IDENTIFICATIONS

9. What are your favorite books?
10. Who is your favorite character? (Ask for each book.)
11. What do you especially like about him/her? (Ask for each character in each book.)
12. What are your favorite videos and movies or TV shows?
13. Who is your favorite character? (Ask for each video, movie, TV show.)
14. What do you especially like about him/her? (Ask for each character in each video, movie, TV show.)
15. What did you dress up as last Halloween?
16. What do you want to dress up as this Halloween?

COGNITIVE UNDERSTANDING OF GENDER (FOR AGES 2½ TO ABOUT 6)

These questions should be asked if the previous interview suggests that the child has significant cross-gender identifications or if parents have reported persistent cross-gender preoccupations and/or behaviors. The examiner can say to the child: Now I'm going to ask you some questions about boy and girl stuff.

17. Are you a boy or a girl?
18. How can you tell the difference between a boy or a girl?
19. If you had long hair and wore a dress, would you turn into a girl?
20. If you played girls' games, would you turn into a girl?
21. When you were a little baby, were you a little boy or a little girl?
22. Were you ever a little girl?
23. When you grow up will you be a mommy or a daddy?

FEELINGS ABOUT ONE'S GENDER

24. Do you think it's better to be a girl or a boy? Why?

25. Tell me some good things about being a boy. Tell me one more.
26. Tell me some not so good things about being a boy? Tell me one more.
27. Tell me some good things about being a girl. Tell me one more.
28. Tell me some not so good things about being a girl. Tell me one more.
29. Is it more fun to go to boys' or girls' birthday parties? Why?

If the child says it is better to be a girl and shows a clear cross-gender preference to the above questions, then ask the following questions:

30. When you were in your mom's tummy, did she want you to be a girl or a boy?
31. When you were in your mom's tummy, did your dad want you to be a boy or a girl?
32. If you had a magic wand, would you like to change yourself into a girl?[1]

Zucker et al. (1993) have factor-analyzed a similar interview and found that both on a cognitive and affective factor, children with GID have more deviant responses than controls.

If the child is denying cross-gender fantasies and behavior, and parents have reported clinically significant current cross-gender behavior, it is sometimes useful to ask questions in the past tense; this can be effective because children are sometimes more able to acknowledge wishes and fantasies at a greater distance. For example, one can ask "Did you ever wish that you were a girl?" or "When you were littler, would you have wanted to change yourself into a girl if you had a magic wand?"

The psychiatric interview of the child also should focus on the child's management of affect with particular focus on depression and the tactics for coping with anger and rage. Children with GID typically struggle with dysphoric affect, are preoccupied with issues of loss, and have difficulties dealing with their own and other's aggression.

Projective psychological testing often is useful in providing information that cannot be elicited easily in a psychiatric interview. For example, a careful analysis of the sequence of a child's responses on a projective measure can bring into relief the content, or associations to the content, that trigger cross-gender fantasies. This in turn provides a fuller picture of the specific meaning of the cross-gender fantasies to an individual child.

The clinician therefore must carefully piece together the multiple interpersonal and intrapsychic factors that, when integrated together, perpetuate the disorder. Each of these multiple factors will be important to address in treatment.

Intervention Strategies

As a multifaceted and multifactorial disorder (Meyer-Bahlburg, 1985), GID of childhood requires a complex and intensive treatment strategy. A sound intervention approach will include both a psychodynamic and an educational component, and will simultaneously address the needs of the parents and those of the child. The ordinary developmental process by which a child normally comes to achieve a sense of gender identity is remarkably robust. For it to become derailed, as it is in GID, a whole host of risk factors must be present simultaneously with each making its own contribution to the condition. And just as it takes a concatenation of risk factors operating together to create and maintain the disorder, effective treatment requires flexible intervention that draws upon techniques and theory found to be most effective in addressing each type of factor.

GID constitutes a psychiatric disturbance requiring rapid intervention. During the evaluation process, attempts to educate the parents about the complex meanings of the behavior are always warranted and, indeed are usually very helpful in motivating them for treatment. Timely intervention is important; the longer the disorder endures, the more intractable it becomes. Once the disorder has become firmly entrenched for more than 2 or 3 years, it is progressively more difficult and much more time-consuming to ameliorate.

INTERVENTION WITH PARENTS

In the toddler, treatment of gender identity disorder must begin first and foremost with efforts at restoring the derailed attachment relationships.

Untreated psychopathology in the parents therefore must be addressed as soon as possible. Most especially, this means identifying and treating current depression and reaction to trauma in the mother and depression and substance abuse in the father. In regard to long-standing character psychopathology in the parents, as soon as it is practical, parents' should be referred for psychotherapy.

In working with the mother, the clinician must understand that the child will not readily engage his core issues in his own treatment until he has reason to believe that his mother is being taken care of and that his own psychotherapy will not adversely affect her. In sum, the child needs to understand that everyone in the family is getting the help needed to make things better. Accordingly, the clinician has to establish a baseline contract about treatment that makes it explicit that everyone, the child and the mother and the father, will each get the help they require.

Addressing the mother's current level of depression is, of course, crucial. Beyond this, it is critical that work with the mother focus on issues of unresolved trauma in her own life that have become organized around gender concepts. For example, on the basis of her previous life experience, a mother may have come to equate masculinity with either aggression or emotional abandonment. It is very common for mothers of boys with GID to confuse healthy rough-and-tumble feistiness with destructive aggression. Conversely, these mothers often construe indications that their boys are sensitive and/or creative as evidence that their sons are not like other boys, whom they believe their sons must be protected from. These mothers must be helped to differentiate between their children's temperament and their own anxious preoccupations.

It is also vitally important for the therapist to help the mother understand that the child's disorder has arisen in the context of a derailment of the attachment relationship with her and that, furthermore, through the cross-gender fantasies and enactments, the child is trying to restore and repair the tie to the mother. This understanding should provide the basis for forming an alliance with the mother that allows her to help the child progress without becoming overly defensive herself about her past contribution to the disorder and without becoming worried that she is losing a vital ally in her own struggles against depression and loss.

Over the course of prolonged treatment, the clinician will have the opportunity to observe repeated instances where the momentary return or upsurge in the child's cross-gender behaviors will occur contemporaneously with fresh instances of withdrawal on the mother's part, or of increased anxiety in the mother about aggression, or of increased inaccessibility or aggression in the father. Addressing these instances as they occur is of the greatest therapeutic import—at once for the child and the mother and father—but this cannot happen until a certain amount of fundamental repair of the primary attachment relationship has already been accomplished.

Occasionally, inexperienced clinicians conclude that the boy's principal need is to establish a relationship with the father. On the basis of this assessment they make the mistake of inadvertently excluding the mothers from treatment or of not addressing the mother's specific needs. This sort of mistaken strategy usually enrages the mother, often increases separation anxiety in the child, and may induce the child to act out the mother's rage at the father. In all these ways it can further exacerbate the child's GID.

In working with the fathers, their own psychopathology needs to be addressed as soon as it is practical to do so. Problems in managing their affect, including anxiety and anger, need to be addressed. The fathers, too, often are attempting to repair multigenerational problems that have remained unresolved. Fathers often feel responsible for their sons' GID and ashamed of their ineffectiveness in being unable to help their sons. It is essential that fathers not be excluded from treatment, whether due to the mother's wishes, the son's rejecting behavior, their own diffidence, or the therapist's failure to establish a working alliance with them. Clinical experience indicates that fathers can be readily engaged in meaningful ways in their children's treatment and often are highly motivated to help their sons. Thus, fathers can make major contributions to clinical improvement, provided their own concerns, anxieties, and perplexities are addressed directly.

A crucial first step in engaging fathers frequently entails coming to terms with their exclusion from the mother-child bond. This requires an understanding of both their role and the role of their wives. Often fathers report that their exclusion happened very early on, while the child was still an infant, and long before symptoms appeared. They also describe how their efforts to establish a relationship with the child, efforts that not infrequently were awkward, had been met with rebuff even to the extreme of father being pushed away. The fathers reacted oversensitively and contributed to the problem by taking the rejection very personally and then withdrawing. Overly sensitive fathers rarely see their son's behavior as indicative of a developmental or interpersonal problem that can be solved.

It is important that mothers be helped to realize that they play an essential role in empowering and vitalizing the relationship between father and son. Mothers must be helped to find a way to become supportive while enjoying their child's forming a relationship with the father if that is to happen. Among the reasons that sons may reject the father is that they are being used by the mother to express her rage at the father.

In some cases sons reject the father because the father is experienced as too rough. These fathers usually have had difficulty adapting their behavior to their sons' sensitive temperament. At times, fathers initiate behaviors such as roughhousing with an intensity that frightens their son and escalates the boy's anxiety. Often they need direct help in learning how to make contact with their shy, inhibited, and often anxious son. Again, clinical experience shows that if they are given the support and guidance they need to develop the skills that will lead to successful engagement with their child, fathers typically become major allies in the treatment process.

Parents of boys with GID rarely have developed an effective parenting subsystem in their relationship. In helping the parents develop this system, the issues of establishing appropriate generational boundaries and of setting appropriate limits on the child's behavior will invariably have to be addressed. The clinician does well to assume, as an initial premise, that the parents know almost nothing about how to set limits. Instead they permissively allow a behavior to escalate until it exceeds their own capacity to tolerate it, at which point they respond with anger and rage. This untenable degree of permissiveness occurs in nearly all domains, including generational boundaries, individual boundaries, aggression, and cross-gender behavior. The possibility of sheer parental ignorance needs to be borne in mind constantly. Where ignorance is the issue, a psychoeducational approach can bring about rapid changes; when this approach does not work, then often psychodynamics must be addressed directly. In either case, parents need and profit from detailed, concrete instruction and discussion of various strategies for setting limits.

In working with the parents, the clinician also should understand that often they are bringing multigenerational issues and unresolved traumas into the therapeutic situation. Not only have the parents frequently been traumatized in their own childhood, but their own parents before them often have experienced severe traumas. Not infrequently, the child's symptoms represent an attempt to repair the damage suffered by more than one generation of his or her family. By the same token, clinical experience has found that when the parents become aware of the child's suffering and can relate it affectively to their "ghosts in the nursery" (Fraiberg, Anderson, & Shapiro, 1975), that awareness then becomes a powerful factor operating on the side of the treatment. It is essential that the family's unresolved conflict around issues of loss or abuse be worked through. To the degree that these issues are fueling the parents' emotional inaccessibility and/or reinforcement of the child's cross-gender behavior, failure to resolve them will have an ongoing negative impact on the child's recovery.

PSYCHOEDUCATION OF THE PARENTS OF BOYS

At the outset, parents need to be educated that GID is neither benign nor something that the child will grow out of spontaneously. They need to be made aware that it will endure, that it will lead to significantly compromised peer relations, and that it often masks intense suffering in the child.

Not infrequently, parents express the concern that the child's behavior indicates that he will grow up to be homosexual and, in the context of that concern, they also fear that the child subsequently will become infected with AIDS. Others will recognize the child's suffering but will fear that helping the child may interfere with a pos-

sible developmental process. We help parents to recognize that our concern is *not* with a child's future sexual orientation, which we feel we cannot predict or even identify when working with children as young as preschoolers. Our concern is with their current distress about their own gender, their unhappiness with themselves, and with their multiple anxieties: about their emotional connection to their parents, about separation, and about the management of aggressive feelings.

We explain to parents that childhood GID and homosexuality are not the same thing. We emphasize that in no individual case is it possible to predict a boy's future sexual orientation based on the presence of childhood GID. Nor do we yet understand the mediating mechanisms between childhood GID and adult sexual orientation. We communicate our belief that, in general, homosexual and heterosexual adult sexual orientation results from a complex interplay of biological and environmental factors operating at multiple levels of development that are not yet well enough understood. We inform parents that no evidence currently exists suggesting that psychotherapy can affect or alter later sexual orientation, but that there is evidence that psychotherapy can reduce gender dysphoria (Zucker & Bradley, 1995).

As the treatment proceeds, the educational function of the therapist evolves. Most parents, for example, are unaware of how they subtly reinforce the disorder, often by being more attentive to the child when the youngster is engaged in cross-gender behavior. Although the parents may show a developing intellectual understanding of how the cross-gender fantasy is compromising the child's creativity and growth, in inattentive moments they still express pleasure in the child's cross-gender enactments.

Similarly, many parents from upper-middle- and upper-class backgrounds come equipped with an ideology that holds that androgyny, however conceived, is to be preferred to traditional gender roles. Exploration of the basis of this ideology often reveals that the parent would like to encourage the son to be a nurturant boy. Often it is helpful for parents to see that taking care of a puppy is more likely to foster nurturance in their son than having Barbie dolls. It is also helpful to explain to parents that initially all children adopt highly stereotyped conceptions of gender, on the basis of their cognitive immaturity, and that they will outgrow them in time unless the family's functioning is itself highly stereotypic.

Education about temperament is also an issue. Fathers need help in learning how to connect with their shy child who tends to be inhibited in novel situations. Mothers need help in not being overprotective and thereby increasing the child's shy behavior. They need to learn how to help the child take risks in small enough doses, so that the child can master anxiety and find successful ways of living with his temperament and even of enjoying it.

Parents often need to be taught how to help their child develop male peer relationships. Often they have no idea who the child plays with in school or how to set up a play date. Parents need to be encouraged to talk to teachers about which same-sex children the child naturally gravitates to or with which children the child might share overlapping interests. It is essential to help parents to set up several play dates a week with peers. This is especially important for boys, since by age 3 to 4, peers play a major role in socializing gender (Fagot, 1993).

Also, as treatment proceeds, parents often need continuing education about the ordinary patterns of development. The toddler's quest for autonomy, like his attempts to widen his circle of relationships, may be experienced as rejection and abandonment. As development proceeds, the vital role of peer socialization is another facet of life not appreciated by many of the mothers; often they are overprotective and feel that their sons are special and not like other boys, and they fear, indeed that the roughhousing of typical boys might be damaging to their sons. From the child's need to establish his own sense of separateness to his need for reasonable and effective limits, there is much about child rearing that these parents will need to learn. The clinician should bear in mind that in important domains, very often neither parent has been exposed to effective parenting models.

INTERVENTION STRATEGIES WITH BOYS

The goal of treatment is neither the suppression of the cross-gender behavior nor its encouragement. The child requires understanding of this behavior, not approval or disapproval. Not infrequently, clinicians inadvertently reinforce the child's cross-gender behavior by focusing too much attention on it, or by providing a playroom with overly enticing stereotypically feminine toys (such as numerous Barbie dolls or wigs and female costumes for cross-dressing). The clinician should not accede to the child's wish that he or she provide additional props for the cross-gender fantasy. Doing so may inadvertently support enactment rather than help the child to begin to represent his conflicts symbolically.

The ultimate goal of the treatment is to provide the child with new coping skills with which to manage his impulses, his anxieties, and his temperament, so that he may draw from a more flexible range of solutions without needing to resort compulsively to the cross-gender enactments. The issues that need to be addressed in any individual child differ from one case to the next and also differ in any given case over the course of treatment, depending on the multiple functions that the cross-gender behavior and fantasies serve. Nor should the therapist restrict his or her interest only to those issues that appear to underlie the cross-gender enactments. In terms of overall levels of symtomatology, children with gender identity disorder are indistinguishable from other children who are referred for psychological problems. Accordingly, the therapist should deal with whatever other psychological problems the child presents with, whether separation anxiety, sleep difficulties, bedwetting, attention deficit disorder, or the like, regardless of their phenomenological or etiological distance from the issue of gender. Incidentally, it should be noted that although almost all of these children are nonpsychotic, a small subgroup will manifest transient psychotic transferences during the treatment.

Two issues are almost invariably salient for these children, although dynamically, their relative weight vis-à-vis one another will vary from one child to the next. The first of these is anxiety about loss and separation. The beginnings and endings of the therapy session provide an immediate occasion for addressing these transference issues, as do the therapist's coming and goings for such things as vacations. As the treatment progresses, and the child comes to have confidence in the stability of the therapeutic relationship, the opportunity for examining the impact of separation will tend to follow more closely events outside the treatment, including, most notably, the oscillations in the mother's and/or father's current emotional availability to the child. Also to be noted is that as the child begins to trust the therapist, he will begin to share some of his inner world, including feelings of abandonment, panic, and psychic disintegration.

The other issue that invariably is salient is aggression: Usually it is a central if not the pivotal issue in the treatment. The intensity of the child's anxiety about aggression derives from multiple sources. Both intrapsychic and interpersonal issues need to be addressed. Often these children have had little opportunity to learn to sublimate their aggressive impulses, with the result that they have not developed internal structures for managing their aggression. This is frequently the case in families where the father has been inaccessible or in families where the parents have had difficulties in managing their own aggression. In such cases, the therapist will be called upon to provide these structures. Yet another major source of anxiety about aggression stems from the fact that much of the child's own anger has been projected onto the environment. Insight into the dynamics of this mechanism and reintegration of these basic impulses is also an essential goal of treatment.

More generally, the child will need help in learning to identify a whole range of feelings in relation to the contexts that evoke them. The therapist can help the older child develop an observing ego with regard to the cross-gender enactments, that is, to begin to see which feelings trigger their employment. Doing this with a toddler is not feasible, owing to the child's cognitive immaturity and difficulty in containing affects. However, it is possible to intuit the underlying feelings via empathic understanding and to encourage the child to explore these indirectly in play. Many preschoolers with GID do not yet have a narrative sense of self and need therapy to help them begin to create stories in which feelings and sequences of events can be related meaningfully.

It is essential that the therapist help the boy to develop relationships with male peers his age by helping the parents to plan weekly play dates with boys who are temperamentally compatible and have overlapping interests. The boy's sense of self and sense of gender are strongly influenced by his ability to have relationships with same-sex peers,

and the inability to do so can have devastating effects on self-esteem.

The child typically brings important assets to the treatment: his capacity to form a productive working alliance, his imaginative capacity, and his potential for creativity. The goal of the treatment is to help free up the child's own capacities, to help him out of compliance and joylessness, and to consolidate a more authentic self.

PSYCHOEDUCATION WITH THE CHILD

Ordinarily education is not considered an important mode of intervention with a toddler. However, clinical experience with children with gender identity disorder suggests that it is a valuable adjunct to play therapy. These children sometimes profit enormously from learning about their own temperament and acquiring effective strategies for coping with it. For example, a child who is fearful of entering a room full of peers at a birthday party can be encouraged to wait and watch at the doorway until he feels ready to go in. A slightly older child, anticipating the same situation, can be encouraged to remember how he coped with a similar situation in the past. Among the most valuable interventions along these lines is to help the child find and interact with peers whose temperament more closely resembles his own. Many of these boys are frankly frightened by the aggressiveness of roughneck boys, but are able to form friendships with boys who have more artistic interests or other interests that do not involve rough and tumble play. By addressing the issue of temperament directly with the child in a way that he can understand, the therapist is not only communicating a basic understanding of the child's multiple social (and familial) predicaments but is also helping the child not to blame himself for characteristics that are out of his voluntary control. Moreover, therapeutic intervention can help the boy to begin to appreciate the strengths and value of his own temperament (such as the positive aspects of sensory sensitivities, or his sensitivity to others' feelings, or his artistic interests) and not just its more vulnerable aspect. Notably, particularly once the boy's sense of security is better established, remarkable capacities for empathy and for creative expression are quite common.

As the child becomes older, an additional area of education that becomes progressively more important is to help him understand the impact of his cross-gender enactment on his peers. While a child still may need to cling to various aspects of his cross-gender fantasy he can be encouraged to choose among them, or to delay their employment, so as not to put off his friends. Little boys are frankly rejecting of cross-gender behavior and little girls merely tolerate it (Fagot, 1993), yet this fact of social life may initially be lost on a boy who has the disorder. One little boy age 4½ was making good progress in forming a close friendship with another boy of similar temperament. However, he needed help in understanding why his friend withdrew and did not want him to play with him after he continually insisted on playing the role of females in fantasy play.

Summary

For a child's positive sense of his own gender to miscarry to the degree that it becomes a source of continuing dysphoria, a great deal must have gone wrong in his life. In a majority of cases, severe stress in the family coupled with preexisting maternal and paternal psychopathology have had a cascading effect upon the family system and upon a temperamentally at-risk child. Successful intervention needs to be proportionally as intensive and extended as the multiple factors that, working together, both brought the disorder into being and are currently perpetuating it. Treatment must be tailored to the specifics of each case; there are multiple pathways to the disorder, and the clinician must be sensitive to these different variations in planning specific treatment strategies.

NOTE

1. Questions 17 to 23 are taken from or are variations of questions from Slaby and Frey's (1975) gender constancy interview. Questions 30 and 31 are from the Zucker et al. (1993) gender identity interview for children.

REFERENCES

Achenbach, T. M., & Edelbrock, C. S. (1983). *Manual for the Child Behavior Checklist and Revised Child Behavior Profile.* Burlington VT: University Associates in Psychiatry.

American Psychiatric Association. (1994). *Diagnostic and statistical manual of mental disorders* (4th ed.). Washington, DC: Author.

Atkins, R. N. (1981). Finding one's father: The mother's contribution to early father representation. *Journal of the American Academy of Psychoanalysis, 9,* 539–559.

Atkins, R. N. (1984). Transitive vitalization and its impact on father representation. *Contemporary Psychoanalysis, 20,* 663–675.

Bates, J. E., Skilbeck, W. M., Smith, K. V. R., & Bentler, P. M. (1974). Gender role abnormalities, An analysis of clinical ratings. *Journal of Abnormal Child Psychology, 2,* 1–15.

Bates, J. E., Skilbeck, W. M., Smith, K. V. R., & Bentler, P. M. (1975). Intervention with families of gender-disturbed boys. *American Journal of Orthopsychiatry, 45,* 150–157.

Bell, A. P., Weinberg, M. S., & Hammersmith, S. K. (1981). *Sexual preference: Its development in men and women.* Bloomington: Indiana University Press.

Bem, S. L. (1989). Genital knowledge and gender constancy in preschool children. *Child Development, 60,* 649–662.

Bradley, S. J. (1985). Gender disorders in childhood: A formulation. In B. W. Steiner (Ed.), *Gender dysphoria: Development, research, management* (pp. 175–188). New York: Plenum Press.

Bradley, S. J. (1990). Affect regulation and psychopathology: Bridging the mind-body gap. *Canadian Journal of Psychiatry, 35,* 540–546.

Bradley, S. J., Doering, R. W., Zucker, K. J., Finegan, J. K., & Gonda, G. M. (1980). Assessment of the gender-disturbed child: A comparison to sibling and psychiatric controls. In J. Samson (Ed.), *Childhood and sexuality* (pp. 554–568). Montreal: Editions Etudes Vivantes.

Bradley, S. J., & Zucker, K. J. (1984, October). *Gender-dysphoric adolescents: Presenting and developmental characteristics.* Paper presented at the joint meeting of the American Academy of Child Psychiatry and the Canadian Academy of Child Psychiatry, Toronto, ON.

Coates, S. (1990). The ontogenesis of boyhood gender identity disorder. *Journal of the American Academy of Psychoanalysis, 18* (3), 414–438.

Coates, S. (1992). The etiology of boyhood gender identity disorder: An integrative model. In J. W. Barron, M. N. Eagle, & D. L. Wolitzky. (Eds.), *Interface of psychoanalysis and psychology* (pp. 245–265). Washington, DC: American Psychological Association.

Coates, S., Friedman, R. C., & Wolfe, S. (1991). The etiology of boyhood gender identity disorder: A model for integrating psychodynamics, temperament and development. *Psychoanalytic Dialogues: A Journal of Relational Perspectives, 1,* 341–383.

Coates, S., Hahn-Burke, S., & Wolfe, S. (1994, June). *Do boys with gender identity disorder have a shy, inhibited temperament?* Coates/GID/Greenspan Paper presented at the International Academy for Sex Research., in Edinburgh, Scotland.

Coates, S. W., Hahn-Burke, S., & Wolfe, S. M. (1994, October). *Do boys with gender identity disorder have a shy, inhibited temperament?* Poster presented at the Annual Meeting of the American Academy of Child and Adolescent Psychiatry, New York.

Coates, S. W., Hahn-Burke, S., Wolfe, S. M., Shindledecker, R., & Nirenberg, O. (1994, October). *Sensory reactivities in boys with gender identity disorder: A comparison with matched controls.* Poster presented at the Annual Meeting of the American Academy of Child and Adolescent Psychiatry, New York.

Coates, S., & Person, E. S. (1985). Extreme boyhood femininity: Isolated finding or pervasive disorder? *Journal of the American Academy of Child Psychiatry, 24,* 702–709.

Coates, S., & Wolfe, S. (1995). Gender identity disorder in boys: The interface of constitution and early experience. *Psychoanalytic Inquiry, 15,* 6–38.

Coates, S., & Zucker, K. (1988). Assessment of gender identity disorders in children. In C. Kestenbaum & D. T. Williams (Eds.), *Handbook of clinical assessment of children and adolescents* (pp. 893–914). New York: New York University Press.

Ehrhardt, A. A., & Meyer-Bahlburg, H. F. L. (1981). Effects of prenatal sex hormones on gender-related behavior. *Science, 211,* 1312–1318.

Emch, M. (1944). On the "need to know" as related to identification and acting out. *International Journal of Psycho-analysis, 25,* 13–19.

Emde, R. N. (1980). Emotional availability: A reciprocal reward system for infants and parents with implications for prevention of psychosocial disorders. In P. M. Taylor (Ed.), *Parent-infant relationships* (pp. 87–115). Orlando, FL: Grune & Stratton.

Emde, R. N. (1983). The prerepresentational self and its affective core. *Psychoanalytic Study of the Child, 38,* 165–192.

Fagot, B. I. (1993, June). *Gender role development in early childhood: Environmental input, internal con-*struction. Paper presented at the International Academy of Sex Research, Pacific Grove, CA.

Fagot, B. I., & Leinbach, M. D., & Hagan, R. (1986). Gender labeling and the adoption of sex-typed behaviors. *Developmental Psychology, 22,* 440–443.

Fast, I. (1984). *Gender identity: A differentiation model.* Hillsdale, NJ: Analytic Press.

Fraiberg, S., Anderson, E., & Shapiro, V. (1975). Ghosts in the nursery. *Journal of the American Academy of Child Psychiatry, 14,* 387–421.

Goldberg, S. (In press). Attachment and childhood behavior problems in normal, at risk, and clinical samples. In L. R. Atkinson & K. J. Zucker (Eds.), *Attachment and psychopathology.* New York: Guilford Press.

Green, A. (1986). The dead mother. In A. Green (Ed.), *On private madness* (pp. 142–173). Madison, CT: International Universities Press.

Green, R. (1974). *Sexual identity conflicts in children and adults.* Baltimore: Penguin Books.

Green, R. (1987). The *"sissy boy syndrome" and the development of homosexuality.* New Haven, CT: Yale University Press.

Green, R., Williams, K., & Goodman, M. (1982). Ninety-nine "tomboys" and "nontomboys": Behavioral contrasts and demographic similarities. *Archives of Sexual Behavior, 11,* 247–266.

Harry, J. (1983). Parasuicide, gender, and gender deviance. *Journal of Health and Social Behavior, 24,* 350–361.

Herzog, J. M. (1982). On affect hunger: The father's role in the modulation of aggressive drive and fantasy. In S. H. Cath, A. K. Gurwitt, & J. M. Ross (Eds.), *Father and child: Developmental and clinical perspectives* (pp. 163–174). Boston: Little, Brown.

Kagan, J. (1989). *Unstable ideas: Temperament, cognition and self.* Cambridge, MA: Harvard University Press.

Kleinbard, D. (1993). *The beginning of terror: A psychological study of Rainer Maria Rilke's life and work.* New York: New York University Press.

Lamb, M. E., & Oppenheim, D. (1989). Fatherhood and father-child relationships: Five years of research. In S. Cath, A. Gurwitt, & L. Gunsberg (Eds.). *Fathers and their families* (pp. 11–26). Hillsdale, NJ: Analytic Press.

Linday, L. (1994). Maternal reports of pregnancy, genital, and related fantasies in preschool and kindergarten children. *Journal of the American Academy of Child and Adolescent Psychiatry, 33,* 416–423.

Lowry, C. B., & Zucker, K. J. (1991). *Is there an association between separation anxiety disorder and gender identity disorder in boys?* Paper presented at the meeting of the Society for Research in Child and Adolescent Psychopathology, Zandvoort, The Netherlands.

Lyons-Ruth, K. (1991). Rapproachement or approachment: Mahler's theory reconsidered from the vantage point of recent research on early attachment relationships. *Psychoanalytic Psychology, 8* (1), 1–23.

Mahler, M. S., Pine, F., & Bergman, A. (1975). *The psychological birth of the human infant.* New York: Basic Books.

Marantz, S., & Coates, S. (1991). Mothers of boys with gender identity disorder: A comparison to normal controls. *Journal of the American Academy of Child and Adolescent Psychiatry, 30,* 136–143.

Meyer-Bahlburg, H. F. L. (1985). Gender identity disorder of childhood: Introduction. *Journal of the American Academy of Child and Adolescent Psychiatry, 24,* 681–683.

Meyer-Bahlburg, H. F. L. (1991). Should the presence of intersexuality in a patient rule out the application of the diagnosis "gender identity disorder"? Unpublished manuscript, *DSM-IV* Subcommittee on Gender Identity Disorders.

Mitchell, J. N. (1991). *Maternal influences on gender identity disorder in boys: Searching for specificity.* Unpublished doctoral dissertation. York University, Downsview, Ontario, Canada.

Rilke, R. M. (1949). *The notebooks of Malte Laurids Brigge.* New York: W. W. Norton.

Saghir, M. T., & Robins, E. (1973). *Male and female homosexuality: A comprehensive investigation.* Baltimore: Williams & Wilkins.

Sandberg, D., Meyer-Bahlburg, H., Ehrhardt, A., & Yager, T. (1993). The prevalence of gender-atypical behavior in elementary school children. *Journal of the Academy of Child and Adolescent Psychiatry, 32,* 306–314.

Slaby, R. G., & Frey, K. S. (1975). Development of gender constancy and selective attention to same-sex models. *Child Development, 46,* 849–856.

Stoller, R. J. (1968). *Sex and gender: Vol. 1. The development of masculinity and femininity.* New York: Science House.

Weissman, M. M., Wickramaratne, P., Warner, V., Karen, J., Prusoff, B. A., Merikangas, K. R., & Gammon, D. (1987). Assessing psychiatric disorders in children: Discrepancies between mothers' and children's reports. *Archives of General Psychiatry, 44,* 747–753.

Winnicott, D. W. (1954). Metapsychological and clinical aspects of regression within the psycho-analytic set-up. In D. W. Winnicott (Ed.), *Through pediatrics to psycho-analysis* (pp. 278–294). London: Hogarth Press, 1975.

Wolfe, S. (1990). *Psychopathology and psychodynamics of parents of boys with a gender identity disorder.* Unpublished doctoral dissertation, City University of New York, New York.

Zucker, K. J. (1985). Cross-gender-identified children. In B. W. Steiner (Ed.), *Gender dysphoria: Development, research, management* (pp. 75–174). New York: Plenum Press.

Zucker, K. J. (1990a). Gender identity disorders in children: Clinical description and natural history. In R. Blanchard & B. W. Steiner (Eds.), *Clinical management of gender identity disorders in children and adults* (pp. 1–23) Washington, DC: American Psychiatric Press.

Zucker, K. J. (1990b). Psychosocial and erotic development in cross-gender identified children. *Canadian Journal of Psychiatry, 35,* 487–495.

Zucker, K. J., & Bradley, S. J. (1995). *Gender identity disorder and psychosexual problems in children and adolescents.* New York: Guilford Press.

Zucker, K. J., Bradley, S. J., & Sullivan, C. B. L. (In press). Traits of separation anxiety in boys with gender identity disorder. *Journal of the American Academy of Child and Adolescent Psychiatry, 35.*

Zucker, K. J., Bradley, S. J., Sullivan, C. B. L., Kuksis, M., Birkenfald-Adams, A., & Mitchell, J. N. (1993). A gender identity interview for children. *Journal of Personality Assessment, 61,* 443–456.

Zucker, K. J., & Green, R. (1992). Psychosexual disorders in children and adolescents. *Journal of Child Psychology and Psychiatry, 33* (1) 107–151.

Zucker, K. J., & Green, R. (1993). Psychological and familial aspects of gender identity disorder. *Child and Adolescent Psychiatric Clinics of North America, 2* (3), 513–542.

41 / Speech, Language, and Communication Disorders in Young Children

Amy M. Wetherby and Barry M. Prizant

Speech, language, and communication disorders are among the most widespread disabilities in early childhood. Research has reported that at least 70% of preschool children with disabilities have identified speech, language, and communication impairments (U.S. Department of Education, 1987), and that 11% of kindergartners have communication disorders (Beitchman, Nair, Clegg,

& Patel, 1986). Early identification and intervention for young children with communication difficulties are important; in particular, communication and language play a significant role in a child's ability to develop relationships, to learn from others within the context of social engagement, and to function with greater independence with increasing age. Early identification and intervention also serve a preventive function against a number of additional difficulties, including socioemotional disturbances and academic difficulties in the early school years, problems that may be closely related to, and possibly result from, early language and communication disorders.

Developmental Framework

In considering the role of communication in the lives of young children, it is important to distinguish between the terms *communication, language,* and *speech.* Communication, the broadest of the three constructs, includes any behavior, whether intentional or unintentional, that conveys meaning to and influences the behavior, ideas, or attitudes of another person. Language can be defined as a conventional system of arbitrary symbols that are combined and used in a rule-governed manner for communication (Lahey, 1988). From a developmental perspective, communication is rooted in social interaction and forms the foundation for the emergence of language (Bloom, 1993). Speech, which is based on auditory input and vocal output, is only one mode for the expression of language. Thus, a child who is not able to speak may be able to benefit from a nonspeech language system, such as sign language or a picture communication board.

A second important distinction is between expressive and receptive skills. Expressive abilities refer to the production of vocal, gestural, or verbal signals, while receptive abilities refer to the process of receiving and comprehending communicative signals of others. Communicative competence requires the ability to develop and use both receptive skills in a listener role and expressive skills in a speaker role.

Communicative interactions are rooted in the early social and affective development of infants (Moore & Dunham, 1995; Prizant & Meyer, 1993). Eye gaze, facial expression and body movement, and orientation are signals that inform the caregiver of a child's physiological and emotional state and thus guide the caregiver's responses to the infant in the service of regulating social interactions. The caregiver's interpretation of and contingent responsiveness to the infant's preintentional communicative signals play an important role in the subsequent development of intentional communication (Dore, 1986; Dunst, Lowe, & Bartholomew, 1990). Early social interactions involving shared affective experiences lead the infant to become aware of the effect that his or her behavior can have on others (Bruner, 1981; Corsaro, 1981; Dore, 1986). Thus, the caregiver's responsiveness to the preintentional communicative behavior of preverbal children plays a critical role in enhancing communication and socioemotional development (Prizant & Wetherby, 1990).

The emergence of communication is a developmental process involving reciprocal interactions between a caregiver and child. Bates and associates (Bates, 1979; Bates, Camaioni, & Volterra, 1975) have provided a theoretical framework to describe the emergence of communication and language. Borrowing terminology from the speech act theory of Austin (1962), they identified three stages in the development of communication. From birth the infant is in the "perlocutionary stage." Although the infant is not yet producing signals with the intention of accomplishing specific goals, the infant's behavior systematically affects the caregiver and thus serves a communicative function.

At about 9 months of age the child moves to the "illocutionary stage" and begins to use preverbal gestures and sounds to communicate intentionally; that is, the child deliberately uses particular signals to communicate for preplanned effects on others. At about 13 months of age the child progresses to the "locutionary stage" and begins to construct linguistic propositions while communicating intentionally with referential words. Thus, communication and language development can be conceptualized as a three-stage ontogenetic process involving movement from perlocutionary or preintentional communication, to illocutionary

474

or intentional preverbal communication, to locutionary or verbal language used intentionally to communicate.

An important assumption of this model is that from birth on, all children communicate in some way. In applying this model to working with young children with communication impairments, the caregiver plays a critical role in interpreting behaviors that are communicative. This model also highlights the broad range of communicative abilities of developmentally delayed preverbal children spanning the perlocutionary and illocutionary stages. Understanding the developmental progression from perlocutionary to illocutionary communication can help the caregiver in enhancing and detecting progress in the communicative abilities of a preverbal child who is developmentally delayed.

The receptive abilities of a preverbal child may be commensurate with or in advance of his or her expressive abilities. Before children comprehend the meaning of words, they use a variety of nonverbal cues to determine a response strategy, and thus they may appear to comprehend specific linguistic information (Chapman, 1981; McLean & Snyder-McLean, 1978). As children move to the illocutionary stage of communication expression, they begin to comprehend *nonverbal cues* provided by their caregivers, including gestures, facial expression, and directed eye gaze (e.g., an adult pointing to or looking at an object "means" the child should give or attend to that object). Children also may respond to paralinguistic cues by using intonation to determine how to respond (e.g., loud voice "means" angry). At this stage children also may respond to *situational cues* by using the immediate environment and knowledge of what to do with objects in order to shape a response (e.g., observe what others do, drink from a cup, put objects in a container). As children progress to the locutionary stage of expression, they begin to comprehend the meanings of familiar words but continue to be guided by the context. It is easy to overestimate a child's comprehension of language if one is not aware of the nonverbal, paralinguistic, or situational cues that the child may be using to determine how to respond. The child's development of comprehension response strategies serves as a bridge to the comprehension of word meanings.

Risk Factors Associated with Language and Communication Disorders

A language disorder is an impairment in the ability to: (1) receive and/or process a symbol system; (2) represent concepts or symbol systems; and/or (3) transmit or use symbol systems (American Speech-Language-Hearing Association, 1982). Childhood language disorders may be classified as primary or secondary, based on contributory factors (Ludlow, 1980). A primary language disorder is present when the language impairment cannot be accounted for by a peripheral sensory or motor deficit, a cognitive and/or social impairment, or adverse environmental conditions; often it is presumed to be due to a dysfunction or impaired development in the central nervous system. Secondary language disorders include language impairments associated with and presumed to be caused by other factors, such as sensory or cognitive impairment or adverse environmental conditions.

Childhood speech and language disorders traditionally have been classified into mutually exclusive categories using a diagnostic model based on etiologic factors. However, a medical model of diagnosis in childhood based on etiologic factors has major limitations. These arise from the high frequency of problems associated with idiopathic or multiple etiologies and the great variability in behavioral presentation, even when a common etiologic factor is known. A diagnostic model based primarily on medical etiology also does not account for the interaction of biological and environmental influences on language development.

Biological and environmental risk factors have been identified that put children at risk for having communication disorders. (For review, see Prizant, Wetherby, & Roberts, 1993). Congenital biological conditions that influence communication development include genetic and metabolic disorders (e.g., Down syndrome, fragile X, cri-du chat), prenatal exposure to toxins, anoxia or asphyxia, and low birthweight. A postnatal biological condition that recently has been a focus of research is recurrent and persistent otitis media with effusion or middle ear infection during early childhood. Some research findings have indicated that certain aspects of speech and language development are delayed in children with a history of middle ear infection (Friel-Patti & Finitzo-Hieber, 1990); others, studying children without a history of middle ear infection, have not reported significant differences (Roberts, Burchinal, Davis, Collier, & Henderson, 1991; Roberts et al., 1995). Environmental factors that have been found to have a significant impact on communication development include living in poverty, being abused and/or neglected, and being exposed to interactional disturbances of caregivers (e.g., adolescent mothers; mothers with depression, bipolar disorder, or cognitive impairments) (Cicchetti, 1989; Tronick, 1989).

The extent or severity of a communication disorder cannot be predicted easily from known risk factors. The combined number of risk factors may be one of the best determinants of outcome (Sameroff, 1987). For example, compared to middle-class families, children of low-income families have been found to have deficient language skills. However, it is the *number* of biological and environmental factors associated with poverty (e.g., poor prenatal health, untreated childhood illnesses) in combination with deficient child-rearing practices that place the exposed children at greater risk for communication disorders.

Impact of Language and Communication Disorders in Early Childhood

Families of young children with communication problems may experience significant stress and confusion related to difficulties in identifying, acknowledging, and understanding their child's problem (Prizant & Meyer, 1993; Prizant & Wetherby, 1993). Determining the existence of communication problems in young children is inherently difficult, due, in part, to the variability both in the age of emergence of first words and in the rate of language acquisition even among normally developing children. When a child begins to dem-

onstrate delays in development of communication skills, it is not uncommon for professionals to disagree as to whether there is any cause for concern. The lack of definitive criteria for communication disorders in infants and toddlers may result in delayed referral by primary care professionals, even when caregivers suspect a problem (Wetherby & Prizant, 1992). Caregivers of children with communication problems also may disagree over whether a problem exists and whether professional guidance should be sought (Gottlieb, 1988). When significant physical, sensory, or cognitive disabilities are present, any of them may lead to earlier identification and more definitive diagnosis of developmental problems. When communication and language delays are not accompanied by such disabilities and when no risk factors (e.g., very low birthweight, perinatal complications) have been identified, significantly delayed referral is more likely to occur.

A significant relationship has been found among preschool language disorders, emotional and behavioral disorders, and later-appearing academic problems. Studies have documented co-occurrence rates of 50 to 60% of language and communication disorders and emotional/behavioral disorders in children and adolescents (Prizant et al., 1990). Although many questions remain regarding causal relationships, it is generally agreed that infants or toddlers with communication delays or disorders are at high risk for the development of emotional and behavioral disorders (Baker & Cantwell, 1987). Socioemotional difficulties impact upon and develop within the context of caregiver-child relationships. The potential for the development of relationship difficulties between young children and their caregivers may be heightened when a child's communicative signals are difficult to read or when a child is unresponsive to the communicative bids of others (Greenspan, 1988; Howlin & Rutter, 1987; Prizant & Meyer, 1993). Children raised in abusive or neglectful environments are at high risk for developmental delays in general and, more specifically, for delays in social and communication development (Cicchetti, 1989).

The behavior of many young children with communication difficulties may pose significant challenges for parents. Among preschoolers, Stevenson and Richman (1976) found that 59% of 3-year-olds with expressive language delays were reported by their parents to have significant behavioral disturbances. Paul (1991a) found that parents of 2-year-old children with slow expressive language development (SELD) perceived greater behavioral disturbance in areas of conduct, activity, and attention in their children compared to parents of age-matched controls, even though the SELD children were within normal limits cognitively on nonverbal measures. Based on extensive family interviews, Bristol and Schopler (1984) identified sources of stress reported by parents of preschool children with significant social and communication disorders. Major sources of stress included the children's lack of effective communication, lack of response to family members, and behavior management problems.

Follow-up studies of preschool children with speech and language problems have consistently demonstrated long-term persistence of speech and language impairments in a substantial proportion of subjects, along with a high incidence of language-learning disabilities (Howlin & Rutter, 1987). Aram and Hall (1989) found that 60% of children who displayed language disorders in the preschool years required special education placement during later childhood. Between 28 and 75% of preschool children with language impairments display speech and language problems that persist in later childhood, and between 53 and 95% show impairments in reading achievement (Scarborough & Dobrich, 1990). Verbal abilities at kindergarten have been found to be moderately predictive of later reading achievement, which provides support for the interrelationship between language impairments and reading disabilities (Catts & Kamhi, 1986; Scarborough & Dobrich, 1990).

In addition to addressing young children's specific communicative limitations, early identification and intervention addressing social and communicative difficulties would likely alleviate stress for caregivers. Bristol and Schopler (1984) found that families were better adapted to their child's disability when there was some clarity and understanding of their child's impairment, early and consistent access to professionals for appropriate services, and contact with other parents who provided psychosocial support. Moreover, early communication/language intervention may prevent or mitigate the persistence of speech and language problems, the development of emotional or be-

havioral disturbances, and the appearance of later learning problems (Baker & Cantwell, 1987; Guralnick & Bennett, 1987).

Potential for Earlier Identification of Communication/Language Impairments

The early identification of children with communication or language impairments continues to pose a dilemma for professionals. Children under age 3 who have communication and language problems may have a specific primary impairment of expressive and/or receptive language, or a secondary impairment due either to a hearing loss or to a more pervasive disturbances in cognitive and/or social development. While these children show very diverse abilities and characteristics, a common feature is that they are late in learning to talk. When other significant disabilities are not present, a delay in or failure to acquire language may be the first evident symptom attended to by parents and professionals. Since the normal range of first word acquisition is between 12 and 20 months of age (Bates, O'Connell, & Shore, 1987), a child may not be referred for a language delay until at best 20 to 24 months, but more typically, after 36 months. A better understanding of specific developmental profiles of relative strengths and weaknesses for young children with communication and language problems is needed to make progress in identifying children at a younger age.

The challenge for professionals evaluating communication and language abilities in very young children is twofold. First, professionals need to be able to distinguish children who are late in beginning to talk but who will catch up spontaneously from those who will have persisting language problems. Second, professionals need to identify children at risk for delayed language development even earlier and hence need to consider other aspects of development in order to detect the risk status for persistent language and communication problems.

Several recent studies indicate that the use of

parental report is a reliable and valid measure of vocabulary development and a sensitive indicator of language delays in children as young as 18 months of age (Bates, Bretherton, & Snyder, 1988; Dale, Bates, Reznick, & Morisset, 1989; Fenson et al., 1993; Rescorla, 1989, 1991). Rescorla (1989) developed the Language Development Survey (LDS), which is a screening vocabulary checklist for parents to complete in a pediatrician's office. Using the LDS, Rescorla reported a mean vocabulary of about 150 words at age 2 and found that about 15% of 2-year-olds across different levels of socioeconomic status had "fewer than 50 words OR no word combinations" (Rescorla, 1989, p. 595). Bates and her colleagues (Bates, Bretherton, & Snyder, 1988; Dale, Bates, Reznick, & Morisset, 1989; Fenson et al., 1993) developed the MacArthur Communicative Development Inventory (CDI), which is a comprehensive parental report instrument that measures vocabulary and grammatical development. Dale and colleagues (1989) reported a mean vocabulary of 372 words at 2 years using the CDI, which contains about twice as many words as the LDS and yielded vocabulary sizes that were about twice the size of the LDS. Several follow-up studies of children who were identified with slow vocabulary development and no other obvious problems at age 2 have been reported (Paul, 1991b; Rescorla & Schwartz, 1990; Thal, Tobias, & Morrison, 1991). These studies, which have used either the LDS or CDI, have consistently reported that about 50% of these children show persisting problems in grammatical development at age 3.

Although the use of a parental report vocabulary checklist has been found to be a sensitive indicator of delayed vocabulary at age 2, this measure alone does not appear to assist in distinguishing children who will catch up spontaneously from those with persisting language problems. Furthermore, relying solely on a measure of vocabulary precludes identifying children at risk for language delays before the emergence of words (i.e., before 18 months of age). An important question to address is whether it is possible to identify children at risk for persisting language problems before a delay in the onset of expressive language is evident (i.e., earlier than 18 to 24 months). A number of patterns have emerged from recent research on children with delayed language that suggest that information about spe-

cific parameters of a child's early communication and symbolic development has important implications for distinguishing between children who will catch up spontaneously from those whose language problems are likely to persist. The identification of patterns predictive of persistent problems should contribute to earlier detection of language problems in infants and toddlers. This literature is reviewed briefly in the next section.

RATE OF COMMUNICATING

Wetherby and colleagues (Wetherby, Cain, Yonclas, & Walker, 1988; Wetherby, Yonclas, & Bryan, 1989) suggested that rate of communicating (ROC), measured by the number of communicative acts (i.e., gestural, vocal, and/or verbal behaviors used communicatively) displayed per minute, is a useful index of communication development for children who have no or few intelligible words. Using semistructured elicitation procedures, Wetherby et al. (1988) found that ROC with gestures and/or vocalizations in normally developing children increased substantially from an average of about 1 act per minute for 1-year olds at the prelinguistic stage to about 5 acts per minute for 2-year-olds at the multiword stage. Based on measures of ROC for preschool children with varying types of language impairments, Wetherby et al. (1989) suggested that increases in ROC are not dependent on advances in expressive language development but may rather reflect a child's sophistication in reciprocity of communication. Children with SELD have been found to show low ROC compared to age-matched peers (Paul, 1991b; Thal & Tobias, 1992), suggesting that this measure may contribute to earlier identification.

RANGE OF COMMUNICATIVE FUNCTIONS

A deficient overall ROC may be an indicator of a delay in communication development. In addition, however, studies of communicative functions (i.e., specific purposes for which children use sounds, gestures, and/or words) provide further important information for early identification.

Research has demonstrated that before the emergence of words, normally developing children acquire communication for three major communicative functions: behavior regulation (e.g., request objects/actions, protest), social interaction (e.g., to request comfort, call, greet, show off), and joint attention (e.g., to comment, request information) (Wetherby et al., 1988). These communicative functions may be placed on a continuum of sociability, with behavioral regulation at the low end and joint attention at the high end. In applying this concept clinically, children with autism in the prelinguistic and early stages of language development were compared to controls at the same language stage. The artistic children showed a predominance of communicative acts for behavioral regulation and a deficient proportion or absence of acts to engage in social interaction and to reference joint attention (Mundy, Sigman, & Kasari, 1990; Wetherby & Prutting, 1984; Wetherby et al., 1989). This pattern of impairments in communicative functions with greater sociability is regarded as one of the hallmarks of autism in young children. When other language-impaired children were tested, their use of the joint attention function was found to be slightly deficient compared to age-matched controls but commensurate with language-matched controls (Leonard, Camarata, Rowan, & Chapman, 1982; Paul, 1991b; Wetherby et al., 1989). Thus, since the expression of joint attention and other social functions emerges before words, significant differences in the use of communicative functions may be evident in young prelinguistic children, and should therefore be of value in the early identification of at-risk infants and toddlers.

QUALITY OF GESTURES AND VOCALIZATION

Differences in the quality of communicative means (i.e., gestures and vocalizations used for communication) have been identified in children with language problems. There have been numerous studies of preschool children with varying types of language impairments, including specific language impairment and autism. It turns out that, compared to language-matched controls, these children use as many or more gestures but fewer vocalizations to express intentions during the prelinguistic and early 1-word stage (Rowan, Leonard, Chapman, & Weiss, 1983; Snyder, 1978; Wetherby & Prutting, 1984; Wetherby et al., 1989). Thal and Tobius (1992) studied the use of presymbolic (e.g., giving, pointing, showing, reaching) versus symbolic (e.g., waving, head nod, depictive or pantomimelike actions) communicative gestures in two groups, namely: children with persisting language delays and those who caught up spontaneously (i.e., late bloomers). They found that the children with persisting language delays did not differ from normally developing children at the same language stage in regard to the number or type of gestures used. Interestingly, the late bloomers used significantly more presymbolic *and* symbolic conventional gestures than the children with persisting language delays, language-matched controls, and age-matched controls. These findings suggest that the late bloomers were compensating for their delayed speech by gesturing more and that increased use of gestures, particularly symbolic gestures, may be a positive prognostic indicator for spontaneous recovery.

Studies of the use of vocalizations for communication in young children who have language impairments have addressed both the coordination of vocalization with gestures and the complexity of vocalizations. Over the second year of life, normally developing children show an increase in the use of vocalizations in coordination with gestural communication, repertoire of consonants, and complexity of syllabic structure of vocalizations. As spoken words become the predominant means of communicating, they also show a gradual increase in the use of vocalizations without gestures (Wetherby et al., 1988). The number of vocalizations accompanied by gestures used by children with language impairments has been found to be similar to those used by language-matched controls (Thal & Tobius, 1992; Wetherby et al., 1989). However, Wetherby et al. found that children with specific language impairment and with autism used fewer vocalizations without gestures than the language-matched controls. Children with specific language impairment compensated for this with the use of coordinated vocalization and gesture, while children with autism relied upon gestures in isolation. In studies of the developmental complexity of vocalizations, children with SELD (Paul, 1991b; Paul & Jennings, 1992; Wetherby et al., 1989) and children with autism

479

(Wetherby et al., 1989) have been found to use a limited consonant inventory and less complex syllabic structure. Thus, reliance on presymbolic gestures and immature phonological development appear to be a common pattern of children with communicative impairments and should be apparent in younger children during the early development of communication.

SOCIAL AND AFFECTIVE ASPECTS OF COMMUNICATION

Research on social aspects of communication development in young children with language problems has identified varying degrees of social impairments among these children. Follow-up studies of 2-year-olds with communicative delays indicate the importance of examining social skills. In a 1-year follow-up study of 2-year-old children with SELD, Paul, Looney, and Dahm (1991) found that at age 3, about half of the children displayed deficits in expressive communication and socialization skills as measured on the Vineland Adaptive Behavior Scales. In a 1-year follow-up study of 2-year-old children referred for possible autism, Lord (1991) reported that over 80% of children who received a diagnosis of autism at age 2 continued to merit the diagnosis at 3. Surprisingly, 28% of children who did not receive a diagnosis of autism at 2 did qualify for this diagnosis at age 3. These findings indicate that the social communicative problems associated with autism are unlikely to resolve spontaneously by age 3; moreover, using current clinical diagnostic tools, they may not be evident until age 3.

Over the first few years of life, the ability to share affective states is an important foundation for communication and language development. Competence in sharing affective states is evident in a young child's ability to coordinate eye gaze between the object of focus and the caregiver, to display positive and negative affect directed to the caregiver, and to read and interpret the affective expressions of the caregiver. Deficits in the ability to share affective states are pronounced in children with autism and may be related to or underlie many aspects of the social deficits associated with autism (Kasari, Sigman, Mundy, & Yirmiya, 1990). Manifestations of deficits in sharing affective states may be evident in young children and contribute to the early identification of children with autism.

SYMBOLIC DEVELOPMENT

The capacity to symbolize entails the ability to make one thing stand for and represent something else. Symbol use is required not only for expressive language but also for language comprehension, play, and other cognitive abilities. Follow-up studies of 2-year-old children with SELD have examined other aspects of symbolic development in relation to expressive language. Paul et al. (1991) found that 1 year later, half of their subjects showed persistent problems in expressive language and one third showed problems in language comprehension. Thal et al. (1991) found that at age 2 those children whose language problems persisted had delays in language comprehension, while those who caught up spontaneously did not show such delays. These preliminary findings suggest that the co-occurrence of delays in language comprehension and production is a poorer prognostic indicator for "catching up" than delays in expressive language alone.

Because of the developmental relationship of language and play, research on play in children with language impairments provides important information for identifying patterns in symbolic development that may contribute to early identification of language impairments. A large number of studies have demonstrated that children with autism show significant deficits in symbolic play (i.e., using pretend action schemes with objects) (Dawson & Adams, 1984; Sigman & Ungerer, 1984; Wetherby & Prutting, 1984; Wing, Gould, Yeates, & Brierly, 1977). Compared to language-matched controls, children with autism perform at lower levels on symbolic play but at higher levels on constructive play (e.g., stacking blocks, combining objects in ordinal relations) (Wetherby & Prutting, 1984). This is presumably because of the greater social demands of symbolic play compared to constructive play. In contrast, symbolic play performance of preschool children with specific language impairments has been found to be deficient compared to age-matched controls but commensurate with or higher than that of language-matched controls (Terrell & Schwartz, 1988; Terrell, Schwartz, Prelock, & Messick, 1984). In their 1-year follow-up study, Thal et al. (1991) found that the children with persisting language problems performed significantly more poorly than those who caught up on the imitation of discrete action schemes and the production of action schemes in sequence within a familiar play script. Rescorla and Goosens (1992) studied symbolic play in toddlers with delay in expressive language only, but with receptive language age based on the Reynell and a Bayley Mental Development Index within a normal range. They found that compared to age-matched controls, these children demonstrated less sophisticated symbolic play in regard to orientation and sequencing of actions schemes and the use of object substitutions.

IMPORTANCE OF PROFILING
COMMUNICATION AND SYMBOLIC ABILITIES

The literature just reviewed suggests that even prior to the emergence of words, a child's profile of communicative and symbolic abilities may be a sensitive indicator of the likelihood of subsequent difficulties in communication and language development. The findings on young children who show persisting language impairments indicate that measures of vocabulary alone are insufficient for early identification. Furthermore, these findings indicate that for earlier identification and differentiation of children who will outgrow their delay from those children who have specific versus more pervasive social or cognitive impairments, *multiple* measures across communicative and symbolic domains are necessary. That is, a child who shows SELD at age 2 and also shows delays in one or more of the other parameters (e.g., rate of communicating, use of joint attention function, symbolic play) would be at higher risk than a child who demonstrates a pattern of SELD and no other delays. These findings suggest greater urgency in initiating intervention that addresses delays not only in expressive language but also in other communicative and symbolic parameters. Because it is not yet possible to consider delays in expressive language for children under 18 months of age, it is therefore even more critical to measure other parameters of communication and symbolic development in at-risk infants and toddlers. Furthermore, patterns of strengths and weaknesses in the parameters just delineated should provide critical information contributing to the early identification of a communication impairment. This in turn should allow placement of a child along a continuum extending from more specific language delays at one extremity to more pervasive social and/or cognitive impairments at the other.

Need for New Emphasis in Direct Child Assessment

Early childhood professionals are beginning to move away from the traditional practice of waiting until a child is talking to evaluate him or her for a communication and/or language impairment. There has been a recent proliferation of research in infant communication and socioemotional development. Nonetheless, current formal tools used for direct assessment of a child's communication and language have major limitations in their capacity to evaluate spontaneous communication during natural interactions (Crais, 1995). Early identification of and intervention with children at risk for developmental disabilities, including language and communication impairments, are now a priority, a fact reflected in the passage of the Education of the Handicapped Act Amendments of 1986 (PL 99–457). However, assessment tools for young children need to go beyond measures of vocabulary, particularly for the identification of children under 2 years of age. As indicated, early communication disorders have far-reaching effects on family well-being, the child's emotional and behavioral development, and later educational achievement; hence, early identification leading to appropriate intervention is crucial.

Meisels and Provence (1989) presented guidelines based on current best practice for the identification and assessment of infants, toddlers, and preschool children in accordance with PL 99–457. According to these guidelines and general practice, assessment in young children may be considered at three levels: (1) developmental screening to identify children who have a high probability of developmental delay or disability and need further assessment; (2) diagnostic assessment to determine the existence of a delay or disability and identify a child's strengths and needs usually using formal assessment instruments; and (3) assessment for individual program planning to determine a child's mastery of skills or tasks. In order to be used with large numbers of children, developmental screening tests need to be very brief and efficient, while diagnostic assessments are more comprehensive and should be based on multiple sources of information. Both developmental screenings and diagnostic assessments need to be scored objectively with demonstrated reliability and validity, need to be culturally unbiased, and, when possible, need to be accomplished with norm-referenced instruments. Assessment for program planning usually entails the use of criterion-referenced assessment instruments. Meisels and Provence (1989) point out that compared to those for preschool children, direct child assessment findings for infants and toddlers have limited predictive validity. Therefore, for very young children, clinicians need to be cautious in making prognostic statements based on assessment findings.

In order to meet the different goals of assessment adequately, speech-language clinicians are faced with the challenge of identifying appropriate assessment instruments for young children. Wetherby and Prizant (1992) delineated several major limitations of the most frequently used formal communication assessment instruments for young children, based on current theories on language development. First, most instruments are not family-centered in that they do not allow for the family to collaborate in decision making about the assessment process or to participate to the extent family members desired. Second, most instruments involving direct child assessment are primarily clinician directed, placing the child in a respondent role and thus limiting observations of spontaneous, child-initiated communication. Third, most formal instruments emphasize language milestones and forms of communication (e.g., number of different gestures, sounds, words, word combinations) rather than the purposes of those forms or the intentions expressed.

Pragmatic/social interactive theories of the past two decades have placed great emphasis on the context of social interaction in language development (Bates, 1976; Bloom, 1993; Bloom & Lahey, 1978; McLean & Snyder-McLean, 1978). Children are viewed as active participants who learn to affect the behavior and attitudes of others through active signaling, and who gradually grasp more sophisticated and conventional means of communication through caregivers' contingent social responsiveness (Dunst et al., 1990). The quality and nature of the contexts in which interaction occurs are considered to have a great influence on the successful acquisition of language and communicative behavior. Proponents of pragmatic theory believe that development cannot be understood simply by focusing solely on the child or the caregivers. Since successful communication involves reciprocity and mutual negotiation, it can be grasped only by analysis of the interactive context (Bates, 1976; Bruner, 1978). Thus, current theories on how children acquire language suggest that the following features are critical to the assessment of language and communication in young children:

1. Communication and language should be assessed within an interactive context in which the child is encouraged to initiate communication.
2. The young child's caregiver should be integrally involved in the assessment in several ways: as an active participant interacting with the child, as an informant about the child's competence and performance, and as a collaborator in decision making.
3. Diagnostic assessment and assessment for program planning should not only identify relative developmental weaknesses but also should provide information about the child's relative strengths in communication and related areas of development.
4. Assessment should be viewed as a dynamic process in which, over time, the child's capacity for achieving communicative competence comes to be understood.

These features are consistent with current trends in assessment strategies for school-age children, which include the use of authentic assessment measures, such as portfolio assessments that evolve dynamically over time (Damico, Secord, & Wiig, 1992). Thus, there is a critical need to move toward *authentic* assessment with infants, toddlers, and developmentally young children by ensuring the ecological validity of assessment practices (Crais, 1995; Damico et al., 1992) and to utilize *dynamic* assessment to explore aspects of contexts that support or impede the child's acquisition of communicative competence (Olswang, Bain, & Johnson, 1992).

Proposed Framework for Direct Assessment of Young Children

We developed the *Communication and Symbolic Behavior Scales* (CSBS) (Wetherby & Prizant, 1993) to provide a more authentic approach to assessment than that offered by the formal assessment tools current available for infants, toddlers, and preschool children. The CSBS is designed to examine communicative, social/affective, and symbolic abilities of children whose capacity for functional communication ranges from prelinguistic intentional communication to early stages of language acquisition (between 8 months and 2 years in communication and language). This assessment instrument is designed to meet the last two levels of assessment identified earlier—diagnostic assessment and assessment for program planning. A developmental screening version of the CSBS is forthcoming.

The CSBS utilizes a standard but flexible format for gathering data. This involves a combination of a caregiver questionnaire and behavior sampling procedures. To begin with, a questionnaire is given to the family ahead of, or on the same day as, the direct child assessment. By posing descriptive questions that solicit examples of typical behaviors, information is gleaned from the caregiver about the child's communicative and symbolic competence. The direct child assessment involves varying degrees of relatively structured and unstructured sampling procedures. These resemble natural, ongoing adult-child interactions and provide opportunities for documenting a child's use of a variety of communicative and symbolic behaviors. During a sample, the CSBS procedures allow for dynamic assessment of the effects of contextual factors on a child's communicative abilities. Dynamic assessment of con-

textual factors also can be considered across samples collected over time. Dynamic assessment is integrated within the CSBS sampling procedures. First, the sample involves both structured communicative opportunities and unstructured play. Thus, parameters of the child's communication can be compared between these contexts. Second, some of the child's communicative attempts are deliberately not responded to as intended so that the child's ability to persist and repair can be examined. Finally, if the child does not initiate communication during structured opportunities, a hierarchy of verbal and gestural cues are offered to support communicative efforts, and the child's response to these can then be examined.

The caregiver is present during the entire sample and is encouraged to respond naturally to the child's bids for interaction. After the sample is collected, the caregiver rates how typical the child's behavior was during the sample along 7 different dimensions—alertness, emotional reaction, level of interest and attention, comfort level, level of activity, overall level of communication, and play behavior. The caregiver's perception rating allows him or her to validate the representativeness of the child's behavior during direct assessment. Thus, the assessment procedures enable the clinician to engage the parent both as an interacter during the direct assessment with the child and as an informant via the caregiver questionnaire and the caregiver perception rating. Having the caregiver present and participating during the sample provides an opportunity for clinician and caregiver to build a consensus on their perceptions of the child's communicative strengths and weaknesses displayed during the sample, and to compare these patterns to information provided on the caregiver questionnaire.

Behaviors collected in the sample are rated along a number of parameters and are converted to scores on 22 5-point rating scales of communication and symbolic behaviors. Seven cluster scores are derived from the 22 scales; the first 6 contribute to the child's profile of communication and the last one to the child's profile of symbolic behaviors:

1. *Communicative Functions*—measures the use of gestures, sounds, or words for behavior regulation and for joint attention, and the proportion of communication used for social functions.
2. *Gestural Communicative Means*—measures the

variety of conventional gestures, use of distal gestures, and coordination of gestures and vocalizations.

3. *Vocal Communicative Means*—measures the use of vocalizations without gestures, inventory of different consonants, and syllabic structure.

4. *Verbal Communicative Means*—measures the number of different words and different word-combinations produced.

5. *Reciprocity*—measures the use of communication in response to the adult's conventional gestures or speech, rate of communicating, and ability to repair communicative breakdowns by repeating and/or modifying previous communication when a goal is not achieved.

6. *Social/Affective Signaling*—measures the use of gaze shifts between person and object, expression of positive affect with directed eye gaze, and episodes of negative affect.

7. *Symbolic Behavior*—measures comprehension of contextual cues, single-word and multiword utterances, the number of different action schemes and complexity of action schemes in symbolic play, and the level of constructive play.

National field testing has been completed on a sample of approximately 300 normally developing children from 8 to 24 months of age and 30 children with developmental disabilities from 18 to 30 months of age.

Assessment of Communication Environment

Assessment of a young child's communicative and symbolic profile provides information about only one half of the communicative interaction. It is also necessary to assess the quality of the communicative environment. Two major dimensions of the communicative environment that need to be assessed include: opportunities for the child to initiate and respond to communication and interactional style of communicative partner(s). Considerations for the assessment of each of these dimensions of the communicative environment are addressed briefly.

Environments may vary a great deal in regard to the quality and quantity of opportunities for communication. The practitioner needs to ask whether situations and persons in the environment provide ample opportunities for the child to initiate and respond to communication for a variety of communicative functions (i.e., behavioral regulation, social interaction, joint attention). That is, does the child have the opportunity to communicate in order to get others to do things, to draw attention to the self, and to direct others' attention to objects or events?

Opportunities to communicate in the service of behavioral regulation generally involve situations in which the child needs to request assistance for objects out of reach, to make choices about desired objects or activities (e.g., food items, toys, games, or play partner), and to indicate undesired objects or activities. Opportunities to regulate behavior should occur throughout activities, not just when materials are first presented or activities are initiated. Evaluation of such opportunities will provide information about the need for environmental arrangements to increase the occasions for such communicating. (See Peck, 1989.)

Opportunities to communicate for social interaction and joint attention are more likely to occur within playful repetitive, turn-taking contexts. (Moore & Dunham, 1995). Bruner (1978, 1981) suggested that joint action routines offer the optimal opportunity for communication development and provide the foundation for learning to exchange roles in conversation. A joint action routine is a repetitive, turn-taking game or activity in which there is mutual attention and participation by both the child and caregiver, exchangeable roles, and predictable sequences. (See Snyder-McLean, Solomonson, McLean, & Sack, 1984.) A prototypical example of a joint action routine is the game of peek-a-boo (Bruner, 1981), which caregiver and child may play endlessly during the first year of life. A joint action routine may involve preparation of a specific end product (e.g., preparing food), organization around a central plot (e.g., pretend play), or cooperative turn-taking games (e.g., peek-a-boo) (Snyder-McLean et al., 1984). Both the quantity and quality of joint action routines engaged in daily with a young child should be evaluated.

A young child's communicative behavior will be influenced not only by the opportunities for communication but also by the interaction style used by communicative partners. Therefore, in order to determine whether the partner is using a facilitative style that fosters communication or a directive style that inhibits communication, it is important to evaluate this aspect of the communicative partner's behavior. The caregiver's contingent social responsiveness to the child's behavior has been found to be a major influence on how successfully the child develops communicative competence (Dunst et al., 1990).

The developmental literature provides guidelines for assessing caregivers' interaction styles (Girolametto, Greenberg, & Manolson, 1986; MacDonald, 1989). Based on developmental guidelines for children at presymbolic stages of communication, the caregiver's interaction style should be evaluated to determine if the following features are present: (1) waiting for the child to initiate communication by pausing and looking expectantly; (2) recognizing the child's behavior as communication by interpreting the communicative function that it serves; and (3) responding contingently to the child's communicative behavior in a manner that is consistent with the child's communicative intention and that matches the youngster's communicative level (MacDonald, 1989).

Thus, if the child is requesting an object, does the caregiver give the desired object immediately? If the child is requesting comfort, does the caregiver provide social and/or physical attention to the child? If the child is commenting, does the caregiver attend to the object or event to which the child is drawing attention?

In addition to being able to follow the child's lead, it is important that the caregiver be able to be a "matched partner" by adjusting behavior so that it matches the child's developmental level, interest, and style (MacDonald, 1989). The practitioner should consider whether the form of the caregiver's communication matches that of the child. MacDonald provides the analogy of being on a staircase with the child in such a way that the partner has one foot on the child's step and the other foot on the next step.

In assessing the communicative partner's interaction style, it is also important to consider the balance between the child and the partner. That is, the practitioner should consider whether both the child and the caregiver take an equal role in participating, and whether the interaction is reciprocal (i.e., each person should influence and respond meaningfully to the other person) (MacDonald, 1989).

In summary, the assessment of the communicative environment should provide information that can be utilized in intervention planning in order to increase opportunities for communicating and enhance the reciprocity of communicative interactions.

Communication Intervention with Young Children

Communication intervention with young children should be one dimension of an integrated intervention plan for the child and his or her family (Prizant et al., 1993). Whether services are provided in a home or center-based program, caregivers possess the greatest potential for actuating positive change in their child's communicative abilities (MacDonald, 1989). However, caregivers must be willing and voluntary participants in such endeavors. This requires that they be respected and supported in setting communication priorities and goals that they value. The degree of successful communication and interaction between a child and his or her caregivers, peers, and siblings is likely to have a significant impact on the parents' sense of competence, the well-being of the family, and the social and emotional well-being of the child (Theadore, Maher, & Prizant, 1990).

Enhancement of communication in young children necessitates a dual focus, one that concentrates on both the child and the communication environment. Once the child's profile of communicative and symbolic abilities has been assessed, it can be used to prioritize communication goals. These will be chosen to enhance the child's readability (i.e., how easy it is to understand what the child means) sophistication of communication. Focus on the communication environment is the other critical aspect of communication enhancement. The two primary components of the communication environment that should be addressed are the quality and quantity of opportunities for communicating, and the interaction strategies used by communicative partners. Next we present guidelines for prioritizing intervention goals for the child and enhancing the communication environment.

FOCUS ON THE CHILD FOR COMMUNICATION ENHANCEMENT

It is important to set optimal goals for communication enhancement in young children. Such prioritizing, however, must be considered in relation to a child's developmental and chronological age. The child's developmental level of communication can be used as a framework for setting up such intervention goals. That is, the communication assessment process should provide information about whether a child is using predominantly preintentional, intentional, or linguistic communication. The child's strengths and needs relative to his or her communication stage should be the basis for decisions about priority goals.

For preintentional children functioning developmentally up to approximately age 8 months the overriding communication goal is to develop a joint attentional focus in reciprocal interactions (Moore & Dunham, 1995). Eventually, the children should gain the capacity to produce signals intentionally in order to affect the behavior of others. This goal is of paramount significance because early reciprocity and intentional communication are the foundations for an expressive communication and language system. This, in turn, will have a great impact on independent functioning and social control. The development of readable, intentional signals occurs in a context of reciprocal play and social interaction involves turn taking and mutual imitation. Therefore, for chronologically and developmentally young children, the early priorities are to establish readiness to engage in social exchange and to participate in turn-taking exchanges and reciprocal play. For preintentional children, two critical goals are to develop the capacity to participate actively in dyadic exchange through vocalization and action and to develop anticipation of events in highly predictable joint action routines. As noted earlier, reciprocal activity or joint action routines are organized

in logical and predictable ways. Children come to anticipate the steps in the routine; eventually they are able to engage in reciprocal activity over extended turns. Initially children are able to fill their turn with subtle signals of attention, affect display, and bodily movement; in time, however, they develop more varied and sophisticated behavioral response repertoires. Their behavior is reinforced by adult imitation and affect attunement.

For very young children, there is no clear point at which intentional communication emerges; however, most investigators agree that developmentally, behavioral evidence for communicative intent is observed at approximately 8 to 9 months (Bates et al., 1987; Wetherby & Prizant, 1989). The expression of communicative intent emerges gradually as children observe the effects of their actions on the behavior of adults. Through this process children are reinforced for their initiatives and develop an awareness of contingency and social causality. Thus, intervention activities that support the development of intentional communication must involve responsive communicative partners reacting consistently and predictably to young children's behavior responding, indeed, as if the children's behavior was intentionally communicative. This is especially true for children with disabilities at emerging intentional levels, for they need much repetition in order to learn to associate their behavior with how it affects others. Furthermore, partners' responses need to be immediate, clear, and naturally reinforcing to the children. Once intent is clearly established, it eventually should involve prompting and modeling of more conventional and readable signals.

Children at a prelinguistic intentional communication stage are clearly using signals to influence the behavior of others. However, initially signals tend to be concrete and idiosyncratic; they may be produced inconsistently, or only in the course of certain routines or within particular contexts. Thus, for children at early prelinguistic intentional levels of communication, expressive communication goals include: (1) developing more consistent and socially acceptable means for expressing intentions; (2) developing more conventional gestural and vocal means for communication; (3) expanding the range of functions or purposes for communication; and (4) developing repair strategies (i.e., persistence in communication) (Prizant & Bailey, 1992; Wetherby & Prizant,

486

1993). The ability to initiate communication within natural social interactions and to communicate spontaneously with different partners and in a variety of situations also continue to be high-priority goals.

Children who have attained the emerging language levels are beginning to use conventional words through speech or signs, but they are still communicating primarily through prelinguistic gestures and vocalizations. The transition from prelinguistic to linguistic communication is at best a gradual process for normally developing children; it is a considerable challenge for children with disabilities. The challenge is due, in part, to the greater motor and cognitive demands inherent in oral language use or the use of other symbol system. Due to motor and cognitive limitations, some children with disabilities will communicate more successfully with nonspeech augmentative communicative means than through speech alone.

When children begin moving into early language stages, they begin to use words to communicate the same meanings and for the same purposes as they were previously transmitting through prelinguistic communicative means (Lahey, 1988). The earliest words code basic semantic relations and refer to a wide spectrum of meanings—for example, the existence or presence of objects, events that recur, objects that reappear or disappear, people acting on objects, actions that change the location of objects, and personal statements of rejection or possession. Children tend to talk more about objects that are moving or changing than about those that are static. These developmental patterns should be considered in making decisions about initial vocabulary selection. It is important to emphasize that appropriate exposure to and modeling of language and communicative behavior in daily interactions is basic to successful acquisition of single- and multiword utterances.

FOCUS ON THE CAREGIVER AND LEARNING ENVIRONMENT FOR COMMUNICATION ENHANCEMENT

Most caregiver-directed approaches concerned with communication development address the following five goals:

1. Sensitize caregivers to their child's level of communication, to their specific strategies in communicating, and to any specific difficulties their children face.
2. Inform caregivers about the sequences and processes of language and communication development.
3. Help caregivers to develop interactive styles that are responsive to their children and supportive of successful communicative interactions.
4. Help caregivers modify daily activities and routines, and develop new activities to support communication development.
5. Improve relationships between caregivers and their young children by helping caregivers to redefine their perceptions of their children's abilities.

Different models for providing services to caregivers have been described both for caregivers of at-risk infants and toddlers (Seitz & Provence, 1990) and for caregivers of developmentally disabled children (Marfo, 1990). These models provide either direct individual caregiver-child therapy or information and support to caregivers through a group educational program. (See Prizant et al., 1993.)

Communication enhancement efforts can be targeted both in a wide variety of daily routines as well as in the context of other activities addressing the child's developmental needs. The value of using naturally occurring events for communication enhancement has been demonstrated repeatedly (McCormick, 1990). However, children with communication delays or disabilities need to be exposed to a special set of learning contexts, contexts that are designed or modified to facilitate, elicit, and support emerging communicative abilities within the framework of reciprocal interactions with caregivers. For children who may become easily distracted or disorganized by high levels of social and environmental stimulation, initially it may be necessary to provide learning activities in protected contexts with minimal distraction.

Activities that young children are exposed to usually are built around some underlying event structure governed by rules of communication and participation that may be more or less flexible (Duchan, 1989). The event structures invoked by caregivers in a child's first 2 years of life create such appropriate interactive contexts, settings that are consistent and predictable for young children learning to communicate. Within action-based routines, children learn about the structure of turn-taking and communicative reciprocity (Bruner, 1981). Examples of routines are familiar social games such as peek-a-boo or "I'm gonna get you," or song routines with verbal and gestural components. Repeated exposure to activities and interactions with predictable formats fosters a child's ability to perceive and internalize the recurring patterns and to take a more active participatory role. During activities with predictable structure, caregivers develop greater expectations for their children's participation through active communicative signaling (Bruner, 1981; Dunst et al., 1990). In planning approaches to communication enhancement, consistency and predictability should be infused into a child's daily experiences. This is best accomplished through the clear marking and highlighting of temporal, spatial, and interactive dimensions of daily routines. (See Prizant & Bailey, 1992.)

Research has demonstrated that the caregiver's style of interaction has an important influence on language and communication development (Mahoney, 1988). The transactional nature of communication development suggests that with appropriate modifications of caregivers' interactive style, children develop a sense of efficacy and competence in communication. This growing sense of efficacy results in ever more active participation in social exchange, which in turn reinforces caregivers' sense of being able parents (Dunst et al., 1990).

Facilitative interaction strategies refer to ways in which communicative partners will spontaneously interact with and respond to children in a manner that is supportive of their communicative growth. These strategies encompass verbal as well as nonverbal behavior. Verbal dimensions include aspects of language structure and use, such as the level of grammatical complexity, vocabulary selection, contingency of turns, and intentions of communication. Interveners must work closely with caregivers to discover interactive styles and strategies that will best support a child's communicative development and that will then enable a child to communicate intentions as independently as possible. The following dimensions of facilitative interaction strategies have been identified as important features when interacting with young children: degree of acceptance of children's communicative bids, degree of directiveness or facilitativeness of partner style, and adjusting the timing and complexity of language and social input (MacDonald, 1989; McCormick, 1990; Prizant & Bailey, 1992).

Summary

Language and communication impairments in young children may have a detrimental impact on a child's emotional and behavioral development, on later educational achievement, and on the family's well being. The early identification of children at risk for language and communication disorders may serve to prevent or mitigate the emergence of such problems and the related difficulties for the child and for the family. Recent research on young children with delayed language suggests that patterns of strengths and weaknesses in communicative and symbolic parameters should provide critical information. This, in turn, will contribute to the early identification of a communication impairment in infants and toddlers. We have suggested that the assessment of language and communication in young children should have several dimensions. For one, it should occur in authentic, interactive contexts; for another, the child's caregiver should be integrally involved as an active participant, informant, and collaborator in decision making. Furthermore, assessment should be viewed as a dynamic process, that is, the child's relative strengths and weaknesses in communication and related areas must be identified and the child's capacity for developing communicative competence understood. Communication enhancement for infants and toddlers should entail a dual focus on both the child and the communication environment. Goals for young children should be prioritized in keeping with their level of preintentional, intentional, or linguistic communication. The primary components of the communication environment that should be addressed include the quantity and quality of opportunities for communicating and interaction strategies used by the caregiver or other communicative partners.

REFERENCES

American Speech-Language-Hearing Association (1982). Definitions: Communicative disorders and variations. *Asha, 24,* 949–950.

Aram, D., & Hall, N. (1989). Longitudinal follow-up of preschool communication disorders: Treatment implications. *School Psychological Review, 18,* 487–501.

Austin, J. (1962). *How to do things with words.* Cambridge, MA: Harvard University Press.

Baker, L., & Cantwell, D. (1987). A prospective psychiatric follow-up of children with speech/language disorders. *Journal of the American Academy of Child and Adolescent Psychiatry, 26,* 546–553.

Bates, E. (1976). *Language and context: The acquisition of pragmatics.* New York: Academic Press.

Bates, E. (1979). *The emergence of symbols: Cognition and communication in infancy.* New York: Academic Press.

Bates, E., Bretherton, I., & Snyder, L. (1988). *From first words to grammar: Individual differences and dissociable mechanisms.* Cambridge: Cambridge University Press.

Bates, E., Camaioni, L., & Volterra, V. (1975). The acquisition of performatives prior to speech. *Merrill-Palmer Quarterly, 21,* 205–226.

Bates, E., O'Connell, B., & Shore, C. (1987). Language and communication in infancy. In J. Osofsky (Ed.), *Handbook of infant development* (pp. 149–203). New York: John Wiley & Sons.

Beitchman, J., Nair, R., Clegg, M., & Patel, P. (1986). Prevalence of speech and language disorders in five-year-old kindergarten children in the Ottawa-Carlton region. *Journal of Speech and Hearing Disorders, 51,* 98–110.

Bloom, L. (1993). *The transition from infancy to language.* New York: Cambridge University Press.

Bloom, L., & Lahey, M. (1978). *Language development and language disorders.* New York: John Wiley & Sons.

Bristol, M., & Schopler, E. (1984). A developmental perspective on stress and coping families of autistic children. In J. Blacher (Ed.), *Families of severely handicapped children* (pp. 91–134). New York: Academic Press.

Bruner, J. (1978). From communication to language: A psychological perspective. In I. Markova (Ed.), *The social context of language.* Chichester: John Wiley & Sons.

Bruner, J. (1981). The social context of language acquisition. *Language and Communication, 1,* 155–178.

Catts, H., & Kamhi, A. (1986). The linguistic basis of reading disorders: Implications for the speech-language pathologist. *Language, Speech, and Hearing Services in Schools, 17,* 329–341.

Chapman, R. (1981). Comprehension strategies in children. In J. Kavanagh & W. Strange (Eds.), *Speech and language in the laboratory, school and clinic* (pp. 308–327). Cambridge, MA: MIT Press.

Cicchetti, D. (1989). How research on child maltreatment has informed the study of child development: Perspectives from developmental psychopathology. In D. Cicchetti & V. Carlson (Eds.), *Child maltreatment: Theory and research on causes and consequences of child abuse and neglect* (pp. 377–431). New York: Cambridge University Press.

Corsaro, W. (1981). The development of social cognition in preschool children: Implications for language learning. *Topics in Language Disorders, 2,* 77–95.

Crais, E. (1995). Expanding the repertoire of tools and techniques for assessing the communication skills of infants and toddlers. *American Journal of Speech Language Pathology, 4,* 47–59.

Dale, P., Bates, E., Reznick, J., & Morisset, C. (1989). The validity of a parent report instrument of child language at 20 months. *Journal of Child Language, 16,* 239–249.

Damico, J., Secord, W., & Wiig, E. (1992). Descriptive language assessment at school: Characteristics and design. In W. Secord (Ed.), *Best practices in school speech-language pathology* (pp. 1–8). San Antonio, TX: Psychological Corp.

Dawson, G., & Adams, A. (1984). Imitation and social responsiveness in autistic children. *Journal of Abnormal Child Psychology, 12,* 209–226.

Dore, J. (1986). The development of conversation competence. In R. Scheifelbusch, (Ed.), *Language competence: Assessment and intervention* (pp. 3–60). San Diego: College-Hill Press.

Duchan, J. (1989). Evaluating adults' talk to children: Assessing adult attunement. *Seminars in Speech and Language, 10,* 17–27.

Dunst, C., Lowe, L. W., & Bartholomew, P. C. (1990). Contingent social responsiveness, family ecology, and infant communicative competence. *National Student Speech Language Hearing Association Journal, 17,* 39–49.

Fenson, L., Dale, P., Reznick, S., Thal, D., Bates, E., Hartung, J., Pethick, S., & Reilly, J. (1993). *Technical manual for the MacArthur Communicative Development Inventories.* San Diego: Singular Press.

Friel-Patti, S. & Finitzo-Hieber, T. (1990). Language learning in a prospective study of otitis media with effusion in the first two years of life. *Journal of Speech and Hearing Research, 33,* 188–194.

Girolametto, L. E., Greenberg, J., & Manolson, H. A. (1986). Developing dialogue skills: The Hanen early language parent program. *Seminars in Speech and Language, 7,* 367–382.

Gottlieb, M. (1988). The response of families to language disorders in the young child. *Seminars in Speech and Language, 9,* 47–53.

Greenspan, S. (1988). Fostering emotional and social development in infants with disabilities. *Zero to Three, 8,* 8–18.

Guralnick, M. & Bennett, F. (1987). *The effectiveness of early intervention for at-risk and handicapped children.* New York: Academic Press.

Howlin, P., & Rutter, M. (1987). The consequences of

language delay for other aspects of development. In W. Yule & M. Rutter (Eds.), *Language development and language disorders* (pp. 272–294). Philadelphia: J. B. Lippincott.

Kasari, C., Sigman, M., Mundy, P., & Yirmiya, N. (1990). Affective sharing in the context of joint attention. *Journal of Autism and Developmental Disorders, 20,* 87–100.

Lahey, M. (1988). *Language disorders and language development.* New York: Macmillan.

Leonard, L., Camarata, S., Rowan, L., & Chapman, K. (1982). The communicative functions of lexical usage by language impaired children. *Applied Psycholinguistics, 3,* 109–127.

Lord, C. (1991, April). *Follow-up of two-year olds referred for possible autism.* Paper presented at the biannual meeting of the Society for Research and Child Development, Seattle, WA.

Ludlow, C. (1980). Children's language disorders: Recent research advances. *Annals of Neurology, 7,* 497–507.

MacDonald, J. (1989). *Becoming partners with children.* San Antonio, TX: Special Press.

Mahoney, G. (1988). Enhancing the developmental competence of handicapped infants. In K. Marfo (Ed.), *Parent-child interaction and developmental disabilities* (pp. 203–219). New York: Praeger.

Marfo, K. (1990). Maternal directiveness in interactions with mentally handicapped children: An analytical commentary. *Journal of Child Psychology and Psychiatry, 31,* 531–549.

McCormick, L. (1990). Intervention processes and procedures. In L. McCormick & R. Schiefelbusch (Eds.), *Early language intervention* (pp. 158–200). Columbus, OH: Merrill.

McLean, J., & Snyder-McLean, L. (1978). *A transactional approach to early language training.* Columbus, OH: Charles E. Merrill.

Meisels, S., & Provence, S. (1989). *Screening and assessment: Guidelines for identifying young disabled and developmentally vulnerable children and their families.* Washington, DC: National Center for Clinical Infant Programs.

Moore, C. & Dunham, P. (Eds.) (1995). *Joint attention: Its origins and role in development.* Hillsdale, NJ: Lawrence Erlbaum.

Mundy, P., Sigman, M., & Kasari, C. (1990). A longitudinal study of joint attention and language development in autistic children. *Journal of Autism and Developmental Disorders, 20,* 115–128.

Olswang, L., Bain, B., & Johnson, G. (1992). Using dynamic assessment with children with language disorders. In S. Warren & J. Reichle (Eds.), *Causes and effects in communication and language intervention* (pp. 187–215). Baltimore: Paul H. Brookes.

Paul, R. (1991a). Language delay and parental perceptions. *Journal of the American Academy of Childhood and Adolescent Psychiatry, 29,* 669–670.

Paul, R. (1991b). Profiles of toddlers with slow expressive language development. *Topics in Language Disorders, 11,* 1–13.

Paul, R., & Jennings, P. (1992). Phonological behavior in toddlers with slow expressive language development. *Journal of Speech and Hearing Research, 35,* 99–107.

Paul, R., Looney, S., & Dahm, P. (1991). Communication and socialization skills at ages 2 and 3 in "late-talking" young children. *Journal of Speech and Hearing Research, 34,* 858–865.

Peck, C. (1989). Assessment of social communicative competence: Evaluating environments. *Seminars in Speech and Language, 10,* 1–15.

Prizant, B., Audet, L., Burke, G., Hummel, L., Maher, S., & Theodore G. (1990). Communication disorders and emotional/behavioral disorders in children. *Journal of Speech and Hearing Disordorders, 55,* 179–192.

Prizant, B., & Bailey, D. (1992). Facilitating acquisition and use of communication skills. In D. Bailey & M. Woolery (Eds.), *Teaching infants and preschoolers with handicaps* (pp. 299–361). Columbus, OH: Charles E. Merrill.

Prizant, B. M., & Meyer, E. (1993). Socioemotional aspects of communication disorders in young children. *American Journal of Speech-Language Pathology, 2,* 56–71.

Prizant, B., & Wetherby, A. (1990). Toward an integrated view of language and socioemotional development in children. *Topics in Language Disorders, 10,* 1–16.

Prizant, B., & Wetherby, A. (1993). Communication and language assessment for young children. *Infants and Young Children, 5,* 20–34.

Prizant, B., Wetherby, A., & Roberts, J. (1993). Communication disorders in infants and toddlers. In C. Zeanah (Ed.), *Handbook of infant mental health* (pp. 260–279). New York: Guilford Press.

Rescorla, L. (1989). The language development survey: A screening tool for delayed language in toddlers. *Journal of Speech and Hearing Disorders, 54,* 587–599.

Rescorla, L. (1991). Identifying expressive language delay at age two. *Topics in Language Disorders, 11,* 14–20.

Rescorla, L., & Goosens, M. (1992). Symbolic play development in toddlers with expressive specific language impairment. *Journal of Speech and Hearing Research, 35,* 1290–1302.

Rescorla, L., & Schwartz, E. (1990). Outcome of specific expressive language delay (SELD). *Applied Psycholinguistics, 11,* 393–408.

Roberts, J., Burchinal, M., Davis, B., Collier, A., & Henderson, F. (1991). Otitis media in early childhood and later language development. *Journal of Speech and Hearing Research, 34,* 1158–1168.

Roberts, J., Burchinal, M., Medley, L., Zeisel, S., Mundy, M., Roush, J., Hooper, S., Bryant, D., & Henderson, F. (1995). Otitis media, hearing sensitivity, and maternal responsiveness in relation to language during infancy. *Journal of Pediatrics, 126,* 481–489.

Rowan, L., Leonard, L., Chapman, K., & Weiss, A.

(1983). Performative and presuppositional skills in language-disordered and normal children. *Journal of Speech and Hearing Research, 26,* 97–106.

Sameroff, A. (1987). The social context of development. In N. Eisenburg (Ed.), *Contemporary topics in development* (pp. 273–291). New York: John Wiley & Sons.

Scarborough, H., & Dobrich, W. (1990). Development of children with early language delay. *Journal of Speech and Hearing Research, 33,* 70–83.

Seitz, V., & Provence, S. (1990). Caregiver-focused models of early intervention. In S. Meisels & J. Shonkoff (Eds.), *Handbook of early childhood intervention* (pp. 400–427), Cambridge: Cambridge University Press.

Sigman, M., & Ungerer, J. (1984). Cognitive and language skills in autistic, mentally retarded and normal children. *Developmental Psychology, 20,* 293–302.

Snyder, L. (1978). Communicative and cognitive abilities and disabilities in the sensorimotor period. *Merrill-Palmer Quarterly, 24,* 161–180.

Snyder-McLean, L., Solomonson, B., McLean, J., & Sack, S. (1984). Structuring joint action routines: A strategy for facilitating communication and language development in the classroom. *Seminars in Speech and Language, 5,* 213–228.

Stevenson, J., & Richman, N. (1976). The prevalence of language delay in a population of three-year-old children and its association with general retardation. *Developmental Medicine and Child Neurology, 18,* 431–441.

Terrell, B. Y., & Schwartz, R. G. (1988). Object transformations in the play of language-impaired children. *Journal of Speech and Hearing Disorders, 53,* 459–466.

Terrell, B. Y., Schwartz, R. G., Prelock, P., & Messick, C. K. (1984). Symbolic play in normal and language impaired children. *Journal of Speech and Hearing Research, 27,* 424–429.

Thal, D., & Tobias, S. (1992). Communicative gestures in children with delayed onset of oral expressive vocabulary. *Journal of Speech and Hearing Research, 35,* 1281–1289.

Thal, D., Tobias, S., & Morrison, D. (1991). Language

and gesture in late talkers: A 1-year follow-up. *Journal of Speech and Hearing Research, 34,* 604–612.

Theadore, G., Maher, S., & Prizant, B. (1990). Early assessment and intervention with emotional and behavioral disorders and communication disorders. *Topics in Language Disorders, 10,* 42–56.

Tronick, E. (1989). Emotions and emotional communication in infancy. *American Psychologist, 44,* 112–119.

U.S. Department of Education. (1987). *Ninth annual report to Congress on the implementation of the Education of the Handicapped Act.* (Prepared by the Division of Innovation and Development, Office of Special Education Programs). Washington, DC: Author.

Wetherby, A., Cain, D., Yonclas, D., & Walker, V. (1988). Analysis of intentional communication of normal children from the prelinguistic to the multiword stage. *Journal of Speech and Hearing Research, 31,* 24–252.

Wetherby, A., & Prizant, B. (1989). The expression of communicative intent: Assessment guidelines. *Seminars in Speech and Language, 10,* 77–91.

Wetherby, A., & Prizant, B. (1992). Profiling young children's communicative competence. In S. Warren & J. Reichle (Eds.), *Perspective on communication and language intervention: Development, assessment, and intervention* (pp. 217–251). Baltimore: Paul H. Brookes.

Wetherby, A., & Prizant, B. (1993). *Communication and Symbolic Behavior Scales—Normed Edition.* Chicago: Applied Symbolix.

Wetherby, A., & Prutting, C. (1984). Profiles of communicative and cognitive-social abilities in autistic children. *Journal of Speech and Hearing Research, 27,* 364–377.

Wetherby, A., Yonclas, D., & Bryan, A. (1989). Communicative profiles of handicapped preschool children: Implications for early identification. *Journal of Speech and Hearing Disorders, 54,* 148–158.

Wing, L., Gould, J., Yeates, S., & Brierly, L. (1977). Symbolic play in severely mentally retarded and in autistic children. *Journal of Child Psychology and Psychiatry, 18,* 167–178.

42 / Sleep Disorders in Infants and Young Children

Klaus Minde

Introduction and Historical Perspective

The phenomenon of sleep and its disturbances has been of interest to clinicians and laypeople since time immemorial. In the Middle Ages, sleep was thought to be a "retreat" of the spirit from the body, permitting other spirits or supernatural forces to enter (Riley, 1985). Rational and scientific thinking changed this perception, and during the past 100 years, two major explanations for the necessity and meaning of sleep have been advanced. The popular one is the restorative theory. It was first developed in 1873 by Dr. William Hammond, a psychiatrist in New York, who defined the purpose of sleep as follows: "The state of general repose which accompanies sleep is of a special value to the organism in allowing the nutrition of the nervous tissue to go on at a greater rate than its destructive metamorphosis" (p. 9). He also stressed that for this reason, "in infants the necessity for sleep is much greater than in adults, and still more so in old persons" (p. 16). While we know today that the brain does not cease to function at night as Hammond suggested, contemporary evidence does support his restorative theory. It is now known, for example, that brain protein synthesis occurs more during sleep or in the customary sleeping periods (Adams, 1980) and that more amino acids are liberated in the late-evening hours than at any other time of the day (Oswald, 1980). In addition, there is evidence that an increase of slow waves during sleep brings about restoration of muscle (Griffin & Trinder, 1978) and that rapid eye movement (REM) sleep restores our emotional well-being (Moruzzi, 1966).

The other theory to explain sleep is often called the ethological or conservation theory. In essence, it states species survival depends on adaptation to the world at large and defense against predators. As this planet is dominated by a circadian rhythm of day and night and most species can find food only during one part of this cycle, it makes ethological sense for the organism to be inactive when feeding is inefficient. Dement (1972) and Kellerman (1981) extended this notion and suggested that the desire for protection against predators has created human beings' sleeping habits, with one person watching to keep others safe. Group sleeping, however, also reinforces bonding and requires a sense of trust in others. Kellerman feels that the fear of losing this protection is the basic cause underlying most sleep disorders. This association between the state of one's relationships and the quality of one's sleep is, of course, the basis of the psychoanalytic and psychodynamic understanding and treatment of sleep problems in children and adults.

The dialogue between those who see sleep solely as a restorative function of the central nervous system and those who understand it to have significant psychological meaning is, as will be seen later, reflected in the way clinicians and parents alike have always diagnosed and treated sleep problems.

This chapter offers an overall summary of sleep problems in young children. First, the biology and development of sleep in young children is described. A discussion of various types of sleep disorders seen in young children, their epidemiology, etiology, and measurement follows. Then the clinical assessment of such a disorder and the impact of specific remedial measures on sleep and waking behaviors are outlined, illustrated by two case descriptions.

The Biology and Development of Sleep

The organization of sleep and waking states proceeds in an orderly fashion from birth onward. At term, infants on average sleep 16.5 hours per 24 hours. This decreases to 14.25 hours at 6 months, 13.75 at 12 months, and 13 hours at 2 years per 24 hours (Ferber, 1985a). At the same time, nocturnal sleep increases from 8 hours at birth to 11 hours at 12 months and 2 years. The sleep state is generally subdivided into periods of active (REM) sleep and quiet (non–rapid eye movement, or NREM) sleep. Cycles of active and quiet sleep alternate regularly (Kleitman, 1963). Newborn infants go from waking into active sleep for 15 to 20 minutes and then into quiet sleep for 8 to 10 minutes (Dreyfus-Brisac, 1979; Parmelee & Stern, 1972). As they mature, their active sleep becomes proportionately shorter, decreasing to 43% at 3 months and 30% of total sleep time by 12 months (Anders, Keener, Bowe, & Shioff, 1983). During the second part of the first year, infants also begin to move from waking to quiet sleep, the pattern observed in adults. At that time they also tend to move less rapidly from REM to NREM sleep (Anders et al., 1983).

While the appropriate development of the ascending reticular formation as well as pontine and forebrain structures are essential for the regulation of REM and NREM sleep, the infant by 12 to 16 weeks gradually acquires other building blocks needed to develop a circadian rhythm. These include appreciation of a day and night cycle as well as the timing of meals or contacts with caregivers (at some times but not at others). The presence of these two systems by 6 to 9 months suggests that sleep patterns of children older than that are qualitatively different from those of neonates. The literature confirms this and suggests that 70% of normal infants sleep through the night by 3 months, increasing to between 78 and 90% by 9 months (Anders, 1979; Moore & Ucko, 1957).

Sleep Disorders

EPIDEMIOLOGY AND MEASUREMENT

Sleep disorders are periodically classified by a special committee of the American Sleep Disorders Association. The last such classification took place in 1990 (Diagnostic Classification Steering Committee, 1990). The recommendations of this committee have been incorporated into the fourth edition of the *Diagnostic and Statistical Manual of Mental Disorders* (*DSM-IV*; American Psychiatric Association, 1994). They focus primarily on sleep disorders in adults, but modifications for pediatric populations have been published (Sheldon, Spire, & Cory, 1992). In general, *DSM-IV* differentiates between disorders of initiating or maintaining sleep (DIMS), also called dyssomnias, (e.g., primary insomnias or hypersomnias, narcolepsy and the sleep-wake schedule disorders, or, using *DSM-IV* terminology, circadian rhythm sleep disorders); and dysfunctions associated with sleep, sleep stages, or partial arousals, also called parasomnias (e.g., sleepwalking, nightmares, or sleep terror disorders).

Some of these disorders (e.g., parasomnias) are rarely seen in infants. Others, such as the insomnias, are common, although estimates of their incidence vary somewhat among investigators because of different definitions of the term *sleep disorder.* Moore and Ucko (1957) defined a good sleeper as an infant who slept without removal from the crib from midnight to 5 A.M. for at least 4 weeks. These authors concluded that 70% of their normative sample of 160 children fulfilled this criterion by 3 months and almost 90% by 9 months. Jenkins and Bax, who followed 360 infants in a central borough of London at specific intervals for 2 years, found that about 20% of their children woke regularly at night (Jenkins, Bax, & Hart, 1980). In a later follow-up report, these same authors provide interesting data on the persistence of sleep problems (Jenkins, Bax, & Hart, 1984). They found that 50 to 70% of poor sleepers at 6, 12, and 18, 30, or 36 months continued to have problems at the next appointment 6 or 12 months later. However, only 20% of children who showed sleep problems at age 6 months still exhibited them at 3 years. Similarly, Beltramini and Hertzig (1983), analyzing the sleep and bedtime behavior of 133 children in the New York Longitudinal Study, directed by Thomas and Chess, reported that 30% of them woke up one or more times every night during the first 4 years of life. More recent studies from Israel and New Zealand confirm these figures (Scher, Tirosh, Jaffe, & Rubin, 1987; Wooding, Boyd, & Geddis, 1990).

All these data are based on parental reports, and there has long been concern about the accuracy of this information. Specifically, two forms of error may distort the estimate of disturbed sleep patterns in children: First, parents may base their judgment on the time an infant wakes up but fail to consider when he or she fell asleep. In other words, an infant who sleeps from 7 P.M. to 2 A.M. may be labeled a "night waker" while the baby who sleeps from 10:30 P.M. to 5:30 A.M. is considered to "sleep through." Yet both infants have an uninterrupted sleep period of 7 hours. Second, many parents either do not notice or do not feel disturbed by their children's night waking (Scott & Richards, 1990). Clearly, an accurate recording system of sleep behavior and well-operationalized clinical criteria are needed to determine the presence and severity of a specific sleep problem.

Richman and her colleagues (1981, 1985) have done much to develop a recording system to define the type and severity of sleep disorders seen in young children. They developed a parental diary in which parents are asked to report the following types of information for 1 week: (1) the time the child went to bed at night; (2) the time he or she went to sleep; (3) the times he or she woke up during the night; (4) the time the child went to sleep again; (5) the frequency with which the parents took the child into their bed; and (6) the time the child woke up in the morning. At the end of the week, the scores are combined, giving the average number or lengths of wakings per night. Each of the 6 items is then rated on a scale of 0 to 4, allowing a Composite Sleep Score of 0 to 24. Richman considers that a score of 12 and above reflects a serious sleep problem if, according to the parents, the child has displayed this behavior for more than 3 months.

This procedure was used to assess the sleep patterns of 771 children ages 1 to 2 years in a London suburb (Richman, 1981). Twenty percent of these children were found to wake up 5 or more times per week. When considering only those who woke up 3 or more times per night, were awake for more than 20 minutes per night, or went into their parents' bed, 9.5% of all these children fulfilled these criteria.

In a later study of 705 3-year-old children, Richman and her colleagues found that 12.1% of the children had difficulties in settling at night, and 14.5% woke at least 3 times per week (Richman, Stevenson, & Graham, 1982). When a subgroup of 94 behavior-disordered youngsters was compared with 91 matched normal controls, the rate of difficulties for settling as well as waking at age 3 was found to be about double (28.7%) among the behavior-disordered children. At age 8, two thirds of the controls and all of the behavior-disordered children who had displayed difficulties in settling at age 3 still showed the same problems. In fact, difficulties in settling at night showed the second highest consistency out of 20 behaviors rated both at the ages of 3 and 8 years in this sample (Richman et al., 1982, p. 91).

In a more recent investigation of a representative sample of 432 German children at ages 5, 20, and 56 months, Wolke obtained very similar results. Thus, 21.5% of children had night waking problems at 5 months, 21.8% at 20 months, and 13.3% at 56 months. One in 4 of 5-year-olds slept regularly in the bed with their parents. Children with night-waking problems had a 2.2 to 2.5-fold increased risk to remain night wakers from one assessment point to the next compared with nonwakers (Wolke, Meyer, Ohrt, & Riegel, 1994).

Scott and his colleagues published the latest estimate of sleep disorders, involving 1,500 1- to 2-year-old children in England (Scott & Richard, 1990). They found that 25% of all 1- to 2-year-old children woke up at least 5 times per week but that only half of these children's mothers considered this to be a serious problem. Not settling at night for more than 30 minutes was the second most common complaint in this sample. It occurred in about 10% of all the children, and in 70% of them it was associated with night wakings. Very early waking, which occurred more frequently in homes where two or more children shared a bedroom, was mentioned least often as a problem.

Very recent work by my own team has added new insights to some of these findings (Minde et al., 1993). We employed a time-lapse infrared video camera in the homes of 30 children with a severe sleep disorder, age's 12 to 36 months, and 28 controls. We compared various sleep parameters as they were reported by the parents and seen on videotape. Our study revealed that parents of poor sleepers recorded on average 2.7 wakings per night while the video camera recorded 3.6 wakings. At the same time, mothers of good sleepers reported them to wake up only 0.5 times per night while film records revealed a surprising average of 3.2 wakings. In other words, there was no difference in the incidence of interrupted sleep experienced by these children. The difference was that the "good sleepers" managed to go back to sleep without waking up their parents. Hence,

494

TABLE 42.1

Factors Associated with Difficulties in Settling and Nighttime Wakings

Type of Problem	Etiological Factors
Disorders of initiating or maintaining sleep (DIMS), or dyssomnias	Mental retardation Epilepsy Medication (e.g., barbiturates, benzodiazepines) Obstructive sleep apnea Social factors Inconsistent limit setting Anxieties and fears Excessive fluid intake at night
Disorders of excessive sleep, or hypersomnia	Mental retardation Obstructive sleep apnea Deprivation and loss
Parasomnias	Family history of sleepwalking or night terrors
Circadian rhythm sleep disorders	Irregular bedtimes Inappropriate bedtimes

it appears that a well-functioning circadian control system requires good state regulation—that is, that the child manages him- or herself when sleep is interrupted (Brazelton, 1984).

In summary, the aforementioned review suggests that:

1. The overall incidence of poor sleepers under 3 years is about 15%.
2. Of children who have problems settling or waking up at 6 months, 80 to 90% will outgrow them within the next 12 to 18 months.
3. Children who have major sleep problems at 36 months are more likely to continue to show these problems in the future, with more than half still manifesting them 5 years later.
4. Children with major sleep problems also have a higher rate of behavior difficulties.
5. A certain number of children wake up several times per night but can get themselves back to sleep without disturbing anyone and hence are not considered problem sleepers.

logical factors within the infant can be differentiated from those that are associated with factors in the infant's environment. The latter category includes the effects of particular medications as well as social and psychological factors, such as parental feelings of anxiety that may be transmitted to young children. Nevertheless, in many cases, environmental stresses act in conjunction with biological vulnerabilities to cause a sleep disturbance in a young child.

Table 42.1 summarizes the most important etiological factors as they affect the dyssomnias, hypersomnias, parasomnias, and circadian rhythm sleep disorders. The table lists only the more common conditions.

Biological Factors Causing Sleep Disorders

MENTAL HANDICAP AND EPILEPSY

There is reason to believe that every type of sleep problem is seen more commonly in children with mental and physical handicaps. Yet in a recent annotation, Stores (1992) points out that despite this apparent association, few studies actu-

Etiology

The causes of sleep disorders in young children are complex and only partially understood. In general, however, sleep problems related to bio-

ally have examined this phenomenon in detail. Nevertheless, there is evidence that intellectually delayed children have a lower percentage of REM sleep and fewer eye movements during REM sleep (i.e., low REM density) (Grubar, 1983). Other authors have pointed out that such children have abnormal sleep spindle activity—sleep spindles may be less common or even absent or are unusually distributed. Spindles are normally seen in Stage 2 of NREM sleep (Shibagaki, Kiyono, & Watanabe, 1982). However, there is no obvious correlation between the type of pathology of the brain function and specific sleep disturbances.

Examining the incidence of disturbed sleep in 155 severely retarded children, Clements, Wing, and Dunn (1986) reported that 56% of the under-5 age group had sleep problems, consisting of frequent night wakings, difficulties in settling, and excessive sleep durations. Nighttime waking was associated with self-injurious behavior during the day. In a study of children up to age 16 with Down syndrome, Quine (1991) found that 44% had sleep problems, but gives no details.

Children with other disorders associated with a mental handicap also have been observed to suffer from sleep problems. For example, in unpublished research from 1992, A. Hunt found settling difficulties in 6 to 8%, night waking in 58%, and early waking in 57% of 201 children with tuberous sclerosis. Most of these children also had seizures. Quine (1991), in the abovementioned study, also showed epilepsy to be associated with severe sleeping problems and suggested that it may, in fact, be one of the contributors to sleep problems in children with other neurological diagnoses. According to Stores (1992), epilepsy is most commonly associated with a reduction of REM sleep, an increase of wakefulness after sleep onset, and unstable sleep states. However, as barbiturates and benzodiazepines, the most frequently used therapeutic agents for seizure disorder, also reduce REM sleep, they may well contribute to the poor sleep pattern of such youngsters (Espie & Tweedie, 1991). Other authors have pointed out that children with cerebral palsy also more frequently have obstructive sleep apnea and show a decreased ability to change body position, which can contribute to disturbed sleep (Kotagal, Gibbons, & Stith, 1994). On the other hand, since organically compromised children have more psychiatric disorders and more stressed parents, problem sleep behavior in these youngsters may also, at least partially, result from compromised or inappropriate parent-child interactions.

NIGHT TERRORS, CONFUSIONAL AROUSALS, AND SLEEPWALKING

Night terrors, confusional arousals, and sleepwalking usually are described as parasomnias, that is, disorders of arousal. They occur during Stage 4 of NREM sleep and are seen most commonly in children ages 5 to 12. They are more frequent in males and run in families. However, there is evidence that toddlers do suffer from night terrors and that true sleepwalking can occur in a toddler confined to a crib (Ferber, 1985b). Clinically, these children present no problem at bedtime but wake crying after 1 to 3 hours and seem inconsolable. Since intense crying, poor responsiveness, and the inability to report dream content are expected at this age, such an event may be misdiagnosed as a bad dream or as another waking. The incidence of this condition in toddlers is not well established, although in one study 9% of 200 mothers with 2½-year-old children considered night terrors and/or sleepwalking to be a problem (Roberts & Schoellkopf, 1951).

OBSTRUCTIVE SLEEP APNEA (OSA)

Obstructive sleep apnea is caused by a collapse of the upper airway following a forceful inspiration against relaxed oropharyngeal muscles during sleep. The sudden hypoxemia disrupts both the sleep pattern and brain metabolism of the infant and also may lead to excessive daytime somnolence. Such children have problems breathing while sleeping (96%), snore excessively (93%), or have direct apneas observed by their parents (80%). Other signs are an overly restless sleep (74%), frequent wakenings (60%), and excessive daytime somnolence and irritability (32%). The condition occurs most frequently in infants who were born prematurely, in children with large tonsils, or in those who have a reduced muscle tone (Hansen, 1987).

BEHAVIORAL ORGANIZATION

The concept of behavioral organization derives from the observation that, from birth onward, children respond to environmental stimuli in an individual style. While some infants react strongly to noise or touch, others are more easily stimulated by smell or by certain textures. The quality of an infant's reaction to stimuli also varies. For example, some infants are less able to cope with normal motor or autonomic stimulation than other; they respond to routine touches by gagging, gasping, or twitching (Als, 1989). It appears as if they are overwhelmed by the stimuli and respond to them in a global, disorganized fashion. While the precise etiology of this condition is not known, medically and neurologically compromised infants are affected more often.

Greenspan and Porges (1984) have extended the concept of behavioral organization to include all the filtering and processing of perceptions and experiences done by the central nervous system in day-to-day life. They have extended the concept of behavioral organization to include all the filtering and processing of perceptions and experiences done by the central nervous system in day-to-day life. In a recently developed diagnostic classification for infants (Zero to Three, 1994), Greenspan and his colleagues identified a group of infants who showed three types of regulatory disorders: hypersensitive infants who can present clinically as either fearful and cautious or negative and defiant; underreactive infants, presenting as either withdrawn and difficult to engage or as self-absorbed; and motorically disorganized, impulsive infants. These infants will have difficulty in processing experiences smoothly, and they will show this difficulty early on in life by being colicky or by having difficulties in organizing their sleep-wake rhythms. Sleep disturbances are common in this population.

OTHER MEDICAL CONDITIONS

Medical conditions outside those just mentioned are rarely responsible for chronic nighttime sleep disruption. However, chronic gastrointestinal and otolaryngeal problems (e.g, gastroesophageal reflux) can at times cause sleep problems, as can chronic otitis.

MEDICATION

Medication can be a source of sleep disturbance for adults and children alike. Drugs with sedating properties, given in an attempt to calm, may have paradoxical effects in children and may hinder their sleep. Nonsedating medication also can disrupt sleep. Bronchodilators (particularly methylxanthine derivatives) and other stimulants are especially problematic as they frequently upset normal sleep patterns.

EXCESSIVE NOCTURNAL FLUID

Intake of excessive fluid at night is common in infancy. Parents report that the child has frequent nighttime wakings and needs 4 to 8 ounces of fluid before being able to go back to sleep. Often the child also has been fed just before bedtime. While parents usually think that the nighttime feedings are in response to an existing sleep disorder, Ferber and Boyle (1983) suggest that more often the feeding itself is the cause of the disorder. Awakenings may be increased because of wetting, learned expectations of feeding, gastrointestinal effects of additional fluid intake, and a disruption of the basic circadian rhythm due to multiple arousals.

Psychological Factors Causing Sleep Disorders

Writers of the psychoanalytic school have long considered sleep disturbances to be a reflection of anxiety and other inner conflicts brought about by problematic parenting. Fraiberg (1950) describes a number of cases in which she felt sleep problems were caused by specific developmental conflicts between infants and their parents. In a long chapter Sperling (1969) saw poor sleep in infants as a first indication of severe later neurotic and possibly even psychotic disturbances. Herzog (1980) reported on a number of toddlers who developed sleep problems after the loss of a loved person. However, none of these reports was based on empirical investigations, and the type and severity of these children's sleep problems were not assessed.

Others have viewed sleep disorders as an interaction between developmental vulnerabilities and specific parental characteristics. For example, Carey (1974), in a study of 60 6- to 12-month-old infants from his consulting practice, found that those 25% who frequently woke up during the night scored significantly lower on the sensory threshold scale of his 9 temperament assessment scales than did good sleepers. He thought that this reflected difficulties these children had keeping outside noises from waking them up. Richman (1981) and Richman et al. (1985) also cite a significant association between sleep problems and a history of perinatal adversity. According to their data on 771 1- to 2-year-old children, nearly 35% of 90 sleep-disordered children were born by cesarean section or had experienced transient asphyxia or other perinatal adversities. On the other hand, it was also found that 38% of the mothers of the poor sleepers had neurotic symptoms and 50% did not confide in their husbands, double the expected rate for the normal population. Lozoff and her group (1984, 1985) made similar suggestions. In a study of 96 toddlers, they found that 85% of mothers with poorly sleeping children were ambivalent toward their infants and 46% had a depressed mood. Among mothers of well-sleeping toddlers, only 35 and 19% of mothers of well-sleeping toddlers showed these characteristics.

Our own data on 28 poor and 30 good sleepers confirm these reports (Minde et al., 1993). Fifty-three percent of our poor sleepers versus 27% of the good sleepers had experienced perinatal problems, including a cesarean section. Poor sleepers also suffered significantly longer from colic (1.7 versus 0.3 months) and more had a difficult temperament (46% versus 13%). Their mothers scored higher on a Malaise Inventory (4.6 versus 2.9) and had more often had previous contacts with a psychiatrist (43% versus 20%). While the reports by Lozoff and Richman are not clear about the direction of the relationship between

the maternal psychological difficulties and their young children's irregular sleep patterns, our data clearly indicate that the mothers' problems preceded those of their infants (Minde et al., 1993). For example, maternal contact with mental health professionals always preceded the birth of the sleep-disturbed infant. Furthermore, in a parallel study by Benoit, Zeanah, Boucher, and Minde (1992), a subgroup of the same mothers ($n = 41$) was administered the Adult Attachment Interview, a structured interview designed to measure an adult's internal working model of attachment (George, Kaplan & Main, unpublished manuscript, 1985). The interviewer inquires about the adult's recollections of early relationships with attachment figures, such as rejections, separations, parental responsiveness, losses, and other relevant attachment experiences. The interview is audiotaped, and verbatim transcripts are rated on seven 9-point scales, measuring the adult's probable experience with his or her attachment figures and his or her current "state of mind" with regard to attachment. In this study, all the mothers of young children with sleep problems were classified as insecurely attached to their own mothers compared with 57% of mothers in the control group. Thus, in this study, mothers whose internal working models of attachment were autonomous/secure were much less likely to have a sleep-disordered infant than were mothers with insecure models. This finding supports the notion that the mother's psychological structures in some way influence how she manages her child's bedtime routines.

SOCIAL FACTORS

Children learn to associate the transition from waking to sleeping time with certain outside events. For example, bedtime may follow a bath, a special story, and a kiss for the teddy bear. Such a routine allows a toddler who as yet has no concept of time to predict the upcoming bedtime—in other words, to feel more in control of his or her life. This sense of control, in turn, eases the separation associated with going to bed and helps the child to sleep. If bedtime routines never get established, settling for sleep can be affected. The same is true if the crib or bed is used as a place for punishment during the day. Sleep problems also can be the result of irregular bedtimes or regular but inappropriate sleep-wake schedules (e.g., putting a toddler to bed at 6 P.M. before he is tired).

EMOTIONAL DEPRIVATION AND LOSS

Children who experience a chronic lack of care often seek out their bed and sleep excessively. It appears as if they try to combat the insensitive caregiving they experience by regressing and using the bed or the sleep process to compensate for shortcomings in their lives. Infants or toddlers who have experienced an acute loss, such as a change of placement, also may exhibit excessively long sleep times. Sleep here becomes a sign of mourning and grief.

In summary then, there is a good deal of evidence that:

1. Sleep disorders in young children can be the result of biological vulnerabilities and/or a sign of a compromised behavioral organization.
2. Sleep problems in children frequently are not identical to the insomnias described in adult populations; frequently the children do not *want* to sleep, while the adults *cannot* sleep.
3. More than in adults, sleep patterns in children reflect the relationship they have with their primary caregivers and others living with them.

The Evaluation of Sleep Disorders

GENERAL CONSIDERATIONS

The evaluation of a family with a sleep-disordered child is complex and must be carried out with tact and sensitivity. In many such families, disturbed nights have been a chronic condition that has existed for several months. These parents and children often present as exhausted, irritable, and feeling helpless. On the other hand, often they are motivated for treatment and prepared to follow advice offered to them if it is within their capabilities.

Some parents express feelings of guilt and anxiety when they talk about wishing to have their evenings to themselves, rather than needing constantly to cuddle their infant or to give the child drinks in the middle of the night. They also may be anxious or overprotective and try to avoid upsetting the child in any possible way. They may be used to checking on the baby frequently because of worries about the child's health; paradoxically by dint of doing so, they interfere with settling patterns.

Our experience suggests that the evaluation of a youngster's sleep problem should be done in the presence of both parents. This establishes from the outset that the child's sleep difficulty is a family matter and gives the interviewer the opportunity to assess both the sleep problem and other family issues.

PROBLEM ANALYSIS

The following questions are useful in assessing a sleep disorder and are based on the Sleep Management Manual developed by Douglas and Richman (1984).

Bedtime and Settling to Sleep: Questions here refer to details about the bedtime of the patient. Is there a bedtime routine? When does this child start getting ready for bed? Where and and at what time does the child fall asleep in the evening and how does the parent gets him or her to settle? For example, does the child fall asleep in mother's arms or in his or her own bed, or has the child any special ways of settling self, such as using a pacifier or a thumb? Does the child come out of the room after being settled? What do parents do at that time?

Waking at Night: It is important to know how many times the child wakes per night and how often it happens per week. How do the parents react to these wakings, who can settle the child more quickly, how long does it take the child to settle again, and how often does he or she end up in the parents' bed?

Daytime Naps: It is important to inquire about daytime naps, their length, and how settling occurs at that time.

Attempted Previous Solutions: Exploration should be directed toward how long the problem has gone on, especially since children show normal variations in sleep patterns; difficulties of less than 3 months' duration do occur in many normal children. What do the parents think started the problem? For example, had there been a particular illness or did the child receive medications? Have the parents consulted other professionals or used sleep medication or particular behavioral methods to calm their youngster?

Other Behavior: We want to know how the youngster behaves during waking hours and whether problems are exhibited then as well. For example, is the child miserable during the day, or can the child amuse him- or herself and get along with others? Has the child been enrolled in any play group or nursery? What are his or her relationships with other children?

The parents are always asked to fill out a sleep diary before the following appointment. (See Table 42.2.) The purpose of this diary is not so much to demand absolute accuracy as to focus the parents' attention on the *behavior.* Such a diary is also helpful in assessing the benefit of specific intervention strategies during treatment.

FAMILY BACKGROUND DATA

It is essential to obtain some objective information about general aspects of the patient's family life—mother, and father's personal background, some account of the families of origin, parents' work, how involved father is in the care of the family, and whether the parents can confide in each other or not. We also want to know about the parents' methods of discipline, their ways of having fun, and their thoughts and ideas about the character and underlying personality of the baby.

OBSERVING THE PARENT-CHILD RELATIONSHIP

Once the formal sleep assessment interview with the parents has been done, it is advisable to evaluate the overall relationship of the infant with his or her caregivers. The rationale here is that difficulties in settling or night sleeping behavior usually also show themselves during daytime interactions between the child and caregivers. Empirical investigations support this association (Minde et al., 1994). Furthermore, these studies suggest that observations of interactions in which parents are encouraged to do things with their babies are most revealing in identifying relationship difficulties in sleep-disordered children.

To learn about the parent-child relationship, it is best to observe the primary caregiver and the problem sleeper both during a free play period and again while they are engaged in a more structured task. This period does not need to exceed 10 minutes for reliable results. The structured task may consist of a having a snack, looking at a book, building something together, or demanding that the older toddler clean up after the playtime. The latter situation often provides especially valuable data because the caregiver-infant dyad is under greater pressure. When looking at the actual behaviors, the interactions of poor sleepers often are characterized by difficulties in the following areas:

1. Joint attention or engagement. The partners are not focused on the same activity or event.
2. Overall reciprocity. There is little verbal dialogue or turn-taking activity in which both partners are engaged in a mutually responsive way.
3. The overall organization or regulation of interactions. The timing and pace of the interactive events between child and parents may not be comprehensible to the observer, since members of the dyad do not participate in and regulate each other's activity.
4. State similarity. The parent's and child's activity levels are poorly matched, as are their moods.
5. General mood during the interaction. Expressions of anger or excessive control appear in either child or caregiver during the play activities. Thus, the parent may attempt to appease the child by not sticking to reasonable demands.

The presence of one or more of these interactive difficulties suggests that the parent finds it hard to set age-appropriate limits. This failure may have a specific motive (e.g., mother may like to have her infant for company in preference to her husband or as replacement during husband's absence), or it may be related to past events in the mother's life.

TABLE 42.2
Sleep Diary

Date: _____

	MONDAY	TUESDAY	WEDNESDAY	THURSDAY	FRIDAY	SATURDAY	SUNDAY
Time went to bed in the evening							
Time went to sleep in the evening							
Time(s) woke during the night							
Time(s) went to sleep again							
How you handled night waking(s)							
Time woke in the morning							
Time of nap(s)							
Time you went to bed							

We find it useful to meet with both parents after these initial evaluations in order to review our findings and assess their willingness to engage in treatment.

The Treatment of Sleep Disorders

After one or two evaluative interviews and a 2-week period in which parents have filled in the sleep diary, we normally begin our treatment sessions. These sessions should include both father and mother and be held at times that are convenient to the work schedules of both. Techniques used for changing children's sleep behavior generally depend on the orientation of the therapist, although most agree that medications are not useful to help children in organizing their sleep. Thus, there are those who suggest children should just cry it out (Spock & Rothenberg, 1985), and others who use a primarily behavioral management approach (Douglas & Richman, 1984). The treatment approach we suggest is based on a behavioral model but acknowledges the dynamic implications of symptoms and behavioral changes. Initially, for example, this means that parents need to be assured that a child who is well loved and stimulated during the day will not be damaged or feel rejected if his or her parents set clear limits about sleep behavior at night.

The general aim of our treatment approach is not necessarily to get the children to sleep more or wake up less often but to teach them to manage their sleep behavior independently without disturbing their parents' sleep. As mentioned earlier, in many young children wake up several times during the night, but they can be encouraged to settle themselves down to sleep again without requiring their parents' presence.

An important aspect of this treatment philosophy is that it does not prescribe how children should behave at night—how many hours of sleep they should get or whether they should sleep in a crib or a regular bed. It is the parents who decide what aspect of the sleep disturbance should be tackled initially. For example, some parents do not mind having their children sleep with them at times, and for others, a midnight breast-feed is an important aspect of their comforting routine. Yet such parents may want to learn how to settle the baby without a fuss in the evening and to get the child to understand that they mean what they say. It is important, therefore, to discuss with parents in detail their hopes and expectations from treatment and to proceed only when there is agreement about the changes the family seeks.

Initially this approach usually precludes the treatment of marital or other psychological difficulties within the couple or the family. While this appears to contradict the substantial data that assert an association between sleep difficulties and various forms of parental psychopathology, we believe the parents' right to select a first target for change should be respected. Doing so often sets the stage for therapeutic suggestions to be heard and implemented so that change can occur. Furthermore, young children often respond very rapidly to minor modifications in their parents' behavior. This is especially likely if the ensuing behavior becomes developmentally more appropriate and/or represents a decrease in the distortions that had colored parental interpretations of the child's disturbed sleep behavior (Lieberman, 1992). For example, if a couple can accept their daughter's frequent waking as a reflection of her somewhat precarious ability to organize her level of arousal and no longer regard it as a hurtful attack on her mother's need to sleep, an entirely new sequence of parent-child transactions may come into being.

In terms of the actual treatment process, we proceed as follows.

Initially, and with an attitude of consistent, responsive support, the sleep difficulties are reviewed. These might include difficulties in first settling down to sleep or repeated awakening at various times during the night or both. This review allows the clinician to form an impression of the settling and bedtime routine of the family (if indeed there is one) and of the routines, interests, and predictability of the child's day in general. Any use the child makes of a transitional object should be noted. During this part of the evaluation, the clinician often can form an impression of the quality of parental motivation to change and of the character of areas of resistance. Often the clinician can sense disagreements between the parents about overall child-rearing practices or issues about the mother's involvement with her child. However, the clinician should not broaden the focus from the sleep behavior but rather try to find areas of agreement and disagreement around this issue.

If the daytime activities of the child (and family) do not occur in a predictable sequence, the therapist should offer information about toddlers' needs for a sense of control and how regular daytime activities can provide this. It is then recommended that the child's day be given a routine, with meals and naps at the same hour, in the same place.

Once daytime routines have been established, the parents are encouraged to create new rituals for bedtime. For example, where a bedtime feeding was part of the ritual, we suggest that this be removed in time and place from bedtime—that it take place earlier and downstairs.

Only then is the sleeping problem itself tackled. Recommendations depend on whether a helpmate (father) is available to the mother or not. Where father is available, it is strongly recommended that he take over most of the bedtime routine (with perhaps a small part of the ritual assigned to mother) or that he take over entirely the night awakenings. We have found that the great majority of fathers are most willing and even enthusiastic collaborators, and that it is often the mothers who seem doubtful, either of their husband's capacity to cope or of their own ability to tolerate the new arrangements.

If the parents agree to such changes, father's thoughts about how he might comfort the child are elicited. He is encouraged to try to keep the child in bed using pats, words, sips of water, and the like.

Parents are encouraged to start their program on a weekend, so that the stresses of work do not await them the next day. They are also warned that they might expect two to three uncomfortable nights but that they would likely see change by the third or fourth night.

In cases where the child cries consistently, it is suggested that the parent in charge of the settling procedure use the "checking" method, wherein the caregiver goes into the child's room and soothes him or her at various *regular* intervals, say every 5 to 10 minutes, until the child falls asleep. Often this is much more tolerable to parents than allowing the child to "cry it out."

If the "checking" approach seems too difficult

for a parent to accomplish on his or her own, a "shaping" technique is employed. For example, if the child was sleeping in mother's bed, she might first move with the child into the child's own bed, then proceed to sit up in the bed, move to sitting at the side of the bed, then move the chair farther away, and so on. This gradual approach provides the child with some externalized "holding," which in turn encourages him or her to find his or her own way of organizing overall behavior.

In our experience, an average of four sessions spaced over an 8-week period will significantly modify the sleep behavior of some 85% of troubled toddlers. Follow-up interviews up to 6 months after the end of treatment reveal virtually no relapses; indeed, there is continuing improvement in the child's overall behavior. Treatment failures occur most often in families where the parents are either unable to establish any kind of routines, or where the problem is only one aspect of ongoing marital discord or other major family disorganization. In addition, the unwillingness of a father or helpmate to participate in restructuring the nighttime routines often spells failure for the treatment. On the other hand, a successful resolution of sleep problems can create a positive impetus to change other troublesome behaviors these children may display. For example, our own work documents that infants ages 12 to 36 months who have overcome their sleep problems after four counseling sessions show much improved interactions with their parents during daytime play and feeding episodes (Minde et al., 1994). This fact suggests that caregivers who learn how to deal with conflict around sleep inadvertently translate these new-skills into their daytime interactions with their child.

CASE EXAMPLES

Case 1: James S.: James was 15 months old at the time of his first interview. His mother began by comparing James's sleep pattern to that of his older brother, Mathew, age 3. Mathew had slept through the night from age 6 months and had never given them any trouble, while James had never slept longer than 4 hours since birth. He had a pattern now of initially sleeping for 4 hours at night and of then waking up every hour thereafter.

Usually in the evening, Mrs. S. would bathe her boys

together and then read a story to Mathew (with James present). After Mathew was in bed, she would carry James into his room, give him a bear and a blanket, then lie down with him and nurse him to sleep. This would usually take between 20 and 25 minutes. Whenever James awakened during the night, Mrs. S. would nurse him again, moving immediately to his bed when he first cried. Up until he was 7 months old, she had had him in her bed at all times. Since that arrangement had disrupted her husband's sleep, as well, she had set up a mattress on the floor for him in another room.

Mrs. S. had never allowed James to cry at all and always quieted him by nursing him. In fact, during the interview, James once walked over to his mother and gave a little knock on her breast. She responded immediately by nursing him, which calmed him, while he twiddled his hair in one hand and put his finger in his mother's mouth.

James naps between noon and 2 P.M. each day; many times this takes place in the car while Mrs. S. picks up Mathew from his nursery school. Occasionally he also sleeps in the late afternoon. This does not appear to affect his sleep at night.

Mr. S. seldom hears James at night, but "once in a blue moon" he will put James to sleep while patting him on the back.

Mrs. S. finds that, without enough sleep herself, she reacts increasingly angrily toward her older boy, Mathew. This has disturbed her and reminded her that as a child, she had great difficulty in falling asleep herself.

Mrs. S. understands James's awakening as an attachment to the particular comfort of nursing at the breast and comments that he has always refused bottles, fingers, or pacifiers. On the other hand, she also sees that his nursing has become a habit rather than being an intense need.

The family history reveals Mrs. S. to be a 39-year old university graduate with an MBA. At 21, she married a U.S. draft dodger but left him after 2 years. She then joined a major bank and within 5 years had become the manager of their international money market operation. Six years ago she married her present husband, a lawyer, who has his own computer consulting firm. She became pregnant shortly thereafter but had a miscarriage. A year later Mathew was born and finally James. Since the birth of Mathew, Mrs. S. has been a full-time mother.

Mr. S. is 41 years old and a lawyer. He has many active hobbies, playing hockey on 3 to 4 nights during the winter and other sports during the summer. He also takes piano and flying lessons.

Treatment Summary: There were 4 interviews, stretching over a 7-week period. Both husband and wife attended all sessions.

In the first interview, there was a tremendous contrast in the couple's appearance and manner. Mrs. S. looked very tired and was dressed in an old parka and mud-covered boots. Mr. S., on the other hand, looked clean, crisp, and alert and was dressed neatly in a dark, formal business suit. While the couple appeared distant during the discussion, Mr. S. was very willing to be part of treatment, and both parents agreed on a plan for James. He would get a new crib; Mrs. S. would nurse James in a rocker beside the crib at bedtime and again at 11 P.M. Thereafter, when he cried during the night, father would go in and reassure him every 15 minutes but would not allow him to get out of the crib.

During the second interview, 2 weeks later, the parents reported that they had carried through their plan but that sickness in the family had interfered to a degree. Yet mother had stuck to her twice-nightly nursing episodes. Lately, the night wakings had decreased from 7 to about 4 and Mr. S. had not taken James out of his bed anymore.

During the third interview, Mrs. S. described the past 2 weeks as a "kind of mixed period." Mr. S. felt that some setbacks were due to his wife's getting away from the habit of putting James down awake. Mrs. S. then described how difficult it was to get James to nap during the day, and how he would do this only in the car. When her husband commented that James would go down for a nap with a bottle, Mrs. S. replied that children get their teeth "rotted out" with bottles. She then said warningly to Mr. S. that James would be weaned only gradually.

During the fourth interview, 3 weeks later, the parents reported that James now slept from about 11:00 P.M. to his early-morning awakening between 5:30 and 6:30 A.M. Mother also reported that he now had a few temper tantrums and was nursing less frequently during the day. Both parents felt they had gone as far in settling James as they could right now. They decided to end treatment at this point, expressing great satisfaction with the results.

Discussion: This case displays some aspects commonly encountered in families with sleep-disordered children. The S. family is a good example of parents who have had children late in life, where mother may try, with the help of her child, to make up for certain hardships and deprivations she has experienced in her own early life. Her abrupt shift from the role of a bank executive to that of a full-time mother, on the one hand, and father's high activity pattern, on the other may signify difficulties the couple have in taking on the parental role and maintaining a sense of intimacy with each other. Mother also showed great difficulty in being authoritative and needed much support in setting limits for this youngster. While the struggle between James and his parents in the S. household continues, there is a sense that the boy has begun to have more control over his behavior and is on his way to a greater degree of individuation and autonomy.

Case 2: Maria M.: Maria, 22 months, was brought to the infant clinic because she was becoming increasingly difficult to settle at night and was demanding more and more stories, drinks of water, or other types of attention. She had learned to "throw up on command" and would do it within seconds whenever her parents refused to attend to her wishes, for example, if they insisted that there was no more story or drink now. The vomiting demanded at least 30 minutes of cleaning-up time, which Maria "seemed to relish." As Maria was able to perform this feat 2 to 3 times per night, both parents were increasingly angry and exhausted but felt helpless in dealing with their daughter.

Maria was the older of two children of a middle-class family. Her mother came from a warm and nurturing family and had worked as a secretary prior to her marriage. She now worked only two days per week, and the family had a trusted full-time housekeeper. Father also claimed that his early life had been untroubled. He worked as a government consultant and appeared to enjoy his family.

Maria was born following a normal pregnancy and had achieved all her milestones at a normal age. She had begun to sleep through the night at 9 months and seemed to have weathered the arrival of her brother 7 months ago without untoward symptoms.

Her present sleep disturbance started 4 months ago, after she had developed a fever, accompanied by diarrhea and vomiting. The parents felt that those episodes of vomiting had "taught her" how to do it.

Treatment Summary: There were three interviews, stretching over a 6-week period. Husband and wife attended all sessions.

In the first interview, Maria came with her parents and actively engaged in playing with the available toys. Both parents were proud of her cognitive achievements. Mother, however, complained a great deal about her own lack of sleep and how, rather than getting up all the time to calm Maria down, she would more and more often permit the child to get into their bed during the night. At the end of the interview, the parents agreed that henceforth father would put Maria to bed. They were also instructed to move the night bottle from the bedroom into the living room and to give it to Maria 45 minutes before her actual bedtime. The parents also were eager to fill in a sleep diary to mark their overall progress. Father agreed to sit with Maria until she was asleep. He was not to engage her in any conversations or games but to function as a calm authority in an attempt to keep Maria relaxed and prevent her from vomiting.

During the second interview two weeks later, father reported that Maria had stopped vomiting. She was now willing to stay in bed on her own in the evening as long as he sat in front of her room with the door somewhat ajar. However, she would still come into her parents' bedroom at least twice a night. Moreover, every second night she would get into her parents' bed, as father did not always hear her and Mrs. M. was too tired to return her to her room. The family was told to carry on with their present regimen, although father was encouraged to take Maria back to her bed as soon as she arrived in her parents' bedroom.

At the third visit 2 weeks later, the parents reported that they initially had found it difficult to return Maria to her bed every night. Instead, they had demanded that she lie down on a blanket next to their bed and sleep there. Maria had done so without objection, and mother had then moved the blanket a little closer toward Maria's door every night. This had encouraged father the past weekend to take Maria and her blanket back to her bed on 4 different occasions. Since then, she had not gotten out of her bed again and now appeared to sleep through the night.

Discussion: In the M. family, the sleep disturbance may have indeed been triggered by Maria's illness and her accidental discovery of her power over her parents through vomiting. Their ingenious way of weaning the girl off her controlling behavior is a good example how parents, with minimal guidance, often can find developmentally appropriate ways to rectify minor developmental aberrations. It is of interest that both parents here came from sound backgrounds and had no trouble making use of the therapist's suggestions.

Summary and Conclusion

This chapter provides an overview of the epidemiology, development, and manifestations of abnormal sleep behaviors in children up to 36 months. It demonstrates that, like other behavioral disturbances in infancy, problems in sleeping often reflect a difficulty within the relationship of the infant with his or her caregivers. It also highlights the contribution biological vulnerabilities in specific developmental parameters, such as behavioral organization, can make to the form and type of symptoms displayed in this disorder. Finally, a treatment program for sleep-disturbed children is described which is based on an understanding of the dynamic and developmental needs of both infants and their caregivers.

REFERENCES

Adams, K. (1980). Sleep as a restorative process and theory to explain why. *Progress in Brain Research, 53*, 289–325.

Als, H. (1989). Self-regulation and motor development in preterm infants. In J. Lockman & N. Hazen (Eds.), *Action in social context. Perspectives on early development* (pp. 65–97). New York: Plenum Press.

American Psychiatric Association. (1994). *Diagnostic and statistical manual of mental disorders* (4th ed.). Washington, DC: Author.

Anders, T. F. (1979). Night waking in infants during the first year of life. *Pediatrics, 63*, 860–864.

Anders, T. F., Keener, M., Bowe, T. R., & Shioff, B. A. (1983). A longitudinal study of night-time sleep-wake patterns in infants from birth to one year. In J. D. Call & E. Galenson (Eds.), *Frontiers of infant psychiatry* (Vol. 1, pp. 150–166). New York: Basic Books.

Beltramini, A. U., & Hertzig, M. E. (1983). Sleep and bedtime behavior in preschool aged children. *Pediatrics, 71*, 153–158.

Benoit, D., Zeanah, C., Boucher, C., & Minde, K. (1992). Sleep disorders in early childhood: Association with insecure maternal attachment. *Journal of the American Academy of Child and Adolescent Psychiatry, 31*, 86–93.

Brazelton, T. B. (1984). *Neonatal Behavioral Assessment Scale.* London: Blackwell.

Carey, W. B. (1974). Night waking and temperament in infancy. *Journal of Pediatrics, 84*, 756–758.

Clements, J., Wing, L., & Dunn, G. (1986). Sleep problems in handicapped children: A preliminary study. *Journal of Child Psychology and Psychiatry, 27*, 399–407.

Dement, W. C. (1972). *Some must watch while some must sleep.* San Francisco: W. H. Freeman.

Diagnostic Classification Steering Committee, M. J. Thorpy (chair). (1990). *International classification of sleep disorders: Diagnostic and scoring manual.* Rochester, MN: American Sleep Disorders Association.

Douglas, J., & Richman, N. (1984). *My child won't sleep.* Harmondsworth: Penguin Books.

Dreyfus-Brisac, C. (1979). Ontogenesis of bioelectrical activity and sleep organization in neonates and infants. In F. Falkner & J. M. Tanner (Eds.), *Human growth* (Vol. 3, pp. 159–182). New York: Plenum Press.

Espie, C. A., & Tweedie, F. M. (1991). Sleep patterns and sleep problems amongst people with mental handicap. *Journal of Mental Deficiency Research, 35*, 25–36.

Ferber, R. (1985a). *Solve your child's sleep problem.* New York: Simon & Schuster.

Ferber, R. (1985b). Sleep disorders in infants and children. In T. L. Riley (Ed.), *Clinical aspects of sleep and sleep disturbance* (pp. 113–157). Boston: Butterworth.

Ferber, R., & Boyle, M. P. (1983). Nocturnal fluid intake: A cause of, not treatment for, sleep disruption in infants and toddlers. *Sleep Research, 12*, 243–249.

Fraiberg, S. (1950). On the sleep disturbances of early childhood. *Psychoanalytic Study of the Child, 5*, 285–309.

George, C., Kaplan, V., & Main, M. (1985). *The Berkeley Adult Attachment Interview.* Unpublished manuscript, University of California, Berkeley.

Greenspan, S. I., & Porges, S. W. (1984). Psychopathology in infancy and early childhood: Clinical perspectives on the organization of sensory and affective-thematic experience. *Child Development, 55*, 49–70.

Griffin, S. J., & Trinder, J. (1978). Physical fitness, exercise and human sleep. *Society Psychophysiological Research, 15*, 447–450.

Grubar, J. C. (1983). Sleep and mental deficiency. *Review of Electroencephalography and Neurophysiology, 13,* 107–114.

Hammond, W. H. (1873). *Sleep and its derangements.* Philadelphia: J. B. Lippincott.

Hansen, C. H. (1987). Obstructive sleep apnea. In A. M. Rudolph (Ed.), *Pediatrics* (18th ed., pp. 1378–1380) Norwalk, CT: Appleton & Lange.

Herzog, J. M. (1980). Sleep disturbances and father hunger in 18- to 20-month-old boys. *Psychoanalytic Study of the Child, 35,* 219–233.

Jenkins, S., Bax, M., & Hart, H. (1980). Behaviour problems in preschool children. *Journal of Child Psychology and Psychiatry, 21,* 5–17.

Jenkins, S., Bax, M., & Hart, H. (1984). Continuities of common behavior problems in preschool children. *Journal of Child Psychology and Psychiatry, 25,* 75–89.

Kellerman, H. (1981). *Sleep disorders: Insomnia and narcolepsy.* New York: Brunner/Mazel.

Kleitman, N. (1963). *Sleep and wakefulness.* Chicago: University of Chicago Press.

Kotagal, S., Gibbons, V. P., & Stith, J. A. (1994). Sleep abnormalities in patients with severe cerebral palsy. *Developmental Medicine and Child Neurology, 36*(4), 304–311.

Lieberman, A. F. (1992). Infant-parent psychotherapy with toddlers. *Developmental Psychopathology, 4,* 559–574.

Lozoff, B., Wolf, A. W., & Davis, N. S. (1984). Cosleeping in urban families with young children in the United States. *Pediatrics, 74,* 171–182.

Lozoff, B., Wolf, A. W., & Davis, N. S. (1985). Sleep problems in pediatric practice. *Pediatrics, 75,* 477–483.

Minde, K., Faucon, A., & Falkner, S. (1996). The effect of treating severe sleep disorders on their daytime behavior. *Journal of the American Academy of Child and Adolescent Psychiatry* 33: 1116–1121.

Minde, K., Popiel, K., Leos, N., Falkner, S., Parker, K., & Handley-Derry, M. (1993). The evaluation and treatment of sleep disturbances in young children. *Journal of Child Psychology and Psychiatry, 34,* 521–533.

Moore, T., & Ucko, L. E. (1957). Night waking in early infancy: Part 1. *Archives of Diseases in Childhood, 33,* 333–342.

Moruzzi, G. (1966). The functional significance of sleep with particular regard to the brain mechanisms underlying consciousness. In J. Eccles (Ed.), *Brain and conscious experience* (pp. 345–355). New York: Springer.

Oswald, I. (1980). Sleep as a restorative process: Human clues. *Progress in Brain Research, 53,* 279–288.

Parmelee, A. H., Jr., & Stern, E. (1972). Development of states in infants. In C. Clemente, D. Purpura, & F. Meyer (Eds.), *Sleep and the maturing nervous system* (pp. 199–228). New York: Academic Press.

Quine, L. (1991). Sleep problems in children with severe mental handicap. *Journal of Mental Deficiency Research, 35,* 269–290.

Richman, N. (1981). A community survey of the characteristics of the 1–2-year-olds with sleep disruptions. *Journal of the American Academy of Child Psychiatry, 20,* 281–291.

Richman, N. (1985). A double-blind drug trial of treatment in young children with waking problems. *Journal of Child Psychology and Psychiatry, 26,* 591–598.

Richman, N., Douglas, J., Hunt, H., Lansdown, R., & Levere, R. (1985). Behavioral methods in the treatment of sleep disorders—a pilot study. *Journal of Child Psychology and Psychiatry, 26,* 581–590.

Richman, N., Stevenson, J., & Graham, P. J. (1982). *Pre-school to school. A behavioral study.* New York: Academic Press.

Riley, T. L. (1985). Historical overview and introduction. In T. R. Riley (Ed.), *Clinical aspects of sleep and sleep disturbance* (pp. 1–7). New York: Butterworth.

Roberts, K. E., & Schoellkopf, J. A. (1951). Eating, sleeping and elimination practices of a group of two-and-one-half-year-old children. *American Journal of Diseases of Children, 82,* 121–152.

Scher, A., Tirosh, E., Jaffe, M., & Rubin, E. (1987). Survey of sleep patterns of Israeli infants and young children. *Sleep Research, 16,* 209.

Scott, G., & Richards, M. P. M. (1990). Night waking in one-year-old children in England. *Child: Care, Health and Development, 16,* 283–302.

Sheldon, S. H., Spire, J. P., & Cory, H. B. (1992). *Pediatric sleep medicine: Differential diagnosis.* Philadelphia: W. B. Saunders.

Shibagaki, M., Kiyono, S., & Watanabe, K. (1982). Spindle evolution in normal and mentally retarded children: A review. *Sleep, 5,* 47–57.

Sperling, M. (1969). Sleep disturbances in children. In J. G. Howells (Ed.), *Modern perspectives in international child psychiatry* (pp. 418–453). New York: Brunner/Mazel.

Spock, B., & Rothenberg, M. B. (1985). *Baby and child care.* New York: Pocket Books.

Stores, G. (1992). Annotation: Sleep studies in children with a mental handicap. *Journal of Child Psychology and Psychiatry, 33,* 1303–1317.

Wolke, D., Meyer, R., Ohrt, B., & Riegel, K. (1994). Incidence and persistence of problems at sleep onset and sleep continuation in the preschool period: Results of a prospective study of a representative sample in Bavaria. *Praxis der Kinderpsychologie und Kinderpsychiatrie, 43*(9), 331–339.

Wooding, A. R., Boyd, J., & Geddis, D.C. (1990). Sleep patterns of New Zealand infants during the first 12 months of life. *Journal of Pediatric Child Health, 26,* 85–88.

Zero to Three. (1994). *Diagnostic classification of mental health and developmental disorders of infancy and early childhood* (pp. 31–38). Washington, DC: Zero to Three—National Center for Clinical Infant Programs.

43 / Regulatory Disorders

Stanley I. Greenspan and Serena Wieder

A New Construct of Regulatory Disorders

Easy babies, fussy babies, quiet babies, self-scheduled babies, sensitive babies, don't-change-the-routine babies, pick-up-and-go babies—these are just a few examples of individual differences in self-regulation that reflect constitutional and maturational variations. Individual differences in sensory reactivity, self-regulation, and behavioral organization in infants have been recognized during the last two to three decades (DeGangi, Di-Pietro, Greenspan, & Porges, 1991; DeGangi, Porges, Sickel, & Greenspan, 1993; Doussard-Roosevelt, Walker, Portales, Greenspan, & Porges, 1990; Escalona, 1968; Greenspan, 1992).

Still, the work describing individual differences in self-regulation has not been integrated into our understanding of behavioral manifestations, symptoms, and problems in adaptation. Because an infant has a limited number of responses or behavioral patterns in relationship to various stresses or difficulties, there has always been considerable overlap in the behavioral symptoms signaling such difficulties. This chapter presents a new diagnostic construct of regulatory disorders (Greenspan, 1992; Diagnostic Classification Task Force, 1994) that considers distinct behavioral patterns, coupled with specific difficulties in sensory, sensorimotor, or processing capacities.

According to the present construct, infants and young children with regulatory disorders present challenging variations in their constitutional and maturational patterns as well as in their interactive and family patterns. These variations, in turn, affect how the children perceive and organize experience. The construct of regulatory disorders emerged from clinical work with a variety of infants and families, where it appeared that some infants had significant constitutional and maturational variations that were contributing to their symptoms. Difficulties with either processing sensations (inflow) or motor planning (outflow)—that is, being able to take in or respond back to the world—compromised some infants' abilities to negotiate with and adjust to their caregivers and environment. (See Greenspan, 1989, for a discussion of constitutional variables.)

Emerging research supports the initial clinical impressions. For example, 8-month-olds with a range of behavioral control difficulties (e.g., in sleeping, eating, self-calming, attention, etc.) evidenced sensory reactivity and motor differences (as assessed via reliable rating scales) as well as measurable psychological and physiological differences. These differences persisted at 18 months and 4 years of age. At 4 years of age, there were also behavioral and learning difficulties (De-Gangi et al., 1993).

The early regulatory patterns can be viewed either as distinct disorders at early developmental stages, in the sense that they constitute maladaptive and often disruptive behavioral patterns, or as intermediary risk patterns for later symptoms and disorders. In considering a developmental pattern, early behavior can be viewed in these two ways, particularly when the early pattern is part of the ongoing interaction with the environment and when this early interaction has later consequences. It may be tempting to view early regulatory differences as simply variations in temperament. The regulatory patterns, however, are determined by "hands-on" assessment (not by parental reports, as with temperament) and are related to specific sensory processing and motor patterns (not simply to general adaptive characteristics, as with temperament). Moreover, as we hope to demonstrate in future research, these regulatory patterns can be altered with proper interventions. Consider these two infants as illustrations of this construct.

CASE EXAMPLES

David and Mark: David, who is 5 months old, sleeps quietly in a darkened room. The phone is turned off.

His parents do not vacuum, play the stereo, or talk loudly. Several months of crying, fussiness, endless rocking sessions, and disrupted sleep have led to this. Every effort is made to make sure that David never misses his nap in his own crib. He cringes when his diaper is changed and cries when he must get dressed, arching away. Although he likes to look around, he is slow to move or turn over. David is also startled by unexpected loud sounds and begins to cry, unable to turn to the sound readily. His parents often feel exhausted and puzzled, trying hard to hide their feelings of disappointment and self-doubt, even from each other. It is not even clear to them that he recognizes they are different from others, since he shows such little pleasure when they approach; yet he clings to them.

In contrast, Mark is 5 months old too. His mother is about to whisk him off to meet a friend at a café, even though it is his naptime. He can always nap there; the noise, lights, and commotion of the café do not bother him. He loves to look around and follow people and sounds, turning eagerly in every direction. As a newborn, when upset, he calmed himself quickly by sucking on his fist, and now he is apt to quiet in response to looking at his mother's face and hearing her voice. In fact, last night he stayed up while his parents had dinner with friends; he joyfully entertained everyone with coos and smiles as he went from hand to hand, while his parents glowed.

These two infants are strikingly different. From birth, every infant must suddenly take in and organize the myriad of sensations of touch, lights, movement, sight, sounds, pain, temperature, and smells of his or her new world. An individual infant's capacity to take in and organize these sensations, as well as the crucial relationships being offered, is obvious early on. Some infants, such as Mark, adapt easily and stay calm and alert. Mark can use vision, hearing, touch, and movement to regulate himself and take an interest in the world. When upset, just looking at his mother helps him become calm and happy, as do her soothing voice and touch. In fact, he brightens and takes in the world with great confidence and security. In contrast, David needs to shut out sounds and vision; he is calmed more by the slow, steady rocking movements of his mother in a quiet, darkened room. When alert, he can take in his parents by looking or listening to one at a time, but too many people or too much stimulation overwhelms him, and he becomes disorganized and fussy. Neither David nor his parents are enjoying this crucial developmental period of his life.

Infants organize themselves in different ways. Clinical observations indicate that to stay calm, some infants suck their fists, gaze at a mobile or face, listen to a soothing voice, or enjoy rocking. Some use one or two sensory modalities, such as vision and movement (rocking), but may become overwhelmed or seem unresponsive to auditory stimuli. Other infants prefer vision and hearing to self-regulate and take an interest in the world, but do not like touch and movement. In contrast to those infants who are hypersensitive and tend to overreact, other infants seem to underreact to what is going on around them, as their parents work harder and harder to get their attention or even a small smile. They tend to be easy and undemanding as babies, not bothered by very much. Later, they may wander around, clutching a familiar object to focus on when too much is going on. These infants appear to be underreactive, hardly noticing the sensations until they become very vigorous and intense, and then overreacting as they insist on restoring a hands-off, quiet state.

A baby who is excessively needy and demanding; fussy or finicky; intermittently angry, labile in his or her moods, or underresponsive and slow to warm up and adapt to new situations—each individual has an impact—on the family, on the nature of interactions among the child and family members, and on the way the child perceives him- or herself and integrates experience. Sometimes one sensory pathway (or two or more) are involved.

When regulatory disorders are evident, they are characterized by difficulties in regulating physiological, sensory, attentional, and motor or affective processes, and in organizing a calm, alert, or affectively positive state. The following classification includes four types of regulatory disorders. The operational definition for each type includes a distinct behavioral pattern, coupled with a sensory, sensorimotor, or organizational processing difficulty that affects the child's daily adaptation and interaction/relationships.

Poorly organized or modulated responses may show themselves in the following domains:

1. The physiological or state repertoire (e.g., irregular breathing, startles, hiccups, gagging)
2. Gross motor activity (e.g., motor disorganization, jerky movements, constant movement)
3. Fine motor activity (e.g., poorly differentiated or sparse, jerky, or limp movements)
4. Attentional organization (e.g., "driven" behavior,

inability to settle down, or, conversely, perseveration about a small detail)

5. Affective organization, including the predominant affective tone (e.g., sober, depressed, happy); the range of affect (e.g., broad or constricted); the degree of modulation expressed (e.g., infant shifts abruptly from being completely calm to screaming frantically); and the capacity to use and organize affect as part of relationships and interaction with others (e.g., avoidant, negativistic, clinging and demanding behavior patterns)

6. Behavioral organization (e.g., aggressive or impulsive behavior)

7. Sleep, eating, or elimination patterns

8. Language (receptive and expressive) and cognitive difficulties

Presenting problems in the behavior of infants and young children may include sleep or feeding difficulties, behavior control difficulties, fearfulness and anxiety, difficulties in speech and language development, and impaired ability to play alone or with others. Parents also may complain that a child gets upset easily or loses his or her temper and has difficulty adapting to changes. (Because the daily routines of caregiving involve continuous sensory, motor, and affective experiences for the infant and young child, handling that is not sensitive to individual differences, irregular conditions in the environment, and/or changes in routine can strongly affect infants and children with regulatory disorders as well as their caregivers.)

Many attentional, affective, motor, sensory, behavioral control, and language problems that traditionally have been viewed as difficulties in their own right may, in certain children, be part of a larger regulatory disorder. Clinicians have used general terms such as *overly sensitive, difficult temperament,* or *reactive* to describe sensory, motor, and integrative patterns that are presumed to be "constitutionally" or "biologically" based, but they have not delineated specifically the sensory pathway or motor functions involved. Growing evidence indicates that constitutional and early maturational patterns contribute to the difficulties of such infants, but early caregiving patterns can exert considerable influence on how constitutional and maturational patterns develop and become part of a child's evolving personality. As interest in these children increases, it is important to systematize descriptions of the sensory, motor, and integrative patterns presumed to be involved.

The diagnosis of regulatory disorder involves both a distinct behavioral pattern and a sensory, sensorimotor, or organizational processing difficulty. When both features are not present, other diagnoses may be more appropriate. For example, an infant who is irritable and withdrawn after being abandoned may be evidencing a predictable type of relationship or attachment difficulty. An infant who is irritable and overly reactive to routine interpersonal experiences, in the absence of a clearly identified sensory, sensorimotor, or processing difficulty, may be evidencing an anxiety or mood disorder. (Sleep or eating difficulties can be symptoms of a regulatory disorder or be part of separate diagnostic categories.)

To make the diagnosis of a regulatory disorder in an infant or young child, the clinician should observe both a sensory, sensorimotor, or processing difficulty from the following list, and one or more behavioral symptoms.

1. Over- or underreactivity to loud, high-, or low-pitched noises

2. Over- or underreactivity to bright lights or new and striking visual images, (i.e., colors, shapes, complex fields)

3. Tactile defensiveness (e.g., overreactivity to dressing, bathing, or stroking of arms, legs, or trunk; avoidance of touching "messy" textures), and/or oral hypersensitivity (e.g., avoidance of food with certain textures)

4. Oral-motor difficulties or incoordination influenced by poor muscle tone, motor planning difficulties, and/or oral tactile hypersensitivity (e.g., avoidance of certain food textures)

5. Underreactivity to touch or pain

6. Gravitational insecurity—that is, under- or overreactivity in a child with normal postural responses (e.g., balance reactions) to the changing sensation of movement involved in brisk horizontal or vertical movements (e.g., being tossed in the air, twirled in a circular motion, or jumping)

7. Under- or overreactivity to odors

8. Under- or overreactivity to temperature

9. Poor muscle tone and muscle stability—for example hypotonia, hypertonia, postural fixation, or lack of smooth movement quality

10. Qualitative deficits in motor planning skills (e.g., difficulty in sequencing the hand movements necessary to explore a novel or complex toy or difficulty climbing a jungle gym)

11. Qualitative deficits in ability to modulate motor

activity (not secondary to anxiety or interactive difficulties)

12. Qualitative deficits in fine motor skills
13. Oral-motor difficulties or incoordination influenced by poor muscle tone, motor planning difficulties, and/or oral tactile hypersensitivity (e.g., avoidance of certain food textures)
14. Qualitative deficits in articulation capacity (e.g., for an 8-month-old, difficulty imitating distinct sounds; for 3-year-old, difficulty finding words to describe an intended or completed action)
15. Qualitative deficits in visual-spatial processing capacities (e.g., for an 8-month-old, difficulty in recognizing different facial configurations; for a 2½-year-old, difficulty in knowing in which direction to turn to get to another room in a familiar house; for a 3½-year-old, difficulty in using visual-spatial cues to recognize and categorize different shapes)
16. Qualitative deficits in capacity to attend and focus, not related to anxiety, interactive difficulties, or clear auditory/verbal or visual/spatial processing problems

Types of Regulatory Disorders

The 4 types of regulatory disorders described in this section are based on the predominant characteristics of children, including behavioral patterns and emotional inclinations, as well as motor and sensory patterns. The first three subtypes are to be used to subclassify the disorder where a tendency toward one predominant pattern is observable. Because some children will not be adequately described by these subtypes, there is an "other" subtype. Note that the description of the first three subtypes includes a discussion of caregiving patterns that promote better regulation and organization in children as well as caregiving patterns that intensify these children's difficulties.

TYPE I: HYPERSENSITIVE

Infants and young children who are overreactive or hypersensitive to various stimuli show a range of behavioral patterns. Two patterns are characteristic, fearful and cautious, and negative

and defiant. In addition, children may be inconsistent in their hypersensitivity. Sensitivities also may vary throughout the day. Most often sensory input tends to have a cumulative effect, so that a child may not be bothered by initial input but have significant difficulty at the end of the day. In addition, response to sensory input seems to interact with the baseline level of arousal. If a child is stressed or tired, less sensory input may be required to trigger a hypersensitive response.

Fearful and Cautious: Behavioral patterns include excessive cautiousness, inhibition, and/or fearfulness. In early infancy, these patterns are manifested by a restricted range of exploration and assertiveness, dislike of changes in routine, and a tendency to be frightened and clinging in new situations. Young children's behavior is characterized by excessive fears and/or worries and by shyness in new experiences, such as forming peer relationships or engaging with new adults. These children may have a fragmented, rather than an integrated, internal representational world and may be distracted easily by different stimuli. Occasionally, they may behave impulsively when overloaded and/or frightened. They tend to be easily upset (e.g., irritable, often crying), cannot soothe themselves readily (e.g., find it difficult to return to sleep), and cannot quickly recover from frustration or disappointment.

Motor and sensory patterns are characterized by overreactivity to touch, loud noses, or bright lights. These children often have adequate auditory-verbal processing abilities but compromised visual-spatial processing ability. They may also be overreactive to movement in space and have motor planning challenges.

Caregiver patterns that enhance flexibility and assertiveness in fearful and cautious children involve empathy, especially for their sensory and affective experience; very gradual and supportive encouragement to explore new experiences; and gentle but firm limits. Inconsistent caregiver patterns intensify these children's difficulties, as when caregivers are overindulgent and/or overprotective some of the time and punitive and/or intrusive at other times.

Negative and Defiant: Behavioral patterns are negativistic, stubborn, controlling, and defiant. These children often do the opposite of what is requested or expected. They have difficulty in making transitions and prefer repetition, absence of change, or, at most, change at a slow pace. Infants tend to be fussy, difficult, and resistant to transitions and changes. Preschoolers tend to be negative, angry, defiant, and stubborn as well as compulsive and perfectionistic. However, these children can evidence joyful, flexible behavior at certain times.

In contrast to fearful/cautious or avoidant children, negative and defiant children do not become fragmented but organize an integrated sense of themselves around negative, defiant patterns. In contrast to impulsive, stimulus-seeking children (Type III, later in this section), negative and defiant children are more controlling, tend to avoid or be slow to engage in new experiences, and are not generally aggressive unless provoked.

Motor and sensory patterns include a tendency toward overreactivity to touch, which may be observed during play in the avoidance of certain textures or manipulation of materials with fingertips. Children with this pattern are also often overreactive to sound. They often show intact or even precocious visual-spatial capacities, but their auditory processing capacity may be compromised. These children may have good muscle tone and postural control but may show some difficulty in fine motor coordination and/or motor planning.

Caregiver patterns that enhance flexibility involve soothing, empathic support of slow, gradual change, and avoidance of power struggles. Caregivers' warmth, even in the face of a child's negativism or rejection, and encouragement of symbolic representation of different affects, especially dependency, anger, and annoyance, also enhance flexibility. In contrast, caregiver patterns that are intrusive, excessively demanding, overstimulating, or punitive tend to intensify children's negative and defiant patterns.

TYPE II: UNDERREACTIVE

Infants and young children who are underreactive to various stimuli may show one of two characteristic patterns: withdrawn and difficult to engage, or self-absorbed, seeming to "march to the beat of their own drummer."

Withdrawn and Difficult to Engage: Behavioral patterns of withdrawn or difficult-to-engage children include a seeming disinterest in exploring relationships or even challenging games or objects. Children may appear apathetic, easily exhausted, and withdrawn. High affective tone and saliency are required to attract their interest, attention, and emotional engagement. Infants may appear delayed or depressed, lacking in motor exploration and responsivity to sensations and social overtures. In addition to continuing these patterns, preschoolers evidence diminished verbal dialogue. Their behavior and play may present only a limited range of ideas and fantasies. Sometimes children will seek out desired sensory input, often engaging in repetitive sensory activities, such as spinning, swinging, or jumping up and down on the bed. The children fully experience these activities through their intensity or repetition.

Motor and sensory patterns are characterized by underreactivity to sounds and movement in space but either over- or underreactivity to touch. Children with this pattern may have intact visual-spatial processing capacities but often experience auditory-verbal processing difficulties. Poor motor quality and motor planning often can be observed, as well as limited exploratory activity or flexibility in play.

Caregiver patterns that provide intense interactive input and foster initiative tend to help underreactive withdrawn children engage, attend, interact, and explore their environment. These patterns involve reaching out, energized wooing, and robust responses to the child's cues, however faint. In contrast, caregiver patterns that are low-key, "laid back," or depressive in tone and rhythm tend to intensify these children's patterns of withdrawal.

Self-Absorbed: Behavioral patterns of self-absorbed children include creativity and imagination, combined with a tendency for the child to tune into his or her own sensations, thoughts, and emotions, rather than being tuned into and attentive to communications from other people. Infants may appear self-absorbed, becoming interested in objects through solitary exploration rather than in the context of interaction. Children may appear inattentive, easily distracted, or preoccupied, especially when not pulled into a task or interaction. Preschoolers tend to escape into fantasy in the presence of external challenges, such as competition with a peer or a demanding preschool activity. They may prefer to play by themselves when others do not actively join their fantasies. Within their fantasy life, these children may show enormous imagination and creativity.

Motor and sensory patterns include a tendency toward decreased auditory-verbal processing capacities coupled with an ability to create a rich range of ideas (receptive language difficulties, coupled with creativity and imagination, make it easier for a child to tune into his or her own ideas than to attend to another person's ideas). Children may or may not show irregularities in other sensory and motor capacities.

Caregiver patterns that are helpful include the tendency to tune into the child's nonverbal and verbal communications and help the child engage in two-way communication, that is, "open and closed circles of communication." Helpful caregiver patterns also encourage a good balance between fantasy and reality and help a child who is attempting to escape into fantasy stay grounded in external reality; for example, they show sensitivity to the child's interests and feelings, promote discussion of daily events and feelings, and make fantasy play a parent-child collaborative endeavor rather than a solitary child activity. In contrast, a caregiver's self-absorption or preoccupation or confusing family communications tend to intensify children's difficulties.

TYPE III: MOTORICALLY DISORGANIZED, IMPULSIVE

Impulsive, motorically disorganized children evidence poor control of behavior coupled with craving sensory input. Some children appear aggressive and fearless. Others simply appear impulsive and disorganized.

Behavioral patterns among motorically disorganized children involve high activity, with children seeking contact and stimulation through deep pressure. The child appears to lack caution. Not infrequently, the motorically disorganized child's tendency to seek contact with people or objects leads to breaking things, intruding into other people's body spaces, unprovoked hitting, and so on. Behavior that begins as a result of poor motor planning and organization may be interpreted by others as aggression rather than excitability. Once others react aggressively to the child, the child's own behavior may in fact become aggressive.

Motorically disorganized infants seek or crave sensory input and stimulation. Preschoolers often show excitable, aggressive, intrusive behavior and a daredevil, risk-taking style as well as preoccupation with aggressive themes in pretend play. When these young children are anxious or unsure of themselves, they may use counterphobic behaviors—for example, hitting before (possibly) getting hit or repeating unacceptable behavior after being asked to stop. When older and able to verbalize and self-observe their own patterns, these children may describe the need for activity and stimulation as a way to feel alive, vibrant, and powerful.

Motor and sensory patterns are characterized by sensory underreactivity, craving of sensory input, and motor discharge. Motorically disorganized children often combine underreactivity to touch and sound, stimulus craving, and/poor motor modulation and motor planning, and evidence diffuse, impulsive behavior toward persons and objects. Similarly, motor activities are unfocused and diffused. Due to their underreactivity, these children may listen fleetingly, attend poorly, and yet crave loud noises or intense music. The craving of stimuli sometimes leads to destructive behavior. These children may evidence either auditory or visual-spatial processing difficulties but also may evidence age-appropriate patterns in these areas.

Caregiver patterns characterized by continuous, warm relating, a great deal of nurturance and empathy, coupled with clear structure and limits, will enhance flexibility and adaptivity. It is helpful for caregivers to provide children with constructive opportunities for sensory and affective involvement, while encouraging modulation and self-regulation. Caregiver patterns that encourage the use of imagination in support of exploration of the external environment will further enhance the child's flexibility. In contrast, caregiver patterns that avoid warm continuous engagement (e.g., changing caregivers), are overly punitive, fail to set clear limits and boundaries on behavior, and either over- or understimulate the child may intensify these difficulties.

TYPE IV: OTHER

The "other" category should be used for children who meet the first criterion for regulatory disorder (i.e., motor or sensory processing difficulty) but whose behavioral patterns are not adequately described by one of the subtypes already discussed.

ADDITIONAL CATEGORIES

Sleeping Difficulties[1]: When a sleep disturbance is the only presenting problem in an infant under 1 year of age, the diagnosis of a primary regulatory-based sleep disorder should be considered. These difficulties in going to sleep, or in waking and returning to sleep, appear related to general difficulties with self-calming and dealing with transitions but do not have clearly associated sensory reactivity, sensory processing, and/or motor difficulties. This type of diagnosis should be used only when the problem is not primarily attributable to anxiety, relationship, or mood disturbances; transient adjustment problems; psychic trauma disorder; or other types of regulatory disorders.

Eating Difficulties[2]: When an eating/feeding disturbance, manifested by difficulties establishing regular feeding patterns with adequate or appropriate intake, is the only presenting problem in an infant under 1 year of age, the diagnosis of a primary regulatory-based eating disorder should be considered. This disturbance is part of an overall pattern of poor self-regulation related to difficulties with self-calming and transitions; again, however, this diagnosis applies only when eating difficulties do not have clearly associated sensory reactivity, sensory processing, and/or motor difficulties.

If the difficulties are accompanied by notable sensorimotor problems, such as tactile hypersensitivity (e.g., a child rejects certain food textures) and/or low oral-motor tone (e.g., a child will eat only soft foods), then the specific regulatory subtypes should be considered instead. If organic/structural problems affect the ability to eat or digest food (e.g., cleft palate, reflux, etc.), this type of diagnosis also does not apply. However, sometimes an eating disturbance may originate in organic or structural difficulties but continues after these initial difficulties have been resolved, in the presence of ongoing finicky or fussy behavior; in such a case, this type may still apply.

When eating disturbances are part of a larger symptom picture, associated with other affective or behavioral disturbances related to primary relationships, trauma, or other adjustment difficulties, one of the other disorders may be a more appropriate diagnosis. If irregular eating patterns or severely constricted food choices are part of multisystem developmental delays and patterns of rigidity and inability to take in new experiences, as in autism or pervasive developmental disorder, this type does not apply.

Therapeutic Approaches for Regulatory Disorders

In a sense, the unusual constitutional and maturational variations evidenced by infants and young children with regulatory problems color all of their experience. In contrast to children whose major difficulties emanate from challenges in the interactional or family patterns, regulatory-disordered infants or young children require major efforts to help them overcome their own constitutional and maturational difficulties with self-regulation; however, the focus on fostering better regulatory capacities cannot and should not occur in isolation from the interactive and family patterns. Three brief case illustrations represent this complex interaction and the therapeutic approaches needed.

CASE EXAMPLES

The Story of Julie: Regulatory Disorder, Hypersensitive Type (Type I): Julie finally fell asleep at her mother's breast as they both lay on the large mattress on the floor. It was after midnight, and the previous hours had been spent pacing, rocking, and finally nursing Julie to sleep. Julie was 13 months old. Her crib had been abandoned 6 or 7 months earlier, when her mother could no longer bear the persistent crying of her first, long-awaited baby. She seemed so helpless, so like a rag doll, so needy, that even the father's anger and dismay could not sway the mother from trying her best to assure her daughter that she could be cared for and would not be abandoned to crying herself to sleep.

Everyone blamed the mother for overprotecting her child. Her pediatrician told her to let the baby cry so that she would learn to go to sleep. The mother's own psychotherapist explored her symbiotic/parasitic needs, fears of separation, or perhaps fears of her daughter's anger if she was not totally there for her. Her husband accused her of rejection as he became more competitive, jealous, and depressed.

Julie was born after a planned, healthy pregnancy and an uneventful delivery. She appeared alert and responsive, quick to look around, and quick to be held so that she felt secure and trusting that someone was always there for her. Although Julie enjoyed being held when dressed, she was sensitive to light touch when stroked and did not like the initial contact with water when bathed, but seemed to adapt. She became vigilant to loud or sudden noises, quickly seeking their source. Frequent feedings and night wakings were routine, and nursing became the way to calm her during early periods of fussy and colicky behavior. Nevertheless, the first 6 months of Julie's life were a pleasure for all. It was not yet apparent that her poor self-regulation of sleeping and eating patterns or her sensitivities or reactivity should be of concern. Her good looking, listening, and vocal responsiveness became the sensory pathways through which she was also able to begin conveying her intentions. Early communication was rich and intense.

At about 6 months, the family moved to a new house; Julie reacted to a DPT (diptheria, pertussis, tetanus) vaccine; and she started waking more frequently. This waking continued over the next half year and worsened whenever she became ill. The parents also noticed that Julie was the last to sit among her peers in the mother's parent group and was not quite crawling at 10 months. Even at 13 months her sitting was still not stable, and the mother recalled that she was slow to hold her head up. It was not apparent to anyone that this pattern indicated low motor tone and motor planning difficulties. Poor postural security and motor delays, however, delayed the active distancing and approach behaviors, and Julie in fact stayed in her mother's symbiotic orbit longer than usual. This was attributed to the overprotective nature of her relationship with the mother.

But Julie vocalized all the time, began speaking at 8 months, and seemed to understand much of what was said to her, following directions and repeating the words. Although she certainly cried to protest, she would not throw objects lest she lose her balance, and had few ways to express anger safely. Nor did she become attached to any transitional objects, preferring to have her mother at her side day and night. Her separation anxiety actually worsened at 1 year of age when the

family housekeeper, whom she knew well, left. After that, no one else was acceptable, and her parents stopped going out during the day and in the evenings, since no one else could get her to sleep. Without mobility either early or later, practicing, individuation, and separation were compromised. Instead, Julie used her precocious verbal abilities to keep her mother close. There was no need to guess what she wanted. Tension, however, began to mount between her parents, and Julie became more intense and verbally demanding, especially at any indication of separation.

The mother did not recognize how quick she was to move in on her baby, offering help before Julie needed it and leading her in activities. This was not done in an intrusive or controlling manner, but in a subdued and rather passive fashion with long pauses. She was an anxious parent who was worried about what to do next, lest she make a mistake. A pattern developed wherein Julie also became passive and permitted herself to be controlled by her mother's overtures and gestures. The mother often looked anxious and hesitant. In this pattern they were highly reciprocal. The father could encourage more assertiveness and activity, putting implicit demands on Julie to respond to him. He tended to retreat, however, in response to his wife's anxiety and began to doubt himself; still, he kept insisting that Julie be allowed to cry at night so that she would finally learn to fall asleep, and yearned for his wife's return.

Thus, when Julie began her second year of life, she was a very bright, verbal child, with strong attachments and relatedness, who appeared happy and responsive to those she knew. However, she was only beginning to stand and walk; her crawling was poor; and she still had difficulty keeping her body upright even for sitting, where she would stretch her legs out far apart and fix her shoulders to stiffen her back in order to maintain her upright posture. She was also quite sensitive to touch and was hesitant to explore unknown objects or spaces. Julie still could not fall asleep without her mother lying next to her and would not be left with anyone.

The parents brought Julie in for an evaluation at 13 months. Observations and parental reports indicated the need for an occupational therapist with expertise in sensory reactivity and processing to examine her poor motor tone, tactile hypersensitivity, and other constitutional variations. Difficulties were indeed confirmed and found to be quite significant, with therapy recommended twice a week. Julie had not been able to establish adequate self-regulation, but did develop a warm and strong attachment in her early months. This attachment became increasingly anxious as she had difficulty with intentional and assertive interactions and with separation. She was able to communicate purposefully and was speaking long before her peers, but it did not help her negotiate the developmental tasks at hand.

Why was Julie not diagnosed earlier? Because she partially attained motor milestones (which have considerable range in infancy) and adapted to the familiar "hands-on" care of her mother, the impact of low tone and tactile hypersensitivity was not fully recognized, as it might have been in a high-risk child with expectable motor problems. Similarly, because Julie was beginning to get up on her feet, it was not as evident that she did not experience the security of strong posture, which could support more active and assertive behavior. She took steps gingerly and did not run off, and was not eager to climb or push. She asked others to do things for her, becoming more verbally controlling, rather than physically experiencing her shakiness and insecurity. When she did walk, the effort appeared so great that she did not notice things underfoot and would quickly lose her balance and fall. Also, she had one parent sending a signal to be careful and another urging her on, but then blaming her for her shortcomings. Thus, when she ordinarily would have been dealing with separation and moving out into the world, she was clinging tightly day and night, even though she was individuating on cognitive and symbolic levels.

If separation anxiety were her only diagnosis and Julie's regulatory difficulties were not addressed, she would not have obtained the treatment she needed to negotiate the next steps of development and, thus, might have become a highly anxious child with major personality constrictions. Simultaneously considering Julie's regulatory difficulties, parental issues, and the specific tasks of each stage of development made it possible to guide Julie's development through the specific challenges this combination presented. At first, treatment responded to the presenting problems by focusing on encouraging mastery through interactive play centered on Julie's assertiveness and focusing on the sleep/separation process and helping the mother see that Julie indeed had the capacities to cope and take charge of her own security at night. More autonomy and assertiveness were also encouraged in day-to-day routines and especially play, making use of Julie's excellent emerging representational capacities. Meanwhile, Julie responded well to occupational therapy, which treated the low motor tone, postural insecurities, tactile defensiveness, and motor planning difficulties. The parents also explored the different meanings this problem had for them and tried to support each other, realizing that their relationship with one another was at least as important as their relationship with Julie. As the next steps were anticipated, it was possible to ameliorate and support the ego functions needed to allow Julie the room to keep growing.

By 2½ years of age, Julie was an assertive, independent toddler, able to separate and go to sleep on her own, fighting her own turf battles with peers, and enjoying her new physical competence. She was a delightful and happy little girl who was taking in more and more of the world in a self-regulated fashion, finding solutions to difficulties when they arose, and happy with her parents and herself. She appeared to welcome new situations, learned and imitated quickly, and when anxious, helped herself by reasoning and thinking. She told others how she felt, using her language and symbolic play capacities to share feelings, to solve problems, and to negotiate her world and relationships.

The Story of Ben: Regulatory Disorder, Motorically Disorganized, Impulsive (Type III): Ben's nursery school teacher called his parents again. Ben was continuing to hit and bite, and the other children were frightened of him. He was calm only in the paint corner, where he worked by himself and created wonderful, colorful images he could describe in detail, even at age 2. As a first child, his parents perceived him as "just fine" until he started nursery school. This occurred shortly after his sister was born, and perhaps this contributed to his outbursts of aggression. As she became more active, so did he, directing his frustration and anger at her by pushing, knocking her over, and even biting. With his parents, Ben could recite all the rules and say what he would do next time, but in reality he was impulsive and appeared unremorseful, making others feel anxious and angry. Many "Sorrys" and time-outs later, Ben's parents sought help.

When first seen, this cute blond little boy appeared terribly anxious. He was clearly very bright but also intense and defensive. Ben was curious and asked a lot of questions about the toys, trying each one out but not organizing any themes. With more support he could elaborate with the doctor kit, cutting off the doll's hurt foot. He then noticed the animals and reported that the zebra was angry and bit because the mother and father hit; he then proceeded to line up all the "biting" animals in one place and the "good" animals in another. Ben could easily elaborate representationally. His characters were always angry, hitting, retaliating, and in trouble unless they could be alone. He was always anxious and could not convey any emotions related to warmth, closeness, or dependency.

More careful observation of Ben over the next few sessions indicated that he usually would respond to questions related to his play but did not interact spontaneously, missing cues and gestures unless they were verbalized. He would have alligators eating people and missiles exploding everywhere. This would alternate with picking safe little figures, such as the Berenstain Bear family, whom he used to reenact his real-life situations as he struggled to be good and find safety in a world fraught with danger and trouble.

Ben's conflicts and anxieties seemed obvious. The initial treatment approach focused on parent guidance, especially because the mother was depressed and the father had withdrawn. The parents were encouraged to get down on the floor every day for "floor time" to play—that is, to interact in a way that followed their child's lead, encouraged symbolic representation, provided cues to support self-regulation, and strengthened their interactive relationship. (See the detailed description of "floor time" in Greenspan, 1992.) Appropriate limits were defined, and individual psychotherapy and teacher consultation were provided. Ben responded quickly as everyone important in his life mobilized to support him and restore his self-esteem. He did especially well in an outdoor summer camp program, where there were few demands and plenty of space and activity. He began to show increased warmth and comfort with closeness and to enjoy life more.

A few months later, when school resumed, severe difficulties began again in Ben's preschool. His new teacher reported hitting, pushing, and the flinging of objects that seemed unprovoked and was again frightening his classmates. He was again isolated and everyone was anxious. In his play sessions, he seemed unusually alarmed by any unexpected movement, and even objected to the therapist's moving a figure without his permission. Although he could now organize a more complex "good guy/bad guy" scene, he insisted on holding both figures and only one (his) could attack. He was always the bad guy and the victor. Ben struggled unsuccessfully to find motives for his figures' actions. If threatened, he would turn red and become agitated and ready to "kill."

Ben's extreme efforts to control everyone in his environment and the degree of panic he exhibited when anything happened that he did not expect (including his own impulsiveness) made it imperative to reexamine the underlying nature of his difficulties. The explanations used so far were not sufficient, although the problems defined to date contributed significantly to his difficulties: He was anxious, aggressive, and impulsive; his family was distressed, with a depressed mother and a distant and blaming father; and his teacher had already

"marked" him as a "bad kid." Because he was so bright and verbal, and promised to be good, rewards and punishments should have gotten him in shape, but had not.

Considering Ben's actions more carefully now suggested several possible underlying processing difficulties. His protection from the outside world was overly fragile. Ben showed alarm when anyone came too close unexpectedly, but when he initiated physical contact he was sufficiently comfortable that he could reach out to be cuddled (e.g., in the early hours of the morning). Even when someone he knew very well made a casual friendly gesture toward him, he would pull back and ask the person not to touch him. If he was in the middle of an action and something was said, he appeared not to attend. He was sensitive to sounds around him, easily distracted but slow to orient himself. He had difficulty recognizing "personal space" and would poke, bump, and seek inappropriate contact with other children. He was also small for his age, tended to toe in, and had low motor tone.

His early history was reexamined, and his mother now reported early regulatory difficulties. Ben had always been a poor sleeper and an erratic eater; as a baby, he had a short fuse and was quick to scream. He hated being picked up or experiencing high or sudden movements; however, he walked early (at 10 months) after a very brief crawling period. Once he was on his feet, these earlier difficulties were less apparent and seemed to be set aside. Further observations (e.g., the difficulty he had manipulating two toy figures in different hands at the same time) confirmed moderate to severe delays in Ben's visual system, resulting in tremendous stress, since Ben received conflicting messages from his two eyes. He could not use vision efficiently to direct his movements or to interpret other people's actions correctly. Difficulties with motor planning, perceptual-motor coordination, and laterality resulted. Reduced motor tone and tactile defensiveness completed this regulatory disorder.

Ben began an intensive therapy program of vision therapy, occupational therapy, and perceptual-motor therapy, in addition to psychotherapy and parent guidance. It was clear that Ben needed to learn how to anticipate and practice in areas where his regulatory system was challenged. Problem-solving discussions (Greenspan & Salmon, 1993) between parents and child were begun to anticipate what would happen the next day at school, focusing on the feelings he would have and the behaviors he would exhibit in response to these feelings. Helping Ben figure out what to expect reduced his sense of surprise and shock, and prepared him for even uncomfortable situations. Psychotherapy also helped Ben experience empathy for his difficulty and get a sense of his assumptions about life, especially how he wanted everything done his way, but at the same time, was frightened of others' competing or being angry with him.

Within several months, Ben appeared more organized, oriented, and focused. He was quick to develop relationships with his additional new therapists (developmental optometrist, occupation therapist, and perceptual-motor therapist) and worked quite hard. He became happier and not only did better with his sister but also made his first friends. In psychotherapy he continued to struggle with whether he was good or bad, frequently and suddenly changing roles within minutes. When his fears and wishes for power were interpreted, he seemed relieved but also very sad, because he also wanted friends. As psychotherapy continued to address his confusion and self-doubt regarding his ability to stay in control, it became apparent that Ben wanted to kill off all the other "good guys" in order to have a second chance to become a "good guy" himself.

The Story of Mark: Regulatory Disorder, Underreactive (Type II): Mark was an easy, undemanding baby who would smile and respond if approached quietly, but did not initiate or seek much contact. In a busy household with tense, working parents and a very demanding 3-year-old sister, it was not readily apparent how underreactive he was. At 18 months he brightened when his parents sang nursery rhymes, danced and moved with him, but left on his own, he would watch his little cars moving back and forth, spin little objects, and often rub a little toy back and forth across his belly. He was also very sensitive to sounds, reacting with alarm to sirens and unexpected noises, and had everyone speaking to him in a near whisper. Yet when he could be engaged, he was related and warm and clearly a bright child. Thus, although he responded to wooing and would reach out when he wanted something specific, he tended to tune out and overfocus on his own little activities, conveying a sense of fragility and constant apprehension as to how the world would impinge on him.

As Mark's second year of life progressed, he appeared to understand what was said when he was listening, but his listening was inconsistent. Noisy and crowded restaurants or shopping malls were distressing, but he sought out vibrating noises. He continued to enjoy swinging, running, chase games, and jumping: These activities made him smile and laugh with pleasure. His motor planning was more uncertain, but he would persist in climbing and getting in and out of small places. Mark always had tended to scan his environment and then overfocus on something small in front of him. Further examination indicated that his eyes did not converge very well, and as a result of developmental immaturities, he employed fragmented visual skills such as fixation, locking in, and tuning out. Activities were started to encourage him to track and use vision to guide his movements.

At 2 years of age, Mark continued to be withdrawn and unfocused. Sensitive and persistent wooing would engage him briefly, but then he would retreat into simple repetitive behaviors with his toys. Pleasure was evident only when strong sensori-motor actions gave him a clearer sense of where his body was in space and allowed him to organize and become aware of his experience. His language and symbolic gestures remained very simple, but Mark started to speak and carry out symbolic acts with dolls. His overall affective quality was still very guarded and subdued. Being with him always meant asking "Will he respond or not?" Anything and everything appeared to overwhelm him as his anxiety fed upon the anxiety of those around him. This little boy lived in a field of tension and fear, selecting bits and pieces of experience he could tolerate.

Living with Mark required exquisite sensitivity to his regulatory difficulties to engage him and help keep him from becoming overwhelmed. His good cognition and receptive language enabled his parents to anticipate and practice the activities that would be difficult for him. Trial runs in new or challenging situations were helpful. The noise and the likelihood of being touched in his nursery school classroom kept him at the edges of the room, but he could still learn from a distance when not pressured. Having him play with one child, in the safety of his own house with his mother present, to situations where he might bump shoulders, deal with aggression, and hear loud noises.

Being empathic was especially difficult because it was not always clear whether he understood, and when he did respond, it was often through rejection. Mark did respond to empathy expressed through facial expressions and gestures, which picked up the child's mood states and conveyed an expectable understanding of them. He especially responded to sources of anxiety (toys breaking, dolls getting hurt or falling, things getting lost or messy, etc.). Mark could engage in conversations centering around these issues as well as vocally object to any interference with the rituals he established to stay safe, such as leaving the door open "just a crack." Mark continued to constrict his world, preferring Sesame Street figures to people. He wanted everything done his way, but at the same time, he was frightened and did not want others to compete with or get angry at him. Setting limits on some of his behavior helped create a sense of security—that his environment could not be totally manipulated or intimidated by him, but also letting him know that he would not be at the mercy of everything.

Mark progressed slowly, showing increased adaptation at nursery school and at home. He also received speech and occupational therapy and attended a speech and language preschool program. His parents included him in all family activities, going many places and arranging many play dates; still, he could not interact readily with other children, preferring the stereotyped world of Sesame Street characters who lent him affect and predictability. Parent-child therapy essentially supported more direct and consistent interaction—gently requiring Mark to respond and challenging him to deal with his anxieties and experiment with aggression. He began with tentatively throwing a puppet behind the couch and rushing to retrieve it, but eventually progressed to throwing it with great delight, knowing he was in charge. He also started to express complex feelings, particularly his anger and distress. He became able to verbalize such abstract feelings as "A terrible thing happened. My grandparents went back to New York," or "I wish I could have it, but I know I can't have it." Once he could express himself and determine what was negotiable and what was not, he became happier and more energetic. New symbolic doors began to open as he felt more secure and could begin to be representational; he was no longer as anxious and defensive.

General Therapeutic Principles for Regulatory Disorders

The foregoing cases suggest a number of therapeutic strategies, including the following:

1. Strengthen the sensory, sensorimotor, or processing vulnerabilities.
2. Work with the way in which the maturational variable influences stage-specific affects, behaviors, and interaction.
3. Help parents correct distortions and projections that are, in part, based on the child's maturational challenges.
4. Facilitate stage-specific, individual-difference-oriented, caregiver-child interaction patterns.
5. Foster higher developmental levels.
6. Foster, as the child becomes representational, understanding of his or her maturational patterns through pretend play and discussions (e.g., "Loud noises make me feel like jumping out of my skin").
7. Foster flexible coping strategies for new challenges.

Conclusion

The new diagnostic concept of regulatory disorders provides a way to assess the individual differences in each child and suggests how these differences may underlie problems in adaptation and learning. This perspective enhances understanding of the other factors influencing the child's life, such as the environment and family dynamics. It also points to the specific intervention approaches needed to support healthier adaptation and development. (See Greenspan, 1992.) As can be seen in all three of the cases described, children with regulatory disorders may seem so overwhelmed, helpless, and unhappy most of the time that clinicians, educators, and parents are at a loss as to how to help them. These children require many small steps, one toe in the water at a time—whether the problems involve sleeping or eating, joining in group time, learning to be more assertive, having fewer tantrums, improving focus and concentration, or learning to use emerging skills.

NOTES

1. This section was formulated in collaboration with Klaus Minde.

2. This section was formulated in collaboration with Irene Chatoor.

REFERENCES

DeGangi, G., DiPietro, J. A., Greenspan, S. I., & Porges, S. W. (1991). Psychophysiological characteristics of the regulatory disordered infant. *Infant Behavioral Development, 14,* 37–50.

DeGangi, G. A., Porges, S. W., Sickel, R., & Greenspan, S. I. (1993). Four-year follow-up of a sample of regulatory disordered infants. *Infant Mental Health Journal, 14*(4), 330–343.

Diagnostic Classification Task Force. Stanley Greenspan, M. D., Chair. 1994. *Diagnostic classification: 0–3: Diagnostic classification of mental health and developmental disorders of infancy and early childhood.* Arlington, VA: ZERO TO THREE/ National Center for Clinical Infant Programs.

Doussard-Roosevelt, J. A., Walker, P. S., Portales, A. L., Greenspan, S. I., & Porges, S. W. (1990). Vagal tone and the fussy infant: Atypical vagal reactivity in the difficult infant. *Infant Behavior & Development, 13,* 352 (abstract).

Escalona, S. (1968). *The roots of individuality.* Chicago: Aldine.

Greenspan, S. I. (1989). *The development of the ego: Implications for personality theory, psychopathology, and the psychotherapeutic process.* Madison, CT: International Universities Press.

Greenspan, S. I. (1992). *Infancy and early childhood: The practice of clinical assessment and intervention with emotional and developmental challenges.* Madison, CT: International Universities Press.

Greenspan, S. I., & Salmon, J. (1993). *Playground politics: The emotional life of your school-aged child.* Reading, MA: Addison Wesley.

44 / Traumatic Stress Disorder of Infancy and Childhood

Bertram A. Ruttenberg

Introduction

The first edition of the *Basic Handbook of Child Psychiatry* (1979) contained only one short reference to "posttraumatic stress disorders" in the chapter by Kessler. It was listed with the reactive disorders, and resulted from a trauma or stress of such suddenness and/or intensity that it overwhelmed the normal protective barrier and the capacity of the ego to maintain its organization and adaptive functions.

The initial reaction was a suspension of full awareness of the danger, often with a concomitant "hypercathexis of some emergency (defensive) functions," followed by regressive "pathological reorganization manifested by defense anxiety, phobic avoidance and increased dependency feelings" (p. 176)—and an ongoing sense of vulnerability.

The second edition of the *Diagnostic and Statistical Manual of Mental Disorders (DSM-II;* American Psychiatric Association [APA], 1968) did not delineate the concept and categorization of traumatic stress disorder or posttraumatic stress disorder (PTSD). The third edition (*DSM-III;* APA, 1980) did include within its anxiety disorders the diagnostic category posttraumatic stress disorder, acute, chronic or delayed. Here characteristic symptoms followed the experience of a psychologically traumatic event that was beyond the range of usual human experience or tolerance.

The characteristic symptoms included (1) re-experiencing the trauma through painful recollection, dreams, or nightmares; (2) psychic numbing or disassociation; (3) a feeling of estrangement or reduced involvement with the outside world; (4) hyperalertness, difficulty sleeping; and (5) dysphoric reaction and disruption of cognitive functioning affecting concentration and memory. While it was stated that the disorder could occur at any age, including childhood, no differentiating descriptions of PTSD in children were offered.

In 1979 Lenore Terr reported the findings of her in-depth study of the 26 schoolchildren ages 5 to 14 who had been kidnapped and buried in a school bus in Chowchilla, California, in 1976. She pointed out that these children had together experienced a trauma that was purely psychological, without concomitant serious physical injury or death on (which eliminated the factor of survival guilt) and that the parents were not present during the traumatic event. She noted several differences between adult (as noted in *DSM-III*) and child reactions to such overwhelming events:

1. In children no amnesia or haziness about the experience was present.
2. The children were not able to deny the actual event, but repetitively relived and reenacted the experience, at will behaviorally and physiologically. "Unbidden" flashbacks did not occur.
3. There were major regressions in ego functioning manifested as destruction of trust, with anticipation of future calamity, misperceptions, overgeneralization of reaction to associated stimuli. These often manifested as startle responses and time confusion, yet such impaired school performance as occurred was not on the basis of cognitive regression but due rather to conduct and personality change factors, motivational and attitudinal.

In 1987 the revised third edition of the *Diagnostic and Statistical Manual of Mental Disorders* (*DSM-III-R*) added a section on age-specific features in PTSD that reflected studies by Terr. The manual noted the nature of the persistent symptoms of increased arousal and associated physical symptoms not present before the trauma—sleep disturbances, nightmares, irritability, and aggressiveness.

Muteness or refusal to talk about the event was seen in some children. It was not to be confused with an inability to remember, but rather as a way of avoiding stimuli associated with the event. Distressing dreams about the event would generalize into dreams of monsters, danger, and rescue. Younger children had no sense that they were reliving the past through their repetitive play. Constricted interest and affect and a sense of foreshortened and hopeless future were also described.

In 1987, the *Basic Handbook of Child Psychiatry* added a fifth volume, *Advances and New Directions*, which contained considerably more material on the posttraumatic stress disorders in children.

In this volume, Terr (1987) reviewed the literature on childhood psychic trauma and her own studies, first citing Freud's 1920 and 1926 definitions and A. Freud's 1967 rejoinder that in order to be a trauma, an external event must take place.

Terr concluded that "Psychic trauma occurs when a sudden unexpected intense external experience overwhelms the individual's coping and defensive operations, creating the feeling of utter helplessness" (p. 263). She further noted that *DSM-III's* qualifier that the traumatic event must be outside the range of usual human experience virtually eliminated such previously designated child traumas as birth of a sibling, a harsh upbringing, and a bad case of a communicable disease. Terr reviewed Anna Freud and Dorothy Burlingham's studies of children in London's bomb shelters; these workers had noted that the presence or absence of stable parents or other adult caregivers determined the traumatic impact of the bombings. Terr stated that these and the Hampstead studies of child holocaust survivors focused more on the presence or absence of the parental protective shield than on the single-blow trauma. She reviewed the differences in the reactions of children and adults, stating that the denial, repression, and numbing used as defenses in adults are not evident in school-age children who have experienced single-blow traumas. In this chapter, Terr first reported observations about the capacity of infants to recall these overwhelming stresses: "Prior to age two or three upsetting life events may not be remembered in words, yet they may be played out in imaginative games or partly recaptured in dreams" (p. 268). She cited cases where toddlers, having experienced particularly shocking intense single episodes, could recall them verbally at a later time.

In the same volume, Goodwin (1987) reporting on the trauma of incest, describing the preschool victim as in a state of "frozen watchfulness and immobility, as well as re-enactment of the sexual abuse, nightmares, ego constriction, anxiety and an irritability and discharge of aggression through tantrums" (p. 108). Regression of ego functioning included inability to sleep alone, clinging, and loss of toilet training and speech.

In the same volume, Justin Call first attempted formally to outline the posttraumatic stress disorder of infancy—acute, chronic, and delayed forms. He noted that the criteria for PTSD in *DSM-III* do not include symptoms that can be identified in infancy, since most of the cited symptoms involved a high degree of cognition and capacity for communication. He felt that the only two criteria that could apply to infants were constricted affect and speech disturbance. He reviewed descriptions of infants who had been severely traumatized through such acute events as severe physical or sexual abuse, animal attack, burns or other physical trauma, or by witnessing the murder of a parent, and noted that in situations of this kind, the infant or small child is overwhelmed with stimuli that cannot be cognitively or affectively organized. Call developed a list of characteristic symptoms of PTSD in infants:

1. A freezing of capacities to adapt to environmental change
2. Disturbances at the physiological level in terms of eating, sleeping, and toileting problems
3. A regression in psychosocial functioning
4. Regression to the state of symbiotic union in relation to the parent
5. Repetitive play patterns in the clinical interview, often including the elements of the traumatic event

Long-term consequences included a tendency to maintain loose contact with the parent figure, a frozen affective development, an inability to experience pleasure, and an extreme degree of cautiousness regarding new experiences.

The Classification of Traumatic Stress Disorders of Infants and Young Children

In 1987 the National Center for Clinical Infant Programs (NCCIP) initiated a Diagnostic Classification Task Force to develop a new diagnostic manual for infants (birth through 3 years), which would address the full range of infant mental health disorders. Other diagnostic approaches (including *DSM-III*) had not attended sufficiently to disorders of infancy and had provided too few categories relevant to and descriptive of infants, their developmental disorders and interaction with their milieu. Infants and young children had to be forced into too few and poorly fitting diagnostic categories, resulting in misdiagnoses, delayed diagnoses, and hesitation in the provision of appropriate therapy.

Recent years have seen an ever burgeoning level of stress and trauma affecting infants and children along with a near disappearance of the traditional parental protective envelope in some quarters. Accordingly, the task force considered this an area of major importance and delineated "psychic trauma disorders" as a major category. Inasmuch as Freud's (1926/1959) definition of psychic trauma emphasized the sense of utter helplessness and the overwhelming of ego functioning quite appropriate to the special vulnerability of infants and small children, and to key elements in the description of *DSM-III*'s Post Traumatic Stress Disorder (PTSD), the term *traumatic stress disorder* was selected over "Psychic Trauma Disorder" with an eye to compatibility with *DSM*. This author was assigned the major responsibility for the development of this category.

In addition to the single overwhelming event (or connected single series, e.g., earthquake and aftershocks; repeated bombings and strafing over a few days), there are chronic and enduring or multiple and unpredictable conditions of major stress and psychic trauma. These impinge on infants and young children with increasing frequency in today's world, and had not been considered in *DSM*'s PTSD. Such events include direct physical and psychological abuse, witnessed violence, the chronic personal and environmental anxiety of living "under the gun," as in worrying when will it strike again, starvation and loss of the protective envelope of the extended family. Experiences of this kind produce symptomatic behavior and dysfunctional and delayed development that differs from the single event, but may have a cumulative debilitating effect as great if not greater than the single overwhelming event. Lenore Terr has described these differences in her Type I and Type II Psychic Trauma Disorders (1989).

The following tables represent my expanded version of my June 1993 working draft of the NCCIP's diagnostic classification manual's categorization of traumatic stress disorders. I chose to adapt this draft because of its richness of clinical description, one that also highlights differences in symptom behaviors resulting from single events and those resulting from chronic enduring stress. The contents of this version were greatly condensed and reorganized by Drs. Charles Zeanah,

Serena Wieder, and Stanley Greenspan for the *Diagnostic Manual* as published (1994). I am particularly grateful to Dr. Zeanah for his contributions to the prior working drafts.

Table 44.1 presents the NCCIP diagnostic classification manual's (June 1993 working draft, with editorial changes by this author) categorization of traumatic stress disorders.

Table 44.2 contrasts symptom manifestations resulting from a single overwhelming event and chronic enduring events.

Examples of Psychosocial Stressors

Table 44.3 lists psychosocial stressors and traumatic events, acute and enduring, that impinge on the infant and young child, arranged in order of severity. This format lends itself to the development of a scale of psychosocial stressors, which could be rated numerically according to occurrence and degree of severity to provide a total stress index. Mild and moderate stressors are included because rapidly developing infants and young children are in a state of relatively unstable, changing equilibria, their adaptive and maturational changes require the outside support that parenting provides. At times of stress, this support is at least momentarily and often chronically unavailable, rendering the child and his or her developing ego functions vulnerable.

Thus, a relatively mild stressor such as the temporary absence, or irritability, or anxiety of a mother, when phase specific—that is, when it occurs at a particularly sensitive time of development—may have a severe impact, especially when an infant is vulnerable to begin with. As we have seen, chronically repeated events or enduring circumstances, each less than overwhelming in itself, may afford the infant some chance to adapt or defend by numbing or denying. In time, however, they also wear down the ego-adaptive and defensive functions and ultimately lead to regression and disorganization.

Recent studies have shown that infants and young children are especially vulnerable to the unpredictability and variety of stressors, which makes it much more difficult for denial and adap-

tation to take place. For instance, 3 or more stressors, even of moderate degree, will combine to reduce functioning IQ to retarded levels in a child with a previously normal or higher basic IQ. This reduction may not be easily reversible.

Again, the *overall* impact (significance or meaning) of any given traumatic event or milieu depends not only on the severity of the psychosocial stressor, but on the ability of the infant (1) to tolerate the stress; (2) to understand it; and (3) to have available outside help in coping as needed. In other words, the ultimate impact of a traumatic event depends on three factors: (1) the severity of the stressor (intensity and duration the stressor is maintained at that level, the suddenness of the initial stress, and the frequency and unpredictability of its recurrence); (2) the developmental level of the child (chronological age, endowment, and ego strength); and (3) the availability and capacity of outside support (adult) to serve as a protective buffer and to help the child understand and deal with the trauma/stress.

Clinical Examples with Discussion of the Long-term Implications and Effects

The common symptoms brought on by extreme events causing psychic trauma include: pervasive anxiety (which may become a more organized panic disorder), nightmares and other sleep problems, irritability, hypervigilance, startle responses, developmental regressions, and avoidance behaviors.

Of longer lasting import are (1) the capacity to recall and relive the incident through visual or other sensory modality memories; these are most clear and less distorted following a single catastrophic experience; (2) repetitive reenactment of both a single incident and enduring events through both behavioral play and physiological reactions; the child may not consciously associate these reenactments with the original traumata; (3) fears of objects, locations, and sensations specifically associated with the original trauma; these

TABLE 44.1

NCCIP Diagnostic Classification Manual—Traumatic Stress Disorders

I. Disorder Resulting from Single Event or Connected Single Series of Events
   A. The infant encounters and reacts to an experienced event or a connected series of events that is unexpected, shocking, and outside the range of usual human experience and that would be markedly distressing to almost anyone; for example, physical assault and/or perceived psychological threat to life or physical integrity, or witnessing serious injury or death of another individual(s) as the result of an accident, catastrophe, or physical violence. This is especially traumatic if there is an emotional attachment or familiarity with the individual(s). (Examples: terrorist attack on family or neighbors, assault rifle attack on preschool nursery, sexual assault, tornado, earthquake and aftershocks, attack or mauling by animal, bombing raids, etc.)

   B. The traumatic event is persistently and symptomatically reproduced or reexperienced in at least one of the following ways:
      1. Posttraumatic play, that is, repetitive play in which themes or aspects of the trauma are expressed. In children above 2½ or 3 years of age, clear verbal recollections of the event are usual. Below that age the memories are more likely to be manifest as somatic symptoms/memories, although instances have been reported where infants traumatized in a pre- or early verbal period can later put their experiences in basic verbal terms.
      2. Recurrent nightmares, even when the content cannot be ascertained.
      3. Intense psychological distress on encountering stimuli recalling some aspect of the traumatic event.
      4. Intense psychological distress at other times (not related to reminder of the trauma).
      Children younger than 18 months, who have limited representational capacities, are less likely to exhibit symptoms indicating a reexperiencing of the traumatic event. Underlying distress would more likely be manifest as disorders or affect, disregulation of behavior, and social disturbance without symbolic representation.

   C. Symptoms not present before the trauma appear in one or both of the forms described below.
      1. Persistent avoidance of stimuli associated with the trauma or numbing of general responsiveness (not present before the trauma), as indicated by at least one of the following:
         a. Loss of recently acquired developmental skills, e.g., language, toilet training.
         b. Marked withdrawal, with cessation of play or social interaction.
         c. Flattening of affect.
      2. Persistent symptoms of increased or decreased arousal (not present before the trauma) as indicated by at least two of the following:
         a. Difficulty falling or staying asleep.
         b. Irritability or outbursts of anger.
         c. Difficulty sustaining attention.
         d. Hypervigilance.
         e. Exaggerated startle response.
         f. Later sadness, withdrawal, preoccupation, anhedonia, or lability of affect.

   D. Onset may be soon after the traumatic event or be delayed as in posttraumatic stress disorders.

II. Disorders Resulting from Continuing, Enduring, or Multiple and Unpredictable Traumatic Events.

   When trauma is prolonged or repeated to the point of representing an enduring condition, the infant or young child may overcome the initial shock reaction and mobilize those defenses and adaptive mechanisms that are available at his or her stage of development.

   These may take the form of withdrawl of cathexis and a general numbing of psychic receptiveness and response. At higher levels of ego organization, the child may display gross repression, denial, primitive reaction formation, identification with the aggressor, and dissociation.

   When infants and young children have suffered from prolonged, repeated, and multiple traumatic events (especially when these are variable and unpredictable), the most prominent manifest symptoms are:
      1. state of confusion, fear, and panic, which may be followed by:
      2. anxiety, irritability, and anger, or sadness, which may then move on to:
      3. depressionlike psychic numbing, withdrawal, or, in the extreme cases, marasmus and failure to thrive in the below 2½- to 3-year-old. In the 2½- to 4-year-old, the adaptive defense pattern may advance to denial through forgetting or "not talking" about it. Another serious outcome can be an apparent indifference to pain or even a masochisticlike reaction formation, manifested by seeking out or pro-

TABLE 44.1

(continued)

voking abuse or traumatic conditions as if having mastered or even enjoying them. The behavior often has a dissociative quality. These reactions may be the precursor of pathologic character formation or multiple personality.

III. Delayed Psychic Trauma Disorder (provisional subtype)

Some clinicians report symptoms such as panic attacks, nightmares, and avoidance behaviors that develop several months after the occurrence of a known trauma. In retrospect, subtle symptoms may be present immediately after the trauma but do not disrupt the child's overall functioning enough to be noticed. These subtle symptoms, however, contribute to maladaptive interactions between child and parent that eventually disturb development and lead to clear-cut significant symptoms. For example, after trauma, a child may become only slightly avoidant and preoccupied. In response, the parent inadvertently pulls away ever so slightly, until one day the child experiences a challenge at nursery school, panics, and refuses to go any more. There also may be a delayed reaction without any intervening process. In some cases the trauma may not be known, but emerging symptoms may lead to further investigation as a result of which an earlier trauma is uncovered.

TABLE 44.2

Traumatic Stress Disorders

Symptom	*Manifestations*
Single or Single Series Event	*Chronic, Enduring, Unpredictable, Traumatic Events*
1. Traumatic event is clearly remembered and persistently reproduced or reexperienced.	1. An initial shock reaction in the form of confusion, fear and panic, followed by denial, and blunting of response.
a. Either repetitive play themes or direct verbal memories—if the incident took place below age 2, the reexperiencing is more likely to be somatic and physiologic form	2. As and if defenses and adaptive mechanisms can be mobilized that are consonant with the infant's developmental age, the child displays the anxiety of anticipation, irritability, anger, sadness, and/or chronic rage often turned on the self
b. Recurrent affect-laden nightmares	
c. Intense anxiety at exposure to reminders of the traumatic event	3. Depressionlike psychic numbing or withdrawal and dissociation or avoidance
2. Regression: Loss of recently acquired developmental skills, such as bowel control along with a withdrawal from play or social interaction; fear of separation	a. Below 2½ years, such a sequence may result in failure to thrive
3. Symptoms of increased or decreased arousal:	b. In the 2½- to 4-year-old, adaptive defenses may advance through "not talking about it" to forgetting, counterphobic behavior, indifference to pain, or even a masochisticlike reaction formation provoking abuse and seeming to enjoy it.
a. Sleep disturbance	
b. Irritability; angry outbursts	
c. Difficulty sustaining attention	
d. Hypervigilance	4. Delayed reaction showing later as a depressive or self-deprecating and self-defeating personality disorder, oppositional disorder, or the ultimate dissociative state, multiple personality. The child may develop profound guilt without conscious connection to or even memory of prior enduring trauma.
e. Exaggerated startle response	
f. Retrospection with sadness, depression, preoccupation, anhedonia	
4. Changing attitudes toward life and future—sense of limited future, hopelessness and loss of basic trust; misperceptions of subsequent events and time distortions.	

TABLE 44.3

Psychosocial Stressors

Notes on the use of this list in the 0- to 3-year infant population:
- In view of rapidly changing progression of developmental steps and the press of biological maturation, for the first year of life "predominantly acute events" should be regarded as those lasting under 1 month (for the first year) and under 3 months in the second and third years of life. "Predominantly enduring circumstances" should be those that last longer.

- In rating the severity of the psychosocial stressor, the following must be considered:
  The nature, intensity, and duration of the stressor and its predictability or unpredictability
  The effects of the trauma, given the infant's biological and developmental level of functioning

- For infants, psychosocial stressors are delineated in terms of the loss of basic safety, security, and comfort—that is, the protective supportive envelope in the infant's proximal microenvironment. The severity of a specific *type* of stressor is to be differentiated from its ultimate impact, which may be modified by the reaction of the environment. Thus, the child's human surrounding may shield and protect and thus lessen the impact, or may compound the impact by offering no protection, or even reinforce the child's distress through anxiety and negative attitudes. These modifying forces are not to be considered in rating the level of severity of the *specific* stressor; they come into play only in assessing its overall impact.
  However, a hostile, negative, rejecting family environment may in itself be a very powerful psychosocial stressor producing psychological battering.

Examples of Stressors

Mild Stressors

Acute Events
- Uneven care with abrupt changes in routine or setting
- Sudden weaning (may also be moderate stress)
- Loss of mother and replacement with foster care when under 4 to 5 months of age

Enduring Circumstances
- Exposure to chronic maternal anxiety
- Overburdened, exhausted mother (may also be to a moderate or severe degree)
- Overstimulation (excessive roughhousing, overfeeding, overburping, tickling)

Moderate Stressors

Acute Events
- Painful procedures and interference with parental bonding, such as may occur in intensive care or hospital procedure
- Acute loss through displacement by new sibling; temporary loss of primary caregiver while remaining in home environment (mother ill or hospitalized); injury (fall, burn, car accident) with mild to moderate injury not requiring hospitalization

Enduring Circumstances
- No bonding via rejecting or severely depressed mother
- Loss through displacement by new sibling (chronic response)
- Stress from insecurity, loss, hostility via: family tensions; jealous, hostile, infantile father; moderate depression or hostile, punitive teasing from mother
- Extended loss of mother and replacement by foster mother when over 5 months
- Overregulation on part of parent
- Overexpectation for performance from a vulnerable, deficient infant, as a denial or narcissistic rejection by parent
- Sexual seductiveness and overstimulation

Severe Stressors

Acute Events
- Retention of the newborn of an addict in intensive care because of a severe withdrawal reaction. (Here the trauma combines physical distress and an absence of "mothering")

Enduring Circumstances
- Retention in hospital and separated from mother (chronic respiratory disorder with infection or other contamination)

TABLE 44.3

(continued)

- Early return to hospital for surgery or anomaly (urethral, pyloric, or tracheal stenosis)
- Sudden loss of family milieu via short-term hospitalization of 2 to 5 days for injury, sepsis, dehydration

- Neglect and stimulus deprivation
- Harsh and negative affect and punishment from family (psychological battering); unpredictability and inconsistency via parental psychosis
- Severe and prolonged maternal depression (maternal unavailability)
- Marital violence (verbal and physical)
- Loss of basic security through disruption of family and creation of anxiety-ridden atmosphere via homelessness, war, famine, hostile or "crack" neighborhood (may also be extreme or catastrophic because of degree and length)

Extreme Stressors

Acute Events

- Sudden inflicted painful injury (battering of a crying infant or child attacked by animal bite or clawing); sexual attack (rape)
- Sudden loss of family or loss of home and security via family panic or disintegration as might be caused by sudden disaster, such as earthquake, fire, or tornado
- Loss through abduction (the reaction may be moderate to extreme) and isolation

Enduring Circumstances

- Continued physical and/or sexual abuse (impact of sexual abuse varies from moderate to extreme depending on phase specificity approach, etc.)
- Prolonged loss and lack of replacement of primary caretaker (separation, divorce, incarceration, death) (dying parent via cancer) (may be moderate to extreme)

Catastrophic Stressors

Acute Events

- Overwhelming anxiety and fear via witnessing parent's torture and/or death
- Sudden loss of family member by murder or drowning, especially when hemorrhage, dismemberment, and mangling of family member or caretaker is involved

Enduring Circumstances

- Chronic, life-threatening situation by virtue of continued physical abuse, battering, etc.
- Family overwhelmed by constant fear and anxiety because their lives are threatened by violence or surrounded by suffering and death or by starvation and disease
- Combined stresses as found in Bosnian, Lebanese,
- Somalian, Ethopian, and Romanian orphanages where hunger, anaclictic depression, and the loss of hope and will to live lead to marasmus and death

---

tend *not* to generalize; (4) loss of trust in the future and in the capacity of the family, school and the like to provide a protective envelope. The child exhibits a long-standing aura of pessimism, vulnerability, and expecting the worst.

Also, as previously noted, young children, more so than infants, experiencing repeated and enduring traumata are more able to make ego-defensive—often maladaptive—adjustments

through denial, often counterphobic, numbing and forgetting, regression and dissociation into fantasy. The following clinical examples illustrate not only the initial reactions but also the longer-lasting posttraumatic personality and characterological manifestations. At times, the child or adult is first seen for these later manifestations, and the original trauma is only later discovered or recalled during therapy.

Clinically, the symptomatic distinction between the single event and repeated enduring traumatic disorders is not always clear cut; over time, we may see crossover and change in the nature of the manifestation.

Case I: At this writing, four young boys ages 2 to 7 have just been seen on an emergency basis. They were referred by Protective Services within 48 hours of having witnessed their father beaten to death by their maternal uncle; this occurred during a drunken brawl that had started out as friendly horseplay. Father and uncle had been close friends who worked together. As was the custom in their Appalachia-like rural area, they had stopped off together at a tavern to have a few on the way home; these became a few too many. After arrival home, the horseplay began, and the tragic escalation took place. After an initial shock reaction, the boys became agitated and totally hyperactive. The older boys showed only minimal availability and ability to exert the "older brother" constraints and protectiveness over the younger ones. Despite their confusion and unfocused anxiety, each could give a clear verbal account of what happened—much less vivid and detailed in the limited language available to the younger two. Mother's account was spare and affectless. She said, "I am very very angry. I have lost a good man. We had a good life and we were very close, and I am two months' pregnant." She was psychically numbed and depressed, and mechanically going through the motions of doing what she had to do. Both mother and children had witnessed a brutal murder and suffered the loss of two adult men they had been very close to and loved, each in their own way. Each was totally overwhelmed so as to be unable to render intrafamilial support; all required intensive treatment and support from the outside.

This vignette illustrates the initial impact of the lack of the protective envelope that might otherwise have mitigated the severity of the impact on the children. External resources had to be mobilized. A long-lasting posttraumatic course for each person may be predicted.

Case II: G., an extremely bright and verbally and motorically precocious 3-year-old, was driving with his mother when their car, slowing down for the car ahead, was rear-ended by a tractor trailer truck at 50 mph. Both mother and child were safety belted and neither was obviously physically traumatized. Because mother was wearing a neck collar (from a previous whiplash neck injury 1½ years before), the rescue squad insisted on carrying her off on a plank stretcher, and, despite her entreaties that they take her child out of the car seat and let him ride with her, he was left in the car seat with the police, crying as he saw her being carried off to the hospital for examination. When he returned home to be reunited with his mother, he was alternatively anxious, clinging and demanding, or hyperactively far ranging in his physical play. His game involved actively playing out different versions of the accident. In one, he smashed his bicycle into a wall or pushed it down the stairs yelling "I'm in an accident." In another, he defensively displaced both the affect and the affected, telling his older brother "My friend J. had an accident. A truck hit him and they had to take his mother out on a board and put her in an ambulance. I'm not scared, but *he* was and worried about his mother." Three days later he was brought for assessment and treatment because of nightmares, problems going to sleep, persistent complaints about pain in his right foot (pediatric examination showed nothing), a need to have mother constantly within sight or hearing, a loss of bowel control (which had been attained 4 months earlier) and general anxious, whiny, clinging behavior, a total change from his preaccident sunny disposition. He displayed a worried, questioning, alertness about what was going on or will be happening. It is interesting that his grandmother referred to his loss of bowel control as his "accidents." When later it was suggested to him that his "pooping" accidents were no accident but an accident *he* could control, their occurrence was reduced considerably.

G. had regressed to an 18- to 24-month-old level in his play; he was filling and dumping, building and smashing. *He* was the truck driver, *he* was the doctor. The theme of his play became one of activity triumphing over passivity—moving from helplessness to being in charge and making things happen.

Issues of loss appeared. When brought to the interview office, he was able to separate from mother with the reassurance that she would be in the waiting room. We dealt with his sleep problems in terms of his fear of waking up and finding her gone. He was able to fall asleep if mother sat in the room, yet the theme "Hold me—I need you" persisted. This was interpreted to him as a way of feeling safer, like a little baby whom mother had to protect and be there for.

When in the car, he continued to have periods of specific phobic anxiety. He was hypervigilant about safety procedures and the route taken, making sure that everyone was belted in, that the speed limit was being observed, and that the road taken could not lead to the expressway, the site of the accident, which he specifically sought to avoid. Upon request, he could recall and talk about the accident in detail, but the intensity of the phobic anxiety and his continued play of smashing what he drove or built led me to inform him that his parents had told me there had been a previous accident when he was a baby of 1½. Although at the time he was unharmed, his mother and brother were hurt. Could it be that the pain in his foot and some of his scared feelings came from that time when he could hardly remember to tell in words, but his body could remember the scared feelings and the pain? The anxiety decreased.

Despite these phobic and regressive tendencies, after the first month he was able to return to nursery school at his own request. Despite some anxiety about the bus having an accident, he was able to go off with only minimal anxiety. He surpassed his preschool peers academically and physically to the point that he was placed in another class where the children were 9 to 12 months older. He adapted quite well, socially and academically. However, he would withhold toileting until his return home.

By the fourth month, his behavior took on characterological qualities, with premature phallic-oedipal explorations interleaved with anal preoccupations. He deployed his body as a whole, diving, jumping, and karate-chopping as if he were a truck. Preoccupation with smells and oppositional testing followed. Possessing mother and controlling her became a wish to marry her, be in bed with Mommy, and have Daddy sleep downstairs. This was countered by the gentle explanation that Mommy is daddy's wife. When he grows up like daddy he can get his own wife. Meanwhile Daddy and Mommy will take care of him and help him grow up. G. thereafter turned his seductive attentions toward the mother of his best friend.

A direct attempt was made to get him weaned from mother and identified with both father and big-boy activities by giving him more time with his father. This was proceeding successfully when, at 5 months' postaccident, it became apparent that mother's neck injuries would require neurosurgical intervention. G. was given careful preparation, including visiting the hospital, meeting mother's surgeon and, on his own initiative, playing out his version of the surgery. Despite this, his sleep and separation problems returned. On visiting his mother postoperatively, he panicked and refused to go home with his father until she promised to come home the next evening, which she did, albeit prematurely. Nightmares resumed, and he would cling to her legs and refuse to separate to the point that several home visits by the therapist were required. Although G. was doing well in his preschool program, it was another month before easy separation from mother was accomplished, and this was associated with the return of her mobility. His play involved being the fireman and the building wrecker. He then became messy and tyrannically demanding of his mother and nasty to the point that mother was referring to herself as the abused one. It reached a peak when he acted out the same behavior in the playroom. He dumped everything on the floor from every container and slogged his feet through the mess, returned from the bathroom incompletely wiped

(which he could do very well), and tracked his feces around the playroom. "I'll hunt you down and poop on you." He refused to gather things up and clean up and listened for the sound of his mother's car. As she was coming up the stairs he went out to greet her and said "I'm scared," but then demanded that she clean up for him. He knew she had to leave to pick up his older brother, and demanded that she pick up for him. Instead, she threatened to leave him in 5 minutes if he hadn't completed the job. Having done this, I suggested she follow through on her promise and sent the next patient away so I could continue with him. G. cried in disbelief when she left. I explained that in reality he wasn't the boss, he was scared of what he had done, and he was relieved that I had taken over and would not let him do so. It scared him that he was out of control of himself. The accidents had made him feel so helpless, he had wanted to be in charge and in control, but in real life his mother and father were the bosses, and as long as he could trust them to be the boss and to be strong and protect him, he would feel better. The accident was something his mother could not help and he has been angry at her because she could not protect him from it. He grudgingly at first, but then with increasing gusto, cooperated as we made a game out of it.

He was relieved when his mother returned to pick him up as promised.

In a hastily called meeting with G.'s parents that night, his behavior was explained to them on several levels—his anger at mother for not being the omnipotent protector, his ambivalent, defensive need to drive her off to guard against his own prematurely evoked oedipal wishes, mixed with his infantile regression. His mother confirmed that his anal-abusive behavior would "like clockwork" follow an oedipal overture. We set up a strict formula of limit setting and the availability of father's presence for superego formation—both of which he needed desperately. Limit setting had been set aside for him out of guilt and compassion of his upset.

G.'s anal sadistic behavior gradually resolved. His play is now of Superman who is invulnerable to bullets and battering and conquers all, goodies and baddies. He has identified with the men building an addition to his house and is himself building roads and bridges. He recently constructed a guillotinelike device that chops off the heads of bad guys. His development seems to be getting back on track.

This case was presented in detail to illustrate the longer-term effects of a catastrophic single event. If it occurs at a sensitive phase, it can throw development off track both by inducing regression and by stimulating premature and pathological character formations. Key to G.'s reactions were the feelings of helplessness that he had experienced and the premature loss of trust because his mother could not be the all-protective envelope under which he had flourished. G.'s parents always had been supportive of and had cheered on his developmental achievements. A well-endowed infant, he had blossomed under this encouragement. One wonders if his reaction to the accident would have been as total if he had been more on his own and in a less supported and prematurely developed state. It is interesting also that early on, he was able to return to nursery school and respond to his father with trust. In his reality they had not failed him. This supports Terr's observation that the fears are trauma specific—in this case, in the child's eyes, it was a specific failure on his mother's part. This case points out that not only the specific trauma must be addressed, but also all the developmental repercussions that it spawned, lest a premature personality and character disorder result.

One suspects also that this accident had called up affects from a previous traumatic accident at 1½, when G. was too young to experience it and later recall it in verbal terms. This may have contributed to the intensity of the affect by setting up a state of heightened vulnerability in respect to just that sequence of events that unfortunately recurred.

Case III: M. was referred by her pediatrician at 3½ years of age for severe behavior problems. These included poor peer relationships, sullen affect, nastiness, and tantrums. Although upset if her mother left the room, she pulled away from attempts to hug her. Mother felt threatened and appalled by her behavior. At 2 years 9 months, however, M. developed cystitis and pyelitis. A month later, her constricted urethra was dilated in the urologist's office without anesthesia. Mother described M.'s terror and pain from the procedure. A month later she was hospitalized for 4 days. Urethotomy was performed under general anesthesia. She was again terrified and would not look at her mother when she visited the next day. Again, a month later, dysuria with cystitis and vaginitis developed and she was unwillingly subjected to vaginal suppositories and frequent catheterizations by the office nurse. These continued for some time, overlapping the early part of her analytic therapy. She would often hide her pain to avoid these procedures.

Her persistent affect was that of anger. She had regressed somewhat, but fixated largely at a "terrible twos" level. Analysis revealed that she blamed her mother for abandoning her at the hospital and not protecting her from the assaults on her genitals. She identified with the aggressor by catheterizing her dolls. In puppet play, horns, noses, fingers, and ears were bitten off. The themes of her play were castration and penetration. Although she could not talk about the traumatic events, she played them out—being prepped and wheeled in on a high cart. She was hyperaware of genital and gender differences and made these differentiations in objects even when they did not exist. A year into her analysis, perhaps fostered by biological maturation, in her fantasy play her father became the surgeon and under the canopy (O.R. lights and hood) his Friday night ritual of cutting the "challa" (bread) became confused with his cutting the "colla" (bride) = her.

The anger at her helplessness in the traumatic play which signifies being in control and the triumph of activity over passivity were important themes for this child and, indeed, seem to appear in the working through of most psychic trauma disorders. For instance, she would spread the biting wolf puppet's jaw wide, and, remarking that she was making it hurt, thus reproduced her own situation in the gynecological stirrup table. She would then snap the wolf's jaw shut on a finger or a doctor puppet head, thus converting helplessness to aggression. The phase-specific appearance of conflicts generated by her repeated and enduring traumas became couched in phallic-oedipal terms.

Her chronic anger and sullenness and need to be in control could gradually be interpreted to her, as was her "be brave, don't cry" theme, which appeared again and again.

Without going into the details of the analysis, it is clear that this example of psychic trauma in infancy had an impact on M.'s subsequent development, causing fixations at the anal-sadistic level. This, in turn, colored the nature of subsequent oedipal development. If left untreated, this pattern could result in undesirable character traits, behavior problems, mistrust of people, and, it can be projected, problems in M.'s sexual adjustment. Although therapy brought much improvement, a quality of mistrust, nastiness, needing to be in control, and a diminished capacity to be carefree and have fun persisted as personality traits. This suggests that to a certain degree the impact of the trauma remains imbedded and difficult to reach through conflict-oriented therapy.

Case IV: A. was referred at age 4 with the diagnosis of infantile autism. This diagnosis was supported by competent psychological testing, and marked by loss of speech, withdrawal, anxiety, and bizarre hand movements developing at age 2.

A detailed history indicated a normal pregnancy and perinatal course, and a level of premorbid development unusual in autistic children. Social and motor milestones had been precocious. He had been very cuddly and breast-fed for 23 months, weaning himself at that time. Speech was precocious. By 14 months he was using 4- and 5-word sentences and had 100-word vocabulary. He was a happy, energetic young child. From 17 to 24 months, A. had had a series of negative babysitting and day care experiences culminating at 24 months in a private home day care situation in which he suddenly developed panicky crying, banging on doors and windows, and refusal to return. He lost his recently achieved toilet training. Anxiety-driven hyperactivity began in which he would run in circles or back and forth, flapping his hands, or twisting and wringing them as he held them over his head. He stopped talking and relating appropriately. By the time I was consulted at age 4, he had begun to jargon and talk in phrases, but with infantile articulation. He had been entered in a series of special preschool programs by which he was described as perseverative, withdrawn, and tuned out most of the time. He would become perseveratively fascinated with all aspects of a particular object, such as lawn mowers or vacuum cleaners, and would repetitiously open and close doors.

In the playroom, his hyperactive behavior and twiddling of pencils and paintbrushes or twisting and wringing of his hands held above his head were prominent and anxiously driven. He perseveratively made unrecognizable scribbles, mostly in red paint, and gave them the names of barnyard animals and birds. He would stare at these, flap, and twiddle the paintbrush. At one point in the midst of these scribbles, a life-size figure of an erect penis could be discerned. When asked what this was, he gave no answer, nor did he display any affection reaction when I commented "It looks like a big man's penis." He, however, became concerned with the tackiness of the paint on his fingers and began compulsive hand washing. His hand wringing took on the character of trying to get something sticky off his fingers. At home he would intermix his twiddling of pencils with direct masturbation, and began to stuff the fingers of one hand into his mouth. Facial tics appeared. In the playroom he discovered a set of 12-inch table legs in a cabinet drawer and began sucking on one. When he explored a closet with an upright vacuum cleaner, he began sucking on the end of the curved handle.

Without referring to his explicit behavior, I asked his mother for more detail about the circumstances of his being withdrawn from the private day care. Mother interjected that an article on child sexual abuse in a parents' magazine had set her wondering. At that time the day care owner's mentally ill grown son had been returned from the state hospital. Mother had seen him wandering around, swathed in a sheet. Could he have been abusing A.? had been growing in her mind, but she tried to suppress it. It had been too awful to think about. She felt guilty for not removing him sooner, but she had needed a day care situation. Mother asked him if he remembers M.'s house (the day care site). His response was to get up, open the back door, cry, and clutch his penis. The next day, after driving by the house, she had asked if F. (the son) had done anything to him. His response was to hop up and down, frenetically babbling about a baby cow and milk in bed with its mommy. He regressed to fecal smearing and called himself a bad boy. She remembered that a few days before his final refusal to go to day care and panic, he had pushed his fingers down his throat until he choked. That day she had come to pick him up and found him locked in a side room, banging on the door with feces in his pants. She also remembered that a number of other parents (mostly professional career women) had removed their children at that time. She contacted several of the families. None wanted to talk about it but implied that things had gone on. One said in parting, "If you go to court I'll back you up."

We spent the next 4 years in gradual reconstruction and working through the events, which had included oral penetration and penile manipulation. The oral trauma was responsible for the sudden cessation of speech. A.'s helplessness and being locked in led to his having to be in control of opening and closing all doors and panicking when he could not. His hyperactivity was anxiety driven, his hand movements were both involvement with the tackiness of the sticky stuff and hand washing. A. had to be in control, be the boss, and gradually deal with his underlying rage. His recall was expressed largely through compulsive behaviors—drawing and acting-out behavior rather than reenactment. Although he has largely recovered his speech, he could verbalize only isolated fragments about his traumata—"F. was bad; taste salty, too big." He remains a provocative, compulsive, unhappy, questioning child who, however, is doing better academically and socially. He plays on words and makes clang associations that have led school consultants to wonder about a nascent thought disorder and schizophrenic process. Medication with clomipramine reduced his obsessive/compulsive symptoms.

This is an example of a child whose early traumatic event went unrecognized or denied. (Parental denial "Say it isn't so" is very common.) It was discovered only when his posttraumatic symptomatology, which had mimicked autism, was assessed and a reconstruction made. Much of his behavior was an attempt to express and undo the overwhelming sensations associated with overstimulation, helplessness, and confinement.

Even when a young child has considerable speech before the trauma, the "unspeakable, unthinkable event" (Winnicott's term for a trauma that is beyond a child's expressive capacity to put into words or thoughts) cannot be expressed verbally, so the child is left with only the somatic, affective pathways for recall. These recollections can sometimes be put into words at a later date when the child has reached a higher adaptive and developmental stage.

Case V: P. was referred at the age of 3½ because of failure to develop communicative speech and to become toilet trained. He was characterized as being in a world of his own. P.'s medical background was negative except for the history of his being scalded at 1½ by boiling water from a pot he had pulled down from the stovetop. In P.'s family the men were weak, alcoholic, and abusive; the women were traditionally strong, but deferred to the men and tolerated the abuse. P. could not communicate verbally but drew strange creatures that had a whimsical human quality about them. Although he spent much time distanced from his peers and seemingly talking to himself in a strange jargon, he grew attached to his child care worker for whom he drew many drawings. Some were of these creatures, some of tunnellike projections from a window to a moonlike body in the sky, and some were words in a strange alphabet. It was several years before he could talk and print English words under the strange script, Rosetta Stone–like, and could verify our impression that these represented his fantasy of escaping the continued stress of experiencing and witnessing abuse by going into his own world. At one point, before this, at about age 4½, mundane TV-screenlike drawings appeared. He was agitated as he drew but could not verbalize an explanation. On inquiry, his mother informed us that his 2-year-old brother had scalded himself in the same manner by pulling down a pot of boiling water, again left unsupervised on the stove. The drawings then had not been of a TV set but of the front of the oven below the burners. What had struck the family was that P. began screaming in pain and verbalizing "Oh my God! Call an ambulance, Joe! Get him to the hospital!" reproducing word for word and affect for affect the anxiety and turmoil of the family's agitated reaction to his original trauma at 1½. It was as if the incident had been tape-recorded in his mind and the new catastrophe had pushed the "play" button.

Indeed it had. A kind of primitive one-time learning found also in other mammals and birds, called "imprinting" by the animal ethologists, results in an indelible memory impression, which is relatively unmodifiable by defensive ego reworking. This seems to be the primary form of affect-associated learning laid down in the first 6 to 9 months of life, closely associated to the limbic-arousal system. It is most certainly activated in older children and adults when the sensory-affect impact of a psychically traumatic event has overwhelmed the ego's capacity to receive, modulate, master, and adapt to the stimuli. The younger the infant or child is maturationally, the more vulnerable he or she is to these overwhelming stresses and, indeed, the more likely it is that a given stress becomes overwhelming. In the preverbal child, or even in the verbal child whose verbal capacity cannot express the intensity and complexity of the experience, it is the nonverbal psychosensorimotor motor experiences that are relived and reenacted.

Second, in the infant, whose body image and body boundaries are not yet well defined, what is remembered and imprinted as *his or her* own experience is the whole undifferentiated gestalt, including the stress reactions and anxiety states of parents and supposedly protective milieu.

With a single catastrophic, overwhelming event, the memories are more likely to remain clear, unchangeable and unforgettable. This may best be explained by this mechanism of imprinting.

A joint study was carried out of the impact of early life traumata on the formation of later pathological aggression and self-destruction (Ruttenberg, Herzog, & Dervian, 1983). This involved both prospective study of 24 premature infants requiring extensive neonatal intensive care featuring massive intrusive physical insult and a retrospective study of 36 autistic children. Both investigations showed a direct correlation between the experiencing of early life traumata (in the second population this also included postnatal abuse and neglect) and the development of self-destructive, self-mutilating behaviors and/or behavior that invited or provoked abuse from adult caregivers.

It was postulated that the impact of the early traumatic intrusion was at the neuronal synaptic level, setting up associative aggressive displays at the subcortical level, which later can be triggered as a patterned response.

Similarly, affective and somatic displays can be set up serving as a primitive memory experienced as pain, a skin reaction, an affect, and so on.

The fact that we may be dealing with actual structural changes in these cases would explain why it is so difficult to modify these displays by psychological means.

We suspect that these early traumatic experiences are in fact early nuclear organismal experiences by the still-forming ego that can shape the way the child later seeks pleasure or pain and, indeed, other aspects of character formation (Ruttenberg, 1985). This sequence can also be set up in later childhood and even in adulthood under circumstances when ego functioning has been shattered or suspended by an overwhelming psychic trauma, allowing actual changes in brain structure to take place. These changes have been documented in cases of torture and long incarceration of political prisoners.

This neuronal level imprinting would explain the classic cases of "shell shock" (World War I) and "battle fatigue" (World War II) in which, after a terrible incident in which his buddies' brains were blown out before his eyes or after a prolonged battle, the soldier is found numbed and confused. After that, for years he is able to function only in a marginal way. He might even be able to talk about the experience in a detached, affectless way. Then, years later, triggered by a single event or stimulus, the former soldier relives the whole flight or battle episode again with intense affect and psychomotor reenactment. This reliving might last for several days, as if every experience and reaction had become his, and with such immediacy that all the observers, staff or family, are caught up in the affective reenactment.

Clearly, then, these traumata will have long-standing, even lifetime impacts on the nature of the person's personality and characterological responses. Such early events have been implicated in the formation of multiple personality disorder.

Case VI: F was a 28-year-old unmarried female when she was referred to me over 35 years ago by her socially prominent sister, because of bouts of odd and outrageous behavior not in keeping with her usual shy, quiet self. At her sister's soirees she might unpredictably become forward and so sparkling that the men would gather around her as if drawn by a magnet. She also would disappear for days at a time and could not account for her whereabouts when she returned. The description of the analysis of her multiple personality dissociative disorder is not the purpose of this vignette. Suffice it to say that each of her 6 named personalities represented an earlier traumatic incident that had been denied. As the analysis progressed, behind each layer, earlier traumata were uncovered that had influenced the setting up of the traumatic situation. For instance, one personality (J.) embodied her seductive behavior that had set up the conditions that led to her being followed off a subway stop and raped in a vacant lot which she had crossed, rather than remaining on the lighted sidewalk. Another (E.) was the name of a girlfriend whose parents she coveted and at 8 years had pushed down a flight of stairs, fantasizing that after E. died the parents would adopt her. Becoming E. was a way of both accomplishing that and undoing the death wish and act. As the analysis reached back to earlier developmental levels, this right-handed, milk-hating girl found herself drinking milk and writing with her left hand. Only then did she remember the kindergarten teacher's prolonged and sadistic methods for forcing her to be right-handed and her mother's tyrannical way of forcing her to drink milk at that time. Her "cockteasing" behavior with men became a crisis situation in that it had provoked violent responses. Her doodles included daggers with a curled twist at the point. She began to complain of a dank, musty odor on the couch, writhe as if pinned down, whine and cry in an infantile voice. Stigmata appeared on her face and neck, on the latter in the form of a handprint. Beyond the complaint "it hurts," she could produce no verbal memory. We reconstructed that she must have been attacked in a dank, musty place—perhaps a back alley. Family contact verified the reconstruction as reported in the papers and hospital records—the culprit was a 15-year-old neighbor, uncircumcized, then diagnosed schizophrenic and committed to a state hospital, where he later died. Her family said she did not have much reaction after the acute fright and marks of the physical trauma had gone. However, in retrospect, she had begun lying and acting strangely—such as letting the dog out of the yard and denying she had done so, or hiding valuable family objects and insisting she did not do it. These were evidently early dissociations. Eventually her various personalities were reintegrated into one total personality and the dissociative behavior disappeared.

F.'s behavior over the years represented an attempt to rework her experience of total helplessness, which occurred during the original ordeal, by dissociation and by being the one who made things happen. Again, a victim of Winnicott's "unthinkable" anxiety, she could not put her original experience into words, and even years later could only act it out, draw a representation, and experience it in a affectosomatosensory motor way.

Her case, as do the others cited, portrays the long-term influence of trauma on the victim's attitudes, behavior, and ability to enjoy life. At times, only through the analysis of the characterological traits and behaviors is the original trauma rediscovered and worked through.

Since the original preparation of this article, *DSM-IV* was introduced (May 1994), and a number of research studies have been reported on the severe and lasting impact of violence, loss, and other severe traumata and acute and chronic stressors on the infant and young child, developmentally, emotionally, psychosocially, and neurobiologically. These studies tend to verify the clinical impressions and hypotheses reported earlier. They illustrate the extreme complexity of the traumatic experience and of the intense mental activity and variety of responses and processes mobilized in the immediate posttrauma period and subsequently as the organism attempts to deal with the overwhelming breach of functioning adaptations, protective ego defenses, and the protective envelope usually afforded by the caregiving milieu.

DSM-IV contains not only an expanded list of overwhelming stressors that can produce PTSD but also lists, for the first time, special developmentally based alternative symptomatology in the young child. *DSM-IV* also adds a category called Acute Stress Disorder; in this disorder, dissociative symptoms, avoidance, and/or arousal and reliving of the trauma take place. If they persist, the disorder becomes PTSD.

Since Perry (1995) and Pynoos (1995) note that there are always repercussions that may not, however, show up until much later, I feel that treating the acute phase as a separate entity could deter the therapist from setting up long-term treatment goals and, in fact, could lead him or her to assume that it has all gone away: "Out of sight, out of mind."

Scheeringa et al. (1995) compared the reliability and validity of the *DSM-IV* criteria with those of the NCCIP's *Diagnostic Classification of Mental Health and Developmental Disorders of Infancy and Early Childhood* (1994) for children under 48 months of age. They found that the NCCIP's criteria were more reliable and valid, and suggested that the standard nosologies will need revision for this age group.

Thomas (1995) concluded that the *DSM-IV* criteria for PTSD were not sensitive enough to be used with the under-4-year-old population; he found those of the NCCIP diagnostic manual (1994), with its developmental orientation, to be much more applicable to infants and young children.

Marans (1995), studying traumatized inner-city children, views exposure to violence as an assault on repression and ego functions in which the child loses the ability to anticipate and to prepare for danger, and to assimilate and to accommodate to the overwhelming stimuli, resulting in neurovegetative dysregulation and subsequent increase in anxiety and new symptomatology.

Scheeringa and Zeanah (1995), studying symptom expression and trauma variables in infants and young children, were surprised to find that PTSD was present more often when the trauma involved threats or injury to caregivers than when the injury was directly experienced by the child. Also, if the parent developed PTSD following a catastrophe, the children were more likely also to develop PTSD—a verification of the original observations made by A. Freud and D. Burlingham in the London subways' bomb shelters in 1944.

Pynoos et al. (1995) have put forth a comprehensive model for integrating the extremely complex interactions involved in the etiology, course, and outcome of traumatic stress on children. They state that assessment should involve the complexity of the traumatic experiences, the secondary stressors, the resilience, the vulnerabilities, and the interactions with the social ecology, the stage of development, and the psychopathology of the child. They present a schematic model of the interacting factors over time.

Perry et al. (1995) discuss the impact of traumatic experiences on the development and functioning of the brain, and postulate that trauma produces neuronal change in the developing brain and in its neurotransmitter systems. They observe that acute adaptive responses, including hyperarousal and dissociation, may, by this means, persist as maladaptive traits ranging from freezing to oppositional-defiant behavior. The authors feel that because the young brain is developing, it is more vulnerable to stressful trauma; we must not use children's so-called resiliency as an excuse to do nothing (i.e., the pediatricians' "Oh, they'll grow out of it" myth).

Finally, Gaensbaur and Siegel (1995), noting the numer of ways that trauma may affect the rapidly developing young child and his or her family, have delineated five levels of impact that have to be addressed in the formulation of therapeutic interventions.

1. The direct impact of the trauma on the child with defensive numbing and heightened arousal with a strong neurobiological base.

2. Associated emotional reactions unique to each child, which derive also from the specific nature of the trauma and its particular content.
3. An interruption or regression from current developmental tasks.
4. The effect on future developmental tasks.
5. The effect of the trauma and the child's symptoms on his or her interaction with the family and on other social interrelationships.

The authors delineate therapeutic principles and stages of therapeutic approach: first soothing and desensitizing the acute reactions, then eliciting and playing through the posttraumatic reenactments, and finally bringing in the parents to work through their reactions to their traumatized child. Medications, while helpful, are to be used with caution and are considered to be adjunctive to the psychotherapeutic interventions.

REFERENCES

American Psychiatric Association. (1980). *Diagnostic and statistical manual of mental disorders* (3rd ed.). Washington, DC: Author.

American Psychiatric Association. (1987). *Diagnostic and statistical manual of mental disorders* (3rd ed., rev.). Washington, DC: Author.

American Psychiatric Association. (1994). *Diagnostic and statistical manual of mental disorders* (4th ed.). Washington, DC: Author.

Call, J. D. (1987). Psychiatric syndromes of infancy. In J. D. Noshpitz (Ed.), *Basic handbook of child psychiatry* (Vol. 5, p. 252). New York: Basic Books.

Freud, A., & Burlingham, D. (1944). *War and children.* New York: International Universities Press.

Freud, S. (1955). *Beyond the pleasure principle.* In J. Strachey (Ed. and Trans.), *The standard edition of the complete psychological works of Sigmund Freud* (hereafter *Standard edition*) (Vol. 18, pp. 1–64). London: Hogarth Press. (Originally published 1920.)

Freud, S. (1959). Inhibitions, symptoms, and anxiety. In *Standard edition* (Vol. 20, pp. 94–129). (Originally published 1926.)

Gaensbauer, T. J., & Siegel, C. H. (1995). Therapeutic approaches to posttraumatic stress disorder in infants and toddlers. *Infant Mental Health Journal, 16* (4), 292–305.

Goodwin, J. (1987). Developmental impacts of incest. In J. D. Noshpitz (Ed.), *Basic handbook of child psychiatry* (Vol. 5, pp. 106–109). New York: Basic Books.

Kessler, E. S. (1979). Reactive disorders. In J. D. Noshpitz (Ed.), *Basic handbook of child psychiatry* (Vol. 2, pp. 175–176). New York: Basic Books.

Marans, S. (1995, December). *Exposure to violence: An assault on repression.* Paper presented at the Vulnerable Child Symposium at the Midwinter Meetings of the American Psychoanalytic Association, New York.

National Center for Clinic Infant Programs. (1994). *Diagnostic classification of mental health and developmental disorders of infancy and early childhood.* Arlington, VA: Author.

Perry, B. D., Pollard, R. A., Blakley, T. L., Baker, W. L., & Vigilante, D. (1995). Childhood trauma, the neurobiology of adaptation, and "use-dependent" development of the brain: How "states" become "traits." *Infant Mental Health Journal, 16* (4), 271–289.

Pynoos, R. S., Steinberg, A. M., and Wraith, R. (1995). A developmental model of childhood traumatic stress. In D. Cicchetti & D. Cohen (Eds.), *Manual of developmental psychopathology. Vol. 2: Risk, disorder and adaptation* (pp. 72–95). New York: John Wiley & Sons.

Ruttenberg, B. A. (1985, December 22). *The origins of masochism.* Paper presented at the midwinter meetings of the American Psychoanalytic Association, New York.

Ruttenberg, B. A., Herzog, J. M., & Derivan, A. T. (1983, April 1). *Association of early life traumata and pathological aggression in children.* Paper presented at the Second World Congress of Infant Psychiatry and Allied Disciplines, Cannes, France.

Scheeringa, M. S., & Zeanah, C. H. (1995). Symptom expression and trauma variables in infants under 48 months of age. *Infant Mental Health Journal, 16* (4), 259–270.

Scheeringa, M. S., Zeanah, C. H., Drell, M. J., & Larrieu, J. A. (1995). Two approaches to the diagnosis of post-traumatic stress disorder in infancy and early childhood. *Journal of the American Academy of Child and Adolescent Psychiatry, 34* (2), 191–200.

Terr, L. C. (1979). Children of Chowchilla—a study of psychia trauma. *Psychoanalytic Study of the Child, 34,* 547–623.

Terr, L. C. (1987). Childhood psychic trauma. In J. D. Noshpitz (Ed.), *Basic handbook of child psychiatry, Vol. 5: Advances and new directions* (pp. 262–272). New York: Basic Books.

Terr, L. C. (1989, December 7). *The sudden shocks and the long-standing terrors of childhood: What's alike and what's different?* First annual Weissman Memorial Lecture, Pennsylvania Hospital, Philadelphia, PA.

Thomas, J. M. (1995). Traumatic stress disorder presents as hyperactivity and disruptive behavior. Case presentation, diagnosis and treatment. *Infant Mental Health Journal, 16* (4), 306–317.

45 / Autism and the Pervasive Developmental Disorders

Ami Klin and Fred R. Volkmar

The pervasive developmental disorders (PDDs) are a group of conditions that share certain core clinical features but that seem to reflect diverse etiologies and natural course. The conditions have their onset in infancy or early childhood and are characterized by typical patterns of delay and deviance affecting primarily the areas of social, affective, and communicative development. Of the various diagnostic concepts included within the overarching class of PDDs, infantile autism, or autistic disorder (American Psychiatric Association [APA], 1987), is the best studied and the paradigmatic condition against which other PDD conditions are defined. Consequently it will be discussed in greatest detail in this chapter. Other conditions within the PDD class are variably included in different diagnostic systems. Despite a recent surge of research studies on these "nonautistic" PDDs, apart from autism their validity still remains controversial (Klin & Volkmar, 1995).

The phenomenological definition of autism remains virtually the same as that initially described by Kanner (1943). However, the wide range of severity, developmental level, and natural course documented in the literature necessitated the creation of the PDD class in order to include disorders with a presentation differing somewhat from Kanner's description of autism. The term *pervasive developmental disorder* emphasizes the pervasiveness of disturbances over a wide range of different domains (in contrast to both the relatively more delineated disabilities of the specific developmental disorders and the anchoring effects of cognitive deficits in primary mental retardation), and the developmental nature of the disorders affecting the normative unfolding of multiple competencies, particularly interpersonal relationships and communication.

In this chapter we provide a historical review of the major diagnostic concepts under the PDD class, then give a clinical description of autism and discuss diagnostic issues, clinical assessment, and interventions.

Diagnostic Concepts

HISTORICAL BACKGROUND

Prior to Kanner's first compendium on child psychiatry (Kanner, 1935), the history of concepts defining early childhood disorders reflected the narrow contemporaneous views of both mental illness and child development. The centuries' old anthropological quest for "the savage in the state of nature" (Zing, 1940) led to descriptions of the so-called feral children, whose bizarre behaviors and absence of language could be explained only by their being reared outside human society (Levi-Strauss, 1949). The most reliable of such accounts, the "Wild Boy of Aveyron," appeared to exhibit the behaviors characteristic of autistic children (Wing, 1978).

The advent of the neurological sciences in the 19th century was accompanied by early taxonomic efforts. The absence of a discipline characterizing children's normative development, however, led to simple extensions of psychopatholgoical concepts derived from work with psychotic adults. In 1867 Maudsley suggested that children could exhibit "insanity." In 1906 De Sanctis extended Kraeplin's concept of dementia praecox (now termed schizophrenia) to describe conditions characterized by an onset in early childhood, social and cognitive deterioration, and stereotypic behavior. In order to distinguish such conditions from disorders with an onset in late adolescence or early adulthood, De Sanctis coined the terms *dementia praecocissima* and *dementia precocissima catatonica.* Heller's (1930), concept of *dementia infantilis* (now termed childhood disintegrative disorder) depicted similar individuals whose condition, however, followed a variable period of normal development in early childhood. Earl's (1934) "primitive catatonic psychosis of idiocy" described a group of severely mentally retarded individuals with no speech and a marked indifference to people as well as absorption in repetitive, purposeless movements. Interestingly, even though the term *idiot* had been used as a classification of mental retardation for over a century, its meaning has the same derivation from Greek as "autistic," meaning a person who lives in his or her own world; originally the term was used in a way similar to the current use of autism (Benda, 1952). Several of Langdon Down's patients described as idiot savants (Down, 1887) presented autistic behaviors, and, in fact, the majority of individuals were so named because of the juxtaposition of their severe mental handicap and an isolated mental ability fulfill criteria for autism (Treffert, 1988).

Some authors suggested that all of these conditions could be considered as childhood variants of schizophrenia (Bender, 1947; Creak, 1961). In 1933 Potter attempted to define childhood schizophrenia on the basis of specific features (e.g., loss of interest in the environment); despite this, the term became synonymous with childhood "psychosis," even though the disorder was clearly less common than in adults and more difficult to characterize. In many ways, the assumption of continuity between child and adult forms of "psychosis" was based on the severity of the conditions (Volkmar & Cohen, 1988). However, various lines of evidence began to suggest that differentiations could be made within the broad group of "psychotic" children on the basis of various features, such as age of onset (Volkmar, Bregman, Cohen, & Cicchetti, 1988), clinical characteristics (Rutter, 1972), family history, and central nervous system dysfunctions (DeMyer, Hingtgen & Jackson, 1981). This body of research convinced most investigators of the pitfalls of simple extension of the term *schizophrenia* to early childhood disorders—particularly the unwarranted assumption of a nosologic relationship with adult disorders and the neglect of developmental factors (Schopler, Rutter, & Chess, 1979). In fact, the term *psychosis* was increasingly seen as less appropriately applied to children, particularly to younger and lower-functioning ones. Nevertheless, despite the current exclusion of "schizophrenia" from official classifications of disorders of childhood (APA, 1980, 1987), a small number of investigators continue to advocate the earlier, broader conceptualization (Cantor, 1988).

During the 1930s the burgeoning field of child psychoanalysis took a developmental perspective in the description of childhood disorders. Both Klein's (1930/1975) clinical descriptions and the elaboration of object-relations theory prepared the ground for later psychoanalytic concepts, the most prominent of which was Mahler's (1952) "symbiotic psychosis." Mahler described a group of children with abnormal social relationships (characterized primarily by an impersonal "clinging" to adults), echolalia, and repetitive speech, and set their symptoms within a framework of developmental theory. This view was influential for many years; it provided not only a conceptualization of childhood disorders but also an etiologic hypothesis and treatment of choice. Although this approach accommodated the possibility that the condition was constitutional in origin (Hobson, 1990), it was taken to suggest primarily that the child's abnormality in personal relations was due to the parents' failure to nurture the child's capacity for relationships: The lack of therapeutic results after long-term analysis along with a vast body of evidence failing to support the suggested abnormalities in parenting resulted in the virtual abandonment of this approach to severely developmentally disordered children, at least in the English-speaking countries.

In contrast to these various approaches, Kanner's "infantile autism" reflected a clinical attitude that emphasized phenomenological description devoid of theoretical preconceptions and that strove to incorporate the findings of the new discipline of child development, as exemplified by the work of Gesell (see Cohen, Volkman, Anderson, & Klin, 1993). Consequently, the term *infantile autism* and his account of its clinical features proved remarkably enduring, surviving almost intact to the present day. In contrast, many, although not all, of the various other forms of "childhood psychoses" are now of only historical interest. The third edition and the third revised edition of the *Diagnostic and Statistical Manual of Mental Disorders* (*DSM-III*, APA, 1980; *DSM-III-R*, APA, 1987) included autism in the PDD class, as well as a "subthreshold" category (termed Atypical PDD in *DSM-III* and PDD-Not Otherwise Specified [NOS] in *DSM-IV*). In addition, *DSM-III* included a Childhood Onset PDD, which differed from autism mainly in terms of its later onset. This subcategory was included following the report of a very few cases (e.g., Easson, 1971; Kolvin, 1971); in view of the dearth of reported cases, it was dropped from *DSM-III-R*. More recently, a renewed interest in variants of autism has resulted in the revival of several different diagnostic concepts. As a result, the tenth edition of the *International Classification of Diseases* (*ICD-10;* World Health Organization, 1990) and the fourth edition of the *Diagnostic and Statistical Manual of Mental Disorders* (*DSM-IV;* APA, 1994) now include Asperger's disorder, Rett's disorder, and childhood disintegrative disorder, in addition to the subthreshold category of PDD-NOS. In most instances, however, some modification of the original concepts has been made on subsequent research.

Autism: Kanner's (1943) original description of infantile autism contained detailed clinical descriptions of 11 children he had seen over a few years. Their most striking clinical feature was their pervasive disinterest in other people, including their parents, an attitude that contrasted markedly with their all-absorbing fascination with the inanimate environment. Kanner conceptualized these cases in terms of a possible congenital disturbance affecting the children's capacity to relate emotionally to others, which resulted in marked withdrawal and social aloneness—or "autism." These children also exhibited a number of unusual developmental and behavioral features, such as a pronounced resistance to change in their environment and routines; stereotypic behaviors including purposeless, repetitive movements; and, often, a specific, isolated interest and proficiency in a trivial task that was endlessly repeated such as block constructions or puzzles. When language developed at all, it was characterized by echolalia (the echoing of another's speech), pronoun reversal, and extreme literalness. Initially Kanner felt that infantile autism was not an early manifestation of schizophrenia; however, his use of the word *autism* suggested unintentional points of similarity. In fact, this term previously had been used to mean active withdrawal from relationships rather than an incapacity to develop them and as a rich fantasy life rather than a lack of imagination. (See Bleuler, 1951.)

By adhering strictly to a description of the clinical phenomena observed, Kanner's account provided a remarkably enduring description of the core features of the disorder; by contrasting the limited social skills of his first patients with normative skills emerging very early on in life, Kanner was careful to place his observations within a developmental context. Nevertheless, certain aspects of his report suggested false leads for research. For example, while his initial report emphasized the apparently congenital nature of the disorder, in his original case series he noted the unusual degrees of personal achievement of the parents and their atypical ways of interacting with the child. This observation appeared to suggest a potential role of parental psychopathology in syndrome pathogenesis. At the time, of course, there was little understanding of the potential contributions of a deviant child to disturbances in parent-child interaction (Bell & Harper, 1977). Early reports emphasized the role of experiential factors in pathogenesis, but subsequent research has shown no evidence of increased parental psychopathology (McAdoo & DeMyer, 1978) and that very adverse experiences early in life do not typically lead to autism (Provence & Lipton, 1962; Rutter, Bartak, & Newman, 1971). Kanner also suggested that autism apparently was not associated with either mental retardation (autistic children seemed to be particularly clever in some narrow respects or with other "organic conditions." Again, research has established that most autistic children also are mentally retarded (Lockyer & Rutter, 1969) and that the condition can be observed in association with diverse medical conditions, such as congenital rubella (Chess, 1971) and fragile X syndrome (Watson et al., 1984). Finally, it became apparent that autistic children commonly develop seizure disorders (Volkmar & Nelson, 1990) and other neurobiological abnormalities consistent with an as-yet unspecified underlying "organic" etiology (Golden, 1987).

The validity of the syndrome proposed by Kanner has been supported by various lines of evidence. A series of studies consistently has revealed that autism differs from childhood schizophrenia in clinical features, such as age of onset (infancy and early childhood vs. later childhood and adolescence), course (relatively unchanged vs. episodic), absence of delusions/hallucinations and social and communicative abilities (markedly more profound in autism), and family history (which is more frequently positive in schizophrenia) (Kolvin, 1971; Rutter, 1972; Volkmar, Cohen, Hoshino, Rende, & Paul, 1988). Another series of studies also has demonstrated that autism differs from developmental language disorders in terms of the pervasiveness of the communicative deficits (in autism the disability encompasses both verbal and nonverbal communication) as well as social (more profound in autism) and cognitive profiles (larger scatter and typical pattern in autism) (Cohen, Caparulo, & Shaywitz, 1976; Rutter, 1978b). Although autism often coexists with mental retardation, autistic children differ from children with primary mental retardation without autism in terms of pattern of scores on IQ tests (scattered vs. even), cognitive processing abilities (less symbolic in autism), and communicative and social skills (unlike the relatively even profile of skills obtained in mental retardation, autistic social dysfunction is in excess of what could be predicted by general cognitive level) (Rutter, 1978a).

NONAUTISTIC PDDS

Childhood Disintegrative Disorder: In 1908 Theodore Heller (1930), a Viennese educator, reported 6 cases of children who had developed normally until 3 to 4 years of age and then exhibited marked developmental and behavioral deterioration with only minimal subsequent recovery. He named this condition *dementia infantilis;* the name of the condition was subsequently changed to Heller's syndrome, and now it usually is referred to as childhood disintegrative disorder.

This disorder probably is extremely rare, with about 100 cases in toto reported in the world literature (Volkmar, 1992). Generally, the early development is entirely normal. The child progresses to the point of speaking in sentences, then a profound developmental regression occurs; once established, the condition is behaviorally similar to autism, although the prognosis is even worse (Volkmar & Cohen, 1989). In some instances the condition has been reported in association with a specific disease process, such as a progressive neurological condition (Corbett, 1987). As a result, the disorder was not included in *DSM-III* (APA, 1980) or *DSM-III-R* (APA, 1987) on the presumption that these cases invariably reflected some other degenerative medical condition. However, it is clear that such a medical condition is observed and/or documented only in a minority of the cases (Volkmar, 1996); accordingly, childhood disintegrative disorder has been included in both *ICD-10* (WHO, 1990) and *DSM-IV* (APA, 1994).

Rett's Disorder: Andreas Rett (1966) described the syndrome now commonly referred to as Rett's disorder. Rett had observed 2 girls in a waiting room who exhibited remarkably similar patterns of deviant behavior and course of development; he subsequently identified a series of 22 cases. Although autisticlike behaviors are observed, particularly during the preschool years, this disorder differs from autism in several ways: It has been reported only in females, the more "autisticlike" phase is relatively brief, it is associated with characteristic stereotyped motor behaviors (resembling "washing" or "wringing" movements) and abnormalities in gait or trunk movement. Breathholding spells and seizures are common, and the associated mental retardation is even more severe than in autism. The early history is remarkable for initially normal early growth and development followed (usually in the first months of life) by developmental regression, deceleration of head growth, and loss of purposeful hand movements.

The apparently normal period of development is much shorter than that observed in childhood disintegrative disorder. Prevalence estimates of Rett's disorder suggest that approximately 1 in 15,000 girls are affected (Trevathan & Adams, 1988). Despite the insidious regression in development and other neurological findings, the pathophysiology of the condition remains unknown (Trevathan & Naidu, 1988). The condition has been included in both *ICD-10* (WHO, 1990) and *DSM-IV* (APA, 1994).

Asperger's Disorder: In the year following Kanner's (1943) report, Hans Asperger (1944/1991), a Viennese physician, described a group of individuals who, despite adequate intellectual skills, exhibited social and behavioral peculiarities that made it difficult for them to participate in group activities and develop friendships (e.g., problems with social interaction and communication, and circumscribed and idiosyncratic patterns of interest). However, Asperger's description differed from Kanner's in that speech was less commonly delayed, motor deficits were more common, the onset appeared to be somewhat later, and all of the initial cases occurred in boys. Asperger also suggested that similar problems could be observed in family members, particularly fathers. Unaware of Kanner's work, Asperger coined the term *autistic psychopathy* to characterize the condition as a personality disorder.

This condition was essentially unknown in the English literature for many years. An influential review and series of case reports by Wing (1981) increased interest in the condition, and since then, both the usage of the term in clinical practice and the number of case reports have been steadily increasing (Klin, 1994). The commonly described clinical features of the disorder include (1) paucity of empathy; (2) naïve, inappropriate, one-sided social interaction, little ability to form friendships and consequent social isolation; (3) pedantic and monotonic speech; (4) poor nonverbal communication; (5) intense absorption in circumscribed topics such as the weather, facts about TV stations, railway tables or maps, which are learned in rote fashion and reflect poor understanding, conveying the impression of eccentricity; and (6) clumsy and ill-coordinated movements and odd posture (Wing, 1981).

Although Asperger originally reported the condition only in boys, reports of girls with the disorder have now appeared. Nevertheless, males are significantly more likely to be affected (Szatmari et al., 1989; Wing, 1991). Although most individuals with the condition function within the average range of intelligence, some have been reported to be mildly retarded (Wing, 1981). The apparent onset of the condition, or at least its recognition, is probably somewhat later than autism; this may primarily reflect the more preserved language and cognitive abilities (Klin and Volkmar, in press). Asperger's disorder tends to be highly stable (Asperger, 1979), and the higher intellectual skills observed suggest a better outcome than is typically observed in autism (Tantam, 1991). Specific learning problems and marked discrepancies between various intellectual skills may be present (Klin et al., 1995a; Ozonoff et al., 1991).

Atypical PDD/PDD-NOS: The term *PDD-NOS* was used in *DSM-III-R* (APA, 1987) to replace the earlier term *atypical PDD;* this latter concept had unintentionally, although probably correctly, been suggestive of Rank's (1949) earlier diagnostic notion of "atypical personality development," a term also used to describe children with some, but not all, features of autism. Such children exhibit patterns of unusual sensitivities, difficulties in social interaction, and other problems suggestive of autism without meeting full criteria for autistic disorder (Volkmar et al., 1994).

The term *PDD-NOS* is problematic in several respects. The category is poorly defined since the definition is essentially a negative one, and although the condition is probably much more common than strictly defined autism (Klin et al., 1995b), research on PDD-NOS has been uncommon. The lack of an explicit definition also means that the concept is used rather inconsistently: for example, some investigators equate it with Asperger's disorder while others view it as on some underlying spectrum with autism, both in terms of developmental functioning and severity of symptomatology. More commonly the term *PDD-NOS* has been used for children with better cognitive and communicative skills and some degree of relatedness. The most common reasons for referral in such cases include parents' concerns about the child's emotional and social devel-

540

opment rather than, as in autism, the failure to develop language.

Over the years, children currently captured by the term *PDD-NOS* have been characterized by numerous diagnostic labels that have been used to provide a taxonomic location and convey the nature of their social and emotional difficulties in relating. While informal descriptions included terms such as eccentric, odd, overanxious, aloof, and weird, formal designations included terms such as borderline, schizotypal, schizoidal disorders, atypical development, childhood psychosis, symbiotic states, and others (Klin, Mayes, Volkmar, & Cohen, 1995). No term, however, has been fully satisfactory nor broadly accepted, and while clinicians have had the sense of a category of such children, there are as yet no clearly defined diagnostic criteria that could guide systematic studies, including those on the basic validity or utility of such a grouping.

There have been several attempts to delineate subgroups within the larger PDD-NOS category, involving terms such as multiplex developmental disorder (Cohen, Paul, & Volkmar, 1987), childhood-onset schizophrenia (McKenna, Gordon, & Lenane, 1994), and others (Szatmari, 1996). No taxonomy of conditions related to children currently assigned by default to the PDD-NOS category is as yet operationally defined or broadly accepted. As pathognomonic symptomatology such as the profound social disability in autism or profound regression as in childhood disintegrative disorder are lacking, it becomes very difficult for investigators to agree on specific clusters of symptoms and deficits that define specific disorders. Given the vast variability in phenomenology, careful studies of profiles of development and adjustment, including quantification of deficits and deviance, are needed in no area of childhood disorders more than in this rather amorphous PDD-NOS category. Future efforts will need to take into account the fact that the pervasive impact inflicted by early disturbances of basic developmental processes, specifically socialization skills and the emergence of a consolidated sense of self, are likely to have a broad range of effects on multiple aspects of development with varied manifestations (Cicchetti & Cohen, 1995).

Autism: Clinical Description

ONSET AND CHARACTERISTICS OF EARLY DEVELOPMENT

In his original description, Kanner (1943) suggested that autism was present from birth. Subsequent research has revealed that the condition sometimes appears within the second or third year of life, but rarely after age 3 (Short & Shopler, 1988; Volkmar, Stier, & Cohen, 1985). As discussed previously, age and type of onset have some value in the differential diagnosis of autism, although various extraneous factors may act to delay case detection, including parental perceptivity, sophistication, or denial, and the level of associated mental retardation in the child. Given such factors, we may refer more correctly to age of "recognition" rather than "onset" of the syndrome.

From a clinical perspective, the early recognition of autism is important, as there is some suggestion that early intervention may reduce subbsequent morbidity (Simeonsson, Olley, & Rosenthal, 1987). Moreover, it is clear that developmental skills at age 5 predict subsequent outcome (Lotter, 1978a). Unfortunately, delays in case recognition remain common. For example, Siegel and colleagues (1988) noted that typically 3 years elapsed between the time parents expressed concern to their child's physician and the time when a definitive diagnosis was made, usually around age 5. Similarly, Ornitz and colleagues (1977) reported that 50% of the families interviewed in their study were concerned about their children at the age of 14 months but that the median age of referral for diagnosis was 46 months, a delay of 32 months. Delays in case detection and referral reflect a lack of knowledge about autism, a dearth of readily applied screening instruments, difficulties in the use of categorical criteria, and the more general lack of awareness of mental health problems by primary health care providers.

A few lists of behavioral criteria intended to alert pediatricians to early signs of autism have been offered (e.g., Prior & Gajzago, 1974); unfortunately, their applicability is problematic as many children with other difficulties (e.g., sensory deficits or global delay) also might present some of the delays and deviations seen in autistic children. Nevertheless, a recent study reported the successful use of a checklist completed by health care providers. This instrument consisted of normative social-cognitive behaviors (e.g., pointing, playing imaginatively) and was used for the early identification of autism among a sample including the siblings of diagnosed autistic children (Baron-Cohen, Allen, & Gillberg, 1992). Even though these results are encouraging, it seems that few if any of the children in the sample (except for the subsequently diagnosed autistic children) suffered from any degree of mental retardation or other significant physical/developmental disorder. Since other developmental disorders are far more common than autism, it remains to be established whether this checklist would be effective in preventing a great number of false positives. Despite these difficulties, and in light of recent federal mandates for extension of services to young children, the issue of early case detection and intervention is now assuming even greater importance.

Given our knowledge of the natural course of the disorder, it may be said that infants and very young autistic children exhibit the "purest" form of the condition (Volkmar & Cohen, 1988). The late detection, however, usually leaves the first 2 to 4 years of life virtually undocumented. As a result, studies of this age group are uncommon. Most studies of early development in autism rely on parental retrospection (e.g., Ornitz et al., 1977) or, less frequently, movies or videotapes made by the parent before the time of their child's diagnosis (Losche, 1990; Massie, 1978). Both of these methods have their limitations. Although parents often have concerns from the first months of the child's life, a referral usually follows later, as parents realize that the child is 18 to 24 months old and still not speaking. Parents may report concern that the child appears not to hear, although paradoxically they also may note that the child is exquisitely sensitive to certain sounds in the inanimate environment, such as the noise of the vacuum cleaner.

Similarly, the child may not respond differentially to parents but be particularly attached to a highly unusual object (e.g., a piece of string or specific magazine). The young autistic child also may have interest in nonfunctional aspects of objects—their smell, taste, or reflection of light—and normal use of materials for play is typically absent; instead, the child may prefer to spin the wheels of a toy truck continuously rather than create a make-believe play sequence with it. Other deviant behaviors include stereotypic, motor mannerisms, such as hand-flapping, twirling, and toe-walking, and a preference for such activities rather than those involving social interaction. Bizarre affective responses may be observed; the child may become highly agitated if the same route or routine is not followed precisely or if an aspect of the environment is not maintained (e.g., furniture arrangement).

Initial studies of the early development of autistic children suggested that their development was erratic and characterized by lags, spurts, and uneven development across domains of functioning, "splinter skills," and the loss of previously acquired skills. Some diagnostic systems (Ritvo & Freeman, 1978) have included unusual rates and sequences of development as a criterion for the condition. Recent research confirms that there may be either islets of special ability or domains in which levels of functioning are relatively higher (Burack & Volkmar, 1991). This apparent developmental unevenness becomes more pronounced past the sensorimotor period (Losche, 1990). However, development within a given domain generally follows expected developmental sequences (Burack & Volkmar, 1991).

SOCIAL DEVELOPMENT

The social disabilities found in autism have been consistently emphasized as an important, if not the most significant central defining, feature of the disorder (Kanner, 1943; Rutter, 1978a). Autistic individuals show a fundamental failure in socialization from early childhood, perhaps even from the first days or weeks of life. Unlike normally developing infants, they display a lack of reciprocity in social contact, inappropriate gaze behavior, tenuous expressions of attachment, and paucity of joint play and communicative skills (Volkmar, 1987). Later in life, symptoms of social impairment persist, even in the case of the highest-functioning individuals, and take the form of a pervasive difficulty in developing friendships, responding empathically to others, and understanding the conventions and expectations inherent in day-to-day social transactions (Volkmar & Cohen, 1985; Volkmar & Klin, 1993).

Paradoxically, the social dysfunction has been the focus of comparatively little systematic study (Fein, Pennington, Markowitz, Braverman, & Waterhouse, 1986). Various factors appear to have contributed to this situation; one is an implicit "cognitive primacy hypothesis" (Cairns, 1979; Rutter, 1983)—an assumption that the condition is primarily cognitive in nature; another is a lack of information on neurobiological systems related to social development (Brothers, 1989); still another is an awareness that some social skills do emerge in these children (Rutter, Greenfield, & Lockyer, 1967); and finally, a lack of truly operational and dimensional definitions of social deficits (Volkmar et al., 1987). More recently, some (primarily) experimental studies have appeared (see Baron-Cohen, 1988, for a review) that focused on different aspects of social development, including attachment behaviors, social interactions, emotional expression, symbolic play, and social cognition.

Although still very limited, the combined data from clinical observations and experimental findings indicate that the social development of young autistic children is qualitatively different from that seen in even very young infants; it differs as well from that observed in mental retardation not associated with autism (Volkmar, 1987). In normative development, a host of perceptual, affective, and neuroregulatory mechanisms predispose young infants to engage in social interaction from very early on in their lives (Cohn & Tronick, 1987; Tronick, 1980). Against this background, the social deficits of autistic infants and young children are striking. For example, the human face appears to hold little interest or have little salience for the autistic child (Volkmar, 1987). Similarly, young autistic children appear to lack a differential preference for speech sounds (Klin, 1991, 1992). Typical forms of early nonverbal interchange are deviant. Very early emerging forms of "intersubjectivity" (Stern, 1985), such as the imitative games of infancy, are absent in these children. They may not seek physical comfort from parents and may be difficult to hold (Ornitz et al., 1977). Similarly, while some may exhibit differential responsivess to familiar adults, the usual robust patterns of attachment do not develop, and autistic children may not respond differentially to their parents un-

til the elementary school years (Mundy & Sigman, 1989).

Social interest and relatively isolated social skills may develop as autistic children enter later childhood and adolescence. However, social responsivity remains a source of considerable disability even for the higher-functioning individuals; their attempts at social interaction fail as a result both of their difficulties in pragmatic communication and empathy and of their failures to integrate various sources of information relevant to interaction. Normal peer relationships do not develop, and even when some social relationships do appear, these tend to be with adults rather than with peers (Volkmar, 1987). In adulthood, even the highest-functioning individuals continue to exhibit significant social deficits. Such individuals are self-described "loners," who may exhibit a desire for social contact, although they are typically incapable of it (Bemporad, 1979; Kanner, Rodriguez, & Ashenden, 1972). In many instances, these individuals are aware of their disability; in response, they develop a number of coping strategies that usually involve learning concrete rules for mediating social interaction. An increased awareness of the disability also might result in some degree of depression (Cohen, 1991).

COMMUNICATIVE DEVELOPMENT

Although autistic children may or may not exhibit problems in speech, their language, and particularly their *use* of whatever linguistic ability is available to them, is almost always deviant (Paul, 1987). About half of autistic individuals never speak; those who do speak exhibit language that is distinctive in numerous ways. (See Paul, 1987, for a review.) Interestingly, numerous studies have revealed that in regard to the less communicative aspects of language, that is, phonology and syntax, autistic individuals' abilities are better than those in IQ-matched controls and often comparable to normative samples (Fay & Mermelstein, 1982). It is in the more functional aspects of language that their degree of communicative disability is shown to be very profound.

For example, autistic individuals's speech often is characterized by inappropriate use of intonational patterns and stress (Menyuk, 1978), conveying the impression of monotonic or pedantic delivery; this abnormality is evidenced also in pre-verbal vocal output (Ricks, 1975). Semantic difficulties often are reflected in the form of extreme literalness as well as a paucity of conceptual words (Fay & Schuler, 1980) and, particularly, terms that express mental states (e.g., beliefs and intentions) in others and in self (Tager-Flusberg, 1993). Yet it is the pragmatic aspects of autistic individuals' speech that is the most universally dysfunctional aspect. (See Baron-Cohen, 1988, for a review.) Even the highest-functioning individuals tend to fail to observe the usual conventions of communication, such as turn-taking, contextualization (i.e., providing background information that is not known to the interlocutor), and so forth. As a result, their conversational style may appear one-sided and, sometimes, incoherent.

Other phenomena commonly observed in autistic individuals' speech include pronoun reversal and immediate and delayed echolalia (Fay & Schuler, 1980). It must be noted, however, that echolalia per se is observed in normally developing children who are acquiring language, and adaptive functions of echolalia in autistic individuals have been noted (Prizant, 1983). Finally, the language deficits in autism differ from those seen in the developmental language disorders, particularly in terms of the communicative, or functional, use of language (Cantwell, Baker, & Rutter, 1978; Paul, 1987).

COGNITIVE DEVELOPMENT

One of the false leads in Kanner's (1943) original description of autism was his impression that autism apparently was not associated with mental retardation, a presumption that lasted for over two decades. This presumption was based on (1) the observation that on certain tasks of traditional IQ tests, for example, in subtests involving rote memory or visual-spatial skills, autistic children often scored within the normal or near-normal range; (2) the notion that the otherwise generally poor performance on IQ tests was a function of volitional noncompliance or negativism, or "untestability"; in other words, such results were due to their "autism"; and (3) the observation that some autistic children exhibited unusual

"splinter skills" or islets of special ability (DeMyer et al., 1981). It is now clear that when tests appropriate to the individuals' developmental level are used and supportive conditions are provided, most individuals with autism score in the mentally retarded range (Lockyer & Rutter, 1969). Subsequent research also revealed that IQ is strongly correlated with severity of the social impairment and other aspects of the disorder (Cohen et al., 1987; Volkmar, Bregman, Cohen, Hooks, & Stevenson, 1989) and is a potent predictor of ultimate outcome (Lockyer & Rutter, 1969; Lotter, 1978a).

Developmental and psychological testing of infants and young children is at best a difficult procedure; with autistic children, such testing usually reveals particular difficulty with tasks requiring language, conceptual reasoning, imitation, or understanding of social conventions and events. Often, nonverbal problem-solving abilities, as in matching shapes or solving inset puzzles, are closer to age-expected levels (Sigman et al., 1987). Deficits in sensorimotor skills, as opposed to more symbolic or communicative skills, are more variably noted (Curcio, 1978; Morgan, Curtrer, Coplin, & Rodrigue, 1989).

A great deal of attention has been given to the cognitive profile and development of autistic children. Even though research studies date primarily from the 1960s and 1970s, particularly studies employing experimental methodologies (Hermelin & O'Connor, 1970), a comprehensive description of autistic children's cognitive abilities and disabilities could be found in Scheerer and colleagues' 1945 monograph reporting an intensive study of an "autistic savant," who was also one of the 11 children described by Kanner. Many of the experimental findings revealed in the 1960s and 1970s studies had been described phenomenologically in this early monograph. In contrast to Kanner's (1943) affective hypothesis, these authors proposed that the disorder affecting their patient (as well as the other 10 children reported by Kanner) was primarily a pervasive impairment of "abstract attitude" (Goldstein, 1948), a term that corresponds to Head's (1926) impairment of "symbolic functions" in the field of traumatic aphasia. This hypothesis is described in exquisite detail, relating symptoms in the areas of social, affective, communicative, cognitive, and behavioral functioning to an underlying inability to symbolize experience and, hence, to profit from the flexibility afforded by conceptual (as against concrete) and generalization (as against context-specific) strategies. These ideas received much corroboration in Hermelin and O'Connor's experimental work (1970) and were summarized and illustrated by Ricks and Wing (1975).

More recently, a new line of research has proposed that the social disabilities in autism reflect a specific, innate, and primarily cognitive incapacity to attribute mental states (e.g., beliefs, intentions, emotions) to others and self and then to use these to explain and predict another person's behavior (the "Theory of Mind" hypothesis; Baron-Cohen, 1990; Leslie, 1987). This hypothesis has grown out of two lines of experimental findings: (1) autistic children's symbolic dysfunction is not generalized; rather, it affects a very specific cognitive capacity; and (2) this cognitive, or social-cognitive, capacity refers to the ability to conceive of other people's subjectivity, or to have a "Theory of Mind." This line of research is of considerable interest as it more parsimoniously accounts for observed deficits in social interaction, communication, and play in autistic children. However, to date, this theory is still limited in several important respects: First, as the postulated early manifestations of a "Theory of Mind" are not exhibited before 1 year of age, at the very earliest, the theory does not account for the very early onset of the condition (Klin, Volkman, & Sparrow, 1992). Second, as the experimental work using this approach tended to focus on verbal subjects, it is unclear how or whether the theory has applicability to lower-functioning (e.g., mute) subjects; in the same vein, higher-functioning and older autistic subjects often are able to conceive other people's intentions cognitively but are nevertheless unable to empathize with them (Klin & Volkmar, 1993). Third, at least some work has suggested that apparent "Theory of Mind" deficits are a function of developmental level rather than diagnostic category (Prior, Dahlstrom, & Squires, 1990).

NEUROBIOLOGICAL STUDIES

Considerable evidence suggests the operation of some as-yet unspecified neurobiological factor or factors in the pathogenesis of autism. For ex-

ample, autistic children are more likely to exhibit physical anomalies, persistent primitive reflexes, various neurological "soft" signs, abnormalities on electroencephalogram, computed tomography (CT) or magnetic resonance imaging (MRI) scan, as well as an increased incidence of seizures (Golden, 1987). As many as 25% of autistic individuals develop seizure disorders; in fact, recent work suggests that the risk of seizure is significantly increased throughout the developmental period—including infancy and early childhood (Volkmar & Nelson, 1990). There is some suggestion of reduced obstetrical and neonatal optimality (Tsai, 1987). Autism is also observed in association with a host of specific medical conditions, such as phenylketonuria, congenital rubella, tuberous sclerosis, and fragile X syndrome (Coleman, 1987); on the other hand, it is much less commonly associated with other conditions, notably Down's syndrome (Bregman & Volkmar, 1988).

There is now evidence of strong genetic contributions in autism (Bailey et al., 1995). For example, there is a higher-than-expected frequency of less severe developmental problems in the relatives of autistic patients. In a study of siblings, August, Stewart, and Tsai (1981) reported that the frequency of autism in siblings was nearly 3%; in other words, the frequency of autism was markedly increased over the expected prevalence in the population. Higher-than-expected rates of cognitive disorder also were present in siblings. Folstein and Piven (1991) reported that monozygotic twins are more likely than dizygotic twins to be concordant for the disorder. Other studies (e.g., Jones & Szatmari, 1988) supported these findings, suggesting that, on balance, the available data to date suggest some role of genetic factors in syndrome pathogenesis, even though a multifactorial etiology is probably very likely (Folstein & Rutter, 1977).

Despite the considerable evidence favoring some neurobiological factor or factors in the pathogenesis of autism, precise and identifiable mechanisms have yet to be specified. Neurobiological findings vary considerably, and findings are often subtle. Neuroanatomical models of the disorder have placed the "site of lesion" at various points on the neuraxis from the brainstem and cerebellum to the cortex (Golden, 1987; Heh et al., 1989). Neurochemical findings are no clearer:

For example, it is evident that, as a group, autistic children exhibit elevated peripheral levels of serotonin, a central nervous system neurotransmitter; however, the significance of this observation is unclear, since the relationship of peripheral to central serotonin levels is not firmly established and individuals suffering from several other conditions also exhibit elevated serotonin levels (Anderson & Hoshino, 1987).

EPIDEMIOLOGY

Various problems pose complications for epidemiological studies: the relative infrequency of autism and associated conditions, difficulties in case identification, changes in diagnostic criteria, and the nature of definitions used. However, most studies of autism have suggested prevalence rates of between 2 and 5 cases in 10,000 children (Zahner & Pauls, 1987). Most studies also suggest that autism is more frequent in males, usually 4 or 5 times as common as in females; however, when girls are affected, they may exhibit a more severe form of the disorder, particularly in terms of having lower IQ. The significance of the observed sex difference is unclear but may reflect the operation of underlying genetic mechanisms (Lord & Schopler, 1987). Although Kanner initially (1943) suggested a preponderance of autism in families of higher socioeconomic status, subsequent controlled research has not confirmed this impression. In fact, autistic children come from families of all social classes (Schopler, Andrews, & Strupp, 1980) and cultures (Lotter, 1978b).

Epidemiological information on other "nonautistic" PDDs is more limited (Klin & Volkmar, 1995). It does appear, however, that "atypical" PDD/PDD-NOS is much more common than more strictly defined autism. Apparently the other pervasive developmental disorders are less common than autism. For example, childhood disintegrative disorders is perhaps 10 times less common than more strictly defined autism.

PSYCHOSOCIAL FACTORS

Studies of parents of autistic children have suggested that they do not differ from parents of other developmentally disordered children in interactional style, in exhibiting unusual personality characteristics, or in exhibiting deviant caretaking practices (DeMyer et al., 1981). The observations that autism is *not often* observed in other siblings and that grossly inadequate emotional nurturing on the part of parents is associated with a different clinical presentation (APA, 1989) are also inconsistent with the notion that parents somehow "cause" autism.

On the other hand, as might be expected, the experience of having an autistic child may have a profound influence on the family (Schopler & Mesibov, 1984). The list of stressors the families must cope with is associated at once with the child's level of cognitive functioning as well as with the severity of the social, communicative, and adaptive impairment and unusual behaviors. For example, at different points of the autistic individual's life, the parents might need to cope with the person's social and affective unresponsiveness, rigidity, and unawareness of social conventions; unusual behaviors may involve absorption in routinized and self-absorbing activities that further the individual's isolation and inaccessibility; when present, stereotypies, self-injurious behaviors, and limited self-sufficiency are particularly taxing on caregivers. Such stressors on parents and other family members vary over the course of the autistic child's development. Over time, different patterns of adaptation are noted, depending on such factors as personal and community resources and the availability of adequate educational and vocational services that are responsive to the child's and family's specific needs (Morgan, 1988).

COURSE AND PROGNOSIS

Several factors act as determinants of course and long-term outcome of the condition, particularly developmental level and communicative and adaptive functioning. Younger children more typically display the "pervasive" unrelatedness alluded to in *DSM-III* (APA, 1980) criteria for autism. Although some evidence of differentiated responsiveness to parents may be observed as the child reaches the elementary school years, patterns of social interaction remain quite deviant and the child's behavior can be quite problematic. For example, enjoyable social interaction may be restricted to circumscribed activities, such as "rough-and-tumble" or "tickling" games, whereas, if left to his or her own devices, the child may be withdrawn or absorbed with trivial aspects of the environment (e.g., light switches) or isolating activities (e.g., puzzles). Attempts at the introduction of structure by placing demands on the child may lead to temper tantrums. Often some gains, such as in terms of communicative and social skills, are observed during the elementary school years. During adolescence, some autistic children exhibit behavioral deterioration, and a smaller number improve (Rutter, 1970). Various interactional styles can be observed, ranging from aloof, to passive, to eccentric (Wing & Attwood, 1987); these styles appear to be closely related to developmental level (Volkmar et al., 1989).

Available information suggests that the outcome for autistic children is quite poor (Kanner et al., 1972), with perhaps only one third able to achieve some degree of personal independence and self-sufficiency as adults (DeMyer et al., 1981). In general, two major factors appear predictive of ultimate outcome: the acquisition of truly communicative speech by age 5 and IQ. It is important to realize that much of the available outcome information is based on data collected during the 1960s and 1970s. During this period fewer services were available, and these often were not provided until the school years. There is some reason to hope that over the past decade, the mandates for earlier intervention, the tendency for earlier detection of the disorder, more intensive and early interventions (e.g., Lovaas, 1987), and the current focus on realistic life skills such as self-sufficiency and vocational training (Hayes, 1987) have improved the long-term outcome for the disorder. Research in this area remains critically needed.

Diagnosis of Autism

CATEGORICAL DEFINITIONS

Categorical definitions of autism typically have emphasized four features essential for diagnosis: (1) early onset, (2) social dysfunction including play, (3) communicative dysfunction, and (4) various unusual behaviors, such as stereotypies and resistance to change, which usually are subsumed under the term *insistence on sameness*. Other features, for example, discrepancies in rates and sequences of development and perceptual abnormalities, are viewed less commonly as central for purposes of definition. Consistent with Rutter's (1978a) influential synthesis of Kanner's original (1943) description and subsequent research, most categorical definitions emphasize that the observed deviance in social and communicative development is not just a function of developmental level. On the other hand, precise metrics for operationalizing this notion have not proven easy to develop. Other factors, such as range in syndrome expression, change with age, and the frequency of "autisticlike" behaviors in individuals with severe mental retardation, have all complicated the development of categorical definitions. The task of diagnosis, particularly with infants and very young children, can be very complicated.

The *DSM-III* (APA, 1980) definition of infantile autism was largely consistent with Rutter's (1978a) synthesis of Kanner's original description. It emphasized the early onset (less than 30 months) of "pervasive" social impairment, gross deficits in language development when speech was present, and bizarre responses to the environment. This definition proved unsatisfactory in several ways: It was most appropriate to younger and lower-functioning individuals, it failed to encompass developmental changes in syndrome expression, and it did not address broader aspects of problems in communication (not just the formal aspects of language) (Volkmar & Cohen, 1988). Major revisions were made in *DSM-III-R* (APA, 1987).

The *DSM-III-R* definition of autistic disorder was intended to be more developmentally oriented and hence more encompassing of expressions of social impairment, more attuned to recent research on symbolic functioning and play in autism, and ahistorical in nature (i.e., a diagnosis could be made based on present examination only). The *DSM-III-R* definition consisted of a set of 16 detailed criteria grouped into 3 categories (deviance in social development, in communication/play/imagination, and restricted range of interests and activities). To achieve a diagnosis of autism, an individual must exhibit at least 8 of the 16 criteria with a minimum number of criteria specified from each category. Although age of onset is no longer a diagnostic criterion, it can be specified as before or after 36 months. Unfortunately, it appears that the attempt to provide a greater developmental orientation resulted in an unintentionally broadened definition, so that many children, particularly those who are both young and retarded, might now inappropriately be termed autistic (Volkmar et al., 1988).

In contrast to *DSM-III-R*, the *ICD-10* (WHO, 1990) draft definition of autism produced results similar to those generated by *DSM-III* (if the *DSM-III* diagnosis was taken in its lifetime sense). The draft definition also appeared to approximate most closely the diagnoses assigned by experienced clinicians (Volkmar, Cicchetti, Bregman, & Cohen, 1992). Another difference between *DSM-III-R* and *ICD-10* was the inclusion in *ICD-10* of various other nonautistic PDDs. The inclusion of additional disorders with some similarity to autism was meant to foster research on these conditions and made it possible to produce a somewhat more stringent definition of autism. The differences between *DSM-III-R* and *ICD-10* were thus further emphasized, and the potential adverse effects of two markedly different official diagnostic systems were clear (Rutter & Schopler, 1992).

As a result of the concerns about *DSM-III-R* and its compatibility with *ICD-10*, a large, multisite, international field trial was undertaken (Volkmar et al., 1994). Goals of this field trial included development of a reliable and efficient diagnostic system for autism (and for other disorders that would be included within the PDD class) and achievement of a reasonable balance of sensitivity and specificity (avoiding overdiagnosis of autism in cases with severe retardation and underdiagnosis in individuals with normal IQ levels). The nature of the *DSM-III-R* overdiagnosis of the condition was to be established, if this indeed was the case, and various alternatives for *DSM-IV* (APA, 1994) were to be outlined. Issues of criterion and disorder convergence with *ICD-10* in the PDD class were also to be addressed explicitly. At the same time, the important differences in *ICD* and *DSM* were noted, most notably in the *ICD-10* approach of having separate guidelines for clinicians apart from research criteria (Volkmar et al., 1994).

For the *DSM-IV* field trial, data were collected on a sample of nearly 1,000 individuals with a diagnosis of autism or other disorders in a range of

settings and sites. Cases were rated by examiners with a range of experience and professional backgrounds; cases typically were rated on the basis of contemporaneous examination and past records (not just on record review). Five sites provided ratings on 100 consecutive cases over the period of a year; other sites provided ratings on a smaller number of cases. Comparison cases included those in which the differential diagnosis would reasonably include autism. Certain cases, such as those with a diagnosis of a nonautistic PDD as included in *ICD-10*, or cases with certain characteristics (e.g., high-functioning females with autism), were intentionally oversampled. Ratings were made of *DSM-III*, *DSM-III-R*, and *ICD-10* criteria as well as of a range of potential new criteria; basic information also was obtained on the case and rater(s) with due attention to issues such as reliability of ratings.

From the results of the field trial, it did appear that the *DSM-III-R* definition was too broad and that it tended to overdiagnose autism in individuals with severe mental retardation. The *ICD-10* approach was noted to have the best overall agreement with clinician diagnosis. Similarly, the available data provided some support for inclusion of other disorders within the PDD class.

A series of alternatives for *DSM-IV* were outlined. In addition, based on these analyses and those related to the development of *ICD-10*, it appeared that several of the 20 detailed *ICD-10* criteria could be eliminated with minimal effect on efficiency of the definition. A decision based both on data and philosophical considerations was made to establish conceptual convergence of *DSM-IV* and *ICD-10* definitions of autism and related PDD disorders.

The *DSM-IV* definition of autism consists of 12 criteria equally divided among the 3 clusters of symptoms (social interaction, communication/play/imagination, and restricted patterns of interest and behavior) and an age-at-onset criterion; the definition is conceptually the same as that employed in *ICD-10*.

DIMENSIONAL DEFINITIONS

In contrast to the categorical approach to diagnosis, an alternative strategy has relied on assessment of dimensions that are relevant to the diagnosis. With the exception of one recently developed instrument (Lord et al., 1989), this approach has focused on either the deviant or normative deficit aspects of the disorder. Most dimensional assessment instruments based on the "deviance" model are designed for somewhat older, school-age children. In a few instances, early development and behaviors are assessed, although usually retrospectively (Parks, 1983). These instruments rely either on parental or teacher report, or on direct observation in structured settings; in most instances highly deviant behaviors are rated or sampled. As a result, several factors have complicated the development and use of such instruments: reliance on parental retrospection brings with it attendant issues of reliability; direct observational procedures may prove less useful for sampling low-frequency behaviors; and assessment of highly deviant behavior similarly raises problems for instrument development and standardization (Parks, 1983). Also, the frequency of apparently "autisticlike" behaviors in infants and young children with other developmental disorders (Adrien, Ornitz, Barthelemy, Sauvage, & LeLord, 1987) raises the specific concern of "false positives" resulting from the utilization of such instruments.

An alternative approach relies on dimensional assessments that are more truly developmental in nature. The utility of normative assessment (e.g., of cognitive or communicative ability) is well established (Cohen et al., 1987; Watson & Marcus, 1988). An instrument that normatively assesses social skills, the Vineland Adaptive Behavior Scales, has become available (Sparrow, Balla, & Cicchetti, 1984); this set of scales circumvents many of the difficult aspects of instruments specifically devised for the assessment of autistic children. Based on a very large, normative sample representative of children in the United States, the Vineland scales focus on the use of behavior to meet the demands of daily life, and provide assessment of, among other areas, communicative and social skills. A series of studies using this instrument (Volkmar et al., 1987) has documented that, consistent with Rutter's (1978a) definition, social skills in autism are indeed deviant relative to mental age. Similarly, based on the Vineland standardization samples, a series of regression equations was derived that appear to predict social and communicative skills on the basis of mental age and other relevant variables (Volkmar, Car-ter, Sparrow, & Cicchetti, 1993). When applied to autistic and nonautistic developmentally disordered samples, social skills in autistic individuals typically were more than 2 standard deviations below the scores predicted on the basis of mental age alone. The discriminative utility of this approach for diagnosis also was suggested in individual item analyses (Klin et al., 1992), which revealed that autistic children typically fail to exhibit a range of social behaviors that normatively are exhibited within the first year of life; the absence of such behaviors was striking even when effects of associated mental retardation were controlled.

Clinical Assessment

By definition, children with autism and other PDDs have delays and deviant patterns in multiple areas of functioning; accordingly, their evaluations often require professionals with different areas of expertise, including communication, overall developmental functioning, and behavioral status. Therefore, the clinical assessment of infants and preschool children with such disorders probably is conducted most effectively by an experienced interdisciplinary team. Three fundamental considerations should guide the assessment process. It is clear that autistic children pose unusual challenges for usual assessment methods (Klin & Shepard, 1994); hence the first consideration concerns the examiner's clinical judgment as to how to obtain the most reliable measures of the child's functioning. For example, as attentional and behavioral difficulties might be a significant obstacle to the evaluation, allowances may be made for small deviations from standardized procedures, if, by doing so, the examiner is able to sample a wider range of the child's abilities while maintaining the general aim of the instrument used. On the other hand, the examiner should be aware that although modifications in usual procedures for administering specific tests sometimes are clinically indicated, results thus obtained must be viewed with great caution. Given the difficulties inherent in the assessment of infants and younger children, several assessment sessions may be required.

Modifications in standard assessment procedures may be helpful to parents (Morgan, 1988); to the extent that it is possible, parents should be encouraged to observe the evaluation of the child. This procedure both helps to demystify assessment procedures and also provides a common set of observations for subsequent discussion. The rationale for specific tests and procedures and the meaning of specific observations then can be reviewed with parents in a more efficient fashion.

Evaluation findings should be translated into a single coherent view of the child, which, in turn, should give rise to a series of easily understood, detailed, concrete, realistic recommendations: Depending on the nature of the child's individual needs, the services of various professionals may be needed. If a multidisciplinary team is providing the evaluation, team members must maintain close communication with each other to avoid fragmentation and duplication of effort. More important, the findings obtained by the different evaluators (e.g., cognitive profile, communicative functioning, clinical presentation) should be integrated with a view to assess not only the implications of each but also to determine the interrelationship of all the abilities and disabilities studied. When possible, the evaluation should be integrated sufficiently that parents receive a single coherent picture of the child and his or her difficulties; a plethora of individual reports is less helpful than a longer report with input from all members of the evaluating team; such a report also has the practical advantage of facilitating discussion among team members who must be able to reconcile or understand apparent discrepancies in their results. When writing their reports, professionals should strive to express the implications of their findings for the child's day-to-day adaptation and learning. In this regard, technical language should be avoided as much as possible.

HISTORY

A careful history should be obtained, including information related to pregnancy and neonatal period, early development, the characteristics of development, and medical and family history. For example, was the baby very "easy" and content to be left alone, was it hard to get a response from the child, did the child smile responsively, was it hard to feed the baby? Information on the nature

and age of apparent onset of the condition can provide important information relevant to differential diagnosis; for example, it is important to know whether the child exhibited a prolonged period of normal development. Questions about development sometimes can be framed for parents around a specific time or well-remembered event, such as the first birthday. The history should include information about normally expected skills (early social interest, babbling and early prelinguistic communicative behaviors, motor development, etc.). The process of taking the history should convey to parents a sense that the information they provide is both helpful and welcome; this can help the clinician establish a collaborative relationship with parents. Whereas the child's history is best obtained during a direct interview with the parents, developmental and behavioral inventories may be mailed to the parents for them to complete prior to their visit in order to elicit information and help them frame observations that can be further elaborated upon during the interview with the help of the examiner.

PSYCHOLOGICAL ASSESSMENT

The psychological assessment aims at establishing the child's overall level of intellectual functioning as well as describing his or her profile in terms of strengths and weaknesses and style of learning. Typically, autistic children have considerable unevenness in functioning. The evaluator should be aware, therefore, that significant deficits in one area might not necessarily predict commensurable deficits in other areas. For example, many tests require linguistic skill and sustained attention, two abilities that children with autism frequently lack. Their failure to perform adequately on some tests may, therefore, reflect deficiencies in these areas rather than more general cognitive impairments. To illustrate this point, one study revealed that when the linguistic and attentional requirements for solution of Piagetian tasks were eliminated, autistic children (ages 4 to 9) performed at levels comparable to normal controls (Lancy & Goldstein, 1982).

Assessment instruments should be selected with an eye to the child's apparent developmental level. For younger children or children whose intellectual skills are markedly delayed, developmental assessment instruments may be used such as the Bayley Scales of Infant Development (Bayley, 1969), or the Uzgiris-Hunt Scales (Uzgiris & Hunt, 1989). For children with an overall mental age of 3 years or above, psychometric batteries should be used, preferably those that are less dependent on verbal abilities, such as the Kaufman-Assessment Battery for Children (Kaufman & Kaufman, 1983). It is important to derive both verbal and nonverbal scores, as a discrepancy favoring the latter often is obtained. For children with nonverbal mental ages over 2 years, nonverbal tests such as the Leiter International Performance Scale (Leiter, 1948) also should be used. (See Cohen et al., 1987, and Watson & Marcus, 1988, for a discussion of assessment instruments.)

In addition to framing the child's overall developmental level, the psychological assessment should provide measures and information of both verbal and nonverbal: problem solving (can the child generate strategies and integrate information?); concept formation (can the child group objects by class, color, etc., or generalize knowledge from one context to another?); style of learning (can the child learn from modeling, imitation, etc.?); and memory skills (how many items of information can the child retain, and is there a difference in the child's ability to recognize inanimate, e.g., geometric forms, as against human faces, stimuli?). Additionally, a measure of visual-spatial and visual-motor integration skills should be obtained to assess the child's sensitivity to the orientation and complexity of objects and ability to write or draw recognizable figures. A description of results should include not only quantified information but also a judgment of how representative of the child's functioning the measure appears to be, and a description of the apparently optimal conditions likely to foster maximal performance on the part of the child.

COMMUNICATIVE ASSESSMENT

The communicative assessment aims at obtaining both quantitative and qualitative information regarding the various aspects of the child's communicative skills. In contrast to some traditional practices, this assessment should include not only the formal aspects of language—articulation, vocabulary, and structure—but also, and

particularly, the suprasegmental aspects of language including intonation and inflection of voice, the use of linguistic skills for communicative purposes and other aspects of pragmatics in speech, and nonverbal forms of communication such as gaze, gestures, or signs. Several language scales are available for very young or very low-functioning children: the Receptive-Expressive Emergent Language Scale (REEL; Bzoch & League, 1971), the Sequenced Inventory of Communicative Development (SICD; Hedrich, Prather, & Tobin, 1975), and the Reynell Developmental Language Scales (Reynell, 1969). It must be noted that, in contrast to the normative population, autistic children's performance on the Peabody Picture Vocabulary Test—Revised (Dunn & Dunn, 1981) or the Expressive One Word Picture Vocabulary Test—Revised (Gardner, 1990) should be seen as measures of receptive and expressive *vocabulary* only, and not as indicators of language comprehension and expression abilities, as autistic children typically are more proficient at naming or pointing to a named picture than communicating with or understanding another person.

For the nonverbal or primarily echolalic child, standardized tests might not be of use. In such instances, the communication specialist should employ informal means to obtain information about the child's communicative resources and prelinguistic skills. These include the child's ability to take turns, to share attention, to vocalize in a consistent fashion, to point to (or gesturally name) objects, to express wishes and protest, to utilize echolalic utterances in a context-appropriate fashion, and so forth. For older and higher-functioning individuals with autism, instruments such as the Clinical Evaluation of Language Fundamentals—Revised (Semel, Wiig, & Secord 1995) may include an assessment of more subtle aspects of communication, such as nonliteral utterances (e.g., metaphor and irony) and ambiguities.

ADAPTIVE FUNCTIONING

An assessment of the child's adaptive skills or capacity for self-sufficiency is an important aspect of the comprehensive evaluation for at least two reasons. First, such an assessment allows the clinician to obtain a representative measure of the child's functioning in real-life situations. The measures and observations obtained during the evaluation in the clinic are inherently affected by extraneous factors, such as the unfamiliarity of the environment and adults, the high degree of structure introduced in order to maximize performance, and the one-to-one approach. It is, therefore, important to acquire information about the child's typical functioning at home and at school, so that possible discrepancies between potential (as measured in the clinic) and actual performance (as expressed in the child's typical environment) can be addressed. Second, several states now condition eligibility for services on both intellectual level (i.e., mental retardation) and adaptive level (capacity for self-sufficiency).

The most widely used instrument to measure adaptive functioning is the Vineland Adaptive Behavior Scales (Sparrow et al., 1984). These scales include measures of Communication (receptive, expressive and written skills), Daily Living skills (personal care, domestic chores, and functioning in the community), Socialization (interpersonal skills, play and coping skills), and Motor functioning (both gross and fine motor skills). Additionally, the Vineland contains a list of maladaptive behaviors that are thought to interfere with the individual's ability to function adaptively. The Vineland has an expanded, a survey, and a classroom edition depending on the objectives and level of detail required (Sparrow & Cicchetti, 1989). One useful aspect of the Vineland scales regards the fact that all of the behaviors included in the semistructured interview can be incorporated immediately as objectives to be achieved within the context of intervention.

PSYCHIATRIC EXAMINATION

The psychiatric examination should include observation during more and less structured periods, such as while interacting with parents and while engaged in assessment by other members of the evaluating team. Areas for observation and inquiry with parents include social development—interest in social interaction, patterns of gaze and eye contact, differential attachments, style of social interaction; communication—receptive

and expressive language, nonverbal and pragmatic communication, communicative intents, echolalia; responses to the environment—motor stereotypes, idiosyncratic responses, resistance to change; and play skills—nonfunctional or idiosyncratic uses of play materials, developmental level of play. The child's capacities for self-awareness—interest in mirror image, awareness of his or her own body, and motor skills—should be observed. Problem behaviors that are likely to interfere with remedial programming should also be noted, such as marked aggression or problems in attention.

FURTHER CONSULTATION

For younger children, consultations with other medical professionals, such as pediatric neurologists or geneticists, may be indicated. History or examination may suggest the need for specific laboratory studies or medical procedures. For example, the presence of severe mental retardation or dysmorphic features in the child, or a family history of mental retardation, suggest the need for genetic screening and chromosome analysis (including screening for fragile X); symptoms suggestive of seizures (e.g., apparent periodic unresponsiveness) suggest the need for electroencephalograms and possible neurological consultation, and so forth. CT or MRI scans may be indicated and sometimes, although not often, reveal disorders such as tuberous sclerosis or degenerative central nervous system disease. A careful history of the pregnancy and neonatal period should be obtained, to ascertain possible pre- or postnatal infections such as congenital rubella. Usually the child's hearing has been tested prior to comprehensive evaluation. If this has not been done, or it was not possible to elicit the child's cooperation, alternative audiometric procedures independent of the child's cooperation should be adopted. In such instances, auditory brainstem evoked responses (BSERs) should be obtained in order to rule out sensory loss (Klin, 1993).

Although autism is associated with a number of other medical conditions, in most instances even extensive medical evaluations fail to reveal an associated medical condition. This fact suggests reasonable caution in seeking additional medical assessments. On the other hand, certain features may suggest the importance of extensive medical investigations, such as the abrupt behavioral and developmental deterioration of a child who was previously developing normally.

DIFFERENTIAL DIAGNOSIS

The differential diagnosis of autism and other PDDs includes language and other specific developmental disorders, mental retardation, sensory impairments (particularly deafness), and reactive attachment disorder. Usually children with language disorders do not exhibit the pattern of serious social deviance and deficit characteristic of autism; often nonverbal communicative abilities are an area of evident strength. In mental retardation, social and communicative skills are usually on a par with overall cognitive skills. Deaf children may exhibit some difficulties in social interaction and some repetitive activities; however, usually they are interested in social interaction and may make use of gestures for communicative purposes. Children with reactive attachment disorders have, by definition, experienced marked psychosocial deprivation, which results in deficits in social interaction, most notably in attachment (expressed as either withdrawal or indiscriminate friendliness). However, the quality of the social deficit is different from that in autism and the disturbance tends to remit after an appropriately responsive and nurturing psychosocial environment is provided.

In young children the task of differential diagnosis is complicated by the inherent difficulties posed by their early developmental level, the frequency of "autisticlike" behaviors in other conditions, and the fact that autism can be present in conjunction with deafness and with mental retardation. In many instances the issues attending diagnosis are clarified with certainty only over time and after a period of intervention. It is appropriate to share with parents a sense of the clinician's degree of confidence in the diagnosis. It is also important to realize that the diagnosis may have important, if not necessarily intended, implications for a host of other purposes: for educational placement and programming, and eligibility for special services in the community. It is critical that the importance of educational and other interventions

be emphasized regardless of how "classically" autistic, or low-functioning, the child appears to be.

Interventions

Despite strong claims by partisans of particular treatment approaches and much dedicated effort that has gone into their implementation, no treatment has been demonstrated to produce major alterations in the natural history of the syndrome (Rutter, 1985; Ward, 1970). In the absence of a definitive cure, there are a thousand treatments. Essentially every conceivable treatment has been utilized for autism, including somatic treatments, drug therapy, psychotherapy, behavior modification, nutritional treatments, and educational interventions (DeMyer et al., 1981; Rutter, 1985). With the exception of a few areas (notably behavior modification and pharmacological intervention and, to a lesser extent, educational interventions), most proposed interventions have not been studied rigorously. Consequently, it has been difficult to assess treatment effects systematically.

Unfortunately, short-term changes readily occur when treaters and/or evaluators are not blind to the hypothesis under study; additionally, short-term changes may be neither sustained nor clinically meaningful. In other instances, particularly in regard to reports of treatment efficacy based on a single case, it may be unclear whether the individual was autistic and what factor or factors were responsible for improvement. The observation that at least a few autistic individuals achieve relatively good outcomes is gratifying, but it also complicates the interpretation of single case studies. To further compound the problem, probably there is no "untreated" autistic child; by the time the diagnosis is definitively made, parents often have tried multiple interventions.

Although there scant is evidence that autism can be "cured," improvement in several aspects of the child's presentation and specific behaviors may be achieved. Simeonsson and colleagues (1987) reviewed 4 comprehensive studies of early intervention for autistic children. The authors concluded that the critical factors in successful programs included structured, behavioral treatment, parent involvement, treatment at an early age, intensive intervention, and focus on generalization of skills to new settings. Other lines of evidence have suggested the importance of appropriate, intensive educational interventions to foster the acquisition of basic social, cognitive, communicative, and adaptive skills (Olley & Stevenson, 1989; Prizant & Schuler, 1987), that are, in turn, related to outcome. Behavior modification techniques can be quite helpful. Early and continuous intervention is highly desirable; some reports (Lovaas, 1987) have suggested marked improvement following early, intensive intervention. Educational programs should be highly structured (Rutter & Bartak, 1973) and oriented around the individual needs of the child. Intervention programs should be comprehensive and include the services of various professionals, including special educators, speech pathologists, and occupational therapists. Parental involvement should be encouraged in order to enhance consistency in approaches at home and at school and to facilitate generalization of skills across settings. Professionals should work with parents to obtain appropriate educational placement and help them become aware of other community resources, such as respite care. Forthcoming federal mandates for provision of remedial services from birth on will increase the availability of services, we hope.

During the 1950s, it was common for professionals to recommend that parents consider institutionalization for severely disabled children. This practice led to the isolation and segregation of children with severe developmental disabilities, and, as a result, many such individuals were prevented from reaching their full potential. An awareness of these issues has produced a marked shift in social policy; most state agencies now attempt to maintain children in their families and communities, although, unfortunately, many necessary services may not be provided. A similar issue has arisen with regard to the integration of autistic children into regular classroom settings. The rationale for this approach is based both on a strongly held philosophical stance (e.g., that "special" educational settings are, by their nature, inferior and discriminatory) as well as on a small body of empirical research (Charlop et al., 1983) that suggests that autistic children can indeed learn from their normally developing peers. Given the nature of social deficits in autism, there is con-

siderable reason to worry that autistic children may not be as able as mentally retarded, nonautistic children to profit from such an approach. In considering various alternative educational placements, the individual needs of the child should be paramount.

In general, pharmacological interventions with infants and young autistic children are probably best avoided. The best-studied agents—the tranquilizers—have some utility in selected cases and in regard to specific maladaptive behaviors, but their many side effects, particularly sedation, may prove problematic (Campbell, Anderson, Green, & Deutsch, 1987). These agents may be indicated in some situations; typically, however, they are given to older children and even then at the lowest effective dose for the shortest period of time. The efficacy of other pharmacological agents has not been clearly established.

Many nontraditional treatments are available. In discussing such treatments with parents, it is helpful to explore the rationale for the proposed treatment, the evidence (if any) of efficacy, and its potential costs (in both financial and human terms) to the child and the family (Klin & Cohen, 1994). Treatments that are minimally disruptive of the child's educational program and that hold little apparent risk to the child are of less concern than those that entail considerable disruption of the child's educational program or the family's life.

Conclusion

Considerable progress in the understanding of the nature of autism and related disorders has been made over the past 50 years. Given the early onset of the condition, it is somewhat paradoxical that our knowledge of autism in infants and very young children remains limited in important respects. Our knowledge of the other pervasive developmental disorders is even more meager. Although it now appears that these conditions arise as a result of some insult to the developing central nervous system, precise and testable pathophysiological mechanisms have not been identified yet.

Nevertheless, autism remains one of the most studied early childhood disorders. Although much of the biological research to date has been un-availing, continued advances in the neurosciences make elucidation of brain pathobiology more likely. The neurosciences can be put to their best use if the current limits of our knowledge concerning phenotype, neurobiology, and etiology are clearly understood. Advances in the understanding of the psychology of autism, both within and across individuals, as well as along behavioral dimensions and with respect to categorical issues should serve to better direct and organize the biological research. Such advances plus the recent nosologic efforts will, it is hoped, result in a better understanding of the syndrome pathogenesis that, in turn, finally might translate into more effective treatment interventions. However, such integration of different lines of research and treatment approaches requires an appreciation of the complexity of the clinical phenomena and the enormous range of each of the salient dimensions. In the process of elucidating such a complex disorder affecting the child's basic capacities for socialization, it is likely that a great deal of light will be shed on the intricacies of every child's development.

REFERENCES

Adrien, J. L., Ornitz, E., Barthelemy, C., Sauvage, D., & Lelord, G. (1987). The presence or absence of certain behaviors associated with infantile autism in severely retarded autistic and nonautistic retarded children and very young normal children. *Journal of Autism and Developmental Disorders, 17,* 407–416.

American Psychiatric Association. (1980). *Diagnostic and statistical manual of mental disorders* (3rd ed.). Washington, DC: Author.

American Psychiatric Association. (1987). *Diagnostic and statistical manual of mental disorders* (3rd ed., rev.). Washington, DC: Author.

American Psychiatric Association. (1989). *Treatment of psychiatric disorders.* Washington, DC: Author.

American Psychiatric Association. (1994). *Diagnostic and statistical manual of mental disorders* (4th ed.). Washington, DC: Author.

Anderson, G. M., & Hoshino, Y. (1987) Neurochemical studies of autism. In D. Cohen & A. Donnellan (Eds.), *Handbook of autism and pervasive developmental disorders* (pp. 166–191). New York: John Wiley & Sons.

Asperger, H. (1991). Autistic psychopathy in childhood. In U. Frith (Ed.), *Autism and Asperger syndrome* (pp. 37–92). Cambridge: Cambridge University Press. (Original work published 1944.)

Asperger, H. (1979). Problems of infantile autism. *Communication, 13,* 35.

August, G. J., Stewart, M. A., & Tsai, L. (1981). The incidence of cognitive disabilities in the siblings of autistic children. *British Journal of Psychiatry, 138,* 416–422.

Bailey, A., Le Couteur, A., Gottesman, I., Bolton, P., Simonoff, E., Yuzda, E., & Rutter, M. (1995). Autism as a strongly genetic disorder: Evidence from a British twin study. *Psychological Medicine, 25* (1), 63–77.

Baron-Cohen, S. (1988). Social and pragmatic deficits in autism: Cognitive or affective? *Journal of Autism and Developmental Disorders, 3,* 379–402.

Baron-Cohen, S. (1990). Autism: A specific cognitive disorder of "mind-blindness." *International Journal of Psychiatry, 2,* 81–90.

Baron-Cohen, S., Allen, J., & Gillberg, C. (1992). Can autism be detected at 18 months? The Needle, the haystack, and the CHAT. *British Journal of Psychiatry, 161,* 839–843.

Bayley, N. (1969). *Bayley Scales of Infant Development.* New York: Psychological Corporation.

Bell, R. Q., & Harper, L. V. (1977). *Child effects on adults.* New York: Lawrence Erlbaum.

Bemporad, J. R. (1979). Adult recollections of a formerly autistic child. *Journal of Autism and Developmental Disorders, 9,* 179–197.

Benda, C. E. (1952). *Developmental disorders of mentation and cerebral palsies.* New York: Grune & Stratton.

Bender, L. (1947). Childhood schizophrenia: Clinical study of 100 schizophrenic children. *American Journal of Orthopsychiatry, 17,* 40–56.

Bettelheim, B. (1967). *The empty fortress.* New York: Free Press.

Bleuler, E. (1951) Dementia praecox of the group of schizophrenia. *Monograph series on Schizophrenia,* No. 1. (J. Zinkin, Trans.). New York: International Universities Press.

Bregman, J. D., & Volkmar, F. R. (1988). Autistic social dysfunction and Down syndrome. *Journal of the American Academy of Child and Adolescent Psychiatry, 27,* 440–441.

Brothers, L. (1989). A biological perspective on empathy. *American Journal of Psychiatry, 146,* 10–19.

Burack, J., & Volkmar, F. R. (1992). Development of low- and high-functioning autistic children. *Journal of Child Psychology and Psychiatry, 33,* 607–616.

Bzoch, K., & League, R. (1971). *Receptive Expressive Emergent Language Scale.* Gainesville, FL: Language Educational Division, Computer Management Corporation.

Cairns, R. B. (1979). *Social development: The origins and plasticity of interchanges.* San Francisco: W. H. Freeman.

Campbell, M., Anderson L. T., Green W. H., & Deutsch S. I. (1987). Psychopharmacology. In D. Cohen & A. Donnellan (Eds.), *Handbook of autism and pervasive developmental disorders* (pp. 545–565). New York: John Wiley & Sons.

Cantor, S. (1988). *Childhood schizophrenia.* New York: Guilford Press.

Cantwell, D., Baker, L., & Rutter, M. (1978). A comparative study of infantile autism and specific developmental receptive language disorder. IV. Analysis of syntax and language function. *Journal of Child Psychology and Psychiatry, 19,* 351–362.

Charlop, M. J., Schreiman, L., & Tryon, A. D. (1983). Learning through observation: The effects of peer modeling on acquisition and generalization in autistic children. *Journal of Abnormal Child Psychology, 11,* 355–366.

Chess, S. (1971). Autism in children with congenital rubella. *Journal of Autism and Childhood Schizophrenia, 1,* 33–47.

Cicchetti, D. V., & Cohen, D. J. (Eds.). (1995). *Developmental psychopathology,* New York: John Wiley & Sons.

Cohen, D. J. (1991). Finding meaning in one's self and others: Clinical studies of children with autism and Tourette syndrome. In F. Kessel, M. Bornstein, & A. Sameroff (Eds.), *Contemporary constructions of the child: Essays in honor of William Kessen* (pp. 159–175). Hillsdale, NJ: Lawrence Erlbaum.

Cohen, D. J., Caparulo, B., & Shaywitz, B. (1976). Primary childhood aphasia and childhood autism. *Journal of the American Academy of Child and Adolescent Psychiatry, 15,* 604–645.

Cohen, D. J., Paul, R., & Volkmar, F. R. (1987). Issues in the classification of pervasive developmental disorders and associated conditions. In D. J. Cohen & A. Donnellan (Eds.), *Handbook of autism and pervasive developmental disorders* (pp. 20–40). New York: John Wiley & Sons.

Cohen, D. J., Volkmar, F. R., Anderson, G., & Klin, A. (1993). Integrating biological and behavioral perspectives in the study and care of autistic individuals: The future ahead. *Israel Journal of Psychiatry, 30* (1), 15–32.

Cohn, J. F., & Tronick, E. Z. (1987). The sequence of dyadic states at 3, 6, and 9 months. *Developmental Psychology, 23,* 68–77.

Coleman, M. (1987). The search for neurobiological subgroups in autism. In E. Schopler & G. Mesibov (Eds.), *Neurobiological issues in autism* (pp. 163–179). New York: Plenum Press.

Corbett, J. (1987). Development, disintegration, and dementia. *Journal of Mental Deficiency Research, 31,* 349–356.

Creak, E. M. (1961). Schizophrenic syndrome in childhood: Progress report of a working party. *Cerebral Palsy Bulletin, 3,* 501–504.

Curcio, F. (1976). Sensorimotor functioning and communication in mute autistic children. *Journal of Autism and Childhood Schizophrenia, 8,* 281–292.

Curcio, F. (1978). Sensorimotor functioning and communication in mute autistic children. *Journal of Autism and Developmental Disorders, 8,* 292–305.

DeMyer, M. K., Hingtgen, J. N., & Jackson, R. K. (1981). Infantile autism reviewed: A decade of research. *Schizophrenia Bulletin, 7,* 388–451.

De Sanctis, S. (1906). Sopra alcune varieta della demenza precoce. *Revista Sperimentale di Freniatria e di Medicina Legale, 32,* 141–165.

Down, J. L. (1887). *On some of the mental affections of childhood and youth.* London: Churchill.

Dunn, L., & Dunn, L. (1981). *Peabody Picture Vocabulary Test—Revised.* Circle Pines, MN: American Guidance Service.

Earl, C. J. C. (1934). The primitive catatonic psychosis of idiocy. *British Journal of Medical Psychology, 14,* 230–253.

Easson, W. M. (1971). Symptomatic autism in childhood and adolescence. *Pediatrics, 47,* 717–722.

Fay, D., & Mermelstein, R. (1982). Language in infantile autism. In S. Rosenberg (Ed.), *Handbook of Applied Psycholinguistics.* Hillsdale, NJ: Erlbaum.

Fay, W., and Schuler, A. L. (1980), *Emerging language in autistic children.* Baltimore: University Park Press.

Fein, D., Pennington, B., Markowitz, P., Braverman, M., & Waterhouse, L. (1986). Towards a neuropsychological model of infantile autism: Are the social deficits primary? *Journal of the American Academy of Child Psychiatry, 25,* 198–212.

Folstein, S., & Piven, J. (1991). Etiology of autism: Genetic influences. *Pediatrics, 87* (5), 767–773.

Folstein, S., & Rutter, M. (1977). Infantile autism: A genetic study of 21 twin pairs. *Journal of Child Psychology and Psychiatry, 18,* 297–321.

Gardner, M. (1990). *Expressive One Word Picture Vocabulary Test.* Los Angeles: Western Psychological Services.

Gillberg, C. (1989). Asperger's syndrome in 23 Swedish children. *Developmental Medicine and Child Neurology, 31,* 520–531.

Gillberg, I. C., & Gillberg, C. (1989). Asperger syndrome—some epidemiological considerations. *Journal of Child Psychology and Psychiatry, 30,* 631–638.

Golden, G. (1987). Neurological functioning. In D. J. Cohen & A. Donnellan (Eds.), *Handbook of autism and pervasive developmental disorders* (pp. 133–147). New York: John Wiley & Sons.

Goldstein, K. (1948). *Language and language disturbances.* New York: Grune & Stratton.

Hayes, R. P. (1987). Training for work. In D. J. Cohen & A. M. Donnellan (Eds.), *Handbook of autism and pervasive developmental disorders* (pp. 360–372). New York: John Wiley & Sons.

Head, H. (1926). *Aphasia and kindred disorders of speech.* London: Cambridge University Press.

Hedrick, D., Prather, F., & Tobin, A. (1975). *Sequenced inventory of communicative development.* Seattle: University of Washington Press.

Heh, C. W., Smith, R., Wu, J., Hazlett, E., Russell, A., Asarnow, R., Tanguay, P., & Buchsbaum, M. S. (1989). Positron emission tomography of the cerebellum in autism. *American Journal of Psychiatry, 146* (2), 242–245.

Heller, T. (1930). Uber Dementia infantilis. *Zeitschrift für Kinderforschung, 37,* 661–667. (Reprinted in *Modern Perspective in International Child Psychiatry,* ed. by J. G. Howell. New York: Brunner/Mazel, 1969, pp. 610–616.)

Heller, T. (1954). About dementia infantilis (translation). *Journal of Nervous and Mental Disease, 119,* 471–477.

Hermelin, B., & O'Connor, N. (1970). *Psychological experiments with autistic children.* New York: Pergamon Press.

Hobson, R. P. (1990). On psychoanalytic approaches to autism. *American Journal of Orthopsychiatry, 60,* 324–336.

Hulse, W. C. (1954). Dementia infantilis. *Journal of Nervous and Mental Diseases, 119,* 471–477.

Jones, M. G., & Szatmari, P. (1988). Stoppage rules and genetic studies of autism. *Journal of Autism and Developmental Disorders, 18,* 31–40.

Kanner, L. (1935). *Child Psychiatry.* Springfield, IL: Charles C. Thomas.

Kanner, L. (1943). Autistic disturbances of affective contact. *Nervous Child, 2,* 217–250.

Kanner, L., Rodriguez, A., & Ashenden, B. (1972). How far can autistic children go in matters of social adaptation? *Journal of Autism and Childhood Schizophrenia, 2,* 9–33.

Kaufman, A. S., & Kaufman, N. L. (1983). *K-ABC: Kaufman Assessment Battery for Children.* Circle Pines, MN: American Guidance Service.

Klein, M. (1975). The importance of symbol-formation in the development of the ego. In M. Klein, *Love, guilt and reparation and other works 1921–1941.* London: Hogarth Press. (Original work published 1930.)

Klin, A. (1991). Young autistic children's listening preferences in regard to speech: A possible characterization of the symptom of social withdrawal. *Journal of Autism and Developmental Disorders, 21,* 29–42.

Klin, A. (1992). Listening preferences in regard to speech in four children with developmental disabilities. *Journal of Child Psychology and Psychiatry, 33,* 763–769.

Klin, A. (1993). Auditory brainstem responses in autism: Brainstem dysfunction or peripheral hearing loss? *Journal of Autism and Developmental Disorders, 23,* 15–35.

Klin, A. (1994). Asperger syndrome. *Child and Adolescent Psychiatry Clinic of North America, 3,* 131–148.

Klin, A., & Cohen, D. J. (1994). The immorality of not-knowing: The ethical imperative to conduct research in child psychiatry. In Y. Hattab (Ed.), *Ethics in child psychiatry* (pp. 217–232). Jerusalem: Gefen Publishers.

Klin, A., Mayes, L. C., Volkmar, F. R., & Cohen, D. J. (1995). Multiplex developmental disorder. *Journal of Developmental and Behavioral Pediatrics, 16* (3), S7–S11.

Klin, A., & Shepard, B. A. (1994). Psychological assessment of autistic children. *Child and Adolescent Psychiatric Clinics of North America, 3* (1), 53–70.

Klin, A., & Volkmar, F. R. (1993). The development of individuals with autism: Implications for the theory of mind hypothesis. In S. Baron-Cohen, H. Tager-Flusberg, & D. J. Cohen (Eds.), *Understanding other minds: Perspectives from autism* (pp. 317–336). Oxford: Oxford University Press.

Klin, A., & Volkmar, F. R. (1995). Autism and the pervasive developmental disorders. *Child and Adolescent Psychiatric Clinics of North America, 4* (3), 617–630.

Klin, A., & Volkmar, F. R. (In press). Asperger's syndrome. In D. J. Cohen & F. R. Volkmar (Eds.), *Handbook of autism and pervasive developmental disorders.* New York: John Wiley & Sons.

Klin, A., Volkmar, F. R., & Sparrow, S. S. (1992). Autistic social dysfunction: Some limitations of the theory of mind hypothesis. *Journal of Child Psychology and Psychiatry, 33,* 861–876.

Klin, A., Volkmar, F. R., Sparrow, S. S., Cicchetti, D. V., & Rourke, B. P. (1995). Validity and neuropsychological characterization of Asperger syndrome. *Journal of Child Psychology and Psychiatry, 36* (7), 1127–1140.

Kolvin, I. (1971). Studies in the childhood psychoses: I. Diagnostic criteria and classification. *British Journal of Psychiatry, 118,* 381–384.

Kraeplin, E. (1919). *Dementia praecox and paraphenia.* Edinburgh: Livingstone.

Lancy, D. F., & Goldstein, G. I. (1982). The use of nonverbal Piagetian tasks to assess the cognitive development of autistic children. *Child Development, 53,* 1233–1241.

Leiter, R. G. (1948). *Leiter International Performance Scale.* Chicago: Stoelting Co.

Leslie, A. M. (1987). Pretense and representation: The origins of "theory of mind." *Psychological Review, 94,* 412–426.

Levi-Strauss, C. (1949). *Les structures elementaires de la parente.* Paris: Presses Universitaires de France.

Lockyer, L., & Rutter, M. (1969). A five to fifteen year follow-up study of infantile psychosis. III. Psychological aspects. *British Journal of Psychiatry, 115,* 865–882.

Lord, C., Rutter, M., Lord, C., Rios, P., Robertson, S., Holdgrafer, M., & McLennan, J. D. (1989). Autism Diagnostic Interview: A semi-structured interview for parents and caregivers of autistic persons. *Journal of Autism and Developmental Disorders, 19,* 363–387.

Lord, C., & Schopler E. (1987). Neurobiological implications of sex differences in autism. In E. Schopler & G. Mesibov (Eds.), *Neurobiological issues in autism* (pp. 192–212). New York: Plenum Press.

Losche, G. (1990). Sensorimotor and action development in autistic children from infancy to early childhood. *Journal of Child Psychology and Psychiatry, 31,* 749–761.

Lotter, V. (1978a). Follow-up studies. In M. Rutter & E. Schopler (Eds.), *Autism: A Reappraisal of concepts and treatment.* New York: Plenum Press.

Lotter, V. (1978b). Childhood autism in Africa. *Journal of Child Psychology and Psychiatry, 19,* 231–244.

Lovaas, O. I. (1987) Behavioral treatment and normal educational and intellectual functioning in young autistic children. *Journal of Consulting and Clinical Psychology, 55,* 3–9.

Mahler, M. (1952). On child psychoses and schizophrenia: Autistic and symbiotic infantile psychoses. *Psychoanalytic Study of the Child, 7,* 286–305.

Massie, H. N. (1978). Blind ratings of mother-infant interaction in home movies of prepsychotic and normal infants. *American Journal of Psychiatry, 135,* 1271–1374.

McAdoo, W. G., & DeMyer, M. Y. (1978). Personality characteristics of parents. In M. Rutter (Ed.), *Autism: A reappraisal of concepts and treatment.* New York: Plenum Press.

McKenna, K., Gordon, C. T., & Lenane, M. (1994). Looking for childhood-onset schizophrenia: The first 71 cases screened. *Journal of the American Academy of Child and Adolescent Psychiatry, 33,* 636–644.

Menyuk, P. (1978). Language: What's wrong and why. In M. Rutter & E. Schopler (Eds.), *Autism: A reappraisal of concepts and treatment.* London: Plenum Press.

Moeschler, J. B., Charman, C. E., Berg, S. Z., & Graham, J. H. (1988). Rett syndrome: Natural history and management. *Pediatrics, 82,* 1–10.

Morgan, S. (1988). The autistic child and family functioning: A developmental-family systems perspective. *Journal of Autism and Developmental Disorders, 18,* 263–280.

Morgan, S., Curtrer, P. S., Coplin, J. W., & Rodrigue, J. R. (1989). Do autistic children differ from retarded and normal children in Piagetian sensorimotor functioning? *Journal of Child Psychology and Psychiatry, 30,* 857–864.

Mundy, P., & Sigman, M. (1989). Specifying the nature of the social impairment in autism. In G. Dawson (Ed.), *Autism: Nature, diagnosis, and treatment.* New York: Guilford Press.

Olley, J. G., & Stevenson, S. E. (1989). Preschool curriculum for children with autism: Addressing early social skills. In G. Dawson (Ed.), *Autism: Nature, diagnosis, and treatment.* New York: Guilford Press.

Ornitz, E. M., Guthrie, D., & Farley, A. H. (1977). Early development of autistic children. *Journal of Autism and Childhood Schizophrenia, 7,* 207–229.

Ozonoff, S., Rogers, S. J., & Pennington, B. F. (1991). Asperger's syndrome: Evidence of an empirical distinction from high-functioning autism. *Journal of Child Psychology and Psychiatry, 32,* 1107–1122.

Parks, S. L. (1983). The assessment of autistic children: A selective review of available instruments. *Journal of Autism and Developmental Disorders, 13,* 255–267.

Paul, R. (1987). Communication in autism. In D. Cohen & A. Donnellan (Eds.), *Handbook of autism and pervasive developmental disorders* (pp. 61–84). New York: John Wiley & Sons, 1987.

Potter, H. W. (1933). Schizophrenia in children. *American Journal of Psychiatry, 89,* 1253–1270.

Prior, M., Dahlstrom, B., & Squires, T. (1990) Autistic children's knowledge of thinking and feeling states in other people. *Journal of Child Psychology and Psychiatry, 31,* 587–601.

Prior, M., & Gajzago, C. (1974, August 3). Recognition of early signs of autism. *Medical Journal of Australia.*

Prizant, B. M. (1983). Language acquisition and communicative behavior in autism: Toward an understanding of the "whole" of it. *Journal of Speech and Hearing Disorders, 48,* 296–307.

Prizant, B. M., & Schuler, A. L. (1986). Facilitating communication: Pre-language approaches. In D. J. Cohen & A. Donnelan (Eds.), *Handbook of autism and disorders of atypical development* (pp. 289–300). New York: John Wiley & Sons.

Prizant, B. M., & Schuler, A. (1987). Facilitating communication: Theoretical foundations. In D. Cohen & A. Donnellan (Eds.), *Handbook of autism and pervasive developmental disorders* (pp. 289–300). New York: John Wiley & Sons.

Provence, S., & Lipton, R. C. (1962). *Infants in institutions.* New York: International Universities Press.

Rank, B. (1949). Adaptation of the psychoanalytic technique for the treatment of young children with atypical development. *American Journal of Orthopsychiatry, 19,* 130–139.

Rett, A. (1966). Uber ein eigenartiges hirntophisces Syndrome bei Hyperammonie im Kindersalter. *Wein Medizinische Wochenschrift, 118,* 723–726.

Reynell, J. (1969). *Developmental language scales.* Windsor, England: N.F.E.R. Publishing Co.

Ricks, D. M. (1975). Vocal communication in preverbal normal and autistic children. In N. O'Connor (Ed.), *Language, cognitive deficits and retardation.* London: Butterworth.

Ricks, D. M., & Wing, L. (1975). Language, communication, and the use of symbols in normal and autistic children. *Journal of Autism and Childhood Schizophrenia, 5,* 191–221.

Ritvo, E. R., & Freeman, B. J. (1978). National Society for Autistic Children definition of the syndrome of autism. *Journal of Autism and Developmental Disorders, 8,* 162–169.

Rutter, M. (1970). Autistic children: Infancy to adulthood. *Seminars in Psychiatry, 2,* 435–450.

Rutter, M. (1972). Childhood schizophrenia reconsidered. *Journal of Autism and Childhood Schizophrenia, 2,* 315–338.

Rutter, M. (1978a). Diagnosis and definition. In M. Rutter & E. Schopler (Eds.), *Autism: A reappraisal of concepts and treatment.* New York: Plenum Press.

Rutter, M. (1978b). Language disorder and infantile autism. In M. Rutter & E. Schopler (Eds.), *Autism: A reappraisal of concepts and treatment.* New York: Plenum Press.

Rutter, M. (1983). Cognitive deficits in the pathogenesis of autism. *Journal of Child Psychology and Psychiatry, 24,* 513–531.

Rutter, M., & Bartak, L. (1973). Special educational treatment of autistic children: A comparative study. II. Follow-up findings and implications for services. *Journal of Child Psychology and Psychiatry, 14,* 241–270.

Rutter, M., Bartak, L., & Newman, S. (1971). Autism: A central disorder of cognition and language. In M. Rutter (Ed.), *Infantile autism: Concepts, characteristics and treatment.* London: Churchill Livingstone.

Rutter, M., Greenfield, D., & Lockyer, L. (1967). A five to fifteen year follow-up of infantile psychosis: II. Social and behavioral outcome. *British Journal of Psychiatry, 113,* 1183–1189.

Rutter, M., & Schopler, E. (1992). Classification of pervasive developmental disorders: Some concepts and practical considerations. *Journal of Autism and Developmental Disorders, 22,* 459–482.

Scheerer, M., Rothmann, E., & Goldstein, K. (1945). A case of "idiot savant": An experimental study of personality organization. *Psychological Monographs, 58* (4).

Schopler, E., Andrews, C. E., & Strupp, K. (1980). Do autistic children come from upper-middle-class parents? *Journal of Autism and Developmental Disorders, 10,* 91–103.

Schopler, E., & Mesibov, G. (Eds.). (1984). *The effects of autism on the family.* New York: Plenum Press.

Schopler, E., Rutter, M., & Chess, S. (1979). Editorial: Change of journal scope and title. *Journal of Autism and Developmental Disorders, 9,* 1–10.

Semel, E., Wiig, E., & Secord, W. (1995). *Clinical evaluation of language fundamentals—3.* San Antonio, TX: The Psychological Corporation. Harcourt Brace.

Short, A. B., & Schopler, E. (1988). Factors relating to age of onset in autism. *Journal of Autism and Developmental Disorders, 18,* 207–216.

Siegel, B., Pliner, C., Eschler, J., & Elliot, G. R. (1988). How autistic children are diagnosed: Difficulties in identification of children with multiple developmental delays. *Journal of Developmental and Behavioral Pediatrics, 9,* 199–204.

Sigman, M., & Ungerer, J. (1984). Attachment behaviors in autistic children. *Journal of Autism & Developmental Disorders, 14,* 231–244.

Sigman, M., Ungerer, J. A., Mundy, P., & Sherman, T. (1987). Cognition in autistic children. In D. J. Cohen & A. M. Donnellan (Eds.), *Handbook of autism and pervasive developmental disorders* (pp. 103–120). New York: John Wiley & Sons.

Simeonsson, R. J., Olley, J. G., & Rosenthal, S. L. (1987). Early intervention for children with autism. In M. J. Guralnick & F. C. Bennett (Eds.), *The effectiveness of early intervention for at-risk and handicapped children.* New York: Academic Press.

Sparrow, S., Balla, D., & Ciccheti, D. (1984). *Vineland Adaptive Behavior Scales.* Circle Pines, MN: American Guidance Service.

Sparrow, S. S., & Cicchetti, D. V. (1989). The Vineland Adaptive Behavior Scales. In C. S. Newmark (Ed.), *Major psychological assessment instruments, Vol. II.* Boston: Allyn & Bacon.

Stern, D. (1985). *The interpersonal world of the human infant.* New York: Basic Books.

Szatmari, P. (1996). Asperger's disorder and atypical pervasive developmental disorder. In F. R. Volkmar (Ed.), *Psychoses and pervasive developmental disorders in childhood and adolescence* (pp. 191–222). Washington, DC: American Psychiatric Press.

Szatmari, P., Bremmer, R., & Nagy, J. N. (1989). Asperger's syndrome: A review of clinical features. *Canadian Journal of Psychiatry, 34* (6), 554–560.

Tager-Flusberg, H. (1993). What language reveals about the understanding of mind in children with autism. In S. Baron-Cohen, H. Tager-Flusberg, & D. J. Cohen (Eds.), *Understanding other minds: Perspectives from autism* (pp. 138–157). Oxford: Oxford University Press.

Tantam, D. (1988). Annotation: Asperger's syndrome. *Journal of Child Psychology and Psychiatry, 29,* 245–255.

Tantam, D. (1991). Asperger syndrome in adulthood. In U. Frith (Ed.), *Autism and Asperger syndrome* (pp. 147–183). Cambridge: Cambridge University Press.

Treffert, D. A. (1988). The idiot savant: A review of the syndrome. *American Journal of Psychiatry, 145,* 563.

Trevathan, E., & Adams, M. J. (1988). The epidemiology and public health significance of Rett syndrome. *Journal of Child Neurology, 3* (Suppl.), S17–S20.

Trevathan, E., & Naidu, S. (1988). The clinical recognition and differential diagnosis of Rett syndrome. *Journal of Child Neurology, 3* (Suppl.), S6–S16.

Tronick, E. (1980). The primacy of social skills in infancy. In D. B. Sawing, R. C. Hawkins, L. Olzenski Waker, & J. H. Penticuff (Eds.), *Exceptional infant, Vol. 4: Psychosocial risks in infant-environment transactions.* New York: Brunner Mazel.

Tsai, L. Y. (1987). Pre-, peri-, and neonatal factors in autism. In E. Schopler & G. B. Mesibov (Eds.), *Neurobiological issues in autism* (pp. 180–191). New York: Plenum Press.

Ungerer, J. A., & Sigman, M. (1981). Symbolic play and language comprehension in autistic children. *Journal of the American Academy of Child Psychiatry, 20,* 318–337.

Uzgiris, I. C., & Hunt, J. McV. (1975). *Assessment in infancy: Ordinal scales of psychological development.* Urbana: University of Illinois Press.

Volkmar, F. R. (1987). Social development. In D. J. Cohen & A. Donnellan (Eds.), *Handbook of autism and pervasive developmental disorders* (pp. 41–60). New York: John Wiley & Sons.

Volkmar, F. R. (1992). Childhood disintegrative disorder: Issues for DSM-IV. *Journal of Autism and Developmental Disorders, 22,* 625–642.

Volkmar, F. R. (1996). The disintegrative disorders: Childhood disintegrative disorder and Rett's disorder. In F. R. Volkmar (Ed.), *Psychoses and pervasive developmental disorders in childhood and adoles-*

cence (pp. 223–248). Washington, DC: American Psychiatric Press.

Volkmar, F. R., Bregman, J., Cohen, D. J., & Cicchetti, D. V. (1988). DSM III and DSM III-R Diagnoses of Autism. *American Journal of Psychiatry, 145,* 1404–1408.

Volkmar, F. R., Bregman, J., Cohen, D. J., Hooks, M., & Stevenson, J. (1989). An examination of social typologies in autism. *Journal of the American Academy of Child and Adolescent Psychiatry, 28,* 82–86.

Volkmar, F. R., Carter, A., Sparrow, S. S., & Cicchetti, D. V. (1993). Quantifying social development in autism. *Journal of the American Academy of Child and Adolescent Psychiatry, 32,* 627–632.

Volkmar, F. R., Cicchetti, D. V., Bregman, J., & Cohen, D. J. (1992). Three diagnostic systems for autism: DSM-III, DSM-III-R, and ICD-10. *Journal of Autism and Developmental Disorders, 22,* 483–492.

Volkmar, F. R., & Cohen, D. J. (1985). A first person account of the experience of infantile autism by Tony W. *Journal of Autism and Developmental Disorders, 15,* 47–54.

Volkmar, F. R., & Cohen, D. J. (1988). Diagnosis of pervasive developmental disorders. In B. Lahey & A. Kazdin (Eds.), *Advances in clinical child psychology* (Vol. 11). New York: Plenum Press.

Volkmar, F. R., & Cohen, D. J. (1989). Disintegrative disorder or "late onset" autism. *Journal of Child Psychology and Psychiatry, 30,* 717–724.

Volkmar, F. R., & Cohen, D. J. (1991). Nonautistic pervasive developmental disorders. In R. Michels (Ed.), *Psychiatry, Vol. 2: Child Psychiatry* (pp. 1–12). Philadelphia: J. B. Lippincott.

Volkmar, F. R., Cohen, D. J., Hoshino, Y., Rende, R., & Paul, R. (1988). Phenomenology and classification of the childhood psychoses. *Psychological Medicine, 18,* 191–201.

Volkmar, F. R., & Klin, A. (1993). Social development in autism: Historical and clinical perspectives. In S. Baron-Cohen, H. Tager-Flusberg, & D. J. Cohen (Eds.), *Understanding other minds: Perspectives from autism* (pp. 40–58). Oxford: Oxford University Press.

Volkmar, F. R., Klin, A., Siegel, B., Szatmari, P., Lord, C., Campbell, M., Freeman, B. J., Cicchetti, D. V., & Rutter, M., Kline, W., Buitelaar, J., Hattab, Y., Fombonne, E., Fuentes, J., Werry, J., Stone, W., Kerbeshian, J., Hoshino, Y., Bregman, J., Loveland, K., Szymanski, L., & Towbin, K. (1994). DSM-IV Autism/pervasive developmental disorder field trial. *American Journal of Psychiatry, 151,* 1361–1367.

Volkmar, F. R., & Nelson, D. S. (1990). Seizure disorders in autism. *Journal of the American Academy of Child and Adolescent Psychiatry, 29,* 127–129.

Volkmar, F. R., Sparrow, S., Goudreau, D., Cicchetti, D. V., Paul, R., & Cohen, D. J. (1987). Social deficits in autism: An operational approach using the Vineland Adaptive Behavior Scales. *Journal of the American Academy of Child and Adolescent Psychiatry, 26,* 156–161.

Volkmar, F. R., Stier, D. M., & Cohen, D. J. (1985). Age of recognition of pervasive developmental disorder. *American Journal of Psychiatry, 142,* 1450–1452.

Ward, A. J. (1970). Early infantile autism: Diagnosis, etiology and treatment. *Psychology Bulletin, 73,* 350–362.

Watson, L. R., & Marcus, L. M. (1988). Diagnosis and assessment of preschool children. In E. Schopler & G. Mesibov (Eds.), *Diagnosis and assessment in autism.* New York: Plenum Press.

Watson, M. S., Leckman, J. F., Annex, B., Breg, W. R., Boles, D., Volkmar, F. R., Cohen, D. J., & Carter, C. (1984). Fragile X in a survey of 75 autistic males. *New England Journal of Medicine,* 1462.

Wing, L. (1978). The wild boy of Aveyron—Book review. *Journal of Autism and Childhood Schizophrenia, 8,* 119–123.

Wing, L. (1981). Asperger's syndrome: A clinical account. *Psychological Medicine, 11,* 115–130.

Wing, L. (1991). The relationship between Asperger's syndrome and Kanner's autism. In U. Frith (Ed.), *Autism and Asperger syndrome* (pp. 93–121). Cambridge: Cambridge University Press.

Wing, L., & Attwood, A. (1987). Syndromes of autism and atypical development. In D. J. Cohen & A. M. Donnellan (Eds.), *Handbook of autism and pervasive developmental disorders* (pp. 3–19). New York: John Wiley & Sons.

World Health Organization. (1990, May). *International classification of diseases* (10th rev.), Chapter 5. Mental and behavioral disorders (including disorders of psychological development). Diagnostic criteria for research (draft for field trials). WHO unpublished manuscript.

Zahner, G. E. P., & Pauls, D. L. (1987). Epidemiological surveys of infantile autism. In D. Cohen & A. Donnellan (Eds.), *Handbook of autism and pervasive developmental disorders* (pp. 199–210). New York: John Wiley & Sons.

Zing, R. M. (1940). Feral man and extreme cases of isolation. *American Journal of Psychology, 53,* 487–517.

46 / Multisystem Developmental Disorder

Stanley I. Greenspan and Serena Wieder

Very young children who have severe relationship and communication problems in addition to motor, sensory, and cognitive difficulties perplex and challenge their families and professionals. A truly integrated approach is needed to treat them.

Not infrequently, parents will report to a professional their concern about a 2½-year-old who is not developing language, does not look at or relate to them, and shows no interest in peers. Asked about the child's earlier development, parents often recall that development in the first year of life was "typical." Their child enjoyed hugging and cuddling and began purposeful gesturing. Family videotapes often document these recollections. (Infrequently, the difficulties began much earlier.) But between 12 and 15 months, the child's preverbal gestural system of communication stopped developing. The toddler did not, for example, grab a parent's hand, lead her to the refrigerator, and vocalize and/or gesture for a certain food. At the same time, parents report, their child began evidencing (or intensifying already existing) oversensitivities to certain sounds or kinds of touch; the child no longer seemed to understand even simple words or gestures. Language stopped developing. Gradually parents noticed that their child became increasingly withdrawn, aimless, and perseverative.

Fortunately, our understanding of these children is growing, and intensive, integrated treatment approaches are helping many children make extraordinary developmental progress, the most remarkable of which is their ability to relate to others with warmth, pleasure, empathy, and growing emotional flexibility.

For reasons not yet entirely clear, but that may go beyond improved early identification services, programs serving infants, young children, and their families are reporting more and more children with severe relationship and communication problems. Many of the behaviors these children evidence were originally described by Kanner as autistic. According to Kanner (1943), "The outstanding 'pathognomonic' fundamental disorder is the children's inability to relate . . . from the beginning of life . . . an extreme autistic aloneness that . . . disregards, ignores, shuts out anything . . . from the outside." These behaviors are systematized in the fourth edition of the *Diagnostic and Statistical Manual of Mental Disorders* (*DSM-IV*) (American Psychiatric Association, 1994) under the category pervasive developmental disorder (PDD). The PDD category has 2 subtypes: autistic disorder (the more classic and severe form) and pervasive developmental disorder not otherwise specified (PDDNOS) (the more general type, which is diagnosed when there is a basic impairment in relating and communicating but all the formal criteria for autistic disorder are not met). Currently, most children with severe relationship and communication problems are diagnosed as having one of these 2 subtypes of PDD.

As we see more children diagnosed as PDD at younger ages, however, clinical features challenge the existing conceptual framework. Children are presenting with a continuum of relationship and affect expression patterns rather than one distinct type. Interestingly, clinicians, because of the lack of more appropriate diagnostic categories, use PDDNOS for many children who have various combinations of social, language, and cognitive dysfunctions, even when there are varying degrees of social relatedness. Parents, however, are very aware that autism and PDDNOS are part of the same broad PDD category.

For the majority of children, the relationship problem is not clearly in evidence in the first year of life (as thought by Kanner), but occurs more often in the second and third years, in connection with difficulties in processing sensations. Furthermore, each child has his or her own unique profile for processing sensations (i.e., "regulatory" profile). This includes differences in sensory reactivity (e.g., tactile, auditory, visual), sensory processing (e.g., auditory/verbal, visual/spatial), and motor tone and motor planning. Most important, the assumption that children with PDD, for the most part, remain relatively unrelated to others, rigid, mechanical, and idiosyncratic (as stated in *DSM-IV*) is not supported by our recent clinical experience. With early diagnosis and a comprehensive integrated relationship-based treatment approach, children originally diagnosed as PDD are learning to relate to others with warmth, empathy, and emotional flexibility—characteristics that run contrary to the very definition of PDD and that have been thought to be possible only for an exceptional few. A number of children we have been working with, diagnosed as autistic or PDDNOS between ages 18 and 30 months, who are now 5 to 7 years old, are fully communicative (using complex sentences adaptively), warm, loving, and joyful. They attend regular schools, are mastering the early academic tasks, are enjoying friendships, and are especially adept at imaginative play. While it is not yet clear what percentage of children ultimately will be capable of these types of cognitive gains, the capacity to become comfortable with closeness and dependency and even become joyful appears to be attainable, often early in the treatment program, no matter what the rate of cognitive and language gains. In addition, cognitive potential cannot be explored until interactive experiences are routine.

The traditional pessimistic prognosis for PDD has been based on experience with children who tend to begin treatment at slightly older ages (later than between 19 and 30 months), and who received more mechanical, structured treatment approaches rather than relationship, affect-cueing based approaches. The possibility must be considered that approaches that do not pull the child into *spontaneous* joyful relationship patterns may intensify rather than remediate the child's difficulty. Even with older PDD-type children who appear quite fixed in their perseverative patterns, as more gestural and/or verbal interactions get going, the perseverative and idiosyncratic behavior decreases and adaptive behavior increases, as does the general sense of relatedness.

The facts that there appears to be a continuum of relationship and communication problems rather than sharp qualitative differences, significant individual differences in each child, and greater potential for emotional growth than formerly thought mandate that we reconsider our long-held assumptions about PDD. It is especially important to reconsider the notions that there is a fixed biological deficit in the capacity to form an interactive relationship, that there is almost always either only minimal progress or chronic deterioration, and that these children are not capable of real emotional warmth, love, and sensitivity in the way other children are.

It is crucial that all diagnostic assessments of young children include careful observation of interactive play between caregiver and child as well as clinician and child. Where this is not done, as has been the case with a number of children whom we have seen recently, clinicians have failed to identify children's emerging capacities to relate warmly and intimately with parents or other familiar caregivers, and misdiagnoses leading to inappropriate treatment recommendations have been made.

A Biopsychosocial Developmental Model

A hypothesis to consider is that while a child's unique, biologically based way of processing and organizing experiences predisposes him or her to relationship and communication difficulties and perseverative and idiosyncratic behaviors, it is the types of interactions, or lack thereof, that bring the child's biology into an experimental context. And it is experiences that determine much of how children feel and behave.

An infant, toddler, or preschooler's auditory/verbal, visual/spatial and/or perceptual/motor processing difficulties may make ordinary relating and communication challenging. The people in the child's immediate environment often will not be able to find some special way to engage and interact with him or her. Therefore, vital social learning may not occur during important periods of development. For example, critical social skills, such as reciprocal gesturing and comprehending the "rules" of complex social interactions are learned at an especially rapid rate between 12 and 24 months. A deficit in these skills could easily look like a biological deficit rather than a reaction to underlying regulatory difficulties (which may have a biological basis).

By the time these children come to professional

attention, their difficult interaction patterns with their caregivers may be intensifying their difficulties. They are likely to perplex, confuse, frustrate, and undermine purposeful, interactive communication of even very competent parents. Parents often rely as much on their child's communicative signals as the child relies on the parents' signals. Parents are not prepared for a toddler who looks away or withdraws. Losing engagement and intentional, interactive relatedness to key caregivers, the children seem to withdraw more idiosyncratically into their own world. This hypothesis suggests, therefore, that there are biologically based regulatory difficulties that contribute to but are not decisive in determining the relationship and communication difficulties. When problems are perceived early, caregivers and children, with appropriate professional help, can learn to work around the regulatory dysfunctions and their associated relationship and communication problems and form varying degrees of warm, empathetic, and satisfying relationships.

In order to recognize the range of different difficulties one observes in children with these regulatory patterns, it may be useful to consider 2 broad types of disorders:

Regulatory disorders are present when children have the regulatory variations described previously, but can nevertheless relate to others and communicate in an age-appropriate fashion.

Multisystem developmental delay describes children who, as part of a severe regulatory dysfunction, also evidence disturbances in relating and communicating. As multisystem developmental delay is a self-evident descriptive term, it does not carry the negative connotations of autism or PDD, and does not rest on a questionable assumption that these types of children are not capable of love, warmth, and comfort with dependency. It may help us take a fresh look at the phenomenon often classified as autism.

Multisystem Developmental Disorder

The defining characteristics of multisystem developmental disorder (MSDD) are:

1. Significant impairment in, but not complete lack of, the ability to engage in an emotional and social relationship with a primary caregiver (e.g., may appear avoidant or aimless but may evidence subtle emergent forms of relating or relate quite warmly intermittently).
2. Significant impairment in forming, maintaining, and/or developing communication. This includes preverbal gestural communication as well as verbal and nonverbal (e.g., figurative) symbolic communication.
3. Significant dysfunction in auditory processing (i.e., perception and comprehension).
4. Significant dysfunction in the processing of other sensations including hyper- and hyporeactivity (e.g., to visual-spatial, tactile, proprioceptive, and vestibular input), and motor planning (e.g., sequencing movements).

These processing, relationship, and communication difficulties described are evidenced in various forms. Next we describe three patterns that are frequently observed, with the caveat that they are not yet intended to suggest specific subtypes but to facilitate clinical identification, treatment planning, and research.

Because children are not expected to evidence certain social behaviors (e.g., simple and complex gestures) until certain ages, the following guidelines should be considered. A classification of Pattern A can be made only in an infant over 5 months of age (when simple gestures and intentional communication can begin to be expected). A classification of Pattern B can be made in an infant over 9 months of age. A classification of Pattern C can be made in a child over 15 months of age.

PATTERN A

Relatedness and Interaction: Pattern A children appear most unrelated and aimless. They can be engaged only via direct sensory involvement where they respond to the sensory challenges as a way of getting involved. For example, they may look at you when you block their path or put your hand on a spot on the rug they are touching. They may crave being squashed underneath pillows, or will hold your hand to jump up and down, or will remove Koosh balls touching their bodies.

Affect: They lack interpersonal warmth or pleasure and usually show flat or inappropriate unmodulated affect.

Communication and Language: These children evidence few, if any, consistent simple intentional gestures, except for sensation-seeking behaviors or for food. They do not use expressive language, do not engage in symbolic play, and do not even seem preoccupied with certain objects.

Sensory Processing: These children show more self-stimulation and rhythmic behaviors than perseverative behavior with objects (as Pattern C does). They constantly seek sensory experiences through their bodies, using motion, touch, pressure, "looking," but are unable to connect these experiences to interpersonal interactions and feelings. On the one hand, they tend to be underreactive to sensation and have low motor tone, requiring more and more intense input to respond. On the other hand, they may be acutely sensitive to certain sensations, to which they overreact and want to avoid. Both under- and overreactivity are typical: for example, children are overreactive to tactile and certain features of auditory input (hypersensitive to certain sounds) and underreactive to vestibular and proprioceptive experiences, resulting in seeking (craving) these inputs from others as well as self-stimulation. These children also have the least sense of where their bodies are in space (often requiring intense physical activity to register feedback) and the most difficulty with motor planning (unable to sequence movements to manipulate toys, build, do puzzles, etc.). Sensation-seeking behaviors provide the openings for intentional communication and language.

Adaptation: These children tend either to show catastrophic reactions to new experiences or changes in familiar routines and environments with extreme tantrums or panic states, or to completely underreact, showing little or no responsiveness and "tuning out."

This pattern should not be diagnosed in children younger than 5 months of age because while the capacity to relate and attend begins earlier, it may not be evident until 5 months, given individual variations.

With interventions that provide the necessary levels of sensory and affective involvement and deal with the underreactivity, hypersensitivities, and motor planning difficulties, these children may evidence gradually increasing relatedness and purposefulness.

PATTERN B

Relatedness and Interaction: Pattern B children are in and out of relatedness, appearing to take flight quickly from moments of connectedness. They will briefly engage in an activity with another, but not directly with the other person. For example, these children can be engaged intermittently via the obstruction of their repetitive activity (e.g., pushing a train back and forth, blocking their path, or hiding the car they want, etc.).

Affect: Affect appears accessible but fleeting, with small islands of shallow satisfaction and pleasure but not deep interpersonal joy and pleasure. These children tend to enjoy repetitive or perseverative activity with objects (rather than only self-stimulation) but also depend on overfocusing on these objects to control and modulate other sensory and interpersonal input.

Communication and Language: These children can intermittently use simple intentional gestures, including motor gestures, vocalization, and affect cues to interact around a mechanical activity; for example, they can take a toy from someone and throw it down repeatedly. Occasionally, constructive interactions are possible, such as handing them a block to build with or adding a car to their line (as long as their "order" is not changed). At around 1 year, these children may begin to speak a few words, such as "bye-bye," "bottle," "mom," or "dad," but then they stop acquiring language and, in fact, between 15 and 24 months begin to "lose" the language they had.

Sensory Processing: These children show more mixed patterns of sensory reactivity and motor tone. They are much more organized than Pattern A children in their seeking of sensation, deliberately running, jumping, wanting to be in the swing, and seeking tactile input. They also show a greater sense of where their bodies are in space, not always stepping on or through things. Visual and spatial skills are often more developed than auditory processing; for example, children may be able to do puzzles or know in which direction to walk. Motor planning is still very difficult, but children can do simple or well-practiced sequences (e.g., go down a slide) or play with toys that roll or have simple cause-and-effect actions.

Adaptations: These children do not tolerate changes and transitions well but can adapt to routines if not overwhelmed by sensory overload. They remain very constricted in the range of experience they can deal with, including limits on what they will eat and wear.

Pattern B should not be diagnosed until 9 months of age because while the capacity of interactive sequences begins earlier, it may not be evident until 9 months, given individual variations.

With interventions that extend interactive sequences, these children may evidence increasingly complex behavioral and affective interactions.

PATTERN C

Relatedness and Interaction: Pattern C children relate to others but still in an in-and-out way, and usually must be in control, both in initiating and ending the interactions. These children can be wooed directly and through objects but can get overloaded easily. If overloaded, they withdraw in an organized way, such as moving to the other side of the room or hiding behind a chair, perhaps resuming eye contact when "safe." These children can be engaged in constructive interactions, building on their interests and favorite objects, such as hiding the car keys or crashing trains with them. Such activities often will bring a smile. They also tend to be very perseverative and preoccupied with certain objects, but will let someone make the perseverative behavior interactive; for example, they will somewhat playfully remove someone's hand from behind the door they keep trying to open and close repeatedly. They can be wooed into interaction and can tolerate more "interference." These children have a sense of what they want and make some effort to help themselves. They will tend to seek some boundaries—separating themselves from others by standing be-

hind a bench—to interact in a more organized manner.

Affect: With these children there are islands of real interpersonal pleasure coupled with more organized avoidance and times of aloofness. Pleasure is evident in spontaneous interaction, very predictable gestural games and songs (nursery rhymes) that have been done repeatedly, and physical activities (e.g., rough-housing).

Communication and Language: These children are consistently capable of simple gestures and some islands of complex intentional communication to get needs and desires met; for example, children will take a parent's hand to help them open the door. These children may gradually learn to use some single words or 2-word phrases intentionally. In many cases, this follows the disruption of spontaneous language (or simple sign language or pointing to pictures) acquisition between 18 and 24 months. These children more easily learn rote verbal patterns such as the alphabet, familiar nursery songs, or video and book scripts. They require a lot of interaction to maintain progress in the intentional use of language and, with such practice, become more spontaneous and adaptive.

These children also may use words "under fire" when their needs or wishes are being blocked and they feel intensely angry. Usually this is accompanied by some motor action. These children also may begin to experiment with simple symbolic play related to their direct experience, recognizing toys for what they are (e.g., may try to eat a toy cookie or get in a toy car, even sitting on a small school bus or toy horse).

Sensory Processing: Pattern C children are beginning to integrate their sensations but still show mixed reactivity with greater preponderance to overreact and get excitable. Motor planning is still difficult but more readily mastered (in contrast to the underreactivity of Pattern A children).

Adaptation: These children are the most adaptive of the three types, but new experiences are difficult. They tend to use organized negative intentional avoidance and withdraw only intermittently. They are better with transitions when given enough time, cues, and gestures to prepare.

Pattern C should not be diagnosed in children

younger than 15 months of age because while the capacity for complex behaviors and gestures begins earlier, it may not be evident until 15 months of age, given individual variations. These children may, at times, become behaviorally (and later on verbally) fragmented and purposefully negative or avoidant (e.g., turning away) when overloaded. With interventions that prolong interactive sequences and foster symbolic elaboration of affects, these children may evidence continuous increases in their intimacy, emotional expressiveness, and level of symbolic thinking.

Treatment Program

A comprehensive treatment program for infants, toddlers, and preschoolers with these problems involves helping them reestablish the developmental sequence that went awry. For many children this means establishing a relationship with two-way communication (simple gestures progressing to complex ones and then symbols). This involves patiently working both with and around their sensory processing and other regulatory difficulties to establish a pleasurable sense of attention and engagement. Following a particular child's lead and supporting his or her spontaneity, internal motivation, and affective expression in free play and unstructured interactions are the vehicles for accomplishing this task. This approach may require enormous ingenuity and persistence when a child's behavior consists of wandering about aimlessly or perseveratively rubbing a favorite object. But such basic strategies as comforting, wooing, and getting in the way of the aimless wanderer or clamping one's own hand on the perseverative rubber's object of desire (so that the child *must* deal with you) may create the spontaneous, self-motivated interaction that will restart the developmental process.

The therapeutic program must begin as soon as possible. The more quickly these children and their parents are reengaged in emotional interactions that use their emerging but not fully developing capacities for communication (initially with gestures rather than words), the better they fare.

The longer such children remain uncommunicative, and the more parents lose their sense of their child's earlier relatedness, the more deeply the children withdraw, and the more perseverative and idiosyncratic they become.

To spend months assessing a child or waiting to see how the child does on his or her own before beginning treatment is to waste critical time. Unless there is strong indication that adaptive development is proceeding on its own or the delay is limited only to a narrow aspect of language or motor behavior, there is not time to "wait and see." When very young children with severe difficulties in relating and communicating come to professional attention, assessment and appropriate intervention must be begun *within days*. Often interventions can be started while assessments are in progress.

A comprehensive program may include interactive play therapy (3 to 5 times a week) often involving both child and parents, speech therapy (3 to 5 times a week), occupational therapy (2 to 5 times a week), and parent counseling. During the preschool years, an important component of such a program is an integrated preschool (i.e., one quarter of the class of children with special needs and three quarters of the class of children without special needs), which has teachers especially gifted in interacting with challenging children and working with them on interactional gesturing, affective cueing, and early symbolic communication, as well as speech/language therapy, occupational therapy, and special education components. In such a program, the children with these patterns interact with children who are fully interactive and communicative. As a child reaches out for relationships, there are peers who reach back.

In order to help in the initiation of or return to an adaptive pattern of social development, a number of important challenges must be met. These involve helping a child learn to attend, relate, interact, experience a range of feelings, and ultimately think and relate in an organized and logical manner. These challenges involve the caregivers' and therapist's awareness of the steps the child needs to master core developmental competencies.

Before looking at how a therapist can help this most challenging group of children master their core developmental processes, it may be useful to

566

identify some of the common strategies that often *do not* work.

One of the most common unhelpful approaches is to lose sight of the developmental progression a child needs and, instead, to zoom in on particular skills in a fragmented or isolated way. For example, a child may be aimless and distracted. A parent or therapist may be trying to get her to put a square block in a square hole. She may do everything but look at the adult and try to copy what the adult is doing. Frustrated by the child's inattentiveness, the therapist or parent (often the parent copies the therapist) may hold the child's face and insist that the child look at him. Next, he may try to get the youngster to listen by talking in a repetitive monotone (much like a computer voice). If the therapist has been influenced by behavioral schools of thought, he may add on a reward every time the child does look at him. The therapist might offer verbal praise (also delivered in a computerized monotone)—"Good girl. Good girl. Good girl"—as well as piece of candy or other treat.

With such mechanical and rigid approaches, it is not atypical for children with autistic spectrum/pervasive developmental disorder patterns to become more stereotyped and more perseverative as they grow. The types of overly rigid and structured interventions that have been organized on behalf of these infants and children may in part support, rather than remediate, their more mechanical behavior.

In addition, there is a tendency, even among the most relationship-oriented therapists, to ignore the delayed child's core needs and developmental level. The therapist assumes that he can form a relationship with the child simply by positioning himself next to the boy and perhaps copying and/or commenting on what he is doing. He might say, "Oh, Johnny is putting one block on top of the other. Oh, Johnny is knocking it down. Now Johnny is building it up again." He may even say, "Oh, boy, Johnny is angry at the blocks," or "Now Johnny likes the blocks." Meanwhile, Johnny may not look at the adult, show little or no emotion, and not necessarily take in what is being said. A therapist and a child may go on in this fashion for weeks or months with very little movement or gain. The problem is that a child who is not yet functioning at a symbolic level, or even at a level that involves complex interactive gestures, is being approached as if he understands more than he does. He will sense some warmth but little else. In such cases what occurs is a type of parallel play between therapist and child, rather than true interactional play.

The tendency to work on "splinter" skills (an isolated, often rote-learned, cognitive capacity) is another way of working developmentally "above" a child. Parents understandably want their cognitively and language-delayed child to appear more normal. The therapist also would like some signs of intellectual brilliance from a delayed youngster. Together, they may help the child master certain splinter skills, such as having her say the days of the week, recognize certain letters or words, or memorize the contents of a book. However, a change of place or context or even of the verbal sequence used to elicit the behavior will take away her ability to recognize the letters or read the book in anything but a concrete and perseverative way. At the same time, more basic interactive skills that would serve as a foundation for true thinking and communicating are ignored.

Principles of Intervention

The primary goal of intervention is to enable children to form a sense of their own personhood—a sense of themselves as intentional, interactive individuals. The sense of one's personhood evolves from the infant's or young child's ability to abstract from a seemingly infinite number of affective interactions with his or her caregivers. This sense of "personhood" seems initially to organize itself around physical sensations, a sense of connection to others and a sense of intentionality (two-way communication involving the use of simple and complex gestures). Next it would define itself in terms of emerging representations or symbols as they became organized and differentiated. As the sense of personhood evolves, earlier and more fundamental levels serve as a foundation for newer levels.

Intervention with children with challenges requires the therapist to remember that their sense of their own being derives not simply from their language functioning, motor functioning, or cognition. Working with each or any of these areas in isolation may only continue a sense of fragmentation. Their sense of themselves derives from how they utilize their bodies as part of intentional engagements and interactions and how they organize the affects these interactions generate. Not only emotional capacities but cognitive ones, such as the ability to think and reason, are based on children's ability to abstract from their own affective experience. Therefore, the therapist must always ask how any intervention affects a child's ability to abstract and organize an emotional, sensation-based experience of who he or she is. Because these children often lack the most basic foundation for interpersonal experiences (i.e., often they are not interactive in the purposeful way that ordinary 8-month-olds are), much of the experience that they might use to abstract a sense of their own personhood is not available to them.

Therefore, for these children, the earliest therapeutic goals must be geared to the first steps in the developmental progression: to foster focus and concentration, engagement with the human world, and two-way intentional communication (and then symbolic levels) in order to create the interactive experiences they can use to abstract a sense of who they are.

As the therapist fosters focus and engagement, he or she must pay attention to the youngster's regulatory difficulties. For example, if a child is overreactive to sound, talking to him in a normal loud voice may lead him to become more aimless and more withdrawn. If she is overreactive to sights, bright lights and even very animated facial expressions may be overwhelming to her. On the other hand, if he is underreactive to sensations of sound and visual/spatial input, talking in a strong voice and using animated facial expressions in a well-lit room may help him attend. Similarly, in terms of her receptive language skills, if she is already at the point where she can decode a complex rhythm, making interesting sounds in complex patterns may be helpful. On the other hand, if she can decode only very simple, two-sequence rhythms, and perhaps understand a single word here and there, using single words (not as symbolic communication, but as gestural communication) and using simple patterns of sound may help her engage.

The therapist may find that a particular child remains relatively better focused in motion, such as being swung. Certain movement rhythms may be more effective than others. For some children, fast rhythms, such as one swing per second, may be ideal. For others, slow rhythms, similar to the breathing rate (one swing every 4, 5, or 6 seconds) may be ideal. Different kinds of tactile input may foster concentration and focus, such as firm pressure on the back, arms, or legs. Large motor movement and joint compressing also may foster attending (i.e., jumping on the bed, or any trampolinelike motion). Each infant and child is unique.

It is especially difficult to foster a sense of intimacy. Here, as the therapist helps children attend and engage, it is critically important to take advantage of their own natural interest. It is vital to follow each child's lead and look for opportunities for that visceral sense of pleasure and intimacy that leads the child to *want* to relate to the human world. Intimacy can be supported as the therapist works on forming simple and then more complex gestural communications.

For example, the father of a very withdrawn child was only verbalizing to his son. The therapist suggested trying simple gestural interactions first. The father put his hand on a toy car very gently, as his son was exploring it, and pointed to a particular part, as if to say "What's that?" But in pointing, the father actually moved the car; the son felt the car moving in his hands and noticed without upset his father's involvement. The son took the car back, but looked at where the father had touched it. This more physical, gestural communication seemed to get at least a faint circle of communication opened and closed—the son's interest in the car, the father's pointing to a spot on the car, moving it a little, and the son's looking at that particular spot, even though he took the car back—which, incidentally, was also a circle-closing response. Opening and closing circles of communication is the primary unit of gestural interaction, and it creates a foundation for all subsequent communication.

After getting this minimal interaction going, as the son moved the car back and forth, the father got another car and started moving it back and forth next to him. The father had his car move toward his son's car but did not crash into it. The son initially pulled his car out of the way but then moved it fast, as his father had, toward his father's car. Now three or four circles were closed in a row and a real interaction was beginning.

Next came the fostering of movement from gestures to symbols. As father and son were using their cars for simple and complex gestures, the father started to describe his own actions. When he moved the car fast, he said "fast," and when he moved it slow, he said "slow." After 4 or 5 repetitions, the boy slammed his car into his father's car and said the word "fast," although he did not pronounce it quite clearly. The father beamed. He was amazed that his son could learn a new word and use it appropriately so quickly. Words and symbols can be learned quickly if they are related to children's actual experiences and built on children's gestures. Words in isolation or as imposed labels have little meaning for the children.

A major challenge for therapists and parents is children's tendency to perseverate. One child would only open and close a door. Another would only bang blocks together. How can therapists work with such patterns? Do they try to get these children to do something else and get into a power struggle? The key is to make the perseveration an interaction; then it is no longer perseverative. Therapists should use these children's intense motivation to their advantage and get gestural circles of communication opened and closed. For example, the therapist can get stuck in the boy's door or get hands caught between the blocks. The therapists must be gentle and playful as the child tries to get them out of the way (like a cat-and-mouse game). Gestural interactions will be occurring, and the child's behavior will be strikingly purposeful and affective, even though the affect may be annoyance or anger. The therapists should welcome *all* human feelings, modulating them, however, and helping to soothe and comfort as well.

Another challenge, as therapists move toward more representational or symbolic elaboration, is to help children differentiate their experiences. Children need to learn cause-and-effect communication and to make connections between various representations or ideas.

Since most children with pervasive and multisystem developmental delays have difficulty with receptive language (i.e., auditory processing), and some also have difficulty with visual/spatial processing, it is much easier for them to pay attention

to their own ideas rather than the ideas of others. A child with this type of pattern has to work perhaps 100 times harder to take in verbal, or at times visual, information from caregivers or therapists than to sense his or her own inner sensations or perceptions.

The way a child categorizes experiences at the level of symbols or representations is through feedback. The parent becomes the representative of what is outside the child and the foundation for reality.

The clinician's or parent's ability to enter children's symbolic world becomes the critical vehicle for fostering emotional differentiation and higher levels of abstract and logical thinking. When, during the pretend play, the youngster ignores the therapist's inquiry about who sits where at the tea party, the therapist should bring the child back to the comment or question until he or she closes the symbolic circle.

The adult might "play dumb" (a little like the TV character Colombo) and bring the child back to the point of confusion. For example, when a child's puppet "bites" the head of the parent's stuffed cat, the parent might say, "Ouch, you hurt me." If the child then looks at the tree outside, the parent may ask, "But what about the cat? What about his ouch?" If she then says, "I'll give another ouch," and bites the cat with the puppet, she has closed the circle of communication. If the parent then says, as her gaze goes back to the tree, "Don't you want to talk more about the cat?" and if the child responds, "No, let's look at the tree," the child has closed yet another circle and also created a logical bridge from one set of ideas to the other. As the parent or therapist helps her create such bridges, always following her lead, the child becomes more and more differentiated. However, letting the child go on her own (and becoming fragmented with her) or becoming too rigid and controlling, may compromise differentiation.

Relating to children when they are feeling strong affects is critical. When children are motivated, for example, in trying to obtain junk food or to go outside, there is often an opportunity to open and close many symbolic circles. A child who is trying to open the door because he wants to go outside and is angry that he cannot may, in the midst of crying and angry shouting, open and close 20 circles of communication. In fact, during these high states of motivation, children often are very differentiated in their thinking. It is important not to frustrate children deliberately, but it is also important to recognize that frustration derived from a difference of opinion is a fine motivator, and one that occurs naturally. The transition times and the periods of negotiation should be stretched. Often a parent or therapist wants to cut short a power struggle over going outside, for example, or gives indirect feedback ("maybe . . . but why don't you look at your book?") because the child is angry and demanding. It is a positive step for a child to be demanding, as long as he or she is gesturally or verbally opening and closing circles. The therapist should endeavor to extend these periods of "motivated" interaction and provide clear and direct feedback ("I want to go out"; "Not now"; "Now"; "Later"; "Not later, now," etc.). The intense affect and motivation, when combined with interactions, help children define themselves emotionally.

Children with multisystem developmental delays often find it especially difficult to shift from concrete modes of thinking or using ideas to more abstract ones, in part because they do not easily generalize from a specific experience to other similar experiences. There is a temptation to teach children answers and repeat the same questions by scripting the dialogue. Sometimes this is justified because the therapist does not want to "confuse" the child with too many new questions. Parents, educators, and therapists who are frustrated by children's slow progress may wish to create an illusion of progress through the mastery of some rote-learned statements.

But children can learn to abstract and generalize only through active experience. The slower the going, the more, not less, spontaneous, active, symbolic interaction a child needs. Often it is helpful to assist children in elaborating their communication, going from the general to the specific, always taking advantage of high states of motivation. Consider, for example, a child at play who has a toy figure sitting on a car; the child is rolling the car toward a toy building. The adult enters the play gesturally, moving another car alongside, and asks, "What's going to happen?" The child is silent. Not getting a response to this most general elaboration, the adult moves to the next level, offering alternatives: "Should we go to the garage or the house over here?" Often, with these more con-

crete alternatives, the child will say "Garage" or "House," or point to one or the other. If the child remains silent, the elaboration may be simplified even further, with the adult still being careful not to tell the child what to do. As the child is moving the car, instead of oversimplifying and saying "Okay, the cars are going into the garage," the adult might say "Okay, the cars are going into my mouth." The child may find this silly and say, "No, the garage," or may just laugh. In either case, a nice symbolic circle has been closed.

Overview of the Steps in the Recovery from Multisystem and Pervasive Development Disorder

As we work with children who are multisystem developmentally delayed and pervasively developmentally disordered, it is important to recognize that their moving from one stage to another can be facilitated only through a certain sequence of steps. Often they begin by being withdrawn, avoidant, and aimless. Next, minimal gestures are used, after the parents, caregivers, and therapists are able to foster enough sense of engagement, concentration, and focus to begin to see simple circles being opened and closed. Initially, the circles are opened and closed in a more reactive way. Slowly but surely, however, children's initiative takes over, particularly if the parents are careful to follow their lead. Simple gestures and an initial level of engagement and focus give way to more complex gestures—first more reactive and then more self-initiated and assertive.

As interactive gestures become routine, children may develop more detail and subtlety in facial expressions and, for the first time, duplicate the expressions and looks of one or both parents. This is a significant step in the development of the children's humanity.

These children move from complex gestures to fragmented symbolic capacities. The capacity will be there one day, then it may not be there for several days; then again, there may be a word to accompany a gesture or an isolated piece of symbolic play, such as putting a puppet on the hand.

As this piecemeal capacity becomes more routine, often there occurs a stage that may not have been described in other accounts of the recovery of children with pervasive development disorder and multisystem delays—a very intense, driven, hypomanic quality in using representation or ideation. The children become needy and cling almost as if they have discovered that the human world is a great place and they do not want to lose it. They can chatter endlessly, but, as indicated earlier, the chatter has a fragmented quality. Islands of representation emerge rather than organized, complete thoughts. Bridges from one set of communication to another often are not clear.

After children go through this driven stage, the intensity often evens out, particularly with more differentiation in their thinking. They become more capable of organized thought as their affect returns to a calmer state; their emotional signaling and gesturing, as well as their use of words, appear to be more and more adaptive. However, even with this progress, children's thinking may tend to be based on their own imagination because they still have more difficulties receiving information from others. It is important for caregivers and therapists to help children open and close symbolic circles so that they can build on other people's information instead of developing more and more idiosyncratic, obsessional, and ritualistic thinking. In fact, the more they are helped through active experience to respond to the ideas and feelings of others, the more flexible they will become.

Parents of children with developmental disabilities share a number of patterns that are critical for the therapist to explore. Sometimes feelings are subtle and beneath the surface. Parents may feel depressed and withdraw from their children; they may deny their sadness and disappointment and become overly perfectionistic and controlling; they may facilitate between withdrawing, states of depression, and intrusive, overcontrolling patterns. In addition, each parent may have his or her own fantasies and related feelings, such as feelings of guilt: "What did I do to make my child so unresponsive?" or of anger: "This is unfair. I've worked too hard for this to be true." The anger may be at the child; it may be at the spouse; it may be at the clinicians and service providers.

An Integrated Intervention Program

The developmental processes described in this chapter are best supported through integrated intervention programs. But in order to support these processes, many communities need to rethink the way in which they organize early intervention and education for children with pervasive and multisystem delays and disorders as well as for all children with disabilities. The following recommendations for a treatment and educational program for infants and young children with pervasive and multiple developmental delays and dysfunctions grow out of the developmental perspective offered herein.

- Each child should have a multidisciplinary team comprised of a mental health professional, a speech pathologist, an occupational therapist, and a special educator. Intensive work with the child and his or her family (e.g., speech therapy, occupational therapy) as described earlier is the core of the program.
- During part of every day, an early intervention program should focus on the interaction patterns of the infant or young child and his or her parents.
- A professional should consult with the parents and other caregivers at least once a week to help with family dynamics and interactive patterns at home.
- Children with disabilities should be integrated into adequately staffed, developmentally appropriate early childhood care and education programs with typically developing children of a similar chronological age or developmental level, with 1 or 2 preschool children with disabilities in a group with 5 typically developing children. Grouping children with disabilities with each other may not be in the interest of any individual child, especially if a child's disability includes difficulties in communication or social interaction. As these children try to communicate, they need someone who can communicate back.
- Early interventionists, child care providers, and teachers should be trained in techniques for mobilizing socially and emotionally appropriate peer-to-peer interaction, particularly between children with disabilities and typically developing children.

A more detailed discussion of the concepts and therapeutic principles and strategies presented in this chapter, along with clinical case studies, can be found in *Infancy and Early Childhood: The Practice of Clinical Assessment and Intervention with Emotional and Developmental Challenges* (Greenspan, 1992).

REFERENCES

American Psychiatric Association Press. (1994). *Diagnostic and statistical manual of mental disorders* (3rd ed., rev.). Washington, DC: Author. (4th ed.)

DeGangi, G., Porges, S. W., & Greenspan, S. I. (1991). Psychophysiological characteristics of the regulatory disordered infant. *Infant Behavior and Development* (April).

Greenspan, S. I. (1989). *The development of the ego: Implications for personality theory; psychopathology; and the psychotherapeutic process.* Madison, CT: International Universities Press.

Greenspan, S. I. (1991). Regulatory disorders in infancy and early childhood. In National Institute of Drug Abuse (Ed.), *Methodological issues in controlled studies on effects of prenatal exposure to drugs of abuse* (Monograph 114). Richmond, VA: Author.

Greenspan, S. I. (1992). *Infancy and early childhood: The practice of clinical assessment and intervention with emotional and developmental challenges.* Madison, CT: International Universities Press.

Kanner, L. (1985). Autistic disturbances of affective contact. In A. Donnellan (Ed.), *Classic readings in autism* (pp. 11–50). New York: Teacher's College Press. (Originally published 1943 in *Nervous Child 2,* 217–250).

Porges, S. W., & Greenspan, S. I. (1991). Regulatory disordered infants: A common theme. In National Institute on Drug Abuse (Ed.), *Methodological issues in controlled studies on effects of prenatal exposure to drugs of abuse.* Richmond, VA: Author.

Zero to Three National Center for Clinical Infant Programs. (1994). *Diagnostic classification: 0–3; Diagnostic classification of mental health and developmental disorders of infancy and early childhood.* Arlington, VA: Author.

NAME INDEX

Name Index

Bakeman, R., 15, 65
Baker, A. J., 92
Baker, L., 476, 477, 544
Baker, W. L., 202, 204, 205, 534
Baker-Ward, L., 128
Bakwin, H., 394
Baldwin, A. L., 204, 206, 231, 236
Baldwin, B. A., 292
Baldwin, C., 204, 206
Baldwin, C. A., 236
Baldwin, C. P., 231
Baldwin, D. A., 17, 63, 66
Baldwin, M. W., 241
Balla, D., 549, 552
Baloh, R. W., 48
Bandura, A., 441
Banis, H. T., 209
Bank, L., 163
Baranowski, M. D., 198
Barlow, D. H., 205
Barnard, K., 194
Barnett, D., 215
Barnhard, J. S., 383
Barocas, R., 202, 207, 228, 229, 230, 236
Baron-Cohen, S., 542, 543, 544, 545
Barr, H. M., 210, 399
Barredo, V. H., 405
Barrera, M. E., 12, 442
Barrett, K. C., 177, 210, 242, 332
Barsch, R. H., 78
Bartak, L., 538, 554
Barthelemy, C., 549
Bartholomew, P. C., 474, 482, 485, 488
Bartlett, E., 73
Barton, M. E., 63, 66
Bartsch, K., 338
Basham, R. B., 201
Baskiewicz, A., 433
Bates, E., 8, 28, 73, 81, 111, 321, 327, 331, 474, 477, 478, 482, 486
Bates, J. E., 162, 164, 251, 252, 253, 262, 269, 315, 462
Bauchner, H., 177, 181, 210
Baudonniere, P.-M., 102
Bauer, B., 46
Bauer, D., 37
Bauer, P. J., 68, 69
Bauman, K. E., 296, 299
Bautista, D., 401
Bax, M., 493
Baxter, J. C., 403
Bayles, K., 162, 164, 253
Bayley, N., 18, 53, 69, 260, 262, 551
Beardslee, W. R., 163, 177, 180, 208
Beck, A. T., 245
Beck, D. C., 422
Becker, J., 379
Beckman, P. J., 420
Beckwith, L., 404, 406, 408
Beebe, B., 27, 178, 179
Beeghly, M., 94, 177, 419
Beezley, P., 170

Begab, M. J., 415
Beilke, R., 406
Beitchman, J., 473, 474
Bejar, R., 402
Bell, A. P., 453
Bell, J. A., 417
Bell, M. A., 272
Bell, R., 170, 538
Bell, S. M., 239, 242, 360, 367
Bellugi, U., 74, 109, 420, 424
Belman, B., 393
Belsky, J., 7, 65, 92, 96, 161, 171, 179, 185, 198, 237, 246, 253
Beltramini, A. U., 493
Bem, S. L., 455
Bemesderfer, S., 288
Bemporad, B., 255
Bemporad, J. R., 543
Benda, C. E., 537
Bendell, D., 181, 182, 183
Bender, L., 537
Benedek, T., 96, 120, 198
Benedict, H., 63
Bengtson, V. L., 192
Benjamin, J., 116
Bennett, D. S., 162, 164
Bennett, F., 477
Bennett, S., 6, 27
Benoit, D., 498
Benson, J. B., 15
Bentler, P. M., 462
Benuth, H., 23
Berg, S. Z., 558
Berger, M., 409
Bergeson, P. S., 433
Bergman, A., 3, 5, 6, 56, 58, 61, 89, 91, 97, 116, 118, 276, 278, 279, 280, 281, 282, 286, 287, 288, 325, 388, 455
Bergmann, A., 192
Berk, R. A., 43, 145
Berko, J., 200
Berlin, L., 243
Berlyne, D. E., 323
Berman, A., 370
Bernbaum, J. D., 370
Berndt, T. J., 306, 308
Bernheimer, L., 421
Bernstein, V. J., 408
Bertalanffy, L. von., 323
Bertenthal, B. I., 12, 13, 14, 36, 37, 102
Berwick, D. M., 367
Besharov, D. J., 397
Best, C. L., 170
Best, K. M., 195, 203, 205, 211, 215, 218
Bettelheim, B., 555
Bettes, B. A., 181
Bhavnagri, N. P., 305
Bibring, E., 245
Bibring, G. L., 199, 295
Biederman, J., 391
Bierman, J. M., 227
Bierman, J. S., 211
Bierman, K. L., 316

SUBJECT INDEX